Pharmacology in the Practice of Anaesthesia

MT

HOM N : HNV
1996
f

Pharmacology in the Practice of Anaesthesia

Leon Kaufman MD, FRCA

Consulting Anaesthetist, University College Hospital and St Mark's Hospital, London and Honorary Senior Lecturer, Faculty of Clinical Sciences, University College London, UK

Peter V Taberner BSc, MSc, PhD

Senior Lecturer in Pharmacology, University of Bristol School of Medical Sciences, Bristol, UK

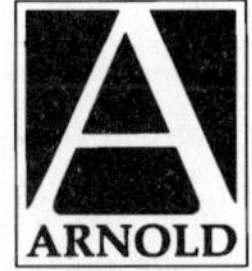

A member of the Hodder Headline Group
LONDON • SYDNEY • AUCKLAND
Co-published in the USA by Oxford University Press, Inc., New York

First published in Great Britain 1996 by
Arnold, a member of the Hodder Headline Group,
338 Euston Road, London NW1 3BH

Co-published in the United States of America by
Oxford University Press, Inc.
198 Madison Avenue, New York, NY 10016
Oxford is a registered tradename of Oxford University Press

Whilst the advice and information in this book is believed to be true and accurate at the date of going to press, neither the authors nor the publisher can accept any legal responsibility or liability for any errors or omissions that may be made. In particular (but without limiting the generality of the preceding disclaimer) every effort has been made to check drug dosages; however it is still possible that errors have been missed. Furthermore, dosage schedules are constantly being revised and new side-effects recognized. For these reasons the reader is strongly urged to consult the drug companies' printed instructions before administering any of the drugs recommended in this book.

British Library Cataloguing in Publication Data
A catalogue record for this book is available from the British Library

Library of Congress Cataloging-in-Publication Data
A catalog record for this book is available from the Library of Congress

ISBN 0 340 55171 2

Typeset in 9pt Sabon by Keyword Typesetting Services Ltd
Printed and bound in Great Britain by The Bath Press, Somerset

Contents

Contributors

Rod F Armstrong FRCA
Consultant in Anaesthesia and Intensive Care, The Middlesex Hospital, London, UK

George R Aronoff MD, FACP
Professor of Medicine and Pharmacology, University of Louisville School of Medicine, Kentucky, USA

Beverley Astley FRCA
Consultant Anaesthetist, Department of Anaesthesia, University College Hospital, London, UK

Wynne Aveling MA, BB BChi, FRCAI
Consultant Anaesthetist, Clinical Directorate of Anaesthesia, Theatres and Day Surgery, The Middlesex Hospital, London, UK

Krishna N. Bakhshi FRCA
Senior Registrar, St Bartholomew's Hospital, London, UK

Richard B Barlow DPhil, DSc
Reader in Pharmacology, Department of Pharmacology, University of Bristol, School of Medical Sciences, Bristol, UK

Colin Beard MB ChB, FRCA
Consultant Anaesthetist, Royal Free Hospital, London, UK

William C Bowman PhD, DSc, FIBiol, FRSE
Professor of Physiology and Pharmacology, University of Strathclyde, Glasgow, UK

Catherine Bullen MB ChB, FRCA
Consultant Anaesthetist, Department of Anaesthesia, The Middlesex Hospital, London, UK

Paul L Cervi MB BCh, MRCPI, MRCPath
Consultant, Department of Haematology, Basildon Hospital, Basildon, UK

Geoff Clarke PhD
Senior Lecturer, Anatomy Department, University of Bristol, School of Medical Sciences, Bristol, UK

Simon JC Cottam MB ChB, FRCA
Consultant Anaesthetist, Department of Anaesthesia, King's College Hospital, London, UK

Helena M Earl MB BS, MRCP, PhD
Senior Lecturer in Medical Oncology; Honorary Director of CRC Trials Unit, CRC Institute for Cancer Studies, Queen Elizabeth Hospital, University of Birmingham, Birmingham, UK

Karen M Erbeck MD
Assistant Professor of Medicine, University of Louisville School of Medicine, Kentucky, USA

M Ehrenstein MD
Senior Registrar, Bloomsbury Rheumatology Unit, London, UK

Robert O Feneck MB BS, LRCP, MRCS, FRCA
Consultant Anaesthetist, St Bartholomew's and London Chest Hospitals, London, UK

John C Foreman MD, PhD
Professor of Pharmacology, University College London, London UK

P Glue MD
Clinical Pharmacist, Schering Plough Research Institute, Kenilworth, New Jersey, USA

Anthony H Goldstone MB BCh, FRCP
Consultant Haematologist and Medical Director, Department of Haematology, University College Hospital, London, UK

David W Green MB BS, FRCA
Consultant Anaesthetist, Department of Anaesthesia, Intensive Care and Pain Relief, King's Healthcare NHS Trust, London, UK

Earnest Grundy MB ChB, MRCP, FRCA
Consultant Anaesthetist, Clinical Directorate of Anaesthesia, Theatres and Day Surgery, The Middlesex Hospital, London, UK

Ian P Hall BM BCh, MRCP
Senior Lecturer, Department of Medicine, University of Nottingham, Nottingham, UK

MJ Halsey MA, DPhil
Head of Anaesthesia, Nuffield Department of Anaesthesia, Radcliffe Infirmary, Oxford, UK

SJ Hill BSc, PhD
Professor of Molecular Pharmacology, Department of Pharmacology, Queen's Medical School, Nottingham, UK

David A Isenberg FRCP, MRCP
Consultant Rheumatologist, Bloomsbury Rheumatology Unit, London, UK

Michael Jordan MB BChir, FRCA
Consultant Anaesthetist, Department of Anaesthesia, St Peter's Hospital, Chertsey, Surrey, UK

L Kaufman MD, FRCA
Consulting Anaesthetist, University College Hospital and St Mark's Hospital and Honorary Senior Lecturer, Faculty of Clinical Sciences, University College London, London, UK

Nigel H Kellow FRCA
Consultant Anaesthetist, Department of Anaesthesia, St Bartholomew's and Royal London Hospitals, London, UK

Anthony B Kurtz MB BS, FRCP,
Consultant Physician, Department of Medicine, The Middlesex Hospital, London, UK

Gillian CL Lachelin FRCOG
Consultant, Department of Obstetrics and Gynaecology, University College London Medical School, London, UK

Richard M Langford MB BS, FRCA
Consultant Anaesthetist, Department of Anaesthesia, St Bartholomew's Hospital, London, UK

Ariel F Lant PhD, FRCP
Professor of Pharmacology and Therapeutics, Charing Cross and Westminster Medical School; and Consultant Physician, Chelsea and Westminster Hospital, London, UK

Hilary J Little BSc, MSc, PhD
Professor of Psychopharmacology, University of Durham, Durham, UK

Alex Livingston PhD, MRCVS
Western College of Veterinary Medicine, University of Saskatchewan, Saskatoon, Canada

Vincent Mak BSc, MB BS, MRCP
Consultant Physician, Department of Thoracic Medicine, Central Middlesex Hospital, London, UK

Robin W Matthews PhD, MDS, BDS
Senior Lecturer in Oral Medicine, University of Bristol Dental School, Bristol, UK

Susan J Milroy MB BS, FRCA
Senior Registrar, Department of Anaesthesia, King's College Hospital, London, UK

B Kevin Park BSc, PhD, MRCP
Professor of Pharmacology and Therapeutics, The University of Liverpool, Liverpool, UK

M Pirmohamed MB ChB, PhD, MRCP
Lecturer, Department of Pharmacology and Therapeutics, The University of Liverpool, Liverpool, UK

Ian Power BSc, MD, FRCA
Associate Professor, University of Sydney, Department of Anaesthesia and Pain Management, Royal North Shore Hospital, Australia

CJ Pycock MB ChB, PhD, DSc, MRCP
Consultant Physician, Worcester Royal Infirmary, Worcester, UK

Andrew G Ramage BSc, MPhil, PhD
Senior Lecturer in Pharmacology, Royal Free School of Medicine, London, UK

Clive JC Roberts MD, FRCP
Senior Consultant Clinical Pharmacologist, Department of Medicine, Bristol Royal Infirmary, Bristol, UK

AD Scott FRCA
Consultant Anaesthetist, Poole General Hospital, Poole, UK

GMS Scott MD, FRCP, MRCPath
Consultant Microbiologist, Department of Microbiology, University College Hospital, London, UK

Michael P Seed BSc, PhD
Research Fellow, Department of Experimental Pathology, St Bartholomew's Hospital, London, UK

Stephen Spiro MD
Consultant Physician, Department of Thoracic Medicine, University College Hospital, London, UK

SC Stanford BSc, DPhil
Senior Lecturer, Department of Pharmacology, University College London, London, UK

Peter V Taberner BSc, MSc, PhD
Senior Lecturer in Pharmacology, University of Bristol School of Medical Sciences, Bristol, UK

Andrew R Webb MB BS, FRCA
Consultant Anaesthetist, Department of Anaesthesia, The Middlesex Hospital, London, UK

Susan J Wilson PhD, EEG Dip
Research Associate, Psychopharmacology Unit, University of Bristol, School of Medical Sciences, Bristol, UK

Paul Yate FRCA
Consultant Anaesthetist, Department of Anaesthetics, The London Hospital, London, UK

Preface

Although this book has been designed to serve as a standard textbook of pharmacology for practising anaesthetists and those studying for postgraduate examinations in anaesthesia, it should also prove valuable to clinical pharmacologists and to clinicians in other specialities, such as intensive care, who wish to understand the mode of action of drugs and how they interact in the patient.

Pharmacology is one of the most rapidly advancing medical sciences in its own right, with several entirely new classes of drugs introduced into clinical use over the last few years. Medical advances in other disciplines have also had a direct effect on drug research; for example, the use of immunosuppressives in transplantation surgery, and the recent rapid development of antiviral agents for the treatment of AIDS.

Drugs are rarely used in isolation and it is therefore increasingly important for clinicians, and anaesthetists in particular, to be aware of their pharmacological properties and potential interactions and adverse reactions. To this end we have adopted a systematic approach, in which the major physiological systems are considered as a whole. In the respiratory and cardiovascular systems, for example, where a very wide range of drugs have important effects, this should facilitate the understanding of the therapeutic use of drugs having different mechanisms of action.

By combining the expertise of research pharmacologists who are at the forefront of their field, investigating the basis of action of drugs, and clinicians who are using these drugs and observing their effects in the patient, we are aiming to provide a sound basis for understanding the general principles behind the use of groups of drugs, and then to illustrate their principles with specific examples from clinical practice.

We are most grateful to the authors for their loyalty and patience, and congratulate them on completing their arduous task. Special thanks to those who were kind enough to update their manuscripts. The publication of this volume coincides with the 150th anniversary of the introduction of anaesthesia with the use of ether (now no longer available in the UK). This book is a testament to the development of anaesthesia which has been of great benefit to mankind.

Leon Kaufman
Peter V Taberner

SECTION ONE

General Principles of Pharmacology

1

Drug Receptors and Mechanisms of Drug Action

PV Taberner

The concept of a drug receptor or binding site is one of the basic tenets of pharmacology. The existence of receptors was originally inferred from the practical observation of the effects of specific chemicals on isolated tissues or intact organisms. Some substances are far more potent at producing a physiological response than other chemically similar compounds. These substances also appeared to be tissue selective in their actions – actions that could be specifically blocked by other chemical entities. The earliest experiments of this type were described by J.N. Langley in 1873, who found that the plant extract, jaborandi, stimulated salivary secretion and that this effect could be blocked with atropine. However, it was not until Ehrlich later postulated the notion of fixed binding sites, based on his experiments with diphtheria toxin, that physiologists began to investigate the quantitative nature of the interaction of drugs with tissues. The first proposal, in 1906, that there were 'receptive substances' present at nerve endings that could receive or transmit signals between nerves, or between nerves and muscles, was also due to Langley. Since then, pharmacologists have been investigating drug–receptor interactions as a means of explaining the mechanisms of drug action and measuring the relative potencies of different drugs. This aspect of pharmacology is termed *pharmacodynamics*.

It is possible to divide drugs into three broad classes in terms of their sites of action:

- drugs that act through receptors (e.g. neuromuscular blockers, opiate analgesics, etc.)
- drugs that act on enzymes, usually as inhibitors (e.g. non-steroidal anti-inflammatory drugs)
- drugs such as the volatile anaesthetics, that appear to have non-specific actions on cell membranes.

THE NATURE OF DRUG RECEPTORS

Drug receptors are now known to be protein structures. With the exception of steroid receptors, they are situated within cell membranes and have a binding site that projects on the outside surface of the cell. Receptor sites can be visualized using autoradiographic techniques that enable the receptor density on a tissue to be determined. Over recent years the protein molecule subunits that make up the receptor structure have not only been isolated and purified from cell membranes but also cloned, using *in vitro* molecular genetic techniques. Different receptor subtypes often consist of the same protein subunits but assembled in different combinations. The protein molecules that make up the receptor structure can also be related to specific identifiable genes, so that the synthesis of artificial receptors is now possible. A genetically expressed defect in a specific protein subunit can lead to the formation of malfunctioning receptors that eventually manifest themselves in the form of an inheritable disorder, often with a well-defined clinical pathology. As new receptor types are characterized an ever-increasing number of drugs are recognized to act through specific extracellular or intracellular receptor molecules. To take one example: the barbiturates, which were until fairly recently thought to be non-specific general depressants, are now known to act at a specific binding site linked to the γ-aminobutyric acid (GABA) receptor.

It is important to distinguish between specific drug-binding sites (e.g. the sites on plasma albumin) and specific receptors, which are linked to a mechanism that produces a physiological response in a tissue or cell. The implication of the existence of any drug receptor in the body is that there must also exist an endogenous ligand that exerts its normal physiological action by binding to the receptor. The presence of specific binding sites for morphine and other opiates thus led directly to the discovery of the endogenous opioids, the enkephalins. Endogenous ligands for the benzodiazepine-, barbiturate- and cannabinoid-binding sites are currently being investigated.

THE DRUG–RECEPTOR INTERACTION

The drug–receptor interaction is sometimes compared to the enzyme–substrate reaction: both involve the binding of a small molecule to a specific site on a protein, but beyond that the analogy breaks down. The enzyme–substrate complex either dissociates to release the substrate or breaks down to form the product of the reaction and free enzyme:

Enzyme–substrate reaction:

$$\mathrm{E} + \mathrm{S} \rightleftharpoons \mathrm{ES} \xrightarrow{\text{Dissociation}} \mathrm{ES\ Product}$$

The formation of the drug–receptor complex leads to the production of a pharmacological signal which may require a cascade of events (transduction) to occur before the eventual physiological response is produced.

Drug–receptor interaction:

$$\mathrm{D} + \mathrm{R} \overset{\text{Affinity}}{\rightleftharpoons} \mathrm{DR} \xrightarrow{\text{Efficacy}} \text{Response}$$

The relative potency of a drug at its site of action is determined first by the affinity of the drug molecule for the receptor. In the simplest situation the size of the response can be related to the proportion of drug receptors occupied by the Law of Mass Action, so that the maximal response is obtained when all the receptors are occupied. This results in a typical hyperbolic saturation binding curve (Fig. 1.1). However, the dose–response relationship is more usually presented as a log concentration–response curve, which has a sigmoidal shape (Fig 1.2).

A drug that produces the maximum response of which the tissue is capable is termed a *full agonist*. A drug that produces a lower maximum response is termed a *partial agonist*. These drugs may bind to the receptor with the same affinity as a full agonist, but the drug–receptor complex that is formed is somehow less efficient at producing the normal response. This property is termed the *efficacy* or *intrinsic activity* of the agonist. A drug that competes with agonists to form a drug–receptor complex which does not result in a physiological response (i.e. has zero efficacy) is termed a *competitive antagonist*. In the presence of a competitive antagonist the log concentration–response curve shows a parallel shift to the right (see Fig. 1.3) so that a higher concentration of agonist is required to achieve the same response as before. In other words, the potency of the agonist is reduced, but the efficacy is unchanged. In the presence of a *non-competitive antagonist* both the potency and the efficacy are

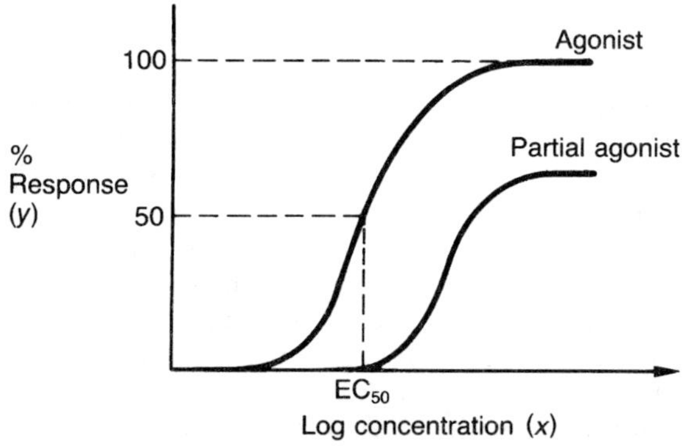

FIGURE 1.2 The log dose–response curve (symmetrical sigmoid).

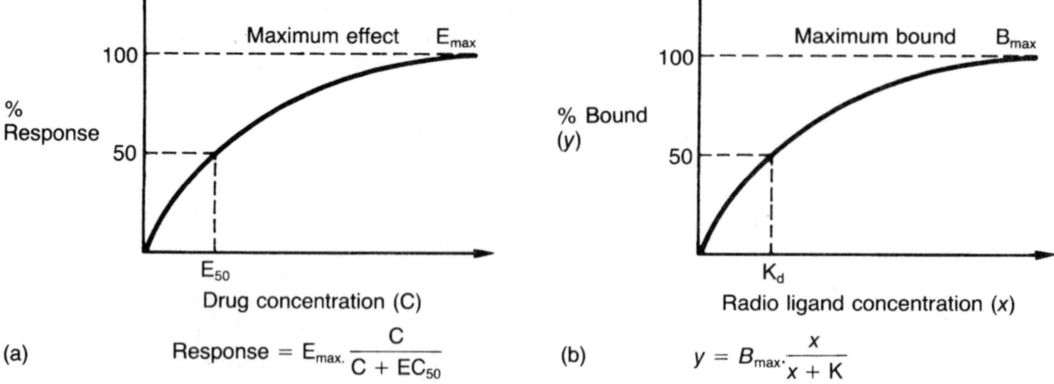

FIGURE 1.1 (a) Dose–response curve (rectangular hyperbola). (b) Receptor-binding curve.

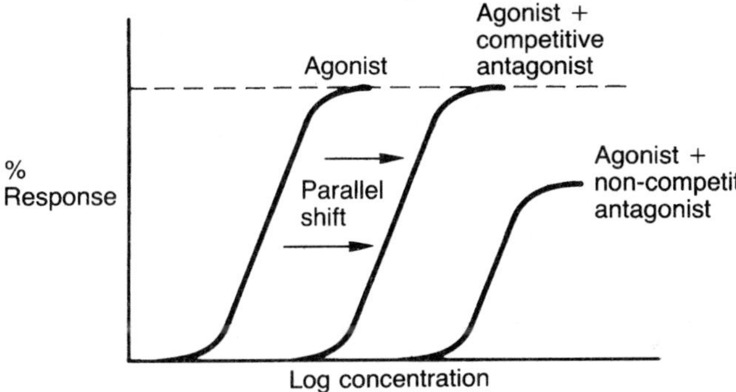

FIGURE 1.3 Effects of antagonists on log concentration–response curves.

reduced, so that the log concentration–response curve is shifted to the right and the maximal response is reduced. It is important to recognize that a partial agonist (such as nalorphine) will resemble a non-competitive antagonist in this situation (see Fig. 1.3) – that is, the displacement of the full agonist (morphine) by nalorphine, will reduce the overall response.

In the case of the benzodiazepine receptor, a further refinement has become necessary with the discovery of anxiogenic compounds, which produce the opposite effect to a normal agonist, even though they bind competitively at the same receptor. These β-carboline compounds have been termed *inverse agonists*. Similarly, some less effective β-carbolines act as *partial inverse agonists*. An entire spectrum of activity can be drawn from full inverse agonists to full agonists, such that all the benzodiazepines and their analogues can be placed at some point between these extremes (see p.69 and also Chapter 21).

In receptor-binding studies the term *ligand* is often employed to describe a compound, usually radiolabelled, which is used to identify a receptor type. A ligand may be either an agonist or antagonist; the only inference is that it binds more or less specifically to a particular receptor type. Since ligand-binding studies using isolated cell membranes do not involve a pharmacological response they will not differentiate agonists from antagonists. In other words, binding experiments cannot measure the efficacy of a drug.

Measuring the potency of agonists

The two parameters that can be derived from plotting concentration–response curves are the affinity of the drug for the receptor, and its efficacy at the receptor. The derivation of equilibrium rate constants for the drug–receptor interaction is shown in Fig. 1.4. It is slightly unfortunate that pharmacologists measuring physiological responses to drugs in isolated tissues have tended to adopt the affinity constant (K_a), which has the dimensions of reciprocal concentration, whereas dissociation constants (K_d) are used in *in vitro* receptor binding studies and enzymology. Since $K_d = 1/K_a$ a high affinity is associated with a low K_d value and vice versa.

If it is assumed that the response measured is in direct proportion to the fraction of the total number of receptors [R] occupied by the drug [DR], then the half-maximal response will be observed when [R] = [DR]. The equation for the drug–receptor interaction:

$$\frac{[D]\,[R]}{[DR]} = K_d \quad \text{then simplifies to : } [D] = K_d$$

where [D] is the concentration of drug producing the half-maximal response; that is, the EC_{50}. For a full agonist the $EC_{50} = 1/K_a$. When comparing the potencies of different drugs the EC_{50} is usually used. In terms of clinical medicine, the relative potency of a drug is probably less important than its efficacy and its specificity of action, since lack of potency can be overcome by increasing the dose. If the efficacy of a full agonist is taken as unity, then the efficacy of a partial agonist will be a fraction of this, related to the relative maximum response obtained, so a partial agonist can never be as effective as a full agonist. An antagonist has zero efficacy.

Measuring the potency of antagonists

Since antagonists do not produce direct responses, their potency has to be measured indirectly. The ratio between the increased concentration of agonist (C') that is required to produce the same response in the presence of a competitive antagonist and the concentration when given alone (C) is related to the dissociation constant of the antagonist (K_i) by the Gaddum–Schild equation, where [I] is the concentration of the antagonist:

$$\frac{C'}{C} = 1 + \frac{[I]}{K_i}$$

This is sometimes expressed using the affinity constant of the antagonist (K_b) so that:

$$\frac{C'}{C} = 1 + [I].\,K_b$$

The concentration of antagonist that necessitates doubling the dose of agonist to achieve the same size of response (i.e. when the dose ratio $\frac{C'}{C} = 2$) is there-

	D Drug	+	R Free receptor	⇌	DR Occupied receptor
Concentrations: N = total number of receptors	x		$N - N_x$		N_x

Rate of forward reaction = $k_{+1}.x.(N - N_x)$

Rate of backward reaction = $k_{-1}.N_x$

At equilibrium the two rates are equal, so $k_{+1}.x.(N - N_x) = k_{-1}.N_x$

The equilibrium rate constant (dissociation constant, K_d) = k_{-1}/k_{+1}
(The affinity constant (K_a) is the reciprocal of this, i.e. k_{+1}/k_{-1})

$$\text{Thus, } x.N = N_x.(K_d + x)$$

Since the fraction of receptors occupied (the occupancy, P_x) = N_x/N

$$P_x = \frac{x}{x + K_d}$$

The dissociation constant K_d is numerically equal to the concentration of drug required to occupy 50% of the receptors at equilibrium. This logistic equation (the Langmuir adsorption isotherm) can be used to describe concentration–response curves or binding curves.

Dose response:

$$y = M \cdot \frac{x}{x + K_d} \quad \text{(Eqn 1)}$$

where y = the response measured, M is the maximum response, and x is the concentration of drug. When the concentration is plotted against the response, the shape of the curve is a rectangular hyperbola (see Fig. 1.1). If the logarithm of the concentration is plotted against the response, the curve is S-shaped (see Fig. 1.2)

Similarly, for binding:

$$B = B_{max} \cdot \frac{x}{x + K_d} \quad \text{(Eqn 2)}$$

where B = amount of bound drug, B_{max} = the maximum binding, and x is the concentration of free (unbound) drug.

FIGURE 1.4 The derivation of equilibrium rate constants.

fore numerically equal to its dissociation constant K_i. The dose ratio method is widely used to compare antagonist potencies. When comparing the potencies of different antagonists in radioligand binding studies, the IC_{50} is usually employed. This is the concentration of antagonist that produces 50% inhibition of agonist binding. It can be related to the K_i value by the Cheng–Prusoff equation:

$$K_i = \frac{IC_{50}}{1 + \frac{[L]}{K_d}}$$

where [L] is the concentration of ligand (which can be an agonist or antagonist), and K_d is its dissociation constant. Methods for estimating equilibrium constants and receptor density (B_{max}) from binding studies are shown in Fig. 1.5.

These relationships all assume that the antagonist is competitive and reversible with respect to the agonist or other ligand. Non-competitive antagonism (or non-specific effects) can be recognized by an alteration in the slope of the dose–response or receptor binding curve.

Although ED_{50} and IC_{50} values are useful for comparing the relative potencies of drugs, they are of less value to the clinician who is more interested in a dose that will be effective in 100% of cases. A large number of other factors need to be taken into account when predicting the effectiveness of a drug *in vivo* from its potency *in vitro*.

REGULATION OF RECEPTORS

Radioligand-binding studies have indicated that the total receptor number in a tissue (estimated from the number of ligand molecules bound per unit weight of tissue or protein) can vary in response to the presence of an agonist and is not necessarily a fixed number. This evidence has provided one explanation for the phenomenon of tachyphylaxis or desensitization. For example, striatal dopamine receptors decrease in number as a consequence of the continued presence of

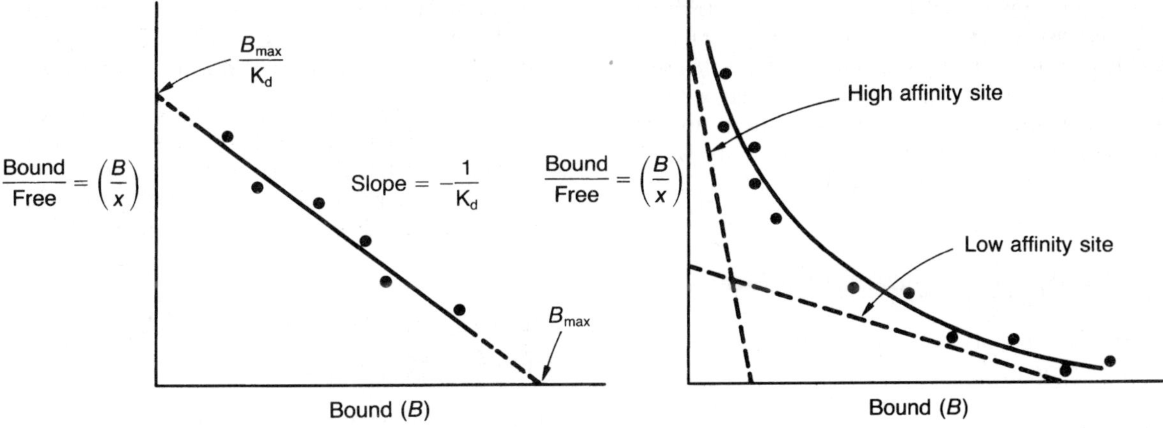

FIGURE 1.5 Derivation of kinetic parameters from binding plots.

dopamine agonists. This *down-regulation* results in a reduced tissue response. Excessive thyroid hormone on the other hand can lead to an increase in the concentration of β-adrenoceptors in the myocardium. This *up-regulation* of receptors can increase the sensitivity of tissues to agonist drugs, particularly where spare receptors are present (see below). Sensitization of the myocardium to circulating catecholamines by general anaesthetics may be due to a similar mechanism. In general, it is the adenylate cyclase-coupled receptors, such as the β-adrenoceptors, that appear to be capable of up- or down-regulation.

RECEPTOR INTERACTIONS (ALLOSTERIC EFFECTS)

It is well known that the binding of a ligand molecule to a receptor site can alter the likelihood of further molecules binding to adjacent sites; the classic example being the binding of oxygen molecules to haemoglobin. When subsequent binding is facilitated by this means (as it is with oxygen and haemoglobin), it is termed positive co-operativity. The converse, which is much less common, is termed negative co-operativity. The presence of co-operativity can be inferred from the shape of the binding plot. By fitting dose–response or binding data to the Hill plot (see Fig. 1.6), a straight line with a slope of 1.0 (the Hill coefficient) will be obtained if no co-operativity is occurring. The Hill coefficient will be >1 if co-operativity is positive and <1 if co-operativity is negative or there are multiple binding sites.

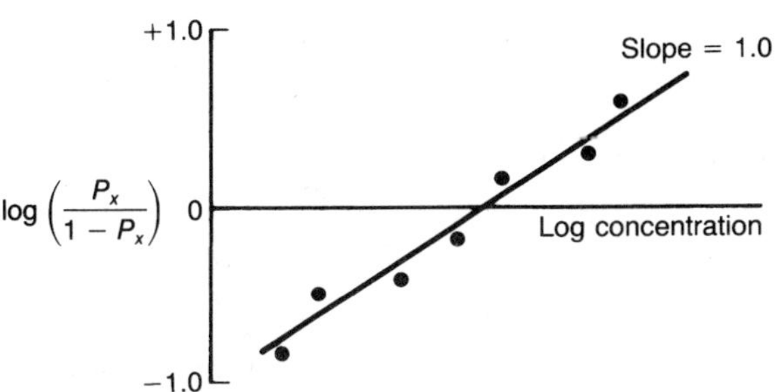

FIGURE 1.6 Detection of receptor subtypes using the Hill plot.

THE SPARE RECEPTOR CONCEPT

It is now recognized, contrary to earlier beliefs, that it is not always necessary for a drug to occupy all the receptors in a tissue in order to produce the maximal response. If only 10% of receptors need to be occupied for a maximal response, the remaining 90% are said to be 'spare'. This is not the same as saying that they are unavailable for binding or in any way different from other receptors; it does not matter which 10% of receptors are occupied at any moment in time, the remainder are, by definition, spare.

The first experimental evidence for the existence of spare receptors came from studies using non-competitive (irreversible) antagonists to block a proportion of the β-adrenoceptors in the heart. Even with the number of receptors available reduced by half, catecholamine agonists were still able to produce the same maximal effect as in the absence of the antagonist. The spare receptor concept can explain why receptor up-regulation can increase the sensitivity of a tissue to an agonist, but without increasing the maximum response. Suppose that the previous figure of 10% occupation represents 50 receptor sites out of a tissue total of 500. If this total is increased to 1000, the 50 receptors required for a maximal response now represent only 5% of the total. We have already seen that the tissue response is proportional to the fraction of receptors occupied (equation in Fig. 1.1(b)), so the concentration of agonist required to occupy only 5% of the total will also be reduced. This is observed as an increase in the apparent affinity of the agonist for the receptor – that is, an increase in tissue sensitivity.

In the case of insulin receptors, it has been estimated that less than 10% need to be occupied in order for the maximum tissue response to be obtained.

Down-regulation of insulin receptors, as in obesity, produces insulin resistance. Conversely, in starvation insulin receptors are up-regulated and insulin sensitivity is increased. A similar situation exists with oestrogen receptors, in which 20% occupation produces the maximum response and tissue sensitivity is regulated by changes in receptor number.

RECEPTOR COUPLING MECHANISMS

The conformational change in a receptor following the binding of an agonist is only the first of several steps necessary before the eventual response is observed. It can be a very rapid chain of events (milliseconds in the case of cholinergic synaptic transmission) or fairly slow – several days in the case of metabolic responses to steroids. It is convenient to divide receptor mechanisms into three broad groups:

- ligand-gated ion channels in which receptor binding produces a rapid change in the permeability of the cell membrane to specific ions; e.g. the GABA receptor and its associated Cl^- channel
- intracellular second messenger systems requiring cyclic AMP, cyclic GMP or Ca^{2+} and often involving protein phosphorylation (Fig. 1.7); e.g. adenylate cyclase dependent dopamine (D2) receptors in the brain
- intracellular receptors which enter the cell nucleus and stimulate DNA transcription and thus protein synthesis; e.g. the oestrogen receptors in the uterus.

A partial list of the different receptor types, their mechanisms of action, and the responses observed is set out in Table 1.1. Drug–receptor interactions will be dealt with in more detail in the later chapters where specific classes of drugs are being described.

DRUG DOSE AND THE CLINICAL RESPONSE

The dose–response relationship described so far relates to the drug effect at its specific site of action. These quantitative relationships are usually investigated in *in vitro* systems in which the concentration of the drug at the receptor is known accurately and is fixed. In the patient it is very unlikely that the circulating level of drug will remain constant, so that the equilibrium situation is never actually achieved. Following either a single or multiple dose of drug, the concentration of drug at its receptor site will depend upon the rate of delivery of drug to that site, usually by the general circulation, and the rate of removal by metabolism and excretion. These factors will be determined by the pharmacokinetic properties of the drug, which cannot be predicted from *in vitro* test systems.

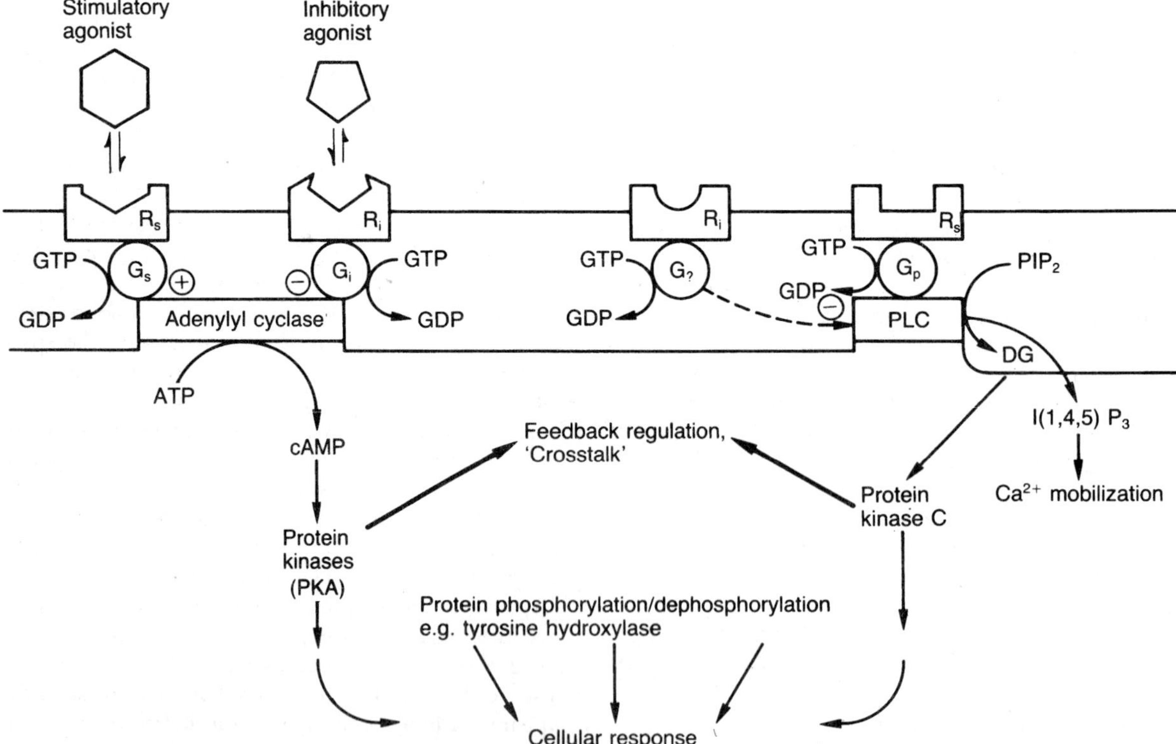

FIGURE 1.7 Adenylyl cyclase and polyphosphoinositide signal transduction mechanisms. R_s, stimulator receptor; R_i, inhibitory receptor; G_s, stimulatory G-protein; G_i, inhibitory G-protein; PLC, phospholipase C; PIP_2, inositol triphosphate; DG, diacylglycerol. Based on Fowler CJ *et al. Trends in Pharmacological Sciences* 1990; 11:84.

TABLE 1.1 Examples of drug receptor mechanisms

DRUG/HORMONE	RECEPTOR TYPE	PERMEABILITY CHANGE	CELL RESPONSE
(a) Ligand-gated ion channels			
Acetylcholine	Nicotinic	Na^+, K^+	Depolarization
GABA	$GABA_A$	Cl^-	Hyperpolarization
	$GABA_B$	K^+	Depolarization
Glutamate	Excitatory amino acid receptors	Na^+, K^+	Depolarization
(b) Receptors with intracellular second messengers			
Acetylcholine	Muscarinic (smooth muscle)	Ca^{2+}	Muscle contraction
Dopamine agonists	Peripheral D_1	cyclic AMP (increased)	Vasodilatation
Histamine	H_1 (smooth muscle)	Ca^{2+}	Muscle contraction
Insulin	Liver plasma membranes	Ca^{2+}, cyclic GMP (?)	Increased glucose uptake
Noradrenaline			
α_1-agonists	α_1 (vas deferens)	Ca^{2+}	Muscle contraction
α_2-agonists	α_2 (sphincters)	cyclic AMP (decreased)	Muscle contraction
β-agonists	β_2 (bronchioles)	cyclic AMP (increased)	Muscle relaxation
Thrombin	Platelets	Ca^{2+}, tri-phosphoinositol	Platelet activation
(c) Intracellular steroid receptors			
Dexamethasone	Glucocorticoid receptors	DNA-directed RNA and protein synthesis	Lipocortin production
Oestradiol	Uterine oestrogen receptors	DNA-directed RNA and protein synthesis	Cell division, tissue growth

To summarize, the affinity of a drug for specific receptor sites can be determined accurately by radioligand binding to isolated membranes *in vitro*. From this information the relative potency and specificity of action of a drug may be inferred. This is of value in judging whether a new drug is likely to present a significant improvement over existing drugs. Then, using isolated tissues *ex vivo*, it is possible to gain knowledge of the efficacy of a drug; that is, its agonist or antagonist properties. However, in order to determine the maximum clinical response and the duration of action it is necessary to carry out whole animal or human studies.

See p. 675 for Glossary of Pharmacological Terms.

FURTHER READING

Furchgott RF, Bursztyn P. Comparison of dissociation constants and relative efficiencies of selective agonists acting on parasympathetic receptors. *Annals of the New York Academy of Science* 1967; **139**: 882.

Kenakin T. The classification of drugs and drug receptors. *Pharmacological Reviews* 1984; **36**: 165.

Laduron PM. Towards a genomic pharmacology: from membranal to nuclear receptors. *Advances in Drug Research* 1992; **22:** 108–48.

Lefkowitz RJ, Caron MG, Stiles GL. Mechanisms of membrane-receptor regulation: biochemical, physiological, and clinical insights derived from studies of the adrenergic receptors. *New England Journal of Medicine* 1984; **310:** 1570.

Molinoff PB, Wolfe, BB, Weiland GA. Quantitative analysis of drug–receptor interactions: II Determination of the properties of receptor subtypes. *Life Sciences* 1981; **29:** 427.

Strickland S, Loeb JN. Obligatory separation of hormone binding and biological response curves in systems dependent on secondary mediators of hormone action. *Proceedings of the National Academy of Sciences USA* 1981; **78:** 1366.

Taylor P, Insel PA. Molecular basis of pharmacologic selectivity. In Pratt WB, Taylor P eds. *Principles of drug action*, 3rd edn. Edinburgh: Churchill Livingstone, 1990, 1–102.

Walaas SI, Greengard P. Protein phosphorylation and neuronal function. *Pharmacological Reviews* 1991; **43:** 299–349

2

Pharmacokinetics – the Absorption, Distribution and Elimination of Drugs

PV Taberner

The pharmacokinetic properties of a drug are as important as its actions on target cells (pharmacodynamics), since they will determine the size and frequency of dosing. The two principal factors which determine the concentration of a drug at its site of action at any time after administration are:

- the rate of absorption and disposition within the body
- the rate of removal by metabolism and excretion.

In many cases the metabolic products are themselves pharmacologically active so drug metabolism does not invariably terminate the therapeutic effects of the drug. Since the aim of drug therapy is to achieve and maintain a blood level of active drug that is above the minimum effective concentration but below the minimum toxic concentration, it is important to understand the pharmacokinetic processes that will affect the bioavailability of an administered drug. This chapter considers the absorption, distribution and excretion of drugs; Chapter 3 addresses the principles of drug metabolism.

BIOAVAILABILITY

This term is commonly used to describe the rate and extent to which an active (free) drug ingredient is absorbed from the administered product to become available at the site of action. The three measurements which are used to describe the bioavailability of a drug are: (1) the total amount absorbed after giving a single dose; (2) the maximum blood or plasma concentration (C_{max}); and (3) the rate of absorption from the site of administration (measured as the time taken for the blood concentration to peak, t_{max}). A drug given by rapid intravenous injection is immediately and completely bioavailable. Administration via other routes leads to incomplete bioavailability; owing either to incomplete absorption, or metabolism of the drug before it reaches the general circulation (*first pass effect*).

A typical blood level/time curve is shown in Fig. 2.1. The total amount of drug absorbed cannot be calculated exactly, but it will be proportional to the area under the curve (AUC). The relative bioavailability of a drug from a particular route of administration can therefore be estimated from the AUC values:

$$\text{Bioavailability} = \frac{\text{AUC} \times \text{Dose}_{\text{iv}}}{\text{AUC}_{\text{iv}} \times \text{Dose}}$$

RATES OF ABSORPTION AND DISTRIBUTION

These will be determined by the route and the rate of administration of the drug, and also by the physicochemical properties of the drug molecule, and by the formulation in which the active drug is presented. In the simplest case, intravenous injection of a bolus of

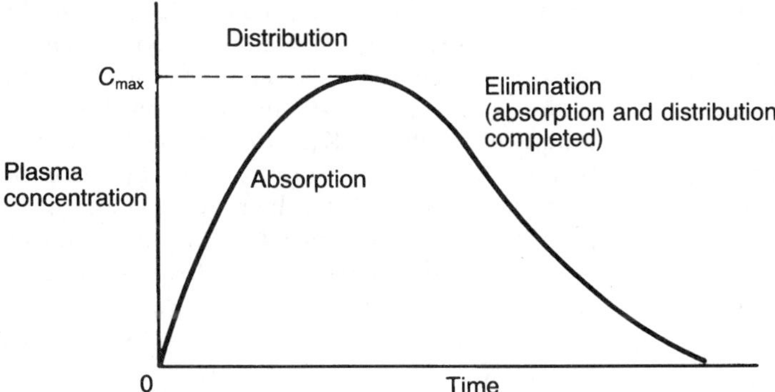

FIGURE 2.1 Typical blood concentration vs. time plot showing absorption, distribution and elimination phases. In the ideal equilibrium situation, where absorption = elimination, the plasma concentration will be constant. This is most nearly achieved by constant iv infusion.

drug, the peak blood level occurs at zero time (t_0) and declines thereafter. The declining part of the curve is sometimes seen to be biphasic; the initial steep part corresponds to the distribution phase, the subsequent slower decline corresponds to the elimination of the drug by metabolism or excretion. Other routes of administration (see below) will produce a gradual rise in blood level to the peak. In these cases the peak concentration will be determined by the net balance between absorption and distribution.

Drug transfer across membranes

The passage of drug molecules into and out of the bloodstream depends upon their ability to cross the lipid barriers presented by the cell membranes separating the bloodstream from the other aqueous compartments of the body. The relative volumes of the various compartments are shown schematically in Fig. 2.2.

Passive diffusion

A lipid-soluble drug (i.e. one that is unionized at physiological pH) will readily cross cell membranes by passive diffusion down the concentration gradient and will also enter the CNS across the blood–brain barrier by the same mechanism. The adipose tissues, which have a high lipid content but low blood perfusion rate, can therefore provide a reservoir in the longer term for highly lipid-soluble drugs. Much of the renal excretory process involves the passive

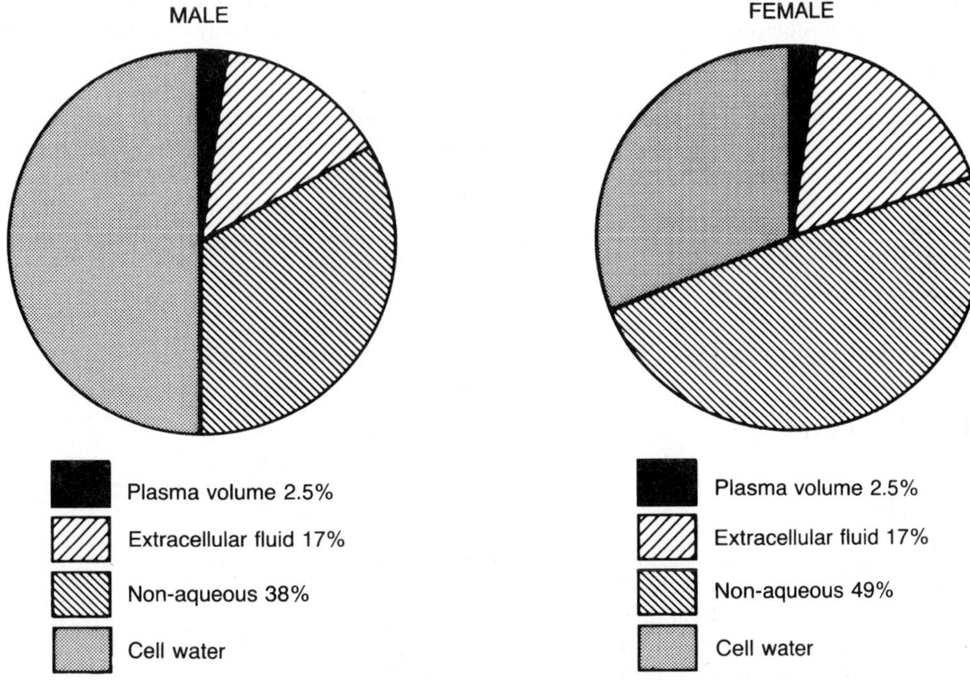

FIGURE 2.2 Relative volumes of the principal body fluid compartments. Total body water (measured by D_2O dilution) averages 62% in males, 51% in females. Extracellular fluid (ECF) (measured by sodium thiosulphate dilution) is similar in both sexes. Plasma volume (measured by Evans blue dye dilution) is slightly greater in males. Cell water (intracellular fluid) is calculated by subtracting ECF from the total water.

transfer of drugs across membranes. The rate of diffusion will depend upon the concentration gradient across the membrane, the surface area of the membrane exposed to the drug, and the relative solubility or partition coefficient of the drug between the aqueous and lipid phases. Historically, the chloroform/water partition coefficient has been used to approximate to the biological situation. It is simple to measure *in vitro* and, from the earliest experiments of Meyer and Overton, has provided a useful predictor of the anaesthetic properties and distribution of drugs *in vivo* (see Chapter 4).

Diffusion through membrane pores

Biological membranes invariably contain small aqueous pores through which small polar molecules may pass. Because of their small size (0.4 nm) only substances of molecular weights less than 150 Da will pass through. Highly polar or ionized molecules are likely to be repelled by ionic charges on the membrane, and they will not pass in spite of their small size.

Lipid solubility, pH and ionization

Since it is only the uncharged species of the drug that can diffuse across a lipid membrane barrier, the relative proportions of ionized and unionized molecules at physiological pH will influence the rates of absorption, distribution, and excretion of a drug. Most drugs are weak acids or bases. Bases will combine with hydrogen ions in solution to form a charged molecule:

$$B + H^+ \rightleftharpoons BH^+$$

The forward ionization reaction will be favoured at acid pH.

Weak acids, in contrast, yield up hydrogen ions when they ionize:

$$AH \rightleftharpoons A^- + H^+$$

This ionization is favoured at alkaline pH.

The ionization constant (pK_a) will determine the proportion of molecules ionized at any given pH:

$$\text{Bases}: \; pK_a - pH = \log_{10} \frac{[BH^+]}{[B]}$$

$$\text{Acids}: \; pK_a - pH = \log_{10} \frac{[AH]}{[A^-]}$$

These Henderson–Hasselbalch equations can be used to calculate the pK_a values for a drug; more often they are used to estimate the proportion of drug that is ionized at any particular pH, when the pK_a value is known. When the pH = pK_a, the drug, whether it be a base or an acid, will be 50% ionized. A change in pH of one unit away from the pK_a will then affect the proportions of ionized and unionized molecules by a factor of 10. For example, quinine (pK_a 8.4) will be about 90% ionized at physiological pH. Small changes in pH can be important for the excretion of a drug from the plasma (pH 7.4) into the urine (pH 6.0–8.0), particularly if the pK_a is close to these physiological values. Drugs with high pK_a values can either be fairly strong bases (atropine, chloroquine, chlorpromazine), or very weak acids (phenytoin, pentobarbitone). Drugs with low pK_a values are either fairly strong acids (dihydroxyphenylalanine (L-DOPA)), or very weak bases (diazepam, librium). Some examples are given in Table 2.1.

Active transport

If an endogenous substrate or drug is to be transported across a membrane against a concentration gradient, then metabolic energy will be required and the process is termed active transport. A carrier protein, or translocase, situated across the cell membrane will bind the substrate and transport it across the membrane, using energy derived from ATP by phosphorylation of the carrier protein (see Fig. 2.3). In some cases (carrier-mediated transport) the carrier acts passively to facilitate diffusion down the concentration gradient; no metabolic energy is required, and the process is termed *facilitated diffusion.*

Active transport can be blocked by metabolic inhibitors such as cyanide and, because there is a specific binding site on the carrier protein, active transport shares many of the properties of the enzyme–substrate interaction: it is stereoselective (only one isomer will be transported) and charge selective, it is saturable, and is subject to competitive inhibition by structural analogues of the normal substrate, or to non-competitive inhibition by ligands that bind to inhibitory sites on the protein. For example, the cardiotonic steroids digitalis and ouabain block the sodium potassium (ATPase-linked) pump in cardiac muscle by inhibiting dephosphorylation of the carrier protein.

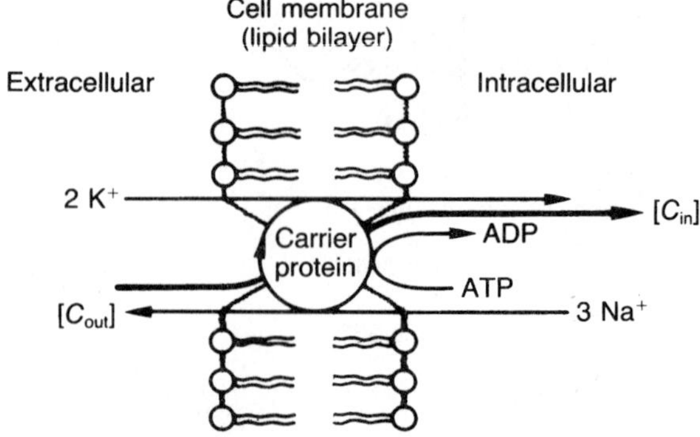

FIGURE 2.3 Mechanism of the active transport process. The cardiac glycoside ouabain blocks the activity of sodium–potassium ATPase by binding specifically to a receptor site on the outside surface of the carrier protein.

TABLE 2.1 Ionization constants (pKa values) of some widely used drugs

WEAK ACIDS		WEAK BASES	
HA DRUG	$H^+ + A^-$ pKa	BH^+ DRUG	$B + H^+$ pKa
Methyl DOPA	2.2, 9.2*	Diazepam	3.3
Ampicillin	2.5	Chlordiazepoxide	4.6
Salicyclic acid	3.0	Methysergide	6.6
Ethacrynic acid	3.5	Pyrimethamine	7.0
Aspirin	3.5	Kanamycin	7.2
Frusemide (furosemide)	3.9	Lidocaine	7.9
Ibuprofen	4.4, 5.2*	Morphine	7.9
Warfarin	5.0	Nicotine	7.9, 3.1*
Tolbutamide	5.3	Scopolamine	8.1
Acetazolamide	7.2	Cocaine	8.5
Phenobarbital	7.4	Isoprenaline (isoproterenol)	8.6
Pentobarbitone	8.1	Procaine	9.0
Theophylline	8.8	Propranolol	9.4
Paracetamol (acetaminophen)	9.5	Desipramine	10.2
		Methyl DOPA	10.6
		Guanethidine	11.4, 8.3*

The pKa value represents the pH at which the drug will be 50% ionized. Some drugs (*) have more than one ionizable group. At 2 pH units *above* the pKa about 99% of an acidic drug will be ionized; at 2 pH units *below* the pKa about 99% of a basic drug will be ionized. The pKa is the negative logarithm of the ionization (dissociation) constant of the molecule.

Important active transport systems from a pharmacokinetic point of view are situated in the gastrointestinal tract, the blood–brain barrier, the biliary tract and the renal tubule. The amino acid transporter in the small intestine epithelium is the route by which L-DOPA is absorbed after oral administration. Tetracyclines are actively transported from serum into bile where they are concentrated. Penicillins are actively pumped from the cerebrospinal fluid to the blood across the choroid plexus. It is the active transport of penicillins across the renal tubule that is responsible for their rapid renal clearance. For therapeutic purposes the carrier can be saturated by a competing substrate in order to inhibit the excretion of a drug. For example, probenecid can be used to achieve a high concentration of penicillin in the circulation.

A number of drugs interact with the specific neuronal active transport systems responsible for terminating the actions of neurotransmitters such as noradrenaline, adrenaline and 5-hydroxytryptamine (5-HT). These are discussed later when the drugs are considered in more detail.

Pinocytosis

Some large molecules (> 1 kDa) can be engulfed by an invagination of the cell membrane and transported into the interior in the form of a vesicle containing extracellular fluid. This mechanism is responsible for the transport of aminoglycoside antibiotics such as gentamicin into the proximal tubule of the kidney. The reverse process, emiocytosis, is the means by which many polypeptide hormones (insulin for example) are secreted into the bloodstream.

VOLUME OF DISTRIBUTION (V_d)

This parameter is usually expressed in litres (l), but is occasionally quoted as l/kg. It relates the total amount of drug in the various aqueous compartments of the body to the blood or plasma concentration (see Fig. 2.2), and so provides a useful relative measure of the distribution of a drug. The apparent V_d is obtained by dividing the total dose by the blood concentration:

$$V_d = \text{Dose}/C_{\text{plasma}}$$

Units: (l) (mg) (mg/l)

It does not represent a real volume, but can be defined as *the volume that would be occupied by the drug if all the drug in the body was at the same concentration as the blood level.* For example, a drug that was entirely confined to the bloodstream would have an apparent V_d equal to the blood volume (5.5 l for a 70-kg man). In practice this is unlikely and the smallest values for apparent V_d are about 7–8 l.

The volume of distribution is determined by:

- the pKa of the drug, and hence its degree of ionization

- the partition coefficient between the blood and other body compartments
- the proportion bound to plasma proteins
- the extent of binding to other proteins and tissues
- the total aqueous volume available.

A highly lipid-soluble drug will leave the blood and tend to accumulate in the fatty tissues, so that very little of the original dose remains in the blood. Consequently, the apparent V_d will be very much greater than the blood volume, and may even exceed the total body volume. Digoxin, for example, distributes readily into muscle, liver and adipose tissue, so the blood level represents a very small proportion of the total dose. Digoxin has an apparent V_d of over 500 l. In contrast, the closely related glycoside digitoxin is highly bound to plasma proteins; a higher proportion of the total dose remains in the plasma, and it has an apparent V_d of 40 l. Some other examples are shown in Table 2.2.

Clearance

This represents the rate of overall elimination or removal of a drug from a specific fluid compartment. It is usually defined in terms of blood (Cl_b), plasma (Cl_p), or renal (Cl_r) clearance:

$$\underset{\text{(ml/min)}}{\text{Plasma clearance } Cl_p} = \underset{\text{(mg/min)}}{\text{Rate of elimination}} / \underset{\text{(mg/ml)}}{C_{plasma}}$$

A plasma clearance rate of 100 ml/min for a drug that is excreted unchanged implies that the kidneys are able to remove the drug from a notional 100 ml of

TABLE 2..2 Distribution volumes (V_d) and plasma protein binding of some widely used drugs

DRUG	% PLASMA PROTEIN BOUND	APPARENT VOLUME OF DISTRIBUTION (l)
Warfarin	99	7.7 ± 0.7
Aspirin	50	11 ± 2
Atracurium	—	11 ± 1.4
Vecuronium	30	15 ± 5
Gentamicin	95	18 ± 6
Indomethacin	90	18 ± 5
Chlordiazepoxide	96	21 ± 2
Tubocurarine	50	21 ± 8
Amoxicillin	18	29 ± 13
Phenobarbitone	50	38 ± 2
Digitoxin	97	38 ± 10
Prazosin	95	42 ± 9
Acyclovir	15	50 ± 17
Lithium	0	55 ± 24
Alfentanyl	92	56 ± 21
Paracetamol (acetaminophen)	10	67 ± 8
Cimetidine	19	70 ± 14
Diazepam	99	77 ± 20
Nifedipine	98	84 ± 35
Tetracycline	65	105 ± 6
Ketamine	12	125 ± 50
Ranitidine	15	130 ± 20
Morphine	35	230 ± 60
Propranolol	93	270 ± 40
Fentanyl	85	280 ± 28
Verapamil	90	280 ± 60
Digoxin	25	640 ± 200
Labetalol	50	700 ± 140
Nortriptyline	92	1300 ± 300
Chloroquine	60	13000

These values, derived from Benet & Williams (Benet LZ, Williams RL Appendix II. Design and optimization of dosage regimens: pharmacokinetic data, In Giilman AG, Rall TW, Nies AS, Taylor P eds. *Goodman and Gilman's The pharmacological basis of therapeutics*, 8th edn. New York: Pergamon Press, 1990: 1650–735) are intended only as a relative guide. They are generally based on a healthy 70-kg subject and may be significantly altered in a disease state.

plasma every minute. This represents *renal clearance* (Cl_r), and it can be estimated from the plasma and urine concentrations of the drug, and the rate of urine production:

$$Cl_r = (C_{urine} \times \text{Urine volume})/C_{plasma}$$

The clearance of a drug that is metabolized wholly by the liver will be limited by the rate of blood flow to the liver. Values of Cl_p can sometimes appear to be non-physiological, especially for drugs such as morphine that are taken up by red blood cells. This is because the plasma concentration will significantly underestimate the total concentration of drug presented to the organ of elimination. Interpatient variations in clearance are larger than variations in absorption or volume of distribution, so clearance rates are the single most important factor in determining the steady-state concentration of a drug and therefore, by inference, the dosing schedule. Renal clearance will depend largely upon the glomerular filtration rate (GFR). This can be assessed by measuring the creatinine clearance (Cr_{Cl}) in a patient. Creatinine is a by-product of normal muscle metabolism and is readily filtered by the glomerulus with little or no secretion or reabsorption by the tubule. If the muscle mass is stable, creatinine production will be constant, and any change in plasma creatinine levels will reflect a change in GFR. The measurement of Cr_{Cl} therefore provides an estimate of the GFR. This is usually done by collecting urine over a 24-h period and taking a plasma sample for creatinine assay sometime in the middle of this period. There are formulae provided for calculating the normal (population average) Cr_{Cl} which take into account the age, weight and sex of the patient. In this way it is possible to determine whether impaired renal function is likely to complicate drug therapy.

Most drugs are eliminated by more than one route, so the overall clearance from plasma represents the sum total of renal, hepatic and other sites of elimination. In almost all cases the rate of elimination of a drug depends upon the blood or plasma concentration, and the clearance will be constant over the normal therapeutic range. The dosing rate can be directly related to clearance by the following equation:

Dose rate	= Clearance	× Steady state plasma concentration
(mg/24 h)	(l/24 h)	(mg/l)

This simplified relationship assumes that the target plasma concentration is well below the equilibrium rate constant (Km) of the metabolizing enzyme and that the GFR is never saturated. One exception to this rule is alcohol (ethanol), which is 95–98% metabolized and saturates its metabolizing enzymes at concentrations well below those obtained by social drinking. As a result, its elimination is independent of the blood level (zero-order kinetics); the fall of the blood concentration with time approximates to a straight line, and the plasma clearance varies with respect to time. Similarly, aspirin at high (toxic) doses will saturate the metabolizing enzymes, thus prolonging the plasma half-life by up to 12 h (see below).

Half-life

The half-life ($t_{1/2}$) of a drug in a body fluid compartment simply represents the time taken for the concentration to fall to half the original concentration. In the absence of any qualification, it can be assumed to refer to plasma half-life.

In the simplest one-compartment pharmacokinetic model in which the drug is instantaneously distributed throughout its V_d (see Fig. 2.4), the decline of the blood concentration will be an exponential decay:

$$-dC/dt = (Cl_p \,.\, C_t) \,/\, V_d$$

where Cl_p is plasma clearance, and C_t = plasma concentration at time t.

Expressed logarithmically:

$$\ln (C_t) = \ln (C_{t=0}) - (Cl_p/V_d) \,.\, t$$

The term Cl_p/V_d is the elimination rate constant k_e. A plot of ln C (the natural logarithm of the plasma concentration) against time will yield a straight line with a slope of $-k_e$:

$$\ln (C_t) - \ln (C_{t=0}) = -k_e \,.\, t$$

Rearranging gives:

$$t = \ln (C_{t=0}/C_t) \,.(1/k_e)$$

Since the plasma half-life represents the time during which the plasma concentration falls by half:

$$t_{1/2} = \ln 2 \,.(1/k_e) = 0.693/k_e$$

In the more commonly encountered two-compartment model (see Fig. 2.5), the rate constant is a hybrid, and includes the rate constants for redistribution into other compartments in addition to the elimination rate constant k_e. Under these circumstances, it is usually designated β; the associated elimination half-life being $t_{1/2\beta}$. Because rate constants have the unit of reciprocal time (i.e. fractions of an hour), it is often easier to think in terms of half-lives, which are in the more familiar units of hours and minutes (see Table 2.3 for examples).

Steady-state kinetics

Although the decline of blood levels of drug following a single dose gives an indication of how long the drug persists in the body, repeated doses will produce fluctuating plasma levels. A gradual accumulation will occur if the previous dose is not completely cleared by the time the next dose is given. The mean plasma level will rise up to the time when the amount entering the bloodstream during each dose interval equals the amount leaving the bloodstream over the same period. This equilibrium is the steady state, and it is important

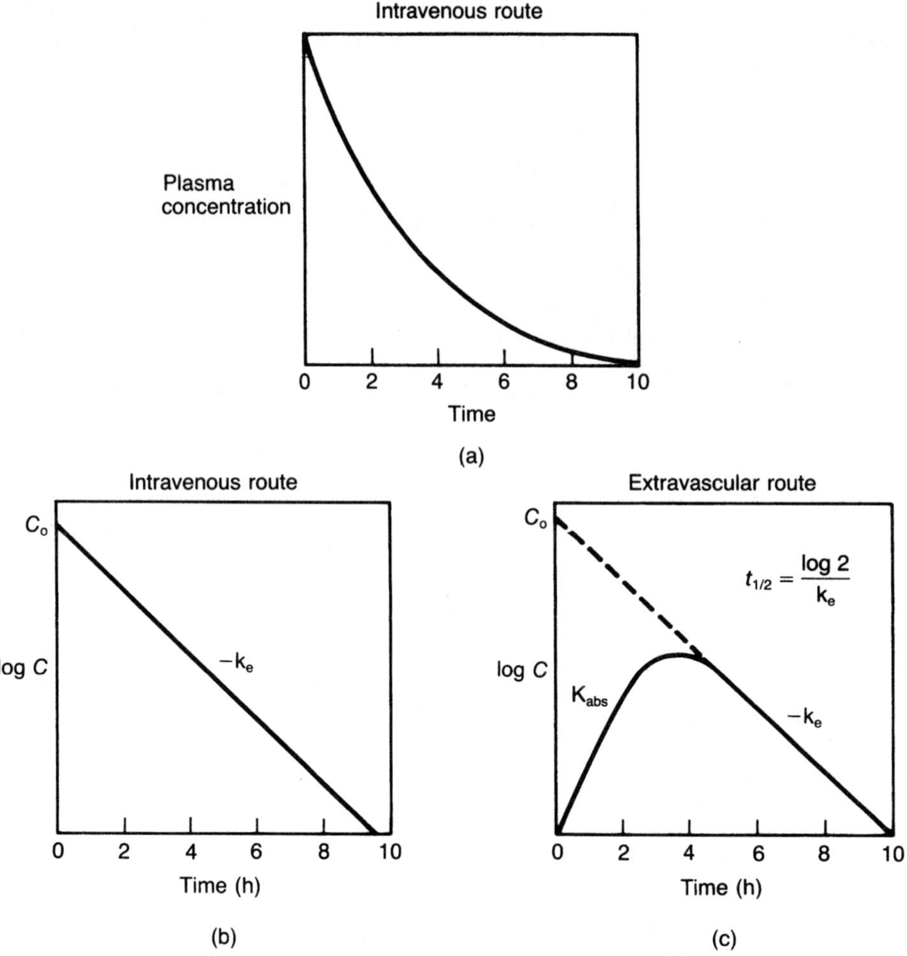

FIGURE 2.4 Exponential decline of plasma drug concentration, single compartment model. (a) Linear plot shows exponential decay (first-order kinetics). (b) and (c) Semi-logarithmic plots yield straight lines.

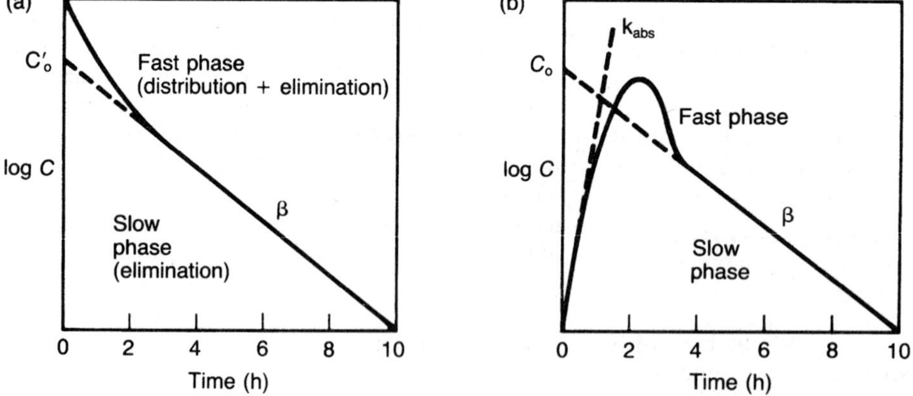

FIGURE 2.5 Two-compartment model of distribution and elimination. (a) Intravenous route. (b) Extravascular route. K_{abs} = rate constant for absorption β = rate constant for elimination.

for the clinician to know when it has been achieved. From a kinetic point of view, a steady state will be attained after four to five half-lives.

It is important to remember that even under steady-state conditions the plasma level will vary with time. It is only the *mean* plasma level during a dosing interval that is constant. If the plasma half-life alters for some reason during dosing, the steady state will be disturbed and the dose or dosing frequency may need to be adjusted to compensate. This is particularly important where drugs either induce or inhibit liver enzymes (see Chapter 3).

TABLE 2.3 Plasma half-lives and clearance rates of some widely used drugs

DRUG	ELIMINATION HALF-LIFE (h)	CLEARANCE (ml/min)	RENAL CLEARANCE (% OF DOSE)
Acetylsalicyclic acid	0.25 ± 0.3	(pH and dose-dependent)	
Atracurium	0.33 ± 0.04	385 ± 70	0
Amoxicillin	1.0 ± 0.1	370 ± 90	50–70
Alfentanyl	1.5 ± 2.0	470 ± 170	>1
Vecuronium	1.5 ± 0.7	210 ± 7	20
Cimetidine	1.9 ± 1.3	540 ± 130	50–70
Paracetamol (acetaminophen)	2.0 ± 0.4	350 ± 100	0
Tubocurarine	2.0 ± 1.1	160 ± 50	40–60
Ketamine	2.3 ± 0.5	1050 ± 350	5
Gallamine	2.5 ± 0.2	84–132	85–100
Morphine	3.0 ± 1.2	1100 ± 140	10
Procainamide	3.0 ± 0.6	350–840	50–70
Triazolam	3.0 ± 1.4	200–500	0
Fentanyl	3.5 ± 0.5	5.5–12.5	6–8
Propranolol	3.9 ± 0.4	840 ± 210	0
Pentazocine	4.5 ± 1.5	1200–1400	<5
Verapamil	4.8 ± 2.4	830 ± 350	<5
Etomidate	5.0 ± 0.8	800–1500	2
Ranitidine	6.2 ± 1.8	730 ± 80	80
Chlordiazepoxide	10 ± 3	38 ± 34	0
Thiopentone	10 ± 2.5	200–250	<1
Pirenzepine	12 ± 2.5	220–300	10
Valproic acid	14 ± 3	7.7 ± 1.4	5
d-Propoxyphene	16 ± 7.5	900 ± 200	0
Desipramine	36 ± 12	2000	<2
Digoxin	39 ± 13	130 ± 67	70–80
Diazepam	43 ± 13	27 ± 4	0
Phenobarbitone	96 ± 24	4.3 ± 0.9	10–20
Digitoxin	5–8 days	3.9 ± 1.3	33

The clearance rates are based on a standard 70-kg subject. Data derived from Benet & Sheiner (1990) – see Table 2.2.
Further pharmacokinetic data is provided in Chapter 29 Appendix (p. 544).

ROUTES OF ADMINISTRATION

The route of administration of a drug will determine the rate at which it enters the bloodstream and, in most instances, its rate of onset of action and clinical efficacy. Since the rate of absorption directly affects the peak plasma concentration, it can be an important factor in reducing the risk of acute adverse reactions due to overdosage. The principal routes of administration are shown diagrammatically in Fig. 2.6. Direct intravenous injection bypasses the absorptive process and achieves the maximum bioavailability of a drug. On the other hand, it can be important for a drug to be excluded from the circulation in order to avoid adverse effects. Some externally applied antibiotics, for example, would be toxic if given systemically and, for orally administered drugs that are intended to act within the gut lumen (laxatives, antilipidaemics, presurgical intestinal antibiotics for instance), absorption from the gut would be a disadvantage. The most widely used routes of administration are oral, sublingual (buccal), inhalational, intramuscular, intravenous, subcutaneous, rectal, topical and transdermal (percutaneous). The intranasal, intrathecal and intracardiac routes are employed more rarely, although the intrathecal route is used in anaesthetics to obtain local effects (see p. 96). The intranasal route is popular amongst abusers of amphetamine and cocaine and may provide an alternative route for administering peptide drugs (see p. 18 for intranasal diabetes, see p. 20 for intrathecal injecitons).

Sublingual administration

For lipid-soluble drugs that are unstable at gastric pH or rapidly metabolized by the liver, this route provides a means of obtaining systemic absorption and high

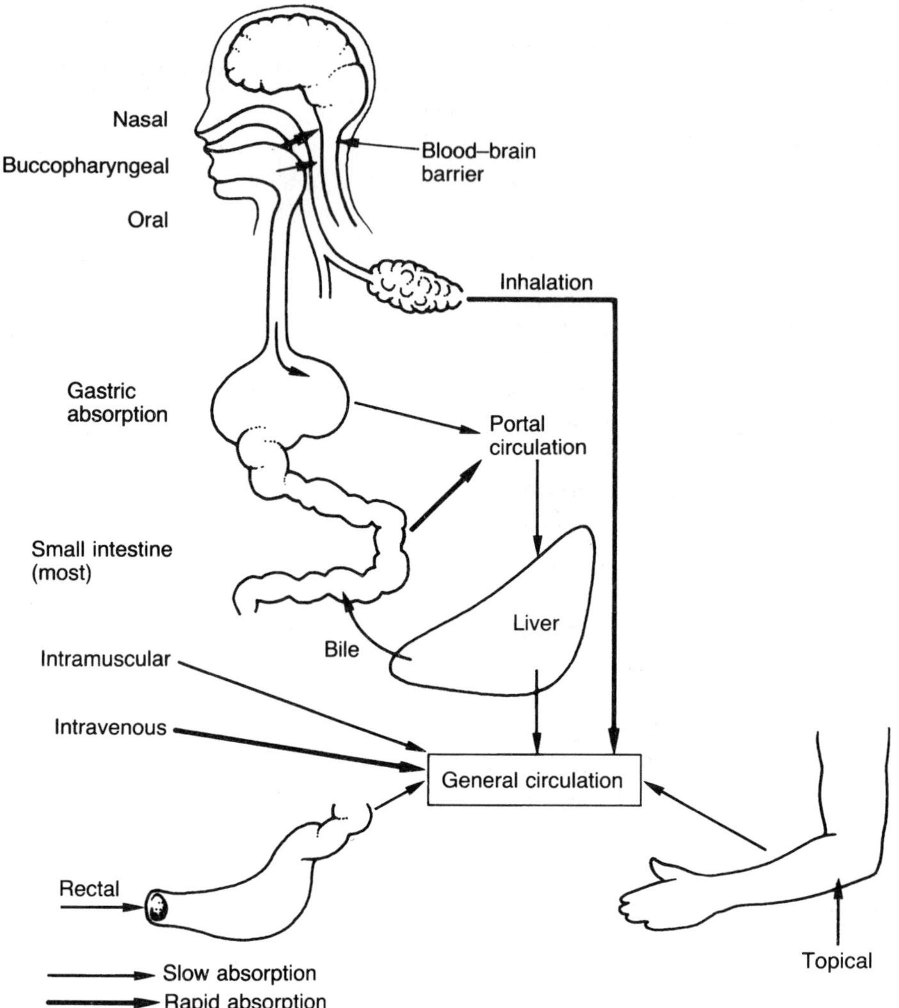

FIGURE 2.6 Routes of administration and the distribution of drugs.

bioavailability by avoiding the portal circulation. Acute treatment of anginal pain with sublingual nitroglycerin is an example.

However, drugs of high molecular weight are not well absorbed by this route, which makes it unsuitable for administering insulin or other large peptides. A recent innovation has been the development of intranasally delivered insulin for diabetics. The nasal mucous membranes present less of a barrier to large molecules than the buccal membranes so that a relatively rapid absorption rate can be achieved.

Inhalational administration

Apart from the inhalation of gaseous anaesthetics and other therapeutic gases, this route can be used for any volatile drug as well as aerosols of liquids or microfined powders. Bronchodilators such as isoprenaline or salbutamol can be inhaled from an aerosol. The antiasthmatic drug sodium cromoglycate, which is water insoluble, is delivered as a fine powder. The large surface area of the lungs and their high blood flow ensure a rapid systemic absorption of lipid-soluble drugs. That this is faster than buccal absorption can be seen by contrasting the greater bioavailability of nicotine in smokers who inhale with those who do not. This route is becoming a clinical option for an increasing number of drugs. The pharmacokinetics of inhalational anaesthetics are described in detail in Chapter 4.

Rectal administration

The veins that drain the rectal region also enter the systemic circulation directly. Consequently, lipid-soluble drugs will be well absorbed from the rectum by passive diffusion across the lipid membranes of the rectal mucosa. This route is used for drugs that are intended to act directly in the rectal and anal regions (local anaesthetic and anti-inflammatory drugs), as well as an alternative to oral administration for drugs used systemically.

Oral administration

This is the most common route of administration for the majority of drugs. The exceptions are those drugs that are destroyed by acid hydrolysis in the stomach or by the action of digestive enzymes in the gut lumen. The use of enteric coatings in drug formulations can overcome this problem by protecting drugs until they have reached the alkaline environment of the small intestine where the coating dissolves, thus releasing the drug. The limiting factor for absorption throughout the gastrointestinal tract is the proportion of unionized drug molecules. Only acidic drugs, such as aspirin, will be absorbed at the gastric pH; for the majority of drugs most absorption occurs in the small intestine. Drugs that are structural analogues of normal metabolites can be transported across the epithelium by the specific active transport process. The cytotoxic drug fluorouracil, for example, is taken up by the non-specific pyrimidine carrier which normally transports thymidine and uracil.

Several additional factors will influence the rate of absorption of a drug following oral administration. These include:

- The presence and nature of any food in the stomach: a fatty meal will absorb any lipid-soluble drug and also slow its absorption by delaying the passage of the drug into the small intestine.
- Gastrointestinal motility. Drugs or dietary components that delay gastric emptying will slow the passage of drugs into the small intestine. Opiate drugs inhibit gastric emptying and peristaltic activity, as do antimuscarinics such as atropine and, perhaps most importantly, alcohol. Conversely, in patients with diarrhoea, the rapid passage of the gut contents will significantly reduce the absorption, and hence the bioavailability, of many drugs.
- Splanchnic blood flow. Drug absorption is severely impaired in hypovolaemia. Portal blood flow, which is reduced in hepatic disease such as cirrhosis, can then become the rate-limiting step in the delivery of drugs into the systemic circulation.
- Formulation of the drug. Acidic drugs, such as aspirin or penicillin, are fairly insoluble at the low pH of the stomach. When given as soluble salts of sodium or potassium in liquid form, the drug precipitates as a fine suspension of the free acid. In this form they are more readily absorbed from the stomach. Conversely, a basic drug such as morphine will not be absorbed until it passes into the small intestine. The difference between liquid and solid preparations of lipid-soluble drugs is well illustrated by the benzodiazepine temazepam. This sedative–hypnotic is much more readily absorbed from a gel-filled capsule than from a tablet. However, the liquid gel form is open to abuse by intravenous drug abusers and is now being withdrawn from sale.
- The importance of the size of drug particles in determining the rate of absorption is well illustrated by the plasma concentration following standard doses of different formulations of aspirin (see Fig. 2.7).

Administration by injection

The intravenous route, as mentioned before, ensures the most rapid delivery of the drug to its site of action. It is the rate of injection or infusion that will determine the rate of delivery of the drug, first to the lungs, then to the systemic circulation. It is advantageous to have the injected material in a soluble form at physiological pH. The intravenous barbiturate thiopentone, for example, is made up with sodium carbonate vehicle to give a pH of 10.5. In this case, extravasation of the vehicle at the site of injection will be painful and can cause tissue necrosis.

If the rate of drug infusion can be adjusted to match the rate of elimination, the plasma level will plateau and an equilibrium state can be maintained. The principal disadvantages of intravenous injection or infusion (the fast onset and offset of action) can be overcome by subcutaneous (sc) or intramuscular (im) injection. The rate of absorption from the site of injection will depend upon the rate of diffusion of the drug away from the injection site and the local blood flow; im injection tends to result in slower absorption than sc. Absorption from the injection site can be increased by the co-administration of hyaluronidase, an enzyme that dissolves the tissue matrix, or reduced by adrenaline or vasopressin analogues, which produce a local vasoconstriction and prevent the escape of the drug into the general circulation. This latter technique is important in the administration of local anaesthetics. The degree of local vasoconstriction or dilatation can

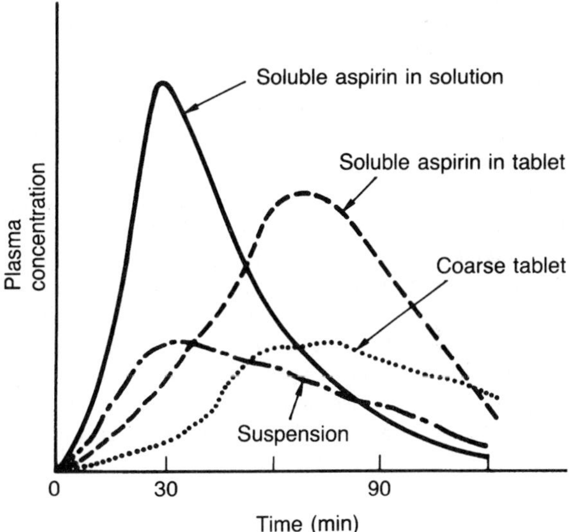

FIGURE 2.7 Influence of drug formulation on absorption of aspirin (acetylsalicylic acid).

also be manipulated by altering the ambient temperature, but care should be taken as the patient's temperature rises and the drug is washed into the bloodstream.

Alternatively, delayed absorption can be achieved by giving the drug in a depot formulation. The numerous preparations of insulin (see Chapter 33) amply illustrate this point. Implanted pellets have been used to achieve a very slow but continuous absorption of a number of drugs – the hormones testosterone and oestradiol have been administered this way; implants of deoxycortone acetate which last up to 6 months have been used to treat cases of Addison's disease.

Intrathecal injection into the subarachnoid space using a lumbar puncture needle has been used to achieve regional anaesthesia (see Chapter 7) and also to deliver antibiotics directly into the CNS, bypassing the blood–brain barrier. Other regional injection methods include the recent introduction of the technique of administering vasodilatory drugs directly into the corpus cavernosum of the penis to treat male patients suffering from erectile impotence.

Topical and transdermal administration

Topical administration is used in ophthalmology, for instilling drugs into the eye, also for treating localized disorders of the skin and mucous membranes, to provide antisepsis, and to achieve a locally high concentration of an antibiotic or other chemotherapeutic agent within an infected area. Drugs that would be too toxic to be tolerated if administered systemically can be given safely in this way. The skin epithelium presents a thicker and less permeable barrier to the entry of drugs compared with other absorptive surfaces and, since the blood perfusion rate is relatively low, there is little likelihood of a locally applied drug appearing at sudden high concentrations in the bloodstream. The exceptions to this rule are highly lipid-soluble organic compounds, particularly if they are dissolved in an organic solvent. Widespread skin exposure can then result in the rapid appearance of symptoms of toxicity. This represents a significant environmental hazard in the case of some pesticides and industrial solvents.

However, transdermal (percutaneous) administration can also be employed for the application of drugs that are sufficiently well absorbed. Clearly, in order to be successful, the drug needs to be unionized and highly lipid soluble. The advantage of this means of delivery is the slow but steady rate of absorption. The earliest example was the anti-anginal drug, glyceryl trinitrate. More recently, antimotion sickness drugs and nicotine have been formulated in adhesive patches. For a given concentration of drug the rate of absorption will be proportional to the size of the patch.

Drug targeting

This technique has been applied particularly to antiviral and antitumour drugs which are generally cytotoxic. The drug is given as an inactive (prodrug) precursor and is only converted to the active principle at the site of action. Enzymes which are specific to the target cells or micro-organisms convert the prodrug to its cytotoxic form. The binding of drugs to tissue-specific antibodies is another means of achieving the same end.

ROUTES OF ELIMINATION

Drugs and their metabolites are largely eliminated through renal excretion, although volatile compounds will be lost through the lungs and by diffusion from the body surface. Other less important routes are the sweat and saliva. A number of drugs are actively excreted in the bile (some cardiac glycosides for example). These can be reabsorbed from the lumen of the duodenum, resulting in the so-called enterohepatic circulation. Apart from the drugs that are not absorbed from the gut, relatively few compounds appear in the faeces. However, in patients with severe diarrhoea, many orally administered drugs will not remain long enough within the gut to be adequately absorbed. This can lead to problems when a consistent blood level is required in order to maintain the clinical effectiveness of a drug. Although many drugs are excreted in the maternal milk, in only a few instances during lactation does the drug reach a therapeutically significant level in the infant. Those drugs that can give rise to problems are: lithium, alcohol, chloral hydrate, opiate analgesics, diazepam, radioactive iodine (^{131}I), chloramphenicol and tetracycline.

FURTHER READING

Bourne DWA, Triggs EJ, Eadie MJ. *Pharmacokinetics for the non-mathematical*, Lancaster: MTP Press, 1986.

Neubig RR. Time course of drug action. In Pratt WB, Taylor P eds. *Principles of drug action*, 3rd edn. New York: Churchill Livingstone, 1990: 297–364.

Pratt WB. The entry, distribution and elimination of drugs. In Pratt WB, Taylor P eds. *Principles of drug action*, 3rd edn. New York: Churchill Livingstone, 1990: 201–96.

Rowland M, Tozer TN. *Clinical pharmacokinetics concepts and applications*, 3rd edn. Baltimore: Williams & Wilkins, 1995.

3

Drug Metabolism

PV Taberner

The biotransformation of drugs into inactive products accounts for the proportion of an administered dose that never reaches the systemic circulation (the *first-pass effect*). Relatively few drugs are excreted unchanged, so that drug metabolism usually determines the duration of action following a single dose. However, some drugs such as acetohexamide or diazepam have one or more pharmacologically active products that prolong their therapeutic effect beyond the time when the parent compound has disappeared from the circulation. Others, such as prednisone, are an inactive prodrug, which has to be converted to the active principal, in this case prednisolone. The principal sites of drug metabolism in the body (in order of exposure) are: the gut lumen, the gastrointestinal mucosa, the plasma, liver, kidneys, skin and lungs. The intestinal flora also play an important role in drug metabolism.

It is important to recognize that drug metabolism is not always synonymous with detoxification. A number of drugs yield toxic products; this toxicity is manifested at the site of metabolism, which is why many adverse reactions to drugs involve the liver. The hepatotoxicity of paracetamol (acetaminophen), for example, is indirectly due to the production of a cytotoxic electrophilic radical within the hepatocytes (see below).

The reactions involved in drug metabolism are traditionally classified as follows:

PHASE I	PHASE II
Oxidation, reduction, hydration, hydrolysis, isomerization	Conjugation reactions with: glucuronide, glutathione, amino acids acetylation, methylation sulphation, etc.

This classification does not imply the sequence in which the reactions occur; for example, conjugation may precede oxidation.

THE MICROSOMAL MIXED FUNCTION OXIDASE

This mixed function oxidase, known also as the cytochrome P-450 system, is the most important enzyme system for oxidizing foreign compounds. Cytochrome P-450 consists of a group of closely related haem-containing isozymes (mixed function oxidases or monooxygenases) situated in the membrane of the endoplasmic reticulum of liver and other tissues. When these membranes are isolated by homogenization and centrifugation they form small vesicles or microsomes. The microsomal P-450 system derives its name from the fact that the cytochrome or pigment, when reduced by reaction with carbon monoxide, has an absorbance peak at 450 nm. This haem protein contains binding sites for oxygen and the substrate for the oxidase reaction. Together with a closely associated flavoprotein reductase (NADPH–cytochrome P-450 reductase) it is able to complete a catalytic oxidation/reduction cycle involving the haem ion, in which the net result is the oxidation of the drug substrate coupled to the reduction of molecular oxygen to water:

$$RH + H^+ + O_2 + NADPH \rightarrow ROH + H_2O + NADP^+$$

where RH is the oxidizable drug substrate and ROH is the oxidized product. NADPH is the reduced form of nicotinamide adenine dinucleotide phosphate. A simplified outline of the P-450 cycle is shown in Fig. 3.1. The rate-limiting step is the reduction of cytochrome P-450 by NADPH.

A number of different oxidative reactions can be catalysed by this system, some specific examples are set out below:

- *aliphatic hydroxylation* – side-chain oxidation of pentobarbitone
- *aromatic hydroxylation* – 3-hydroxylation of the benzene ring of lignocaine

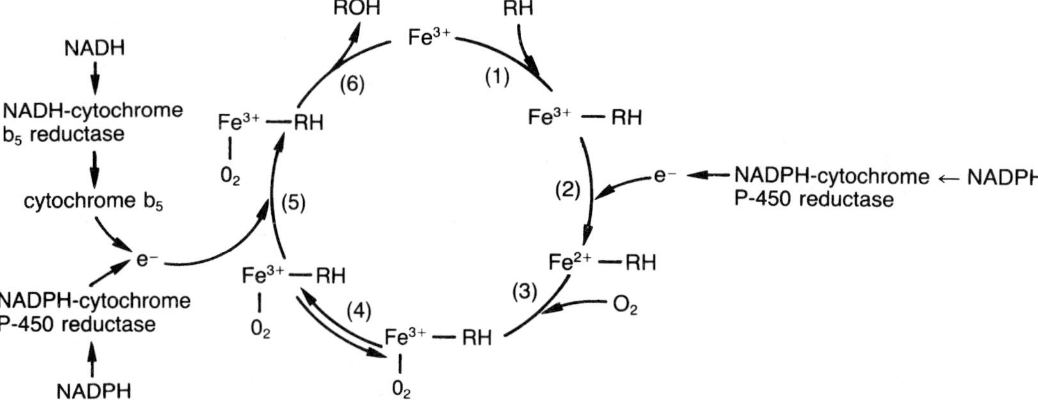

FIGURE 3.1 The cytochrome P-450 cycle. RH represents the drug substrate, ROH the corresponding hydroxylated metabolite. (Adapted from White R, Coon MJ. *Annual Review of Biochemistry* 1980; **49**: 315–56.)

- *epoxidation* – epoxides are unstable intermediates which may be carcinogenic; e.g. the 4,5-epoxide of benzo[α]pyrene
- *oxidative deamination* – the metabolism of amphetamine to phenylacetone and ammonia
- *N-dealkylation* – the demethylation of diazepam to N-desmethyldiazepam
- *O-dealkylation* – the demethylation of codeine to yield morphine
- *N-oxidation* – this can result in the production of putative carcinogens, e.g. the N-oxidation of 2-acetylamino-fluorene
- *S-oxidation* – the oxidation of chlorpromazine to a sulphoxide
- *dehalogenation* – this is an important metabolic route for the halogenated general anaesthetics; e.g. the oxidative dechlorination and debromination of halothane to yield trifluoroacetic acid.

The common factor to all these reactions is that the product is more polar than the original drug, so that urinary excretion is facilitated. Also, the metabolites can be more readily conjugated by subsequent enzymic action.

The multiple forms (isozymes) of cytochrome P-450 have important pharmacological and toxicological implications. First, they may account for the differences in drug metabolism between species, as well as individual variations observed as a function of race, sex, age and environment. Second, many cancer-producing chemicals and teratogens are only activated by P-450 isozymes. More important from a clinical point of view is the ability of certain drugs or chemicals to induce (i.e. increase the specific activity of) cytochrome P-450.

Liver microsomes also contain the enzymes diamine oxidase, which metabolizes the endogenous diamines histamine, cadaverine and putrescine, and xanthine oxidase, which metabolizes a number of endogenous purines as well as xanthine-containing drugs (e.g. caffeine, theophylline, theobromine) to their corresponding uric acid derivatives. The immunosuppressant drug, mercaptopurine, is also inactivated by xanthine oxidase.

The liver cytosolic enzyme epoxide hydrolase, in addition to its role in the metabolism of endogenous steroids, has an important function in the detoxification of many of the active epoxide intermediates produced by the mixed function oxidase, most notably the metabolites of carbamazepine, cyproheptidine and protriptyline. It can be induced by phenobarbitone and other xenobiotic compounds. The principal enzymes involve in phase I reactions are listed in Table 3.1.

PHASE II (CONJUGATION) REACTIONS

Both parent drugs and their metabolites produced from phase I metabolism can undergo coupling reactions with endogenous compounds or active groups to yield conjugates. The principal reactions (acetylation, glucuronidation, glutathione conjugation, glycine conjugation, methylation, ribosylation and sulphation) together with examples of the drugs involved, are summarized in Table 3.2. The transferase enzymes that catalyse these reactions are present in both microsomes and the cytosol of the cell. The endogenous substrates are initially activated, often by a high energy phosphate bond, before conjugation with the drug. The products of these conjugation reactions are pharmacologically inactive and, being more polar than the parent compound, are more readily excreted via the kidney.

One exception to this rule is morphine 6-glucuronide, which is at least as potent as morphine as an analgesic. If a drug is taken in overdose it is possible to overwhelm the conjugation process by exhausting the available conjugate. This is seen in acute paracetamol poisoning in which the highly reactive free radical arising from cytochrome P450 oxidation reaches levels

TABLE 3.1 The principal drug-metabolizing enzymes

ENZYME	SUBSTRATES (specific examples)	DISTRIBUTION
Microsomal mixed function oxidase (P-450 system)	Broad spectrum (see text)	Liver, intestinal mucosa, lung, skin, kidney
Alcohol dehydrogenase	Primary alcohols (ethanol, methanol)	Liver, brain, gastric mucosa
Aldehyde dehydrogenase	Aldehydes (acetaldehyde, formaldehyde)	Liver, kidney, lung
Acetylcholinesterase	Acetylcholine	Cholinergic synapses, brain and periphery
Pseudocholinesterase (non-specific esterase)	Esters (procaine, succinylcholine, pethidine)	Blood plasma
Hydroxysteroid oxidoreductase	Steroids (testosterone)	Widespread
Diamine oxidase	Diamines (histamine, putrescine)	Widespread
Monoamine oxidase	Amines, catecholamines (dopamine, noradrenaline, 5-HT, tyramine)	Intestinal mucosa, liver, sympathetic nerve endings
Xanthine oxidase	Purines (allopurinol, theophylline, hypoxanthine, caffeine)	Widespread
Amidase	Amides (indomethacin, lidocaine, procainamide)	Liver

The principal enzymes that catalyse the conjugation reactions (phase II) are summarized in Table 3.2)

TABLE 3.2 Phase II (conjugation) reactions

CONJUGATION (CONJUGATE)	ENZYME (LOCATION)	SUBSTRATES	DRUG EXAMPLES
Acetylation (acetyl-CoA)	N-acetyl transferase (cytosol)	Amines	Clonazepam, isoniazid, sulphonamides
Glucuronidation (UDP glucuronic acid)	UDP glucuronyl transferase (microsomes)	Alcohols, phenols, carboxylic acids, sulphonamides	Digitoxin, digoxin, diazepam, morphine, paracetamol, etc.
Glutathione conjugation	GSH-S-transferase (cytosol and microsomes)	Hydroxylamines, epoxides, nitro-compounds	Ethacrynic acid, paracetamol epoxide
Glycine conjugation	AcylCoA glycine transferase (mitochondria)	AcylCoA derivatives of carboxylic acids	Salicylates, benzoic acid, nicotinic acid
Methylation (S-adenosyl methionine)	Transmethylases (cytosol)	Amines, catecholamines, phenols	Adrenaline, dopamine, histamine, thiouracil
Sulphation (P-adenosyl phosphosulphate)	Sulphotransferase (cytosol)	Alcohols, phenols, aromatic amines	Coumarins, oestrone, methyl DOPA, paracetamol

UDP: uridine diphosphate; GSH: reduced glutathione; AcCoA: acetyl-coenzyme A.

which are cytotoxic, leading eventually to liver failure (see Fig. 3.2).

The enterohepatic circulation

The molecular weight of a drug or its conjugate has an important influence on its route of excretion from the liver: compounds with a molecular weight below 300 tend to appear mostly in the urine, those of higher molecular weight are largely excreted in the bile and so re-enter the intestine. Once in the gut lumen the glucuronide may be hydrolysed to release the parent drug by the action of β-glucuronidase enzymes present in bacteria in the gut. The deconjugated drug may then be reabsorbed into the portal circulation and begin the cycle over again. This physiological process, shown diagrammatically in Fig. 3.3, tends to conserve endogenous steroids and the bile salts. It has the effect of prolonging the half-life of drugs such as chloramphenicol.

Non-microsomal drug metabolism

Although the liver microsomal enzymes are the principal site of drug metabolism, a number of other enzymes, notably alcohol dehydrogenase, non-specific plasma esterase and monoamine oxidase, are also important (see Table 3.1).

Dehydrogenases

Alcohol dehydrogenase, in the gastric mucosa and liver, oxidizes a wide range of primary alcohols including ethanol, methanol, chloral hydrate and ethylene glycol. The toxic aldehyde products are rapidly oxidized to the appropriate acid by a non-specific aldehyde dehydrogenase. These two enzymes are important in the treatment of alcoholism and alcohol or glycol poisoning (see Chapter 37).

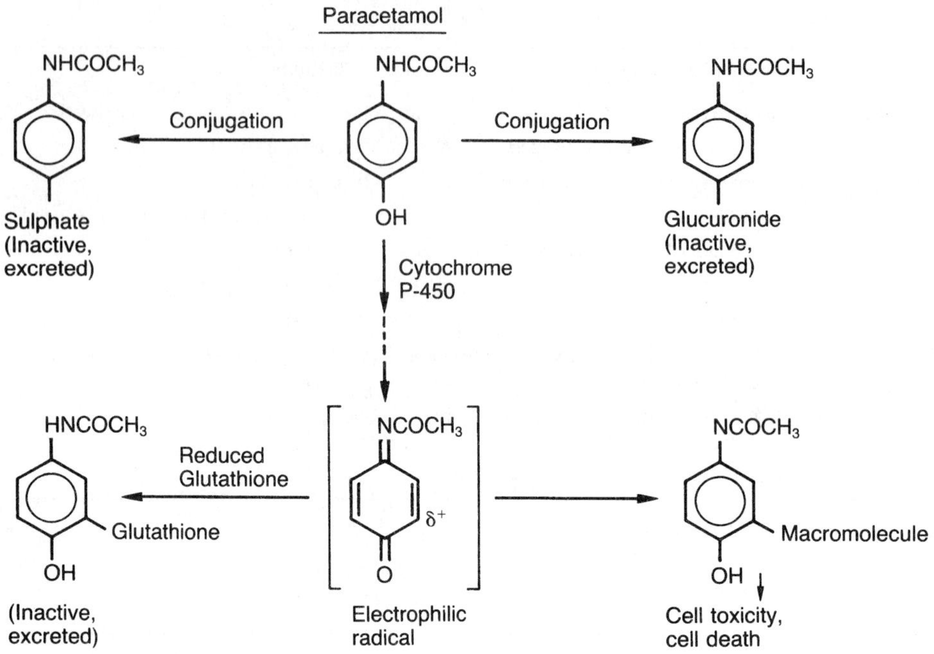

FIGURE 3.2 The metabolism of paracetamol.

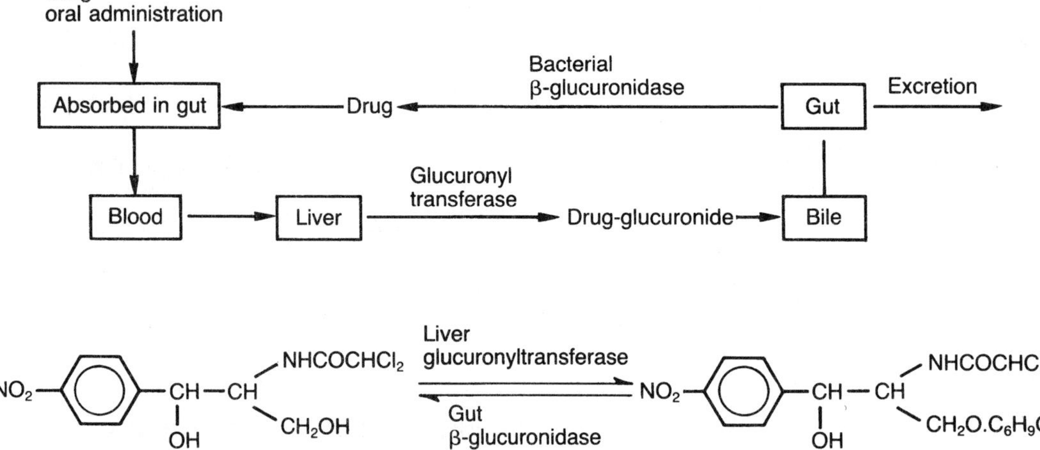

FIGURE 3.3 The enterohepatic recirculation of drugs. (From Gibson GG, Skett P. *Introduction to drug metabolism*. London: Chapman & Hall, 1986.)

Hydrolases

These enzymes catalyse the hydrolysis of ester links in a number of drugs. Acetylcholinesterase (AChE) present in the synaptic cleft of cholinergic synapses hydrolyses the released transmitter and thereby terminates its action. It is relatively specific for acetylcholine. Butyrylcholinesterase (known also as pseudocholinesterase or plasma esterase) consists of a family of enzymes distributed widely throughout the body and possessing a broad spectrum of activity. The plasma enzyme has an important role in the inactivation of procaine, suxamethonium and propanidid. Some amides can also by hydrolysed albeit more slowly than the corresponding ester. For example, procainamide, the amide analogue of procaine, persists sufficiently long in the circulation to have a marked antiarrhythmic effect on the myocardium whereas procaine has negligible activity.

Amine oxidases

Monoamine oxidase (MAO) is present in sympathetic nerve terminals where it inactivates the endogenous catecholamine neurotransmitters although, unlike

AChE, it is not immediately responsible for terminating their synaptic actions. It will also metabolize exogenous amines that have similar structures. For example, MAO in the intestinal mucosa prevents the entry of ingested amines into the systemic circulation. In patients treated with MAO inhibitors (MAOIs) this action is compromised, so that the potentially dangerous cardiovascular effects of tyramine, which is present in a number of foods, become evident. Under normal circumstances tyramine can be ingested without risk, but patients on MAOI therapy have to avoid tyramine-containing foods.

FACTORS AFFECTING DRUG METABOLISM

Individual differences in drug metabolism are a function of age, sex, genetic background and the patient's nutritional state. Exogenous factors including environmental hazards such as smoking, diurnal variation, and the presence of other drugs can also influence the ability of an individual to inactivate a drug. In consequence, the effects of a given dose of a drug may be significantly enhanced or attenuated from what one expects.

Genetic factors

Defects in a number of drug-metabolizing enzymes can be inherited as autosomal recessive traits. In these cases the homozygote inherits an isozyme that is less effective than the normal enzyme. The most frequently occurring enzyme defects are summarized in Table 3.3. About 1 in 3000 patients possess a pseudocholinesterase which metabolizes suxamethonium (succinylcholine) at a far slower rate than normal. In these subjects the neuromuscular blockade following succinylcholine is inordinately prolonged. About 50% of caucasians can be described as 'slow acetylators'; they possess a low affinity N-acetyltransferase isozyme that is responsible for the potentiation of drugs such as isoniazid, sulphonamides and clonazepam. Isoniazid toxicity is more likely in slow acetylators, whereas hepatotoxicity due to the acetylated metabolite of isoniazid is more frequent in fast acetylators.

A low affinity aldehyde dehydrogenase is present in a high proportion of Asian peoples and, as a consequence, they are intolerant to alcohol and will experience a disulfiram reaction (flushing, palpitations, headache) in response to fairly low doses of alcohol. A proportion of African negroes have very low levels of the liver enzyme glucose-6-phosphate dehydrogenase. Although not directly involved in drug metabolism, this enzyme is responsible for maintaining the level of NADPH, an important cofactor for a number of dehydrogenase reactions in the liver. Patients lacking this enzyme are intolerant of antimalarial drugs and some non-steroidal anti-inflammatory compounds. The inherited condition, Gilbert's disease, is characterized by an abnormally low level of UDP glucuronyl-transferase activity. This enzyme, normally responsible for the conjugation of endogenous bilirubin, is also responsible for the inactivation of a number of drugs including narcotic analgesics and paracetamol (see Table 3.2).

Exogenous factors

The working environment or lifestyle can lead to chronic exposure to toxic chemical entities that affect drug metabolism; benzpyrene in cigarette smoke, for example, is a potent inducer of cytochrome P-450 (see below). Microsomal oxidation of ethanol normally accounts for only a small proportion of the total ethanol metabolized, but in regular drinkers this proportion can be markedly increased, at the expense of the metabolism of other drugs which may be competing for the same enzyme.

TABLE 3.3 Genetic enzyme deficiencies affecting drug metabolism

ENZYME DEFICIENT OR DEFECTIVE	FREQUENCY	DRUGS AFFECTED	SYMPTOMS
Non-specific plasma esterase	0.03%	Suxamethonium (succinylcholine)	Prolonged muscle relaxation, apnoea
Cytosolic N-acetyl transferase	≈50%	Isoniazid Procainamide Hydralazine	Peripheral polyneuropathy, hepatitis lupus erythematosus
Glucose-6-phosphate dehydrogenase	Wide racial variation (0–50%)	Antimalarials Nalidixic acids Sulphonamides	Susceptibility to drug-induced haemolysis
NADH methaemaglobin reductase Cytochrome b_5 Phenacetin O-de-ethylase	<2%	Nitrates Nitrites Quinones	Methaemaglobinaemia
Cytochrome P-450 (debrisoquine 4-hydroxylase)	8% (UK)	Debrisoquine Guanoxan	Prolongation of drug action

Induction of cytochrome P-450

Two principal mechanisms of induction of specific isozymes of cytochrome P-450 are now recognized. The first, exemplified by phenobarbitone, involves an increase in the cellular concentration of the translatable polysomal messenger RNA for cytochrome P-450b (LM_2), so that the synthetic capacity for P-450 is increased. A partial list of drugs that can induce cytochrome P-450, and the drugs particularly affected, is given in Table 3.4. In contrast to drug-induction, environmental exposure to polycyclic aromatic hydrocarbons (e.g. benzo[α]pyrene) induces cytochrome P-450c (P-448 or LM_4) by a mechanism that involves binding to a cytosolic receptor. The process is thought to be analogous to the mechanism by which steroids act on target cells to induce protein synthesis. Although P-450c represents only about 5% of the total P-450, induction can increase its concentration by up to sixteen times. This results in a significant increase in drug metabolizing capacity and a reduction in the clinical efficacy of any drugs that are inactivated by this enzyme.

TABLE 3.5 Inhibitors of cytochrome P-450 and other drug-metabolizing enzyme activity

Cytochrome P-450	
Drugs	
Amantadine	(Antiviral agent)
Cimetidine	(H_2 antagonist, anti-ulcer drug)
Chloramphenicol	(Broad-spectrum antibiotic)
Cyclophosphamide	(Immunosuppressant and anticancer drug)
Ethchlorvynol	(Sedative, hypnotic)
Indomethacin	(Non-steroidal anti-inflammatory)
Metyrapone	(Diagnostic agent for pituitary dysfunction)
Tilorone	(Antiviral agent)
Hazardous chemicals (xenobiotics)	
Carbon disulphide	(industrial reagent)
Carbon tetrachloride	(industrial solvent)
Parathion	(insecticide)
Aldehyde dehydrogenase	
Disulfiram, cyanamide (used in alcohol aversion therapy)	
Drugs affected: coumarin anticoagulants	
Cholinesterases	
Ecothiopate, edrophonium, neostigmine, physostigmine	
Drugs affected: procaine, propanidid, suxamethonium	
Monoamine oxidase (MAO)	
Phenelzine, tranylcypromine, isocarboxazid	
Drugs affected: sympathomimetics, pethidine, dietary tyramine	

INHIBITION OF CYTOCHROME P-450

A number of drugs and xenobiotic chemicals are capable of inhibiting cytochrome P-450 by a variety of mechanisms (see Table 3.5). Compounds containing an olefinic (—C=C—) or acetylenic (—C≡C—) function can be porphyrinogenic; by binding covalently to the haem protein they produce green porphyrin-based pigments that are enzymically inactive. Drugs that can destroy cytochrome P-450 by this means include allobarbital, ethchlorvynol, ethinylestradiol, fluroxene, norethindrone, secobarbital and vinyl chloride. Several drugs that are substrates for cytochrome P-450 yield intermediates that bind tightly to the enzyme, so that it is prevented from completing the oxidative cycle. This causes a reduction in drug-metabolizing capacity with the consequent potentiation and prolongation of the effects of any other drug that is inactivated by the P-450 system. Drugs of this type includ cimetidine, fenfluramine, isoniazid, methadone, propoxyphene and sulphanilamide. All these drugs are contraindicated in patients with a history of acute porphyria because of the risk of precipitating an acute porphyric crisis.

Phase I drug metabolism is also reduced in cases of severe burns and, as a result, the actions of lignocaine and pethidine in particular may be prolonged.

Induction and inhibition of other drug metabolizing enzymes

Several substances capable of inducing NADPH cytochrome P-450 reductase have also been shown to induce other enzymes; for example, phenobarbitone increases the activity of epoxide hydrolase, glucuronyltransferase and glutathione-S-transferase. Pesticides such as aldrin and dieldrin also induce a range of liver enzymes.

TABLE 3.4 Inducers of cytochrome P-450 activity

INDUCER	DRUGS AFFECTED
Phenobarbitone and most other barbiturates	Barbiturates, chloramphenicol, cortisol, coumarin anticoagulants (including warfarin), digitoxin, phenylbutazone, phenytoin, quinine, testosterone
Phenylbutazone	Aminopyrine, cortisol, digitoxin
Griseofulvin, ethchlorvynol	Warfarin
Rifampicin	Coumarin anticoagulants, digitoxin, glucocorticoids, methadone, oral contraceptives, propranolol

FURTHER READING

Alvares AP, Pratt WB. Pathways of drug metabolism. In Pratt WB & Taylor P, eds. *Principles of drug action*, 3rd edn. London: Churchill Livingstone, 1990; 365–422.

Gibson GG, Skett P. *Introduction to drug metabolism*, London: Chapman & Hall, 1986.

Murray M. Mechanisms of the inhibition of cytochrome P-450-mediated drug oxidation by therapeutic agents. *Drug Metabolism Reviews* 1987; **18**: 55–78.

Nerbert DW, Weber WW, Pharmacogenetics, In Pratt WB & Taylor P, eds. *Principles of drug action* 3rd edn. London: Churchill Livingstone, 1990; 469–532.

Schenkman JB, Kupfer D (eds.). *Hepatic cytochrome P–450 mono-oxygenase system.* Oxford: Pergamon Press, 1982.

SECTION TWO

Anaesthetic drugs

4

Principles of Anaesthesia

MJ Halsey

DEFINITIONS OF ANAESTHESIA

General anaesthesia must be defined as a loss of awareness and (possibly) recall of a noxious stimulus. This contrasts with the absence of sensation of pain. For example, a patient with high spinal cord transection has a loss of sensation in his or her body but this is not general anaesthesia. Analgesia on the other hand means a reduction in the perception of pain but not its abolition (sometimes the expression 'total analgesia' is used for abolition of pain). 'Analgesia' implies the presence of consciousness whereas the characteristics of 'general anaesthesia' include unconsciousness. The relationships between anaesthesia and analgesia are not fully understood. Some general anaesthetics at subanaesthetic concentrations (e.g. 50% nitrous oxide) have good analgesic effects, others appear to be relatively ineffective.

A further complication is local or regional anaesthesia which, in its simplest definition, means a loss of sensation in one part of the body. However, it may be more accurate to use the term 'analgesia' (e.g. epidural analgesia, spinal analgesia) because not all sensation is necessarily abolished. Thus patients subjected to the regional anaesthetic techniques may be warned 'you will feel no pain but you may feel the surgeon touching you'.

On the other hand, a local anaesthetic administered around the site prior to stitching a minor wound usually abolishes not only the pain but also any sensation of the process. However, in general, different kinds of sensation are conveyed separately and are not necessarily lost together. For example, compression caused by pressure on the sciatic nerve by the edge of a chair can result in a foot 'going to sleep'. In this case the sense of touch usually is lost before that of pain – in contrast to the effect of local anaesthetics, for example.

The essential characteristic of drug-induced anaesthesia is the reversible loss of perception of, and response to, a noxious stimulus. General anaesthesia also includes the loss of consciousness although this characteristic has become difficult to define with some of the new non-narcotic intravenous anaesthetics. For example, ketamine produces a state of unconsciousness described as dissociation anaesthesia. Patients appear cataleptic and have complete analgesia and amnesia but appear to be only mildly sedated.

A case can be made that 'unconsciousness' can only be defined in terms of absence of recall. The problem with such a definition is that a patient could be fully 'conscious' during an operation but have no recall of it. Although this is theoretically possible, the practical issue is that such a state would be accompanied during the operation by obvious signs of excessive autonomic activity.

THE RELATIVE POTENCIES OF ANAESTHETICS

The potencies of the inhaled general anaesthetics are the essential basic data for all the studies on their site and mode of action. For example, a number of potential cellular sites of action have been rejected because they are affected only by very high partial pressures of anaesthetics (sometimes as much as ten times greater than the clinical range). Currently one of the most useful estimates of the potency of an anaesthetic in humans is MAC – the minimum alveolar concentration of the agent which just prevents a gross muscular response to a surgical incision in 50% of patients (Table 4.1). In this case (since the total pressure is known and constant) the concentration is a measure of the partial pressure of the agent. Although we do not know the exact site of action, the partial pressure of the anaesthetic will be the same throughout the part of the system at equilibrium. When determining MAC it is necessary only to attain equilibrium between the anaesthetic partial pressure in the alveoli and in the site in the central nervous system. It has been determined empirically that the arterial partial pressure comes into equilibrium with that at the site of action within 10–15 min. It is obviously impossible to verify equilibrium conditions directly but convincing indirect evidence comes from the fact that the MAC value is the same after 8 h equilibration period as after the normal 15-min period. However, during the equilibration period the general uptake of anaesthetic into the other organs and tissues in the body is continually changing and so the inspired to alveolar partial pressure difference is never constant. It is therefore necessary to decrease the inspired concentration to maintain constant the alveolar partial pressure (Fig. 4.1). The use of alveolar anaesthetic samples (as determined by end-tidal sampling techniques) is one of the major advantages of the MAC concept over some other potency measurements – particularly those in smaller animals – because many problems of the uptake and distribution of the agents are overcome relatively easily.

MAC has been an established technique for over 25 years but there are still some subtleties that continue to be investigated. A current example is the determination of the alveolar to arterial partial pressure gradient. If this gradient is significant during anaesthesia it will distort the MAC value. To avoid the problem the general approach is to minimize the alveolar to inspired partial pressure differences by the use of over-pressure initially but it is now recognized that unless such precautions are taken, the alveolar partial pressure is not an adequate representation of the partial pressure at the site of action.

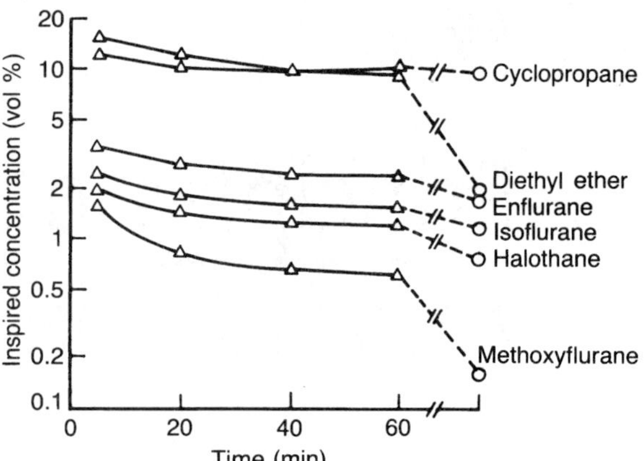

FIGURE 4.1 The inspired concentrations of five agents (in oxygen) which theoretically would be required to maintain surgical anaesthesia over discrete periods of time (solid lines; Δ symbols). These are the *anaesthetizing inspired concentrations* equivalent to the minimum alveolar concentration (MAC); the latter correspond to the data at complete equilibration; that is, at time '∞' (dotted line; o symbols). This plot includes the effects of the uptake and distribution of the agents and illustrates that if one were to rely on knowledge of the anaesthetizing inspired concentration one would also have to take into account the variation with time which in turn would vary between agents. It is interesting to see that these effects can be so large that for equilibration periods up to 20 min, not even the ranking order of the anaesthetizing inspired concentrations is the same as that of the equivalent MAC values. (Reproduced with permission from Halsey MJ. In: Nunn JF, Utting JE, Brown BR. eds. *General anaesthesia*. London: Butterworths, 1989: 19–29.)

The MAC concepts have been applied to many different species, although the techniques have to be adapted. Thus the rat and dog MACs do not use surgical stimuli, but instead use a noxious stimulus on the tail. The response appears to be integrated with time and consistent results are obtained only if the stimulus is maintained for 1–2 min. The use of the rat is also associated with the problem that usually inspired concentrations are determined. It is of course possible to use special techniques such as tracheostomies to facilitate end-tidal sampling but a more practical solution is the approach to the MAC value from both higher and lower anaesthetic partial pressures to reverse any inspired to alveolar gradients. An analogous problem occurs when mice are used. In this case the traditional end-point is the loss of righting reflex – a complex reflex consisting only in part of a postural effect. The major conceptual problem with the mouse – or tadpole – loss of righting reflex is that these are not responses evoked by noxious stimuli.

TABLE 4.1 Anaesthetic potencies (MAC) of various anaesthetics in different species (vol %) in oxygen

	HUMAN	DOG	RAT
Halothane	0.76	1.00	1.24
Isoflurane	1.15	1.43	1.45
Enflurane	1.68	2.2	2.2
Sevoflurane	2.05	2.5	2.8
Fluroxene	3.4	6.3	4.22
Desflurane	6.0	7.2	7.71
Cyclopropane	9.2	18.00	16.00
Xenon	71.00	119.00	—
Nitrous oxide	105.00	205.00	148.00

An example of the ratios of MAC values in different species is provided in Table 4.2. Although the coefficients of variation of these ratios are not large (relative to the errors involved in the determination of the potencies themselves) the ratios for a pair of species do differ significantly. This fact has an important implication for the correlation studies to determine the molecular site of action, which will be discussed later.

STRUCTURE–ACTIVITY RELATIONSHIPS

In the past it has been argued that there are no relationships between chemical structures of the inhaled general anaesthetic agents and their pharmacological functions. Thus the gaseous and volatile agents range from the halogenated ethers and hydrocarbons, through nitrous oxide to the so-called inert gases (e.g. argon and xenon). Under specific circumstances, the physiological gases oxygen and carbon dioxide are anaesthetics. It is, of course, clear that there is no single spatial arrangement of atoms in a molecule that is essential for anaesthetic activity. The search for the 'anesthesiophore', as the supposed critical structure of an anaesthetic molecule was termed, was finally abandoned in the early 1960s. However, chemical structures influence the physical properties of molecules which, in turn, appear to be one of the primary factors in anaesthetic potencies. In the former case it is the structure of the entire molecule that is important rather than the structure of a particular group of atoms. There is evidence from the anaesthetic 'cut-off' phenomenon that physical properties may not be the sole determinant of anaesthetic potency. When ascending a homologous series of compounds like the alkanes, or alkanols, the anaesthetic potency increases, in line with the hydrophobic solubility, but then suddenly the compounds cease to have any anaesthetic activities. This 'cut-off' as it has been termed has been ascribed to the molecules being too large for the anaesthetic site of action. Such a crude explanation is recognized as being an oversimplification and it may well be that this area of anaesthetic research will provide alternative approaches to the study of membrane mechanisms.

TABLE 4.2 Ratios of MAC values between different species in oxygen

	RAT/DOG	RAT/HUMAN	DOG/ HUMAN
Halothane	1.24	1.63	1.32
Isoflurane	1.01	1.26	1.24
Enflurane	1.00	1.31	1.31
Sevoflurane	1.12	1.28	1.20
Fluroxene	0.70	1.24	1.85
Desflurane	1.07	1.28	1.20
Cyclopropane	0.89	1.74	1.96
Nitrous oxide	0.72	1.41	1.95
Mean ratio	0.97	1.40	1.50
SD	0.19	0.19	0.35

CHIRALITY

Halothane has *d*- and *l*-optical isomers (the clinically available agent is the racemic mixture of the two). Some years ago the isomers were partially separated out and their anaesthetic potencies were found to be identical. It should be noted that the experiment was difficult, the isomers were not optically pure, and as yet the other inhalational agents with asymmetric centres (e.g. enflurane and isoflurane) have not had their *in vivo* potencies determined. However, molecular and cellular perturbations with the optical isomers of anaesthetics are now being actively studied in a range of model systems.

The reason for studying this aspect of an agent's pharmacological behaviour is that there is a fundamental controversy in the anaesthetic mechanisms field as to whether the agents act directly on the proteins of excitable membranes or indirectly via the lipids that surround them. Stereoisomers are compounds that have the same molecular formula and geometrical arrangement when viewed in two dimensions. However, they differ in their arrangement of the substituents around an asymmetric or 'chiral' carbon atom. The two isomers are mirror images of each other and exhibit optical activity. They have identical physical properties such as solubilities and as such their anaesthetic potencies related to their lipid solubilities would be predicted to be identical. However, there are some macromolecular sites of action that exhibit stereoselective binding and the demonstration of stereospecific potencies of an anaesthetic is a strong indication of a specific interaction, probably with a protein. It is only possible to say 'probably' because in addition to proteins both the rigid ring structure of cholesterol and the headgroups of lipids have chiral centres. In contrast the hydrocarbon core of a membrane's bilayer is achiral and, as such, drug interactions in these non-polar centres are usually non-selective. The usual example of stereoselectivity of a narcotic agent with lipids is the adsorption of morphine to phosphatidylserine, which is strongly influenced by the morphine aligning with the charged phospholipid head groups. Interactions with protein sites may not necessarily be stereospecific but, in general, the more specific the interaction (with binding involving more than two points of 'attachment') the higher the chances of stereoselectivity.

A current example of a stereoselective action on anaesthetic potencies is provided by D-medetomidine, an α-adrenoceptor agonist, which can decrease halothane MAC dose dependently to less than 10%

of the control value. This effect appears to be highly specific for the α_2-adrenoceptor since the optical isomer L-medetomidine had little or no effect on the halothane MAC. The interaction between halothane and D-medetomidine appears to be additive rather than synergistic and it has been argued that it may be mediated presynaptically by decreasing norepinephrine release and postsynaptically by depressing neuronal excitation. The α-adrenoceptor agonists clearly have a number of actions in addition to their direct anaesthetic effects and the burgeoning studies in this area are probably relevant only to this specific agent rather than to anaesthesia in general.

Ketamine is a good example of a stereoselective intravenous agent. The initial alternative mechanisms for the differences in potencies included the possibility of stereoselective metabolism. Although such an effect would be very interesting from the point of view of mechanism of metabolism, the relevance of the *in vivo* observations to mechanism of anaesthesia would be reduced. However, the differences in pharmacological potencies between the two optical isomers were demonstrated not to be due to marked differences in biodisposition. The brain levels and plasma concentrations of the less potent (−) isomer were in general equal to those of the (+) isomer. Interestingly, the potency ratios between the two isomers appears to be greater for ketamine's action as an analgesic than as an anaesthetic. The ratio varies from 1.5 to 3.0. The variation may represent the suspected concentration dependence of any stereospecific saturable interaction or it may reveal different molecular mechanisms associated with analgesia and anaesthesia.

The (+) ketamine isomer may be a more useful anaesthetic than either the racemic mixture or the (−) isomer. The arguments are not overwhelming clinically but the recognition of differential effects of ketamine isomers has led to a number of mechanistic studies. The (+) isomer is approximately four times more potent than the (−) isomer on catecholamine high affinity transport in synaptosomes. In contrast the (−) isomer is approximately twice as effective as the (+) isomer against serotonin transport. The anaesthetic implications of such *in vitro* studies are not yet clear but the data lend support to the general hypothesis that specific monoaminergic pathways may be involved in selective pharmacological actions of the drug. A more recent study has demonstrated the stereoselective effect of ketamine isomers on neuronal and extraneuronal catecholamine uptake mechanisms in selected tissues. The overall evidence on ketamine stereoisomers suggests that the differences in potencies may be clinically relevant to relative side-effects rather than to the critical mechanisms of general anaesthesia.

UPTAKE AND DISTRIBUTION

The pharmacokinetics of inhalational anaesthetics have been extensively studied over the last 30 years. The underlying principles of pharmacokinetics have been set out in Chapter 2, while specific examples of inhalation agents are covered in Chapter 5 (see Further Reading). The uninitiated would be forgiven for concluding that there is nothing new in this area other than the application of established principles to new inhalational agents. However, recent developments indicate that major advances in the topic are currently underway.

The first development is the practical application of new techniques for studying anaesthetic distribution *in vivo*. Although direct methods of determining drug distributions, such as autoradiography, were applied to the inhaled anaesthetics some time ago, it is only more recently that non-invasive observations have been possible. A range of nuclear magnetic resonance techniques have been developed that are based on the signal analysis of ^{19}F nuclei. These, of course, are applicable to all fluorinated anaesthetics and enable the kinetics of cerebral distributions of those agents to be followed directly.

The second development is the renaissance of alternative concepts in the interpretation of uptake and distribution data. The kinetics of anaesthetic uptake and distribution have been interpreted in the past as being *perfusion* limited rather than *diffusion* limited. Thus the emphasis has been on the solubilities of the different agents and the relative blood flows and capacities of the different tissues. However, there is increasing recognition that, in addition to perfusion-based distribution, there is both intertissue diffusion of the agents as well as diffusion through the skin and other tissue–gas interfaces. Moreover, the simple fixed capacity concepts of the different compartments have to be modified to allow for the metabolism of the anaesthetic. The latter aspect is well established for the intravenous anaesthetics but has been regarded as a relatively minor effect for the inhalation agents (in the case of uptake and distribution studies rather than toxicity investigations).

The difference between the classical and current studies on the kinetics of inhalation anaesthetics is illustrated by the water analogue shown in Fig. 4.2.

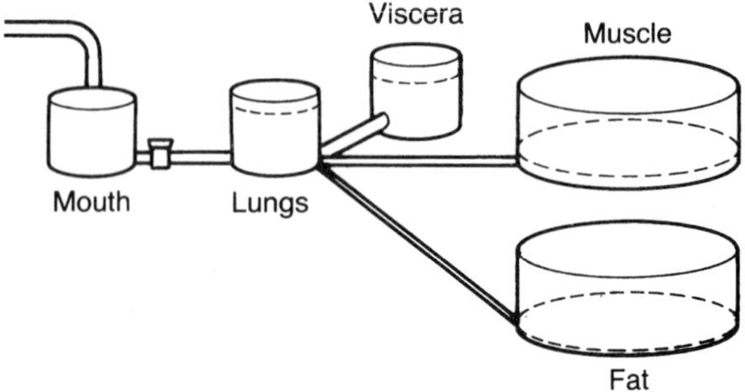

FIGURE 4.2 Water analogy of uptake and distribution of agents illustrating the classical approach to the topic. (Reproduced with permission from Mapleson WW. In: Nunn JF, Utting JE, Brown BR. eds. *General anaesthesia*. London: Butterworths, 1989: 44–59.)

This describes the uptake and distribution of an inhaled anaesthetic from a non-rebreathing system in terms of water flowing directly to a series of cylindrical containers. The water represents the anaesthetic itself, with the depth of water in any container representing the anaesthetic partial pressure. The containers represent the various groups of organs and tissues and their different volumes represent the storage capacities of those groups for a particular anaesthetic. The size of the pipes connecting to the containers represents the relative perfusions of the different compartments. This hydraulic analogy can be developed into a quantitative approach for the interpretation of uptake and distribution of different anaesthetics.

It is clear that this model (at least in its simplest form) considers each compartment to be self-contained with ingress or egress of the agent via the connecting pipe. As described in detail in the next section, more recent studies have included the probability of direct interconnections between the containers representing intertissue diffusion. In addition, metabolism can be represented by a variable leak in the visceral container. Modelling the effect of metabolism is complicated by the fact that the absolute rates may only be partial pressure dependent up to a certain value, and hence the 'leak' has to be variable.

The water analogue is particularly helpful in determining the circumstances when intertissue diffusion will become important. For example, the phenomenon could not be a significant factor during the initial uptake of the agent because the partial pressure gradients between the different compartments will be relatively small. On the other hand it will be significant when, for example, the visceral compartment is almost saturated while the other two compartments have much lower *partial pressures* (although the absolute amounts in the compartments may or may not be comparable). Finally any intertissue diffusion will become less important towards the end of the anaesthetic uptake because the partial pressure *gradients* will again be reduced.

A similar analysis of the maximum impact of metabolism indicates that its effects will be more marked during recovery from anaesthesia. Thus comparisons between induction and eduction of anaesthetics may reveal more than the expected mirror image pattern.

INDUCTION vs. EDUCTION

Nearly all the factors controlling the uptake of inhaled anaesthetics also apply to recovery from anaesthesia. Thus the characteristic uptake curves relating alveolar to inspired concentrations have their counterparts in the recovery curves relating the alveolar concentration to the alveolar concentration immediately preceding the cessation of anaesthetic administration.

The major difference between induction and eduction of the agent is the variable equilibration of the different tissue groups at the end of the anaesthetic. Whereas at the start of induction all tissues have the same partial pressure (namely zero), at the start of eduction each tissue has a different degree of saturation depending on the length of the prior period of anaesthesia.

Figures 4.3 and 4.4 illustrate some recent 'washin' and 'washout' data for desflurane, isoflurane and halothane in humans. The observations were made with the concomitant administration of the three agents (at approximately one-third MAC for each) in addition to a 'basal' anaesthetic of nitrous oxide plus thiopentone and midazolam. It is interesting that, as predicted from the relative solubilities, both washin and washout rates for the volatile agents were most rapid for desflurane followed by isoflurane and halothane. However, although isoflurane washed in more rapidly than halothane, its washout rate was similar. Since the agents were being studied simultaneously this apparent anomaly cannot be related to agent-specific differences in ventilation or cardiovas-

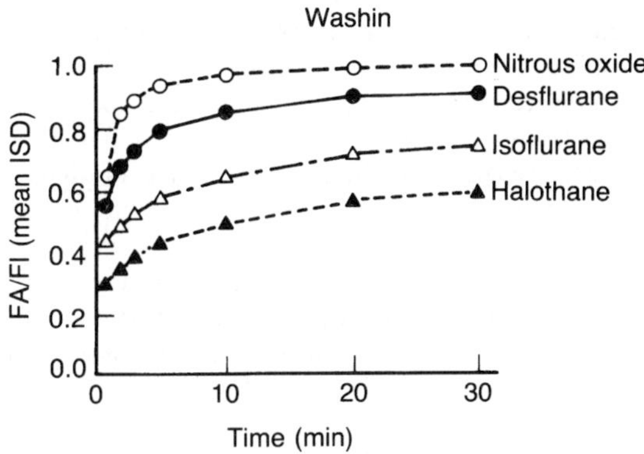

FIGURE 4.3 The comparative uptake curves for four anaesthetics relating the alveolar concentration (FA) to the inspired concentration (FI). (Reproduced with permission from Yasuda N, Lockhart SH, Eger EI, Weiskopf RB, Johnson BH, Fassoulaki A. *Anesthesia and Analgesia* 1990; 70: S444.)

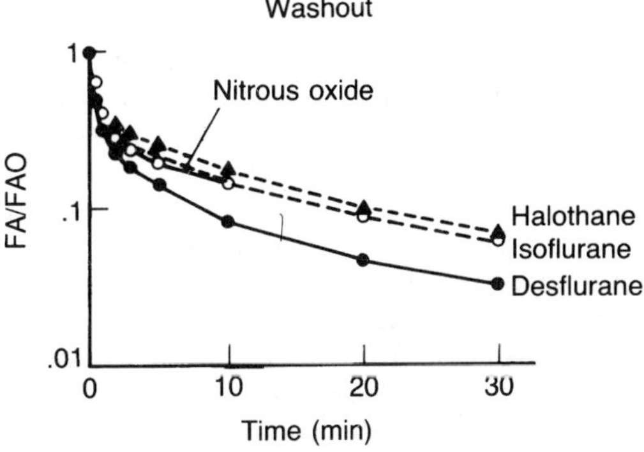

FIGURE 4.4 The comparative washout curves for four anaesthetics relating the alveolar concentration (FA) to the initial alveolar concentration prior to cessation of anaesthetic equilibration (FAO). (Reproduced with permission from Yasuda N, Lockhart SH, Eger EI, Weiskopf RB, Johnson BH, Fassoulaki A. *Anesthesia and Analgesia* 1990; 70: 5444).

cular perturbations. One explanation is that the closeness of the halothane and isoflurane washout curves is related to the greater metabolism of halothane. This is consistent with the observation that although the washout observations were continued over 5–7 days, the overall recovery of halothane was less than that of desflurane or isoflurane.

There are other interesting comparisons between the agents but the most relevant to uptake and distribution is the increasing evidence for intertissue diffusion. This is revealed by the quantitative analysis of the eduction data in terms of equations based on five compartments with different time constants. This and previous studies indicate that the first, second, third and fifth compartments represent lungs, vessel-rich group, muscle group and the fat group respectively. However, it is the fourth group which has all the characteristics of an intertissue diffusion component. The fact that this fourth group is essential for an adequate fit between predicted and observed data is one of the reasons for the current interest in intertissue diffusion.

Intertissue diffusion has long been recognized as a component of uptake and distribution of anaesthetic gases but, despite some excellent mathematical modelling and direct autoradiographic evidence, the phenomenon has been regarded as non-rate limiting. The new work demonstrates that the exclusive perfusion-based models are an over-simplification and have to be replaced by perfusion–diffusion models. The diffusion component of anaesthetic distribution includes percutaneous losses. These have been measured and it would appear that the absolute magnitude of the percutaneous loss is a trivial fraction of the total amount of anaesthetic taken up. However, visceral losses from the abdomen or thorax during surgery may be considerably larger and studies are in progress to determine if this prediction is correct.

CEREBRAL UPTAKE OF ANAESTHETICS

The advent of *in vivo* ^{19}F nuclear magnetic resonance (NMR) has made possible non-invasive measurements of anaesthetic kinetics at the biophase itself. This is potentially a considerable advance on the traditional approach of measuring alveolar concentrations. The NMR techniques do have limitations and the early experiments in the anaesthesia field were over-enthusiastically interpreted. The initial studies purported to demonstrate that anaesthetics were eliminated very slowly from the brain. This was at variance with the classical concepts of anaesthetic pharmacokinetics. It now appears that there was a technical error in the earlier work and that the NMR detector was sensing anaesthetic in adjacent fat tissues rather than in the brain itself.

A current study on cerebral washout of desflurane, isoflurane and halothane illustrates the new approach. The assumption was made that end-tidal, arterial and cerebral partial pressures were equal at the end of the 30-min equilibration period. The relative curves for the three agents are in accordance with the solubility predictions (Fig. 4.5). In addition, the respective brain concentration decay curves parallel the alveolar washout curves. However, the most interesting aspect is the clear demonstration of a temporal lag between cerebral and alveolar washout. The alveolar partial pressure will increase more rapidly than the cerebral concentration during induction and decrease more rapidly during eduction. This leads to the prediction that plotting the fraction of maximum cerebral concentration against the fraction of maximum alveolar concentration will reveal a hysteresis curve.

The current work on uptake and distribution of inhalational agents is advancing in terms of both theoretical concepts and practical measurements. There is now good reason for optimism that future research will be able to delineate more details of cerebral pharmacokinetics. This in itself will not answer the question as to how the anaesthetics work but their elucidation will provide a framework for the molecular and cellular investigations of anaesthetic action.

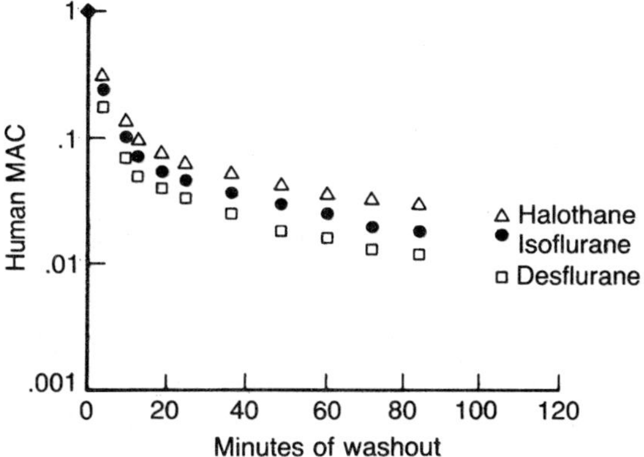

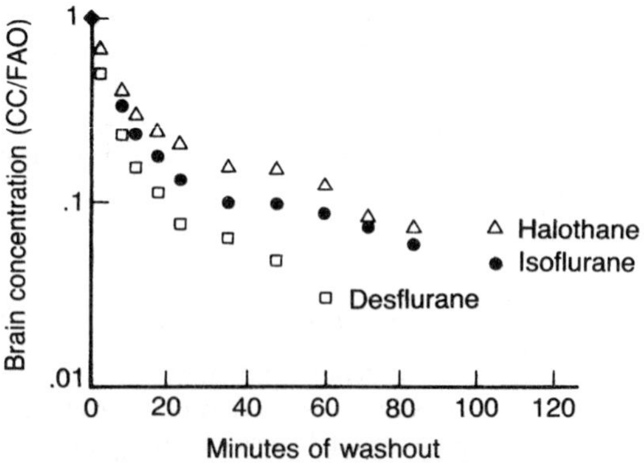

FIGURE 4.5 The brain concentrations (CC) and alveolar concentration (FA) as fractions of the initial alveolar concentration prior to cessation of anaesthetic equilibration (FAO). (Reproduced with permission from Lockhart SH, Cohen Y, Yasuda N, Friere BA, Eger EI. *Anesthesia and Analgesia* 1990; 70: S244.)

HISTORY OF ANAESTHETIC MECHANISMS

Meyer and Overton described the relationship between anaesthetic potency and hydrophobicity at the turn of this century and postulated that the critical site of action was the cell membrane. This is often regarded as the first major unifying theory of anaesthetics' mode of action. Their hypothesis originated from the work on 'cell fat dissolution' by von Bibra and Harless over 50 years earlier and almost immediately after the initial clinical demonstration of anaesthesia. Subsequent hypotheses, all of which predate Meyer and Overton, include 'membrane echymosis' and 'cell wall induration', and the attempt at a water solubility correlation by Richet. In 1920 K. H. Meyer and Gottlieb-Billroth extended the lipid theory of narcosis to experiments performed on mice and, like Meyer and Overton, did not restrict their study simply to one homologous series of compounds. They appear to have been aware of some of the experimental artefacts associated with the variable uptake and distribution of anaesthetics. For example, they measured the concentration of narcotic in the 'respiratory' air at 1 atmosphere necessary to anaesthetize lightly mice within three-quarters of an hour. They also determined the solubility coefficients of the gaseous narcotics in vegetable oil (olive or sesame) and concluded that anaesthetic potency increased with lipid solubility. They restated the 'Lipid Theory of Narcosis' as 'There will always occur narcosis, whenever a chemically indifferent substance infiltrates in a determined molar concentration into the cell lipoids'.

Olive oil has been the traditional model solvent although it is in fact an inconsistent mixture of various lipids. Subsequently it was argued that the best site of action was represented by more polar solvents such as *n*-octanol. There have also been studies in which various membranes *per se* have been used as representative of the anaesthetic site of action.

CORRELATION STUDIES

The correlation between anaesthetic potency and hydrophobic solubility can be expressed as:

$$\text{MAC} \times \text{Solubility} = \text{a Constant}$$

Varying the solvent clearly can increase or decrease the standard deviation of the mean constant for a group of compounds. This is illustrated in Fig. 4.6 which presents several correlation plots for seven inhalational anaesthetics representing a 12-fold variation in anaesthetic potencies – all of which have been determined by the same method in humans. The absolute solubilities in the different solvents are in the order:

Benzene < *n*-Octanol < Olive Oil < Lecithin < Intralipid

The relationship described by MAC × solubility is consistent over the wide range of MAC values but the degree of consistency differs between the solvents. Of the model solvents, *n*-octanol, benzene, olive oil and intralipid were inferior to lecithin. Despite its desirable solubility parameter, benzene was no better than olive oil in predicting potency. Intralipid was selected because of its additional aqueous component but variability of the correlation did not differ significantly from that for olive oil. *n*-Octanol, which has been favoured by other investigators, also had a coefficient of variation that was not significantly different from that for olive oil. Why should lecithin solubilities produce the lowest coefficient of variation? In biological terms, it is one of the known constituents of the neuronal membranes. In physicochemical terms, it has both a polar and a non-polar region, again a property of all neuronal membranes. However, lecithin may not be the most representative site of anaesthetic action and other components or combination of components may be even more representative.

The lecithin correlation has demonstrably approached the limit imposed by biological variation and the capacity to measure accurately both potency and solubility. The implication is that no single solvent can precisely mimic the site of action of anaesthesia in all species. As has already been discussed, the ratios of rat, dog and human MACs are themselves not consistent (Table 4.2). If there is a single site of anaesthetic action in a given species, its physical properties must vary from species to species, suggesting we can only

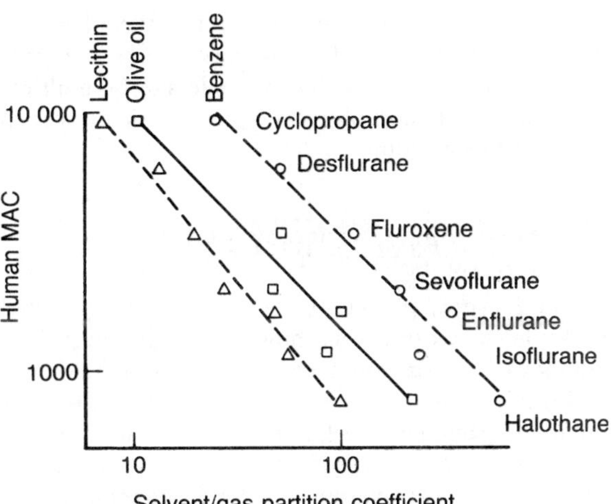

FIGURE 4.6 The logarithms of human MAC values for halothane, isoflurane, enflurane, sevoflurane, fluroxene, desflurane and cyclopropane (given in order of decreasing potency) correlate closely with the logarithms for their respective solubilities in olive oil, benzene and lecithin. The highest correlation (largest r^2) is found with lecithin ($r^2 = 0.979$), and lower correlations are found with olive oil (0.946) and benzene (0.944). More important, the slope of the relationship for lecithin is −0.987 (i.e. it approaches 1.0), whereas the slopes for olive oil (−0.834) and benzene (−0.780) are distinctly less than 1.0. (Reproduced with permission from Taheri S, Halsey MJ, Liu J, Eger EI, Koblin DD, Laster MJ. *Anesthesia and Analgesia* 1991; **34**: 627–34.)

hope to find a model solvent for the site of action within a given species. This, of course, presumes that the neuronal membrane has a single site or multiple sites with a common physical characteristic critical to the anaesthetic action.

PRESSURE REVERSAL OF ANAESTHESIA

Pressure reversal of anaesthesia was first demonstrated in the 1940s when it was shown that light emitted by luminous bacteria could be dimmed by anaesthetics and restored by the application of high pressure. The luminous bacteria model system was chosen because the rates of the underlying intracellular biochemical reactions could be determined from the direct measurements of light ouput. The concentrations of anaesthetics which inhibited the light output correlated with those required for surgical anaesthesia in both absolute and relative terms. The phenomenon of pressure reversal of anaesthesia was confirmed 20 years later in newts and mice. The data were interpreted in terms of the critical volume hypothesis which postulated that anaesthesia occurs when the volume of the site of action has expanded beyond a critical amount. This was effectively a unitary hypothesis in that it was assumed that all anaesthetics acted at the same single site. Subsequent studies with a wide range of different types of anaesthetics led to an alternative hypothesis that different anaesthetics have different molecular sites of action (Fig. 4.7). This 'multi-site hypothesis of anaesthetic action' was controversial when first proposed because it challenged the unitary concepts of all anaesthetics acting in the same way. However, it is now accepted generally and much of the current mechanistic data is interpreted as being agent specific. The unitary concept probably still applies within a closely related group of anaesthetics but falls down when a broader pharmacological range of different types of agents are considered.

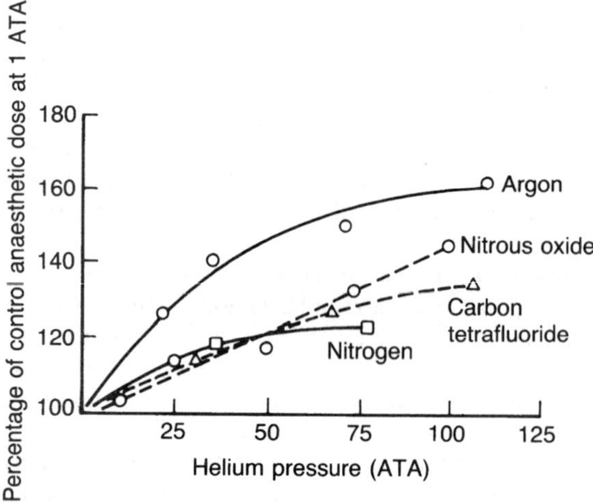

FIGURE 4.7 Pressure reversal data for different gaseous anaesthetics on mice. Anaesthesia was assessed in terms of the percentage of control anaesthetic dose at 1 atmosphere absolute (ATA) required to reduce the righting reflex of mice to 50% of control value. (Original data from four groups of authors referenced in, and reproduced with permission from Wardley-Smith B, Halsey MJ. *British Journal of Anaesthesia* 1985; 57: 1248–56.

Experiments based on the intact nervous system of whole animals – including humans – cannot have as detailed hypotheses as one would like. There is, however, a greater degree of confidence in stating that the experiments are directly relevant to general anaesthesia than is the case with the studies using isolated components – whether cellular or molecular – of the central nervous system. The molecular interpretations of the pressure-reversal data are consistent with the neurophysiological and neuropharmacological approaches to studying the mechanisms of the agents, which in general conclude that different anaesthetics act on different structures in neuronal membranes to produce anaesthesia. For example, the effects of althesin and methohexitone have been compared on synaptic excitation and inhibition in the spinal cord; the results showed clear differences between the agents suggesting that each anaesthetic has an individual spectrum of neurophysiological effects that contributes to its own anaesthetic properties. Studies in intact animals and in synaptic preparations of the olfactory cortex demonstrated that althesin and methohexitone had synergistic, rather than additive effects, which again is evidence consistent with the multi-site hypothesis. The potassium-stimulated γ-amino-butyric acid (GABA) and D-aspartate release from cortical brain slices was inhibited by methohexitone but not by althesin. There are also dissimilar influences of the barbiturates and steroid anaesthetic on the responses of the lamprey reticulospinal neurones to GABA, glycine and L-glutamate. Not all studies show major differences between the agents. For example, both barbiturates and althesin enhanced depolarizing responses to GABA and muscimol in the rat cuneate nucleus slice with little effect on responses to glycine, which has been interpreted in terms of the interactions with the $GABA_A$-receptor complex.

It is important to have the complementary evidence of the overall anaesthetic behavioural responses which in the pressure reversal experiments also reveal differences between agents. In summary, the pressure reversal data indicate that there is no universal linear relationship between anaesthetic potencies and environmental pressure. This is in agreement with the predictions of the multi-site hypothesis and provides further support for the concept of different sites of anaesthetic action with differing physical properties and with both finite capacities and compressibility.

NEURONAL MEMBRANES

Biological membranes are complex and diverse, both in structure and function, yet all consist of a lipid bilayer of the Görter–Grendel type with protein and other non-lipid components. Much of the work on molecular mechanisms of general anaesthesia has, for pragmatic reasons, concentrated on the lipid components. It is currently fashionable to invoke neuronal proteins as the primary target for anaesthetics and to suggest, for example, that lipid fluidity hypotheses are naive. While this may be true, many of the ideas on anaesthetic protein perturbations are based on macromolecules which are only models for the site of action. This situation may be rectified by the developing work on reconstituted neuronal proteins.

LIPID SITES OF ACTION

The effects of anaesthetics on phase transitions and fluidity in lipid bilayers have been studied using similar techniques to those used for investigating the basic structure of membranes. These have included electron spin resonance and NMR spectroscopy, differential scanning calorimetry, fluorimetry, light scattering, and permeability measurements.

A vast amount of data has been obtained over the last decade concerning the effects of anaesthetics on lipid bilayer fluidity and lipid transition temperatures. The best available summary is for halothane (Table 4.3). What appears certain and has been verified by a variety of techniques is that high concentrations of anaesthetic, both inhalational and non-inhalational, can produce large perturbations in lipid bilayers. However, it is at clinically relevant concentrations that one has to be more critical of the results. As far as fluidity changes are concerned, where a change has been seen at clinically relevant concentrations of anaesthetic it has generally been an increase in fluidity. It seems likely that the small fluidity increases at clinical concentrations of anaesthetic are real, although the magnitude of the changes is probably so small as to test the sensitivity of the various techniques. In fact it has been estimated that, in terms of fluidity, a general anaesthetic dose is equivalent to a 0.32°C rise in temperature. If fluidity changes are important in producing anaesthesia, it is difficult to reconcile this with the fact that such small changes in temperature do not produce anaesthesia in man. Decreases in lipid phase transition temperatures are invariably seen with inhalational anaesthetic agents but non-gaseous anaesthetics such as the alkanols appear to produce either increases or decreases in transition temperature, with a possible dependence on lipid chain length.

Techniques other than those indicated in Table 4.3 which have been used to examine the effects of anaesthetics on bilayer structure have generally indicated a lack of effect. They have included Raman spectroscopy, X-ray and neutron diffraction. The technique of ^{31}P-NMR has been applied to lipid membranes in the investigation of non-bilayer lipid structures. In pure lipid systems it is known that, when hydrated, certain phospholipids such as unsaturated phosphatidylethanolamines and cardiolipin preferentially adopt non-bilayer configurations. These can take the form of a hexagonal phase in which the lipid molecules orientate to form cylinders in which the headgroups surround a channel of

TABLE 4.3 Effect(s) of halothane on lipid fluidity and transition temperature

TECHNIQUE	LIPID MEMBRANE	CONCENTRATION OF ANAESTHETIC	FLUIDITY CHANGE	CHANGE IN Tc
ESR	PLPC	0.16–0.32 mM	↓	
	PLPC	9.3 mM	↑	
ESR	DPPC	0.32–1.6 mM	↓	
	DPPC	9.3 mM	↑	
ESR	PC/Chol (1.0 : 0.6)	49–490 mmol/mol lipid	↑	
ESR	PC/Chol (1 : 1)	5 mmol/l lipid	↑	
ESR	4% PA/PC	11 mM	↑	
	20% PA/PC		↑	
	4% PA/33% chol/PC		↑	
NMR	DPPC	30–170 mM	↑	
DSC	DPPC	0.003–0.150 atm		↓
DSC	DPPC	80–450 mM		↓
Fluorescence anisotropy	DMPC	14.4–44.0 mM		↓
Fluorescence anisotropy	Synaptosomal plasma membranes	0.5–3% (v/v) (gaseous concentration used for equilibration)	↑	
Light scattering	DPPC	0.65 mM		↓

(Reproduced with permission from Dluzewski AR, Halsey MJ, Simmonds AC. Membrane interactions with general and local anaesthetics: a review of molecular hypotheses of anaesthesia. *Molecular Aspects of Medicine* 1983; **6**: 459–573.)
PLPC, DPPC, etc., are different types of lipids.

water and the hydrocarbon tails are displayed radially, or inverted micelles in which the headgroups again surround an aqueous compartment and the hydrocarbon tails are displayed radially. Both general and local anaesthetics can affect the formation of non-bilayer phases. Whether this has any relevance to the mechanism of anaesthesia is yet to be seen, especially as a definite role for non-bilayer phases has yet to be established in biological membranes. It has been suggested that such lipid phases are likely to participate in membrane fusion; indeed it has been demonstrated in a model system using Ca^{2+}-induced fusion of liposomes that uncharged anaesthetics enhance fusion whereas the charged tertiary amine anaesthetics inhibit fusion, although the concentrations required were higher than those used clinically.

The biophysical studies determine how anaesthetics affect the physical properties of lipid bilayers. However, the functional aspects of these systems are related to the movement of ions across the membrane either passively or when driven by an electromotive force. The experiments with anaesthetics and bimolecular lipid membranes (BLM) have given rise to many interesting and sometimes conflicting results. Perhaps this is to be expected in view of the diversity of both the anaesthetic agents and the lipid systems used, but in spite of this, certain trends do seem to be emerging. For example, certain alcohols, chloroform, trichloroethylene and halothane all produce an increase in the conductance of BLMs but the concentration of anaesthetic required to do this is substantially greater than that required to produce general anaesthesia. In absolute terms the conductance increases produced by anaesthetics are quite insignificant (as are the permeability changes in liposomes) and so the feeling is that they are more an indication of a change in some other physical property of the bilayer (e.g. changes in fluidity and/or thickness in the hydrocarbon region of the lipid).

The possibility now exists of the anaesthetic acting on a membrane channel either by direct action or indirectly, as might be mediated by a change in the state of the lipid that surrounds it. This has led to an interest in direct anaesthetic–macromolecule interactions as discussed in the next section.

PROTEIN SITES OF ACTION

One approach to studying the structure–activity relationships of the general anaesthetics is to investigate the detailed manner in which they interact with potential sites of action in macromolecules. If the anaesthetic was simply loosely bound to the molecule surface (as is the case with the Langmuir absorption of gases, for example), then it is unlikely that there would be much structural dependency. On the other hand, interactions with internal hydrophobic areas are potentially more critically dependent on the size, geometry, structure and composition of the individual agents.

Various proteins have been used to study anaesthetic interactions; haemoglobin has proved to be a very useful model protein which can be studied in detail in solutions using NMR. NMR is a technique that is sensitive to small structural changes in protein, while haemoglobin is large enough to have a series of internal hydrophobic areas that provide an opportunity for the study of site preferences determined by the structure–activity relationships of the anaesthetic molecule, if they exist.

It is now established that anaesthetics at clinical concentrations interact with haemoglobin in solution and, by inference, are capable of interacting with other proteins, such as those associated with synaptic transmission in the central nervous system, or those associated with the 'side-effects' of anaesthesia. At clinical concentrations (1 MAC), the interactions with haemoglobin are localized and specific, and quite different for different agents. Additional effects are related to the partial pressure of the anaesthetic agent. More extensive investigations revealed that consistent perturbations could be observed in only a very few NMR peaks over wide ranges of pH and solution composition and occurred at clinical concentrations (i.e. 1 MAC) of halothane.

Although the perturbations are observed on surface residues, it does not necessarily imply that the interaction is a surface one. A more plausible conclusion is that the surface perturbations monitor the expansion of hydrophobic pockets within the protein that have been invaded by the hydrophobic anaesthetic molecules. Volatile anaesthetics appear to have two types of interaction with proteins. First there is occupancy of hydrophobic pockets, which is a function of hydrophobic solubility rather than molecular structure. This type of action by itself could not explain the differences in side-effects found with different anaesthetics. However, there is a second type of interaction, which is influenced by additional factors such as molecular size, shape and charge, which are specific for different anaesthetics. It would appear that this provides a basis for the selective effects of different anaesthetics on particular physiological functions. Haemoglobin is not the only model protein that has been studied in the investigation of anaesthetic mechanisms and examples of other studies are included in Table 4.4.

CALCIUM CHANNELS

An alternative approach to the study of lipid and protein model systems *in vitro* is to study the pharmacological manipulation of ion channels *in vivo*. An example is the use of dihydropyridine calcium channel antagonists and the Bay K 8644 agonist as probes to investigate the potential roles of calcium channels in mechanisms of anaesthesia.

It has been demonstrated that the calcium antagonists (in micromolar brain concentrations) increase the anaesthetic potencies of inhalational and intravenous agents. The antagonists do not possess anaesthetic properties themselves, and are not sedative at the doses used. In general, Bay K 8644 antagonizes anaesthesia. Calcium antagonists and Bay K 8644 do not affect blood or brain anaesthetic concentrations. Nitrendipine prevents the development of tolerance to nitrous oxide anaesthesia and the sedative effects of ethanol.

TABLE 4.4 Effect of anaesthetics on secondary structure of membrane proteins

MEMBRANE	ANAESTHETIC	% DECREASE IN MOLAR ELLIPTICITY
Erythrocyte membrane	Butanol 10 mM	−14
	Ketamine 1 mM	−13
	Isoflurane 0.38 mM	−25
	Enflurane 0.38 mM	−1.7
Halobacterium halobium purple membrane	Butanol 0.35 mM	−39
	Ketamine 4.3 mM	−36
Bovine brain synaptic membranes	Butanol 40 mM	−7
	Ketamine 0.35 mM	−8
Sarcoplasmic reticulum-reconstituted ATPase	Butanol 100 mM	−20

(Reproduced with permission from Curatola G, Lenay G, Zolese G. In: Aloia RC, Curtain CC, Gordon LM eds. *Drug and anesthetic effects on membrane structure and function*. New York: Wiley Liss, 1991; 35–70.)

CONCLUSION

Anaesthetics interact with both proteins and lipids of the neuronal membrane. The functional perturbations that result are either due to direct disruption of ion channel or receptor function, or related to indirect actions via the lipids that are associated with these macromolecules. It is inappropriate to attempt to provide an all-embracing definitive hypothesis of the mechanisms of anaesthesia but the integration of the different effects of anaesthesia at a molecular level is the ambitious long-term goal of the mechanistic studies. The results are relevant to an understanding not only of these types of drugs but also of the neurobiology of the brain.

FURTHER READING

Aloia RC, Curtain CC, Gordon LM, eds. *Drug and anesthetic effects on membrane structure and function*. New York: Wiley-Liss, 1991.

Eger EI. *Anesthetic uptake and action*. Baltimore: Williams & Wilkins, 1984.

Halsey MJ. Molecular mechanisms of anaesthesia. In: Nunn JF, Utting JE, Brown BR, eds. *General anaesthesia*. London: Butterworths, 1989: 19–29.

Lockhart SH, Cohen Y, Yasuda N, Friere BA, Eger EI. Cerebral washout of desflurane vs. isoflurane and halothane from rabbit brain. *Anesthesia and Analgesia* 1990; 70: S244.

Mapleson WW. Pharmacokinetics of inhalational anaesthetics. In: Nunn JF, Utting JE, Brown BR. eds. *General anaesthesia*. London: Butterworths, 1989: 44–59.

Overton CE. In: Lipnick RL ed. *Studies of narcosis*. New York: Chapman & Hall, 1991.

Papper EM, Kitz RJ. *Uptake and distribution of anesthetic agents*. New York: McGraw-Hill, 1963.

Taheri S, Halsey MJ, Liu J, Eger II EI, Koblin DD, Laster MJ. What solvent best represents the site of action of inhaled anesthetics in humans, rats and dogs? *Anesthesia and Analgesia* 1991; **34**: 627–34.

Wardley-Smith B, Halsey MJ. Mixtures of inhalational and intravenous anaesthetics at high pressure: a test of the multi-site hypothesis of general anaesthesia. *British Journal of Anaesthesia* 1985; 57: 1248–56.

Yusada N, Lockhart SH, Eger EI, Weiskopf RB, Johnson BH, Fassoulaki A. Desflurane, isoflurane and halothane pharmacokinetics in humans. *Anesthesia and Analgesia* 1990; 70: S444.

5

General Anaesthesia

HISTORICAL BACKGROUND

From time immemorial the relief of pain has been foremost in the mind of mankind. Various mixtures of herbs, alcohol, opium, mandrakes and hemlock have been advocated by inhalation often in a form of a sponge or 'apple' applied to the patient's face. It was only with advances in inorganic chemistry with the discovery of nitrous oxide by Priestley, carbon dioxide by Black and oxygen by Lavoisier that gases became available for inhalation.

The analgesic properties of nitrous oxide were known to Humphrey Davy in 1800, but it was left to Horace Wells in 1844 to appreciate its value for dental anaesthesia; its sole use for major surgery proved disastrous and it was not until 1846 in Boston that W. T. G. Morton demonstrated the first successful use of ether anaesthesia for major surgery, an agent which had been manufactured in the 16th century. The first public demonstration of ether anaesthesia in the UK took place in University College Hospital on 21 December 1846 when the anaesthetist was a medical student. Chloroform was introduced in 1847 and cyclopropane in 1934. The Second World War saw the introduction of trichloroethylene in 1941 and halothane was first used clinically in 1956. Enflurane was introduced 10 years later followed by isoflurane in 1971, and more recently by sevoflurane and desflurane.

PART I INHALATIONAL ANAESTHETICS

M Jordan

The inhalational anaesthetics are a group of gases and vapours capable of bringing about a reversible abolition of the perception of all external stimuli if inhaled in an appropriate concentration. Throughout the history of anaesthesia numerous inhaled agents have been used, although less than twenty have been eventually accepted into clinical practice, and fewer than half that number are in use anywhere today. The withdrawal of trichloroethylene in 1989 and cyclopropane in 1990 reduced to four the number of inhalational anaesthetics in regular clinical use in the UK, bringing the UK in line with North America and much of Western Europe.

The extensive toxicity studies required before the introduction of any new drug has slowed the pace at which new pharmaceuticals are introduced, increased development costs and reduced the period in which the patent holder may recover investment before the compound may be manufactured in generic form. None the less, the search for the ideal inhalational anaesthetic continues. Such an agent would need to have certain characteristics:

- It must have an extremely stable molecule. This implies non-inflammability, resistance to degradation by UV light or soda lime, and resistance to biotransformation within the body.
- It must be free of toxic effects on any organ, in anaesthetic or trace concentrations.
- It must have a low blood : gas partition coefficient, allowing for rapid induction, recovery and changes of anaesthetic depth.
- It must have minimal side-effects on the cardiovascular and respiratory systems.
- It should not increase cerebral blood flow or intracranial pressure, or have any stimulant/convulsant properties.
- Its vapour should be pleasant and non-irritant to breathe.
- Its mean alveolar concentration (MAC) should be sufficiently low to allow the use of high concentrations of oxygen.

None of the currently available inhalational anaesthetics fulfils all these requirements.

NITROUS OXIDE – DINITROGEN MONOXIDE – N_2O

Physical chemistry

Molecular weight	44.016
Boiling point at 1 bar (°C)	−89.0
Critical temperature (°C)	36.5
Critical pressure (kPa)	7265

Although usually referred to as a gas, below its critical temperature nitrous oxide is technically a vapour, and can be liquefied by the application of pressure alone. In the UK it is supplied in liquid form in steel cylinders painted French Blue. At 21°C, the pressure inside a nitrous oxide cylinder is 5060 kPa, its vapour pressure at that temperature. As long as there is both liquid and gaseous nitrous oxide in the cylinder, the measured pressure depends only on its temperature. When in use, the latent heat of vaporization of liquid nitrous oxide will cause the cylinder to cool and the pressure within will tend to fall. The only reliable guide to the cylinder's contents is therefore the weight. At 15°C, nitrous oxide weighs 1.87 g/l (approximately 1.5 times the weight of air), and the weight of the empty cylinder ('tare weight') is stamped on the valve.

Chemistry

Nitrous oxide supports combustion as vigorously as oxygen. Inflammable anaesthetics such as diethyl ether, ethyl chloride or cyclopropane may be ignited at lower concentrations in nitrous oxide than in oxygen.[1] It is a very stable molecule at lower temperatures, stable in soda lime, and not significantly metabolized. Nitrous oxide in the stratosphere, however, acts as a catalyst in ozone destruction and contributes to the production of acid rain, although the part played by waste anaesthetic nitrous oxide in these processes is insignificant beside the quantities released in the manufacture of fertilizers.[2]

Manufacture

Although produced as a by-product in a number of industrial processes, including the manufacture of nylon, medical nitrous oxide is usually derived from the thermal decomposition of ammonium nitrate. The reaction is strongly exothermic and potentially explosive. Significant quantities of nitric oxide and nitrogen dioxide are also produced and are removed by scrubbing with sodium hydroxide and potassium permanganate. Contamination of medical nitrous oxide with other nitrogen oxides was responsible for the deaths of two patients in the UK in 1966.[3]

Anaesthetic characteristics

Blood : gas partition coefficient	0.47 (37°C)
Oil : gas partition coefficient	1.4 (37°C)
MAC (%)	105

Nitrous oxide is unique among commonly used inhalational anaesthetics in having a MAC of greater than 100%. It follows that it is seldom possible to produce a state of general anaesthesia using nitrous oxide alone at atmospheric pressure. It can be used as the sole general anaesthetic under hyperbaric conditions, and this was described as long ago as 1879.[4] A recent study of hyperbaric nitrous oxide anaesthesia in eight male volunteers discovered a variety of effects not normally seen at lower partial pressures, including tachypnoea, tachycardia, rises in arterial pressure, clonus and opisthotonus.[5] Pressure chamber techniques have been used for accurate determination of the MAC of the agent in man.[6] Estimation of the additive contribution of nitrous oxide to halothane MAC in routine anaesthesia in children has produced a very similar value for MAC.[7] The MAC in animals is considerably higher than in man. The value in the dog is 188%, and in the rat 150%, although differences in methodology between studies in different species make direct comparisons difficult. Its low solubility in blood confers speed of induction and recovery. When used in conjunction with potent inhaled anaesthetics, their speed of onset is hastened by the second gas effect and the anaesthetic contribution of nitrous oxide can reduce the concentration of the volatile agent needed by up to 60%.

Nitrous oxide is a good analgesic, possibly because it induces release of brain opioid peptides,[8] although such rapid tolerance to this effect occurs that it has been shown to be without analgesic properties after less than 150 min when inhaled by volunteers.[9]

Circulation

The effects of nitrous oxide on the circulation are much less marked than those of the volatile agents. *In vitro* studies of guinea pig myocardium show that 50% nitrous oxide will depress contractility by 10–15%,[10] but its high MAC has complicated studies of its effects on physiology under general anaesthesia. These are usually determined by adding it to the inspired mixture during anaesthesia maintained by another inhaled or intravenous agent, and in chronically instrumented dogs[11] it produces significant myocardial depression superimposed on sufentanil or isoflurane anaesthesia. This effect is also seen in humans, particularly in patients with poor left ventricular function. Meretoja *et al.*[12] found that introduction of 70% nitrous oxide decreased systemic arterial pressure by an average of 10% during high-dose fentanyl-oxygen anaesthesia.

In several studies in dogs with critical coronary narrowing[13–16] nitrous oxide consistently produced global depression of myocardial function, and worsened myocardial dysfunction in ischaemic areas, although this seems to be less of a problem in man.[17] Moreover, nitrous oxide does not appear to worsen pulmonary hypertension or ventricular dysfunction in patients with mitral valve disease.[18]

A study of adrenaline-induced arrhythmias in humans undergoing hypophysectomy showed nitrous oxide to have a slight tendency to increase AV dissociation.[19]

In practice, the myocardial depression of nitrous oxide is usually offset by its tendency to increase sympathetic outflow and circulating noradrenaline,[20,21] such that cardiac output, systemic and pulmonary vascular resistance and arterial pressure actually rise slightly.[22] High doses of opiates may block this effect, and the results of research involving high-dose opiate techniques must be interpreted with this in mind.

Nitrous oxide will produce a change in distribution of cardiac output and its addition to halothane anaesthesia in the rat produces a decrease in blood flow to kidneys, liver, small bowel and spleen, but an increase in cerebral blood flow.[23] Its effects on cerebral blood flow and intracranial pressure in man are considered below.

Respiration

Nitrous oxide was long considered to have a negligible effect on respiratory drive, based on its observed effect on P_aCO_2 in conscious volunteers. In dogs, it has been suggested that nitrous oxide actually counteracts the respiratory depression produced by halothane,[24] but in man, its addition to a volatile anaesthetic produces unequivocal further depression,[25] similar to that produced by an equipotent concentration of halothane, but rather less than enflurane.[26] There is depression of the response both to hypercarbia and hypoxia, and the tendency of emerging nitrous oxide to displace oxygen from the alveoli during recovery (diffusion hypoxia) makes supplementary oxygen advisable during this time.

Central nervous system

Nitrous oxide has long been known to increase cerebral blood flow when added to a halothane anaesthetic.[27,28] It acts as a cerebral metabolic stimulant (although a recent study[29] failed to demonstrate this) and partially reduces the cerebral protective effect of thiopentone (see discussion under isoflurane). Introduction of nitrous oxide in isoflurane anaesthesia will increase intracranial pressure even in the presence of hyperventilation.[30] Although these effects are relatively mild and discounted by many, its tendency to worsen the effects of air embolism and pneumocephalus (see below) together with the advent of isoflurane and propofol have led to a decline in its use in neuroanaesthesia in North America.

Other systems

Nitrous oxide will diffuse into air-filled spaces within the body at a faster rate than nitrogen can leave, resulting in an increase in pressure in the bowel and middle ear. The effects of pneumothorax, pneumocephalus (such as commonly occurs after craniotomy) and air embolism are all worsened, and its diffusion into the cuff of a tracheal tube will increase the pressure therein.

Toxicity

Nitrous oxide inactivates vitamin B_{12}, inhibiting methionine synthetase, thus affecting DNA synthesis. Megaloblastic changes in bone marrow similar to those seen in folate deficiency can follow its prolonged administration (in excess of 24 h),[31] although folinic acid ameliorates these effects.[32–34] A study in twenty dental surgeons who routinely employed nitrous oxide sedation showed three to have an abnormal response to a deoxyuridine suppression test. Chronic abuse of nitrous oxide can lead to a myeloneuropathy similar to that seen in pernicious anaemia.[35]

In view of the above the possible toxic effects of nitrous oxide on the fetus have been extensively investigated. Prolonged exposure in early pregnancy produces malformations in the offspring of laboratory animals,[36,37] but its use in general anaesthesia for cervical cerclage and other procedures during the first two trimesters of pregnancy[38,39] has not been found to have adverse effects, although the sample sizes were small. Larger-scale retrospective research on the outcome of pregnancy in operating theatre staff show an increased susceptibility to spontaneous abortion,[40] although the mechanisms involved are unclear, and may not be related to nitrous oxide, or indeed inhaled anaesthetics at all. Nitrous oxide does not affect the success rate for *in vitro* fertilization.[41]

Malignant hyperpyrexia may be triggered by nitrous oxide.[42] In this inherited condition, due to an underlying defect of the sarcoplasmic reticulum, sustained contraction of skeletal muscle may be triggered by a variety of compounds, including the volatile anaesthetics and suxamethonium. A hypermetabolic state results, with a massive rise in body temperature, production of carbon dioxide and acidosis, leading to death. Prompt treatment with dantrolene will reverse the situation.

Status

Despite its low potency, nitrous oxide remains, after nearly 150 years, the basis of most general anaesthetics in the developed world. In use, it is almost odourless, non-irritant, has only mild effects on circulation and respiration, does not contribute significantly to postoperative nausea and is relatively cheap.

HALOTHANE – 2-BROMO-2-CHLORO-1,1,1-TRIFLUOROETHANE

```
     F   Br
     |   |
 F — C — C — H
     |   |
     F   Cl
```

Halothane

History

The development of halothane was facilitated by advances in fluorine chemistry made in the course of the development of nuclear weapons during the Second World War, although it was not itself synthesized until 1951, by Suckling of ICI, with the first clinical trials reported in 1956.

Physical chemistry

▪ Molecular weight	197.38
▪ Boiling point (°C)	50.2
▪ Vapour pressure at 20°C (kPa)	32.53
▪ Maximum vapour concentration at 20°C	32%

At atmospheric pressure halothane is a colourless clear volatile liquid with a non-irritant vapour.

Chemistry

Although non-inflammable in air at any concentration, 4.75% halothane vapour will ignite in a 30% oxygen–70% nitrous oxide mixture.[43] In pure nitrous oxide, 1% halothane will ignite. In practice, however, halothane may be regarded as non-inflammable in clinically used gas mixtures.

The halothane molecule, an alkane, is less stable than enflurane or isoflurane, and requires the addition of 0.01% thymol as a stabilizer. It must also be kept cool and protected from UV light. Although there is theoretical possibility of accumulation of breakdown products of halothane in a closed circuit, they are only present in very low concentrations[44] and are not thought to represent a risk.[45] In the presence of moisture, halothane vapour is mildly corrosive to aluminium, tin and brass.

Anaesthetic characteristics

▪ Blood : gas partition coefficient	2.3 (37°C)
▪ Oil : gas partition coefficient	224 (37°C)
▪ MAC (%)	0.75

Halothane has a non-irritant vapour allowing the administration of high concentrations with minimal risk of coughing, breath-holding or laryngospasm. In terms of speed and smoothness of induction of anaesthesia this outweighs the lower blood-gas solubility coefficients of enflurane and isoflurane, particularly in inhalational induction of anaesthesia in children.

Halothane possesses no significant analgesic properties.

Circulation

Halothane is a profound myocardial depressant, producing a dose-related fall in arterial pressure. Cardiac output, stroke volume, left ventricular stroke work and myocardial contractility are all depressed and right atrial and left ventricular end-diastolic pressures are increased. Heart rate may decrease but systemic vascular resistance is unchanged.[46–48] *In vitro* studies confirm that the major site of action of halothane on the circulation is the myocardium itself, the mechanism being a reduction in intracellular Ca^{2+} by inhibition of ion transport in the myocardial sarcoplasmic reticulum,[49] possibly with a reduction in responsiveness of the myofibrils to calcium.[50] Meanwhile, there is a depression of baroreflex control of systemic vascular resistance[51] and of heart rate,[52] allowing vagal predominance and bradycardia (which is easily reversed by atropine).

Other alkane anaesthetics such as halopropane, teflurane and norflurane were withdrawn as a result of their tendency to produce cardiac arrhythmias, and a variety of arrhythmias are seen in association with halothane anaesthesia, junctional rhythms being relatively common. Halothane slows conductive tissue allowing escape and re-entry type phenomena, as well as increasing automaticity of the myocardium and sensitizing it to the arrhythmogenic effects of catecholamines, endogenous or exogenous. Premature ventricular extrasystoles are often seen, and high circulating levels of catecholamines can occasionally precipitate ventricular tachycardia or fibrillation.

Although the overall systemic vascular resistance is unaltered by halothane, there are marked changes in the distribution of cardiac output. Flow to the skin and the cerebral circulation is increased, splanchnic, renal and hepatic flow decreased, particularly during hypotension. The coronary circulation is not directly affected (see further discussion under isoflurane).

Respiration

Spontaneous respiration under halothane anaesthesia is rapid and shallow.[53,54] In the absence of surgical stimulation, hypercarbia almost always results; 1.5 MAC may be expected to increase P_aCO_2 to 6.5 kPa or more. In common with enflurane and isoflurane, halothane depresses the ventilatory response to both hypercarbia and hypoxia,[55–57] effects that seems to be mediated largely on the respiratory centres themselves,[4] although halothane does exert an action on the carotid bodies.[58] In addition to its effects on the neural control of respiration, halothane inhibits hypoxic pulmonary vasoconstriction,[59,60] causing a deterioration in gas exchange.

Halothane is a powerful bronchodilator, and is a drug of last resort in the treatment of status asthmaticus.[61,62] Its antagonism of histamine-induced bronchospasm may persist for 24 h following anaesthesia.[63] Although ciliary movement is depressed by halothane, recovery of function is rapid.

Central nervous system

Halothane has long been known to increase cerebral blood flow and thus intracranial pressure, particularly in the presence of low intracranial compliance.[64] At normocarbia, 1 MAC of halothane will increase cerebral blood flow by 150%; 2 MAC will quadruple it.[30] Hyperventilation greatly reduces this effect, but hypocarbia must be established before the introduction of halothane. Autoregulation of the cerebral circulation is abolished by 1 MAC halothane.

Other systems

In common with enflurane and isoflurane, halothane is a significant skeletal muscle relaxant, and will potentiate the effects of neuromuscular blocking agents, apparently by a postsynaptic action. In patients with myasthenia gravis, depression of the train-of-four response may be seen.[65]

Halothane is a uterine relaxant and may contribute to uterine laxity and increased blood loss after delivery at Caesarean section or following therapeutic abortion. In the past, worries about haemorrhage and depression of the fetus led to the use of very low concentrations of halothane in obstetric patients, with a resulting high incidence of awareness. It is now appreciated that at inspired concentrations of up to 0.5%, halothane does not materially affect blood loss,[66] and fetal depression blamed on anaesthetic agents may have been due to undiagnosed aortocaval compression.

Higher concentrations of halothane may be a useful uterine depressant in anaesthesia for external version of the fetus, and have been used to relax the uterine constriction ring, although there is a considerable risk of haemorrhage, and the concentrations needed may produce undesirable hypotension.

Metabolic fate

In vivo, at least 20% and possibly as much as 40%[67] of absorbed halothane undergoes biotransformation to a variety of metabolites, including trifluoroacetic acid. This process is enhanced by enzyme induction, and is thought to hold the key to halothane hepatotoxicity (see below).

Toxicity

In a very small proportion of patients (approximately 1 in 10 000 administrations), halothane will initiate a form of acute hepatic necrosis similar to that caused by viral hepatitis. The syndrome carries a 50% mortality. Over 80% of cases are associated with multiple exposures to halothane. Repeat exposure within a short period of time seems to be disproportionately hazardous but there is no clear 'safe interval'. It is more common in obese patients and women are more often affected than men. It is very rare in children. The underlying mechanism is not entirely clear, but certainly has an immunological basis and may be related to biotransformation of halothane. Animal models involving enzyme induction and a period of hypoxia will produce a similar pathological picture, but opinions differ as to their relevance to the condition in man. It is now recommended that halothane should be avoided in patients who have received it within the previous 3 months, or who have a history of unexplained disturbance of liver function following its use. For a full account of 'halothane hepatitis' the reader is referred to the reviews of Stock and Strunin[68] and Ray and Drummond.[69]

Halothane may trigger malignant hyperpyrexia in susceptible patients.

Status

The combination of non-inflammability, high potency, low solubility and lack of pungency made halothane a huge advance on the available anaesthetics at the time of its introduction in 1956. Although fears over halothane hepatitis and the frequency of arrhythmias during its administration have resulted in a marked reduction in the use of halothane in adult anaesthesia, it remains the pre-eminent volatile agent in paediatric practice, the most effective bronchodilator, and the most appropriate volatile agent in the presence of ischaemic heart disease. Since the withdrawal of cyclopropane, it is unrivalled among commercially available agents for the inhalational induction of anaesthesia in child or adult. Among emerging compounds, only desflurane offers substantially quicker induction and recovery. In 1991 it was estimated by one of its principal manufacturers to have a market share by volume of 47% in the UK, 14% in the USA and 22% worldwide.

ENFLURANE – 2-CHLORO-1,1,2-TRIFLUOROETHYL DIFLUOROMETHYL ETHER

```
     F   F       F
     |   |       |
H —  C — C — O — C — H
     |   |       |
     Cl  F       F
```

Enflurane

History

During the early 1960s a team of chemists at Ohio Medical Products led by Ross Terrell synthesized over 700 compounds in an attempt to find a successor to halothane that did not suffer from its disadvantages. From this programme emerged enflurane (Compound 347), isoflurane (Compound 469) and desflurane (Compound 653).

Physical chemistry

- Molecular weight 184.5
- Boiling point (°C) 56.5
- Vapour pressure at 20°C (kPa) 23.6
- Maximum vapour concentration at 20°C 23%

At atmospheric pressure enflurane is a colourless clear liquid with a sweet, mildly pungent smell.

Chemistry

Enflurane, like halothane, may be regarded as non-inflammable in any concentration encountered in clinical practice, although 5.75% enflurane will ignite in 30% oxygen–70% nitrous oxide (a mixture equivalent to 8.9 MAC).[43]

Enflurane is very stable at room temperature and does not require the addition of a chemical stabilizer. It does not attack metals, nor is it chemically altered by soda lime. Although presented in brown bottles, it has been shown to be stable for at least 5 years in clear glass.[70]

Manufacture

Details of the manufacturing process of many of the current volatile agents are industrial secrets, but production of enflurane involves the reaction of a halogenated alcohol with chlorine and hydrofluoric acid, via chlorotrifluoroethylene. Multiple distillation yields 99.9% pure enflurane.

Anaesthetic characteristics

- Blood:gas partition coefficient 1.91 (37°C)
- Oil:gas partition coefficient 98.5 (37°C)
- MAC (%) 1.68

The MAC of enflurane is 40% higher than its structural isomer isoflurane, reflecting the fact that it has excitatory as well as anaesthetic properties (see Central nervous system). The mild pungency of enflurane, its respiratory depressant effects and its high MAC render it rather less easy to use than halothane in inhalational induction of anaesthesia. Another handicap is that, in terms of MAC, most enflurane vaporizers deliver less than their halothane or isoflurane versions. Following intravenous induction, however, maintenance and emergence from enflurane is usually smooth. A slight increase in secretions may be seen.

Enflurane in subanaesthetic concentrations has been used as an obstetric analgesic. In labouring patients, enflurane outscored 50% nitrous oxide, although its recipients were drowsier.[71]

Circulation

At concentrations of up to 1.5 MAC, the effects of enflurane on arterial pressure, stroke volume and right atrial pressure are similar to those of halothane,[72–74] although cardiac output is better maintained because enflurane consistently reduces systemic vascular resistance (by about 16% at 1 MAC).[75] It was claimed that at deeper levels of anaesthesia it is a more profound myocardial depressant – the administration of 2 MAC enflurane to unstimulated volunteers produced profound hypotension[75] – but subsequent studies have provided conflicting evidence. Both agents attenuate baroreflex control of the circulation, but unlike halothane, enflurane may increase the heart rate. Enflurane does not increase adrenergic outflow.

Disturbances of cardiac rhythm are less common under enflurane than halothane anaesthesia. In a study of children undergoing adenoidectomy, a procedure associated with a high incidence of arrhythmias, a group receiving enflurane had a 32% incidence of arrhythmias of all types, compared with 72% in a group receiving halothane.[76] Animal studies have shown that, at 1.2 MAC halothane, the mean intravenous dose of adrenaline needed to provoke ventricular extrasystoles is 5 μg/kg. The corresponding figure for 1.2 MAC enflurane is 17 μg/kg.[77]

Enflurane is a coronary vasodilator,[78] and in the presence of experimentally induced myocardial ischaemia in the dog, appears to have a beneficial effect on the ischaemic region, improving lactate extraction and preserving subendocardial blood flow.[79] In patients undergoing coronary artery grafting, enflurane did not alter myocardial lactate extraction or cause ST changes.[80]

In vitro and in animal preparations, enflurane is a splanchnic vasodilator,[81–83] although the results of these studies do not guarantee the preservation of flow during hypotension *in vivo*. Renal blood flow, glomerular filtration rate and urine output are depressed slightly less by enflurane than by halothane or isoflurane.

Respiration

It is now accepted that enflurane is the most powerful respiratory depressant among the current volatile anaesthetics. At 1 MAC, higher $PaCO_2$ levels are seen under enflurane than halothane[84] and hypoxic and hypercapnic drive are reduced more by enflurane than halothane.[57] The administration of more than 1.5 MAC enflurane usually necessitates respiratory support. Unlike halothane, enflurane does not cause a tachypnoea.

Enflurane is an effective bronchodilator, though less so than halothane.[85] It is usually said to impair hypoxic pulmonary vasoconstriction,[4] although at least two studies have failed to demonstrate this.[73,86]

Central nervous system

Early studies of enflurane[87] noted its tendency to produce tonic–clonic activity in some patients, and it was soon discovered that in high concentrations, spike-and-wave seizure EEG activity is seen. This effect is particularly pronounced in the presence of hypocarbia. EEG changes may persist for a number of hours postoperatively and may be linked to delayed seizures,[88,89] although these are a very rare occurrence. Enflurane is, however, not recommended for use in epileptic patients.

Enflurane produces a dose-related increase in cerebral blood flow, but this is less marked than that seen with halothane. Similar MAC values of halothane and enflurane in 70% N_2O, equivalent to 1.5 MAC, were found to increase cerebral blood flow (CBF) by 166% and 35% respectively.[90] Prior to the introduction of isoflurane, low concentrations of enflurane had become popular in neuroanaesthesia and had been shown to have very little effect on intracranial pressure in patients with cerebral tumours,[91] although the same study drew attention to the difficulty of maintaining adequate cerebral perfusion pressure in some patients due to hypotension.

Other systems

Enflurane greatly enhances the effects of neuromuscular blocking drugs,[92] an effect seen particularly with tubocurarine and pancuronium. In a study comparing equivalent concentrations of halothane and enflurane in 60% nitrous oxide, their effects on the potency of atracurium were similar, but its duration of action was 34% longer with enflurane.[93] As with halothane, the site of action appears to be postjunctional, but there is a CNS element.

Like halothane, enflurane relaxes the pregnant uterus. At low concentrations, there is little to choose between the agents in this respect, but at 1.5 MAC, a concentration seldom used in the obstetric patient, enflurane has a greater effect.[94]

Metabolic fate

Enflurane is much less easily metabolized than halothane, and the fraction of absorbed enflurane undergoing biotransformation is between 2 and 8.5%.[67] Among the breakdown products identified are difluoromethoxydifluoroacetic acid and free fluoride ions, which are relevant in the context of possible renal effects (see below).

Toxicity

Enflurane-induced hepatitis has been reported[95] but it is an exceedingly rare event. One case was reported in a patient who had survived halothane hepatitis, suggesting cross-sensitization,[96] but the condition is certainly over-diagnosed.[97] A rat model of enflurane hepatitis exists,[98] but as with halothane, the relevance of animal models involving enzyme-induction and hypoxia has been questioned.[99]

The liberation of free fluoride ions as a metabolic product raised concern about possible nephrotoxic effects, akin to those caused by methoxyflurane. High-output renal failure is associated with plasma fluoride concentrations above 40 μmol/l but this level is at least double that seen after even prolonged enflurane anaesthesia, and the risk would appear to be slight. None the less, there are case reports of renal damage after enflurane.[100]

Enflurane is capable of triggering malignant hyperpyrexia in susceptible individuals.

Status

Enflurane was introduced in the USA in 1972, at the time of widespread concern over halothane hepatitis. It rapidly became the most popular anaesthetic for adult anaesthesia in North America, and remained so until the introduction of isoflurane. Its release in the UK was delayed by lengthy toxicity studies until 1978. Perhaps because of the greater popularity of spontaneous respiration techniques among British anaesthetists, enflurane has never been as popular in the UK. Throughout the developed world, the use of enflurane is declining in favour of isoflurane.

ISOFLURANE – 1-CHLORO-2,2,2-TRIFLUOROETHYL DIFLUOROMETHYL ETHER

```
     F   H        F
     |   |        |
  F—C—C—O—C—H        Isoflurane
     |   |        |
     F   Cl       F
```

History

Isoflurane was synthesized by Ross Terrell in 1965, shortly after enflurane. It was appreciated at the time that its manufacture would be more difficult and expensive than enflurane, but its introduction was planned for 1975. It was, however, delayed by research findings that appeared to demonstrate a carcinogenic effect of isoflurane in laboratory mice.[101] This was eventually traced to contamination of the animals' laboratory feed, but the delays involved in repetition of the research[102] put back its introduction until 1981 in the USA and to 1982 in the UK.

Physical chemistry

■ Molecular weight	184.5
■ Boiling point (°C)	48.5
■ Vapour pressure at 20°C (kPa)	33.4
■ Maximum vapour concentration at 20°C	33%

At atmospheric pressure isoflurane is a colourless clear liquid with a pungent ethereal smell.

Chemistry

As with the other modern volatile anaesthetics, isoflurane is non-inflammable under all conditions likely to be encountered clinically. It is not inflammable in air or oxygen at any concentration. In 30% oxygen–70% nitrous oxide, 7.0% isoflurane can be ignited by a 900 W spark,[43] but this is well above the maximum power output of most electrosurgical apparatus.

Isoflurane has an extremely stable molecule, and does not require the addition of a chemical stabilizer. It is not degraded by exposure to ultraviolet light, is stable in soda lime except at high temperatures, and does not react with metals.[103]

Manufacture

Isoflurane may be synthesized via a number of different pathways, but in the commercial process trifluoroethanol is reacted with CF_2HCl and the product chlorinated to produce 98% isoflurane. The contaminant is $CF_3CHClOCF_2Cl$, which is rendered water-soluble by acetone and separated by the addition of water.[104]

Anaesthetic characteristics

■ Blood : gas partition coefficient	1.4 (37°C)
■ Oil : gas partition coefficient	90.8 (37°C)
■ MAC (%)	1.15

The pungency of isoflurane vapour renders it more difficult to use than halothane in inhalational induction of anaesthesia and outweighs its lower blood : gas solubility coefficient in this respect.[105] Once anaesthesia is established, however, control of depth is rapidly accomplished, awakening is more rapid than with halothane[106] and is accompanied by less shivering and nausea than is seen with enflurane.[107,108]

Circulation

Like enflurane and halothane, isoflurane produces a fall in arterial pressure, but this is largely as a result of a reduction of systemic vascular resistance.

Myocardial depression, so much a feature of halothane anaesthesia, is much less marked with isoflurane.[109–112] Although stroke volume may fall, this is offset by an increase in heart rate as a result of better preservation of baroreflexes[113–115] and cardiac output is thus better preserved than with the other agents.[116–118] This is also the case in the presence of haemorrhage.[74]

One of the most controversial aspects of isoflurane pharmacology concerns its action as a coronary vasodilator, an effect which is maximal at 2 MAC.[119] In the presence of normal coronary anatomy, this serves to maintain coronary flow at increased depths of anaesthesia conferring a greater margin of safety on isoflurane as compared with enflurane and halothane. In patients with ischaemic heart disease, however, there exists the potential for 'coronary steal', as maximally dilated normal coronary arteries 'steal' flow from stenosed vessels, worsening ischaemia. Although some animal studies have been equivocal,[120–122] there is good experimental evidence that isoflurane does induce a maldistribution of coronary flow in animal models[123] and in patients with coronary heart disease.[124] Patients with a total occlusion of a major coronary branch with a collateral supply to the distal segment are at risk, particularly if the collaterals arise from an artery that is itself stenosed. This anatomy exists in about a quarter of patients with coronary heart disease.[125] In such patients, care must be taken to maintain coronary perfusion pressure and avoid tachycardia. Isoflurane is probably best avoided in patients with multiple vessel disease,[126] and one study showed a higher incidence of myocardial infarction in patients undergoing coronary artery surgery under isoflurane than in a matched group receiving enflurane.[127]

Isoflurane does not increase the incidence of arrhythmias, and minimally sensitizes the myocardium to catecholamines, which may be used safely in three times the dose permissible with halothane. Dental patients suffer fewer ventricular arrhythmias under isoflurane than under halothane,[128] and it may be a safer agent in the presence of intraventricular conduction defects.[129]

Respiration

Early studies of isoflurane concluded that it was a profound respiratory depressant,[130] but later work has shown it to be at worst little different from halothane[131] and an improvement on enflurane.[132,133] Specifically, in terms of alteration of the response to hypoxia or hypercarbia, isoflurane is actually less of a depressant than either of the other agents.[57] Isoflurane may increase the respiratory rate, though less than halothane.[131,133]

Isoflurane is an effective bronchodilator and has been used in status asthmaticus.[134,135] Although it is slightly less effective than halothane in this application, its reduced tendency to cause arrhythmias offers increased safety in patients receiving sympathomimetics or in the presence of hypercarbia.

Isoflurane has been shown not to interfere with pulmonary hypoxic vasoconstriction in humans at inspired concentrations of around 1 MAC,[136,137] although an effect has been shown in animal studies.[138]

Central nervous system

Possibly the most important area in which isoflurane is superior to other inhalation agents is in its effect on CBF and metabolism. In contrast to halothane, isoflurane at concentrations up to 1 MAC has very little effect on CBF at normal arterial carbon dioxide tensions,[139] and is a better preserver of cerebral autoregulation.[140] Patients for intracranial surgery are usually hyperventilated in order to reduce CBF, cerebral blood volume and intracranial pressure, and it is important that the CO_2 responsiveness of the cerebral circulation is preserved by the anaesthetic agent. Isoflurane is better in this respect than nitrous oxide,[140] vascular responsiveness being preserved at concentrations of up to 2 MAC.[141] Isoflurane does not increase the rate of cerebrospinal fluid (CSF) production, unlike enflurane.[142]

Isoflurane does not induce seizures or EEG changes of the type seen with enflurane,[143] and indeed has been used in status epilepticus.[144] As the alveolar concentration of isoflurane is increased, cerebral metabolic rate is markedly reduced to a point, at about 2 MAC, where electrical silence occurs – a state that cannot safely be attained with enflurane or halothane. It follows that, alone among the volatile agents but similar to the barbiturates, isoflurane provides useful protection of the brain during hypoxic or ischaemic insults.[145,146] The use of isoflurane for the deliberate induction of hypotension, as well as reducing cerebral metabolic oxygen demand, favourably affects the cerebral oxygen supply–demand balance,[147] maintains tissue PO_2 values[148] and preserves normal energy stores.[30]

Other systems

Even more than halothane, isoflurane augments the effect of skeletal muscle relaxants, particularly tubocurarine and pancuronium, but also alcuronium[149] and the newer agents, atracurium, vecuronium[150] and mivacurium.[151] Myasthenic patients may demonstrate significant reduction in train-of-four ratio with isoflurane alone.[152]

Isoflurane relaxes the pregnant uterus but may cause less bleeding and uterine relaxation at Caesarean section than an equivalent concentration of halothane.[153] Hepatic artery blood flow is similarly reduced by isoflurane or halothane, but the better preservation of portal flow by isoflurane results in a higher hepatic oxygen delivery than under halothane.[154]

Metabolic fate

Isoflurane is very resistant to biotransformation, less than 0.2% of absorbed isoflurane being recoverable from urine as free fluoride or organic fluorine.[155] Enzyme induction may increase this figure slightly, but isoflurane is the most inert of the current volatile agents.

Toxicity

The unfounded fears referred to above concerning possible carcinogenicity of isoflurane resulted in the agent being subjected to the most stringent examination for possible toxicity. It appears to be entirely without nephrotoxic or hepatotoxic effects and may be used in safety in patients with hepatic or renal disease. Successive studies have shown it to be without mutagenic or teratogenic effects. Isoflurane has in fact been shown to reduce the teratogenic effects of nitrous oxide in rats.[156]

Malignant hyperpyrexia has been reported following isoflurane anaesthesia.[157]

Status

Isoflurane has established itself as the pre-eminent volatile agent in adult anaesthesia in North America, and its use is increasing throughout the developed world despite its cost, adjusted for MAC, being up to twenty-five times that of halothane.

SEVOFLURANE – FLUROMETHYL 2,2,2-TRIFLUORO-1-(TRIFLUOROMETHYL)ETHYL ETHER

```
        F
        |
    H — C — H
        |
    F   O   F
    |   |   |
F — C — C — C — F
    |   |   |
    F   H   F
```

Sevoflurane

History

Sevoflurane was first synthesized in the early 1970s by BM Regan at Travenol Laboratories, Illinois and its clinical use reported in 1975.[158] Sevoflurane was introduced in the United Kingdom and North America in 1995.

Physical chemistry

▪ Molecular weight	200.05
▪ Boiling point (°C)	58.5
▪ Vapour pressure at 20°C (kPa)	21.33
▪ Maximum vapour concentration at 20°C	21%

Sevoflurane is a clear, pleasant smelling volatile liquid.

Chemistry

Although non-inflammable, sevoflurane is not as stable as isoflurane, particularly in soda lime. One study found sevoflurane vapour exposed to soda lime degraded at the rate of 6.5% per hour at 22°C and was even less stable at higher temperatures.[159]

Anaesthetic characteristics

▪ Blood : gas partition coefficient	0.68 (37°C)
▪ Oil : gas partition coefficient	47.2 (37°C)
▪ MAC (%)	1.71[160] to 2.05[161]

The low blood-gas solubility coefficient coupled with a pleasant smell confers fast induction characteristics on sevoflurane, confirmed in a comparative study against enflurane.[162] Emergence times, however, were found to be similar for the two agents, and although sevoflurane is rapidly cleared from the blood and, initially, from the brain, the slower β-elimination characteristics from brain and adipose tissue are similar to halothane.[163]

Circulation

Studies in swine imply that sevoflurane may be less of a cardiovascular depressant than either halothane or isoflurane, 1.5 MAC sevoflurane lowering systolic pressure by 36% compared with 43% and 46% for isoflurane and halothane respectively. Cardiac index was decreased 53% by halothane and 43% by isoflurane, yet was unchanged from the awake value by sevoflurane.[164] In dogs, sevoflurane produced very similar effects on cardiac function and coronary flow to isoflurane.[165]

In volunteer studies, sevoflurane caused a decrease in systolic pressure but little effect on heart rate.[166]

Respiration

A comparison of the respiratory effects of sevoflurane and halothane showed them to have similar characteristics at 1.1 MAC, but at 1.4 MAC sevoflurane was a more profound depressant.[167]

Central nervous system

In the rabbit, the effects of sevoflurane on CBF, cerebral metabolic rate, intracranial pressure and the EEG are indistinguishable from those of isoflurane.[168]

Other systems

Sevoflurane potentiates non-depolarizing muscle relaxants, although it may be less potent in this respect than halothane, enflurane or isoflurane.[169]

Toxicity

Any toxicity study of sevoflurane must take into account possible breakdown products. A study of hepatotoxicity in a hypoxic enzyme-induced rat model[170] showed sevoflurane passed through soda lime to be no more hepatotoxic than isoflurane, but in general the toxicity of a volatile anaesthetic is often related to its molecular stability.

Status

Its instability in soda lime remains an obstacle to the more widespread introduction of sevoflurane, as the independent actions of the breakdown products have yet to be elucidated, and toxicity studies are complicated. In any event, the agent cannot be considered suitable for low-flow or closed-circuit anaesthesia.

DESFLURANE – DIFLUOROMETHYL 1-FLUORO-2,2,2-TRIFLUOROETHYL ETHER

```
    F   F       F
    |   |       |
F — C — C — O — C — F
    |   |       |
    F   H       H
```

Desflurane

Formerly known as I-653, desflurane, too, was originally synthesized by Terrell but was not at the time selected for further evaluation as it was difficult to produce and could not be administered from standard vaporizers because of its low boiling point. However, in the quest for lower solubility compounds it was re-evaluated, and eventually released commercially in the United States and UK in 1993.

Physical chemistry

- Molecular weight 168.04
- Boiling point (°C) 23.5
- Vapour pressure at 20°C (kPa) 88.53
- Maximum vapour concentration at 20°C 88%

Desflurane is close to its boiling point at room temperature, and cannot be administered from conventional vaporizers. A temperature-compensated vaporizer, the Tec 6, was specially developed. The device is electrically heated and pressurized, with accurate concentrations being maintained by a differential pressure transducer which matches the delivered pressure from the vaporizing chamber to that in the bypass.[171] Desflurane vapour is mildly irritant.

Chemistry

Desflurane is non-inflammable and has a very stable molecule, not significantly degraded by soda lime at 80°C,[172] a temperature at which even isoflurane is unstable. Recent reports, however, have suggested that it and other volatile agents can be degraded in very dry soda lime or Baralyme (a barium-based carbon dioxide absorbent) resulting in the production of toxic levels of carbon monoxide.[173] Ordinarily this situation would only occur if high flows of dry gas were vented to the atmosphere through a soda lime canister for many hours, and significantly most of the case reports relate to cases anaesthetized on equipment that had lain unused with gases flowing over a weekend.

Anaesthetic characteristics

- Blood : gas partition coefficient 0.4 (37°C)
- Oil : gas partition coefficient 19.0 (37°C)
- MAC (%) 6.0

Although desflurane has an even lower blood : gas solubility coefficient than nitrous oxide, conferring speed of induction, the brain : blood partition coefficient is intermediate between the value for nitrous oxide and that for isoflurane. The predicted recovery characteristics would therefore be rather slower than nitrous oxide, and this has proved to be the case.

Although desflurane alone was successfully used for induction of anaesthesia in early studies,[174] in a clinical setting inhalational induction is accompanied by a high incidence of coughing, breath-holding and apnoea.[175] Recovery is significantly faster than from other volatile agents after short or intermediate exposure,[176, 177] although the difference is less marked after prolonged anaesthesia. Desflurane may cause less vomiting than isoflurane.[178]

Circulation

Desflurane and isoflurane have very similar effects on the cardiovascular system. In normocarbic volunteers, desflurane decreases systemic vascular resistance and arterial pressure, raising right heart filling pressure[179]. Stroke volume index falls, but cardiac output is well maintained, in fact rather better than with isoflurane. Although desflurane is a coronary vasodilator, it has not been shown to increase morbidity in patients with coronary disease, and canine models have provided no evidence of coronary steal.[180] Unusually among modern inhalational anaesthetics, desflurane produces a marked sympathetic response if inhaled concentrations are increased rapidly,[181,182] presumably due to the irritant effect of the vapour. The incidence of arrhythmias and the sensitisation of the myocardium to exogenous catecholamines under desflurane is very similar to that seen with isoflurane.[183]

Respiration

Desflurane produces a dose-dependent increase in respiratory rate and reduction in tidal volume resulting in moderate hypercarbia in the spontaneously breathing volunteer. At 1 MAC the arterial carbon dioxide tension is increased by about 20%.[166] At deeper levels of anaesthesia, the respiratory depression seen with desflurane seems to be intermediate between that of isoflurane and enflurane.

Central nervous system

Studies in the dog showed desflurane to be a cerebral vasodilator, even at concentrations as low as 0.5 MAC.[184] However, measurement of CSF pressure in dogs showed little difference between the effects of isoflurane and desflurane during hypocarbia.[185] In humans undergoing surgery for intracranial mass lesions, the effects of desflurane and isoflurane on cerebral blood flow were very similar.[186]

Toxicity

No disturbances of hepatic or renal function have been seen in animal or volunteer studies.[187] Biotransformation appears to be less than with isoflurane.[188]

Status

Desflurane has become a popular agent in the field of day-case anaesthesia where it offers significantly better recovery characteristics. In the in-patient setting, however, it has yet to displace isoflurane.

OTHER INHALATIONAL ANAESTHETICS

Cyclopropane – C_3H_6

Cyclopropane is a colourless gas with a sweet odour, whose anaesthetic properties were first described in 1929 by Henderson and Lucus of Toronto. It was introduced in the UK in 1933. Like nitrous oxide, it is, at room temperature, below its critical temperature and was supplied under pressure as a liquid in orange cylinders. At room temperature the pressure inside the cylinder is about 500 kPa and thus sufficiently close to the working pressure of a modern anaesthetic machine for a reducing valve to be unnecessary. A MAC of 9.2% and a blood : gas partition coefficient of 0.46 made it a useful agent for inhalational induction of anaesthesia, particularly in children. Its principal hazard is that, mixed with oxygen, it is explosive in any concentration between 2.5 and 50%. It is also a powerful respiratory depressant, and the resulting hypercarbia, coupled with a tendency to increase circulating levels of catecholamines, makes arrhythmias a very common occurrence during its administration. It was withdrawn from production in 1990.

Trichloroethylene – CCl_2CHCl

Trichloroethylene is a colourless volatile liquid, long used as an industrial solvent and degreasing agent, but first used in anaesthesia by Lehmann in 1911 and popularized in the UK by Langton Hewer following its introduction in 1941. Non-inflammable in clinical concentrations, 10% trichloroethylene will ignite in oxygen, although this is far above the clinically used range of concentrations (MAC is 0.17%). The molecule is unstable in soda lime, producing highly toxic breakdown products including phosgene. It produces such a marked tachypnoea that its use was largely limited to ventilated patients. Dysrhythmias are common during trichloroethylene administration, and recovery, which is prolonged as a result of a high blood : gas solubility coefficient, is accompanied by a high incidence of nausea and vomiting. It has analgesic properties inhaled intermittently in concentrations of 0.35–0.5% and was used as an obstetric analgesic in drawover-type inhalers before the widespread introduction of nitrous oxide–oxygen mixtures. It was withdrawn in the UK in 1989.

Methoxyflurane – 2,2,-dichloro-1,1-difluoroethyl methyl ether

Methoxyflurane is a liquid agent first used by Artusio and Van Poznak in 1960. It can barely be described as volatile as its boiling point is 104°C and the maximum vapour concentration obtainable at room temperature is only 3%. However, the MAC is very low at 0.16%. A high blood : gas solubility coefficient (12.0) slows induction and recovery, but it is non-inflammable, has good analgesic properties, does not commonly cause dysrhythmias and does not depress respiration unduly, being comparable to halothane in this respect. Unfortunately, up to 70% of absorbed methoxyflurane undergoes biotransformation releasing dichloroacetic acid, oxalic acid, difluoroacetic acid and free fluoride ions. This greatly limits its use as administration in excess of 2 MAC-hours may produce nephrotoxic plasma fluoride levels. It is no longer available in the UK.

Diethyl ether – $C_2H_5OC_2H_5$

Diethyl ether was the agent used by Morton in the first public demonstration of anaesthesia at Boston in 1846, although it is known to have been used by Crawford Long, unreported, as early as 1842. It was a fortunate choice as the first general anaesthetic, its properties making it particularly safe in unskilled hands. It is a respiratory stimulant in normal use, and the increase in sympathetic outflow seen with the agent tends to maintain arterial pressure until deep levels of anaesthesia. However, it has an irritant vapour and a high blood : gas solubility coefficient (12.0), making inhalational induction slow and prone to interruption by coughing and laryngospasm. Profuse salivation makes antisialogogue premedication necessary. Nausea and vomiting are very common following its administration, and awakening is prolonged. It is highly inflammable and is explosive in oxygen in concentrations as low as 2% (MAC is 1.92%). Being soluble in water, it has been given as an intravenous infusion, with the patient breathing oxygen from a closed circuit, a technique which overcomes a number of the problems associated with its administration.

Anaesthetic diethyl ether for human use has not been available in the UK since 1988, although it remains popular in many parts of the world.

THE FUTURE OF INHALATIONAL ANAESTHESIA

Despite the development of intravenous anaesthetics with suitable pharmacokinetics for the maintenance of anaesthesia, inhalational agents seem likely to remain the basis of most general anaesthetics for the foreseeable future. The current generation of inhaled agents are of low toxicity and have acceptable cardiovascular and respiratory characteristics. Although apparatus for their administration is more complex, during maintenance of anaesthesia the volatile agents are easier to use and cheaper than intravenous drugs. Disconnections of breathing systems are reliably detected by pressure failure alarms and capnography, but extravasation or disconnection of an intravenous infusion may pass unnoticed for long enough for awareness to result.

REFERENCES

1. Blackburn JP. Explosions. In: Scurr, C, Feldman, S, eds. *Scientific foundations of anaesthesia.* London: Heinemann, 1976: 516–18.
2. Waterson CK. Recovery of waste anaesthetic gases. In: Brown B ed. *Future anesthesia delivery systems.* Philadelphia: F. A. Davis, 1984: 109–24.
3. Howell RS. C. Medical Gases (1) – manufacture and uses. In: Kaufman L ed. *Anaesthesia review* 7. London: Churchill Livingstone, 1990: 87–103.
4. Marshall BE, Longnecker DE. General anesthetics. In: Goodman LS, Gilman A, Rall TW, Nies AS, Taylor P, eds. *Goodman and Gilman's The pharmacological basis of therapeutics.* New York: Pergamon, 1990: 285–310.
5. Russell GB, Snider MT, Richard RB, Loomis JL. Hyperbaric nitrous oxide as the sole anesthetic agent in humans. *Anesthesia and Analgesia* 1990; **70**: 289–95.
6. Winter PM, Hornbein TF, Smith G. Hyperbaric nitrous oxide anesthesia in man: determination of anesthetic potency (MAC) and cardiorespiratory effects. *Abstracts American Society of Anesthesiologists Meeting* 1972: 103–4.
7. Murray DJ, Mehta MP, Forbes RB, Dull DL. Additive contribution of nitrous oxide to halothane MAC in infants and children. *Anesthesia and Analgesia* 1990, **71**: 120–4.
8. Quock RM, Kouchich FJ, Tseng LF. Does nitrous oxide induce release of brain opioid peptides? *Pharmacology* 1985; **30**: 95–9.
9. Rupreht, J, Dworacek, B, Bonke, B, Dzoljic MR, van Eijndhoven JH, de Vlieger M. Tolerance to nitrous oxide in volunteers. *Acta Anesthesiologica Scandinavica* 1985; **29**: 635–8.
10. Lawson D, Frazer MJ, Lynch C. 3rd. Nitrous oxide effects on isolated myocardium: a reexamination *in vitro*. *Anesthesiology* 1990; **73**: 930–43.
11. Pagel PS, Kampine JP, Schmeling WT, Warltier DC. Effects of nitrous oxide on myocardial contractility as evaluated by the preload recruitable stroke work relationship in chronically instrumented dogs. *Anaesthesiology* 1990; **73**: 1148–57.
12. Meretoja OA, Takkunen O, Heikkil H, Wegelius U. Haemodynamic response to nitrous oxide during high-dose fentanyl pancuronium anaesthesia. *Acta Anaesthesiologica Scandinavica* 1985; **29**: 137–41.
13. Philbin DM, Foex P, Drummond G, Lowenstein E, Ryder WA, Jones LA. Postsystolic shortening of canine left ventricle supplied by a stenotic coronary artery when nitrous oxide is added in the presence of narcotics. *Anesthesiology* 1985; **62**: 166–74.
14. Ramsay JG, Arvieux CC, Foex P, Philbin DM, Jeavons P, Ryder WA, Jones LA. Regional and global myocardial

function in the dog when nitrous oxide is added to halothane in the presence of critical coronary artery constriction. *Anesthesia and Analgesia* 1986; **65**: 431–6.

15 Leone BJ, Philbin DM, Lehot JJ, Foex P, Ryder WA. Gradual or abrupt nitrous oxide administration in a canine model of critical coronary stenosis induces regional myocardial dysfunction that is worsened by halothane. *Anesthesia and Analgesia* 1988; **67**: 814–22.

16 Nathan HJ. Nitrous oxide worsens myocardial ischemia in isoflurane-anesthetized dogs. *Anesthesiology* 1988; **68**: 407–15.

17 Mitchell MM, Prakash O, Rulf EN, van Daele ME, Cahalan MK, Roelandt JR. Nitrous oxide does not induce myocardial ischemia in patients with ischemic heart disease and poor ventricular function. *Anesthesiology* 1989; **71**: 526–34.

18 Konstadt SN, Reich DL, Thys DM. Nitrous oxide does not exacerbate pulmonary hypertension or ventricular dysfunction in patients with mitral valvular disease. *Canadian Journal of Anaesthesia* 1990; **37**: 613–17.

19 Lampe GH, Donegan JH, Rupp SM, Wauk LZ, Witendale P, Fouts KE, Rose BM, Litt L, Rampil IJ, Wilson CB. Nitrous oxide and epinephrine-induced arrhythmias. *Anesthesia and Analgesia* 1990; **71**: 602–5.

20 Ebert TJ. Differential effects of nitrous oxide on baroreflex control of heart rate and peripheral sympathetic nerve activity in humans. *Anesthesiology* 1990; **72**: 16–22.

21 Ebert TJ, Kampine JP. Nitrous oxide augments sympathetic outflow: direct evidence from human peroneal nerve recordings. *Anesthesia and Analgesia* 1989; **69**: 444–9.

22 Hornbein TF, Martin WE, Bronica JJ, Freund FG, Parmentier P. Nitrous oxide effects on the circulatory and ventilatory responses to halothane. *Anesthesiology* 1969; **31**: 250–60.

23 Seyde WC, Ellis JE, Longnecker DE. The addition of nitrous oxide to halothane decreases renal and splanchnic flow and increases cerebral blood flow in rats. *British Journal of Anaesthesia* 1986; **58**: 63–8.

24 Hall LW. Effects of nitrous oxide during halothane anaesthesia in the dog. *British Journal of Anaesthesia* 1988; **60**: 207–15.

25 Wren WS, Meeke R, Davenport J, O'Griofa, P. Effects of nitrous oxide on the respiratory pattern of spontaneously breathing children during anaesthesia. *British Journal of Anaesthesia* 1984; **56**: 881–98.

26 Murat I, Le Bret F, Chaussain M, Saint-Maurice C. Respiratory effects of nitrous oxide during halothane or enflurane anesthesia in children. *Acta Anaesthesiologica Scandinavica* 1988; **32**: 186–92.

27 Barker J. Nitrous oxide in neurosurgical anaesthesia (editorial). *British Journal of Anaesthesia* 1987; **59**: 146–7.

28 Todd MM. The effects of P_aCO_2 on the cerebrovascular response to nitrous oxide in the halothane-anesthetised rabbit. *Anesthesia and Analgesia* 1987; **66**: 1090–5.

29 Reasoner DK, Warner DS, Todd MM, McAllister A. Effects of nitrous oxide on cerebral metabolic rate in rats anaesthestized with isoflurane. *British Journal of Anaesthesia* 1990; **65**: 210–15.

30 Frost EA. M. Inhalation anaesthetic agents in neurosurgery. *British Journal of Anaesthesia* 1984; **56**: 47S–56S.

31 Amos RJ, Amess JA, Hinds CJ, Mollin DL. Investigations into the effect of nitrous oxide anaesthesia on folate metabolism in patients receiving intensive care. *Chemotherapy* 1985; **4**: 393–9.

32 Amos RJ, Amess JA, Nancekievill DG, Rees GM. Prevention of nitrous oxide-induced megaloblastic changes in bone marrow using folinic acid. *British Journal of Anaesthesia* 1984; **56**: 103–7.

33 Nunn JF, Chanarin I, Tanner AG, Owen ER. Megaloblastic bone marrow changes after repeated nitrous oxide anaesthesia. Reversal with folinic acid. *British Journal of Anaesthesia* 1986; **58**: 1469–70.

34 Gillman MA. Folinic acid prevents megaloblastic changes associated with nitrous oxide (letter). *Anesthesia and Analgesia* 1988; **67**: 1018–19.

35 Lunsford JM, Wynn MH, Kwan WH. Nitrous oxide-induced myeloneuropathy. *Journal of Foot Surgery* 1983; **22**: 222–5.

36 Fujinaga M, Baden JM, Mazze RI. Susceptible period of nitrous oxide teratogenicity in Sprague–Dawley rats. *Teratology* 1989; **40**: 439–44.

37 Mazze RI, Fujinaga M, Baden JM. Halothane prevents nitrous oxide teratogenicity in Sprague–Dawley rats; folinic acid does not. *Teratology* 1988; **38**: 121–7.

38 Crawford JS, Lewis, M. Nitrous oxide in early human pregnancy. *Anaesthesia* 1986; **41**: 900–5.

39 Aldridge LM, Tunstall ME. Nitrous oxide and the fetus. A review and the results of a retrospective study of 175 cases of anaesthesia for insertion of Shirodkar suture. *British Journal of Anaesthesia* 1986; **58**: 1348–56.

40 Vessey MP. Epidemiological studies of the occupational hazards of anaesthesia – a review. *Anaesthesia* 1978; **33**: 430–8.

41 Rosen MA, Roizen MF, Eger EI, Glass RH, Martin M, Dandekar PV, Dailey PA, Litt L. The effect of nitrous oxide on *in vitro* fertilization success rate. *Anesthesiology* 1987; **67**: 42–4.

42 Waite PD, Ballard JB, Yonfa A. Malignant hyperthermia in a patient receiving nitrous oxide. *Journal of Oral and Maxillofacial Surgery* 1985; **43**: 907–9.

43 Leonard PF. The lower limits of flammability of halothane enflurane and isoflurane. *Anesthesia and Analgesia* 1975; **54**: 238–40.

44 Sharp JH, Trudell JR, Cohen EN. Volatile anesthetics and decomposition products in man. *Anesthesiology* 1979; **50**: 2.

45 Eger EI. Editorial. *Anesthesiology* 1979; **50**: 1.

46 Bahlman SH, Eger EI, Halsey MJ, Stevens WC, Shakespeare TF, Smith NT, Cromwell TH, Fourcade, H. The cardiovascular effects of halothane in man during spontaneous ventilation. *Anesthesiology* 1972; **36**: 494–502.

47 Eger EI, Smith NT, Stoelting RK, Cullen DJ, Kadis LB, Whitcher CE. Cardiovascular effects of halothane in man. *Anesthesiology* 1970 ; **32**: 396–409.

48 Sonntag H, Donath U, Hillebrand W, Merin RG, Radke, J. Left ventricular function in conscious man and during halothane anesthesia. *Anesthesiology* 1978; **48**: 320–4.

49 Komai H, Rusy BF. Direct effect of halothane and isoflurane on the function of the sarcoplasmic reticulum in intact rabbit atria. *Anesthesiology* 1990; **72**: 694–8.

50 Housmans PR, Murat I. Comparative effects of halothane, enflurane and isoflurane at equipotent anesthetic concentrations on isolated ventricular myocardium of the ferret. I. Contractility. *Anesthesiology* 1988; **69**: 451–63.

51 Ebert TJ, Kotrly KJ, Vucins EJ, Pattison CZ, Kampine JP. Halothane anesthesia attentuates cardiopulmonary

baroreflex control of peripheral resistance in humans. *Anesthesiology* 1985; **63**: 668–74.

52 Duke PC, Fownes D, Wade JG. Halothane depresses baroreflex control of heart rate in man. *Anesthesiology* 1977; **46**: 184–7.

53 Murat I, Delleur MM, MacGee K, Saint-Maurice, C. Changes in ventilatory patterns during halothane anaesthesia in children. *British Journal of Anaesthesia* 1985; **57**: 569–72.

54 Lindahl SS, Yates AP, Hatch DJ. Respiratory depression in children at different end-tidal halothane concentrations. *Anaesthesia* 1987; **42**: 1267–75.

55 Murat I, Chaussain M, Saint-Maurice C. Ventilatory responses to carbon dioxide in children during nitrous oxide halothane anaesthesia. *British Journal of Anaesthesia* 1985; **57**: 1197–203.

56 Knill RL, Gelb AW. Ventilatory responses to hypoxia and hypercapnia during halothane sedation and anaesthesia in man. *Anesthesiology* 1978; **49**: 244–51.

57 Hirshman RE, McCullough RE, Cohen PJ, Weil JV. Depression of hypoxic ventilatory response by halothane, enflurane and isoflurane in dogs. *British Journal of Anaesthesia* 1977; **49**: 957–63.

58 Knill RL, Clement JL. Site of selective action of halothane on the peripheral chemoreflex pathway in humans. *Anesthesiology* 1984; **61**: 121–6.

59 Johnson D, Hurst T, Mayers, T. Halothane affects regional hypoxic pulmonary vasoconstriction. *Canadian Journal of Anaesthesia* 1990; **37**: S167.

60 Johnson D, Mayers I, To T. The effects of halothane in hypoxic pulmonary vasoconstriction. *Anesthesiology* 1990; **72**: 125–33.

61 Bayliff CD, Koch JP, Faclier G. The use of halothane in the treatment of status asthmaticus. *Drug Intelligence and Clinical Pharmacy* 1985; **19**: 307–9.

62 Saulnier FF, Durocher AV, Deturck RA, Lefebvre MC, Wattel FE. Respiratory and haemodynamic effects of halothane in status asthmaticus. *Intensive Care Medicine* 1990; **16**: 104–7.

63 Jones RM. Inhalational and intravenous agents. In: Nimmo WS, Smith, G. eds. *Anaesthesia*. London: Blackwell, 1989: 34–59.

64 MacDowell DG. Effects of drugs on cerebral blood flow and cerebral metabolism. *British Journal of Anaesthesia* 1965; **37**: 236.

65 Eisenkraft JB, Papatestas AE, Sivak M. Neuromuscular effects of halogenated agents in patients with myasthenia gravis. *Anesthesiology* 1984; **61**: A307.

66 Moir DD. Anaesthesia for caesarean section: an evaluation of a method using low concentrations of halothane and 50 per cent oxygen. *British Journal of Anaesthesia* 1970; **42**: 136–42.

67 Carpenter RL, Eger EI, Johnson BH, Unadkat JD, Sheiner LB. The extent of metabolism of inhaled anaesthetics in humans. *Anesthesiology* 1986; **65**: 201–5.

68 Stock GL, Strunin L. Unexplained hepatitis following halothane. *Anesthesiology* 1985; **63**: 424–39.

69 Ray DC, Drummond GB. Halothane hepatitis. *British Journal of Anaesthesia* 1991; **67**: 84–99.

70 Vitcha JF. A history of Forane. *Anesthesiology* 1971; **35**: 4–7.

71 McGuinness, C Rosen, M. Enflurane as an analgesic in labour. *Anaesthesia* 1984; **39**: 24–6.

72 Van Trigt P, Christian CC, Fagraeus L, Spray TL, Peyton RB, Pellom GL, Wechsler AS. Myocardial depression by anesthetic agents (halothane, enflurane and nitrous oxide): quantitation based on end-systolic pressure–dimension relations. *American Journal of Cardiology* 1984; **53**: 243–7.

73 Marshall BE, Cohen PJ, Klingenmaier CH, Neigh JL, Pender JW. Some pulmonary and cardiovascular effects of enflurane (Ethrane) anaesthesia with varying P_aCO_2 in man. *British Journal of Anaesthesia* 1971; **43**: 996–1002.

74 Seyde WC, Longnecker DE. Anesthetic influences on regional hemodynamics in normal and hemorrhaged rats. *Anesthesiology* 1984; **61**: 686–98.

75 Calverley RK, Smith NT, Prys-Roberts C, Eger EI, Jones CW. Cardiovascular effects of enflurane anesthesia during controlled ventilation in man. *Anesthesia and Analgesia* 1978; **57**: 619–28.

76 Sigurdsson GH, Lindahl, S. Cardiac arrhythmias in intubated children during adenoidectomy. A comparison between halothane and enflurane anaesthesia. *Acta Anaesthesiologica Scandinavica* 1983; **27**: 484–9.

77 Munson ES, Tucker WK. Doses of epinephrine causing arrhythmia during enflurane, methoxyflurane and halothane anaesthesia in dogs. *Canadian Anaesthetists Society Journal* 1975; **22**: 495–501.

78 Reiz S, Rydvall A, Haggmark S. Coronary haemodynamic effects of surgery during enflurane–nitrous oxide anaesthesia in patients with ischaemic heart disease. *Acta Anaesthesiologica Scandinavica* 1985; **29**: 106–12.

79 van Ackern K, Vetter HO, Bruckner UB, Madler C, Mittman U, Peter K. Effects of enflurane on myocardial ischaemia in the dog. *British Journal of Anaesthesia* 1985; **57**: 497–504.

80 Moffitt EA, Imrie DD, Scovil JE, Glenn JJ, Cousins CL, Del Campo C, Sullivan JA, Kinley CE. Myocardial metabolism and haemodynamic responses with enflurane anaesthesia for coronary artery surgery. *Canadian Anaesthetists Society Journal* 1984; **31**: 604–10.

81 Kobayashi Y, Yoshida K, Noguchi M, Wakasugi Y, Ito H, Okabe E. Effect of enflurane on contractile reactivity in isolated canine mesenteric arteries and veins. *Anesthesia and Analgesia* 1990; **70**: 530–6.

82 Henriksson BA, Biber B, Lundberg D, Martner J, Ponten J, Sonander H. Intestinal vascular effects of inhaled and locally administered enflurane in the cat. *Acta Anaesthesiologica Scandinavica* 1985; **29**: 294–9.

83 Henriksson BA, Biber B, Lundberg D, Martner J, Nilsson H, Ponten J. Vasodilator response to enflurane in the small intestine. *Acta Anaesthesiologica Scandinavica* 1985; **29**: 287–93.

84 Murat I, Le Bret F, Chaussain M, Saint-Maurice C. Respiratory effects of nitrous oxide during halothane or enflurane anaesthesia in children. *Acta Anaesthesiologica Scandinavica* 1988; **32**: 186–92.

85 Echeverria M, Gelb AW, Wexler HR, Ahmad D, Kenefick P. Enflurane and halothane in status asthmaticus. *Chest* 1986; **89**: 152–4.

86 Carlsson AJ, Hedenstierna G, Bindsley L. Hypoxia-induced vasoconstriction in human lung exposed to enflurane anaesthesia. *Acta Anaesthesiologica Scandinavica* 1987; **31**: 57–62.

87 Virtue RW, Lund LO, Phelps M, Vogel J, Beckwith H, Heron M. Difluoromethyl 1,1,2-trifluoro 2-chloroethyl ether as an anaesthetic agent: results with dogs and a preliminary note on observations with man. *Canadian Anaesthetists Society Journal* 1966; **13**: 233.

88 Nicholl JM. Status epilepticus following enflurane anaesthesia. *Anaesthesia* 1986; **41**: 927–30.

89 Jenkins J, Milne AC. Convulsive reaction following enflurane anaesthesia. *Anaesthesia* 1984; **39**: 44–5.
90 Eintrei C, Leszniewski W, Carlsson C. Local application of ^{133}Xe for measurement of regional cerebral blood flow during halothane, enflurane and isoflurane anesthesia in humans. *Anesthesiology* 1985; **63**: 391–4.
91 Moss E, Dearden NM, MacDowell DG. Effects of 2% enflurane on intracranial pressure and cerebral perfusion pressure. *British Journal of Anaesthesia* 1983; **55**: 1083–8.
92 Schuh FT. Differential increase in potency of neuromuscular blocking agents by enflurane and halothane. *International Journal of Pharmacology Therapeutics and Toxicology* 1983; **21**: 383–6.
93 Rupp SM, McChristian JW, Miller RD. Neuromuscular effects of atracurium during halothane–nitrous oxide and enflurane–nitrous oxide anesthesia in humans. *Anesthesiology* 1985; **63**: 16–19.
94 Forrest JB. Comparative pharmacology of inhalational anaesthetics. In: Nunn JF, Utting JE, Brown BR eds. *General anaesthesia*. London: Butterworths, 1989: 60–72.
95 Paull JD, Fortune DW. Hepatotoxicity and death following two enflurane anaesthetics. *Anaesthesia* 1987; **42**: 1191–6.
96 Sigurdsson J, Hreidarsson AB, Thjodleifsson B. Enflurane hepatitis. A report of a case with a previous history of halothane hepatitis. *Acta Anaesthesiologica Scandinavica* 1985; **29**: 495–6.
97 Eger EI, Smuckler EA, Ferrell LD, Goldsmith CH, Johnson BH. Is enflurane hepatotoxic? *Anesthesia and Analgesia* 1986; **65**: 21–30.
98 Lind RC, Gandolfi AJ, Sipes IG, Brown BR. Comparison of the requirements for hepatic injury with halothane and enflurane in rats. *Anesthesia and Analgesia* 1985; **64**: 955–63.
99 Mazze RI. Metabolism of the inhaled anaesthetics: implications of enzyme induction. *British Journal of Anaesthesia* 1984; **56**: 27S–41S.
100 Eichhorn JH, Hedley-Whyte J, Steinman TI, Kaufmann JM, Laasberg LH. Renal failure following enflurane anaesthesia. *Anaesthesiology* 1976; **45**: 557–60.
101 Corbett TH. Cancer and congenital anomalies associated with anesthetics. *Annals of the New York Academy of Science* 1976; **271**: 58–66.
102 Eger EI, White AE, Brown CL, Biava CG, Corbett TH, Stevens WC. A test of the carcinogenicity of enflurane, isoflurane, halothane, methoxyflurane and nitrous oxide in mice. *Anesthesia and Analgesia* 1978; **57**: 678–94.
103 Eger EI. The pharmacology of isoflurane. *British Journal of Anaesthesia* 1984; **56**: 71S–99S.
104 Terrell RC. Physical and chemical properties of anaesthetic agents. *British Journal of Anaesthesia* 1984; **56**: 3S–7S.
105 Phillips AJ, Brimacombe JR, Simpson DL. Anaesthetic induction with isoflurane or halothane. Oxygen saturation during induction with isoflurane or halothane in unpremedicated children. *Anaesthesia* 1988; **43**: 927–9.
106 Wren WS, McShane AJ, McCarthy JG, Lamont BJ, Casey WF, Hannon VM. Isoflurane in paediatric anaesthesia. Induction and recovery from anaesthesia. *Anaesthesia* 1985; **40**: 315–23.
107 Hovorka J, Korttila K, Erkola O. Nausea and vomiting after general anesthesia with isoflurane, enflurane or fentanyl in combination with nitrous oxide and oxygen. *European Journal of Anaesthesiology* 1988; **5**: 177–82.
108 McCulloch PR, Milne B. Neurological phenomena during emergence from enflurane or isoflurane anaesthesia. *Canadian Journal of Anaesthesia* 1990; **37**: 739–42.
109 Lynch C. Differential depression of myocardial contractility by halothane and isoflurane *in vitro*. *Anesthesiology* 1986; **64**: 620–31.
110 Luk HN, Lin CI, Chang CL, Lee AR. Differential inotropic effects of halothane and isoflurane in dog ventricular tissues. *European Journal of Anaesthesiology* 1987; **136**: 409–13.
111 Lynch C. Effects of halothane and isoflurane on isolated human ventricular myocardium. *Anesthesiology* 1988; **68**: 429–32.
112 Wolf WJ, Neal MB, Mathew BP, Bee DE. Comparison of the *in vitro* myocardial depressant effects of isoflurane and halothane anesthesia. *Anesthesiology* 1988; **69**: 660–6.
113 Seagard JL, Elegbe EO, Hopp FA, Bosnjak ZJ, Von Colditz JH, Kalbfleisch JH. Effects of isoflurane on the baroreceptor reflex. *Anesthesiology* 1983; **59**: 511–20.
114 Takeshima R, Dohi S. Comparison of arterial baroreflex function in humans anesthetized with enflurane or isoflurane. *Anesthesia and Analgesia* 1989; **69**: 284–90.
115 Kotrly KJ, Ebert TJ, Vucins E, Igler FO, Barney JA, Kampine JP. Baroreceptor reflex control of heart rate during isoflurane anesthesia in humans. *Anesthesiology* 1984; **60**: 173–9.
116 Bastard OG, Carter JG, Moyers JR, Bross BA. Circulatory effects of isoflurane in patients with ischemic heart disease: a comparison with halothane. *Anesthesia and Analgesia* 1984; **63**: 635–9.
117 Cromwell TH, Stevens WC, Eger EI, Shakespeare TF, Halsey MJ, Bahlman SH, Fourcade HE. The cardiovascular effects of compound 469 (Forane) during spontaneous ventilation and CO_2 challenge in man. *Anesthesiology* 1971; **35**: 17–25.
118 Stevens WC, Cromwell TH, Halsey MJ, Eger EI, Shakespeare TF, Bahlman SH. The cardivascular effects of a new inhalation anesthetic, Forane, in human volunteers at constant arterial carbon dioxide tension. *Anesthesiology* 1971; **35**: 8–16.
119 Gelman S, Fowler KC, Smith LR. Regional blood flow during isoflurane and halothane anesthesia. *Anesthesia and Analgesia* 1984; **63**: 557–65.
120 Cason BA, Verrier ED, London MJ, Mangano DT, Hickey RF. Effects of isoflurane and halothane on coronary vascular resistance and collateral myocardial blood flow: their capacity to induce coronary steal. *Anesthesiology* 1987; **67**: 665–75.
121 Tatekawa S, Traber KB, Hantler CB, Tait AR, Gallagher KP, Knight PR. Effects of isoflurane on myocardial blood flow, function and oxygen consumption in the presence of critical coronary stenosis in dogs. *Anesthesia and Analgesia* 1987; **66**: 1073–82.
122 Larach DR, Schuler HG, Skeehan TM, Peterson CJ. Direct effects of myocardial depressant drugs on coronary vascular tone: anesthetic vasodilation by halothane and isoflurane. *Journal of Pharmacology and Experimental Therapeutics* 1990; **254**: 58–64.
123 Buffington CW, Romson JL, Levine A, Duttlinger NC, Huang AH. Isoflurane induces coronary steal in a canine model of chronic coronary occlusion. *Anesthesiology* 1987; **66**: 280–92.
124 Khambatta HJ, Sonntag H, Larsen R, Stephan H, Stone JG, Kettler, D. Global and regional myocardial blood flow and metabolism during equipotent halothane and

isoflurane anesthesia in patients with coronary artery disease. *Anesthesia and Analgesia* 1988; **67**: 936–42.

125 Buffington CW, Davis KB, Gillispie S, Pettinger, M. The prevalence of steal-prone coronary anatomy in patients with coronary artery disease: an analysis of the Coronary Artery Surgery Study Registry. *Anesthesiology* 1988; **69**: 721–7.

126 Reiz S, Balfors E, Sorensen MB, Ariola S, Friedman A, Truedson H. Isoflurane – a powerful coronary vasodilator in patients with coronary artery disease. *Anesthesiology* 1983; **59**: 91–7.

127 Inoue K, Reichelt W, el-Banayosy A, Minami K, Dallman G, Hartmann N. Does isoflurane lead to a higher incidence of myocardial infarction and perioperative death than enflurane in coronary artery surgery? A clinical study of 1178 patients. *Anesthesia and Analgesia* 1990; **71**: 469–74.

128 Cripps TP, Edmondson RS. Isoflurane for anesthesia in the dental chair. A comparison of the incidence of cardiac arrhythmias during anaesthesia with halothane and isoflurane. *Anaesthesia* 1987; **42**: 189–91.

129 Ozaki S, Nakaya H, Gotoh Y, Azuma M, Kemmotsu O, Kanno, M. Effects of isoflurane on conduction velocity and maximum rate of rise of action potential upstroke in guinea pig papillary muscles. *Anesthesia and Analgesia* 1990; **70**: 618–23.

130 Fourcade HE, Stevens WC, Larson P, Cromwell TH, Bahlman SH, Hickey RF, Halsey MJ, Eger EI. The ventilatory effects of Forane, a new inhaled anesthetic. *Anesthesiology* 1971; **35**: 26–31.

131 Alagesan K, Nunn JF, Feeley TW, Heneghan CP. Comparison of the respiratory depressant effects of halothane and isoflurane in routine surgery. *British Journal of Anaesthesia* 1987; **59**: 1070–9.

132 Johannesson GP, Lindahl SG. Pulmonary ventilation and gas exchange in children anaesthetized with halothane, enflurane and isoflurane. *Acta Anaesthesiologica Scandinavica* 1987; **31**: 375–80.

133 Wren WS, Allen P, Synnott A, O'Keeffe D, O'Griofa P. Effects of halothane, isoflurane and enflurane on ventilation in children. *British Journal of Anaesthesia* 1987; **59**: 399–409.

134 Bierman MI, Brown M, Muren O, Keenan RL, Glauser FL. Prolonged isoflurane anesthesia in status asthmaticus. *Critical Care Medicine* 1986; **14**: 832–3.

135 Johnstone RG, Noseworthy TW, Friesen EG, Yule HA, Shustack, A. Isoflurane therapy for status asthmaticus in children and adults. *Chest* 1990; **97**: 698–701.

136 Carlsson AJ, Bindsley L, Hedenstierna, G. Hypoxia-induced vasoconstriction in the human lung. The effect of isoflurane anesthesia. *Anesthesiology* 1987; **66**: 312–16.

137 Rogers SN, Benumof JL. Halothane and isoflurane do not decrease P_aO_2 during one-lung ventilation in intravenously anesthetized patients. *Anesthesia and Analgesia* 1985; **64**: 946–54.

138 Domino KB, Borowec L, Alexander CM, Williams JJ, Chen L, Marshall C, Marshall BE. Influence of isoflurane on hypoxic pulmonary vasoconstriction in dogs. *Anesthesiology* 1986; **64**: 423–9.

139 Murphy FL, Kennel EM, Johnstone RE. The effects of enflurane, isoflurane and halothane on cerebral blood flow and metabolism in man. In: Abstracts of Scientific Papers, American Society of Anesthesiologists Meeting 1974: 61.

140 Drummond JC, Todd MM, Shapiro HM. CO_2 responsiveness of the cerebral circulation during isoflurane anesthesia and N_2O sedation in cats. *Anesthesiology* 1982; **57**: A333.

141 McPherson RW, Briar JE, Traystman RJ. Cerebrovascular responsiveness to carbon dioxide in dogs with 1.4% and 2.8% isoflurane. *Anesthesiology* 1989; **70**: 843–50.

142 Artru AA. Isoflurane does not increase the rate of CSF production in the dog. *Anesthesiology* 1984; **60**: 193–7.

143 Ito BM, Sato S, Kufta CV, Tran D. Effect of isoflurane and enflurane on the electrocorticogram of epileptic patients. *Neurology* 1988; **38**: 924–8.

144 Kofke WA, Young RS, Davis P, Woelfel SK, Gray L, Johnson D, Gelb A, Meeke R, Warner DS, Pearson KS. Isoflurane for refractory status epilepticus: a clinical series. *Anesthesiology* 1989; **71**: 653–9.

145 Newberg LA, Michenfelder JD. Cerebral protection by isoflurane during hypoxemia or ischemia. *Anesthesiology* 1983; **59**: 29–35.

146 Michenfelder JD, Sundt TM, Fode N, Sharbrough FW. Isoflurane when compared to enflurane and halothane decreases the frequency of cerebral ischemia during carotid endarterectomy. *Anesthesiology* 1987; **67**: 336–40.

147 Newman B, Gelb AW, Lam AM. The effect of isoflurane-induced hypotension on cerebral blood flow and cerebral metabolic rate for oxygen in humans. *Anesthesiology* 1986; **64**: 307–10.

148 Seyde WC, Longnecker DE. Cerebral oxygen tension in rats during deliberate hypotension with sodium nitroprusside, 2-chloradenosine or deep isoflurane anesthesia. *Anesthesiology* 1986; **64**: 480–5.

149 Keens SJ, Hunter JM, Snowdon SL, Utting JE. Potentiation of the neuromuscular blockade produced by alcuronium with halothane, enflurane and isoflurane. *British Journal of Anesthesia* 1987; **59**: 1011–16.

150 Rupp SM, Miller RD, Gencarelli PJ. Vecuronium-induced neuromuscular blockade during enflurane, isoflurane and halothane anesthesia in human. *Anesthesiology* 1984; **60**: 101–5.

151 Weber S, Brandom BW, Powers DM, Sarner JB, Woelfel SK, Cook DR, Foster VJ, McNulty BF, Weakly JN. Mivacurium chloride (BW B1090U)-induced neuromuscular blockade during nitrous oxide–isoflurane and nitrous oxide–narcotic anesthesia in adult surgical patients. *Anesthesia and Analgesia* 1988; **67**: 495–9.

152 Nilsson E, Muller K. Neuromuscular effects of isoflurane in patients with myasthenia gravis. *Acta Anaesthesiologica Scandinavica* 1990; **34**: 126–31.

153 Ghaly RG, Flynn RJ, Moore J. Isoflurane as an alternative to halothane for caesarean section. *Anaesthesia* 1988; **43**: 5–7.

154 Hursh D, Gelman S, Bradley EL. Hepatic oxygen supply during halothane or isoflurane anaesthesia in guinea pigs. *Anesthesiology* 1987; **67**: 701–6.

155 Holaday DA, Fiserova-Bergerova V, Latto IP, Zumbiei MA. Resistance of isoflurane to biotransformation in man. *Anesthesiology* 1975; **43**: 325–32.

156 Fujinaga M, Baden JM, Yhap EO, Mazze RI. Reproductive and teratogenic effects of nitrous oxide, isoflurane, and their combination in Sprague–Dawley rats. *Anesthesiology* 1987; **67**: 960–4.

157 Jensen AG, Bach V, Werner MU, Nielsen HK, Jensen MH. A fatal case of malignant hyperthermia following

isoflurane anaesthesia. *Acta Anaesthesiologica Scandinavica* 1986; **30**: 293–4.

158 Wallin RF, Regan BM, Napoli MO, Stern IJ. Sevoflurane: a new inhalation anesthetic agent. *Anesthesia and Analgesia* 1975; **54**: 758.

159 Strum DP, Johnson BH, Eger EI. Stability of sevoflurane in soda lime. *Anesthesiology* 1987; **67**: 779–81.

160 Katoh T, Ikeda K. The minimum alveolar concentration (MAC) of sevoflurane in humans. *Anesthesiology* 1987; **66**: 301–3.

161 Scheller MS, Saidman LJ, Partridge BL. MAC of sevoflurane in humans and the New Zealand white rabbit. *Canadian Journal of Anaesthesia* 1988; **35**: 153–6.

162 Saito S, Goto F, Kadoi Y, Takahashi T, Fujita T, Mogi K. Comparative clinical study of induction and emergence time in sevoflurane and enflurane anaesthesia. *Acta Anaesthesiologica Scandinavica* 1989; **33**: 389–90.

163 Stern RC, Towler SC, White PF, Evers AS. Elimination kinetics of sevoflurane and halothane from blood, brain, and adipose tissue in the rat. *Anesthesia and Analgesia* 1990; **71**: 658–64.

164 Lerman J, Dyston JP, Gallagher TM, Miyasaka K, Volgyesi GA, Burrows FA. The minimum alveolar concentration and hemodynamic effects of halothane, isoflurane and sevoflurane in newborn swine. *Anesthesiology* 1990; **73**: 717–21.

165 Bernard JM, Wouters PF, Doursout MF, Florence B, Chelly JE, Merin RG. Effects of sevoflurane and isoflurane on cardiac and coronary dynamics in chronically instrumented dogs. *Anesthesiology* 1990; **72**: 656–62.

166 Jones RM. Desflurane and sevoflurane: inhalation anaesthetics for this decade? *British Journal of Anaesthesia* 1990; **65**: 527–36.

167 Doi M, Ikeda K, Respiratory effects of sevoflurane. *Anesthesia and Analgesia* 1987; **66**: 241–4.

168 Scheller MS, Tateishi A, Drummond JC, Zornow MH. The effects of sevoflurane on cerebral blood flow, cerebral metabolic rate for oxygen, intracranial pressure and the electroencephalogram are similar to those of isoflurane in the rabbit. *Anesthesiology* 1988; **68**: 548–51.

169 Kobayashi O, Ohta Y, Kosaka F. Interaction of sevoflurane, isoflurane, enflurane and halothane with non-depolarizing muscle relaxants and their prejunctional effects at the neuromuscular junction. *Acta Medica Okayama* 1990; **44**: 209–15.

170 Strum DP, Eger EI, Johnson BH, Steffey EP, Ferrell LD. Toxicity of sevoflurane in rats. *Anesthesia and Analgesia* 1987; **66**: 769–73.

171 Andrews JJ, Johnston RV Jr. The new Tec 6 desflurane vaporizer. *Anesthesia and Analgesia* 1993; **76**: 1338–41.

172 Strum DP, Eger EI. The absorption and degradation of isoflurane and I-653 by dry soda lime at various temperatures. *Anesthesia and Analgesia* 1987; **66**: 1312–15.

173 Fang ZX, Eger EI. UCSF research shows CO comes from CO_2 absorbent. *Anesthesia Patient Safety Foundation Newsletter* 1994; **9**: 25–28.

174 Jones RM, Cashman JN, Mant TGK. Clinical impressions and cardiorespiratory effects of a new fluorinated inhalation anaesthetic, desflurane (I-653), in volunteers. *British Journal of Anaesthesia* 1990; **64**: 11–15.

175 Van Hemelrijck J, Smith I, White PF. Use of desflurane for outpatient anesthesia. A comparison with propofol and nitrous oxide. *Anesthesiology* 1991; **75**: 197–203.

176 Ghouri AF, Bodner M, White PF. Psychomotor recovery after desflurane versus isoflurane in outpatients. *Anesthesiology* 1990; **73**: A9.

177 Tsai SK, Lee C, Kwan WF, Chen BJ. Recovery of cognitive functions after anaesthesia with desflurane or isoflurane and nitrous oxide. *British Journal of Anesthesia* 1992; **69**: 255–8.

178 Zahl K, Prasad K, Mingus M, Shapiro A. Desflurane versus isoflurane with or without N_2O for outpatient laparoscopy. *Anesthesiology* 1990; **73**: A11.

179 Weiskopf RB, Cahalan MK, Eger EI, Yasuda N, Rampil IJ, Ionescu P, Lockhart SH, Johnson BH, Freire B, Kelley S. Cardiovascular actions of desflurane in normocarbic volunteers. *Anesthesia and Analgesia.* 1991; **73**: 143–56.

180 Hartman JC, Pagel PS, Kampine JP, Schmeling WT, Warltier DC. Influence of desflurane on regional distribution of coronary blood flow in a chronically instrumented canine model of multivessel coronary artery obstruction. *Anesthesia and Analgesia* 1991; **72**: 289–99.

181 Calahan M, Weiskopf R, Ionescu P, Yasuda N, Eger E, Rampil I, Lockhart S, Freire B, Caldwell J, Koblin D, Kelly S, Johnson B, Holmes M. Cardiovascular effects of I-653 and nitrous oxide in humans. *Anesthesiology* 1989; **71**: A26.

182 Weiskopf RB, Moore MA, Eger EI, Noorani M. McKay L, Chortkoff B, Hart PS, Damask M. Rapid increase in desflurane concentration is associated with greater transient cardiovascular stimulation than with rapid increase in isoflurane concentration in humans. *Anesthesiology* 1994; **80**: 1035–45.

183 Weiskopf RB, Eger EI, Holmes MA, Rampil IJ, Johnson, B, Brown JG, Yasuda N, Targ AG. Epinephrine-induced premature ventricular contractions and changes in arterial blood pressure and heart rate during I-653, isoflurane and halothane anesthesia in humans. *Anesthesiology* 1989; **70**: 293–8.

184 Lutz LJ, Milde JH, Milde LN. The cerebral functional, metabolic and hemodynamic effects of desflurane in dogs. *Anesthesiology* 1990; **73**: 125–31.

185 Artru AA, Powers K, Doepfner P. CSF sagittal sinus and jugular venous pressures during desflurane or isoflurane anaesthesia in dogs. *Journal of Neurosurgical Anesthesiology* 1994; **6**: 239–48.

186 Ornstein E, Young WL, Fleischer LH, Ostapkovich N. Desflurane and isoflurane have similar effects on cerebral blood flow in patients with intracranial mass lesions. *Anesthesiology* 1993; **79**: 498–502.

187 Weiskopf RB, Eger EI 2d, Ionescu P, Yasuda N, Cahalan MK, Freire B, Peterson N, Lockhart SH, Rampil IJ, Laster M. Desflurane does not produce hepatic or renal injury in human volunteers. *Anesthesia and Analgesia* 1992; **74**: 570–4.

188 Koblin DD, Weiskopf RB, Holmes MA, Konopka K, Rampil IJ, Eger EI, Waskell L. Metabolism of I-653 and isoflurane in swine. *Anesthesia and Analgesia* 1989; **68**: 147–9.

PART II INTRAVENOUS ANAESTHESIA

P Yate

Although a wide variety of drugs are capable of rendering a patient unconscious when injected intravenously, the term 'intravenous anaesthetic agent' is usually restricted to those drugs used clinically to produce anaesthesia by the intravenous route. These compounds are characterized by a rapid onset of action, recovery from unconsciousness within a few minutes and acceptable side-effects.

HISTORY

The first modern report of intravenous anaesthesia was by Professor Ore, a professor of physiology in Bordeaux, who reported the use of intravenous chloral hydrate in sixty-five patients with only one death; however, this report does not seem to have been taken up. Perhaps the true beginning of modern intravenous anaesthesia was the synthesis of barbituric acid by von Bayer in 1864, and although barbituric acid itself has no intrinsic hypnotic activity, it did lead to the synthesis of the first clinically useful barbiturate, phenobarbitone, in 1903 by Fischer and von Meering. In 1921 the first intravenous barbiturate, somnifene, became available, a long-acting barbiturate with a slow onset of action. In 1932, hexobarbitone (evipan) synthesized by Weese in Dusseldorf, was the first short-acting barbiturate. This advance was largely overtaken by the synthesis of thiopentone in 1932. Thiopentone rapidly became the standard drug for induction and maintenance of anaesthesia. However, in 1942 after problems with thiopentone in the management of casualties, the risks of large doses of thiopentone in shocked patients became apparent and thiopentone began to be used more conservatively and its use was largely restricted to the induction of anaesthesia.

Since then a large number of compounds have been investigated as induction agents; however, only a few have made it to the market and over half of those that did are now no longer available.

PRINCIPLES

The requirements of an ideal intravenous anaesthetic agent are well described and include:

- water solubility
- stability in solution
- no venous or tissue damage
- sleep in one arm–brain circulation time
- short duration of action
- non-cumulative
- inactivation by metabolism to inactive metabolites
- no cardiovascular effects
- analgesia
- no histamine release or adverse immunological effects
- no increase in muscle tone or involuntary movements
- painless injection
- absence of metabolic effects.

Sleep in one arm–brain circulation time

The speed of onset is largely determined by delivering sufficient quantity of potent hypnotic to the target organ, in this case the brain. This is achieved by using compounds with a high lipid solubility. For example, substitution of a thio group on to pentobarbitone, a relatively slow onset barbiturate, turns it into thiopentone and increases its lipid solubility by a factor of around 60. To a certain extent speed of onset can be modified by increasing the concentration gradient by administering larger doses. However, this will increase the peak plasma concentration of the drug resulting in exaggerated side-effects and delayed recovery.

Rapid recovery, absence of accumulation and no hangover

This is largely determined by pharmacokinetic factors. Immediate recovery from a bolus of intravenous anaesthetic agent is, in virtually all cases, due to redistribution of the drug rather than metabolism or excretion. In particular, the drug is distributed from the so-called vessel-rich group which is considered to include organs such as the brain, to the so-called muscle-group. The drug is then later distributed into fat, fat playing little part in the initial redistribution due to its low blood flow (Fig. 5.1).

The fall in total drug in the body over time is due to metabolism and excretion. This can be easiest studied by following the plasma concentration of the drug over time and is most commonly done as a semi-log plot (see Chapter 2). If a drug is considered to be given as an intravenous dose into a one-compartment volume and eliminated at a fixed rate (Fig. 2.4(a)) assuming elimination is proportional to concentration gradient,

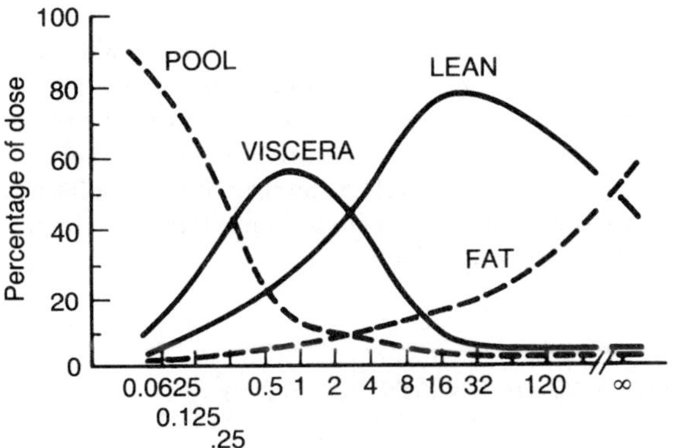

FIGURE 5.1 The distribution of thiopentone following a single intravenous injection. (Reproduced with permission from Price HL, Covnat PJ, Safer JN, Corner EH, Price ML. *Clinical Pharmacology and Therapeutics* 1990; **1**:)

that is first-order elimination, when this is plotted out a simple exponential plot is seen (Fig. 2.4(b), p.16).

However, most intravenous induction agents cannot be described in such simple terms and more complex models have to be considered to describe their behaviour. Occasionally drug behaviour can be described by a two-compartment model (Fig. 2.5, p.16). In this case the plasma concentration after a single intravenous dose can be described by a biexponential curve with an initial rapid redistribution phase and a slower elimination period (Fig. 5.1). These curves are, of course, a hybrid of distribution and excretion (Fig. 5.2).

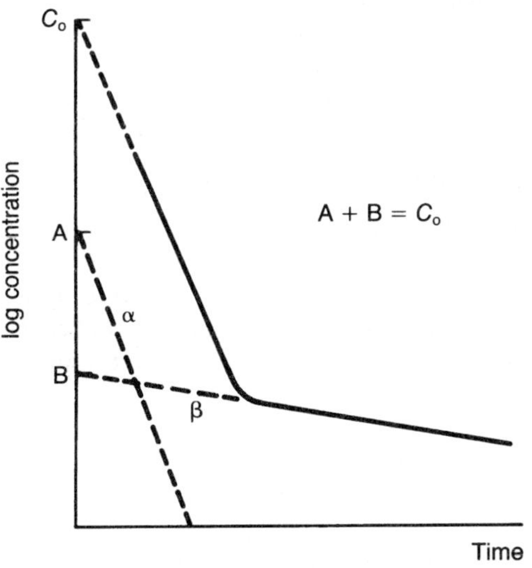

FIGURE 5.2 A biexponential curve describing the decline of plasma concentration of a drug against time when injected into a two-compartment model. α represents the slope of the distribution phase and β that of the elimination phase. Extrapolating the curve back to time zero gives the concentration at time 0 (C_0). A, Concentration in the central compartment; B, concentration in the peripheral compartment at time 0, assuming full distribution.

From this, two hybrid rate constants can be measured, α and β, and an equation:

$$\text{Concentration at time } t\ (C_t) = \text{A}e^{-\alpha t} + \text{B}e^{-\beta t}$$

To work out α and β it is assumed that A + B = concentration at time 0. The kinetics of most intravenous anaesthetic agents are, however, best described by a three-compartment model (Fig. 5.3). This model, known as a mammillary model, assumes that all drug clearance takes place from the central compartment and is best described by a tri-exponential curve.

$$\text{Concentration at time } t\ (C_t) = \text{A}e^{-\alpha t} + \text{B}e^{-\beta t} + \text{D}e^{-\delta t}$$

Aside from the half-lives, two other important descriptions of drug disposition can be determined.

Clearance

This can be defined as the volume of a compartment completely cleared of drug per unit time. Clearance itself is independent of concentration, but if concentration is increased as there is more drug in the blood and as clearance is described as the volume totally cleared, more drug is removed. Thus, it can usually be described as a first-order phenomenon – that is, rate is proportional to concentration. The concept of clearance is most familiar when related to the kidney, but for intravenous anaesthetics hepatic clearance is usually more important. Drugs may be described in terms of their extraction ratio as a measure of hepatic efficiency. The ER_h = hepatic clearance/hepatic blood flow. Thus a drug with an extraction ratio approaching 1 – that is, a clearance of around 22 ml/kg/min (normal liver blood flow) would be very susceptible to changes in liver blood flow as the limiting factor here is liver blood flow. For a drug with a low clearance such as thiopentone, with an extraction ratio of about 0.2, clearance can be described as largely flow independent. As stated above, clearance of intravenous agents is usually first order; that is, clearance is proportional to concentration. However, on occasions, clearance may be capacity limited; that is, liver enzymes are now overwhelmed. In this situation clearance is no longer dependent on concentration and becomes fixed (zero-order kinetics). All the currently used intravenous agents exhibit first-order kinetics in normal clinical practice. However, when the

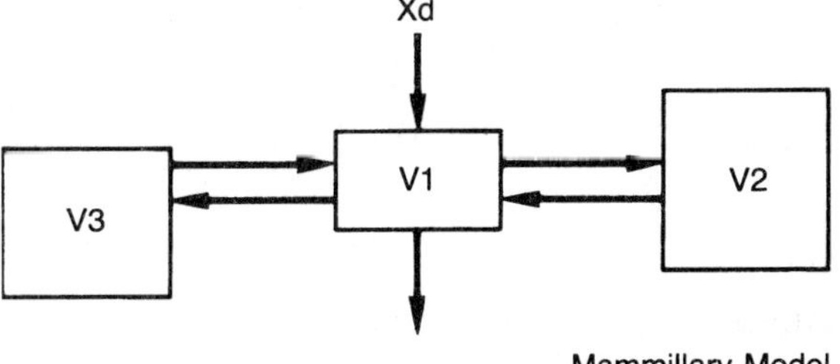

FIGURE 5.3 A graphical representation of a three-compartment model with three compartments V1, V2 and V3.

doses are significantly increased kinetics may change. When high dose thiopentone is used for cerebral protection, if the dose exceeds 500 mg/kg/24 h, the elimination half-life increases as the capacity of the excretory system becomes saturated. As the plasma concentration falls, so the half-life decreases until the kinetics become linear again.

Volume of distribution

This is a theoretical concept of a calculated volume through which the drug is evenly distributed and may frequently exceed total body volume (see Chapter 2). It equals the dose of drug given divided by the concentration achieved (dose/C_{plasma}). This for multicompartment models, however, will give an underestimate of the total volume of distribution as the drug is not fully distributed at time zero. A more accurate volume of distribution is the volume of distribution at a steady-state concentration achieved by infusing a drug.

Volume of distribution can be related to the other variables as

$$\text{Volume of distribution} = \frac{\text{Clearance} \times \text{half-life}}{0.693}$$

The ideal intravenous agent should be rapidly redistributed to give a rapid awakening followed by a fast clearance from the body to prevent any residual hangover and to avoid accumulation if repeated dosing is used. As can be seen from Table 5.1, the intravenous anaesthetics have a large volume of distribution due to their high lipid solubility. The differences are largely due to variations in clearance which may have a significant effect on the duration of the 'hangover' seen with the different agents. As the redistribution half-life is very similar between the various agents immediate recovery is very similar.

Water solubility and stability in solution

This is desirable but has proved problematic. By their nature, intravenous anaesthetics are highly lipid soluble rather than water soluble and hence the need for special solvents, some of which are associated with problems – most notably, the association between cremophor EL and adverse reactions. Alternatively, water solubility has been achieved by manipulating the pH of the solution, for example by using highly alkaline solutions of barbiturates. The stability of these solutions is important not only for convenience but also to facilitate the setting up of infusions.

Absence of metabolic effects

Any metabolic effect is probably undesirable; however, two particular problems are known to be associated with intravenous anaesthesia: the suppression of adrenal steroid synthesis which achieves clinical significance with etomidate, and precipitation of porphyric crises, especially by the barbiturates.

The porphyrias are a relatively rare group of conditions caused by defects in the enzymes responsible for the synthesis of haem. The synthesis of haem is controlled by a negative feedback on the enzyme aminolaevulic acid (ALA) synthetase. If P-450 hepatic enzyme system activity is increased by induction, ALA synthetase activity is increased. In patients with porphyria due to enzyme deficiencies this will result in the increased production of haem precursors or porphyrins. Two types of porphyria are important to the anaesthetist: acute intermittent porphyria in which an acute attack is characterized by neurological and gastrointestinal symptoms, and variegate porphyria, which is clinically similar but with the addition of photosensitivity. Although this problem is mainly associated with the barbiturates neither midazolam nor etomidate nor the steroid induction agents should be considered safe. Propofol is probably safe.

No histamine release or adverse immunological effects

Adverse reactions to intravenous anaesthetic agents may be due to an exaggeration of their normal effects such as cardiovascular depression with thiopentone or

TABLE 5.1 Summary of mean pharmacokinetics of popular intravenous anaesthetic agents

DRUG	TERMINAL HALF-LIFE (h)	CLEARANCE (ml/kg/min)	VOLUME OF DISTRIBUTION (l/kg)
Thiopentone	11.6	3.4	2.5
Methohexitone	3.9	10.9	2.2
Etomidate	5	11.5	4.5
Midazolam	1–4	6–11	1–2
Ketamine	2–3	19	3
Propofol	2–3	18–25	12

as an idiosyncratic effect usually thought to have an immunological basis. The incidence of severe adverse reactions is difficult to assess but is thought to occur in approximately 1 in 50 000 administrations with fatalities in 1 in 500 000 administrations.

There appear to be three main mechanisms. Some agents, such as thiopentone and morphine, are capable of a direct effect on mast cells and basophils leading to degranulation and histamine release – a true Type I hypersensitivity reaction mediated by IgE – this is believed to be the mechanism of severe reactions to thiopentone. Otherwise, these reactions are initiated via the complement system leading to an inflammatory response. This latter may occur either via the classical complement pathway activated by the combination of an antigen (the drug) and an antibody, or by the so-called alternative complement pathway in which the drug, notably althesin and other cremophor-containing compounds, directly stimulates the conversion of C_3 resulting in C_5 activation and histamine release.

CLINICAL USES OF INTRAVENOUS ANAESTHETIC AGENTS

For induction of anaesthesia

The main indication for these drugs is the induction of anaesthesia. This is achieved by injecting either a pre-calculated dose or, more commonly, by slow intravenous injection titrating the dose against clinical signs. The useful clinical signs of satisfactory induction of anaesthesia include loss of lash reflex, loss of verbal contact, loss of muscle tone and loss of pupillary response to light.

For maintenance of anaesthesia

In recent years there has been the development of intravenous anaesthetic agents with short half-lives, notably althesin, etomidate and propofol, enabling anaesthesia to be maintained by repeated administration of these drugs without fear of excessive accumulation and delayed recovery. There are several theoretical advantages to this. The prime stimulus for the development of this technique was the perceived need to reduce atmospheric pollution of the operating theatre environment with anaesthetic gases and, in particular, the avoidance of the use of nitrous oxide. This indication was paralleled by a desire to avoid the risks of hepatotoxicity believed to be associated with repeated halothane administration. Subsequently other indications have become apparent:

- avoidance of atmospheric pollution with anaesthetic gases
- anaesthesia for laryngeal surgery
- anaesthesia for pulmonary surgery when abolition of the hypoxic pulmonary vasoconstrictor response may be harmful
- anaesthesia for malignant hyperpyrexia sensitive patients
- maintenance of anaesthesia on cardiopulmonary bypass
- anaesthesia for neurosurgery where the effects of some intravenous anaesthetic agents in reducing cerebral metabolic rate and CBF may be beneficial
- to facilitate computer control of anaesthesia.

The use of an intravenous agent by itself has been found to be unsatisfactory due to the excessive dosage required leading to delayed recovery and cardiovascular depression. A more satisfactory approach requires supplementation with either nitrous oxide or, if pollution is to be avoided, with an opioid or regional anaesthesia.

Administration may be by repeated intravenous injection or by continuous infusion. The advantages of infusions include more stable anaesthesia, greater cardiovascular stability, reduced total dose, better recovery, reduced postoperative sedation, convenience for a long operation, and less risk of awareness. Disadvantages include the need for complex equipment and risk of overdosage if depth of anaesthesia is not monitored and this may be very difficult to measure. In an effort to enable comparisons to be made between the various agents, the minimum infusion rate (MIR) has been described. This is the minimum infusion rate required to prevent movement in 50% of subjects on surgical incision. It can also be described under various conditions, for example the MIR of a drug in the presence of 60% nitrous oxide. The MIR should not be considered a direct minimum alveolar concentration (MAC) equivalent as it reflects the administration rate not the plasma concentration.

To control seizures

Parenterally or rectally administered benzodiazepines are now first choice for controlling seizures. Thiopentone, in particular, has proved very useful in controlling resistant status epilepticus. Propofol is probably not an anticonvulsant. Ketamine should not be used to treat convulsions owing to its effect on cerebral metabolism and haemodynamics and low dose methohexitone may stimulate seizure activity on the EEG although it has been used successfully to treat fits.

Sedation in the intensive care unit

Many of the shorter-acting intravenous agents have been used for sedating patients in the intensive care unit. This technique has not been without problems, most seriously after etomidate infusion where suppression of steroid synthesis had serious consequences.

THE INDIVIDUAL DRUGS

Barbiturates

The basic compound for all the barbiturates is barbituric acid and this was synthesized in 1864 by von Bayer from urea and malonic acid (Fig. 5.4). This compound has no hypnotic activity and it was not until 1903 with the synthesis of phenobarbitone that the hypnotic potential of these compounds became realized. The early barbiturates are characterized by a slow onset and a long duration of action. These oxybarbiturates are formulated by the addition of carbon-containing chains at the C_5 position (Fig. 5.5).

Substitution of carbon containing chains at the R_1 and R_2 positions is essential for hypnotic activity. The R_1 and R_2 chains of the clinically useful barbiturates range in length from four to eight carbon atoms. Drugs such as phenobarbitone and barbitone have elimination half-lives of around 50–90 h and pentobarbitone has a half-life of 40 h. Subsequently, two important modifications were discovered which led to the introduction of the rapid onset, rapid recovery barbiturates suitable for use as intravenous induction agents. First, the addition of a methyl group at position 1 to produce a methyl barbiturate. This is characterized by a rapid onset of action, excitatory movements at induction and 'convulsant' activity. Second, the substitution of a sulphur for oxygen at position 2 produces thiobarbiturates, again with a rapid onset of action, but this time with a smooth onset of anaesthesia. This rapid onset of action is due to an increase in the lipid solubility, thiopentone is sixty-six times more lipid soluble than its oxybarbiturate pentobarbitone.

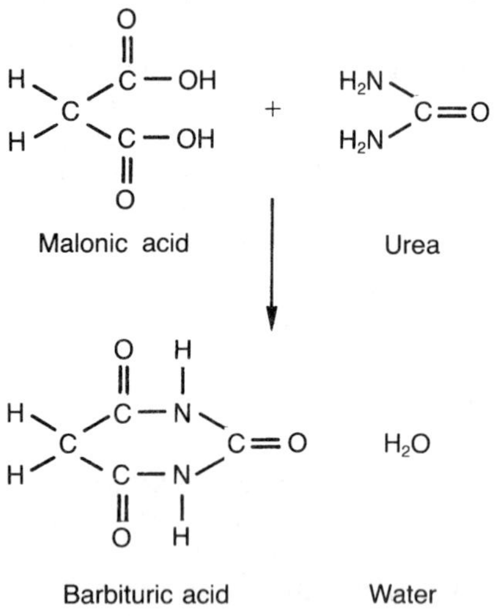

The mode of action of the barbiturates is, as yet, not fully resolved; however, recent developments have brought the answer tantalizingly close. Barbiturates, like all intravenous anaesthetic agents and also inhalational agents, can have their effect at least partially reversed by the effects of high pressure. This is believed to indicate a general non-specific effect of barbiturates on membranes, the relative stereospecificity of their action suggesting that their main mechanism of action is to react with specific receptors rather than have a general effect on membranes. The most likely site for this is at the γ-amino-butyric acid ($GABA_A$) receptor. This is a protein complex that acts by modifying transmembrane potential by altering chloride conductance. The action of GABA at this receptor can be modified allosterically by both benzodiazepines and barbiturates although almost certainly at separate sites as they have different effects. Benzodiazepines increase the frequency of the chloride channel opening and barbiturates prolong the duration of the opening.

FIGURE 5.4 The synthesis of barbituric acid from malonic acid and urea.

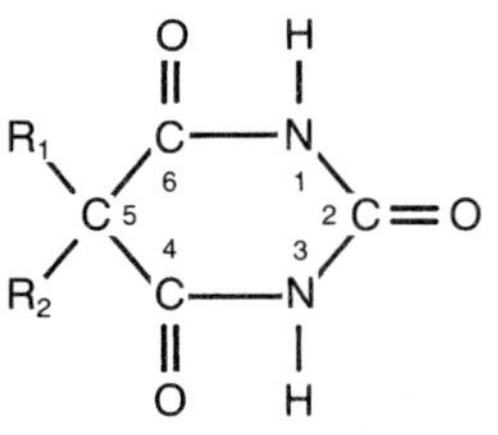

FIGURE 5.5 The barbiturate ring.

Thiopentone

Thiopentone was originally synthesized by Tabern and Volwieler at Abbott Laboratories in the USA in 1932. The first recorded administration was by Ralph Waters at Wisconsin Hospital, Madison in 1934 and was first described and popularized by Dr John Lundy at the Mayo Clinic. The drug still remains the most popular intravenous induction agent in the world today.

Physical chemistry

The molecule is pentobarbitone with the substitution of sulphur for oxygen at the C_2 carbon atom and is also known as thionembutal (Fig. 5.6). It is a powder which is made up with water as a 2.5% solution and occasionally in Europe as a 5% solution. It smells of hydrogen sulphide. The drug is presented as the sodium salt to solubilize it and can only be safely assumed to remain stable in solution for 48 h. The solution also contains 6% sodium carbonate to prevent the formation of free acid and has a pH of 10.8.

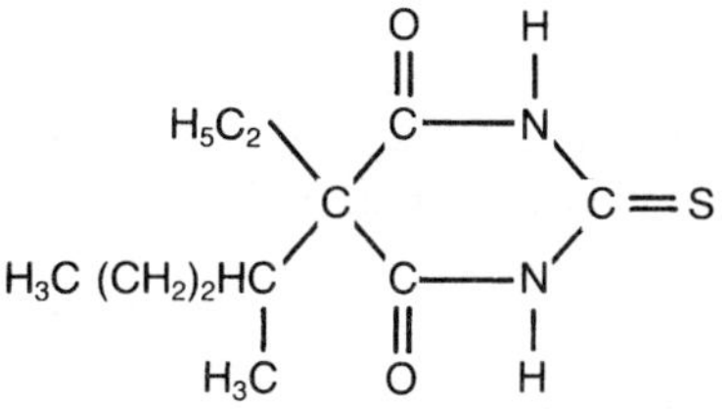

FIGURE 5.6 Thiopentone.

Pharmacokinetics and pharmacodynamics

Thiopentone has a distribution half-life of 8.5 min and an elimination half-life of 697 min. The volume of distribution at steady state is 1.3–3.3 l/kg. Clearance is slow at between 1.6 and 4.3 ml/kg/min. The drug is 65–75% protein bound mainly to albumin, which is reduced in hepatic and renal failure. Pregnant patients and children have increased clearance. The effective thiopentone concentration for anaesthesia is around 6 μg/ml free drug or 40 μg/ml total drug.

Metabolism and excretion

The drug is mainly excreted by the liver as its high lipid solubility leads to tubular reabsorption. As its clearance is low compared with liver blood flow, normally about 21 ml/kg/min, it has a hepatic extraction ratio of 0.08–0.2 and thus can be described as having a capacity-limited binding sensitive elimination; that is, clearance is largely unaffected by changes in liver blood flow as the limiting factor is the liver's ability to metabolize the drug. It is metabolized by the P-450 system to thiopentone carboxylic acid. A small percentage of the drug, around 3%, is metabolized to pentobarbitone which has a distribution half-life of 4 h and an elimination half-life of 17–50 h. This is not normally clinically significant, but may become so when very high doses are used. Excretion of the drug is normally first order, but may, if excessive doses are used such as in the Intensive Therapy Unit (ITU/ICU), become zero order. This usually occurs when the plasma concentration of free drug exceeds 50 μg/ml and half-lives of 70 h and more have been reported. This usually requires doses greater than 500 mg/kg over 24 h.

Clinical features

Nervous system

The drug is a potent cerebral depressant causing up to a 50% reduction in cerebral metabolism, CBF and hence intracranial pressure although tolerance to this effect will develop with time. Cerebral autoregulation and vascular responsiveness to carbon dioxide are unchanged. The pupils dilate and then constrict and intraocular pressure falls. The drug is a potent anticonvulsant. Changes in the EEG following intravenous injection initially show reduced activity especially in the α-band with an increase in slow θ- and δ-activity and some low voltage β. Later the activity is predominantly mixed α and β. With overdosage burst suppression occurs. It is said to increase sensitivity to pain. It has no significant effect on the neuromuscular junction. Patients with dystrophia myotonica are said to be especially sensitive to thiopentone.

Cardiovascular system

Thiopentone, like most intravenous anaesthetic agents, is a potent cardiovascular depressant. In healthy patients after a standard induction dose systolic blood pressure will fall by around 15%, cardiac output by up to 25%, and contractility by up to 15%. The drug causes myocardial depression and peripheral vasodilatation. This is to a certain extent compensated for by a reflex tachycardia; the heart rate may rise by up to 30%, mediated by the baroreceptors. These changes may result in a steep rise in myocardial oxygen consumption and a consequent increase in coronary blood flow. On occasions the induced cardiovascular depression may be severe and even life threatening. This is particularly seen in those patients where the cardiovascular system is already stressed. High-risk patients include shocked patients with hypovolaemia and those with a fixed cardiac output such as patients with valvular heart disease and constrictive pericarditis. In all these situations thiopentone has been used successfully, providing consideration is given to reducing the dose. The cardiovascular systems of children appear to have particular resistance to the effect of thiopentone.

Respiratory system

Mild depression of ventilation is routinely observed. Thiopentone is associated with the development of laryngospasm and bronchospasm, particularly at induction of anaesthesia. Thus, thiopentone is relatively contraindicated in patients with asthma.

Other effects

Thiopentone is not associated with postoperative vomiting. Urticaria is common, particularly around the site of injection. Thiopentone is particularly toxic to skin and subcutaneous tissues. If extravasated, local tissue damage is common. Local venous thrombosis occurs in about 10% of cases and is worse if 5% solution is used. The most serious local complications are seen after inadvertent intra-arterial injections. This is characterized by pain, but not always; arterial spasm; blanching of the limb; disappearance of the radial pulse; and later, oedema and gangrene. Long-term sequelae are seen in 31% of patients if 5% thiopentone is injected intra-arterially, but only in 7% if 2.5% solution is used. It is postulated to be due to the formation of thiopentone crystals in the blood, causing a chemical endarteritis and noradrenaline release. Treatment is largely symptomatic and includes the injection through the same needle of a vasodilator such as papaverine or tolazoline, heparin 10 000 units to prevent thrombosis and the institution of a brachial plexus block for pain relief and to produce a sympathetic block.

The drug is associated with a 350% rise in plasma histamine concentration. Clinically insignificant hypokalaemia and hyperglycaemia may occur. The drug is absolutely contraindicated in patients suffering from porphyria.

Thiopentone freely crosses the placenta and may cause fetal depression; however, in clinical practice the degree of fetal depression produced by a single induction dose of thiopentone does not represent a hazard to the fetus.

Serious adverse reactions are reported to occur in approximately 1 in 14 000 to 1 in 20 000 administrations and may be severe. It appears to be a true Type I IgE-mediated hypersensitivity reaction.

Clinical uses of thiopentone

Induction of anaesthesia

This is usually smooth and rapid occurring in one arm–brain circulation time. Involuntary movements are rare as is pain on injection. Recovery of awareness after a single dose takes about 5 min and is due to redistribution of the drug. However, on psychometric testing impairment may still be detected the following day. Provided care is taken to titrate the dose of thiopentone to the patient, thiopentone is a satisfactory agent for most patients. The induction dose ranges from 3.5 to 5 mg/kg. Induction of anaesthesia can also be achieved by rectal administration.

Maintenance of anaesthesia

Although it is possible to maintain anaesthesia with intermittent doses of thiopentone or even infusions, the pharmacokinetic profile of thiopentone is such that significant accumulation will occur with a consequence of a very slow recovery.

Anticonvulsant therapy

Thiopentone is a potent anticonvulsant and may be life saving in resistant cases of status epilepticus although care must be taken to secure the patient's airway and, if repeat doses are used, to monitor both the serum thiopentone and pentobarbitone concentrations to avoid overdosage.

Methohexitone

Methohexitone was first described in 1957.

Physical chemistry

This is a methylated oxybarbiturate (Fig. 5.7). It is prepared as a 1% solution containing sodium carbonate and has a pH of 11.1.

Pharmacokinetics and metabolism

Methohexitone has an elimination half-life of around 3 h. The volume of distribution is similar to that of thiopentone of 1–2 l/kg, but its clearance of 10–12 ml/kg/min is approximately three times that of thiopentone and it is this that is responsible for its shorter half-life. However, with a higher clearance, the excretion of methohexitone is more sensitive to changes in liver blood flow and the elimination of methohexitone may be reduced if anaesthetic techniques are used that reduce liver blood flow.

Clinical features

Methohexitone is essentially very similar to thiopentone. There are, however, a few important differences. The drug may initiate epileptiform activity on the EEG although methohexitone has also been used successfully as an anticonvulsant.

Its use is also associated with abnormal excitatory movements during induction of anaesthesia. These are increased by premedication with hyoscine or promethazine and can be reduced by pretreatment with fentanyl.

Although methohexitone is less irritant to tissues than thiopentone, injection of methohexitone is associated with severe pain in approximately 60% of administrations if veins on the back of the hand are used. This can be reduced to 17% if a forearm vein is used. The pain can also be reduced by premixing the methohexitone with lignocaine. Approximately 8% of patients will experience postoperative venous sequelae after methohexitone. Severe allergic reactions are rare after methohexitone and it is difficult to make a true estimate of their incidence.

Clinical use

Methohexitone is an effective induction agent at a dose of around 1.5 mg/kg. Induction of anaesthesia is

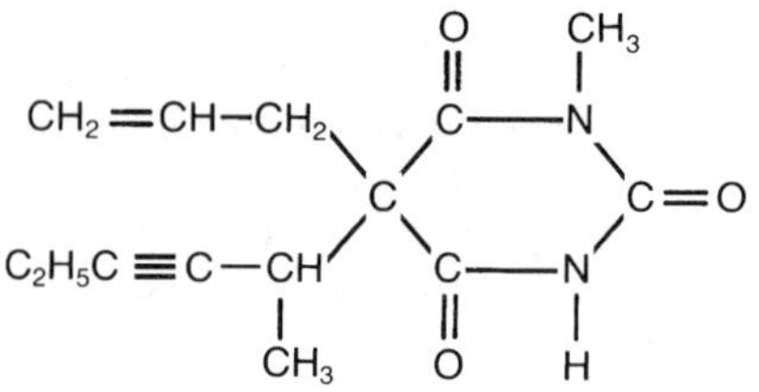

O CH$_3$
$CH_2{=}CH{-}CH_2$ C—N
C C=O
$C_2H_5C{\equiv}C{-}CH$ C—N
CH$_3$ O H

FIGURE 5.7 Methohexitone.

characterized by a painful injection, followed by a rapid onset of sleep often associated with excitatory phenomena. Recovery from methohexitone is rapid, and due to its shorter half-life so is any postoperative mental impairment compared with that seen after thiopentone. This rapid recovery has led to methohexitone's popularity as an induction agent for day case surgery. The kinetics of methohexitone also mean it can also be used for maintenance of anaesthesia by infusion. However, these kinetics are not ideal and accumulation tends to occur if this technique is used for operations lasting more than half an hour and the recovery time may then become unacceptably long.

Methohexitone is used clinically by clinical neurophysiologists at very low doses to uncover seizure activity during EEG recordings.

Etomidate

Physical chemistry

Developed in 1971, etomidate is a carboxylated imidazole and is structurally related to imidazole antifungal agents such as ketoconazole. The compound is soluble in water and is presented either in solution (2 mg/ml) with 35% propylene glycol or as a concentrated form (125 mg/ml) dissolved in absolute alcohol designed for use by infusion – a technique not now recommended. A second formulation of etomidate was required when the drug was used for infusion as there is an upper limit on the maximum safe dose of propylene glycol as excessive doses may precipitate haemolysis (Fig. 5.8).

Pharmacokinetics and metabolism

Etomidate has a relatively short elimination half-life of approximately 75 min with a clearance of 11.7 ml/kg/min. The drug is rapidly hydrolysed by the liver to 5-imidazocarboxylic acid and thus its duration is prolonged by liver disease. Approximately 2% is excreted unchanged, the rest as glucuronide conjugates. It is 77% bound to albumin in the plasma. An effective plasma concentration is around 150–250 μg/1.

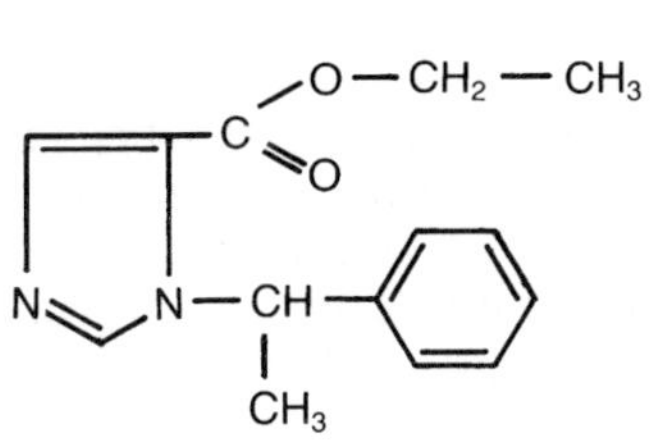

$O-CH_2-CH_3$, C, O, N, N—CH, CH_3

R–(+)ethyl-1-(1-phenylethyl)-1H-Imidazole-5-Carboxylate

FIGURE 5.8 Etomidate.

Clinical features

Nervous system

Etomidate has an effect on cerebral metabolism similar to that seen with thiopentone. CBF, cerebral metabolic rate of oxygen consumption and intercranial pressure are all reduced as is intraocular pressure. Etomidate is associated with excitatory myoclonic movement in around 30% of patients, particularly during induction of anaesthesia. These movements are not associated with any abnormal activity on the EEG and an increase in the plasma concentration does not prevent them. It is an effective anticonvulsant. The drug has a mild depressing effect on plasma pseudocholinesterase and may slightly prolong the effect of suxamethonium.

Cardiovascular effects

Etomidate is believed to have a less depressant effect on the cardiovascular system than thiopentone. Cardiac output falls by around 10% due to a fall in stroke volume of 13% and systolic blood pressure falls by 13%. The myocardial depression is to a certain degree compensated for by a 6% rise in heart rate.

Other effects

The drug is not particularly irritant to tissues although approximately 10% of patients may suffer from local thrombophlebitis. About 10% of patients also complain of pain on injection. Postoperative nausea and vomiting may prove a problem after etomidate.

Metabolic effects

Etomidate does not routinely provoke the release of histamine and is believed to be either not at all, or at the most, very rarely associated with severe adverse reactions and thus is highly suitable for use in atopic patients. It is not safe for use in patients with porphyria. The major problem with etomidate is its effect on the adrenal cortex. Owing to its short elimination half-life, etomidate became popular for sedation in intensive care units. An audit of trauma patients in Glasgow identified a dramatic rise in deaths from sepsis and this was tracked back to the introduction of etomidate. It is now known that this was probably due to the potent inhibitory effects of etomidate on steroid synthesis. Etomidate blocks the seventeen α-hydroxylase and eleven β-hydroxylase enzymes causing reduction in both cortisol and other steroid production (Fig. 5.9).

Clinical uses

Etomidate is an effective induction agent at a dose of 0.3 mg/kg producing anaesthesia in one arm–brain circulation time. Its pharmacokinetic profile makes it suitable for day case anaesthesia; however, despite this, due to its effect on steroid synthesis it is contraindicated for use by infusion apart from maintenance for very short

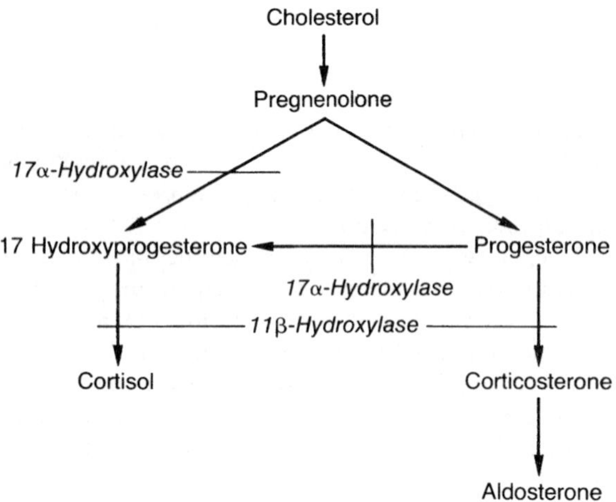

FIGURE 5.9 The steps in the synthesis of cortisol and aldosterone from cholesterol illustrating the sites in which enzyme activity is inhibited by etomidate.

cases. Today, its primary indication is as induction agent for patients at risk from cardiovascular depression.

Ketamine

Ketamine, an arylcyclohexylamine, is a derivative of phencyclidine, a drug that was originally developed as an anaesthetic agent, but was rapidly abandoned due to its potent hallucinogenic effects. Phencyclidine is also encountered as a drug of abuse and it is known by a variety of names including angel dust and PCP. It is now restricted to veterinary use.

Chemistry

Ketamine or 2-(O-chlorophenyl)-2-methylamino cyclohexanone (Fig. 5.10) is supplied as a 1%, 5% and 10% solution for administration either intravenously or intramuscularly. It is a racemic mixture but separating out the isomers offers no advantages, the S(+) being the most potent.

Pharmacokinetics and metabolism

Ketamine has a terminal half-life of around 150–240 min, a clearance of 19 ml/kg/min and a volume of distribution of 3.1 l/kg. Ketamine is *n*-demethylated in the liver to norketamine and then hydroxylated to hydroxynorketamine compounds which are then excreted as glucuronide derivatives. Norketamine also has hypnotic and analgesic properties, having approximately one-third the potency of the parent ketamine. Ketamine is an analgesic at blood concentrations of greater than 150 μg/ml and a hypnotic at greater than 640 μg/ml.

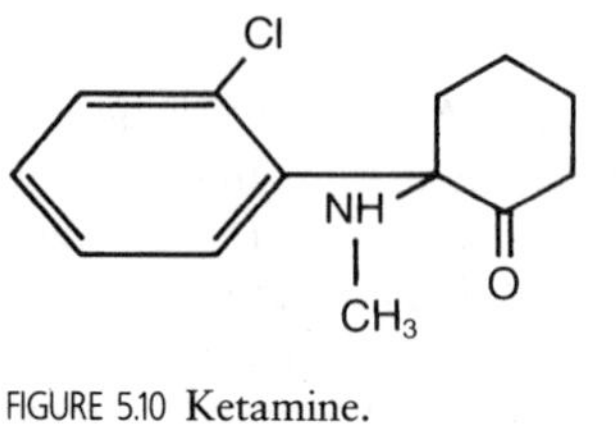

FIGURE 5.10 Ketamine.

Clinical effects

Nervous system

Ketamine produces a state known as dissociative anaesthesia. This is observed even when low doses are used to produce analgesia and then the patient describes a sensation of floating. At high doses the patient is unconscious, but appears awake, may move, have their eyes open, remaining hypertonic with intact corneal reflexes. They may even make purposeful movements. On recovery, the patient may complain of hallucinations or more properly illusions as the patients do have insight. These are experienced by the vast majority of adult patients receiving ketamine and can be very disturbing. Flashback hallucinations have been reported persisting in patients for up to a year postoperatively. Most patients who experience them are reluctant to repeat ketamine anaesthesia. They are said to be less common in the young and elderly, or at least less troublesome. The incidence is increased by atropine and may be severe in patients with personality problems. Originally these patients were managed in the postoperative period by isolating them in a quiet location with low light; this is now known to be unsatisfactory and patients are best managed in the normal recovery area with reassurance from a friendly nurse. The frequency can be reduced by pretreatment with droperidol although, at a cost of further dysphoria, the most effective method is prophylactic treatment with preoperative warning and a benzodiazepine, particularly lorezepam.

Ketamine appears to work by depressing the sensory relay nuclei in the brain and at the same time stimulating the limbic system; that is, direct inhibition of telencephalic function with stimulation of diencephalic structures. At a cellular level ketamine almost certainly works by acting as an antagonist at the NMDA (N-methyl-D-aspartate) receptor probably at the postsynaptic site, possibly binding to a site within the ion channel. The EEG shows marked activity in the θ and β bands. The overall effect is marked central nervous system stimulation which will result in an increase in cerebral metabolic rate of around 20%, increased CBF by as much as 50%, and raised intercranial pressure. A modest rise in intraocular pressure is also observed. Ketamine does have the potential to become a substance of abuse.

Despite the rigidity observed with ketamine, it is almost certainly safe to use in malignant hyperpyrexia susceptible subjects.

Cardiovascular system

The drug is a potent cardiovascular stimulant. Following induction of anaesthesia a significant, but transient, rise in both heart rate and blood pressure is seen, normally of the order of 30% which last about 5 min. This is probably due to two factors: (1) central nervous system stimulation and an increase in circulating catecholamines; and (2) ketamine may also have a cocaine-like effect at the adrenergic receptors. Applied to the isolated heart, however, it is a negative inotrope. Peripherally, ketamine is a vasodilator.

Arrhythmias are rare as ketamine has antiarrhythmic properties. The cardiovascular changes are not sustained if an infusion is used or if a second increment of ketamine is given.

Respiratory system

The laryngeal reflexes are partially preserved, but airway patency cannot be relied upon, nor can protection from aspiration. Ketamine is a potent bronchodilator and has been used in the treatment of status asthmaticus. Respiratory depression is not a feature.

Other effects

Vomiting is not uncommon after ketamine and copious salivation may prove a problem during anaesthesia. Erythematous skin rashes are seen in 20% of patients. Ketamine itself is not irritant to tissues and can be safely injected intramuscularly. Severe adverse reactions are very rare. Ketamine freely crosses the placenta and may cause fetal depression and increases uterine tone. For these reasons it is not recommended for routine use in obstetrics although it has been used successfully in difficult situations. Its use should be avoided in pregnant patients with hypertensive disease. Hypokalaemia and hyperglycaemia may be observed.

Clinical uses of ketamine

The psychological effects of ketamine have made it unsuitable for use as a routine agent for induction of anaesthesia. Ketamine has proved very useful, however, in more difficult circumstances, such as field anaesthesia, in developing countries in wartime, for operator anaesthetists and is particularly useful in children where the psychological effects appear to be less important and it is here that the main indications occur, notably for anaesthesia for radiotherapy and burns dressings. The induction dose of ketamine is 2mg/kg intravenously and 5–10 mg/kg intramuscularly. Increasing the dosage does not intensify the effect; it merely prolongs the duration of action.

Benzodiazepines

These compounds have many of the features of the ideal anaesthetic agent. They are hypnotic, muscle relaxants, anticonvulsant anxiolytic, amnesics, cause minimal cardiac and respiratory depression, and potentiate analgesics.

This relative specificity of action is due to the augmentation of the action of the inhibitory neurotransmitter GABA at $GABA_A$ receptors in the CNS (see p. 38 and Chapter 21). The discovery of these benzodiazepine receptors also led to the development of the specific benzodiazepine antagonist, flumazenil. Benzodiazepines act allosterically to increase the affinity of the $GABA_A$ receptor for GABA. This increases the number of chloride ion channels opened by a given concentration of GABA. This leads to sedation and anticonvulsant activity.

Most of the benzodiazepines (see p. 38 and Chapter 21) are long acting, have a relatively slow onset of action and are rather unpredictable, making them unsuitable for use as an induction agent. Only two benzodiazepines, diazepam and midazolam, are used as induction agents and only midazolam can be considered to fill the criteria for a modern induction agent.

Diazepam

This agent was for many years the only available benzodiazepine suitable for use as an intravenous induction agent, although its unpredictability and long duration of action limited its use. Until recently, diazepam was only available dissolved in propylene glycol; this preparation was associated with pain on injection and a very high incidence of local venous complications. Now reformulated as a lipid emulsion, pain on injection and venous sequelae are rare. The drug is 99% bound to albumin thus any change in protein binding such as in hypoalbuminaemic states may result in a large change in effect. The volume of distribution at steady state has been measured at 0.7–1.6 l/kg. The long elimination half-life of 20–70 h leads to a long duration of action and considerable accumulation if repeat dosing is used. This long half-life is due to a very slow clearance of around 0.5 ml/kg/min. This long duration of action is further compounded by its metabolism. Diazepam is oxidized in the liver to desmethyldiazepam and oxazepam both with hypnotic activity. Clinically, the onset of action with diazepam is smooth but both the speed of onset of sleep and the dose required are unpredictable. The main advantage of induction with diazepam is the cardiovascular stability associated with its use. Recovery of consciousness after diazepam will take significantly longer than after other intravenous anaesthetic agents and evidence of psychomotor impairment may persist into the following day. For these reasons diazepam as an intravenous induction agent has been largely superseded by midazolam.

Midazolam

This compound was first synthesized in 1976 by Freyer and Welser and has achieved considerable popularity, both as an induction agent and as a sedative for endoscopic procedures.

Chemistry

The drug (Fig. 5.11) exists in a pharmacologically inactive form in the ampoule where it is water soluble. When it enters the patient and the pH rises above 4 the imidazole ring closes and it becomes lipid soluble. The drug is much more lipophilic than the other benzodiazepines, hence it is able rapidly to penetrate the brain. It has twice the affinity for benzodiazepine receptors than that of diazepam. The drug is 96% protein bound. Midazolam has an elimination half-life of 1–4 h and is relatively rapidly cleared. This is believed to be due to the vulnerability of the imidazole ring to metabolism, the clearance 6–12 ml/kg/min is about ten times that of diazepam. Midazolam is hydroxylated by hepatic microsomal oxidative enzymes in the liver to a variety of metabolites including small amounts of weakly pharmocologically active 1 and 4 hydroxyl metabolites. These metabolites are then conjugated to glucuronides and excreted via the kidney.

The elimination half-life may vary enormously in the clinical setting. In patients in intensive care it may be as long as 18 h. This may be partly due to the discovery that there is a group of poor metabolizers, as the half-life of midazolam appears to have a bimodal distribution, with approximately 6% of the population having a half-life greater than 8 h. The half-life of midazolam is also increased by old age and obesity, but not by renal failure.

Clinical features

Nervous system

A dose of 0.15 mg/kg produces 20–30 min of amnesia, which is longer than diazepam but shorter than lorazepam. It reduces cerebral oxygen consumption, CBF by 34% and intracranial pressure. It is a central muscle relaxant but has no effect on the neuromuscular junction.

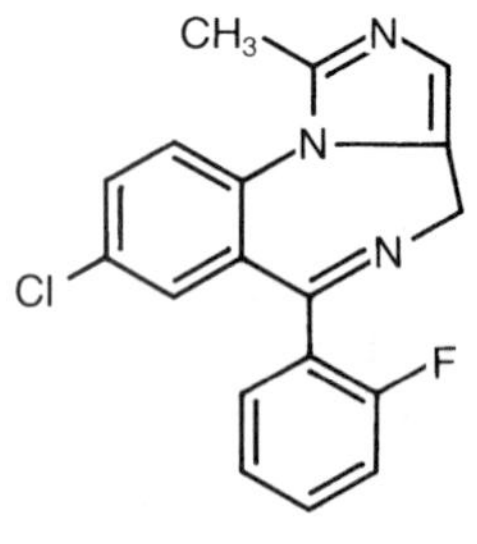

CH_3 N N N Cl F

FIGURE 5.11 Midazolam.

Cardiovascular system

The drug is associated with good cardiovascular stability, although a dose of greater than 0.15 mg/kg will produce a fall in blood pressure due to a reduced systemic vascular resistance, reduced venous return and myocardial depression. These effects are greater than those seen with diazepam.

Other effects

At doses greater than 0.15 mg/kg given intravenously, transient apnoea may occur especially after opiate premedication. Nausea and vomiting are rare after midazolam, which is remarkably non-irritant to tissues. The incidence of major adverse reactions is negligible. There is some doubt about its safety in patients with porphyria. The drug crosses the placenta, but not as fast as thiopentone. Infants of mothers given midazolam may exhibit signs of poor body tone.

Clinical uses

The standard induction dose is 0.2–0.3 mg/kg, which is reduced by opiate premedication. The response is very variable and the induction time is slower than thiopentone, but may be increased by increasing the speed of injection. Its main use is for the induction of anaesthesia in patients in whom good cardiovascular stability is required. The drug has also become popular for sedation for endoscopy and in the intensive care unit.

Opioids

The use of opioids for the induction of anaesthesia has achieved some popularity for induction in high-risk patients, such as for patients prior to cardiac surgery. The doses required are very large, for example 100–200 μg/kg of fentanyl.

The proposed advantages of this technique are cardiovascular stability and possible suppression of the metabolic response to surgery. Disadvantages include rigidity on induction, awareness under anaesthesia and postoperative respiratory depression. For further information on these compounds see Chapters 25 and 26.

Propofol

Propofol is one of a group of alkyl phenols investigated at ICI Laboratories. It was originally investigated as ICI 35868 when it was formulated with cremophor. Concerns about adverse reactions to cremophor led to this preparation being withdrawn and propofol is now presented as an emulsion.

Chemistry

Propofol is 2,6-diisopropylphenol (Fig. 5.12). It is produced as a 1% solution formulated in a mixture of

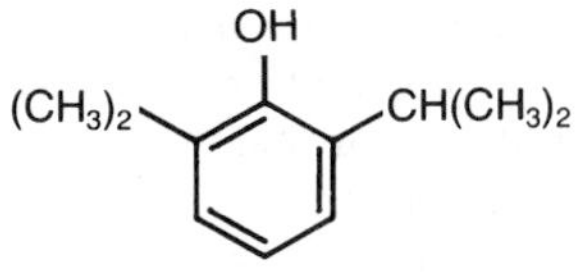

OH
$(CH_3)_2$ $CH(CH_3)_2$

2-6-diisopropylphenol

FIGURE 5.12 Propofol.

10% w/v soya bean oil, 1.2% w/v egg phosphatide and 2.5% w/v glycerol. Propofol is rapidly metabolized in the liver to 1 and 4 glucuronide and 4 sulphate conjugates. Only 0.3% is excreted unchanged. The elimination half-life is approximately 90 min and it has a clearance of 22–35 ml/kg/min; this is greater than liver blood flow which suggests that extra hepatic metabolism takes place probably in the lungs, kidney and gastrointestinal tract. The rate of clearance is unaffected by mild degrees of hepatic or renal impairment. The effective plasma concentration for anaesthesia is 2–8 μg/ml.

Clinical pharmacology

Nervous system

Propofol is a potent cerebral depressant producing profound depression of the EEG, burst suppression occurring readily. Movement is often seen at induction, but is not associated with epileptiform changes on the EEG and may be reduced by increasing the dose. It is suggested these may be due to imbalance between the cortex and the medulla during induction. Therapeutic concentrations of propofol reduce cerebral metabolic rate of oxygen by 35% and CBF by 50% and reduces intraocular pressure. The cerebral vascular resistance is increased by 50%. Propofol is not an anticonvulsant, although if compared with methohexitone a shorter seizure duration is observed during electroconvulsive therapy. There are several reports of 'epilepsy' following propofol administration and also of seizures being controlled by propofol. Experimental data from both animal and human research strongly suggests that propofol is not convulsant and can be safely used in patients with epilepsy. Recovery from propofol anaesthesia is quick and smooth and often characterized by euphoria, hunger and even amorous feelings. There is some evidence that propofol has antiemetic properties.

Despite the impression of muscle relaxation propofol appears to have no effect on the neuromuscular junction nor to interact with neuromuscular blocking agents.

Cardiovascular system

Propofol is a potent cardiovascular depressant. A 20–30% fall in systolic blood pressure is routinely seen after induction of anaesthesia. The cardiac output is reduced by a maximum of 10% and may not change at all. A modest increase (2–10%) in heart rate may transiently be observed although not as great as would be expected for such a marked fall in blood pressure. The main mechanism for this fall seems to be a 20% reduction in systemic vascular resistance associated with a shift in the slope, but not sensitivity of the baroreceptor response and a central vagotonic effect. This can be contrasted with thiopentone where the major effect is myocardial depression and tachycardia thus resulting in a greater increase in myocardial oxygen consumption than would be expected with propofol, when induction of anaesthesia is associated with a 30% fall in the rate pressure product which can be considered a crude indicator of myocardial oxygen consumption. Conversely, the cardiovascular effects of propofol do result in a significant modification of the potentially adverse haemodynamic effects of tracheal intubation.

At clinical concentrations propofol has no effect on cardiac electrophysiology. Infusions of propofol for maintenance of anaesthesia are associated with reasonable cardiovascular stability. The systolic arterial pressure falls by up to 30%, the heart rate by up to 15% and the cardiac output by as much as 30%. The cardiovascular effects of propofol can be minimized by slow intravenous injection or by the prophylactic administration of an anticholinergic agent, particularly glycopyrrolate 5 μg/kg intravenously.

Respiratory system

Paralleling its effect on the cardiovascular system, propofol given as a bolus is a potent respiratory depressant and periods of apnoea of up to 1 min may routinely be seen after induction of anaesthesia. This effect is not a problem during maintenance of anaesthesia although mild elevations of end-tidal carbon dioxide concentration will be observed especially after opiate premedication.

Other effects

Propofol is not toxic to tissues and venous sequelae are rarely seen; however, injection may be painful. Approximately 50% of patients will complain of pain if propofol is injected into a vein on the dorsum of a hand. This pain may be reduced to 10% by injecting into a forearm vein, eliminated by injecting into a fast running intravenous infusion, modestly diminished by cooling the propofol to 4°C, or significantly modified by premixing the propofol with 20 mg of lignocaine. It is recommended by the manufacturers that mixing of drugs should only take place immediately prior to their use. Vomiting is rare after propofol. Propofol is safe to use in patients with malignant hyperpyrexia susceptibility and in patients with porphyria. At clinical doses, propofol has no *in vivo* effect on adrenal steroid genesis. Adverse reactions to propofol have been estimated to occur with an incidence of 1 in 60 000 administrations. Propofol does cross the placenta, but has been safely used for anaesthesia for Caesarian section.

Clinical use

Propofol is an effective induction agent inducing anaesthesia in one arm–brain circulation time. It is particularly useful for day case anaesthesia and for administration by infusion due to its rapid clearance. It appears to suppress the pharyngeal and laryngeal reflexes, allowing for early insertion of an airway, a laryngeal mask or even an endotracheal tube. Its cardiovascular profile means that it has to be used with caution in high-risk patients. The standard induction dose is approximately 2.5 mg/kg. This needs to be modified to account for the patient's condition and age. The cardiovascular effects can be minimized by induction by infusion. For maintenance of anaesthesia an infusion rate of 6–12 mg/kg/h is required depending on the presence of other anaesthetic agents. In view of its effect of shortening seizure duration, propofol is not an ideal agent for electroconvulsive therapy, and probably it is best avoided in patients with known epilepsy.

Propofol has proved a very effective agent for use by infusion to sedate patients in the Intensive Care Unit. Propofol, however, should not be used for the sedation of children in Intensive Care Units as there have been several reports of fatalities following prolonged propofol infusions, these children developing severe acidosis and profound bradycardia. It is not recommended that propofol should be used under any circumstances in children under the age of three. Recent work has explored the possibility of using propofol as an antiemetic prior to cancer chemotherapy, as an antipuritic and as an anxiolytic.

INTRAVENOUS INDUCTION AGENTS OF INTEREST, BUT NOT CURRENTLY AVAILABLE

Steroid anaesthetics

These were developed following the observation of the hypnotic activity of metabolites of progesterone in 1957. The first compound used clinically was hydroxydione, a relatively slow-onset induction agent. One of the original compounds discovered, pregnanalone, is now undergoing investigation as an intravenous anaesthetic after recently being reformulated. Prior to this, two other intravenous steroid anaesthetic preparations have been extensively investigated one of which, althesin, was marketed for several years.

Althesin

Althesin is a mixture of two steroid anaesthetics, the more potent alphaxalone 9 mg/ml and alphadalone 3 mg/ml. The latter is added to help solubilize the former. Despite the mixing, the agent is still insoluble in water and was formulated in cremophor EL. With althesin, induction of anaesthesia is painless. It is non-irritant and its cardiovascular effects are similar to thiopentone although involuntary movements are common. Its elimination half-life is 29 min and recovery from anaesthesia is quick and smooth and the drug became popular both as an induction agent and for use by infusion both for maintenance of anaesthesia and for sedation in the intensive care unit.

The drug was withdrawn by the manufacturers after concern about the high incidence of adverse reactions estimated at 1 in 900 administrations and due to the solvent cremophor El. This was not a true IgE-mediated anaphylaxis but believed to be mediated by the alternative pathway involving complement activation.

Minaxolone

Minaxolone is a water-soluble steroid induction agent with an elimination half-life of 40–80 min but otherwise similar to althesin. Investigation was discontinued after toxicological problems.

Eltanolone (pregnanalone)

Pregnanalone has now been reformulated in an oil/water emulsion and is being investigated under the name Eltanolone. Eltanolone has a high therapeutic index. Clinically the induction dose is in the range of 0.5 – 0.9 mg/kg. The drug causes a transient increase in heart rate and a maximum reduction in blood pressure of around 20%; ventilatory depression is modest. Recovery from Eltanolone appears to be somewhat slower than that seen after propofol. Eltanolone has a high clearance with a hepatic extraction ratio close to 1, suggesting that it is cleared from the body via other tissues aside from the liver. The drug is still undergoing investigation and has not yet been released for general use.

Propanadid

Propanadid is a eugenol derivative. Its use is characterized by a very rapid recovery. It is the only agent in which metabolism plays a significant part in the initial reduction in plasma concentration precipitating recovery of conciousness. Induction of anaesthesia was associated with hyperventilation followed by apnoea and marked cardiovascular depression. Postoperative vomiting and venous irritation was common and adverse reactions were estimated to occur in approximately 1 in 500 administrations. For this reason the drug was withdrawn.

FURTHER READING

Berkowitz DE, Schinne DA. New advances in receptor pharmacology. *Current Opinion in Anaesthesiology* 1991; **4**: 486–96.

Cullen PM, Turtle M, Prys-Roberts C, Way WC, Dye J. Effect of propofol on baroflex activity in humans. *Anesthesia and Analgesia* 1987; **66**: 1115–20.

Dundee JW, Sear JW. Intravenous anaesthesia – What is new? *Bailliere's Clinical Anaesthesiology* Vol 5, No 2. London: Bailliere Tindal, 1991.

Dundee JW, Wyant GM. *Intravenous anasthesia* 2nd edn. London: Churchill Livingstone, 1988.

Franks NP, Lieb WR. Molecular and cellular mechanisms of general anaesthesia. *Nature* 1994; **367**:607–14.

Hull CJ. Pharmacokinetics and pharmacodynamics. *British Journal of Anaesthesia* 1979; **51**: 579–94.

Jensen NF, Fiddler DS, Stripe V. Anaesthetic considerations in porthyrias. *Anaesthesia and Analgesia* 1994; **80**: 591–9.

Reeves JG, Fragen RJ, Vinik HR, Greenblatt DJ. Midazolam: pharmacology and uses. *Anesthesiology* 1985; **62**: 310–24.

Sebel PS, Lowdon JD. Propofol: A new intravenous anaesthetic. *Anesthesiology* 1989; **71**: 260–77.

Smith I, White PF, Nathanson M, Gouldson R. Propofol, an update on its clinical use. *Anaesthesiology* 1994; **81**: 1005–43.

White PF. Kinetics of anaesthetic drugs in clinical anaesthesiology. *Bailliere's Clinical Anaesthesiology* Vol 5, No 3. London: Bailliere Tindal, 1991.

White PF, Way WL, Trevor AJ. Ketamine – Its pharmacology and therapeutic uses. *Anesthesiology* 1982; **56**: 119–36.

6

Therapeutic Gases

RF Armstrong

That oxygen is of fundamental importance to the mammalian organism is clear from a consideration of cellular metabolism. Oxidative phosphorylation taking place in the mitochondria consumes oxygen with the production of ATP, a source of readily accessible energy. At critically low levels of oxygen tension in the mitochondria (0.3 kPA) oxidative phosphorylation fails and cellular respiration becomes anaerobic.

This inefficient process produces a poor yield of ATP, capable of supporting voluntary muscle for a short time but unable to fuel the high-energy using tissues such as the brain and kidney. In addition, lactic acid production causes a rapid reduction in tissue pH with deleterious effects on cellular function. Maintenance of appropriate oxygen tensions is therefore one of the body's most important homeostatic functions. At the same time the system of oxygen uptake and transport is highly vulnerable to interference, a problem made worse by the inability of the body to store oxygen.

The process by which oxygen is taken up by the lung and directed to the body can be represented by a cascade in which oxygen moves down a gradient of partial pressures from air (PO_2 21 kPa), alveoli (13.7 kPa), arterial blood (13.2 kPa) and capillary (6.8 kPa) to the mitochondria (0.5–3.0 kPa). Alternatively, this process can be viewed as a circular system in which oxygen is taken up at the pulmonary capillaries, onloaded on to a transport system and distributed around the body (Fig. 6.1).

During disease states, oxygen flow to the tissues may be impaired at several levels. Respiratory disorders may interfere with oxygen uptake at the lungs and cardiovascular failure may hinder oxygen transport.

In order to improve oxygenation, consideration needs to be given to the process of oxygen uptake and how it can be manipulated. Points of access to the oxygen cascade range from the inspired mixture, through pulmonary ventilation to the oxygen transport system itself. Clearly it is important to identify where any defect exists in the system. This may require simple blood gas measurements or the more complex assessment of cardiac output.

THE INSPIRED MIXTURE AND OXYGEN TENSION

Approximately 20.9% of dry inspired air is oxygen. Given a normal barometric pressure of 100 kPa (760 mmHg) at sea level the inspired oxygen tension (P_iO_2) of dry inspired gas in the trachea will be 20.93/100 × 100 = 20.93 kPa. Owing to the presence of water vapour exerting a pressure of approximately 6 kPa, there is a slight reduction in oxygen tension in tracheal air. At alveolar level a further reduction in tension occurs according to the simplified alveolar air equation

$$P_AO_2 = F_iO_2(P_b - PH_2O) - \frac{P_aCO_2}{RQ}$$

where F_iO_2 is fractional inspired oxygen concentration; P_b is atmospheric pressure; RQ is the respiratory quotient; PH_2O is water vapour pressure and P_AO_2 = alveolar oxygen tension.

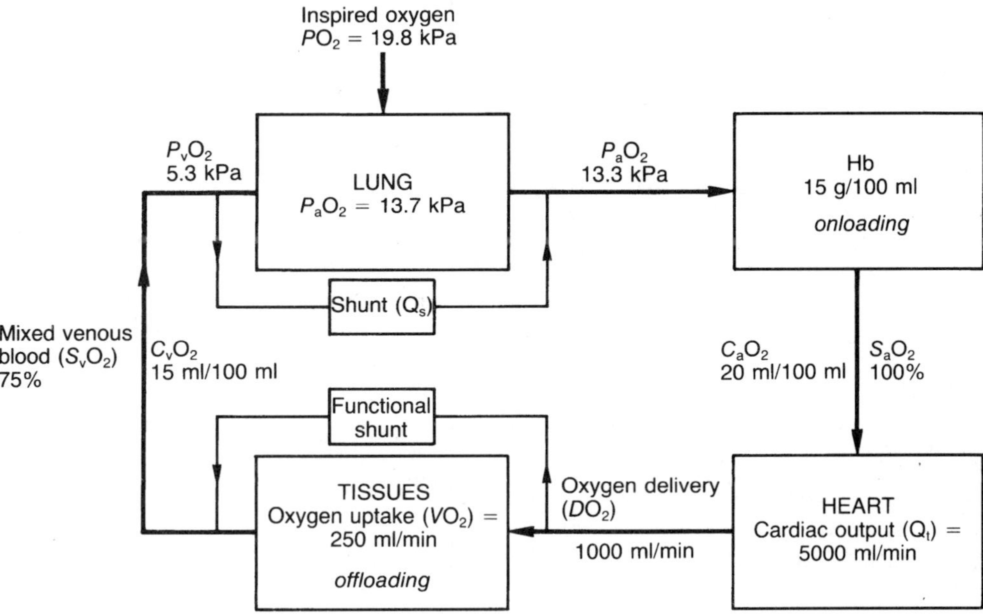

FIGURE 6.1 Oxygen flow. A circuit diagram.

From the alveolar air equation it can be seen how a period of hypoventilation will affect oxygenation. Assuming an arterial PCO_2 of 13.0 kPa in a patient breathing air, the alveolar air equation can be substituted as follows.

$$P_AO_2 = 0.21(100 - 6) - \frac{13}{0.8} = 3.49 \text{ kPa}$$

Given the slight drop in oxygen tension from alveolus to arterial blood, the consequences of such a low alveolar oxygen tension are likely to be serious. However, by increasing the inspired oxygen concentration to as little as 30% a significant improvement occurs, for example

$$P_AO_2 = 0.3(100 - 6) - \frac{13}{0.8} = 12 \text{ kPa}$$

With the aid of this equation it is also obvious that a reduction in PCO_2, for example by artificial ventilation, will of itself improve oxygenation.

The alveolar arterial difference

In the normal lung there is a difference of approximately 2 kPa between alveolar and arterial PO_2 (P_aO_2). With increasing age this may rise to 5.0 kPa. The difference is due to the presence of channels allowing mixed venous blood to percolate via Thebesian veins or bronchopulmonary anastomoses, across the pulmonary circuit without exposure to alveolar gas. In pathological states this difference may be markedly increased by the presence of shunts (areas of perfusion without ventilation) or by ventilation perfusion mismatch. Both these abnormalities may exist at the same time causing a flow of imperfectly oxygenated blood to reach the left atrium, with an inevitable reduction in P_aO_2. Common causes of this are pneumonia oedema or neoplasm producing areas of collapse and consolidation.

Management of the hypoxaemic patient is directed at improving the P_aO_2 with oxygen. In the case of a large shunt (over 30% of the cardiac output), oxygen therapy will not be very effective. This is illustrated by the isoshunt diagram (Fig. 6.2). In Fig. 6.2 an arteriovenous oxygen difference of 5.0 ml is assumed, as in the clinical situation mixed venous oxygen levels may not be available. Although in practice a trial and error approach is often used to choose the right inspired oxygen concentration, the virtual shunt diagram provides a useful insight into the relationship between F_iO_2 and P_aO_2 at different shunt levels.

EVALUATION OF BLOOD GASES

An important step in the management of the hypoxaemic patient is to ascertain the degree of respiratory impairment. Measurement of blood gases is the cornerstone of this process but not before evaluation of the F_iO_2. If the oxygen mask is of the type giving a known concentration then the alveolar tension can be easily calculated using the alveolar air equation. From this the arterial tension that should be present if the lungs were normal, can be derived. To illustrate this point

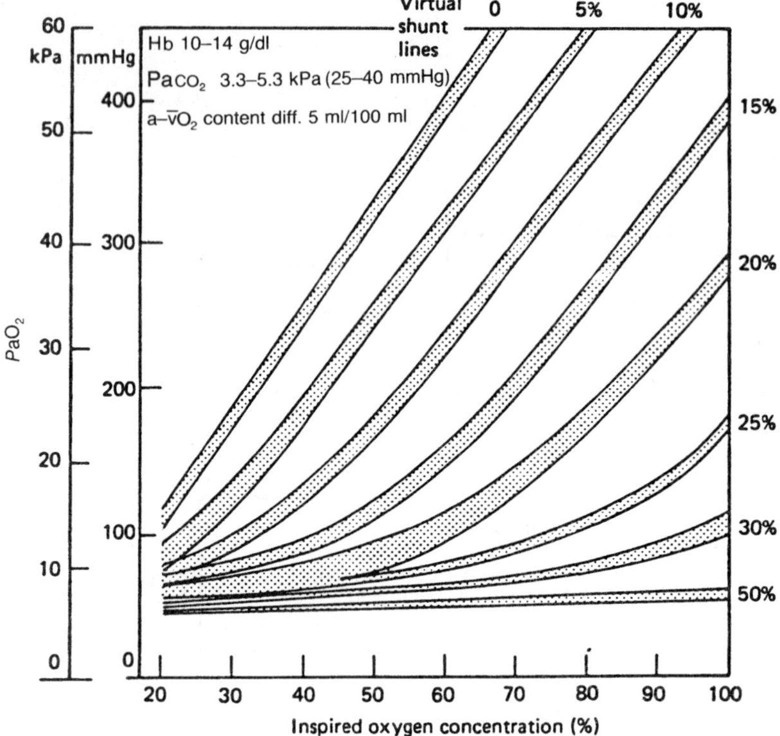

FIGURE 6.2 Isoshunt lines (Reproduced with permission from Benatar SR, Hewlett AM, Nunn JF. *British Journal of Anaesthesia* 1973; 45: 711).

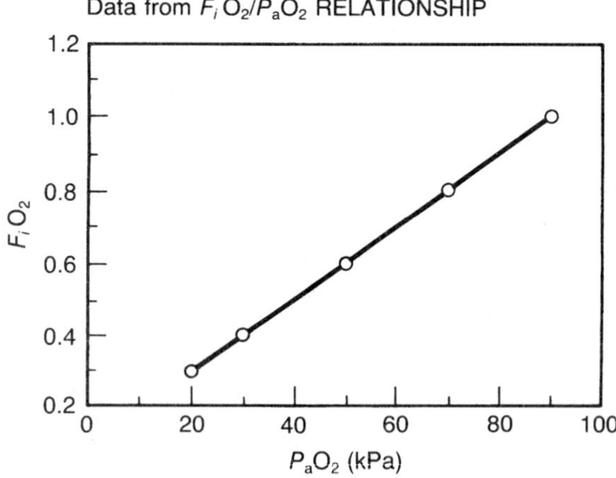

FIGURE 6.3 Relationship between inspired oxygen concentration and calculated alveolar oxygen tension.

consider the blood gases of a fireman rescued from a smoke filled room:

P_aO_2 13.5 kPa
P_aCO_2 5.0 kPa
pH 7.38
HCO_3 24 mmol
Saturation 100%

At first sight these results seem normal. However, when the inspired oxygen concentration is noted to be 60% the degree of respiratory impairment becomes clear. Consideration of the alveolar air equation reveals that the P_aO_2 should be approximately 50 kPa. In general terms the fireman's respiratory function could be described as only being 25% of normal. Figure 6.3 demonstrates the relationship between F_iO_2 and calculated alveolar PO_2.

Thus by comparing the expected P_aO_2 with the actual P_aO_2 the clinician can gain a useful insight into the state of the patient's lungs. At the same time an apparently normal saturation value can be kept in perspective knowing that on oxygen therapy a saturation of 100% does not exclude severe lung disorder.

A useful clinical guideline is that if the P_aO_2 is less than one-third of expected then the patient has a serious degree of respiratory impairment, possibly indicating positive pressure support.

OXYGEN THERAPY

Once the decision to give oxygen is made, then an appropriate administration system has to be chosen. Leigh[1] has divided oxygen masks into two groups, namely fixed performance and variable performance. The former give accurate inspired oxygen concentrations independently of patient factors, the latter are inaccurate low flow devices giving concentrations which vary according to patients' respiratory characteristics.

FLOW RATES DURING SPONTANEOUS VENTILATION

During spontaneous breathing in the healthy adult, inspiratory flow rates reach a peak of approximately 40 l/min. At end expiration a pause occurs during which there is no flow (Fig. 6.4). During exertion or tachypnoeic states flow rates increase to levels of 50 l/min and the expiratory pause decreases. It is these factors that will affect the inspired oxygen concentration.

Variable performance masks receive 4–6 l/min from the flow meters into the small reservoir space between face and mask. This space is minimized to prevent rebreathing of expired carbon dioxide. The effect of this low quantity of oxygen flowing into the inspired airstream can be compared to the effects of the River Fleet flowing into the Thames. There is immediate dilution by the greater airflow so that the final inspired oxygen concentration is not only low, it is not known. Furthermore, it is likely to vary from breath to breath and from minute to minute. These masks are therefore only suitable for giving 'some' oxygen to patients with low oxygen demands and whose exact F_iO_2 is not likely to be needed. Fixed performance masks are usually based on a venturi system. In this arrangement oxygen from the flowmeter entrains air at a venturi. As a result a high flow of oxygen-enriched air of known concentration is directed at the patient's face. This rapid flow matches the patient's own inspiratory flow so that no extraneous air is sucked around the sides of the mask and the final concentration is known. Masks of this type give a range of concentrations from 24 to 60%, depending on the size of the venturi (Fig. 6.5).

When higher concentrations are needed, as for example in carbon monoxide poisoning, a system that includes a reservoir bag is needed. If adequate arterial oxygen tensions are still not achievable then positive pressure ventilation with high inspired oxygen concentrations should be instituted.

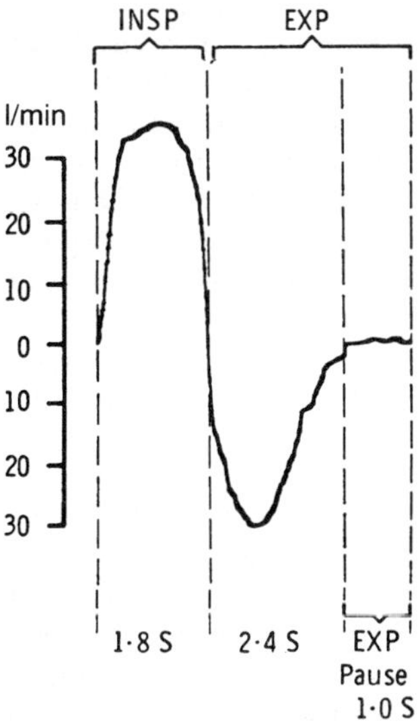

FIGURE 6.4 One respiratory cycle from pneumotachograph of a resting healthy male subject. (Reproduced with permission from JM Leigh. In: Scurr C, Feldman S, Soni N eds. *Scientific foundations of anaesthesia*, 4th edn. Oxford: Butterworth Heinemann.)

OXYGEN CONTENT AND THE DISSOCIATION CURVE

Although oxygen tension is of undeniable importance, oxygen content must also be considered. A look at the oxygen dissociation curve (Fig. 6.6) reveals that a saturation of 100% normally corresponds to an oxygen content of 20.9 ml.

Several points emerge from a study of the dissociation curve. With worsening respiratory function, oxygen saturations and therefore content are well maintained until an oxygen tension of approximately 8.0 kPa is reached. At this point the steep slope of the curve results in a rapid fall off in oxygen content from 18 ml to 5.0 ml for a drop in P_aO_2 of only 6.0 kPa. Clearly it is important to keep saturations above 90% (P_aO_2 8 kPa) if serious hypoxaemia is to be avoided.

The shape of this curve can be utilized in the management of patients with chronic hypercarbic respiratory failure. The technique of controlled oxygen therapy[2] relies on the use of only minor increases in inspired oxygen concentrations (24–28%) to generate small improvements in P_aO_2. This avoids suppression of any hypoxic respiratory drive but at the same time achieves a large incremental increase in oxygen content (Fig. 6.7).

Unfortunately the deserved popularity of this approach can result in some hypoxic patients receiving

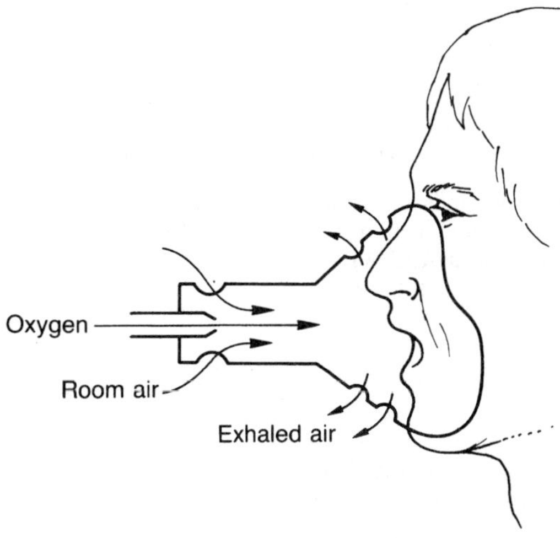

FIGURE 6.5 Venturi system of oxygen delivery. (Reproduced with permission from Adams AP, Cashman J. *Anaesthesia, analgesia and intensive care*. London: Edward Arnold, 1991.)

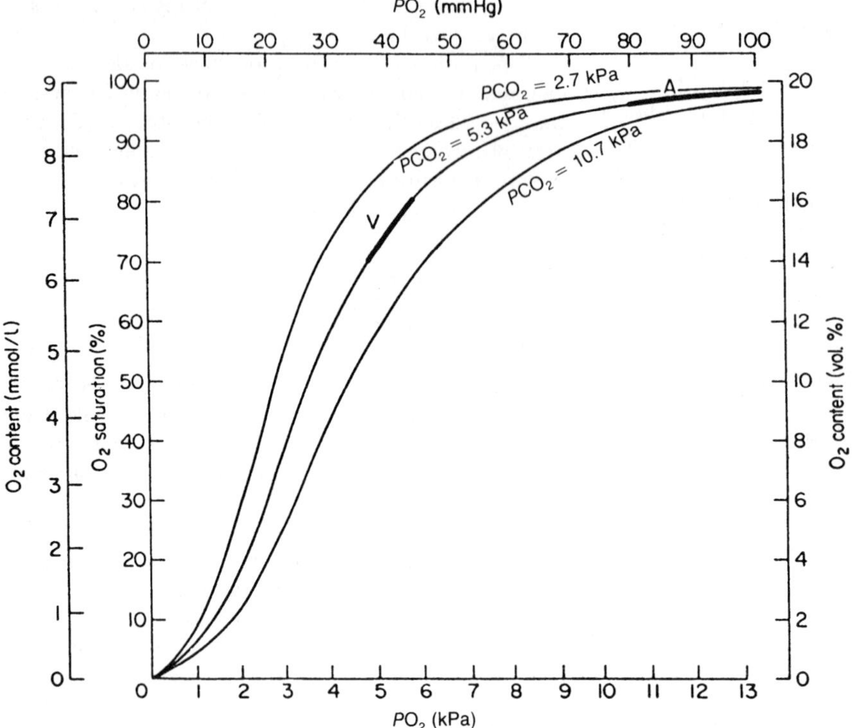

FIGURE 6.6 The oxyhaemoglobin dissociation curve. (Reproduced with permission from Sykes MN. *Respiratory failure.* Oxford: Blackwell Scientific.)

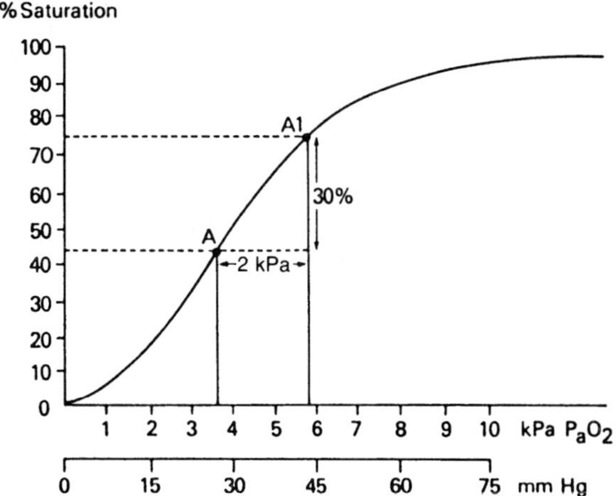

FIGURE 6.7 The significant effect of a small increment in oxygen tension on oxygen saturation. (Reproduced with permission from Aitkenhead AR, Smith G. *Textbook of anaesthesia.* Edinburgh: Churchill Livingstone.)

unnecessarily low inspired oxygen concentrations even though they do not fall into the category of chronic hypercarbic respiratory failure and are not reliant on a hypoxic drive. In these circumstances it is only by frequent monitoring of blood gases that mistaken choices of inspired oxygen concentration can be recognized and corrected.

MONITORING OXYGENATION

While blood gas measurement is the gold standard of oxygenation monitoring, the growing use of oximetry deserves attention. In this technique two wavelengths of light, red and infrared, are transmitted from light-emitting diodes and passed through an arterial bed such as the finger. Part of the light is absorbed by haemoglobin, part by oxyhaemoglobin, and part by the tissues. Because there is a slight increase in the volume of the tissues due to the pulsation of arteries and arterioles with each heartbeat, light absorption varies during the pulsatile and non-pulsatile phases of blood flow. By subtracting the transmitted signals during the non-pulsatile phase from the total signal the light absorption caused by the arterial blood can be differentiated from that produced by the tissues, bones and skin.[3]

While errors may occur in this sort of system[4] oximeters have now become accepted as a means of monitoring oxygenation and have proved to be a major advance in patient safety. Minor problems are a tendency to inaccuracy at low saturations and a delayed response in poorly perfused skin. On occasions interpretation of the readings may cause confusion, particularly in patients receiving oxygen therapy. In the case of deteriorating respiratory function the P_aO_2 may be steadily falling having started at perhaps 30 kPa on an F_iO_2 of 0.6. However, there will not be a fall in saturation until the P_aO_2 reaches approximately 10 kPa. Over 11 kPa, the saturation remains a reassuring 95–100%. Staff caring for patients with respiratory problems should be warned that recognition of developing hypoxaemia can be delayed when oximetry is combined with oxygen therapy.

OXYGEN TRANSPORT

Although a low arterial oxygen content provides a serious threat to the integrity of the organism, there are several compensatory mechanisms by which the effects of oxygen lack can be forestalled. The ability of the healthy body to compensate for hypoxia can be illustrated by the adaptation to altitude. During their oxygen-free Everest climb in 1978, Messner and Habeler experienced alveolar oxygen tensions which as a result of the low barometric pressure at that altitude (8847 m) have been calculated to be in the region of 4.8 kPa. At alveolar pressures of this order, the P_aO_2 will be in the region of 3 kPa and corresponds to an O_2 content of 9.0 ml/100 ml of blood. While there are other compensatory mechanisms including polycythaemia, oxygen dissociation curve shifts and vasodilatation, a major factor in the body's ability to deal with such low oxygen contents is the ability to increase cardiac output and organ blood flow. By mimicking this response the clinician can support the body's attempts to function in conditions of oxygen lack. Manipulation of the oxygen flux[5] has recently been demonstrated to be of importance in the management of shock.[6]

Normal levels of oxygen flux or delivery (DO_2) are 1000 ml/min and can be calculated as follows:

$$\text{Cardiac output (l/min)} \times \text{oxygen content (ml/l)} = \text{oxygen delivery}$$

$$\text{i.e. } 5 \text{ l/min} \times 200 \text{ ml } O_2/\text{l} = 1000 \text{ ml/min}$$

Given a normal oxygen consumption of 250 ml/min, it is clear that an adequate oxygen flux or delivery can be maintained in the face of low oxygen content by raising cardiac output. In routine clinical care this is done by ensuring proper filling of the intravascular space, correcting a low haemoglobin and by use of inotropes.

For the clinician responsible for supervision of oxygen therapy it is important not to neglect cardiac output. Omitting to support this vital transport system can be compared to a relief agency that loads its planes with vital supplies but fails to check they are capable of flying. Adequate intravascular filling, correction of anaemia and support of cardiac output are all part of the process of giving oxygen to the patient.

INDICATIONS FOR OXYGEN THERAPY

Assuming the patient under consideration does not belong to that small subset whose respiratory drive is dependent on hypoxia, a general indication for oxygen therapy is a P_aO_2 below 10 kPa, a saturation less than 95%, or a respiratory rate above 25 or below 10 per minute. Where oxygen measurements are unavailable certain clinical situations demand the use of oxygen. These include the whole range of acute and chronic lung disorders, postoperative patients, particularly the old and obese, myocardial infarction and acute hypotension. The growing use of potent pain therapy techniques utilizing intravenous and epidural opiates may also indicate O_2 therapy if hypoxaemia consequent upon respiratory depression is to be avoided. In carbon monoxide poisoning the high affinity of carbon monoxide for haemoglobin (200 times that of oxygen) results in a dangerous reduction in oxygen carrying capacity. At levels of over 50% carboxyhaemoglobin the effects are lethal. Oxygen administration at high F_iO_2 with the possible addition of intermittent positive pressure ventilation increases the rate of elimination of carbon monoxide and will reduce lethality and long-term cerebral injury.

HYPERBARIC OXYGEN

At pressures of two atmospheres (2 ATA) the P_iO_2 of humidified oxygen is approximately 190 kPa. Although the arterial PO_2 rises to over 170 kPa in these circumstances, the inability of haemoglobin to carry more oxygen results in a meagre oxygen content increase to 23.4 ml/100 ml.[7] Nevertheless, allowing for a normal AV oxygen difference of 5.0 ml this gives a venous oxygen content of 18.4 ml and a venous PO_2 of 9.1 kPa. Because tissue PO_2, corresponds more closely to venous PO_2 this improvement has been the basis for using hyperbaric oxygen therapeutically.

In particular, various authorities have recommended this treatment for gas gangrene and carbon monoxide poisoning.[8] However, the logistic difficulty involved in getting ill patients to centres with these facilities and the controversy that surrounds their results has resulted in a poor take up of this treatment option.

OXYGEN TOXICITY

During the administration of high oxygen concentrations deleterious effects have been reported on brain, immature retina and lung. Convulsions occurring at partial pressures over 2 ATA have proved a major hazard in diving work but do not constitute a clinical problem. Retrolental fibroplasia in the premature infant has been attributed to the use of high inspired oxygen concentrations. The pathophysiological process produced by hyperoxia ($P_aO_2 > 27$ kPa) is initially a constriction of the retinal vessels which develops if unchecked to a vaso-obliterative process, with retinal scarring, detachment and blindness. Infants below 1500 g body weight suffer the highest incidence of retrolental fibroplasia with described frequencies of 16–34%.[9] Prevention of this disorder requires strict monitoring of arterial blood gases or transcutaneous oxygen.

Pulmonary oxygen toxicity remains an ever-present concern in both adult and neonatal intensive care though its pathogenesis is still unclear. Early work in rats[10] demonstrated damage to the capillary endothelium with increasing permeability. Later, replacement of the Type 1 epithelial cells by Type 2 cells occurs. Subsequent work on humans has been complicated by the difficulty in differentiating potential oxygen damage from the condition that preceded its use. Current practice is to minimize the use of concentrations above 60% by the judicious use of bronchodilators and techniques of assisted breathing such as positive end expiratory or constant positive airway pressure. In general, an oxyhaemoglobin saturation of 90% is considered the lowest acceptable level and efforts should be made to keep the F_iO_2 as low as possible commensurate with this objective.

The source of oxygen's toxicity may lie in the capacity of the oxygen molecule to change into a reduced form by the addition of a single electron to its outer shell. The resulting highly reactive and unstable free radical known as superoxide anion is not only toxic but may form other dangerous chemicals including hydrogen peroxide and hydroxyl free radical. Oxygen-derived free radicals are important biologically as bactericidal agents in neutrophils and macrophages. In certain circumstances these substances may be released into the surrounding cellular environment, a process that has been hypothesized as a contributing factor in the adult respiratory distress syndrome. During administration of high oxygen concentrations, oxygen partial pressures in the tissues may reach levels over 60 kPa causing oxygen free radicals to be released. This may be the basis of pulmonary oxygen toxicity. Free radical scavengers such as ascorbic acid, vitamin E and the enzymes superoxide dismutase and catalase afford the body protection against free radicals. However, as yet, these chemicals have no useful clinical place in therapy.

RESPIRATORY FAILURE

Failure to maintain normal blood gases is a fairly stringent definition of respiratory failure yet it affords the medical and nursing team the advantage of allowing identification of the at-risk patient. This allows their proper placement, the choice of monitoring systems and the correct method of oxygen administration. Under certain circumstances oxygenation or carbon dioxide excretion becomes so deranged that alternative forms of oxygen therapy have to be introduced:

CRITERIA FOR INTRODUCTION OF RESPIRATORY SUPPORT	
Respiratory rate	>30/min
Vital capacity	<10–15 ml/kg
P_aO_2	<11.0 kPa on 40% O_2
or P_aO_2	<one-third expected
P_aCO_2	high enough to lower pH to below 7.2

CONSTANT POSITIVE AIRWAY PRESSURE (CPAP)

In the spontaneously breathing, co-operative and conscious patient whose oxygenation criteria meet those above, constant positive airway pressure via a tight-fitting mask provides effective treatment, reducing respiratory rate (with its associated high energy demands) as well as improving P_aO_2. In the unconscious patient this system can be used via an endotracheal tube. The technique allows the patient to breathe from a high flow, high concentration source of oxygen and exhale against a valve opening at pressures from 2.5 to 10 cmH_2O. During the inspiratory cycle the resistance to gas flow is so low that no fall occurs in airway pressure.

Problems associated with CPAP stem from the application of pressure to the airway. They range from damage to the bridge of the nose caused by the tight application of the mask, or distension of the stomach with oxygen, to the more serious problems of pulmonary barotrauma and depression of cardiac output.

NASAL CPAP AND VENTILATION

Recognition by clinicians of the problems associated with obstructive sleep apnoea stimulated interest in methods of respiratory support that were non-invasive and simple enough to be used in the home. Nasal CPAP using pressures of 5–10 cmH_2O was found to be capable of splinting the upper airway in this group of patients,[11] with significant clinical improvement. Subsequently nasal ventilation was introduced using the same type of mask. This technique needed the development of a new generation of cheap simple ventilators capable of responding rapidly to the patient's inspiratory efforts with a delivered tidal volume as well as having the facility to take over ventilation in the absence of spontaneous breaths.

Several types of machine are now available, some battery driven, others with their own compressor (Bromptonpac). An increasing number of publications[12] bear witness to their value in acute and chronic respiratory failure both in the hospital and the home.

INTERMITTENT POSITIVE PRESSURE VENTILATION (IPPV)

Once the non-invasive forms of respiratory support fail to arrest any decline in the patient's condition, intubation of the airway and institution of mechanical ventilation must follow. The variety of machines available, including flow or pressure generated, time or volume cycled, electronic or pneumatic, makes choice difficult. Apart from considerations of cost and reliability, the growing use of ventilatory modes incorporating spontaneous breaths by the patient means that circuitry resistance must be minimized. In this way excessive work of breathing[13] due to low gas flows, slow responding demand valves and poorly designed patient circuits, can be reduced.

INTERMITTENT MANDATORY VENTILATION (IMV)

In this sophistication of IPPV, the patient breathes spontaneously through the ventilator circuit but receives at set intervals a machine breath.[14] These mandatory breaths can be synchronized to fit in with the patient's respiratory pattern so that extra breaths are not 'stacked' on top of a spontaneous tidal volume – a process likely to cause dangerous rises in intrathoracic pressure.

IMV has not been shown to reduce weaning time from IPPV but there is some evidence that respiratory muscle retraining may occur and that sedation needs are lowered. Given the many drawbacks of sedation, such as reduction in blood pressure, difficulty in establishing enteral nutrition, and persisting effects, any technique that can claim to minimize drug usage is to be encouraged.

POSITIVE END-EXPIRATORY PRESSURE (PEEP)

The application of a positive pressure (normally 5–10 cmH_2O) during the expiratory phase of the ventilator's respiratory cycle has been shown to improve arterial oxygen tension, increase functional residual capacity and lung compliance. There is no evidence, however, that it does much else. Early claims of preventing acute respiratory distress syndrome (ARDS), reducing lung water, and hastening lung recovery have never been proved.

Nevertheless, it has a very definite place in modern intensive care,[15] usually being introduced at saturations below 90% on inspired oxygen concentrations above 0.6. This allows reduction in F_iO_2 and with it the danger of pulmonary oxygen toxicity. Drawbacks include pulmonary barotrauma and depression of cardiac output. Above PEEP levels of 10 cmH_2O intensive haemodynamic monitoring is advisable. Current practice favours the use of sufficient PEEP to support oxygenation, avoidance of lung damage by restricting airway pressure and tidal volume, permitting moderate hypercarbia and, when necessary, using reversal of inspiratory and expiratory times to recruit the 'slow' alveoli.

CARBON DIOXIDE

Whether carbon dioxide can be described as a therapeutic gas is arguable. Nevertheless, its effects are of such profound importance in the body (regulating respiratory minute volume, cardiac output, peripheral vascular resistance and cerebral blood flow) that its inclusion as such may be forgiven.

Carbon dioxide is an end product of metabolism. At rest approximately 200 ml/min are produced by the body rising to much higher levels (>1000 ml/min) during exercise. From its cellular origin carbon dioxide is transported to the lung where in the steady state its

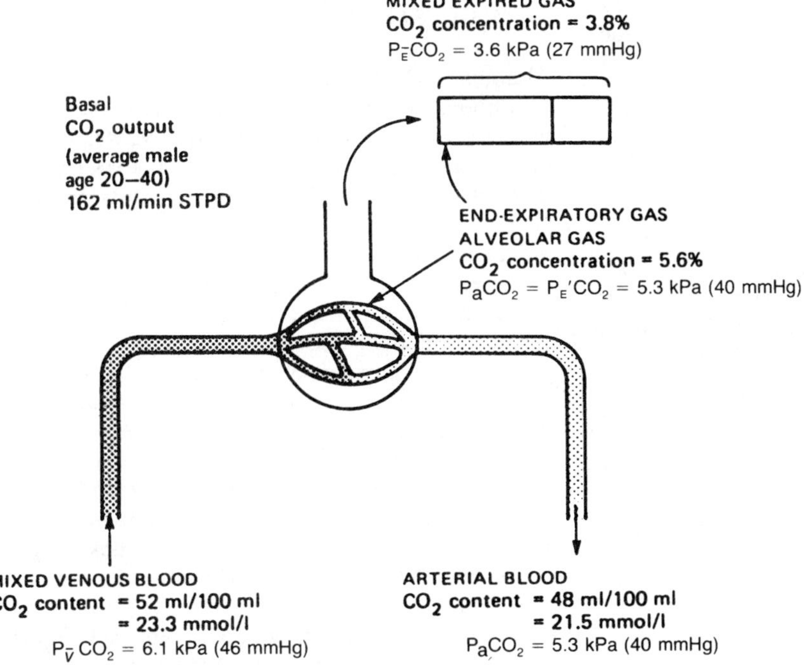

FIGURE 6.8 Normal values of CO_2 levels. (Reproduced with permission from Nunn JF. *Applied respiratory physiology*, 3rd edn. London: Butterworths.)

elimination by pulmonary ventilation equals the rate of production. Most CO_2 is carried in the plasma as bicarbonate (50%) with smaller amounts travelling in solution, some in combination with plasma proteins, and the rest (25%) in the red cell as carbamino-haemoglobin.

Carbon dioxide stores in the body are very large, approximating 120 l[7] and situated in blood, organs, muscle and bone. One of the benefits of this large storage facility is the ability of the asphyxiating or hypoventilating patient to accommodate retention of CO_2 without marked increases in PCO_2. At respiratory arrest the rate of rise of P_aCO_2 is only of the order of 0.4–0.8 kPa/min. The normal physiological levels of CO_2 are shown in Fig. 6.8.

Effects on the respiratory system

Groups of cells in the medulla respond to a variety of stimuli to control respiration. The dominant stimulus is carbon dioxide acting on chemoreceptors, both at the medullary centre as well as peripherally at chemoreceptors in the carotid and aortic bodies. Surrounded by cerebrospinal fluid (CSF) the central chemoreceptors respond to changes in hydrogen ion concentration. Although the cell membrane of the blood–brain barrier is impermeable to hydrogen ions, there is rapid equilibration between CO_2 in the blood and the CSF as CO_2 can rapidly diffuse across the blood–brain barrier. Thus changes in arterial CO_2 produce immediate respiratory responses as CO_2 reacts with water in the CSF to form carbonic acid, bicarbonate and hydrogen ions. With increasing inspired concentrations, the minute volume increases rapidly, reaching levels as high as 70 l/min when breathing 10% CO_2. After some time this response fades as bicarbonate ions from the plasma cross the blood–brain barrier to act as a buffer. It is for this reason that chronically raised levels of CO_2 produce a diminishing ventilatory drive as CSF pH returns to normal.

The peripheral chemoreceptors situated in the carotid and aortic bodies are sensitive to both carbon dioxide and oxygen and are stimulated by both hypoxia and hypercarbia to increase ventilatory drive. Together with central receptors and pulmonary stretch receptors they are co-ordinated by higher centres to stimulate inspiratory and expiratory neurones driving intercostal and diaphragmatic muscle. By this organized, interactive and sensitive system the body maintains its internal milieu, keeping pH and blood gas tensions within the normal range.

Effects on the circulatory system

The overall effects of carbon dioxide on cardiovascular function are the result of several conflicting actions. Acting directly, carbon dioxide depresses cardiac output and causes vasodilatation. Indirectly, however, there is marked stimulation of the sympathetic nervous system with release of adrenaline and noradrenaline. The overall result is an increase in cardiac output, a rise in blood pressure and a fall in systemic vascular resistance.

Effects on the cerebral circulation

The cerebral blood flow (CBF) usually approximates to 50 ml/100 g of brain/min and shows a linear response to carbon dioxide rising steadily with increasing PCO_2 to a maximum of around 100 ml/100 g.[16] As PCO_2 is reduced towards 2.5 kPa CBF decreases to around 20 ml/100 g/min. Below this level, cerebral vasoconstriction becomes so intense that tissue hypoxia may occur producing cerebral vasodilatation.

These responses are utilized in the management of head injury, when hyperventilation techniques are used to reduce intracranial pressure (ICP). In these circumstances, arterial PCO_2 levels of between 3.5 and 4.0 kPa are recommended. However, because CSF bicarbonate readjusts to this low value, the duration of cerebral vasoconstriction is unpredictable. Furthermore, over-enthusiastic ventilation by producing alkalosis may provoke tissue hypoxia and consequent vasodilatation. Finally, a too rapid rise of PCO_2 to normocapnia may cause a rapid increase in CBF (and ICP) as CSF pH falls in the presence of a low bicarbonate. Because of these uncertainties there is a strong case for measuring ICP where expertise and facilities allow.

Uses of carbon dioxide

Although CO_2 has some historical reputation as an anaesthetic (Henry Hill Hickman 1824) the dangers of acidosis and convulsions have outweighed any other considerations. However, in the UK cylinders of CO_2 have been used by anaesthetists for many years, being used to stimulate respiration during the administration of inhalational anaesthetics and thus to hasten uptake. More commonly, CO_2 administration has been popular as a means of raising PCO_2 at the end of an anaesthetic involving hyperventilation techniques. Following a study by Razis[17] and a subsequent editorial in the *British Journal of Anaesthesia*[18] it emerged that over 60% of UK anaesthetists used CO_2 on a daily basis and that 77% of respondents objected to its removal from the machine. Two hundred respondents knew of CO_2 related accidents, of which 29% were fatal. Most of these cases were due to the rotameter bobbin floating unrecognized at the top of the flowmeter.

Present recommendations are to remove CO_2 cylinders from machines until required and to alter the design of CO_2 flowmeters so that only low flows (500 ml/min) are possible. In this respect it is of note that the British Anaesthetic and Respiratory Equipment Manufacturers' Association is currently devising a flow limitation device on the CO_2 flowmeter. The impression is that the use of CO_2 by anaesthetists is on the wane. Clearly, the Association of Anaesthetists of Great Britain and Ireland thinks this is a trend to be encouraged. Professor AP Adams sums it up 'It is best reserved for putting out fires'.[19]

Measurement of carbon dioxide as a monitoring technique

Since the concept of minimal monitoring was introduced by hospitals associated with the Harvard Medical School and applied by the American Society of Anesthesiologists, end-tidal CO_2 analysis has become standard in many countries.[19]

In the UK, also, infrared absorption capnography is now widely used in modern anaesthetic and intensive care environments. Continuous sampling of inspiratory and expiratory gas produces the typical saw tooth pattern seen on the capnogram. The baseline represents inspired gas. Normally there should be no CO_2 measured at this stage unless rebreathing is present. The upstroke marks the rise in expired concentration as expiration begins, first emptying the anatomical deadspace (no CO_2) then displaying alveolar CO_2 as it rises to a plateau. Increases in the slope of the plateau suggest maldistribution of inspired gas. Air embolism or acute falls in cardiac output produce reductions in end-tidal readings due to poor perfusion of the lung and an increase in dead space. Finally the downstroke represents the arrival of the next breath. A checklist (Fig. 6.9) demonstrates the usefulness of this type of monitoring.

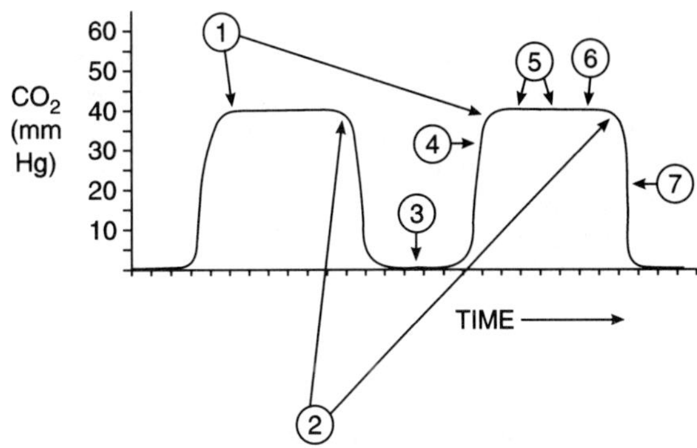

FIGURE 6.9 The checklist for a capnogram. 1. Plateau/onset. Is there a pattern giving evidence of ventilation? 2. Plateau/peak. Are peak values appropriate? Are the ventilator settings and the patient's respiratory pattern consistent with the capnogram and capnographic findings? 3. Baseline: Is the inspired carbon dioxide tension zero (normal baseline), or is there evidence of rebreathing (elevated baseline)? 4. Upstroke. Is there evidence of slow exhalation (slanted upstroke)? 5. Plateau/horizontal. Is there evidence of uneven emptying of lungs? 6. Plateau/smooth. Is expiration interrupted by inspiratory efforts? 7. Downstroke. Is the downstroke steep, or is there evidence of slow inspiration or partial rebreathing? (Reproduced with permission from Gravenstein JS, Paulus DA, Hayes TJ. *Capnography in clinical practice.* Stoneham, MA: Butterworths, 1989.)

HELIUM

The presence of helium in group VIII of the Periodic Table suggests its lack of chemical reactivity. Like the other noble gases, helium is present in air but undergoes no known chemical change in the body. Its uses in medicine are based on its low density and its extreme insolubility in water. In investigative respiratory physiology, known volumes and concentrations of helium breathed from a closed circuit can be used to measure functional residual capacity (FRC) and its derived values, residual volume and total lung capacity. Because it is not absorbed, its equilibrium concentration is proportional to the volume of air in the lung at end exhalation.

During prolonged diving at depths of greater than 50 m (pressures of 6 ATA) several problems manifest themselves. Breathing air the alveolar PO_2 will be approximately 120 kPA, possibly high enough to cause pulmonary oxygen toxicity, though not high enough to provoke convulsions. At this pressure nitrogen has a narcotic effect, dissolving in body tissues sufficiently to release bubbles on decompression, and because of its high density making breathing difficult. For these reasons helium has been introduced as a diluent gas, having no narcotic properties, a much lower density and being far less soluble in tissues.

The low density of helium allows it to flow through an orifice three times as fast as air. This has proved useful in certain respiratory disorders. During normal circumstances, air flow in the lung is predominantly laminar though turbulence is present in the larger airways. Once high flow rates or high resistance to gas flow is experienced the flow becomes increasingly turbulent. This situation commonly exists in conditions producing upper airway obstruction such as croup, postextubation stridor, or thermal injury. Because flow rates in turbulent conditions are inversely related to density and because helium has only one-seventh the density of air there is a case for the administration of helium and oxygen mixtures to these patients. Several publications bear testimony to the value of this approach[20] using 80/20% mixtures of helium and oxygen. However, drawbacks exist. In the case of a hypoxaemic patient, 20% oxygen may not suffice and the advantages gained by reducing the work of breathing may be offset by unacceptably low oxygen levels in the blood. Increasing the F_iO_2 will reduce the concentration of helium and thus increase the density.

NITRIC OXIDE

The recognition that nitric oxide (NO) was a potent endogenous vasodilator led to intensive study of this gas and its eventual synthesis from L-arginine.[21] Subsequently it was shown to be a powerful systemic and pulmonary vasodilator, producing its effect by activating cyclic guanosine monophosphate to cause relaxation of vascular smooth muscle. In the blood, nitric oxide binds rapidly to haemoglobin, becoming inactivated with a half life of only a few seconds.

Uses

The clinical uses of nitric oxide stem from its vasodilatory effects on the pulmonary circulation. In particular it is used in the treatment of pulmonary hypertension in the paediatric cardiac patient and in the Adult Respiratory Distress Syndrome (ARDS). In this latter group of patients with the typical non-homogeneous disorder of lung function, inhalation causes vasodilatation in the aerated zones of the lung resulting in reduced intrapulmonary shunt and improving V/Q ratios. In addition there is bronchodilation and a reduction in pulmonary artery pressures which facilitates right ventricular function. Because of its short half life systemic hypotensive effects are minimal and of no significance.

Toxicity

There is a theoretical possibility that oxidation of NO during the use of high F_iO_2 may lead to the formation of nitrogen dioxide and thus nitric acid. This highly toxic product is capable of causing an acid pneumonitis. However in the concentrations used in clinical practice (1–50 ppm) and with in-line monitoring of both nitric oxide and nitrogen dioxide levels toxic effects have not been reported. Neither has the formation of methaemoglobin been a clinical problem.

WATER VAPOUR

Normally the alveolar air is 100% saturated with water vapour. At 37°C this vapour exerts a pressure of approximately 6.25 kPa. A litre of inspired gas contains about 44 mgH_2O. Humidification and warming of the inspired air is carried out by the nasal passages and upper airway so that by the time gas reaches the trachea it is fully saturated. This process promotes the efficient performance of the respiratory cilia whose ability to clear mucus becomes progressively reduced below saturations of 75%. During respiratory therapy administration of dry gases, or bypassing the nose by intubation/tracheostomy can impair the function of this important defence system, reducing resistance to infection and the ability to expectorate particles and sputum. By adequately humidifying the inspired mixture, tenacious secretions are liquified, crusting and blockage of artificial airways is prevented and mucociliary clearance facilitated. Warming the inspired gas will not only increase water vapour pressure but prevent heat loss via the airway.

Techniques

Water humidifiers are a popular adjunct to respiratory care. Because saturation by water vapour is dependent on temperature, cold water baths are inefficient providing only 50–60% saturation. Most units now use heated humidifiers at temperatures of about 40°C, so that by the time the warmed and moist gases reach the patient the cooling effect of the delivery tubing will have reduced the inspired temperature to body heat. The drawbacks of this type of system are three-fold. First, there is bound to be condensation in the inspiratory limb of the circuit as the gases cool. If this is allowed to collect it may drain into the patient's respiratory passages causing coughing. Introducing water traps to collect this condensate increases junctions and the risk of leaks from disconnections. Second, heating systems have been known to malfunction resulting in thermal injury to the patient. Efforts to resolve this problem have been largely successful due to the introduction of thermostats in the baths and thermistors close to the patient. Feedback circuitry can then be used to maintain the bath temperature at desired levels. Finally, water baths may be a potent source of nosocomial infection if not properly cleaned and maintained.

Droplet humidifiers

These function by ultrasonic- or venturi-induced breakup of water films into clouds of fine droplets, some small enough to produce a colloidal suspension in air (aerosol). The droplets are carried into the lung to vaporize there or to be deposited as liquid. The site of deposition will depend on the particle size, smaller ones (2–10 μm) reaching the small bronchi or even alveoli. In intubated patients, this type of system can result in significant water overload. In non-intubated patients, it is doubtful whether any droplets reach the trachea.

Heat and moisture exchangers (HMEs)

These are plastic filters through which the patient breathes or is ventilated. Heat and moisture from the exhaled air are retained at the filter so that the next inspiration is warmed and humidified. Claims that they may act as bacterial filters allied with their simplicity and disposability have increased usage, but humidification is not very efficient. Reports of increased incidences of tube blockage associated with the use of HMEs have led to some reservations about their use. It is noteworthy that both heated water systems and HMEs can cause increases in circuitry resistance.

REFERENCES

1 Leigh JM. Variation in performance of oxygen therapy devices. *Anaesthesia* 1970; **25**: 210.

2 Campbell EJM. A method of controlled oxygen administration which reduces the risk of CO_2 retention. *Lancet* 1960; ii: 12.

3 Gravenstein JS. *Gas monitoring and pulse oximetry.* Stoneham, MA: Butterworth Heinemann, 1990.

4 Ralston AC, Webb RK, Runciman WB. Potential errors in pulse oximetry. *Anaesthesia* 1991; **46**(3): 202–6.

5 Nunn JF, Freeman J. Problems of oxygenation and oxygen transport during haemorrhage. *Anaesthesia* 1964; **19**: 206.

6 Shoemaker WC, Appel PL, Kram HB, Waxman K, Lee TS. Prospective trial of supranormal values of survivors as therapeutic goals in high risk surgical patients. *Chest* 1988; **94**: 1176–86.

7 Nunn JF. *Applied respiratory physiology*, 3rd edn. London: Butterworths, 1987.

8 Broome JR, Pearson RR, Skrine H. Carbon monoxide poisoning, forgotten not gone. *British Journal of Hospital Medicine* 1988; **39**: 298–305.

9 Merenstein JB, Gardner SL. *Handbook of neonatal intensive care.* USA: C.V. Mosby, 1989.

10 Weibel ER. Oxygen effect on lung cells. *Archives Internal Medicine* 1971; **128**: 54.

11 Sullivan CE, Issa FG, Berthon Jones M, Eves L. Reversal of obstructive sleep apnoea by continuous positive airway pressure applied through the nares. *Lancet* 1981; i: 862–5.

12 Elliot MW, Stevens MJ, Phillips GD, Branthwaite MA. Non invasive mechanical ventilation for acute respiratory failure. *British Medical Journal* 1990; **300**: 358–60.

13 Bersten AD, Rutten AJ, Vedig AE, Skowronski A. Additional work of breathing imposed by endotracheal tubes, breathing circuits and intensive care ventilators. *Critical Care Medicine* 1989; **17**: 671–7.

14 Kirby RR. Synchronised intermittent mandatory ventilation versus assist control: Just the facts ma'am. *Critical Care Medicine* 1989; **17**: 706–7.

15 Civetta JM. After quibbles and contrasts, concepts and caveats. *Chest* 1988; **93**: 897–8.

16 Reivich M. Arterial PCO_2 and cerebral haemodynamics. *American Journal of Physiology* 1964; **206**: 25.

17 Razis PA. Carbon dioxide – a survey of its use in anaesthesia in the UK. *Anaesthesia* 1989; **44**: 348–51.

18 Nunn JF ed. Carbon dioxide cylinders on anaesthetic apparatus. *British Journal of Anaesthesia* 1990; **65**: 155–6.

19 Adams AP. Safety in anaesthetic practice. In: Atkinson RS, Adams AP eds. *Recent advances in anaesthetics and analgesia* **17**. Edinburgh: Churchill Livingstone, 1992.

20 Kemper KJ, Ritz RH, Benson MS, Bishop MS. Helium oxygen mixture in the treatment of post extubation stridor in paediatric trauma patients. *Critical Care Medicine* 1991; **19**: 356–9.

21 Bone RC. A new therapy for the Adult Respiratory Distress Syndrome. *New England Journal of Medicine* 1993; **328**: 431–2.

7

Local Anaesthesia

Part I Pharmacology of Local Anaesthesia

RW Matthews

INTRODUCTION

By definition, anaesthesia implies loss of consciousness whereas the term 'analgesia' refers to pain control. By usage, when the term 'local' is applied to anaesthesia no loss of consciousness is implied. Strictly speaking a more correct term would be local analgesia. However, 'local anaesthesia' is in such universal common use that this term will be used throughout this text.

Local anaesthesia may be produced by:

- application of cold
- application of pressure
- ischaemia, and
- drug action upon neural conduction.

This chapter deals with the drugs used to produce local anaesthesia.

The first chemical local anaesthetic, the ester cocaine, was introduced into clinical practice by Koller in 1884 who described its topical anaesthetic properties for ophthalmological use. Injection of cocaine to produce local anaesthesia was pioneered in America in the same year by Halstead and by Nash who independently described the use of cocaine for dental purposes. In England, the dentist William Hunt first described the use of injectable cocaine in 1886. The use of cocaine, however, was not without problems chiefly as a result of its addictive potential, the variability of its effectiveness (it being a plant derivative and subject to climatic variations) and an adverse effect upon tissues which resulted in sloughing.

It was in 1905 that Einhorn synthesized the first injectable local anaesthetic of clinical value – procaine. Shortly afterwards, amethocaine and chloroprocaine became available. These synthetic agents were superior to cocaine in that they had a known strength (unaffected by biological factors), were better tolerated by tissues and did not possess addictive potential. In 1943, Lofgren synthesized lignocaine, a new class of local anaesthetic agent, which with its close relations, forms the basis of modern local anaesthesia.

STRUCTURE OF LOCAL ANAESTHETICS

Generally, local anaesthetics conform to a common structure consisting of three components: a lipophilic aromatic portion, an intermediate chain and a hydrophilic amine group (Fig. 7.1). The linkage between the aromatic and intermediate components can be an ester or amide type and each forms a distinct chemical group. Those with an amino-ester linkage include procaine, amethocaine, benzocaine and chloroprocaine

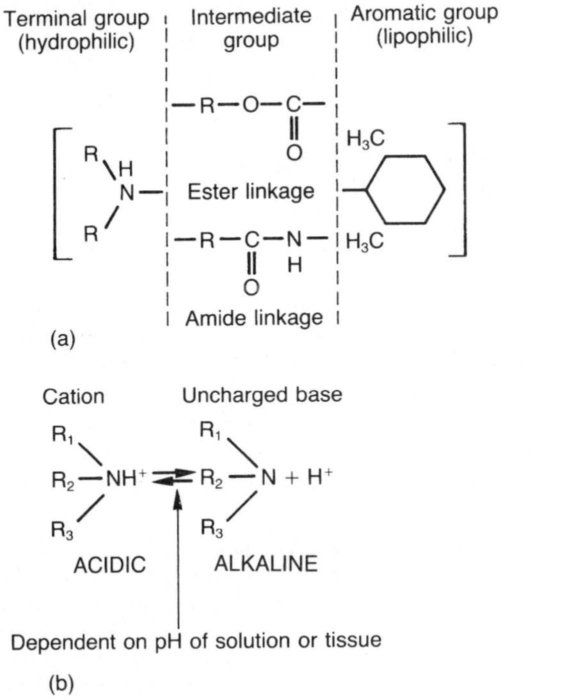

Terminal group (hydrophilic) | Intermediate group | Aromatic group (lipophilic)

—R—O—C(=O)—
Ester linkage
—R—C(=O)—N(H)—
Amide linkage

(a)

Cation | Uncharged base

$R_1R_2R_3NH^+ \rightleftharpoons R_1R_2R_3N + H^+$

ACIDIC | ALKALINE

Dependent on pH of solution or tissue

(b)

FIGURE 7.1 (a) Molecular configuration of local anaesthetics. (b) pH effect upon dissociation of local anaesthetic molecule.

and are ester derivatives of para-aminobenzoic acid. Those with an amide linkage include lignocaine, mepivacaine, prilocaine, bupivacaine and etidocaine.

Ester types of local anaesthetic are relatively unstable in solution and are readily metabolized by plasma and tissue esterases which are ubiquitous. Thus, duration of anaesthesia is short. Amide types, however, are metabolized exclusively by liver amidases. Recovery from anaesthesia with amide agents is by redistribution of the agent from the injected site into the blood circulation. Ester-type agents are rarely used as injectable local anaesthetic agents today, the amide types having replaced them. Esters, such as amethocaine and benzocaine, still have limited use as topical agents.

The chemical grouping of an agent has other important considerations. Esters are highly allergenic, which limits their clinical usefulness. Operators readily developed contact allergy to ester agents when they were in common use. Patient allergy to these agents was a serious problem too and still limits their usefulness as topical agents. Being derivatives of para-aminobenzoic acid, ester types of local anaesthetic agents can, theoretically, interfere with the bacteriostatic action of sulphonamides because the latter act as competitive antagonists for para-aminobenzoic acid which is required by organisms sensitive to sulphonamides. Thus, ester agents in these circumstances would inhibit sulphonamide action allowing bacterial proliferation. Amide agents do not antagonize sulphonamides.

Many other amine drugs possess anaesthetic properties. Examples include antihistamines, atropine, pethidine and quinidine. The anaesthetic action of these agents cannot be made use of clinically but does explain why sufficiently large doses of these drugs produce untoward effects upon the electrical processes in the heart.

IDEAL PROPERTIES OF A LOCAL ANAESTHETIC

In reality, no 'ideal' agent exists. By comparison with the 'ideal', the various advantages and disadvantages of currently available agents may be highlighted. The ideal requirements are as follows.

Reversibility

The action of a local anaesthetic drug upon nerves and nerve endings should be specific and totally reversible. All current agents allow complete recovery and resumption of normal neural activity by redistribution from the site and metabolic inactivation. There is no drug that will safely reverse local anaesthetic action. Many different substances can interfere with neural transmission and produce anaesthesia (e.g. phenol or alcohol), but to be clinically useful a drug must have a totally reversible action at a concentration that does not significantly damage the tissues. This latter feature of a local anaesthetic agent is related to the *potency* of that drug.

Rapidity of onset (latency)

The drug should produce an anaesthesic effect rapidly and without any initial excitation.

Stability

The drug must be soluble and stable in solution, to give a relatively long shelf-life, as well as being capable of sterilization by heat. Cocaine is unstable when heated but lignocaine is very stable and solutions may be sterilized by this means.

Versatility

The drug should have penetrating properties so that it may be used topically or by injection and therefore be applicable to a wide variety of clinical situations. Procaine is extremely ineffective topically whereas lignocaine is effective.

Duration

The duration of anaesthesia must be sufficient to permit completion of the planned operation. Duration varies considerably with different agents. It has already been noted that ester agents are susceptible to plasma and tissue esterases, making their duration of action very short compared with amide agents, which are unaffected by esterases. Compatibility of agents with vasoconstrictor agents is important in prolongation of their anaesthetic effect by delaying absorption of the anaesthetic drug into the circulation. The effect of vasoconstrictors (e.g. adrenaline) is more pronounced in amides than esters, again due to the differing susceptibility of these agents to tissue esterases.

Unwanted effects

There should be freedom from unwanted effects. Any agent can become involved in idiosyncratic, allergic or other unwanted reactions. Currently used amide preparations, however, have a good safety record.

An index of safety of a drug may be expressed as a therapeutic ratio; that is, the ratio of the $LD_{50} : ED_{50}$ (LD_{50} = dose that kills 50% of animals injected with drug; ED_{50} = dose that produces desired effect in 50% of animals injected). The higher the therapeutic ratio the greater the safety margin of the drug. The method used to determine these ratios is important. Values reached by subcutaneous injection of drugs into experimental animals are of limited use as the most serious effects of injection are most likely after intravenous injection, which in the case of injectable local anaesthetic agents is only likely to occur inadvertently. However, this can occur and must be considered. Ideally, the therapeutic ratio should be determined in man but obviously such values have to be determined in animals. Objective testing of agents may be carried out using *in vitro* isolated nerve preparations.

The therapeutic ratios given in Table 7.1, therefore, represent a compromise having been calculated from the acute intravenous LD_{50} values in rabbit and the relative potency values (ED_{50}) determined in frog sciatic nerve preparations.

Readily metabolized

Solutions of local anaesthetic must be able to be metabolized to inactive and relatively harmless compounds that are readily excretable. The liver is the primary site of detoxification of local anaesthetic drugs by virtue of amidases, which split amide-type drugs, and as the source of plasma cholinesterases, which are important in the metabolism of esters. Thus, patients with impaired liver function present the risk of overdosage from the use of normal dosages. Products of metabolism are excreted via the kidney. Impaired renal function, therefore, must be considered too.

PHARMACOLOGICAL ACTIONS OF LOCAL ANAESTHETICS

- reversible block of neural conduction in nerve fibres and nerve endings
- relaxation of smooth muscle (e.g. vasodilatation)
- reversible block of skeletal muscle motor end-plate transmission (this is usually clinically insignificant)
- quinidine-like action upon the heart
- mixed features of both stimulation and depression of the central nervous system due to a common action of local anaesthetic drugs on cell membranes.

THEORIES OF ACTION OF LOCAL ANAESTHETICS

The precise mechanism whereby local anaesthetic drugs block neural conduction is still theoretical. The conduction of nerve impulses along a nerve depends upon changes in electrical activity within a nerve resulting from ion movement across nerve membranes. In the resting state, a nerve membrane is permeable to potassium ions but relatively impermeable to sodium ions. There is a resting potential difference between the inside and outside of a nerve cell of approximately −70 mV (see Figure 7.2). To maintain this, the outward flow of sodium ions across the nerve membrane is maintained by an active process, which utilizes ATP, termed the 'sodium pump'. Potassium ions are maintained on the interior of the nerve cell principally by electrical gradient forces whereby the negative charge of the nerve cell membrane holds the positively charged potassium ions intracellularly by electrostatic action. In addition, a minor, active 'potassium pump' mechanism may contribute.

During depolarization, sodium ions rapidly flood intracellularly across the nerve membrane from the extracellular fluid. This leads to a temporary reversal of polarity across the cell membrane (see Fig. 7.2). There is also an outward flow of potassium ions from the cell along their concentration gradient. The outward movement of potassium ions initiates repolarization during which there is a brief 'hyperpolarization' phase. The sodium pump action rapidly reverses the situation and, with inward movement of potassium ions, the resting membrane potential is restored by the end of repolarization (see Figs 7.2 and 7.3).

Local anaesthetic agents produce neural inhibition by interfering with the sodium channels in the nerve membrane, preventing the influx of sodium ions that initiates depolarization and impulse transmission. This action may be produced by physically blocking sodium channel pores at either their extracellular end or at their intracellular (axoplasmal) end (see Fig. 7.4).

TABLE 7.1 **Physicochemical characteristics of clinically useful local anaesthetics**

ANAESTHETIC	REL-POTENCY (ISOLATED NERVE) (a)	REL-TOXICITY (LD50 IV RABBIT) (b)	THERAPEUTIC RATIO (b)/(a)	pKa (25°C)	APPROX. % AS BASE AT pH 7.4	ONSET	APPROX. LIPID SOLUBILITY (PARTITION COEFFICIENT)	CLINICAL POTENCY*	PROTEIN BINDING (%)	DURATION
Procaine HCl (allocaine; synacine; ethocaine)	0.26	0.47	1.8	8.9	2	Slow	0.6	1	6	Short
Amethocaine HCl (dicaine; pontocaine; tetracaine)	9.5	4.3	0.45	8.5	5	Slow	80.0	8	76	Long
Lignocaine HCl (lidocaine; xylocaine)	1.0	1.0	1.0	7.9	35	Fast	2.9	2	65	Intermediate
Prilocaine HCl (propitocaine, Citanest)	0.65	0.77	1.18	7.7	35	Fast	1.5	2	55	Intermediate
Mepivacaine HCl (carbocaine)	0.55	0.81	1.47	7.5	40	Fast	0.8	2	75	Intermediate
Etidocaine HCl	—	—	—	7.7	35	Fast	140.0	6	94	Prolonged
Bupivacaine HCl	—	—	—	8.1	20	Intermediate	30.0	8	95	Prolonged

*1 = weak; 10 = excellent.

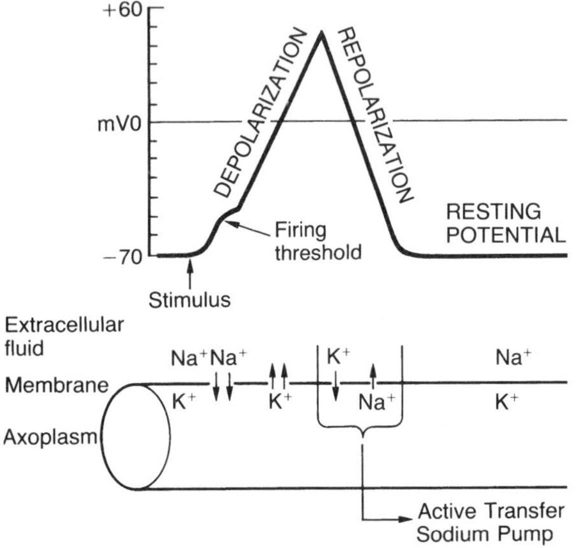

FIGURE 7.2 Ion movement during an action potential.

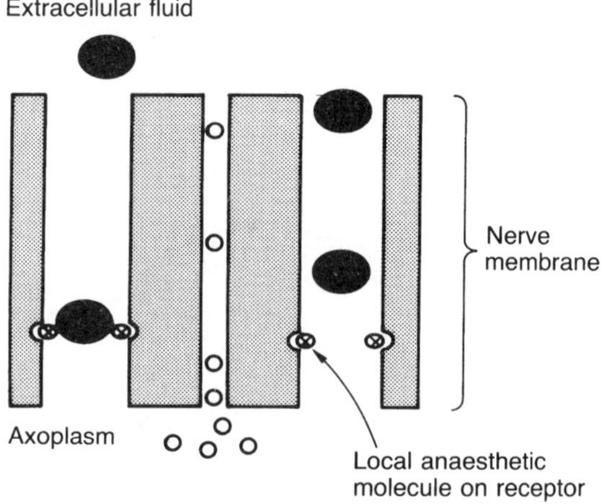

FIGURE 7.4 Local anaesthetic molecular blocking sodium channels at the inner surface of the nerve membrane. ● = Na^+; ○ = K^+.

An alternative theory proposes that local anaesthetic agents act by binding to a receptor which prevents molecular conformational changes that allow sodium channels to change from a resting closed state, holding sodium ions extracellularly, to an open state permitting influx and depolarization (see Fig. 7.5). In the latter theory, the binding site's availability to local anaesthetic molecules depends upon the channel's molecular conformation and the molecular characteristics of the drug. Further, once bound, a drug will differentially limit the sodium channel's permeability. Small anaesthetic molecules may enter and leave the available sites relatively quickly giving rapid onset and short duration anaesthesia. Larger molecules may enter and leave more slowly and be unable to

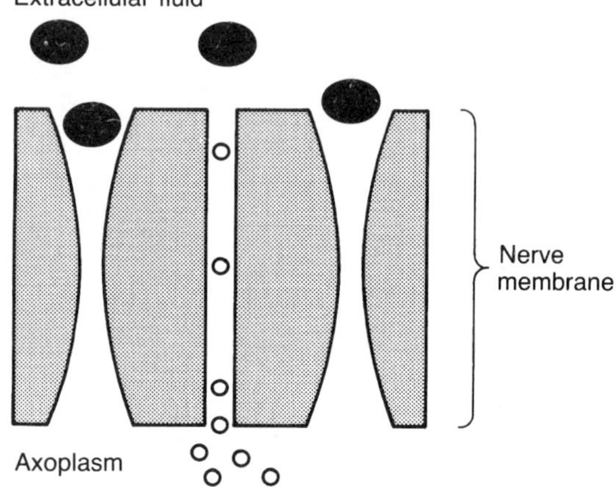

FIGURE 7.5 'Swelling' of the walls of the sodium channels preventing depolarisation. ● = Na^+; ○ = K^+.

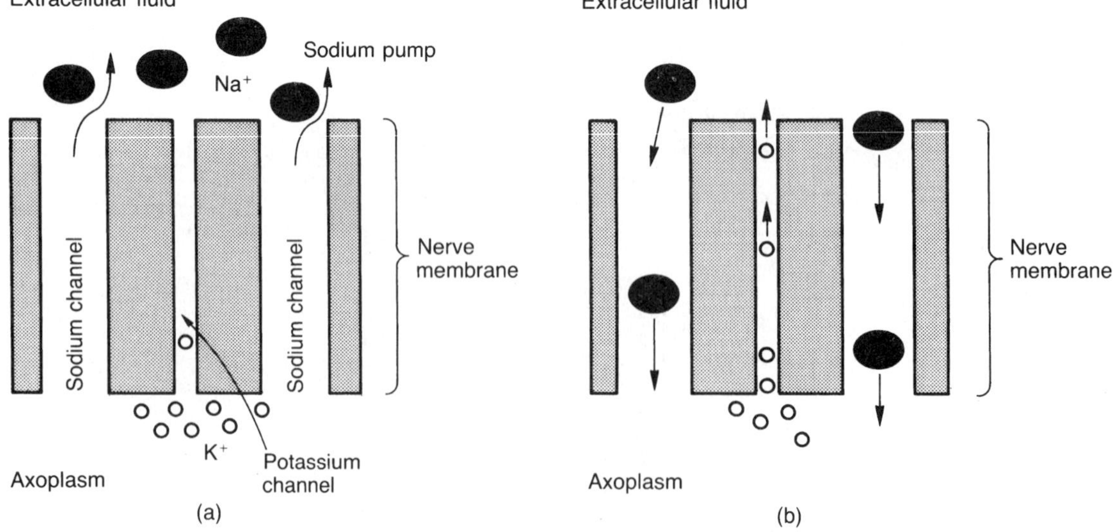

FIGURE 7.3 (a) Resting nerve membrane. ● = Na^+; ○ = K^+. (b) Depolarising nerve membrane. ● = Na^+; ○ = K^+.

reach the deeper receptors closer to the axoplasm. Intermediate sized molecules may enter relatively rapidly, bind to sites relatively deep into the nerve membrane towards the axoplasm and leave at rates dependent upon the drug's molecular shape and structural flexibility. Such a theory would explain the differing effects of agents and forms an alternative theory to the earlier simplistic physical blockade of open channels.

The degree of blockade produced by a given concentration of anaesthetic drug is very much dependent upon the recent activity of the nerve. A resting nerve is much less susceptible to blockade than one that has recently been firing. Further, the higher the frequency of recent stimulation the greater the blockade. Thus, the concept of *tonic* and *phasic* inhibition has arisen:

- tonic inhibition is measured during infrequent stimulation
- phasic inhibition results when the frequency of depolarization increases.

These frequency and use-dependent characteristics of local anaesthetic action may be accounted for by differences in the accessibility of the sodium channel receptors in the two states as well as by differences in the affinity of drug molecules for the receptors, which are thought to be voltage dependent.

In summary, the theories of local anaesthetic drug action try to account for the following sequence of events which produce blockade of nerve conduction and pain control:

- binding of drug to receptors in the nerve membrane
- reduction of membrane permeability to sodium ions
- prevention of depolarization and nerve impulse propagation
- release of drug from receptor sites and resumption of normal neural activity.

Nerve membranes are 7–80 Å thick, composed of layers of phospholipid molecules between outer and inner layers of protein molecules: some of the protein molecules extend across the phospholipid layer. Except for very small fibres, all human nerves possess a myelin sheath that forms an insulating and protective layer for the nerve. Such a layer forms a diffusion barrier for the action of local anaesthetic agents by preventing access to the nerve membrane. Fortunately, every 0.5–3.0 mm the myelin sheath is interrupted exposing the nerve membrane and it is at these 'nodes of Ranvier' where local anaesthetic drugs act. In such myelinated nerves, conduction of an impulse is from one node to the next (saltatory conduction) and effective neural block by local anaesthetics requires that two or more neighbouring nodes be blocked.

PHYSICOCHEMICAL CHARACTERISTICS

Three features of local anaesthetic drugs are clinically important in the production of neural blockade and reflect the ability of drug molecules reaching and entering the nerve membrane sodium channels. These features are:

- potency
- duration
- speed of onset.

Access to sodium channels is dependent upon the molecular structure and physicochemical characteristics of a drug (as well as the recent firing history of the nerve described earlier). These characteristics are:

- lipid solubility (partition coefficient)
- protein binding ability
- pKa values
- vasodilator properties, and
- diffusability of the drug through non-neural tissues.

Potency

The inherent ability of a drug to produce neural blockade without tissue damage is an index of its potency. *In vitro*, the potency of a local anaesthetic is directly related to its lipid solubility. As 80% of the nerve membrane structure is lipid, those drugs that have a high lipid solubility are readily absorbed into the membrane and effect conduction blockade. For example, mepivacaine and prilocaine are the least lipid-soluble amide anaesthetics with resultant low potency and weaker anaesthetic effect than etidocaine which has high potency due to its high lipid solubility. Lignocaine in the same *in vitro* system shows a lipid solubility and potency which is twice that of prilocaine or mepivicaine but inferior to etidocaine (see Table 7.1).

In vivo studies in man, however, indicate that the relationship between lipid solubility and potency is not so clear, as despite the differences in observed lipid solubility *in vitro* between lignocaine, prilocaine and mepivicaine, the clinical anaesthetic effect of each agent shows little difference. The difference between *in vitro* and *in vivo* studies is thought to be related to the vasodilator properties of each drug. Lignocaine is a more potent vasodilator than prilocaine or mepivicaine which results in a more rapid wash-out effect of lignocaine from nerves, compared with the other two agents, resulting in a clinical shorter anaesthetic effect. The highly lipid-soluble etidocaine, which has high potency *in vitro*, is thought to become bound to adipose tissue thereby theoretically reducing the amount available for neural blockade giving it reduced clinical potency (see Table 7.1). However, clinically etidocaine is still superior in potency to lignocaine, prilocaine and mepivacaine.

Bupivacaine *in vitro* is less potent than etidocaine which matches its lipid solubility but *in vivo* it is superior to etidocaine, probably reflecting the lesser adipose tissue absorption effect compared with etidocaine. The greater lipid solubility of bupivacaine compared with lignocaine, prilocaine and mepivacaine makes it superior in potency to these agents in both *in vivo* and *in vitro* situations (see Table 7.1).

Duration of anaesthesia

The degree of protein binding of anaesthetic agents is the main factor affecting duration of anaesthetic effect each produces. Following attachment of drug molecules to receptors in the sodium channels of nerve membranes, the degree of protein binding determines the rate of release of the drug from these sites permitting resumption of normal neural activity. Those with a high degree of protein binding will remain on the receptors longer and thereby prolong the anaesthetic effect. The degree of receptor binding of anaesthetic drugs is estimated by their ability to bind to plasma proteins. It is thought that this value represents the actual binding affinity that exists in a nerve membrane. Procaine *in vitro* shows a short duration of anaesthetic effect which matches its poor protein-binding ability. The long duration of anaesthesia in both *in vitro* and *in vivo* testing of etidocaine and bupivacaine compared with lignocaine, prilocaine and mepivacaine may be related to their higher protein-binding ability (see Table 7.1). The vasodilator effects mentioned above should be borne in mind when comparing the *in vivo* results of duration of anaesthesia.

Speed of onset (latency)

The speed of onset of conduction block in isolated nerve preparations is determined principally by the pKa (dissociation constant) value of the drug. This is defined as the pH at which the ionized and unionized forms of the drug are present in equal amounts. Since local anaesthetics are weak bases, it follows that they will exist partly in a unionized and partly in an ionized form. It is the lipid-soluble uncharged form of a local anaesthetic drug that is important for penetration into the nerve sheath. The more uncharged form of the drug that is available at a given pH, the more rapid the onset of anaesthesia. In the *in vivo* situation where tissue pH is normally 7.4, the lower the pKa value of a drug, the quicker the onset of anaesthesia. The percentage of a drug that is present in the unionized form at normal tissue pH of 7.4, is inversely proportional to the pKa value of that drug (see Chapter 2). For example, lignocaine, prilocaine and etidocaine all have a pKa value of 7.7. At pH 7.4, approximately 35% of the drug is present in the unionized form, the rest being in the ionized form (65%). Amethocaine has a pKa of 8.6 and that of procaine is 8.9, which at pH 7.4 gives the percentage unionized form of each drug as 5.0% and 4.8% respectively accounting for these agents' slow onset time. Bupivacaine, with a pKa of 8.1 has 15% of the drug in the unionized form at pH 7.4 giving it an intermediate rate of onset of action compared with the previous examples.

Vasodilator properties

The potency and duration of anaesthesia are affected by the inherent vasodilator activity of anaesthetic drugs. Absorption of anaesthetic molecules from the site into the circulation reduces the amount available for penetration into the nerve membrane. Thus, drugs with similar potency and protein-binding ability have vastly different clinical effects due to, among other factors, their vasoactivity. Conversely, drugs with widely differing characteristics have similar clinical effects because of these vascular effects. In the concentrations used clinically, most local anaesthetic drugs (except cocaine) tend to have vasodilator properties. The least vasodilator agents are mepivicaine and prilocaine, while lignocaine is a powerful vasodilator. The clinical consequences of this are seen by comparing the *in vitro* with *in vivo* activity of these drugs. Using isolated nerve preparations, lignocaine is significantly more potent than mepivacaine while the duration of blockade of each is similar. However, *in vivo* there is little difference in their potency but mepivacaine produces a slightly longer anaesthetic effect than lignocaine. These differences may be related to the greater vasodilator effect of lignocaine *in vivo*.

Addition of vasoconstrictors to local anaesthetic solutions containing lignocaine or mepivacaine eliminates these differences, which tends to confirm the vasodilator theory for the observed differences *in vivo* using plain solutions.

Cocaine possesses inherent vasoconstrictor activity due to its effect in preventing catecholamine re-uptake into postganglionic nerve endings ('amine pump' inhibition) thereby promoting vasoconstriction.

Non-neural diffusion

Diffusion through non-neural tissue is not related to pKa values which govern the penetration of a drug into nerve membranes. Thus, the onset of action of two similar drugs (e.g. lignocaine and prilocaine each with a pKa of 7.7) is similar in isolated nerve preparations, but *in vivo*, lignocaine has a faster onset thought to be due to the increased ease with which ligocaine can diffuse across non-neural tissues. Another important factor affecting non-neural diffusion of a drug is the tissue concentration because of the concentration gradient.

Differential sensitivity of nerves

An important clinical consideration of a local anaesthetic drug is its selectivity in blocking sensory nerves whilst motor fibres are unaffected. As a general rule, the sensitivity of nerves to local anaesthetics is inversely proportional to their diameter. Thus, smaller nerve fibres are more susceptible to blockade than larger diameter fibres. Smaller nerve fibres appear more sensitive to sodium lack. General visceral afferent and general visceral efferent (autonomic) nerves are very susceptible to local anaesthetic drugs due to their fineness. Since somatic sensory information is carried by smaller fibres than those that convey somatic motor impulses, sensory loss is achieved before motor blockade. Further, the order of sensory loss is generally pain–temperature–touch–pressure.

Bupivacaine and etidocaine are both long-acting local anaesthetics with useful characteristics of differential sensory and motor blocking ability. Bupivacaine at concentrations of 0.25% and 0.5% may be used to provide postoperative pain relief with good sensory blockade and minimal motor effects. Epidural injection of these concentrations enables pain-free childbirth with the advantage that the mother still has lower limb motor control. At 0.75%, bupivacaine produces more effective sensory anaesthesia with a more rapid onset but motor blockade then becomes significant. Etidocaine, on the other hand, shows little differential sensitivity between sensory and motor blockade. To provide effective anaesthesia there is always accompanying motor blockade. This makes etidocaine a useful local anaesthetic agent where profound, long-acting anaesthesia of rapid onset is required with motor blockade but this agent is not applicable for epidural anaesthesia in labour where motor function with pain control is desirable.

Vasoconstrictors

Duration of anaesthesia is directly related to the contact time of the drug with nerves. Vasoconstrictors perform a dual function. First, such agents decrease the rate of dilution of a drug from a nerve into the circulation. Second, the rate of absorption of the drug from the injection site is reduced which thereby makes available more anaesthetic molecules which can enter the nerve membrane. Both these actions serve to increase the neural contact time and thus the depth and duration of anaesthesia. The most common vasoconstrictor is adrenaline. Powerful vasoconstrictors, like adrenaline, should be avoided in situations where vascular insufficiency would result in necrosis. Such situations are digital or penile local anaesthesia as well as areas of osteoradionecrosis.

Local anaesthetic solutions usually contain adrenaline at a concentration of 1 part in 20 000 which is equivalent to 5 μg/ml of solution. This concentration is the optimum when used with lignocaine for epidural or intercostal anaesthesia. For dental use, the optimum concentration of adrenaline (in the UK) is 1 part in 80 000 (12.5 μg/ml). In poorly vascular regions such a concentration of adrenaline can lead to delayed healing, tissue oedema or necrosis – effects that probably occur due to adrenaline causing increased oxygen consumption of tissue which leads to hypoxia and subsequent tissue damage.

There is a differential effect upon prolongation of anaesthesia by the addition of adrenaline depending upon the base drug involved. For lignocaine and mepivacaine, there is great benefit from adrenaline in the duration of anaesthesia when used for epidural, regional or peripheral nerve block anaesthesia. Similarly, prilocaine, bupivacaine and etidocaine with adrenaline show prolongation of anaesthetic effect with infiltration and peripheral nerve block, but for epidural use the addition of adrenaline with these agents does not prolong anaesthesia. The weak vasodilator property of prilocaine is probably the cause of the reduced effect of adrenaline in this situation whereas bupivacaine and etidocaine have a high lipid solubility which probably accounts for the reduced adrenaline effect of these agents in epidural blocks. The concentration of the base drug used also has an effect in the duration of anaesthesia with adrenaline.

The worst effects of local anaesthetics, with or without adrenaline, will be manifest if inadvertent intravascular injection is made. In dentistry, this is of particular relevance due to the high vascularity of the region. Use of the Astra 'self-aspirating' system of injection almost totally eliminates this risk.

Where inadvertent adrenergic stimulation is inadvisable, such as for those with severe cardiac dysfunction, the alternative felypressin may be used. Felypressin is an analogue of the pituitary hormone oxytocin and produces vasoconstriction by local hormonal rather than by adrenergic means. In dental solutions it is available at a concentration of 0.03 iu/ml of a 3% prilocaine solution (Astra Pharmaceuticals, Sweden). Comparing this concentration with adrenaline (which in dental cartridges is normally at a concentration of 1:80 000) felypressin represents a concentration of approximately 1:2 000 000. At this level, it is thought that the local vasoactivity of felypressin is virtually insignificant and the mode of action to prolong anaesthesia is proposed to be by catalysing the absorption of the base drug (in this case prilocaine) into neural membranes.

Noradrenaline and its analogues (e.g. levonordefrin) are common vasoconstrictors added to prolong local anaesthetic action, particularly in the USA. However, dental use of these principally α-adrenergic agonists has recently been discouraged following fatalities due to a profound peripheral vasoconstriction effect without β-adrenergic cardiac stimulation, which has resulted in circulatory collapse in healthy individuals. In these instances it is probable that inadvertent intravascular injection was made. Noradrenaline and its analogues are, therefore, contraindicated for use in local anaesthesia.

UNTOWARD EFFECTS OF LOCAL ANAESTHETICS

Owing to anaesthetic drug

- central nervous system
  mixed stimulatory and depressive effects especially of cortex, medulla, respiratory centre, vasomotor centre
- cardiovascular system
  direct cardiac and vascular effects
- hypersensitivity
  rare (often due to preservatives which should be avoided, e.g. methylparabens)
- intolerance
- idiosyncrasy

Not owing to anaesthetic drug

- psychomotor (e.g. vasovagal syncope)
- vasomotor (e.g. due to vasoconstrictor effect).

PART II LOCAL ANAESTHETIC AGENTS

EM Grundy

GENERAL CONSIDERATIONS

Uptake, distribution and elimination

Uptake of local anaesthetic from a tissue site depends on the fat solubility of the drug. The more lipid soluble the drug the greater the potency, the longer the duration of action and the smaller the amount of free drug available for systemic absorption. Absorption itself is dependent on the local blood supply at the tissue site, thus local anatomy is obviously important. Systemic absorption from tissue sites occurs in the following descending order: intercostal, caudal, epidural, peripheral nerve with least absorption following subcutaneous infiltration. Drug effects on the local blood vessels are also important with both the intrinsic vasoactivity of the local anaesthetic (lignocaine is a more potent vasodilator than prilocaine and carbocaine) and the presence of vasoconstrictors such as adrenaline contributing to the overall picture. Peak blood levels after regional blocks are usually seen 10–30 min after the tissue injection of the local anaesthetic.

Protein binding of local anaesthetic drug can be to either plasma proteins or to the membrane proteins of the neuronal membrane. It correlates well with both potency and duration of action.

The pharmacokinetics of lignocaine after systemic administration are well documented and illustrative of local anaesthetic agents. It has a volume of distribution (steady state) of 91 l, a terminal half-life of 1.6 h and a plasma clearance of 0.95 l/min. After an intravenous bolus the elimination of lignocaine is well described by a two-compartment open kinetic model with a distribution half-life ($t_{\frac{1}{2}}\ \alpha$) of 8 min and an elimination half-life ($t_{\frac{1}{2}}\ \beta$) of 100 min in normal humans.

Elimination of local anaesthetics is primarily by metabolism with less than 5% being excreted unchanged by the kidney.

The ester group undergoes rapid hydrolysis by hepatic-derived esterases both in the liver and in the plasma (by plasma cholinesterases). The rate of hydrolysis varies markedly between the esters, with chlorprocaine 16× and procaine 4× the rate that amethocaine is hydrolysed. Reduced hydrolysis is seen in newborns and patients with impaired liver function.

The amide group is rapidly metabolized in the liver and undergoes 'first pass metabolism'. The drug lignocaine undergoes de-ethylation to give monoethyl glycine xylidine (MEGX) which in turn undergoes either further de-ethylation to glycine xylidine (GX) or hydrolysis to give 2,6 xylidine. Impaired metabolism occurs in patients with reduced hepatic blood flow, such as those in heart failure.

Systemic effects and toxicity

Systemic toxicity of local anaesthetics is directly related to blood levels of the drug. High blood levels can be achieved by either an accidental intravascular injection or by an administration of an overdose into a relatively vascular tissue site with subsequent rapid uptake. Both of these mechanisms are more likely in a vascular area such as the epidural space.

The systemic effects of lignocaine are described as an example of a typical local anaesthetic agent. [1]

At low systemic blood levels (1.5 mcg/ml) lignocaine has an action on the fast Na^+ channels in the heart, which results in an increase in the duration of the action potential and an increase in the effective refractory period of the Purkinje system and the ventricles. No detectable changes are produced in the ECG. This action as a Class Ib antidysrhythmic agent makes it probably the agent of choice for the suppression of ventricular arrhythmias. As expected from the pharmacokinetics of lignocaine, it dissociates rapidly from its site of action and thus intravenous infusions are necessary to maintain therapeutic blood levels.

With increasing blood levels (> 5 mcg/ml) central nervous system disturbances become apparent with perioral anaesthesia, agitation, dysarthria, disorientation, confusion and eventually culminating in full *grand mal* convulsions at blood levels around 10 mcg/ml. The administration of anticonvulsants significantly increases the blood level at which convulsions occur. Benzodiazepines are the anticonvulsant of choice, and are frequently administered as an adjuvant to a regional anaesthetic technique for their amnesic, anxiolytic and sedative effects and incidentally raise the convulsive theshold.

With much higher blood levels (> 20 mcg/ml) increasing cardiorespiratory depression becomes apparent. Initial respiratory depression is followed by bradycardia and hypotension. Lignocaine is not known to have any autonomic activity but has both intrinsic vasodilator activity and its action on Na^+ channels, including those in the heart. This combination accounts for the circulatory collapse associated with extremely high blood levels.

Idiosyncrasy

Allergic drug reactions to the ester group of local anaesthetics are well recognized, and not uncommonly follow skin or surface contact. True allergic drug reactions have been reported with amide local anaesthetic agents; however, they are excessively rare. High sympathetic block or systemic effects are the usual explanation of events that patients report as allergy.

Local toxicity

Extensive laboratory testing ensures that the local anaesthetics, in the concentration used clinically, have no direct neurotoxic activity (i.e. their activity is truly fully reversible). However, this may not be true if the drug ends up other than where intended. Recently there were reports that chlorprocaine intended for epidural space (400 mg in 20 ml) but accidentally administered into the subarachnoid space had resulted in a permanent, although subtle, neurological deficit.[2]

However additions to the injected local anaesthetic solution are a more likely source of neurotoxicity. Multidose vials usually contain methylparaben as a bacteriostatic agent. Bisulphite is present as an antioxidant in some agents and adrenaline is often present as a vasoconstrictor.

The presence of a vasoconstrictor such as adrenaline produces a reduction in local tissue vascularity, thus decreased systemic absorption and hence a higher local concentration of local anaesthetic agent. This results in a lower peak blood level of drug, increased density of block and increased duration of block. The magnitude of the effect will depend on the local vascularity around the nerve, the intrinsic vasodilator activity of the local anaesthetic drug and, lastly, the concentration and the vasoconstrictor used. For subcutaneous infiltration and peripheral nerve block, adrenaline in a concentration of 5 mcg/ml (1 in 200 000) is best but around the face a higher concentration of 12.5 mcg/ml (1 in 80 000) is better. The addition of vasoconstrictors is contraindicated where blocks involve an end artery such as penile or digital arteries.

Increasingly, opiates are being added to local anaesthetic solutions to produce mixtures to be administered into the epidural space.

In clinical practice, multidose vials are best avoided because of the risk of cross-infection and the presence of bacteriostatic agents. Ampoules should be checked carefully and a new needle used for drawing up the drug (drug residue lurking in the hub of a needle may be benign injected intravenously but neurotoxic if injected alongside a nerve). Additions to local anaesthetic solutions, such as opiates and vasoconstrictors, should be carefully monitored for dilution errors. Ideally a commercially prepared mixture is to be preferred. Lastly, use of special regional block needles reduces the remote risk of direct needle trauma producing a permanent neuronal deficit.

SITES OF ADMINISTRATION

Subcutaneous infiltration and peripheral nerve block

The surrounding tissues are least vascular with these sites and thus the intrinsic vasoactivity of the local anaesthetic has the most influence on duration of action. The addition of adrenaline produces significant prolongation of duration of action. The concentration required is the minimum shown in the Table 7.2, as only sensory blockade is achieved.

Epidural and caudal blocks

The epidural space is highly vascular, with a large epidural venous plexus, and requires a relatively large volume of local anaesthetic to produce a block. Thus systemic toxicity is most likely with this block and

TABLE 7.2 Maximum doses and clinically used concentrations of local anaesthetics

	MAX. DOSE (mg/kg)		CONCENTRATION USED CLINICALLY			
	PLAIN	WITH ADRENALINE	LOW	HIGH	TOPICAL	SPINAL
Amethocaine	1.5	—	—	—	—	1%
Cocaine	3	—	—	—	5%	—
Chlorprocaine	11	13	1%	3%	—	—
Bupivacaine	2	3	0.25%	0.75%	—	0.5%
Lignocaine	3	7	0.5%	2%	4%	5%
Etidocaine	4	6	0.5%	1.5%	—	—
Mepivacaine	6	7	0.5%	2%	—	—
Prilocaine	6	8	0.5%	2%	—	—

maximum recommended dosages are derived for this block and extrapolated to all situations.

Because of the high vascularity of this site, the duration of block is much shorter and the addition of vasoconstrictor makes little difference to the duration of action. The concentration required is the maximum shown in Table 7.2, as motor blockade is desirable for surgical anaesthesia.

Spinal (subarachnoid) block

The local anaesthetic is applied directly to the nerve roots as they cross the subarachnoid space and are bathed in cerebrospinal fluid (CSF) before they acquire their protective connective tissue coatings. The absence of the connective tissue sheaths permits a much smaller dose of local anaesthetic to produce an intense block. The amount of systemic absorption of this tiny dose from the relatively avascular subarachnoid space is trivial.

Amethocaine, and bupivacaine and lignocaine in (hyperbaric) dextrose solutions, are the only drugs currently available for spinal administration.

Topical to mucosa

Application of local anaesthetics to mucosae, especially those with marked intrinsic vasodilator activity such as lignocaine, results in rapid systemic absorption. Indeed uptake is so rapid that blood levels achieved are similar to those achieved with intravenous injection. Intratracheal instillation of lignocaine with absorption from tracheobronchial mucosa is now recommended during resuscitation if venous access is not immediately available.

Cocaine is an exception among the local anaesthetics in that it has intrinsic vasoconstrictor activity. Its sole remaining clinical use is on the nasal mucosae where the combination of local anaesthetic activity and vasoconstrictor activity is particularly used for nasal surgery.

Topical to skin

Normally high concentrations of local anaesthetic are required in order to penetrate skin, with topical emulsions having at most 20% of local anaesthetic in the base form. The advent of eutectic mixture local anaesthetic (EMLA) cream provides a cream with the local anaesthetic present in greater concentration than possible with either alone. A eutectic mixture is one that has a melting point lower than either of its constituents. EMLA cream has lignocaine and prilocaine present and is an oil above 16°C and has a very high concentration of local anaesthetic in these droplets. EMLA cream is finding extensive indications in paediatric practice to cover venepuncture and minor surgical procedures. It has the disadvantage that it has to be applied at least an hour before to achieve optimum analgesia.[3]

IVRA (intravenous regional anaesthesia)

With this technique a limb is isolated with a tourniquet and a high volume of a low concentration of local anaesthetic (without adrenaline) introduced into the empty venous compartment. With the passage of time, progressive tissue binding of the local anaesthetic occurs such that after 30 min over half the dose of local anaesthetic is tissue bound and thus not released on tourniquet deflation. Early inadvertent tourniquet deflation will release toxic doses into the systemic circulation. Prilocaine (0.5%) is the least toxic local anaesthetic and thus the agent of choice for IVRA. Bupivacaine is contraindicated because of its adverse cardiac effects with systemic toxicity.

OBSTETRIC ANAESTHESIA

There is understandable nervousness that any drug that achieves significant systemic levels in the mother will pass transplacental and produce similar fetal levels with unpredictable consequences.

In the labour ward epidural analgesia is administered to labouring parturients either as frequent bolus doses or increasingly as a continuous infusion. Current practice is to use bupivacaine in a concentration of 0.1–0.25% which will provide a differential block with pain relief and some sensory block and no or minimal loss of motor power and proprioreception. The blood levels achieved in the fetus are low. Subtle impairment in neurobehavioural assessment in the first 24 h of neonatal life has been reported following lignocaine and mepivacaine,[3] which is why bupivacaine is preferred. Although this neurobehavioural impairment has not been shown to be of any clinical significance in the mature healthy neonates studied, there are no good data for the premature or distressed neonate and extrapolation of data to this situation must be with reservation. It must be remembered that the drugs in the doses used in other forms of pain relief in labour may well produce even less desirable effects on the fetus.

Similar considerations apply to neonates delivered at Caesarian section under epidural analgesia.

INDIVIDUAL DRUGS

Cocaine

This is a naturally occurring alkaloid that is an ester of benzoic acid. In addition to its local anaesthetic activity, it blocks the re-uptake of noradrenaline into nerve endings. Peripherally this results in local vasoconstriction and if systemic blood levels are achieved central stimulation is produced and this is the root of its addictive potential.

- CNS: in low doses a sense of euphoria and well being are produced. In higher doses emesis, agitation, restlessness progressing through to excitement, delirium and convulsions. Late medullary depression is associated with respiratory failure and death.
- CVS: initially increased sympathetic activity increases capacity to perform physical work and produces mydriasis. This progresses to the 'sympathetic storm' picture of tremor, peripheral vasoconstriction, tachycardia, hypertension, hyperpyrexia and eventual death.

Clinically, the use of cocaine is restricted to topical application to the mucosa of the upper airway. In the nose the combination of local anaesthetic activity with vasoconstriction is particularly valuable and it is used either as a 25% paste or as a 5% solution with a maximum recommended dose of 3 mg/kg. Addition of adrenaline to cocaine is unnecessary because of its intrinsic vasoconstrictor activity, and undesirable because cocaine sensitizes the heart to the action of catecholamines.

Chlorprocaine

This is an ester and an halogenated derivative of procaine. Rapid hydrolysis by plasma esterase means that after a rapid onset it has a short duration of action (30–60 min). It is available as 1%, 2% and 3% solution and the maximum recommended dose is 11 mg/kg (13 mg/kg with adrenaline). Epidural use of the drug has declined since reports of neurotoxicity following accidental subarachnoid injection,[2] although the role of additives in this situation has been questioned.

Etidocaine

Etidocaine is a long-acting amide local anaesthetic. It possesses a high degree of lipid solubility and is three times more potent than lignocaine.

It is available as a 0.5%, 1% and 1.5% solution and motor block is a prominent feature with epidural use. Maximum recommended dose is 4 mg/kg (6mg/kg with adrenaline).

Lignocaine

Lignocaine was the first of the amide family of local anaesthetic agents and it remains the yardstick by which the others are assessed.

Cardiovascular and neurological effects are as described above under systemic effects.

It is available as 0.5%, 1% and 2% solutions and the maximum recommended dose is 3 mg/kg (7 mg/kg with adrenaline). It is used extensively for subcutaneous infiltration, peripheral nerve blocks and epidural use, as a general rule adrenaline is added.

Lignocaine is also used as a 4% topical solution applied to the mucosa of the upper respiratory tract. The absorption from this vascular site of this vasodilating drug is as rapid as after intravenous injection and intratracheal administration is advocated as an alternative to vascular access during resuscitation.

For subarachnoid use, a hyperbaric solution containing 5% lignocaine in 7.5% dextrose is available and a dose of 50–200 mg is employed. This only provides around 90 min of surgical anaesthesia time.

Mepivacaine

Mepivacaine is an amide with very similar properties to lignocaine. It is available as 0.5%, 1% and 2% solutions and although it is equipotent with lignocaine it is less toxic with a maximum recommended dose of 6 mg/kg (7 mg/kg with adrenaline). It is said to have a slightly longer duration of action than lignocaine and it is used widely in the USA.

Prilocaine

This amide is equipotent to lignocaine and is available as 0.5%, 1% and 2% solutions. It is less toxic with a maximum recommended dose of 6 mg/kg (8 mg/kg with adrenaline). It is the drug of choice for IVRA where accidental or inadvertent cuff deflation with subsequent acute systemic toxicity can occur.[5]

Prilocaine undergoes rapid hepatic metabolism to *o*-toludine and this metabolite is thought to cause the methaemoglobinaemia that can be seen following high doses (10 mg/kg) of prilocaine.

Amethocaine (tetracaine USP)

This is an ester drug with a maximum recommended dose of 1.5 mg/kg. It is a long-acting drug used extensively in the USA for spinal anaesthesia. It is presented as amethocaine crystals which are dissolved in either sterile water (hypobaric) or CSF (isobaric) or 10% dextrose (hyperbaric) and the solution injected in a dose of 5–20 mg.

Bupivacaine

Bupivacaine is an amide drug that is available as 0.25%, 0.5% and 0.75% solutions and the maximum recommended dose is 2 mg/kg (3 mg/kg with adrenaline). With infusion or repeated dose it is recommended that 2 mg/kg is not exceeded over any 4-h period.

It is the longest-acting local anaesthetic agent currently available and is extensively used for regional techniques where a prolonged block for surgery will help with postoperative analgesia in the early postoperative period or where the block technique is being used for pain control, for example postoperative or labour pain.

Sudden cardiovascular collapse has occurred following accidental systemic administration from which resuscitation has been difficult or unsuccessful. Systemic administration in a sheep model has shown two patterns of cardiovascular collapse – one very similar to that seen with lignocaine with respiratory depression, bradycardia and hypotension without arrhythmia and the other with sudden onset ventricular tachycardia or fibrillation without hypoxia or acidosis.[6] High tissue binding of bupivacaine means that once bound to the myocardium a prolonged effect can be expected. Consequently bupivacaine is not recommended for IVRA (where accidental tourniquet deflation is an ever-present risk) and the 0.75% solution is not recommended for obstetric use.

For spinal use a 0.5% solution in 8% dextrose (hyperbaric) is available and a dose of 5–20 mg is employed.

Ropivacaine

Ropivacaine is a long-acting amide drug that is currently undergoing clinical trials. It is thought to be equipotent with bupivacaine but less toxic.

REFERENCES

1 Mather LE, Cousins MJ. Local anaesthetics and their current clinical use. *Drugs* 1979; **18**: 185–205.
2 Moore DC, Spierdiijk J, Van Kleef J D, Coleman RI, Love GF. Chlorprocaine neurotoxicity: four additional cases. *Anesthesia and Analgesia* 1982; **61**: 155–9.
3 Evers H., Von Darde O, Juhlin L, Ohlsen L, Vinnars E. Dermal effects of compositions based on eutectic mixtures of lignocaine and prilocaine (EMLA). *British Journal of Anaesthesia* 1985; **57**: 997–1005.
4 Scanlon JW, Brown WU, Weiss JB. *et al.* Neurobehavioural responses of newborn infants after maternal epidural anaesthesia. *Anesthesiology* 1974; **40**: 121–8.
5 Editorial: Cardiotoxicity of local anaesthetic agents. *Lancet* 1986; **ii**: 1192–3.
6 Nancarrow C, Rutten AJ, Runciman WB, Mather LE, Carapetis RJ, McLean CF, Hipkins SF. Myocardial and cerebral drug concentrations and the mechanisms of death after fatal intravenous doses of lidocaine, bupivacaine and ropivacaine in sheep. *Anesthesia and Analgesia* 1989; **69**: 276–83.

SECTION THREE

Drugs Acting at Synaptic and Neuroeffector Junctional Sites

8

The Principles of Peripheral Cholinergic and Adrenergic Transmission

WC Bowman

PERIPHERAL SYNAPTIC AND NEUROEFFECTOR TRANSMISSION

The development of the concept that the nerve impulse is transmitted across synapses and neuroeffector junctions by chemical mediators arose largely from a study of autonomic nervous function, particularly in experiments in which the effects of drugs were compared with the effects of nerve stimulation. The effects of stimulating autonomic nerves are given in Table 8.1.

In 1869, Schmiedeberg showed that the actions of the alkaloid muscarine (Fig. 8.1), from the toadstool *Amanita muscaria*, closely resembled the effects of stimulation of the vagus nerve; the incorrect explanation offered was that muscarine stimulated the vagus nerve endings. Then Dixon, in 1907, found that a muscarine-like substance was released from the frog's heart when the vagus nerve was stimulated and he suggested that excitation of a nerve induces the local liberation of a chemical mediator. Choline, which is present in body tissues, has actions like those of muscarine but it is much weaker. However, the acetyl ester of choline, acetylcholine (Fig. 8.1), also has muscarine-like actions and is much more potent than choline. Studies on acetylcholine were begun in the USA by Hunt (1900–6), who came across it as a depressor substance in adrenal extracts (that were free from adrenaline), and in Britain by Dale (1906–14), who had identified it as the depressor substance present in an extract of ergot. Dale found that responses to acetylcholine mimicked most of the effects of parasympathetic nerve stimulation (Table 8.1). These actions of acetylcholine became known as muscarinic actions or parasympathomimetic actions. Dale further showed that after the injection of atropine the muscarinic actions of acetylcholine were abolished. The muscarinic actions of acetylcholine include vasodilatation and bradycardia with a consequent fall in blood pressure. After atropine, these muscarinic effects were no longer evident, but larger doses of acetylcholine then produced a pronounced rise in blood pressure and in heart rate. The injection of the alkaloid nicotine (Fig. 8.1), from the tobacco plant, also produced these latter effects by exciting sympathetic ganglion cells. Actions of acetylcholine that resemble those of nicotine became known as nicotinic actions. After large doses of nicotine, ganglionic transmission was blocked and this prevented the action of acetylcholine in the atropinized animal. These results suggested that acetylcholine, like nicotine, stimulated ganglion cells.

TABLE 8.1 Effects of stimulating some autonomic nerves

TISSUE	SYMPATHETIC NERVES	PARASYMPATHETIC NERVES
Eye and associated structures:		
Dilator pupillae (i.e. radial muscle of iris)	Contraction giving dilated pupil, i.e. mydriasis	Not innervated
Constrictor pupillae (i.e. circular muscle of iris)	Not innervated	Contraction giving constricted pupil, i.e. miosis
Smooth muscle of eyelid	Contraction. Lid is elevated	Not innervated
Ciliary muscle	Relaxation	Contraction. Accommodation for near vision
Lacrimal glands and conjunctiva	Vasoconstriction	Secretion and vasodilatation
Salivary glands	Vasoconstriction. Sparse, thick mucinous secretion of saliva	Vasodilatation. Profuse watery secretion
Lung	Inhibits parasympathetic, therefore smooth musle of bronchi relaxed. Pulmonary vasoconstriction	Smooth muscle of bronchi contracted. Mucous glands stimulated
Heart	Rate, force and conduction velocity increased	Rate slowed. Refractory period reduced
Stomach	Motility and tone decreased. Sphincters contracted	Motility and tone increased. Sphincters relaxed
Intestine	Motility and tone decreased. Sphincters contracted. Vasoconstriction	Motility and tone increased. Sphincters relaxed. Secretions stimulated
Omentum and other fat depots	Fatty acids released into blood	Not innervated
Liver	Glucose released into blood	Not innervated?
Pancreas	Secretory cells not innervated. Vasoconstriction	Increase in exocrine and endocrine secretion
Kidney and juxtaglomerular apparatus	Vasoconstriction. Renin secretion	Not innervated
Bladder:		
Detrusor	Relaxed?	Contracted
Trigone and sphincters	Contracted	Relaxed
Ureter	Increased tone and motility	Not innervated
Sweat glands		
Eccrine	Secretion of sweat	Not innervated
Apocrine	Not innervated	Not innervated
Pilomotor muscles	Contraction	Not innervated
Blood vessels:		
Skin	Vasoconstriction	Mostly not innervated. Some areas vasodilatation
Skeletal muscle	Vasoconstrictor and vasodilator nerve fibres present	Not innervated?
Brain	Vasoconstriction	Not innervated?

Oliver and Schäfer in 1894 reported that the injection of an extract of adrenal glands raised the blood pressure of an animal. The active principle, named adrenaline (Fig. 8.1), was confined to the medulla. Langley later showed that the actions of an adrenal extract closely resembled the responses resulting from stimulation of sympathetic nerves (Table 8.1). The actions remained after the sympathetic nerves had been sectioned and allowed to degenerate; hence it was concluded that the extract acted on the effector cells and not on the nerves. Elliott, in 1904–7, was the first to suggest that adrenaline is liberated from sympathetic nerve endings when they are stimulated, and that the released adrenaline then acts on the responsive cells. However, in 1910, Dale emphasized that the responses to adrenaline were not always identical with those resulting from stimulation of sympathetic nerves. He studied the actions of a large series of compounds related chemically to adrenaline and pointed out that noradrenaline (Fig. 8.1) mimicked the effects of sympathetic stimulation more closely. von Euler and his colleagues later proved that (−)-noradrenaline (henceforth simply called noradrenaline) is in fact the transmitter at most sympathetic nerve endings in mammals. A few utilize dopamine as their transmitter. Substances whose actions resemble responses to sympathetic nerve stimulation were termed sympathomimetic drugs. Among these, those amines containing a catechol nucleus are termed catecholamines. Three catecholamines, (−)-adrenaline, (−)-noradrenaline and dopamine (Fig. 8.1), occur in tissues. On a point of nomenclature, in the USA adrenaline and noradrenaline are called epinephrine and norepinephrine respectively, in order to avoid the use of an American tradename. These terms are similarly derived. Thus, adrenaline is so named because it comes from the adrenal gland which is close to the kidney. Hence 'ad' (Latin = near) renes (Latin = kidney). Epinephrine has a similar derivation; thus 'epi' (Greek = above) 'nephros' (Greek = kidney).

The first conclusive evidence that neuroeffector transmission is mediated by chemicals was provided by Loewi in 1921. He irrigated two isolated frog hearts with Ringer's solution in such a way that the fluid flowed from one heart

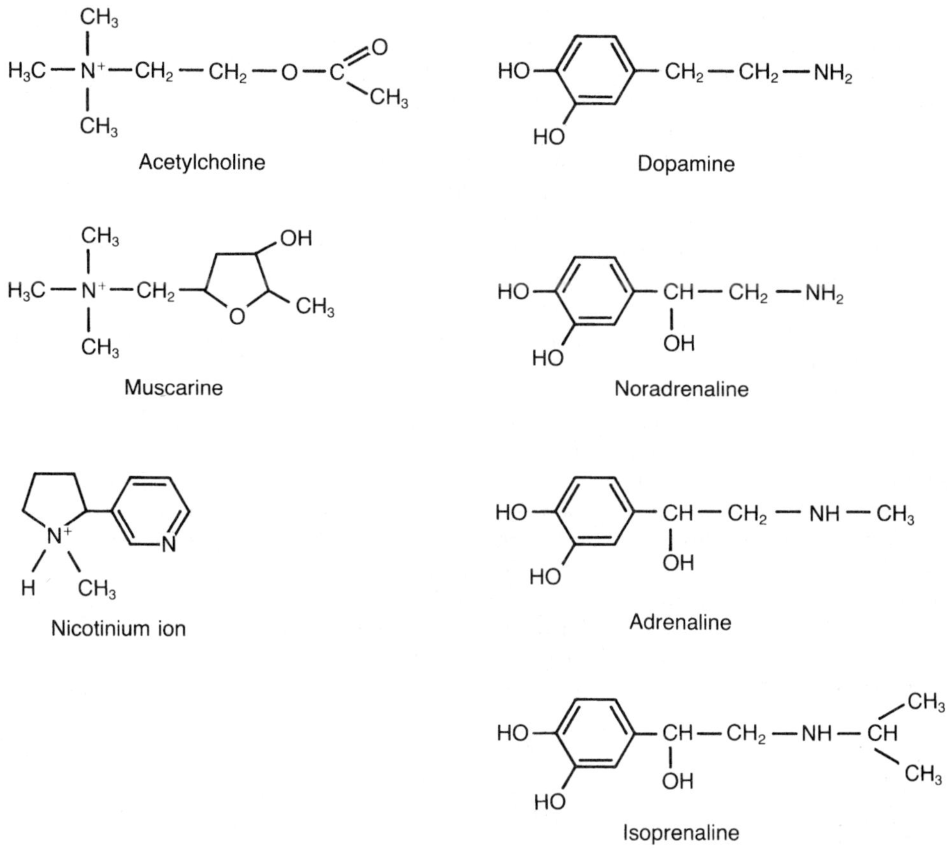

FIGURE 8.1 Structures of acetylcholine and noradrenaline and of related compounds. Nicotine is shown as the protonated nicotinium ion, which is the active form. Most molecules of nicotine exist in this form at body pH.

and then on to the other. When the parasympathetic nerve (the vagus) to the first heart was stimulated, the heart slowed and its beats became weaker, and shortly afterwards the second heart responded in a similar manner. He postulated that a substance, then termed Vagusstoff, was released from the nerve endings in the first heart and carried in the perfusion fluid to the second heart. Later he showed that a much greater effect of Vagusstoff could be obtained in the presence of physostigmine, an inhibitor of the enzyme cholinesterase, and also that the effects of acetylcholine were greatly increased by physostigmine. It is now clear that Vagusstoff is in fact acetylcholine.

Loewi also showed that when the sympathetic nerve (the nervus accelerans) to the first heart was stimulated, the frequency of beating became faster and the beat became more powerful, and then the second heart responded in a similar way, indicating that another substance, then termed Acceleranstoff, was released from the sympathetic nerve endings. The actions of Acceleranstoff closely resembled those of adrenaline, and it is now known that it is in fact adrenaline, which is the transmitter of cardiac sympathetic nerves in frogs and toads. In mammals, however, the transmitter is noradrenaline. Subsequent to Loewi's early work a vast amount of evidence has been obtained to show that acetylcholine is responsible for chemical transmission at autonomic ganglia, and acetylcholine or noradrenaline at most neuroeffector junctions.

Dale, in 1933, designated those nerve fibres that release acetylcholine, and the associated transmission mechanisms, as cholinergic, and those that make use of adrenaline-like substances as adrenergic. In mammals, most peripheral 'adrenergic' transmission events are more correctly described as noradrenergic. Dale was much concerned that the terminology should not be degraded and hence lose precision. The British Pharmacological Society attempts to maintain Dale's original meaning by restricting the ending 'ergic' to adjectives describing nerve fibres and the transmission mechanism. Thus, for example, a dopaminergic fibre is one that functions by releasing dopamine as its transmitter. The term should not be used simply to mean 'pertaining to'. Terms such as 'cholinergic receptor' and 'cholinergic drugs' are not within Dale's restricted meaning. For the former, acetylcholine receptor is more appropriate. Current research shows, however, that there is a problem in naming nerve fibres in this way, for many nerve fibres, perhaps most, release more than one transmitter. This matter is mentioned again later. Transmission events may well involve only one transmitter and are therefore correctly described as cholinergic, noradrenergic or dopaminergic, etc. but caution is now necessary in applying the terms to nerve fibres, although the practice continues for the time being.

The short latency and brevity of the contraction of a striated muscle in response to a single nerve impulse led many early investigators to doubt the possibility of a chemical transmission mechanism at the neuromuscular junction in skeletal muscle. However, Dale, Feldberg and Vogt, in 1936, demonstrated the release of acetylcholine on stimulation of a somatic motor nerve. They perfused the blood vessels of the tongue of a cat and when they stimulated the hypoglossal nerve, producing contraction of the striated muscle in the tongue, acetylcholine was identified in the perfusion fluid leaving the tongue. In other experiments, the gastrocnemius muscle in the leg of the dog or the cat was perfused and the motor roots of the sciatic nerve were stimulated inside the spinal column, so as to avoid stimulating nerve fibres other than motoneurones. The substance appearing in the perfusate behaved qualitatively and quantitatively in the same way as a standard solution of acetylcholine when assayed biologically. The presence of the substance was detected only when physostigmine was added to the perfusion fluid to inhibit cholinesterase. Dale and his coworkers then showed that the release of acetylcholine was not due to the contraction of the muscle. First, curare abolished the contractions although acetylcholine was still present in the perfusate after nerve stimulation. Second, direct electrical stimulation of the chronically denervated muscle elicited contractions, but no acetylcholine was detected in the perfusion fluid.

These experiments showed that acetylcholine was released when the motor nerves were stimulated, and further work showed that it mimicked the effect of nerve stimulation in causing contraction. In succeeding years, overwhelmingly convincing evidence was obtained that the transmission of excitation from the motor nerve endings to the striated muscle fibres in the muscles, not only of mammals, but also of birds and amphibia, is mediated by acetylcholine. Acetylcholine is synthesized within the motor nerve endings and stored within the synaptic vesicles (see p. 110). When released from the nerve endings by nerve impulses, acetylcholine diffuses across the narrow junctional gap and depolarizes the postjunctional membrane to produce an endplate potential. This action of acetylcholine is mimicked by nicotine, and in accordance with Dale's classification (p. 103, this chapter) is therefore described as a nicotinic action of acetylcholine.

Figure 8.2 illustrates the sites of cholinergic and noradrenergic transmission in both the autonomic and somatic branches of the peripheral nervous system. Until about 15 years ago, such a diagram would have been regarded as essentially accurate and complete. However, more recent research has indicated that it is necessary to modify this relatively simple picture to a substantial extent for three main reasons:

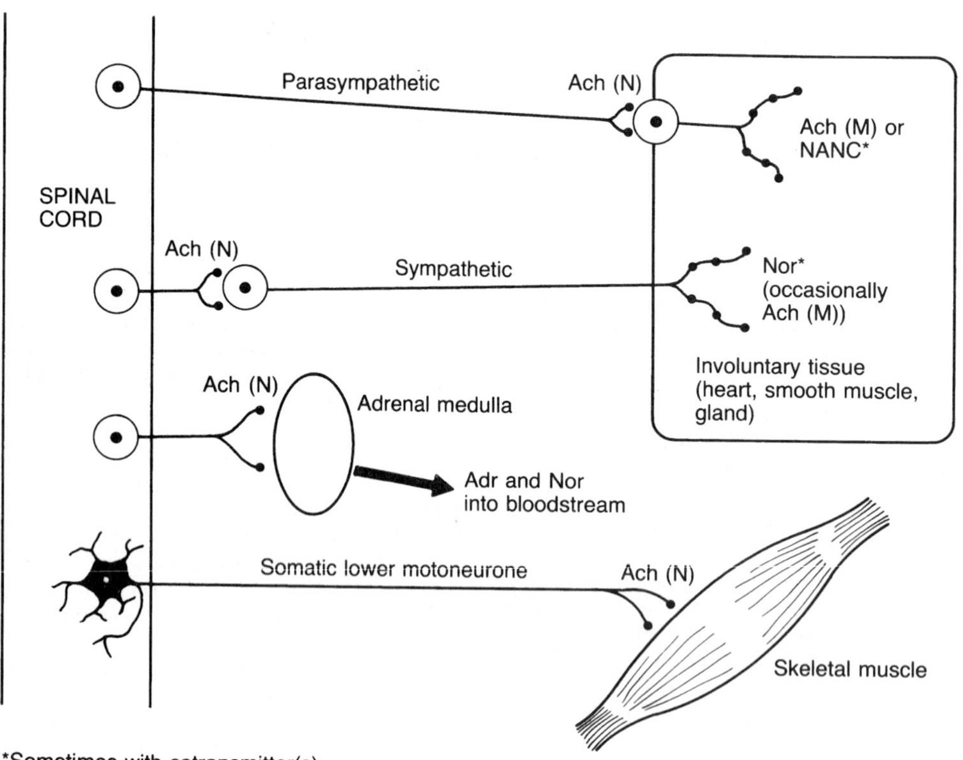

FIGURE 8.2 Diagrammatic representation of the peripheral efferent nervous system. Many involuntary organs are innervated by both branches of the autonomic nervous system – sympathetic and parasympathetic – but there are important exceptions (see Table 8.1). Skeletal muscle is innervated by the lower motoneurones of the somatic nervous system. Ach (N), acetylcholine with a nicotinic action; Ach (M), acetylcholine with a muscarinic action; Nor, noradrenaline; Adr, adrenaline. Note that this diagram takes no account of NANC (non-adrenergic, non-cholinergic) transmitters, cotransmitters, or prejunctional receptors (see text). Nor does it include the likelihood that sensory nerve fibres conduct not only in an afferent direction, but also antidromically along branches that may release vasodilator transmitters on to the smooth muscle of arterioles, or bronchoconstrictor transmitters into the lungs. This is the so-called sensory-efferent role of sensory nerve fibres. *Sometimes with cotransmitter(s).

(1) the discovery of peripheral transmitters in addition to noradrenaline (or dopamine) and acetylcholine; (2) the discovery that some (perhaps many) nerve fibres release two, or maybe more, transmitters; and (3) the discovery of receptors on nerve endings that modulate the release of the transmitter(s).

SYNTHESIS OF NORADRENALINE AND ACETYLCHOLINE

In noradrenergic neurones, noradrenaline is synthesized from tyrosine (Fig. 8.3). Tyrosine is actively taken up into the nerve fibre where it is first hydroxylated to produce *d*ihydr*o*xy*p*henyl*a*lanine (DOPA) under the influence of the cytoplasmic enzyme tyrosine hydroxylase. DOPA is then decarboxylated to produce dopamine (3-hydroxytyramine) under the influence of the enzyme aromatic amino acid decarboxylase (or DOPA decarboxylase). Dopamine is actively taken up into granular storage vesicles in the varicosities of the nerve endings, and there, in most instances, a β-hydroxyl group is added by the enzyme dopamine β-hydroxylase to produce noradrenaline. In a very few cases (e.g. in some nerve fibres innervating certain blood vessels and in interneurone-like structures in sympathetic ganglia), synthesis stops at dopamine, which itself functions as the neurotransmitter. In the adrenal medulla a further step, the *N*-methylation of noradrenaline to produce adrenaline, occurs. This step is catalysed by the enzyme phenylethanolamine-*N*-methyl transferase.

Acetylcholine is synthesized in the axoplasm of the terminals of cholinergic nerve fibres from choline and acetylcoenzyme A, under the influence of the enzyme choline-O-acetyltransferase. It is then actively loaded into small vesicles, the synaptic vesicles (see p. 110), ready for release.

PERIPHERAL INACTIVATION OF NORADRENALINE AND ACETYLCHOLINE

The main mechanism by which transmitter noradrenaline is inactivated after being released is by re-uptake into the varicosities of sympathetic nerve endings. The process is known as *neuronal re-uptake* or *uptake 1*. It is a high affinity active transport system that is capable of sequestering noradrenaline against a substantial concentration gradient. Once inside the axoplasm, the noradrenaline may be reloaded into vesicles and re-used as the neurotransmitter. Uptake 1 serves to maintain an adequate supply of transmitter by augmenting that produced by *de novo* synthesis. However, there is an additional uptake process, *uptake 2* or *non-neuronal uptake*, into smooth and cardiac muscle and endothelium, that serves to remove any excess. Uptake 2 has a much lower affinity than uptake 1 for noradrenaline. Thus, the Michaelis–Menten constant or dissociation constant (K_m) for uptake 2 (*c.* 250 μmol/l) is around 800 times greater than that for uptake 1. On the other hand, the maximum rate of uptake (V_{max}) of noradrenaline by uptake 1 (around 1–1.5 nmol/g/min) is much lower (around 80 times lower) than that for uptake 2. The two uptake mechanisms are not selective for noradrenaline. Adrenaline and even isoprenaline are also substrates. Both have least affinity for isoprenaline. Uptake 1 has greatest specificity for noradrenaline whereas uptake 2 has the greatest specificity for adrenaline. Other substrates

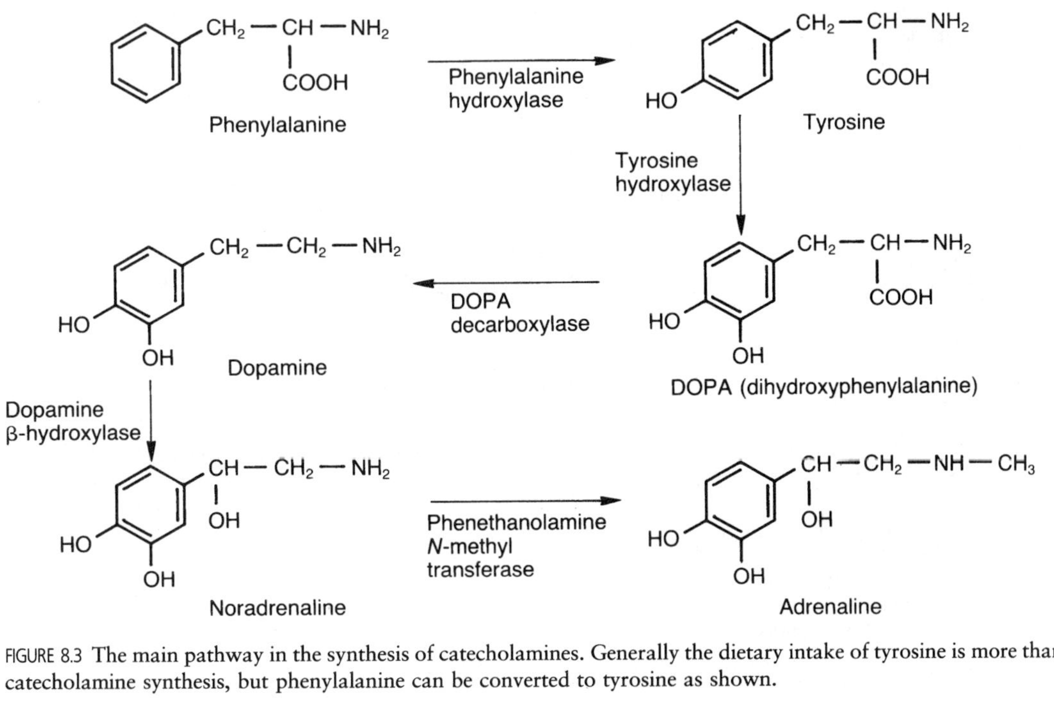

FIGURE 8.3 The main pathway in the synthesis of catecholamines. Generally the dietary intake of tyrosine is more than adequate for catecholamine synthesis, but phenylalanine can be converted to tyrosine as shown.

for both uptake processes include dopamine and 5-hydroxytryptamine.

The uptake processes may be inhibited by certain drugs which are dealt with in detail elsewhere (Chapter 14). Phenoxybenzamine, (p. 193) the main action of which is to block α-adrenoceptors, also blocks both uptake 1 and uptake 2. The local anaesthetic drug cocaine (pp. 97, 190) selectively blocks uptake 1, as do the tricyclic antidepressant drugs (p. 344), such as desipramine. The metabolite of noradrenaline, normetanephrine, and steroid hormones, such as oestrogens and corticosterone, block uptake 2, but not uptake 1. Surprisingly perhaps, the neuromuscular blocking drug pancuronium, which is also a steroid, is said to block uptake 1 rather than uptake 2.

Noradrenaline and adrenaline may also be inactivated by metabolic degradation, although this is of secondary importance in the periphery as far as neuronally released noradrenaline is concerned. Two main enzymes are involved: *monoamine oxidase* (MAO), which occurs in two forms known as MAO-A and MAO-B, and catechol-O-methyltransferase (COMT) (Fig. 8.4). MAO is located on the outer membranes of mitochondria, and is present in many organs such as liver and intestine, but especially in the varicosities of noradrenergic nerve endings. Noradrenaline and adrenaline (and 5-hydroxtryptamine) are substrates for MAO-A, whereas dopamine may be acted upon by both MAO-A and MAO-B. COMT acts on many substrates that contain a catechol group, including the catecholamines. As its name indicates, the result of its activity is methylation of one of the two catechol-OH groups.

Within the sympathetic varicosities, MAO controls the content of dopamine and noradrenaline, and hence the releasable store of the transmitter. MAO catalyses the conversion of catecholamines to their corresponding aldehydes, which are then rapidly metabolized by aldehyde dehydrogenase to the carboxylic acid; that is, to dihydroxymandelic acid (DOMA) in the case of

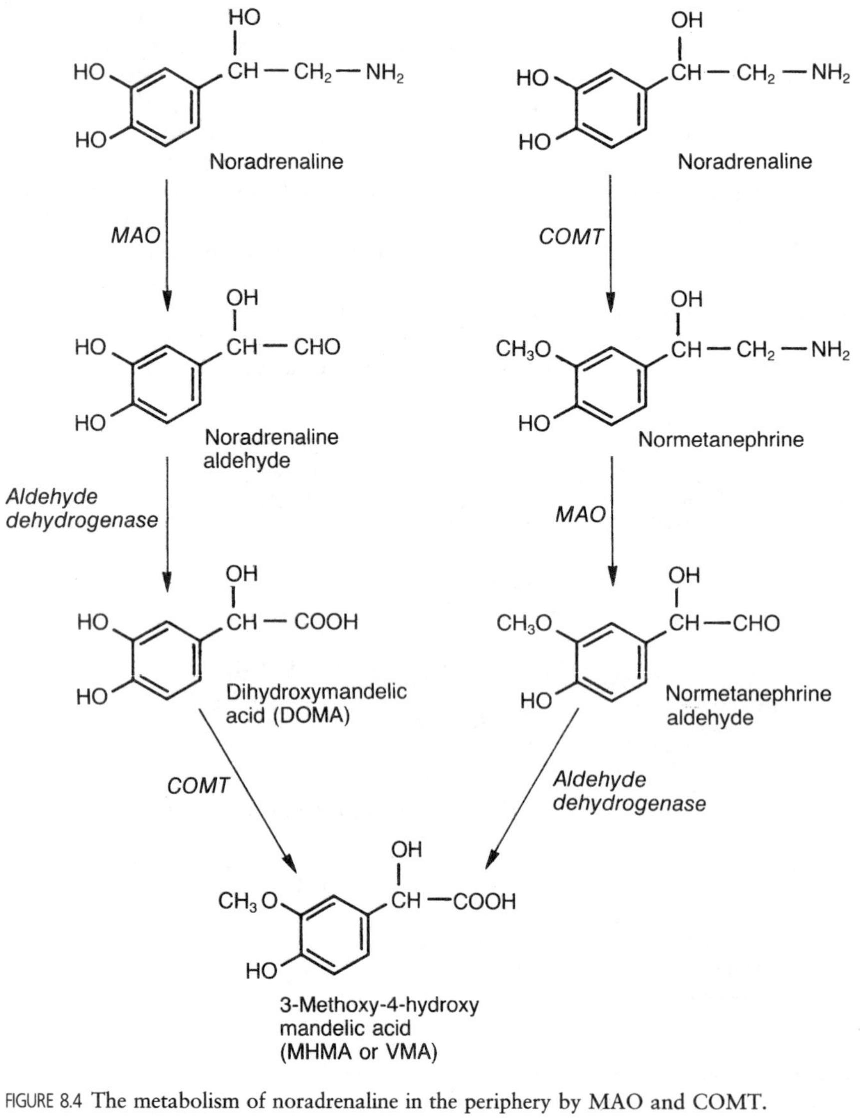

FIGURE 8.4 The metabolism of noradrenaline in the periphery by MAO and COMT.

noradrenaline. DOMA is still a catechol and can be acted upon by COMT to produce 3-methoxy-4-hydroxymandelic acid (MHMA – often incorrectly referred to as VMA).

COMT acts on noradrenaline to produce its O-methylated derivative normetanephrine. Normetanephrine may then be acted upon by MAO and aldehyde dehydrogenase, so that MHMA is again the final metabolite that appears in the urine.

Acetylcholine released from nerve endings is inactivated by hydrolysis, with the production of choline and acetate, under the influence of the enzyme acetylcholinesterase which is located in the junctional gap. This enzyme is dealt with in detail in Chapter 10. A special high affinity transport mechanism for the uptake of choline for acetylcholine synthesis exists at cholinergic nerve endings. Some of the choline produced from acetylcholine hydrolysis is taken up again by this mechanism. Choline is also derived from the diet and is synthesized in the liver.

RELEASE OF ACETYLCHOLINE OR NORADRENALINE BY NERVE IMPULSES

When a nerve impulse reaches a nerve ending, the fall in terminal membrane potential causes the opening of voltage-operated calcium channels. Calcium ions then enter the terminal axoplasm along their concentration gradient and, through a mechanism that is not yet fully understood, cause the transmitter storage vesicles to fuse with the terminal membrane and discharge their contents into the junctional gap. One mechanism that does seem to play a part in vesicle fusion at many synapses involves three types of integral vesicular membrane proteins called *synaptotagmin, synaptobrevin* and *synaptophysins*, together with small GTP-binding proteins, such as that known as *rab 3a*; the precise role of each is not yet clear. Synaptobrevin binds to a receptor protein known as *syntaxin* in the terminal axonal membrane, the binding requiring the presence of additional soluble proteins and factors. In this way, the vesicles may dock at the release sites. Synaptotagmin and synaptophysins are calcium-binding proteins. It is thought that calcium ions that enter the terminal axoplasm on the arrival of a nerve impulse bind to these proteins. The binding induces a conformational change that is transmitted through the whole complex with the docking proteins, so that a fusion channel or pore is formed that allows the transmitter and other vesicle contents to escape into the synaptic or junctional cleft. The vesicle membranes remain transiently fused with the terminal axonal membrane but are shortly recovered by endocytosis and reformed into vesicles.

Another vesicular protein has been shown by Greengard and his coworkers to be concerned more with the availability of transmitter for release (i.e. with mobilization) than with the release process itself; it is called *synapsin I*. Synapsin I molecules are bound to the surface of the vesicles by their tail regions forming a cage-like structure around each vesicle. Synapsin I has the property of binding to the protein actin. Hence, it is thought to anchor vesicles to the cytoskeleton of the nerve endings. Synapsin I is a substrate for phosphorylation by various kinase enzymes (cyclic AMP-dependent protein kinase, calcium-calmodulin activated protein kinases I and II). Phosphorylation of the tail region of synapsin I by calcium-calmodulin activated protein kinase II decreases the affinity of synapsin I for the vesicle surface. Hence, it may be that, in the presence of Ca^{2+}, the vesicles dissociate from the cytoskeleton and thereby move freely in the axoplasm, becoming available for the release process. Cyclic AMP-dependent protein kinase acts to phosphorylate the head region of synapsin I. The role of this process is not yet understood, although the fact that processes that elevate the axonal content of cyclic AMP (e.g. β-adrenoceptor stimulation) enhance mobilization or release of transmitter, may indicate that phosphorylation of the head region of synapsin I is important in the vesicular release process. Figure 8.5 represents what is known of the roles of synapsin I synaptobrevin, synaptotagmin and synaptophysin in transmitter mobilization and release.

A transmitter substance, once released from the axon terminal, interacts with specific components of the membrane of the postjunctional cell which are termed receptors. The interaction between the transmitter and its receptors then sets in train a series of events which culminate in the observable response (e.g. depolarization of a ganglion cell; contraction or relaxation of smooth muscle; secretion in glandular tissues; an alteration in cardiac activity; see Table 8.1).

RECEPTORS

As long ago as 1878, Langley in Cambridge formulated the concept of receptors as a result of his experiments demonstrating the opposing actions of pilocarpine and atropine on salivary flow in the cat. He assumed that there was some substance in the physiological system with which atropine and pilocarpine were capable of forming compounds. Later, in 1905, he introduced the idea of a 'specific receptive substance' as the site of action of nicotine and curare in the myoneural junction. The actual term 'receptor' was first used around 1910 by Paul Ehrlich whose experiments led him to the idea, based on his experience of immunochemistry, that drugs act by combining with specific chemical groupings on larger molecules of cells. He called these groupings receptors.

Several types of receptors have now been isolated in a pure form but, for many years, although an indispensable concept for discussion and for understanding mechanisms of action of neurotransmitters and drugs, they remained no more than hypothetical entities. A

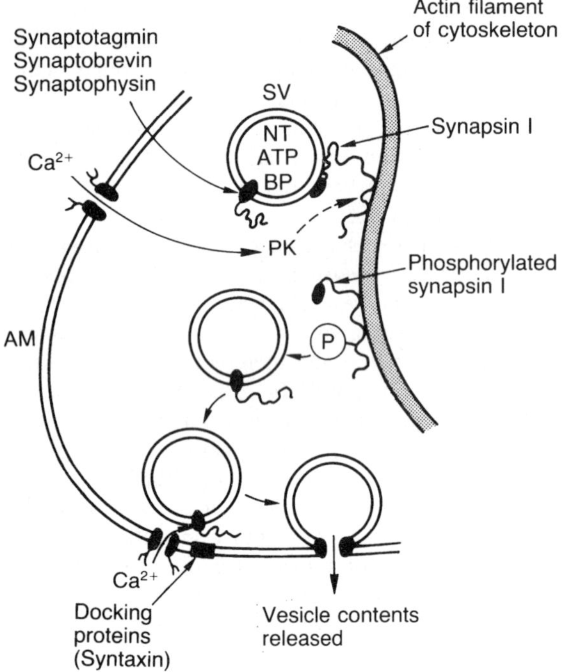

FIGURE 8.5 The release of neurotransmitters. The vesicle membrane incorporates three different types of integral proteins (synaptotagmin, synaptobrevin and synaptophysins) although only one is shown in the diagram. These proteins are involved in docking of the synaptic vesicle with its release site which contains docking proteins including syntaxin. Ca^{2+} that enters the axoplasm through voltage-operated calcium channels in the terminal axonal membrane (AM) is shown as having two effects: (1) It combines with calmodulin and the calci-calmodulin complex then activates a protein kinase (PK) that phosphorylates the tail region of synapsin I. This frees the synaptic vesicle (SV) from its anchor with the cytoskeleton so that it can move towards the release sites. (2) It binds to the integral membrane proteins synaptotagmin and synaptophysin causing the opening of a fusion channel. The vesicular contents, i.e. the neurotransmitter (NT: acetylcholine or noradrenaline), a transmitter binding protein (BP: chromogranins in the case of noradrenaline and possibly vesiculin in the case of acetylcholine), ATP, and often ions such as Ca^{2+} and Mg^{2+}, are released into the junctional gap.

vast literature describes deductions concerning them based on pharmacological experiments in which mechanical cellular responses, many steps removed from the actual drug–receptor interaction, were measured. Studies of structure : action relations in such experiments, with both agonists and antagonists, have given some insight into the complementary nature of the binding groups that comprise the receptor recognition sites and have provided information for defining receptor types, including subtypes of receptors within a larger group. Related studies, initiated by Clark and Gaddum (50–60 years ago) allowed the derivation of mathematical descriptions of concentration–response relations based on and developed from the mass action law. In relatively recent years, important forward steps in protein chemistry and in molecular gene cloning studies have led to the elucidation of the complete structures of many types and subtypes of receptor.

Receptor nomenclature is dealt with in some detail below. For the present, suffice to say that, in accordance with Dale's concept, those acetylcholine receptors that respond to nicotine (i.e. in muscle and in autonomic ganglion cells) are called *nicotinic acetylcholine receptors*; those that respond to muscarine (e.g. in the heart, in glands and in smooth muscle) are called *muscarinic acetylcholine receptors*; and those that respond to adrenaline or noradrenaline, or both, are called *adrenoceptors*.

The nicotinic acetylcholine receptors of muscle and of autonomic ganglia are alike in that they are each composed of five protein subunits or protomers arranged like a rosette with a central pore that can be in the closed, or, when acted upon by acetylcholine, in the open, conformation. In fetal muscle, the five protomers of the receptor have been designated α, β, γ and δ, there being two subunits of the α-type. In adult muscle, the protomer corresponding to the fetal γ-subunit is slightly different and is designated ε. Muscle nicotinic acetylcholine receptors are discussed more fully in Chapter 12. In autonomic ganglia, the receptors are composed of α- and β-type subunits only (2α and 3β), although these are not identical in composition with the α- and β-subunits of muscle receptors. Nicotinic acetylcholine receptors are generally similar in structure to other types of receptors in which an ion channel is an integral part of the receptor complex (e.g. glycine receptors, most subtypes of glutamate receptors, γ-aminobutyric acid ($GABA_A$) receptors, 5-HT_3 receptors and ATP receptors of the P2X type). These also are composed of four or five protomers surrounding an ion channel.

Muscarinic acetylcholine receptors and adrenoceptors, although differing from each other in relation to the particular agonists and antagonists with which they combine, are nevertheless related to each other, being members of the same superfamily of G-protein coupled receptors (p. 8). They are composed of about 500 amino acid residues with the N-terminal to the outside and the C-terminal to the inside. Receptor proteins of this group do not surround an ion channel. There are seven α-helices which cross the membrane from side to side and which show a high degree of homology in all G-protein coupled receptors. Surprisingly, the binding site for ligands is not on the external N-terminal end of the protein. Rather, it is located on the external surface ends of one or more of the transmembrane α-helices. The third of the cytoplasmic loops of the chain (joining the fifth and sixth transmembrane helices) is longer than the other two and contains the site that couples to the G-protein. The structure and functioning of G-protein coupled receptors is dealt with more fully in Chapter 1.

SITES AND CLASSIFICATION OF PERIPHERAL ACETYLCHOLINE RECEPTORS AND ADRENOCEPTORS

Pharmacologists have traditionally named and classified receptors and their subtypes in terms of their recognition sites for specific ligands (i.e. for molecules with which they bind; Latin ligare: to bind). Today, modern techniques of cell biology, including the purification and cloning of genomic fractions of cell surface receptors, have led to the discovery of a range of receptor subtypes that have hitherto escaped classical pharmacological techniques. It must be ascertained of course, before therapeutic importance is assigned to them, that subtypes of receptor discovered by gene-cloning studies are actually expressed *in vivo*. Receptors are not classified in accordance with their method of functioning, although it is the case that different subtypes of receptor often (though not invariably) do function by different second messenger systems. The main name of a broad receptor group, for example acetylcholine receptors, and adrenoceptors, is derived from the endogenous chemical that is its specific agonist – that is, acetylcholine and noradrenaline respectively in these cases. It has long been clear from the use of exogenous agonists and antagonists that receptors within a broad group are not homogeneous, even though the endogenous agonist is common for all receptors within the group. Thus, for example, all acetylcholine receptors respond to acetylcholine, yet Dale's early observations with muscarine and nicotine showed that subtypes of acetylcholine receptor, called muscarinic (or M) acetylcholine receptors and nicotinic (or N) acetylcholine receptors, exist within the broad group. From the therapeutic point of view, the more subtypes that can be detected, the better, since it becomes more and more possible to synthesize drugs with relatively selective actions on particular receptor subgroups, and hence often on particular organs. To state the obvious as an example: because atropine selectively blocks muscarinic acetylcholine receptors without affecting nicotinic acetylcholine receptors, it is possible to dry up a patient's secretions without simultaneously causing paralysis.

It is now known that the broad subdivision into muscarinic and nicotinic subtypes, though useful, is far from the whole story. Subclassifications into at least three subtypes of muscarinic receptors (M_1, M_2 and M_3 – gene cloning suggests five subtypes), and at least two and probably many more subtypes of nicotinic receptors ($N_{muscle\ type}$, $N_{neuronal\ type}$) have been described (Table 8.2).

In 1948, Ahlquist compared the relative potencies on different tissues of a number of sympathomimetics including noradrenaline, adrenaline and isoprenaline. He found that the order of potency on smooth muscle that responded with contraction was adrenaline > noradrenaline > isoprenaline, whereas on smooth muscle that responded with relaxation the order of potency was isoprenaline > adrenaline > noradrenaline. The order of potency for stimulation of the heart was similar to that for relaxation of smooth muscle. In order to explain these findings, he postulated that there are two subtypes of adrenoceptor which he designated α-adrenoceptors and β-adrenoceptors. Effector cells with α-adrenoceptors have a high sensitivity to adrenaline and noradrenaline but are practically insensitive to isoprenaline, whereas those with β-adrenoceptors have a higher sensitivity to isoprenaline than to other catecholamines and are usually more sensitive to adrenaline than to noradrenaline. Ahlquist's concept of α- and β-receptors has been universally adopted. However, it is now recognized that noradrenaline is often more potent than adrenaline on α-receptors, but it may appear to be less potent because it is removed more rapidly than is adrenaline from the region of the receptors. Therefore, the greater potency of noradrenaline can only be demonstrated satisfactorily when the removal process is eliminated by sympathetic denervation or is inhibited by cocaine or other drugs. Selective α- and β-adrenoceptor antagonists are available. Phenoxybenzamine is an example of the former, and propranolol of the latter.

A clear indication that β-adrenoceptors are not homogeneous is provided by the observation that noradrenaline, an effective stimulant of cardiac β-adrenoceptors, has little or no ability to stimulate β-adrenoceptors mediating vasodilatation in the smooth muscles of blood vessels. Lands and his colleagues in 1967 divided β-adrenoceptors into two distinct subtypes on the basis of the differential sensitivity of various tissues to a series of β-adrenoceptor agonists. The β-adrenoceptors of the heart were of one type, designated β_1-adrenoceptors; those of bronchial, vascular and uterine smooth muscle were of another type and were designated β_2-adrenoceptors.

More recently, many relatively specific β_1-adrenoceptor agonists and antagonists have been developed and several of them have been put into clinical use. β_3-adrenoceptors (formerly called atypical β-adrenoceptors) have also recently been designated; they are present in adipose tissue (adipocytes) and stimulate lipolysis and non-shivering thermogenesis.

α-Adrenoceptors also have been shown not to be homogeneous. They were first classified into two subtypes, α_1- and α_2-adrenoceptors. α_2-Adrenoceptors were originally thought to occur only on noradrenergic nerve terminals where they function in a negative feedback mechanism. However, they are now known to be present also on some effector cells. Further subclassification of adrenoceptors has become evident more recently, and at least five subtypes (α_{1A}, α_{1B}, α_{1D}, α_{2A}, α_{2B}) are now recognized. Table 8.2 includes the main subtypes and the characteristics of adrenoceptors. Receptors formally designated α_{1C} were found to be α_{1A} receptors, and α_{1C} is therefore now omitted from the series.

TABLE 8.2 Subtypes of peripheral acetylcholine receptors and adrenoceptors

MAIN TYPE	SUBTYPES	MECHANISM (SECOND MESSENGERS)	SELECTIVE AGONISTS	SELECTIVE ANTAGONISTS	TYPICAL LOCATION
	M_1	$InsP_3$/DG – closure of K^+ M channels	McN/A 343 AH 6405	Pirenzepine, telenzepine	Sympathetic ganglion cells
	M_2	cAMP reduction or K^+ channel operated via G-protein	—	Methoctramine, gallamine (but non-competitive)	SA node of heart, some autoreceptors including airways
Acetycholine receptors	M_3	$InsP_3$/DG	—	Hexahydrosiladifenidol	Smooth muscle generally e.g. gut, bronchi
	$N_{\text{muscle type}}$	Directly opens cation channel	—	Pancuronium, vecuronium, atracurium, α-bungarotoxin	Motor endplate
	$N_{\text{neuronal type}}$	Directly opens cation channel	Dimethylphenyl-piperazinium; nicotine. Both only relatively selective	Trimetaphan; neuronal bungarotoxin	Autonomic ganglia
	α_{1A}		Phenylephrine, methoxamine and cirazoline are selective for α_1 class as a whole	WB4101; (+)niguldipine; 5-methyl-urapadil; abanoquil prazosin	Smooth muscle
	α_{1B}	$InsP_3$/DG for all α_1		Spiperone prazosin	Heart, liver, spleen
	α_{1D}			BMY 7378	CNS Prostate (human)
Adrenoceptors	α_{2A}	cAMP reduction or K^+ channel opened via G-protein	Oxymetazoline (partial agonist)	Yohimbine and rauwolscine are selective for α_2 as a whole	Smooth muscle, some autoreceptors, platelets, lipocytes
	α_{2B}	cAMP reduction	Clonidine selective for α_2 as a whole		Atria, kidney CNS
	β_1	cAMP increase for all β-adrenoceptors	Noradrenaline, xamoterol (relative to β_2)	Atenolol	Heart
	β_2		Procaterol	ICI 11851	Bronchi
	β_3		BRL 37344	SR 59230A	Lipocytes

The second messenger mechanisms are described fully in Chapter 1.
$InsP_3$/DG = the production of inositol trisphosphate and diacylglycerol by activation of the enzyme phospholipase C. cAMP = cyclic adenosine monophosphate. McN/A343 = 4(*m*-chlorophenylcarbamoyloxy)-2-butyn trimethylammonium bromide. AH 6405 = 1,4,5,6-tetrahydro-5-phenoxypyrimidine. BRL 37344 = sodium-4-2-[2-hydroxy-(3-chlorophenyl)ethylaminopropyl phenoxyacetate]. ICI 11851 = erythro-DL-1-(7-methylindan-4-yloxy)-3-isopropylamine butane-2-ol. WB4101 is N-[2-(2,6-dimethoxyphenoxy)ethyl]-2,3-dihydroxo-1,4-benzodioxan-2-methaneamine. BMY 7378 is 8-{2-[-2 methoxyphenyl-1-piperazinyl]ethyl}-8-azaspiro [4,5] decal-7,9-dione dihydrochloride. SR 59230A is (3-(2-ethyl-phenoxy)-1-[(IS)-1,2,3,4-tetrahydronaphth-1-ylamino]-(2S)-2-propanol oxalate. These compounds have no therapeutic uses but are useful pharmacological tools for differentiating receptor subtypes.

NONADRENERGIC NONCHOLINERGIC (NANC) TRANSMISSION

There is clear evidence, especially from experiments by Burnstock and his colleagues, for the existence of inhibitory autonomic nerves that liberate neither acetylcholine nor a catecholamine. Burnstock has long believed that ATP or some other purine nucleotide functions as the neurotransmitter in some of these instances, and has described such nerve fibres or the transmission event as *purinergic*. In these instances the nucleotide functions in a pharmacodynamic rather than a biochemical sense. In recent years, antagonists of the pharmacological actions of ATP have been developed and experiments with these antagonists have added support to Burnstock's proposal. The problem is complex, however, and the full picture has not yet emerged. Difficulties include the fact that all cells synthesize ATP, and many neurones release small amounts of ATP along with their conventional transmitters. In some instances, although not all, ATP functions as a cotransmitter rather than the main transmitter as described below.

Some peripheral NANC nerve fibres clearly do not release a purine nucleotide as their transmitter. In some instances, largely in the gut, but also in the airways, a polypeptide may fulfil the role of neurotransmitter and the neurone is described as *peptidergic*. Polypeptides that may function in this way include substance P, neuropeptide Y, cholecystokinin, calcitonin gene-related peptide, and vasoactive intestinal peptide (VIP) among others.

In a few instances, the inhibitory nerves have been found to make use of nitric oxide (NO), derived from L-arginine, in the transmission mechanism. The synthesizing enzyme, nitric oxide synthase, is activated by Ca^{2+}. Presumably Ca^{2+}, entering the axon terminal on the arrival of a nerve impulse, activates the enzyme and nitric oxide is generated from L-arginine. Nitric oxide is a very small diffusible molecule. It cannot be stored in vesicles but must be synthesized on demand. It presumably diffuses across the junctional gap and penetrates the effector cell, where it acts intracellularly to stimulate the activity of a soluble cytosolic guanylate cyclase enzyme, and the cyclic GMP produced activates a protein kinase that brings about relaxation of smooth muscle. It is not in fact yet absolutely clear whether nitric oxide is released from the nerve ending as such, or whether it is liberated after release of a larger molecule. There is clear evidence in the central nervous system for a trans-synaptic action of nitric oxide. The term *nitrergic* has been suggested to describe the transmission mechanism when the effects of nerve impulses are mediated by nitric oxide. Instances in the periphery where transmission has been shown to be nitrergic include relaxation of the bovine retractor penis muscle and rat anococcygeus muscle in response to inhibitory nerve stimulation, penile erection in some species, and some components of gastrointestinal and airways relaxation. However, it would be surprising if the transmission mechanisms to these few tissues were unique. Nitric oxide is a powerful vasodilator substance. It is in fact identical with the so-called endothelium derived relaxing factor (EDRF) of blood vessels (see p. 222). It may well be that inhibitory 'nitrergic' transmission mechanisms will be discovered at sites in addition to the few referred to above.

There are clear instances in which afferent nerve fibres not only transmit signals to the central nervous system, but also release transmitters locally by antidromic excitation of peripheral branches. For example, part of the so-called triple response and aspects of neurogenic inflammation depend on such a local release mechanism. Evidence has been obtained that in the lungs, vagal afferents release substance P, and possibly other so-called neurokinins, by antidromic impulses in local branches. Substance P is a powerful bronchoconstrictor. The bronchoconstriction that follows chemical irritation of vagal sensory nerve endings probably depends on such a mechanism.

COTRANSMITTERS

Many nerve fibres contain ATP or a polypeptide, or both, in addition to what has been regarded as their main transmitter. At some peripheral neuroeffector junctions, traditionally regarded as noradrenergic, evidence has been obtained that noradrenaline is released together with ATP or a polypeptide such as neuropeptide Y, and that these so-called cotransmitters mediate part of the transmission event, or modulate the activity or release of the main transmitter. There may also be cotransmission in parasympathetic nerves. For example, VIP is often stored together with acetylcholine. In the cat salivary gland, low frequency stimulation evokes the release of acetylcholine from parasympathetic nerves causing salivary secretion and some vasodilatation. At higher frequencies of stimulation, the nerves release VIP together with acetylcholine to produce marked vasodilatation and indirect enhancement of acetylcholine release by stimulation of prejunctional VIP receptors. Future evidence may indicate that cotransmission is more prevalent than presently available evidence suggests.

PREJUNCTIONAL RECEPTORS

Although there is some controversy over their physiological function, there is clear evidence for the existence, near the nerve endings of most and possibly all axons, of receptors that respond to endogenous chemicals. These presynaptic or prejunctional receptors mediate either an increase or a decrease in the release of transmitter in response to nerve impulses. Nerve terminal receptors that respond to the same transmitter as that released from the associated nerve endings are called autoreceptors. Autoreceptors are usually, although not invariably, of a different subtype from that of the postjunctional receptors. Many physiologists and pharmacologists believe that autoreceptors function in complex negative or positive feedback control systems that modulate transmitter release. Such autoreceptors at the neuromuscular junction in skeletal muscle are referred to on p. 139.

Nerve terminal receptors that respond to different transmitters released from adjacent nerve endings or to other endogenous chemicals or autacoids, such as prostaglandins or adenosine, are called heteroreceptors. In several instances, parasympathetic cholinergic nerve endings have been shown to possess inhibitory heteroreceptors for noradrenaline. The converse, sympathetic noradrenergic nerve endings with inhibitory acetylcholine heteroreceptors, has also been demonstrated. This provides a mechanism whereby, in reciprocally innervated tissues, one branch of the autonomic nervous system not only produces the opposite effect to the other branch, but at the same time depresses any activity of the opposing branch.

Autacoids, such as prostaglandins and adenosine (derived from ATP), may be produced by the activated tissue rather than released from nerves. They may then act back on specific receptors on the adjacent nerve endings to depress transmitter release, hence functioning in a negative feedback control mechanism that ensures against overreactivity of the innervated tissue.

FURTHER READING

Bell C ed. Novel perpheral neurotransmitters. *International encyclopedia of pharmacology and therapeutics*, Section 135. New York: Pergamon Press, 1991.

Burnstock G, Hoyle CHV eds. *Autonomic neuroeffector mechanisms*, Vol. 1. Chur, Switzerland: Harwood Academic, 1992.

Kalsner S, Westfall TC eds. Presynaptic receptors and the question of autoregulation of neurotransmitter release. *Annals of the New York Academy of Sciences* 1990; **604**: 1–652.

Rand MJ. Nitrergic transmission: nitric oxide as a mediator of non-adrenergic, non-cholinergic neuro-effector transmission. *Clinical and Experimental Pharmacology and Physiology* 1992; **19**: 147–69.

Südhof TC, Jahn R. Proteins of synaptic vesicles involved in exocytosis and membrane recycling. *Neuron* 1991; **6**: 665–7.

Watson SP, Girdlestone D. Receptor and ion channel nomenclature supplment. 6th edn. *Trends in Pharmacological Sciences* 1995.

9

Muscarinic and Nicotinic Agonists

RB Barlow

To understand the title of this chapter it helps to look at an experiment made by Dale in 1914, which has already been referred to in Chapter 8 and illustrated in Fig. 8.2. Dale was studying the effects of acetylcholine on blood pressure in an anaesthetized cat. Small doses (5 μg: 25 nmol) of acetylcholine produced vasodilatation and a fall in pressure. With slightly larger doses (50 μg: 250 nmol) the heart slowed also. In very much larger doses (5 mg: 2.5 μmol) there was a rise in blood pressure. This rise was easier to see if the animal had been given atropine, which blocked the fall in blood pressure. Depending on the dose, acetylcholine could lower or raise the blood pressure. Dale then tested other compounds. These included (+)muscarine, one of the alkaloids in *Amanita muscaria* and (−)nicotine, obtained from tobacco. He found that (+)muscarine always lowered the blood pressure whereas (−)nicotine always raised it: thus he divided the properties of acetylcholine into 'muscarine-like' and 'nicotine-like'. These must be brought about by different mechanisms because there are drugs that block one property and not the other. For example, atropine blocks the (muscarinic) fall in pressure but not the (nicotinic) rise. The rise could be blocked by an extract of 'curare' and this did not affect the fall. Unfortunately curare also produced paralysis of voluntary muscle so the animal stopped breathing and had to be put on a ventilator, but the effects on respiration and on blocking the rise in blood pressure are distinct. The rise in blood pressure produced by (−)nicotine can be blocked by hexamethonium without affecting the respiration.

Dale's division of the properties of acetylcholine into muscarine-like and nicotine-like was later explained by supposing that there are different types of acetylcholine receptor. Muscarinic receptors occur on blood vessels. They produce vasodilatation when stimulated by an agonist (muscarine or acetylcholine) and are blocked by atropine. Muscarinic receptors occur also in the heart and stimulation of them produces a hyperpolarization with a decrease in the rate and force of the atrial beat. It was vagal slowing of the frog heart that was used by Loewi in 1921 to demonstrate that nerve impulses caused the release of chemical transmitters, and the material he called 'vagus-stoff' is acetylcholine and acts at muscarinic receptors. Most effects of stimulating parasympathetic nerves involve the release of acetylcholine and its action on muscarinic receptors. Note, however, that in Dale's experiment the fall in blood pressure is largely due to lowered peripheral resistance (and not to the effect on the heart) and the receptors involved are not part of the parasympathetic nervous system.

The rise in blood pressure produced by the nicotine-like actions of acetylcholine involves stimulation of receptors in sympathetic ganglia, with the subsequent release of noradrenaline from postganglionic nerve endings. Nicotine can also stimulate receptors in the adrenal medulla, with the resulting release of adrenaline and noradrenaline into the bloodstream. Because the use of curare extracts to block the rise in blood pressure produced by (−)nicotine was associated with paralysis of voluntary muscles, these too should have nicotinic receptors but they are of a different type.

Nicotinic receptors can therefore be divided into 'ganglionic' and 'neuromuscular'. There is an important practical difference between drugs that are primarily ganglion-blocking (such as hexamethonium) and those that are primarily neuromuscular blocking. While it is true that curare alkaloids, of which (+)tubocurarine chloride is the most commonly available, have ganglion-blocking activity it is important to realize that the main effect is to produce paralysis. Ganglion-block can, however, occur when (+)tubocurarine chloride has been given as a relaxant to a patient undergoing surgery (and who is on a ventilator!).

The sites where the receptors involved in the muscarinic and nicotinic actions of acetylcholine are located can be summarized:

- nicotinic:
  - ganglia (sympathetic and parasympathetic)
  - neuromuscular junction
- muscarinic:
  - parasympathetically innervated smooth muscle and organs
  - sympathetically innervated smooth muscle where acetylcholine is the transmitter.

Pure proteins from many types of nicotinic and muscarinic receptor have been isolated and the amino-acid sequence has been calculated so the classification starting with Dale's experiment and based on what compounds do could in theory be replaced by a classification based on what the receptors are. Molecular biologists have identified many distinct types of nicotinic and muscarinic receptor so logically the terms 'muscarinic' and 'nicotinic' should disappear. They are unsatisfactory because one needs to have studied Dale's experiment to understand how the terms came to be chosen and also because, even today, it is very difficult to obtain pure (+)muscarine. Receptors are more likely to be classified as 'muscarinic' because they are blocked by atropine rather than because they are known to be activated by (+)muscarine.

At present, the molecular biologist can distinguish five subtypes of muscarinic receptor and three of these can be identified by pharmacologists:

- M_1 receptors occur in sympathetic ganglia, where they are linked to a slow depolarization, as opposed to the rapid depolarization produced by nicotine
- M_2 receptors are found in the heart where they are involved in the decrease in the rate and force of beating, and
- M_3 receptors are involved in glandular secretion, in the contraction of intestinal smooth muscle and also in the vasodilatation and fall in blood pressure observed by Dale — though this is now known to be brought about by nitric oxide (NO).

Studies on nicotinic receptors obtained from the electric organs of fish such as *Electrophorus electricus* have made it possible to obtain pictures of what they look like and it is possible to distinguish many subtypes in muscle and brain. The pharmacologist, however, is limited by the selectivity of the drugs that are available so the distinction must be between neuromuscular and ganglionic receptors. With muscarinic receptors there are reasonably selective drugs for M_1 receptors, the compound McNeil A 343 as agonist and pirenzepine as antagonist, and there are anatagonists that distinguish between M_2 and M_3 receptors, but no really selective agonists as yet.

It is not yet time for a classification of receptors based on structure to replace the older classification of drugs into muscarine-like or nicotine-like agonists or antagonists, depending on what they do to tissues.

SUBSTANCES THAT PRODUCE ACETYLCHOLINE-LIKE EFFECTS

There are few substances that act like acetylcholine at both muscarinic and nicotinic receptors. Propionylcholine, for instance, is weaker than acetylcholine at muscarinic receptors but stronger than acetylcholine at nicotinic receptors. Because the action of acetylcholine at many sites, however, is limited by its hydrolysis by acetylcholinesterase, inhibitors of this enzyme, such as physostigmine (also called eserine), will prolong the effects of endogenous acetylcholine and so have (indirectly) both muscarinic and nicotinic activity. Note, however, that such compounds only have acetylcholine-like effects at sites where acetylcholine is being produced and hydrolysed and they do not produce the vasodilatation and fall in blood pressure obtained with small doses of muscarine or acetylcholine, which involve receptors where this does not seem to be occurring. These compounds are described as 'anticholinesterases' and are discussed in Chapter 10.

MUSCARINIC AGONISTS

These would be expected to produce effects similar to those of parasympathetic stimulation. They cause smooth muscle to contract and stimulate secretion and in the gastrointestinal tract this promotes digestion. Similar effects are seen in the bronchial tree and the increase in fluid and narrowing of the air passages may be dangerous. The effects on blood pressure have already been noted. The vasodilatation, however, is not an effect seen by stimulating the parasympathetic, though the slowing or even arrest of the heart can be produced by stimulating the vagus nerve. Muscarinic agonists will constrict the pupil of the eye (miosis) and cause the ciliary muscle to contract, allowing the lens to become more spherical and setting the focus for near vision. Most muscarinic agonists are quaternary salts (see below) and do not cross the blood–brain barrier but when applied to the central nervous system in an experiment, they produce an arousal, similar to that seen with acetylcholine.

Muscarinic agonists have only limited uses: to promote contraction of the gut when there is constipation or contraction of the bladder when there is retention of urine. In either situation it is important to be sure first that there is no mechanical obstruction. The effect of contracting the ciliary muscle should open up the Canal of Schlemm, which is adjacent (Fig. 9.1), and this has been made use of to lower the intraocular pressure in an attack of glaucoma. For the same

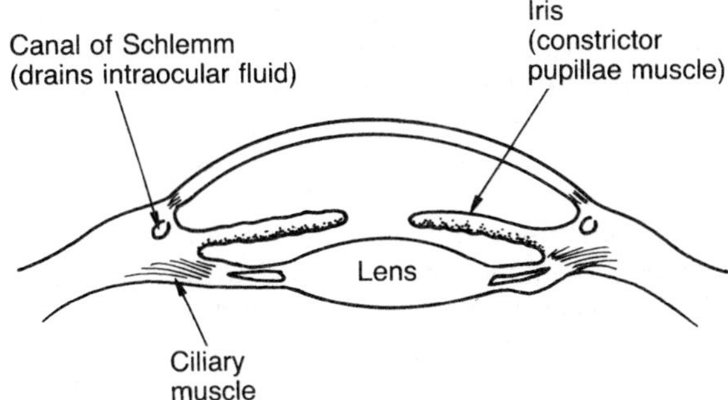

FIGURE 9.1 Anterior of the eye showing ciliary muscle and Canal of Schlemm.

reason, muscarinic blocking drugs are contraindicated in glaucoma. The effects of a muscarinic agonist are not pleasant and may be life-threatening – a profound fall in blood pressure, cardiac arrest, bronchoconstriction, excessive bronchial secretion, as well as extensive intestinal movement. Their therapeutic use is almost entirely confined to the eye, where the drug can be applied to the cornea and does not reach the general circulation.

Drugs

Two chemical features found in acetylcholine (see Fig. 9.2) are particularly important for muscarinic agonists because they determine what the body does to the drug and hence what the drug does to the body. If it contains a quaternary ammonium group (a nitrogen atom with four bonds to carbon) the compound is permanently ionized. Strictly, the negative ion should be specified, for example, acetylcholine iodide, but this is often omitted. Such a compound is likely to have difficulty crossing membranes, because it is not likely to be lipid soluble. It probably does not produce central effects because it has difficulty crossing the blood–brain barrier. There will also be problems with its oral absorption and it will have to be given by injection.

If it contains an ester group the compound may be a substrate for cholinesterases (see Chapter 10) and readily broken down. Alternatively the compound may inhibit acetylcholinesterase and produce pharmacological effects indirectly. The replacement of acetyl (CH_3CO–) by carbamyl (H_2NCO–) produces an ester that is stable to cholinesterases, and carbamylcholine (carbacholine) is often used experimentally as a stable form of acetylcholine. Its effects last longer than those of acetylcholine when cholinesterases are present, though it is actually slightly weaker than acetylcholine in its action at receptors. Muscarinic effects are produced by lower concentrations of acetylcholine than nicotinic effects, for example around 10 nM compared with around 1 μM, and carbachol has more of the nicotine-like activity of acetylcholine than of the muscarine-like activity so the concentrations may be around 50 nM (muscarinic) compared with 2 μM (nicotinic).

Resistance to cholinesterase can also be obtained by adding a methyl group next to the ester. This produces an asymmetric carbon atom so the compound acetyl-β-methylcholine exists as (+) and (−) isomers but is usually only available as the racemate. This is hydrolysed at about 25% of the rate of acetylcholine by acetylcholinesterases and even more slowly by butyrylcholinesterases. The (+) isomer has much of the muscarine-like activity of acetylcholine: the (−) isomer has only about 0.5% of the muscarine-like activity of the (+) isomer and both isomers have only weak nicotine-like properties. (±) Acetyl-β-methylcholine (methacholine chloride, mecholyl) has therefore appreciable muscarine-like activity. Further resistance to acetylcholinesterase can be obtained by combining a carbamyl group with the β-methyl group in the compound carbamyl-β-methylcholine (bethanechol). Like methacholine, this compound has little nicotinic activity.

The history of the chemistry of (+)muscarine, the compound originally used by Dale, is a muddled story. It was not until 1957 that the correct structure was discovered and confirmed by chemical synthesis (Hardegger and Lohse) and X-ray crystallography (Kogl, Salemink, Schouten and Jellinek). The molecule contains three asymmetric carbon atoms so there are eight possible isomers and the naturally occurring (+)muscarine is much the most active. It is a quaternary

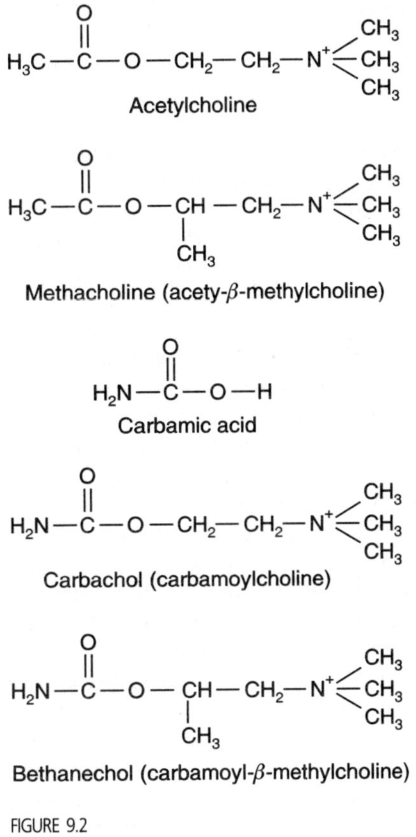

$$H_3C-C(=O)-O-CH_2-CH_2-N^+(CH_3)_3$$

Acetylcholine

$$H_3C-C(=O)-O-CH(CH_3)-CH_2-N^+(CH_3)_3$$

Methacholine (acety-β-methylcholine)

$$H_2N-C(=O)-O-H$$

Carbamic acid

$$H_2N-C(=O)-O-CH_2-CH_2-N^+(CH_3)_3$$

Carbachol (carbamoylcholine)

$$H_2N-C(=O)-O-CH(CH_3)-CH_2-N^+(CH_3)_3$$

Bethanechol (carbamoyl-β-methylcholine)

FIGURE 9.2

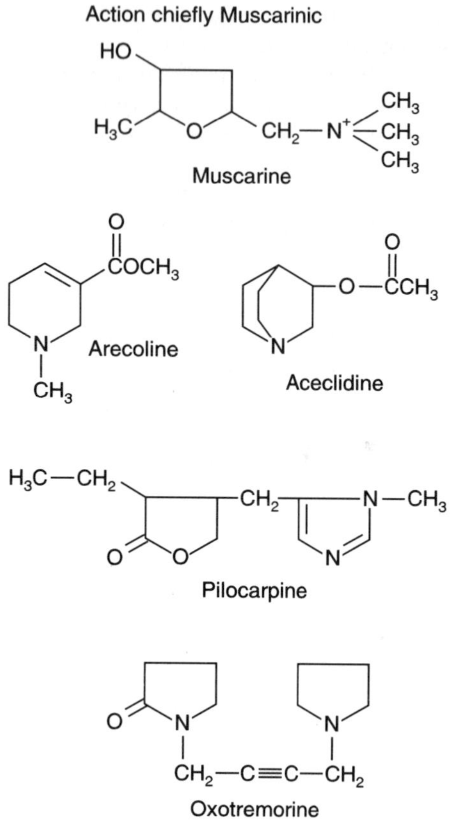

Action chiefly Muscarinic

Muscarine

Arecoline

Aceclidine

Pilocarpine

Oxotremorine

FIGURE 9.3

salt and is not an ester and although it is a highly active substance, it is almost certainly not the material responsible for poisoning with *Amanita muscaria* as it does not occur in quantity and is not well absorbed by mouth (Fig. 9.3).

There are two other naturally occurring compounds with muscarinic activity that are important – arecoline and pilocarpine. Arecoline occurs in the betel nut, which is widely chewed in the Indian subcontinent. Pilocarpine comes from the leaves of shrubs growing in South America and these are also chewed. Although the structures are different, both alkaloids are tertiary bases and so exist as an equilibrium mixture of charged (protonated) and uncharged forms and can cross membranes. Their absorption will be increased if the pH is alkaline and the betel nut is often mixed with lime. The most obvious pharmacological effect of arecoline and pilocarpine is to produce salivation, but it is not impossible that there are also central effects which may make the habit pleasurable. Both substances are weaker than acetylcholine and are esters but they are not substrates for cholinesterases so their effects are not as transient as those of acetylcholine. Their ability to cross membranes means that they can be applied to the cornea and produce effects in the eye.

Although acetylcholine is highly active at muscarinic receptors and is the 'natural' ligand, there are many synthetic compounds with high or even greater activity. Possibly the most active found so far is F2268, which resembles (+)muscarine and is a quaternary salt. The two synthetic compounds oxotremorine and aceclidine are of interest because they are not quaternary and cross membranes. Oxotremorine produces tremors by an action at muscarinic receptors in the central nervous system.

In the peripheral nervous system M_1 receptors are relatively unimportant and as yet there are no agonists that satisfactorily distinguish between muscarinic M_2 and M_3 receptors. For effects on gut or bladder in the clinic the choice is between methacholine and bethanechol, given by injection. For effects on the eye the choice is between pilocarpine and aceclidine. Radioligand binding experiments show that there are M_1 as well as M_3 receptors in the central nervous system but the effects of selective muscarinic agonists are not fully known.

NICOTINIC AGONISTS

As has already been mentioned, the pressor effect of (−)nicotine is produced by its stimulation of sympathetic ganglia and possibly also (depending on the dose) of receptors in the adrenal medulla. However, it stimulates parasympathetic ganglia as well as sympathetic ganglia, so the overall effect depends on the balance between the two divisions of the autonomic nervous system. In the gastrointestinal tract, in contrast to the cardiovascular system, it is the parasympathetic effects that predominate, so there is increased movement.

The actions of nicotine itself, like those of (+)tubocurarine chloride, however, are not confined to ganglia; it also affects the neuromuscular junction. They are further complicated by changing from stimulation to block. This phenomenon, described as 'tachyphylaxis' or 'desensitization', was first noted when it was found that if you gave repeated doses of (−)nicotine the rise in blood pressure progressively declined. The neuromuscular junction seems to be particularly susceptible to desensitization and the effects of (−)nicotine are seen as paralysis, even though the compound initially acts as an agonist (see Chapter 12). Nicotine itself can cross the blood–brain barrier and stimulate the central nervous system. It can produce tremor and convulsions, stimulate the vomiting centre and stimulate and then depress the respiratory centre. This central action combined with paralysis of the muscles involved in respiration is life-threatening but not part of its effects on ganglia. Many readers will be familiar with the effects of nicotine. Enough is absorbed, if a smoker inhales, to produce a detectable effect on blood pressure, at least with the first cigarette of the day. For some people the pleasurable effects (which may be central) outweigh the unpleasant effects and lead to addiction. Nicotine is well-absorbed through the skin and this is exploited in skin patches, which can deliver nicotine and provide an alternative to cigarettes as an aid to giving up smoking. Toxic doses of nicotine can be absorbed through the skin by contact with pesticide products that contain high concentrations of the free base.

Ganglion-stimulants have no therapeutic value. It is more satisfactory to use drugs that act at α-adrenergic receptors, in order to raise the blood pressure, or at muscarinic receptors, in order to contract smooth muscle or stimulate secretion. Ganglion-stimulants, however, have a long history as useful tools in research, starting in 1889 with the work of Langley and Dickinson who applied solutions of nicotine to tissues with a small brush so as to locate the position of ganglia in tissues.

Drugs

Nicotine consists of a pyridine ring attached to a pyrrolidine ring and it is the naturally occurring (−) isomer that is commercially available. The nitrogen in the pyridine ring is only weakly basic but the pyrrolidine nitrogen, which has a methyl group attached, has a pK_a of about 8. About two-thirds is therefore protonated at body pH and it is this form that acts at nicotinic receptors. It does not look very much like acetylcholine but the quaternary salt, nicotine mono-methiodide has similar effects on the peripheral nervous system (Fig. 9.4). DMPP (dimethyl-phenyl-piperazinium) is a quaternary salt with ganglion-stimulant properties but also blocks muscarinic receptors. Nicotinic agonists can also be obtained by methylating phenolic amines, such as *m*-tyramine or dopamine: the quaternary salts occur naturally as leptodactyline, from the skin of a South American lizard, and coryneine, from a Mexican cactus. These are potent ganglion stimulants and are also agonists at the neuromuscular junction, though this effect is seen as a block.

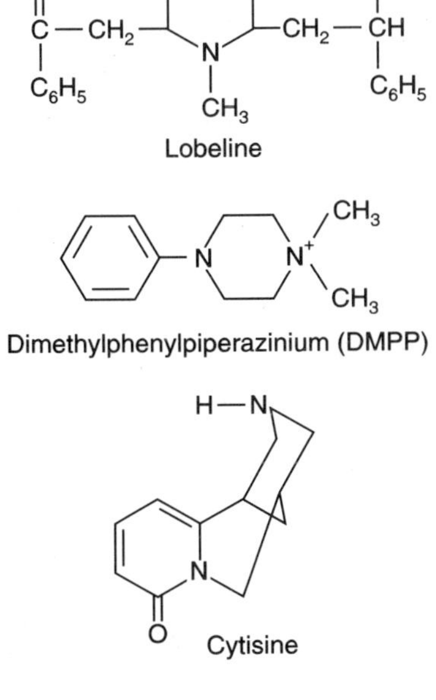

The alkaloid cytisine, which occurs in laburnum, has many of the properties of nicotine, which it resembles in structure, and the alkaloid lobeline, from lobelia, has sometimes been used as a respiratory stimulant and as a substitute for nicotine in herbal remedies. Until recently this has been the only, and very limited, clinical use for nicotinic agonists but it has been found that there are nicotine-binding sites in the brain and their numbers are reduced in certain diseases. It has been suggested that effects of impaired memory may be offset by smoking and it may even be possible that a more selective centrally acting nicotinic agonist may be produced for this purpose.

Action chiefly Nicotinic

Nicotine

Lobeline

Dimethylphenylpiperazinium (DMPP)

Cytisine

FIGURE 9.4

GANGLION-BLOCKING AGENTS

It has already been mentioned that although Dale used an extract of 'curare' to block the effects of nicotine on blood pressure, this also produced respiratory paralysis but that the effects of nicotine on the blood pressure can be blocked by hexamethonium without affecting the respiration. Because of the dominance of the sympathetic in the control of blood pressure, ganglion-blocking agents lower blood pressure and were used extensively in the 1950s to treat hypertension. With quaternary compounds, such as hexamethonium and pentolinium, there are problems with absorption from oral doses but this does not occur with mecamylamine (a secondary amine) and pempidine (a tertiary amine). All the compounds available block parasympathetic ganglia as well as sympathetic ganglia, so they block digestive processes that are largely under parasympathetic control.

This undesirable effect resembles that of atropine (p. 128). It is the direct consequence of using a ganglion-blocking agent, rather than an incidental 'side-effect', and could only be avoided if drugs were developed which specifically blocked sympathetic ganglia. It is not surprising, therefore, that ganglion-blocking agents have been superseded by drugs that are more selective and affect only sympathetic postganglionic synapses (p. 182). Another direct and undesirable consequence of ganglion-blockade (or of any form of sympathetic block) is the occurrence of postural hypotension: when the subject stands up after lying down, the rise in blood pressure necessary to pump the blood to the head is blocked and the subject collapses. This effect can sometimes be useful, however, because it can be a way of controlling bleeding in surgery. After a short-acting ganglion-blocking agent, such as trimetaphan, has been given, blood will pool under gravity in a limb lowered over the operating table or more generally if the table is tilted. This reduces the circulation, and therefore bleeding, in areas where the surgeon is operating – though there is a need to ensure that tissues do not become anoxic.

SUMMARY

Acetylcholine has muscarine-like and nicotine-like properties. It lowers blood pressure by dilating blood vessels, it slows (or even stops) the heart, promotes gastric and salivary secretion and stimulates smooth muscle. These effects are imitated by muscarine and antagonized by atropine. In higher doses it causes a rise in blood pressure that is imitated by nicotine and antagonized by ganglion-blocking agents such as hexamethonium. It is also the transmitter substance at the neuromuscular junction but at this site the effects of nicotine are seen as a desensitizing block.

Muscarine-like compounds (methacholine, bethanechol) have limited uses for contracting the smooth muscle of intestine or bladder and non-quaternary compounds (pilocarpine, aceclidine) may be applied to the cornea to contract the ciliary body and lower intraocular pressure in glaucoma.

Nicotine-like ganglion stimulants (DMPP, coryneine, cytisine) are research tools but lobeline is sometimes used as a respiratory stimulant.

FURTHER READING

Bebbington A, Brimblecombe RW. Muscarinic receptors in the peripheral and central nervous system. *Advances in Drug Research* 1965; **2**: 143–72.

Goyal RK. Muscarinic receptor subtypes: physiology and clinical implications. *New England Journal of Medicine* 1989; **321**: 1022–9.

Kosterlitz HW. Effects of choline esters on smooth muscle and secretions. In: Root, W. S., Hofmann, F. G. eds. *Physiological pharmacology*, Vol 3. *The nervous system – Part C: Autonomic nervous system drugs*. New York: Academic Press, 1967, 97–161.

Leopold IH, Duzman E. Observations on the pharmacology of glaucoma. *Annual Review of Pharmacology and Toxicology* 1986; **26**: 401–26.

Nathanson NM. Molecular properties of the muscarinic acetylcholine receptor. *Annual Review of Neuroscience* 1987; **10**, 197–236.

10

Cholinesterase and Anticholinesterases

PV Taberner

CHOLINESTERASES

There are a number of esterase enzymes in the body that catalyse the hydrolysis of ester links to release an organic acid and an alcohol moiety. The most important enzymes from a pharmacological point of view are the specific acetylcholinesterase, which is found in synapses of cholinergic neurones and at skeletal muscle motor nerve endplates, and the non-specific acylcholine acyl hydrolase (also known as pseudocholinesterase or butyrylcholinesterase), which is found in the liver and plasma. They belong to a superfamily of serine hydrolases.

Acetylcholinesterase

Acetylcholinesterase is responsible for the rapid destruction of released acetylcholine, thus terminating the depolarizing actions of this neurotransmitter. A striking feature of the enzyme is its very high turnover number – it requires only 40 ms to hydrolyse a molecule of acetylcholine to acetate and choline. This is important if the postjunctional membrane is to repolarize rapidly after each nerve impulse, and makes it possible for cholinergic neurones to transmit up to 1000 impulses per second. Such is the efficiency of the enzyme that it is usually necessary to block the enzyme in order to be able to detect free acetylcholine in nerve or muscle tissue. The enzyme is made up of four subunits ($\alpha 2\beta 2$) and is bound to the postsynaptic cell basement membrane within the synaptic cleft (Fig. 12.3b, p. 137). The molecular architecture of the active site is well understood as is the catalytic mechanism. The active site is negatively charged, attracting the positively charged quaternary group of acetylcholine to an anionic subsite containing a glutamate residue. The acetylcholine molecule binds covalently to a serine residue at the adjacent esteratic site, the choline moiety is cleaved and released; the labile acetyl-enzyme intermediate then reacts with water to yield acetate and free enzyme (Fig. 10.1). This mechanism is important for understanding how the anticholinesterases act to block the enzyme (see below).

Acetylcholinesterase is highly substrate selective; small structural changes in a choline ester will render it resistant to enzymatic hydrolysis.

Since acetylcholine was the first neurotransmitter to be identified, it was originally thought that the rapid enzymatic inactivation process was a prerequisite for a neurotransmitter. This has subsequently been found not to be the case, and acetylcholinesterase is almost unique in this respect. Inhibition of the enzyme has immediate and profound effects on cholinergic nerve function.

Pseudocholinesterase

Pseudocholinesterase is far less specific than acetylcholinesterase and probably has a detoxifying role. A number of drugs are inactivated by hydrolysis catalysed by pseudocholinesterase, notably the neuromuscular blocking agent succinylcholine and the local anaesthetic procaine. The very short duration of action of succinylcholine (suxamethonium) is due to this hydrolysis reaction (Fig. 10.2). A single gene codes for pseudocholinesterase and in some individuals an atypical isozyme is expressed which has a 100-fold lower affinity for suxamethonium. The concentrations of suxamethonium used clinically to produce muscular paralysis do not saturate the enzyme, so that in subjects with the atypical enzyme, metabolic inactivation will be

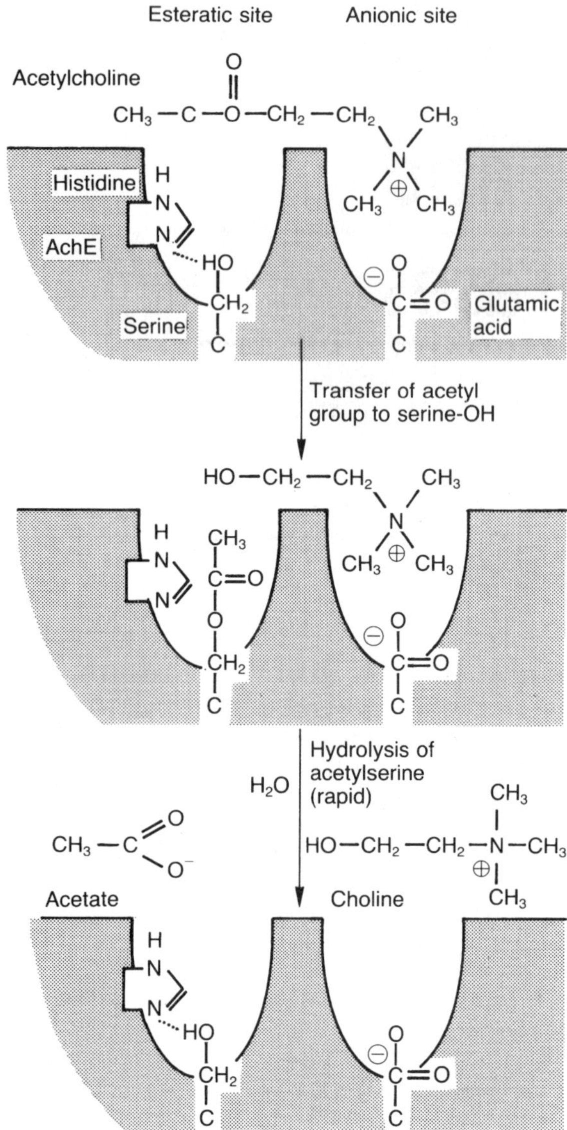

FIGURE 10.1 Catalytic reaction mechanism of acetylcholinesterase.

very much slowed. These individuals will experience an exaggerated response to suxamethonium with symptoms of prolonged muscular paralysis and apnoea.

The presence of the atypical enzyme can be determined by a simple blood test in which the rate of hydrolysis of benzoylcholine in the presence of dibucaine is measured *in vitro*. Dibucaine inhibits the normal enzyme by about 80% under the assay conditions chosen, but the atypical enzyme remains unaffected. The percentage inhibition is termed the dibucaine number, which provides an index of normal enzyme activity. Overall, about 1 in 3000 patients possess this atypical enzyme, but the incidence will be much higher in families where cases occur. The abnormal gene is widespread throughout the world although it is rare in negroid and oriental races and absent in the Japanese.

Other drugs whose metabolic degradation will be influenced by pseudocholinesterase activity include heroin (diacetylmorphine) and cocaine. This may have implications in the recreational use and abuse of these drugs.

ANTICHOLINESTERASES (ANTI-ChE AGENTS)

These compounds have found uses as chemical warfare agents and insecticides as well as therapeutic drugs. They inhibit both acetylcholinesterase (AChE) and pseudocholinesterase about equally, although it is the AChE block that is therapeutically important. Anti-ChE agents can be divided into three groups, based on the mechanism of their inhibition at the active site (Fig. 10.3). This mechanism determines only their duration of action, their therapeutic or toxic effects are qualitatively the same.

Quaternary compounds such as edrophonium compete directly with acetylcholine for binding to the anionic subsite. Edrophonium contains no ester linkage and is not metabolized by the enzyme. It is short acting because it binds reversibly and is rapidly eliminated by renal clearance.

Eserine (physostigmine) and neostigmine contain carbamyl ester linkages which are hydrolysed by AChE, but more slowly than a simple ester link. Neostigmine contains a quaternary amine group; physostigmine is a tertiary amine. In addition to competing with acetylcholine for binding at the anionic site, the carbamyl-enzyme intermediate is more resistant to hydrolysis than the normal ester intermediate. This has the effect of preventing the access of acetylcholine molecules to the active site for several hours.

The organophosphorous inhibitors such as the insecticide tetra-ethyl pyrophosphate (TEPP) and the nerve gas sarin (isopropyl methylphosphonofluoridate) react directly with the esteratic subsite to form highly stable intermediates. The phosphorylated or phosphonylated enzyme is effectively inactivated and the recovery of AChE activity is dependent on synthesis of new enzyme. Some quaternary organophosphorous compounds (echothiopate for example) interact with both the anionic and esteratic subsites. This makes them extremely potent and selective inhibitors.

Our extensive knowledge of the mode of action of anti-ChE agents and their structure–activity relationships probably owes more to their military rather than medical applications. However, the widespread use of organophosphorous compounds as commercial insecticides makes accidental poisoning an important aspect of their pharmacology and toxicology.

PHARMACOLOGICAL PROPERTIES OF ANTI-ChE AGENTS

These drugs will potentiate the actions of acetylcholine released from presynaptic nerve endings. In the

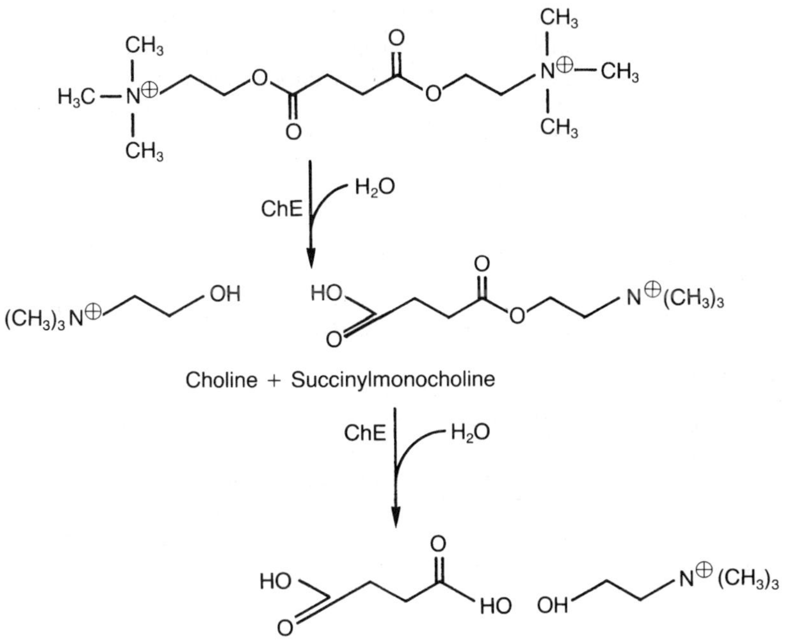

ChE H_2O

Choline + Succinylmonocholine

ChE H_2O

FIGURE 10.2 Metabolism of suxamethonium by pseudocholinesteras.

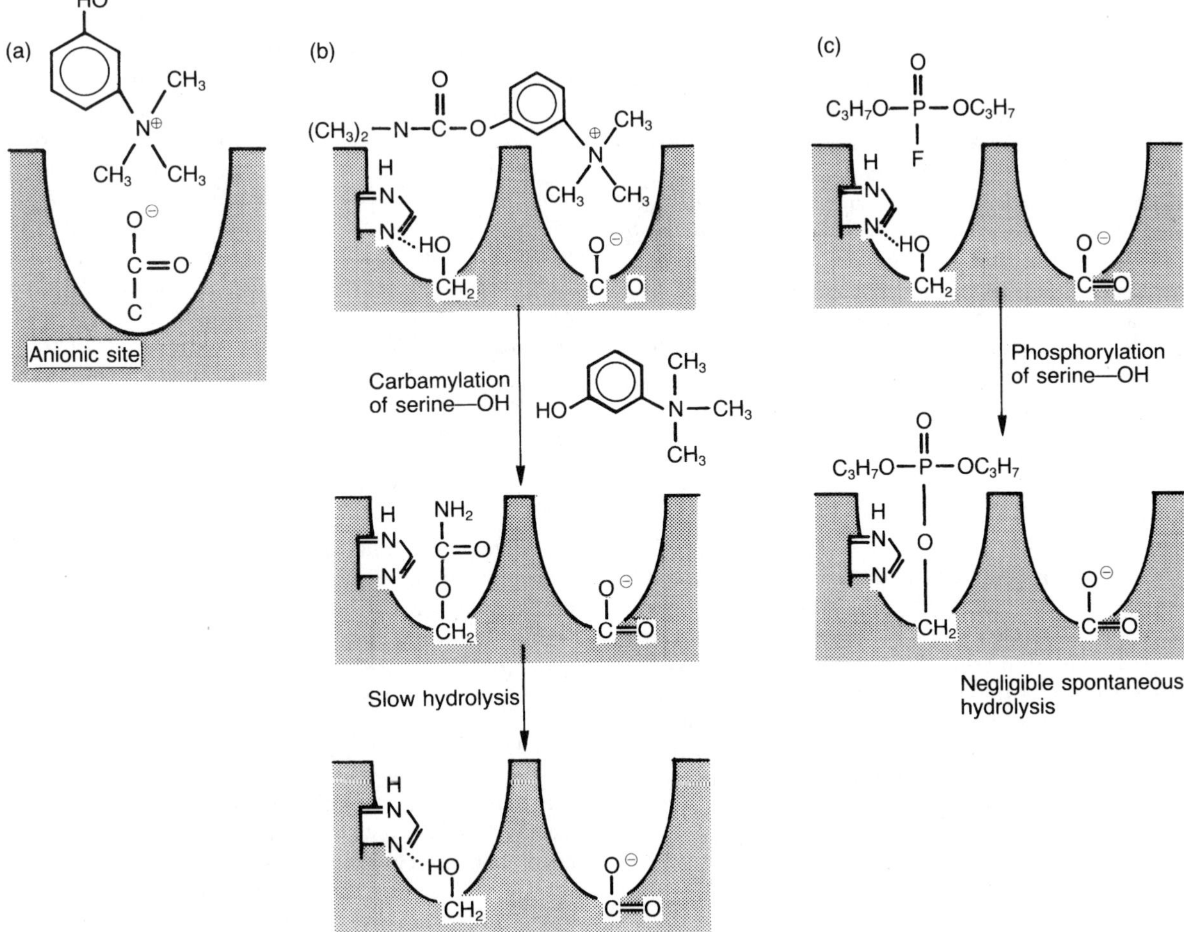

FIGURE 10.3 Mechanism of cholinesterase inhibition. (a) Edrophonium – reversible ionic binding. (b) Carboxylation (neostigmine). (c) Action of an organophosphate (Dyflos).

autonomic nervous system they will facilitate ganglionic transmission at both sympathetic and parasympathetic ganglia and at postganglionic parasympathetic endings. Neuromuscular transmission at voluntary muscles will also be facilitated. In addition to these peripheral sites, central neurones receiving an input from cholinergic neurones will also be stimulated. These CNS effects are restricted to the lipid-soluble anti-ChE agents; the quaternary compounds cannot penetrate the blood–brain barrier and are also less well absorbed from the gastrointestinal tract due in part to gastric acid hydrolysis. This apart, the effects of the different agents are qualitatively similar. The overall physiological response will be an increase in acetylcholine-mediated functions. This will be manifested by stimulation of smooth muscle, glandular secretions and, in the first instance, voluntary skeletal muscle. The parasympathetic smooth muscle and glandular secretion effects (which can be life-threatening) can be controlled by prophylactic treatment with a muscarinic antagonist such as atropine. The skeletal muscle effects are more difficult to control or prevent (see below).

Gastrointestinal tract

Oesophageal peristalsis, gastric motility and gastric acid secretion are increased by anti-ChEs. Intestinal motility and peristalsis is increased along the length of the alimentary tract, due to potentiation of acetylcholine released from the parasympathetic ganglia present in Auerbach's plexus and at the postganglionic endings on the smooth muscle fibres. Regurgitation of gastric contents may occur at high doses. The increase in smooth muscle motility can be of value in the treatment of atony of gut smooth muscle as well as the bladder, although the specifically acting muscarinic agonists are normally preferred (see Chapter 9).

Cardiovascular system

The autonomic ganglionic effects of anti-ChEs on both sympathetic and parasympathetic pathways, combined with the direct effects at parasympathetic muscarinic nerve endings of the vagus nerve in the heart, make the gross actions of these drugs on the heart and vasculature difficult to predict. The overall response is normally of bradycardia with a consequent fall in blood pressure due to increased vagal stimulation of the myocardium. The peripheral vasculature is unaffected.

The eye

If an anti-ChE is applied locally to the conjunctiva an almost immediate constriction of the pupil (miosis) will be observed, followed by blockade of the accommodation reflex. This is due to contraction of the sphincter pupillae and the ciliary muscles respectively. The miosis can be very long lasting and this phenomenon can be exploited to advantage in the management of glaucoma. The prolonged contraction of the pupil facilitates the drainage of aqueous humour through the canal of Schlemm and relieves intraocular pressure.

Glandular secretions

Postganglionic parasympathetic fibres innervate salivary, sweat, bronchial, lachrymal and parietal gland cells. Excessive cholinergic stimulation leads to increased production and secretion of saliva, tears and sweat. Increased bronchial secretion can lead to significant respiratory problems including pneumonia or even asphyxiation. This is a characteristic feature of poisoning by the more toxic anti-ChE agents.

Skeletal neuromuscular junction

The acetylcholine released by a single nerve impulse is normally sufficient to produce an endplate potential which results in a fast or slow twitch response (see Chapter 12). In the presence of an anti-ChE the acetylcholine remains longer than the refractory period following the twitch. This means that the normal development and decay of individual endplate depolarizations is lost so that asynchronous excitation and fibrillation of individual muscle fibres occur. Eventually, a depolarization block will be produced as a direct consequence of cholinergic overactivity. Although anti-ChEs can overcome the effects of competitive neuromuscular blocking agents, it is important to realize that they will exacerbate a depolarizing block. Neostigmine is notable for the fact that, in addition to its anti-ChE activity, it can stimulate the contraction of skeletal muscle fibres directly. This action is quite distinct from its anti-ChE activity.

Contraindications for the use of anti-ChEs would certainly include respiratory insufficiency and asthma, bradycardia or hypotension, myocardial infarction, peptic ulceration, epilepsy or Parkinsonism.

Central nervous system

The central effects of lipid-soluble anti-ChE agents are usually less apparent than the peripheral actions outlined above. However, animal experiments have shown that cholinergic neurones in the cortex and hippocampus in particular are involved in the memory processes of consolidation and recall. Muscarinic agonists tend to inhibit memory and learning, whereas anti-ChEs can improve these functions. This suggests that these drugs might be of value in restoring the memory deficits associated with various neurological conditions such as Wernicke–Korsakoff syndrome and Alzheimer's disease. The anti-ChE drug tacrine has undergone clinical trials for this purpose, but the results are still rather equivocal.

ANTICHOLINESTERASES IN THERAPEUTIC USE

As mentioned above, the principal difference between the individual anti-ChE agents used clinically is in their duration of action. Systemic administration is always likely to lead to unwanted (and largely unavoidable) side-effects so that they are often applied locally for a specific effect. Alternatively, the muscarinic side-effects can be controlled by concomitant treatment with muscarinic antagonists. The pharmacological properties and therapeutic uses of the drugs currently available are summarized in Table 10.1 and described more fully in Chapter 11.

Edrophonium chloride is a very short-acting (less than 10 min) quaternary base with no central actions. It is normally used either for the diagnosis of myasthenia gravis or the determination of the appropriate dosage of a cholinergic drug in myasthenia. The edrophonium test distinguishes between muscular weakness due to insufficient medication and muscular weakness resulting from a depolarizing block induced by an excessive dose of a cholinergic or anti-ChE drug.

Neostigmine bromide (Prostigmin) is used orally for the chronic treatment of myasthenia gravis. It has a specific application to restore the control of voluntary muscle tone in the treatment of competitive neuromuscular block, but care must be taken as it has a longer duration of action (30 min) than edrophonium. A muscarinic antagonist would normally be given to diminish or block the parasympathetic side-effects (see p. 164).

It is essential to monitor the pulse rate as the duration of action may outlast that of atropine and profound bradycardia may develop (see Chapter 11). *Pyridostigmine*, which is similar in structure to neostigmine (Fig. 10.4), is rather more potent than neostigmine and has a longer duration of action. It is used mostly in the treatment of myasthenia gravis.

Edrophonium

Neostigmine

Physostigmine (Eserine)

Pyridostigmine

Dyflos

Ecothiopate

Parathion

Paraoxon

Carbaryl

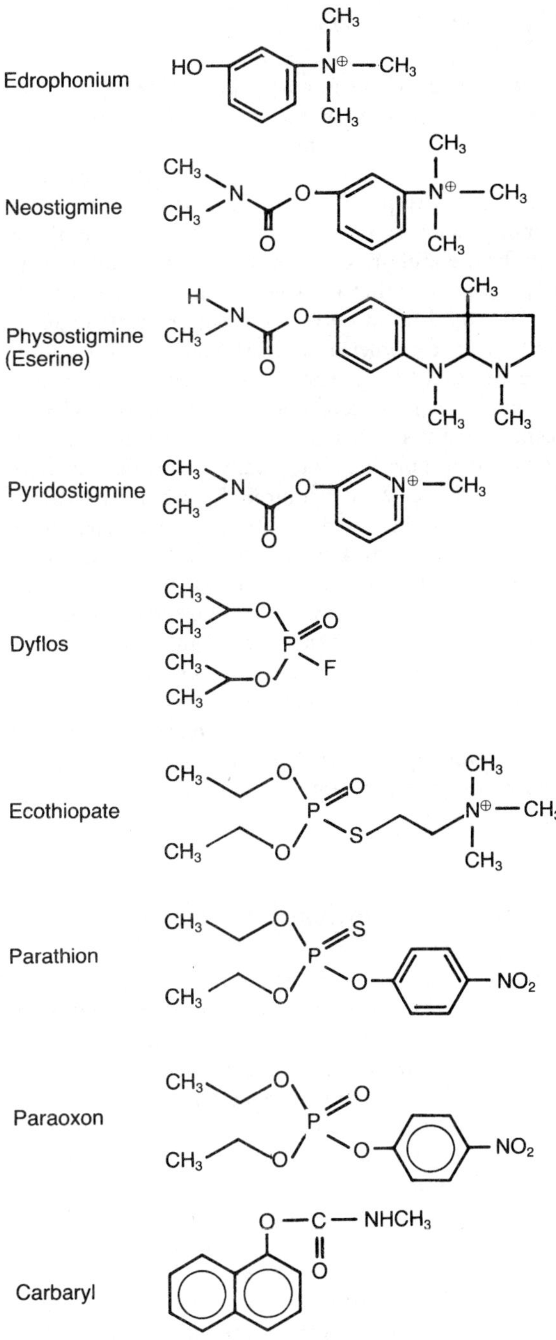

FIGURE 10.4 Chemical structures of some anticholinesterases.

TABLE 10.1 Therapeutic applications of anticholinesterases

DRUG	DOSE/ROUTE OF ADMINISTRATION	DURATION OF ACTION	APPLICATION
Edrophonium	5–10 mg iv	10 min	Diagnosis of myasthenia gravis
Neostigmine	2.5–5 mg iv	0.5–1.0 h	Reversal of neuromuscular blockade
Neostigmine	15 mg oral	2–4 h	Myasthenia gravis
Pyridostigmine	60 mg oral	3–6 h	Myastehnia gravis
Ambenonium	10 mg	3–8 h	Myasthenia gravis
Physostigmine sulphate (eserine)	1 drop (0.25%) instilled into the eye		Glaucoma

Myasthenia gravis

Myasthenia gravis is an autoimmune disease in which there is a reduction in the number of acetylcholine receptors at the neuromuscular junction. There are many clinical subgroups such as ocular myasthenia which readily respond to steroids such as prednisolone. Immunosuppressant therapy involving azathioprine may be helpful in patients who have moderate to severe weakness that does not respond to steroids. In the UK the drug in current use is pyridostigmine, 30 mg four to five times a day, although the dose can be increased to 120 mg. The concomitant colic and diarrhoea are usually controlled by the antimuscarinic agent propantheline. Patients with early myasthenia, whose symptoms are not readily controlled by anticholinesterases, may require thymectomy. Muscle weakness may be due not only to an exacerbation of the myasthenia (myasthenic crisis), but also to an excess of anticholinesterase drugs which, in high doses, can cause neuromuscular blockade (cholinergic crisis). The signs of toxicity from anticholinesterases can be detected by the presence of increased secretions, sweating, tears, nausea, colic and vomiting, and constriction of the pupil. The bis-quaternary compound *ambenonium* is also used in some countries outside the UK. Its properties are essentially similar to neostigmine.

Other uses of anticholinesterases

Anticholinesterases have been used in the management of patients with urinary retention associated with atony of the bladder detrusor muscle and in the management of paralytic ileus. It is essential to monitor the ECG when, for example, neostigmine is administered. This therapy is not recommended for ileus following resection of the bowel, as dehiscence of the anastomosis is likely to ensue.

Physostigmine (eserine) is a natural product found in Calabar beans. These were originally used by West African peoples in trials by ordeal in which the accused was required to eat the beans. Death was interpreted as an indication of guilt. Perhaps the innocent individual would consume a large dose, sufficient to induce vomiting, whereas the guilty subject would be more tentative and absorb a potentially lethal dose of the active principle. This drug is no longer used clinically except for topical application in the treatment of glaucoma. *Pyridostigmine* has similar properties but with rather less muscarinic effects, so that it is better tolerated when given by mouth.

Ecothiopate iodide (Phospholine) is used in the USA. It is a long-acting anti-ChE which is only used in ophthalmic applications. The very potent organophosphorous compound *isoflurophate* (DFP) is used similarly to provide long-term relief from glaucoma. Neither of these compounds should ever be administered orally. It is not often appreciated that the instillation of drugs on the conjunctiva can lead to systemic absorption resulting in inhibition of pseudocholinesterase. This may result in potentiation of drugs such as succinylcholine and local anaesthetics containing an ester linkage, such as procaine, amethocaine and cocaine.

Organophosphorous insecticides such as *parathion*, *paraoxan* (the active metabolite of parathion), *malathion* and *diazinon* are all used commercially and can produce toxic effects in mammalian species. Chronic exposure of farmers to organophosphate-containing sheep dips is believed to be responsible for some long-term neurological disorders. *Malathion* is probably the safest agent since it is efficiently detoxified by higher organisms and can be used for the topical treatment of head lice (pediculosis) and scabies (*Sarcoptes scabiei*). Similarly, the insecticide *Carbaryl* is a carbamylating inhibitor of ChE that is poorly absorbed through the skin and can be regarded as selectively toxic towards arthropoda.

The nerve gases (sarin, tabun) are volatile organophosphorous compounds with low molecular weights. The extreme toxicity of these compounds is due both to their lipid solubility, which facilitates skin absorption, and the rapid and irreversible block of AChE. They will readily penetrate the skin and cross the blood–brain barrier.

REACTIVATION OF ACETYLCHOLINESTERASE

Having said that many anti-ChE agents produce an irreversible inhibition of the cholinesterases, the search for antidotes to the nerve gases has led to the development of reactivator compounds that can accelerate hydrolysis of the covalent bond between the anti-ChE and the enzyme. The first compound, pyridine-2-aldoxime methyl chloride (*pralidoxime mesylate*, 2-PAM, P2S), was introduced in 1955. The nucleophilic oxime group is highly reactive towards the phosphorus atom in the enzyme–inhibitor complex. An oxime-phosphonate is formed which then breaks away from the enzyme leaving a regenerated active site (Fig. 10.5). A number of other oximes with similar properties have since been developed including *obidoxime* (Toxogonon), which is several times more potent than pralidoxime, and *trimedoxime* bromide (TMB-4).

Phosphorylated AChE molecules undergo a chemical 'ageing' process that makes them resistant to reactivation. This phenomenon limits the usefulness of oxime reactivators. They are less effective against carbamylated ChE and are not therefore recommended for overcoming physostigmine or neostigmine overdosage. Also, and perhaps not surprisingly, the oximes themselves do possess some anti-ChE activity. They are most effective at overcoming organophosphorous poisoning at the neuromuscular junction.

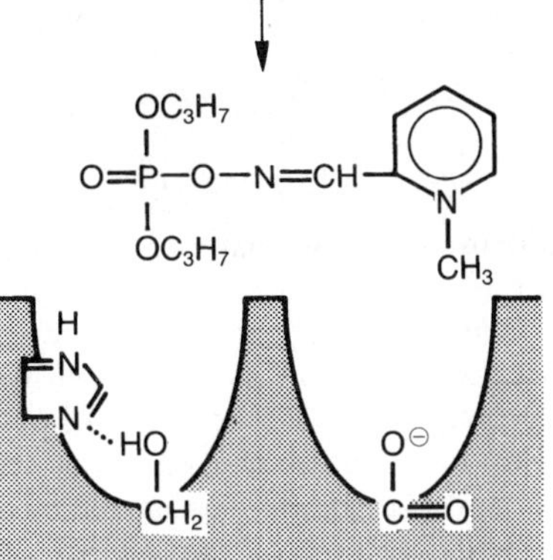

FIGURE 10.5 Reactivation of cholinesterase by pralidoxime.

FURTHER READING

Davis KL, Thal LJ, Gamzu ER *et al.* A double-blind placebo controlled multicenter study of tacrine for Alzheimer's disease. *New England Journal of Medicine* 1992; **327**: 1253.

Drachman D. ed. Myasthenia gravis: biology and treatment. *Annals of the New York Academy of Sciences* 1987; *555*.

Farrar HC, Wells TG, Kearns GL. Use of continuous infusion of pralidoxime for treatment of organophosphate poisoning in children. *Journal of Pediatrics* 1990; **116**: 658.

Hobbiger F. Pharmacology of anticholinesterase drugs. In: Zaimis E. ed. *Neuromuscular junction. Handbuch der Experimentellen Pharmakologie*, Vol 42. Berlin: Springer-Verlag, 1976; 487–581.

Lehmann H, Liddell J. Genetical variants of human serum pseudocholinesterase. *Progress in Medical Genetics* 1964; **3**: 75.

Leopold IH, Duzman E. Observations on the pharmacology of glaucoma. *Annual Review of Pharmacology and Toxicology* 1986; **26**: 401.

Rosenberry TL. Acetylcholinesterase. *Advances in Enzymology* 1975; **43**: 103.

Solana RP, Harris LW, Carter WH, Talbot BG, Carchman RA, Gennings C. Evaluation of a two-drug combination pretreatment against organophosphorus exposure. *Toxicology and Applied Pharmacology* 1990; **102**: 421.

Thompson JC, Whittaker M. A study of the pseudocholinesterase in 78 cases of apnoea following suxamethonium. *Acta Genetica et Statistica Medica* 1966; **16**: 209.

Wachtel RE. Comparison of anticholinesterases and their effects on acetycholine-activated ion channels. *Anesthesiology* 1990; **72**: 496.

11

Antimuscarinic Drugs

RB Barlow

INTRODUCTION

In Dale's original experiment (p. 103) the fall in blood pressure produced by very small doses of acetylcholine – or muscarine – was blocked by atropine. This alkaloid occurs in *Atropa belladonna* (deadly nightshade) and also in *Hyoscyamus niger* (henbane) and *Datura stramonium* (thornapple, Jimson weed). The natural material is (–)hyoscyamine but this racemizes easily and some methods of extraction deliberately produce the racemate, atropine, rather than partially racemized material. The (–) isomer is over 200 times as potent as the (+) isomer, thus atropine is almost exactly half as active as (–)hyoscyamine. A closely related alkaloid, hyoscine, is also known as scopolamine (this is the name used in the USA). The multiplicity of names is unfortunate but it is important to realize that atropine is a mixture of (–) and (+) hyoscyamine and also that hyoscine and scopolamine are two names for the same compound (Fig. 11.1).

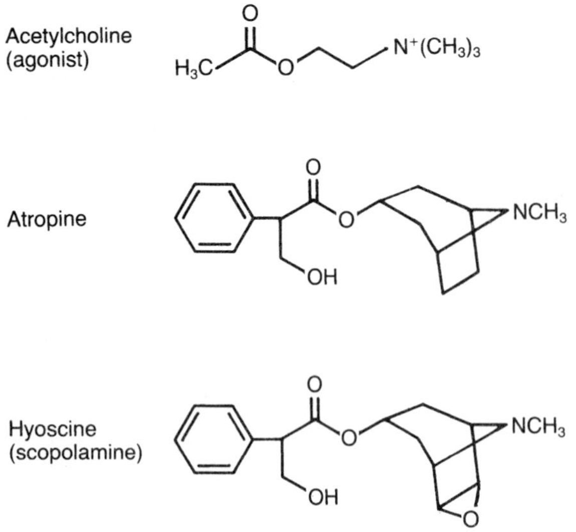

This chapter, then, is about atropine-like drugs; that is, substances that block muscarine-sensitive acetylcholine receptors. They block the effects of parasympathetic stimulation and also those effects of acetylcholine that do not involve the parasympathetic, such as the cholinergic section of the sympathetic. Although it is now clear that there are subclasses of muscarinic receptors, drugs acting selectively at one type rather than another are only recently emerging. Most antimuscarinic drugs affect a range of muscarinic receptors and their effects are typified by those of atropine.

Acetylcholine (agonist)
H_3C O O $N^+(CH_3)_3$

Atropine
O O NCH_3 OH

Hyoscine (scopolamine)
O O NCH_3 OH O

FIGURE 11.1

ATROPINE

Atropine has been widely used as premedication before administering a volatile anaesthetic and its effects have been experienced by many people at some time or another. When substances such as chloroform or diethyl ether are inhaled, they irritate the bronchial passages and produce copious secretions. This can be sufficient to produce death by drowning and atropine was used to prevent this. It will also prevent vagal arrest of the heart, which could occur as a result of vagal stimulation produced by the stress of the operation, and it will stop intestinal movement, which may be beneficial in abdominal surgery. The dose administered preoperatively is around 0.02 mg/kg and the compound is distributed through the total body fluid so the expected concentration is roughly 0.02/700 mg/ml which is 0.02/700/350 = 82 nM. This seems very low but atropine, which acts competitively, has a very high affinity for muscarinic receptors (the pA_2 or log affinity constant is 9), so this concentration produces a dose-ratio of 83 (pp. 5–6), which is a very large effect. Whatever the amount of acetylcholine needed to stop the heart or drown the patient, with this concentration of atropine you would need 83 times that amount to produce the same effect.

Although this small dose produces a large effect, and in spite of the trivial name 'deadly nightshade', the patient usually only experiences slight discomfort. The most noticeable effect is dryness of the mouth. There may also be a sensation of warmth, associated with inability to lose heat by sweating, because the sympathetic innervation of sweating is cholinergic. The effect on the heart rate depends on the sympathetic tone. If this is high the heart will beat faster because there are no opposing vagal effects but if it is low there should be little change in rate. There is little effect on blood pressure. Respiration may be slightly stimulated by a central mechanism and bronchial relaxation may be apparent in patients with bronchoconstriction. The inhibition of secretion and movement in the gastro-intestinal tract and the effects on the eye, dilatation of the pupil and paralysis of accommodation, are unlikely to be noticed by a patient immediately before an operation but may be apparent afterwards with possible constipation or retention of urine.

The effects of atropine and atropine-like compounds on gastrointestinal secretion and movement have long been recognized. Tincture of bella donna is a traditional and effective treatment of the painful spasm associated with various forms of colic. The treatment of ulcers of the gastrointestinal tract has been less successful, requiring the administration of the compounds over a long period. Bella donna cigarettes have been used to relieve some forms of bronchospasm and are effective if this is caused by acetylcholine, but ineffective if, as is usually the case, some other agent is responsible, such as histamine or leukotrienes. Bella donna alkaloids have also been widely used in ophthalmology to dilate the pupil and allow inspection of the retina.

Atropine-like drugs are also an essential part of the treatment of poisoning by anticholinesterases: they prevent the muscarinic effects, which would otherwise cause victims to drown in their own secretions and their heart to stop, but must be supplemented by treatment for the nicotinic effects which would otherwise lead to respiratory paralysis (see previous chapter).

Atropine-like drugs which can cross the blood–brain barrier have also been used in the treatment of Parkinson's disease. With dopamine deficiency and lowered inhibitory control, a balance may be achieved by reducing the excitatory cholinergic output with an atropine-like compound. Different drugs have been developed for particular uses and now that substances are appearing that act preferentially at one type of muscarinic receptor rather than another, further developments are likely. It would be particularly desirable to have drugs which exclusively affected airways or bladder or gut.

Because many behave competitively as antagonists at muscarinic receptors and give results that fit the Gaddum–Schild equation, their activity can be expressed as a dissociation or affinity constant, or

TABLE 11.1 Affinity for muscarinic receptors (guinea-pig ileum): values of log K (affinity), pA_2 or –log K (dissociation), 37°C. Note that the scale is logarithmic and a difference of 1 unit indicates a 10-fold difference in activity

(–) Hyoscyamine	9.38
(+) Hyoscyamine	6.86
Atropine	9.00
(–) Hyoscine (scopolamine)	9.36
(–) Hyoscine methiodide	
(N-methyl scopolamine)	9.70
Quinuclidyl benzilate (QNB)	>10
(±) Homatropine	7.22
Procyclidine	7.95
Benzhexol	8.45
Oxyphenonium	9.80

more conveniently as the logarithm of this (pA_2). For atropine and receptors in guinea-pig ileum this is 9 (the dissociation constant is about 1 nM). Not only does this make it possible to compare drugs (Table 11.1), it makes it possible to compare binding to receptors in different tissues and so assess selectivity.

DRUGS

Atropine is the ester of tropine with (±)tropic acid. Tropine contains a six-membered piperidine ring fused to a five-membered pyrrolidine ring. This system (tropane) occurs also in cocaine and as an amino-alcohol it can be compared with choline but is rigid instead of flexible. Hyoscine is the tropic ester of scopine (or oscine), which has an extra oxygen atom bridging the methylene groups of the five-membered ring; this makes the compound a weaker base. Its peripheral properties are very similar to those of hyoscyamine and it is about twice as active, but its central properties are purely depressant and more marked (Table 11.2). It lacks the slight stimulant effects of hyoscyamine, for example on respiration, and is supposed to be more

TABLE 11.2 Differences between atropine and hyoscine

	ATROPINE	HYOSCINE (SCOPOLAMINE)
Heart	+	
Bronchial Tone	+	
Intestine	+	
Secretions		+
Eye		+
Amnesia		+
Antiemetic		+

+ Indicates more effective block at this site.
Atropine has no effect on amnesia or vomiting.

effective in producing amnesia. Atropine-like compounds block the actions of acetylcholine and drugs have been successfully developed from this compound by changing the acetyl group of this compound into something larger, such as benziloyl ($Ph_2C(OH)$-COO-), which has affinity for muscarinic receptors but lacks efficacy and is a potent antagonist. Compounds of this type include lachesine and *propantheline*. The choline part (-CH_2CH_2-NMe_3) can be replaced by a pyrrolidine ring, such as in glycopyrronium, or by a piperidine ring, as in *pipenzolate* and *mepenzolate*. The ester with the particularly rigid 3-hydroxy-quinuclidine ring, quinuclidinyl benzilate (QNB) is particularly potent and can be obtained radiolabelled and used in experiments to locate muscarinic-binding sites. Hyoscine methiodide (N-methyl scopolamine) is also very potent and can be obtained radio-labelled. The structures of some clinically used antimuscarinic drugs are shown in Fig. 11.2.

When applied to the eye, the effects of atropine are so powerful that the pupil may be dilated and the accommodation paralysed for days. It is this mydriatic action that accounts for the name 'bella donna' but the paralysis of accommodation is the price that must be paid for the beauty of dilated pupils! There is also the possibility of precipitating an attack of glaucoma, by preventing the ciliary muscle contracting, there may be decreased drainage through the canal of Schlemm and a rise in intraocular pressure. There is a need for weaker drugs that produce transient effects and which cross the cornea and can be applied as eye-drops (so quaternary salts are usually unsuitable). Homatropine, the ester of tropine with mandelic acid, has long been used in ophthalmology and tropicamide is another example.

For premedication before an operation the central effects of hyoscine may make it preferable to atropine. In the elderly it can cause disorientation. In patients with heart disease, the tachycardia associated with the vagal effects of atropine may be undesirable. There are substances that have been found experimentally to be less active at M_3 receptors than at M_2 receptors and these may be available before long.

For the relief of acute spasm in smooth muscle some drugs have advantages over atropine, although these are not often great advantages. Quaternary compounds will have fewer central effects but will not be well absorbed orally. An aerosol form of *ipratropium*, the quaternary *iso*propyl derivative of atropine, is available for the treament of asthma (see p. 291). This lacks the central effects of atropine but has the vagal-blocking effect. It has also some ganglion-blocking activity, however, and because it affects sympathetic transmission as well as parasympathetic, there may be less tachycardia. The same is also supposed to be true of propantheline, another quaternary compound that is sometimes used (given by injection) for the treatment of renal colic.

In the treatment of gastric and duodenal ulcers drugs must be given for a long period and the effects of atropine on the heart, salivation, sweating, on the central nervous system and on the eye, which may be tolerable in the short term, are no longer acceptable. Many compounds were developed during the 1950s but if they were quaternary and lacked central actions, their absorption was not always reliable and if they entered the bloodstream in concentrations that affected secretion and motility, they also affected the heart. The H_2 antihistamines, such as cimetidine and ranitidine, were a big improvement. Recently, however, there has been renewed interest in the use of drugs blocking muscarinic acetylcholine receptors. The drug, pirenzepine, developed from the tricyclic antidepressants, is very effective clinically and it was found to be acting by blocking acetylcholine receptors. It blocks M_1 receptors more than M_2 or M_3 receptors and its effects on healing are not accompanied by the effects on heart and vision seen with the atropine-like compounds previously available.

The use of atropine-like drugs in the treatment of Parkinson's disease started with the observation that, when atropine was given to control the excessive salivation associated with postencephalitic Parkinsonism, there was also a reduction in tremor. Other substances that have been used include procyclidine, benzhexol and benztropine. These are non-quaternary compounds that cross the blood–brain barrier and they are not esters – benztropine is the benzhydryl ether of tropine – and so are not broken down rapidly. However, as with all other uses of atropine-like compounds, in the long term they are unpleasant and there is a need for compounds without the effects on heart, salivation, sweating and intestine. Their beneficial effects in Parkinson's disease are also limited to the early stages (p. 375).

SELECTIVITY OF ATROPINE-LIKE COMPOUNDS

Molecular biologists have shown that there are several subclasses of muscarinic receptors and, although few selective agonists have yet been obtained, antagonists with considerable selectivity have been found; some are shown in Fig. 11.3. Pirenzepine and telenzepine are reasonably specific for M_1 receptors. Hexahydro-sila-diphenidyl and its *p*-fluoro derivative are more active at M_3 receptors than at M_2 receptors, as is 4-diphenylacetoxy N-methylpiperidine (4DAMP) methobromide. The alkaloid himbacine and the compound AFDX-116 (developed from pirenzepine) have the reverse selectivity, being more active at M_2 receptors in the heart than at M_3 receptors in the ileum. The selectivity of some compounds can be seen from the values shown in Table 11.3. Not all compounds are competitive, however. The neuromuscular-blocking agent gallamine triethiodide and similar compounds have long been known clinically to have vagal-blocking effects as well as producing paralysis of voluntary muscle. Results obtained with these compounds and muscari-

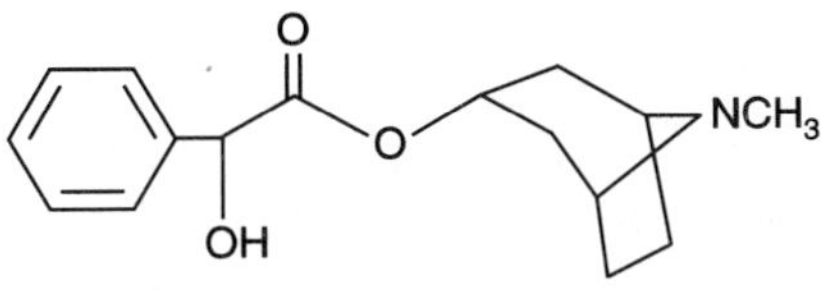

Homatropine*

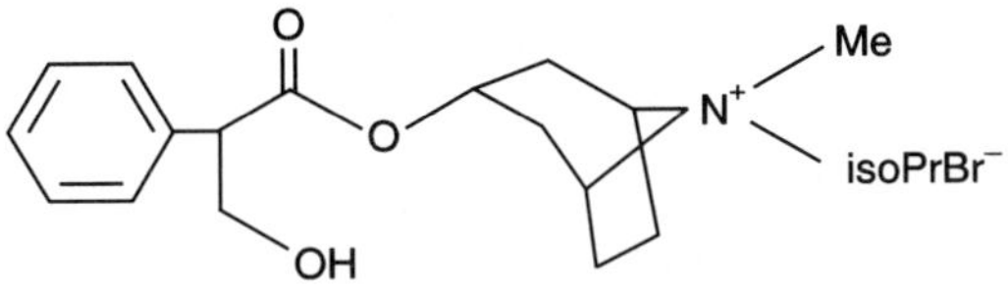

Ipratropium bromide

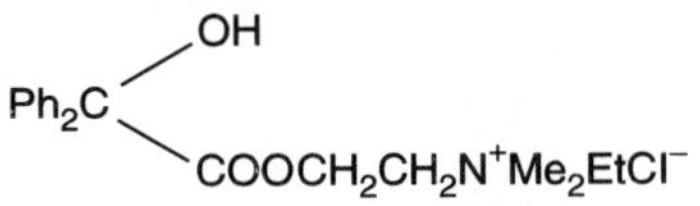

$Ph_2C(OH)COOCH_2CH_2N^+Me_2EtCl^-$

Lachesine chloride

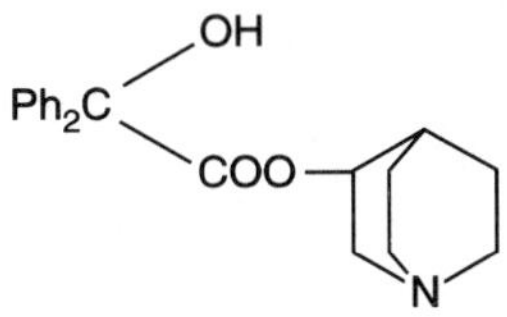

Quinuclidyl benzilate
QNB

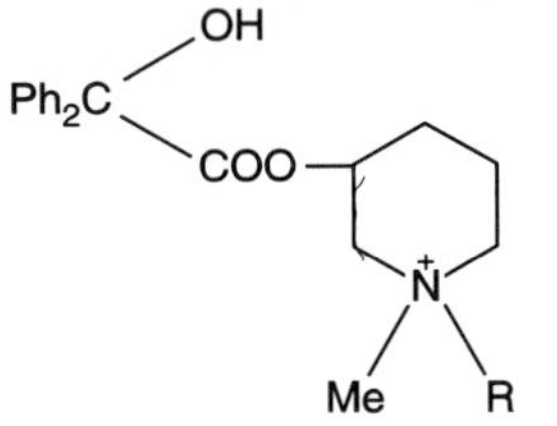

R = Me: Mepenzolate bromide
R = Et: Pipenzolate bromide

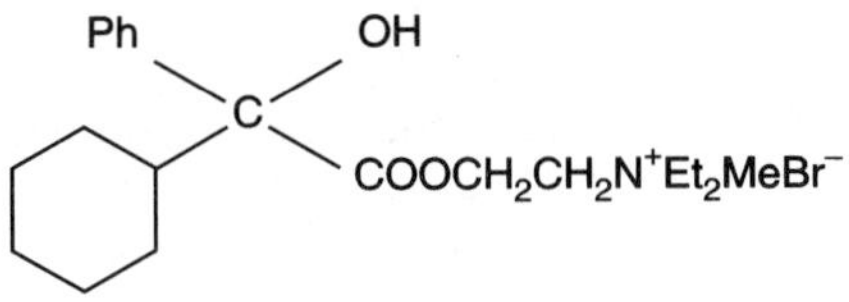

Oxyphenonium bromide

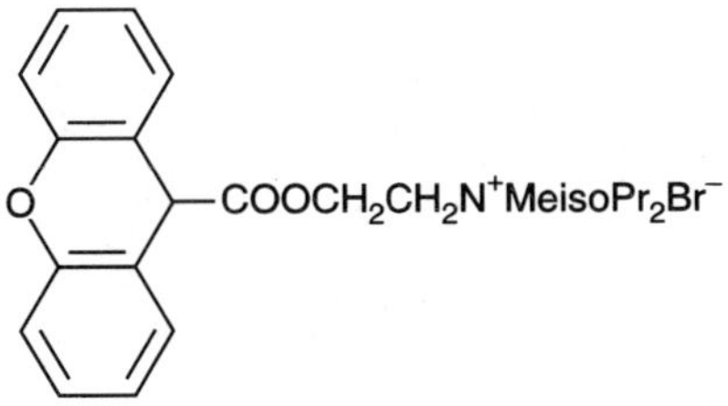

Propantheline bromide

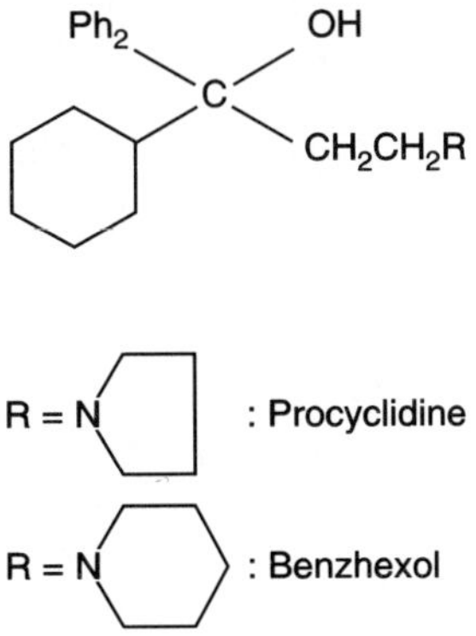

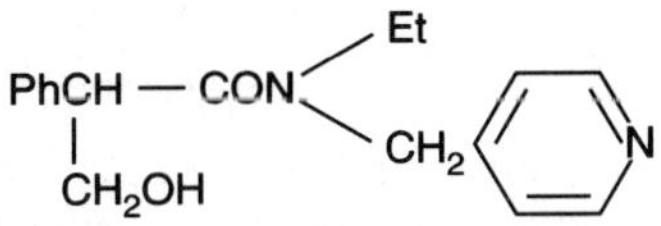

R = N(pyrrolidine) : Procyclidine

R = N(piperidine) : Benzhexol

Tropicamide*

FIGURE 11.2 Antimuscarinic drugs in clinical use: * indicates used on the eye.

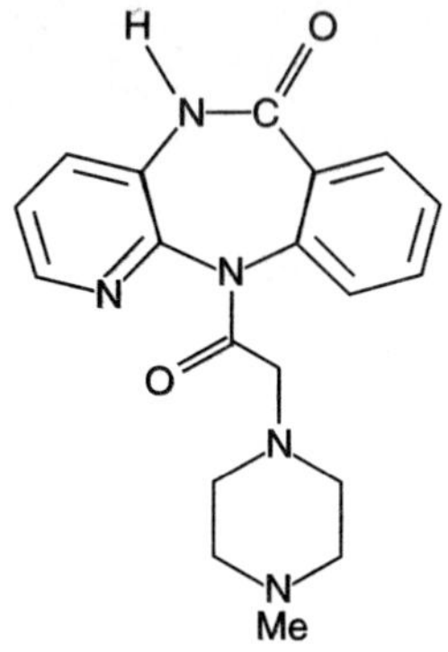

Pirenzepine

M1 selective

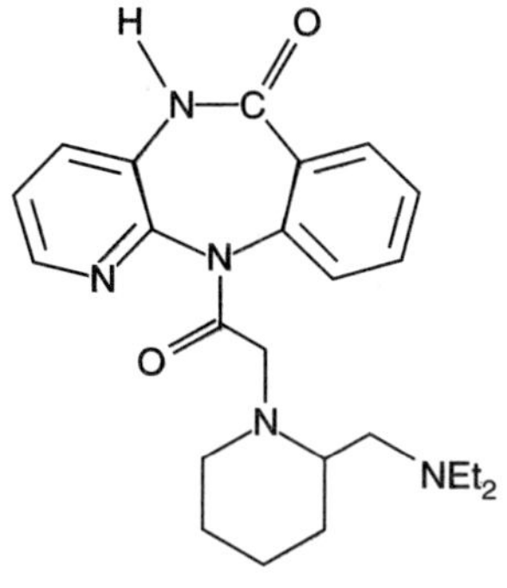

AF–DX 116

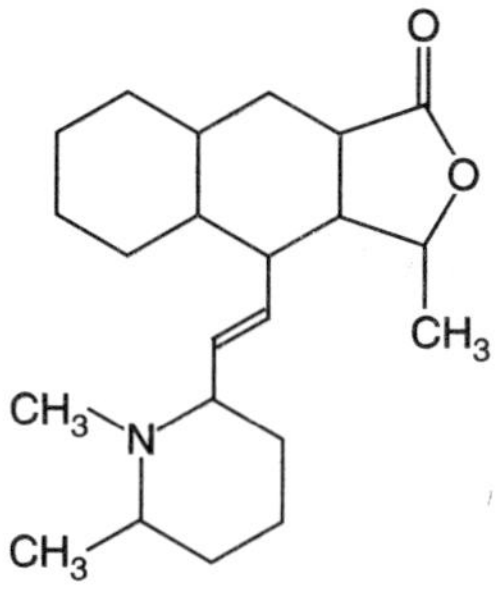

Himbacine

M2 selective

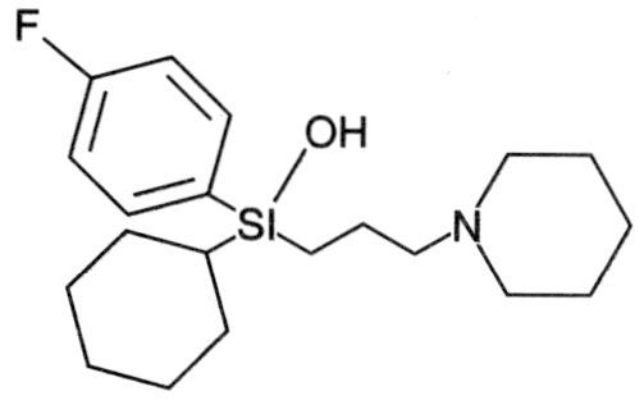

p-fluoro-hexahydro-diphenidyl

M3 selective

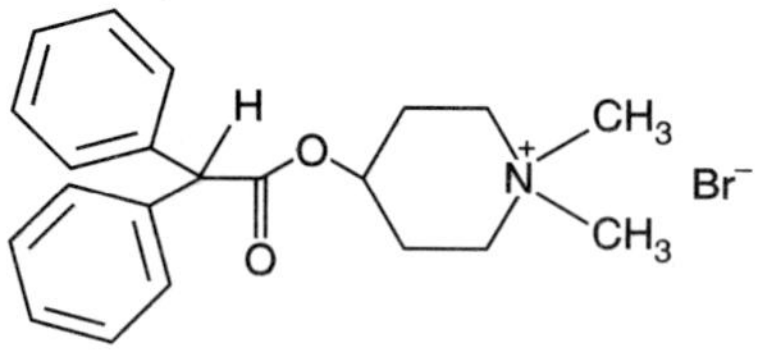

4-DAMP methobromide

FIGURE 11.3 Selective antimuscarinic drugs.

nic agonists do not fit the Gaddum–Schild equation and the compounds appear to be acting at an allosteric site. It is possible, therefore, that in addition to the emergence of more selective competitive agonists, compounds may be developed that act at the allosteric site.

SUMMARY

The short-term use of atropine-like compounds includes preoperative medication and the treatment of various forms of colic and of bronchospasm. Short-lasting drugs (homatropine) that can cross the cornea are available for inspection of the eye. The long-term use of atropine-like drugs for the treatment of peptic ulcers is only successful with more recently introduced drugs (pirenzepine), which have some selectivity. There is a limited use for some centrally acting compounds (benzhexol, procyclidine) in the treatment of Parkinson's disease. The compounds are essential for dealing with the muscarinic effects of acetylcholine in poisoning with an anticholinesterase (but must be supplemented by treatment for the nicotinic effects).

The emergence of more selective antimuscarinic drugs is to be expected. Therapeutic applications of antimuscarinic drugs are summarized in Table 11.4.

TABLE 11.3 Selectivity: values of log K for muscarinic receptors in guinea-pig atria (M_2) and ileum (M_3)

	M_2	M_3
Atropine	9.1	9.3
Pirenzepine	6.4	6.6
AFDX-116	7.3	6.2
4DAMP methobromide	8.0	9.0
p-Fluoro-hexahydro-sila-diphenidol	5.7	7.6

TABLE 11..4 Therapeutic applications of antimuscarinic drugs

PRE-MEDICATION	ANTI-SPASMODIC ANTI-ULCER	BRONCHODILATORS	OPHTHALMOLOGY	PARKINSONISM
Atropine Glycopyrronium Hyoscine (also called scopolamine)	Pirenzipine (Atropine)	Ipatropium Oxitropium (Atropine)	Homatropine Tropicamide (Atropine)	Benzhexol Benztropine Procyclidine

The pharmacology of individual agents is described in detail within the relevant chapters.

12

Neuromuscular Transmission

Part I Neuromuscular Transmission and Neuromuscular Blocking Agents

WC Bowman

INTRODUCTION

The term 'neuromuscular blocking agent' might be applied to any substance that interrupts transmission from nerve to muscle. However, it is generally restricted to those agents, and related substances, that are used by anaesthetists to produce striated muscle relaxation during surgical anaesthesia, and that act essentially by reversibly blocking the interaction of the neurotransmitter acetylcholine with its receptor sites (nicotinic acetylcholine receptors, Chapter 8) on the postjunctional face of the motor endplate. The drugs tubocurarine and suxamethonium are the prototype drugs of this broad class.

The widespread use of neuromuscular blocking drugs in anaesthetic practice stems from 1942 when two Canadian anaesthesiologists, Drs Griffith and Johnson, demonstrated the efficacy of 'Intocostrin', an extract of a South American plant (*Chondrodendron tomentosum*) that contains tubocurarine, in producing muscle relaxation in anaesthetized patients. It is the case that about 30 years earlier, a German surgeon called Läwen had successfully used a partially purified extract called curarine in a similar way, but his description of his technique was largely ignored, probably because at that time anaesthesia was not a specialist branch of the medical profession. Griffith and Johnson's observations, and Cullen's soon thereafter, were in fact those that set the stage for the modern and universal technique of inducing muscle relaxation with neuromuscular blocking agents, thereby permitting easy tracheal intubation, and achieving abdominal relaxation while allowing the dose of anaesthetic agent to be reduced well below toxic levels.

Although the clinical use of neuromuscular blocking agents is only just over 50 years old, the history of these drugs goes back to much earlier times. Exaggerated stories about the effects of South American Indians' arrow poisons, or *curares*, were brought back to Europe by early explorers, including Sir Walter Raleigh, after Columbus' voyages. Two main poisonous plants were used in the preparation of the arrow poisons. Those from the forest regions of Ecuador and Peru contained ingredients derived from the vines of species of *Chondrodendron*, especially *C. tomentosum*, and those from the more easterly regions in the Guianas and the lower Orinoco contained ingredients from species of *Strychnos*, especially *S. toxifera*. Three types of curare were described, named after the containers in which the Indians packed them. Tube curare was packed in tubes made from sections of bamboo, pot curare in earthenware pots, and calabash curare in small calabashes or gourds. Game, paralysed or killed by curares, was harmless on ingestion because any active principles that survive cooking are absorbed from the gut to no more than a trivial extent. The curares contain a great many alkaloids and these were extracted and studied chemically in the mid 1930s by a number of chemists, prominent amongst whom was Harold King in Oxford. King purified and characterized the first sample of (+)-tubocurarine (called *d*-tubocurarine in the USA) from tube curare in 1935. He almost got the structure correct. His trivial error was to designate both nitrogens as quaternary, whereas, as Everett and his colleagues showed 35 years later, one of the nitrogens is in fact tertiary (Fig. 12.1), although strongly protonated at body pH. In the UK the official name of (+)-tubocurarine is simply tubocurarine, there being no other form readily available.

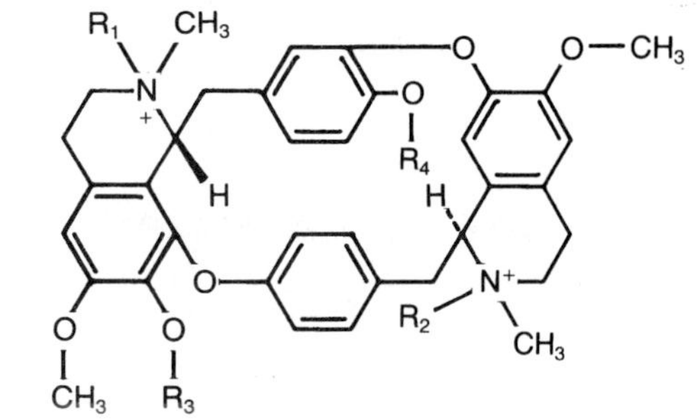

The only other naturally occurring curare alkaloid of importance is toxiferine I (Fig. 12.1), isolated from *S. toxifera* by King in 1949. Toxiferine I is rather unstable in solution and is not used in anaesthetic practice. However, the semisynthetic compound alcuronium is derived from it. Alcuronium (diallylnortoxiferine) has allyl radicals ($-CH_2-CH_2{=}CH_2$) in place of methyl groups attached to the quaternary nitrogens of toxiferine.

In the middle of the 19th century, the famous French physiologist, Claude Bernard, carried out simple but elegant experiments on frogs demonstrating that the site of action of curare lies somewhere between the motor nerve axons and the contractile apparatus of the muscle; that is, somewhere at the neuromuscular junction. Thus, he showed that curare has no effect on conduction of the nerve impulse nor on the ability of muscle to contract, yet it prevents the former from evoking the latter. The upper section of Fig. 12.2 illustrates an experiment that is no more than a more modern version of Claude Bernard's experiment. In a dose that blocked muscle twitches evoked by stimulating the motor nerve, the neuromuscular-blocking agent was without effect on the action potentials in the motor nerve; nor did it affect the contractility of the muscle as shown by the normal twitches evoked by direct muscle stimulation (Fig. 12.2(a)). The neuromuscular-blocking agent used in the experiment of Fig. 12.2 was vecuronium rather than tubocurarine, but similar results are obtained with tubocurarine and, indeed, with all drugs of this class. At the time of Claude

	R_1	R_2	R_3	R_4
(+) − Tubocurarine (protonated form)	CH_3	H	H	H
Metocurine	CH_3	CH_3	CH_3	CH_3

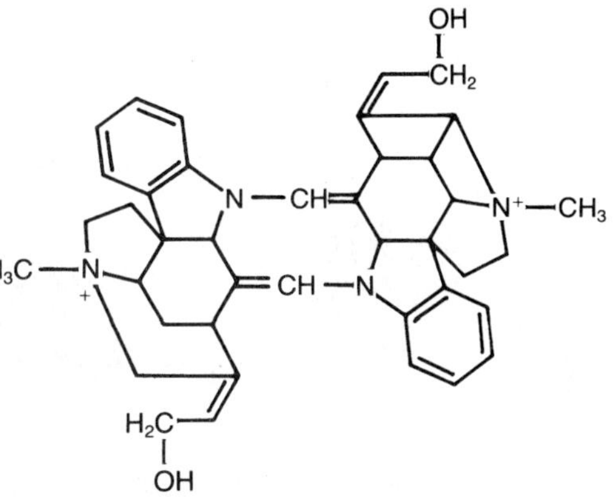

Toxiferine I, in alcuronium, the methyl groups attached to the quaternary nitrogens are replaced by allyl groups ($-CH_2-CH{=}CH_2$)

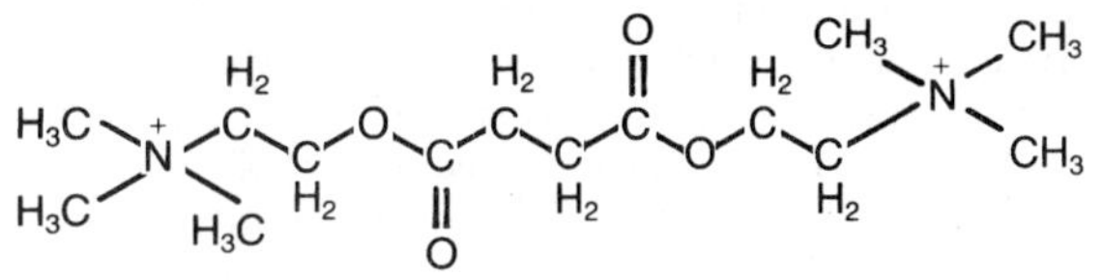

Succinyldicholine (suxamethonium)

FIGURE 12.1 Structures of prototype neuromuscular-blocking drugs. Succinyldicholine is a depolarizing blocking drug, and the only one to be retained in anaesthetic practice. As a chemical it has been known since 1906, but it was only introduced into anaesthetic practice in 1951. The other drugs illustrated are non-depolarizing blocking drugs either obtained directly from plants or derivatives of those obtained from plants.

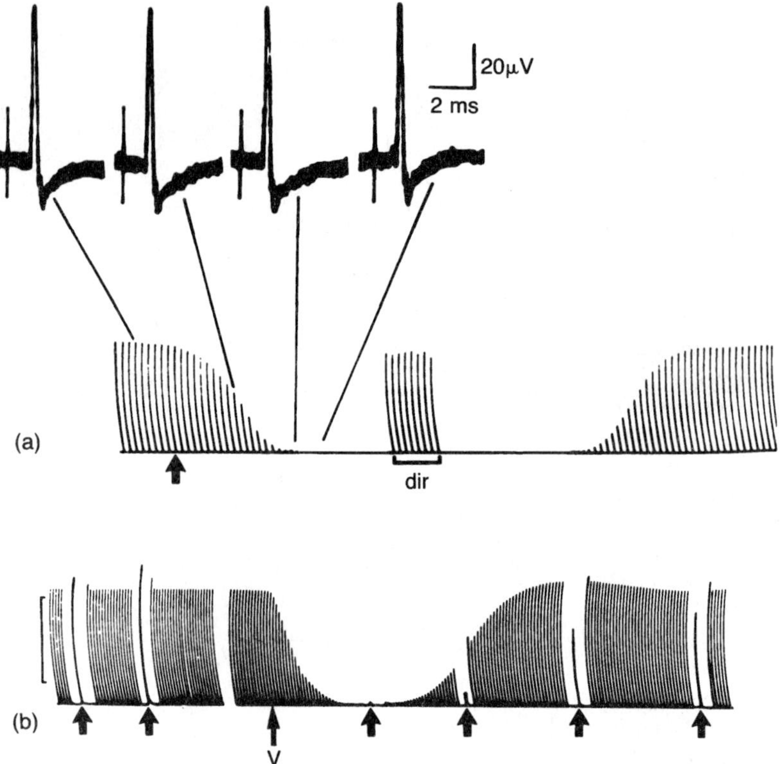

FIGURE 12.2 Cats anaesthetized with chloralose. Maximal twitches of tibialis anterior muscles were evoked by stimulating the motor nerve (0.1 Hz). (a) Antidromic nerve action potentials were recorded from a ventral root simultaneously with the twitches. The representative action potentials were associated with the twitches indicated by the oblique lines. At the arrow, a neuromuscular-blocking drug (vecuronium 100 µg/kg) was injected intravenously. This dose caused complete block of the twitches evoked by nerve stimulation, but was without effect on the nerve action potentials. During the block, the muscle responded normally to direct stimulation (dir). (b) At intervals, electrical simulation was temporarily stopped and acetylcholine (8 µg) was injected close-arterially into the muscle (unlabelled arrows). The contractions above the unlabelled arrows are the responses to acetylcholine. At V, vecuronium (30 µg/kg) was injected iv. During the block of the twitches evoked by nerve stimulation, the contractions produced by close-arterially injected acetylcholine were also blocked. Tension calibration: 5N (Reproduced with permission from Baird WLM, Bowman WC, Kerr WJ, *British Journal of Anaesthesia* 1982; **54**: 375–85.)

Bernard's experiments around 1850 the concepts of chemical transmission and of specific receptors had not been proposed. Experiments of the type illustrated in the lower section of Fig. 12.2 (Fig. 12.2(b)) were first carried out more than 80 years later by Sir Henry Dale and his co-workers. In the experiment illustrated in Fig. 12.2(b), the muscle was made to contract in two ways: either by stimulating the motor nerve, or by injecting acetylcholine directly into its arterial supply. The neuromuscular-blocking agent blocked both types of contraction because, as is now known, it blocks the receptors on the motor endplate with which acetylcholine interacts.

Neuromuscular-blocking agents, as exemplified by curare or tubocurarine, are unusual and perhaps unique among clinically useful drugs in that knowledge of their mechanism of action preceded their widespread clinical use by almost a century. The converse is the case with most drugs of ancient origin (e.g. morphine, digitalis, cinchona) in that their therapeutic uses long preceded the discovery of their mechanisms of action. Curare and tubocurarine played important parts as tools in physiological experiments concerned with cholinergic transmission and the neuromuscular junction, long before their use as muscle relaxants during surgical anaesthesia was contemplated.

The mechanism of action of neuromuscular-blocking drugs is closely bound up with the anatomy and physiology of the neuromuscular junction. Hence it is convenient to deal with these latter aspects before or alongside the pharmacology of the drugs that modify the process.

NEUROMUSCULAR TRANSMISSION

The neuromuscular junction

The large, fast-conducting myelinated (Aα) axons of the motoneurones that innervate skeletal muscle (Fig. 12.3(a)) have their cell bodies in the anterior horn cells of the spinal cord or the brain stem. They pass, without interruption, to the skeletal muscles where each axon

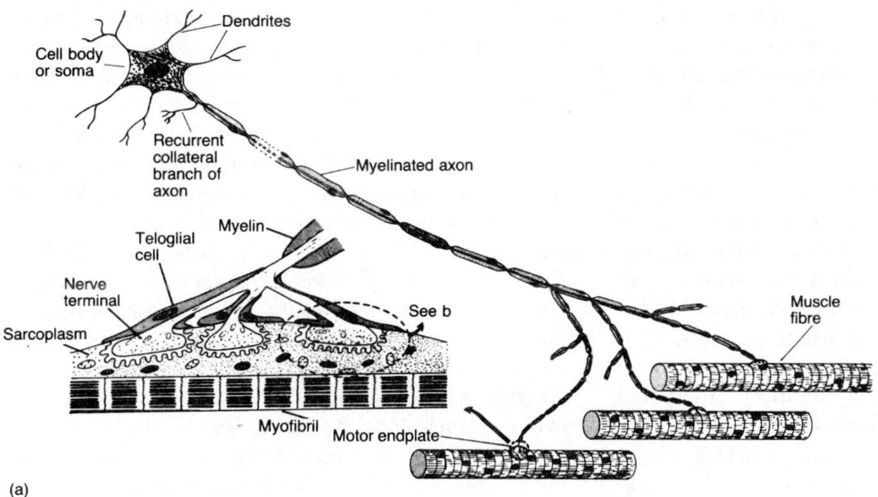

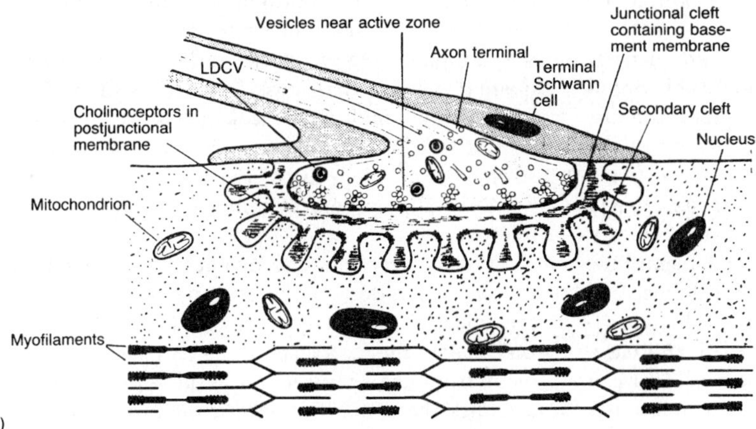

FIGURE 12.3 (a) Diagram of a motor unit containing focally innervated muscle fibres. A motor endplate is enlarged as the inset on the left. (Reproduced with permission from Bowman WC, Rand MJ. *Textbook of pharmacology*, 2nd edn. Oxford: Blackwell Scientific Publications, 1980.) (b) A neuromuscular junction enlarged from the motor endplate of (a). The axon terminal contains mitochondria, microtubules and acetylcholine-containing vesicles. LDCV is a large dense-cored vesicle containing calcitonin gene-related peptide.

branches many times. Each individual branch loses its myelin, and then ends in a small bunch of three or four swellings within each of which are visible all the subcellular organelles characteristic of a cholinergic synapse, especially thousands of electron lucent spherical vesicles (*c*. 45 nm in diameter) that contain about 80% of the acetylcholine that is contained within each nerve terminal. A small proportion of the vesicles is lined up alongside electron-dense bars (so-called active zones) in the terminal membrane opposite to the endplate membrane of the muscle fibre. These vesicles are thought to contain the readily releasable or immediately available store of transmitter. The remaining vesicles are thought to contain the reserve store of releasable transmitter. The processes that replenish the immediately available store from the reserve store are collectively known as *mobilization*.

In addition to the numerous small translucent acetylcholine-containing vesicles, there are a few larger dense-cored vesicles that have been shown to contain calcitonin gene-related peptide (CGRP). Whether CGRP functions as a cotransmitter is a matter of some controversy; indeed some authors believe that it is not present in mammalian motor nerve terminals at all, but rather is confined to sensory terminals. However, the majority of experts are convinced of its presence in both motor and sensory terminals, including those of man. It has a number of effects on the neuromuscular system as described below.

Each nerve terminal swelling lies in an indentation, a junctional cleft, in the muscle fibre membrane. The postjunctional membrane of the junctional cleft, that is, of the motor endplate, is greatly expanded by junctional folds to form secondary clefts, and the whole neuromuscular junction is encapsulated by the terminal Schwann cells (teloglia) which fuse with the muscle fibre membrane. In most mammalian muscles, each muscle fibre receives its innervation from a single branch of a motor axon at a central point on the muscle surface. Such muscle fibres are said to be focally innervated. A single axon, together with the group of muscle fibres that it innervates, comprise a motor unit. Only the area of muscle fibre membrane that comprises the motor endplate is sensitive to acetylcholine. In many of the muscles of birds and amphibia, the muscles contain a large number of multiply innervated fibres; that is, the muscle fibre receives its innervation from many axon branches, and motor endplates are widely distributed over the muscle fibre surface. Consequently, such muscle fibres are sensitive to acetylcholine over most of their surfaces, and this leads to a different kind of response to nicotinic agonists from that exhibited by focally innervated fibres. In mammals, including humans, multiply innervated fibres are present in only a few muscles (extraocular muscles, internal ear muscle, striated muscle in upper oesophagus). The presence of such fibres in the extraocular muscles accounts for, or at least contributes to, the increase in intraocular pressure produced by suxamethonium.

The nicotinic acetylcholine receptors are densely located on the shoulders of the junctional folds opposite to the active zones of the nerve terminal. The distance from the active zones to the receptors across the junctional gap is about 60 nm. Receptors are virtually absent from other parts of the endplate membrane and from the rest of the muscle fibre. The space between the nerve terminal and the postjunctional membrane contains a collagen-like, mucopolysaccharide material called the basement membrane. Most of the acetylcholinesterase of the junction is attached to the basement membrane (see Chapter 10). Figure 12.3(b) is a diagrammatic representation of the neuromuscular junction.

Prejunctional events in neuromuscular transmission

Acetylcholine is synthesized in the axoplasm of the nerve endings from choline and acetylcoenzyme A, the reaction being catalysed by the enzyme choline-O-acetyl transferase. The choline is derived from the extracellular fluid, and is transported through the axon terminal membrane by a special high affinity, carrier-facilitated transport system. Much of the choline is obtained from the diet or synthesized in the liver, but at least some of the choline derived from the breakdown of released acetylcholine is taken up and re-used in transmitter synthesis. The acetate is produced in the mitochondria from pyruvate obtained from glucose in the Embden–Meyerhof glycolytic pathway. However, the acetate derived from acetylcholine breakdown is also taken up again and re-used. The acetylcholine formed in the axoplasm is loaded into the vesicles by an active transport mechanism in the vesicle walls.

In the absence of nerve impulses, acetylcholine is released spontaneously and at random intervals in small uniform amounts thought to correspond to the amount contained in each vesicle. The mean frequency of release of these small packets of acetylcholine differs in different species, but is generally less than one per second in human muscles. The amount of acetylcholine released in this way is far too small to initiate the contractile sequence, but it can be detected by the small endplate depolarizations, the miniature endplate potentials (MEPPs), that it produces. A MEPP is thought to arise whenever a vesicle randomly collides with a release site and discharges its contents. In addition to spontaneous vesicular release, a considerably greater amount of acetylcholine (more than 100-fold greater) is spontaneously released in a non-quantal manner, apparently by direct leakage from the axoplasm through the membrane to the extracellular fluid. This, so-called, molecular leakage is still too small to cause muscle contraction, although it maintains a small and continuous depolarization of the endplate membrane relative to the membrane outside the endplate region. One difference between the quantal release that gives rise to MEPPs and the non-quantal molecular leakage is that the latter is not Ca^{2+} dependent, whereas the former is strongly Ca^{2+} dependent, the necessary calcium ions mostly being present within the axoplasm and the mitochondria.

When a nerve impulse invades the nerve terminals, the depolarization of the terminal membrane causes the opening of voltage-operated Ca^{2+} channels, and Ca^{2+} enters the axoplasm along its concentration gradient from the extracellular fluid. Intracellular Ca^{2+} activates the process of exocytosis in which vesicular membranes transiently fuse with the terminal membrane, and around fifty vesicles in the active zones thereby discharge their acetylcholine into the junctional gap to initiate the series of events that leads to muscle contraction. Release evoked by a nerve impulse is strongly dependent on the presence of extracellular Ca^{2+} and its ability to enter the axoplasm. It is worthwhile noting that the disease Lambert–Eaton myasthenic syndrome is associated with an autoantibody that is thought to be directed against the nerve terminal calcium channels. Hence, in this disease, insufficient Ca^{2+} enters the terminals to activate the release mechanism fully, and consequently transmitter release is inadequate, although it builds up to become more adequate with repeated stimulation (contrast myasthenia gravis in which repetitive stimulation causes enhanced failure).

A high local concentration of Ca^{2+} is necessary to induce vesicle fusion in the active zones. At those junctions, including the neuromuscular junction, that discharge an effective amount of transmitter in response to a single nerve impulse, the calcium channels concerned with release must be adjacent to the active zones in order to achieve the appropriate high local concentration.

The docking and release mechanisms involve the integral vesicular membrane proteins, synaptobrevin, synaptotagmin, synaptophysins, and the docking protein syntaxin, as described on page 110. The synapsin I mechanism (p. 110) is probably also involved in the release and mobilization of vesicles anchored to the cytoskeleton. Vesicles that have discharged their contents, quickly reform and are refilled with freshly synthesized acetylcholine. Hence, although vesicles are originally synthesized in the cell body, from which they pass to the terminals by transport along the microtubules, once they reach the terminals they may be recycled many times. Freshly synthesized acetylcholine is the first to be released, suggesting that during low frequencies of nerve impulses the vesicles that are already docked at the active zones are repeatedly refilled and discharged.

The prejunctional events in transmission are susceptible to pharmacological attack, and the effects of drugs and other agents that act prejunctionally are summarized in Table 12.1. With few exceptions, prejunctional sites of drug action are not clinically important. However, they should be borne in mind because of occasional intentional relevance (e.g. 4-aminopyridine to facilitate transmission), because of accidental drug interaction (e.g. streptomycin together with a neuromuscular-blocking drug), or because of toxicity (e.g. botulism).

Botulinum toxin (type A) is not only of toxicological importance, for it is also used therapeutically, by precise localized injection, to alleviate certain muscle dystonias (e.g. strabismus, blepharospasm, hemifacial spasm, torticolis) by blocking acetylcholine release. Hence, interaction with muscle relaxants must be borne in mind.

Cotransmission

The possibility that CGRP contained in dense-cored vesicles plays a cotransmitter role at the neuromuscular junction is referred to above. CGRP is released by nerve impulses, the necessary frequency of stimulation being higher than that necessary to release acetylcholine, which is of course released even by a single isolated impulse. Release of CGRP is also Ca^{2+} dependent, although the axonal calcium channels involved are different from those that mediate acetylcholine release. Because the dense-cored vesicles are not anchored at the active zones, the general rise in axoplasmic Ca^{2+} concentration required to discharge them can be achieved only by repetitive stimulation. CGRP exerts a number of postjunctional effects on the neuromuscular system. Its acute effects include an increase in contractility, prolongation of post-tetanic potentiation, stimulation of an electrogenic Na^+/K^+ pump that elevates the membrane potential, and enhanced nicotinic receptor desensitization. Its chronic effect is to increase the synthesis of acetylcholine receptors.

Feedback control of transmitter release

There is increasing evidence that many released neurotransmitters, both in the periphery and in the central nervous system, exert part of their action back on their own nerve terminals, through so-called autoreceptors, to modulate the release of stored transmitter by subsequent nerve impulses. The neuromuscular junction is

TABLE 12.1 Some drugs and toxins that modify prejunctional mechanisms

PREJUNCTIONAL EFFECT	DRUG OR TOXIN: MODE OF ACTION
Inhibition of acetylcholine synthesis	*N-Methyl-4-(1-naphthylvinyl)pyridinium (NVP+)*: directly inhibits choline-O-acetyltransferase but non-specific in its actions
	Hemicholinium-3 (HC-3): inhibits transport of choline into axoplasm, hence depriving synthetic enzyme of its substrate
	The triethyl analogue of choline (triethylcholine): behaves similarly to HC-3, but may itself be transported, acetylated and released as a false transmitter
Inhibition of vesicle loading	*Vesamicol (AH 5183)*: inhibits the transport of acetylcholine into vesicles in the nerve endings
Inhibition of evoked acetylcholine release	*Adenosine*: acts on terminal membrane A_1 receptors to reduce Ca^{2+} influx in response to action potential (There are also A_{2A} receptors which under some circumstances mediate an increase in acetylcholine release)
	Botulinum toxin: binds to specific acceptor in terminal membrane and is taken up into axoplasm, probably via the vesicle recycling process. It then inhibits exocytosis of acetylcholine by inactivating the vesicular membrane protein synaptobrevin
	Aminoglycoside antibiotics: act like Mg^{2+} ions to inhibit the release mechanism. Site of action may be the voltage-operated Ca^{2+} channels in the terminal membrane
Enhancement of evoked acetylcholine release	4-Aminopyridine, tetraethylammonium, and dendrotoxins (from the green mamba) prolong the action potential by blocking the delayed rectifier K^+ channels. Consequently more Ca^{2+} enters the terminals and more acetylcholine is released. Tetraethylammonium and charybdotoxin (from a scorpion venom) also block certain other types of K^+ channels, an action that also serves to facilitate acetylcholine release

no exception. The best evidence is in favour of prejunctionally located nicotinic autoreceptors that facilitate not the actual release mechanism but rather the mobilization of stored transmitter into the immediately available situation (Fig. 12.4). In this way availability of transmitter for release is made to match the demand for it. In the absence of such a mechanism, availability for release could not keep up with the demands of high frequency stimulation. Hence, transmitter output would fall off during rapid rates of stimulation, and so the muscle response would fade.

This positive feedback control mechanism is referred to again during the discussion of the actions of non-depolarizing neuromuscular-blocking drugs (p. 145). There is also evidence for the presence of two populations of muscarinic receptors on the nerve endings, one that inhibits and the other that facilitates transmitter release. However, the physiological importance and the conditions under which these muscarinic receptors are activated have not yet been ascertained.

Postjunctional events in neuromuscular transmission

Studies of nicotinic acetylcholine receptors in the motor endplate have been greatly aided by two important zoological contributions: the presence of a rich source of receptor material of the motor endplate

(a)

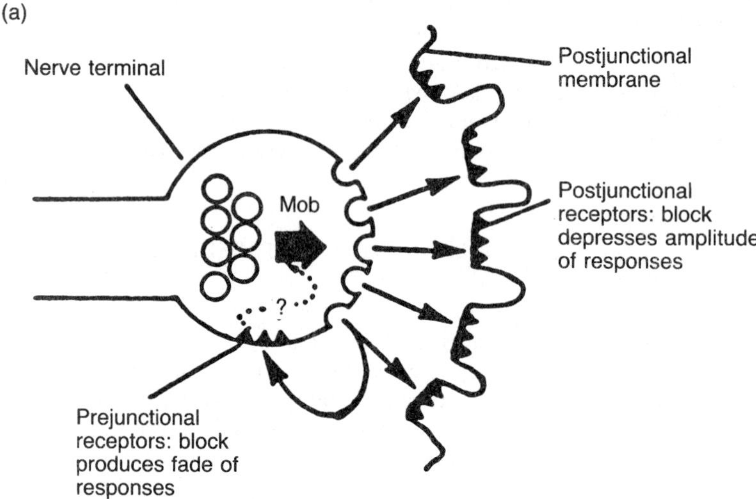

(b)

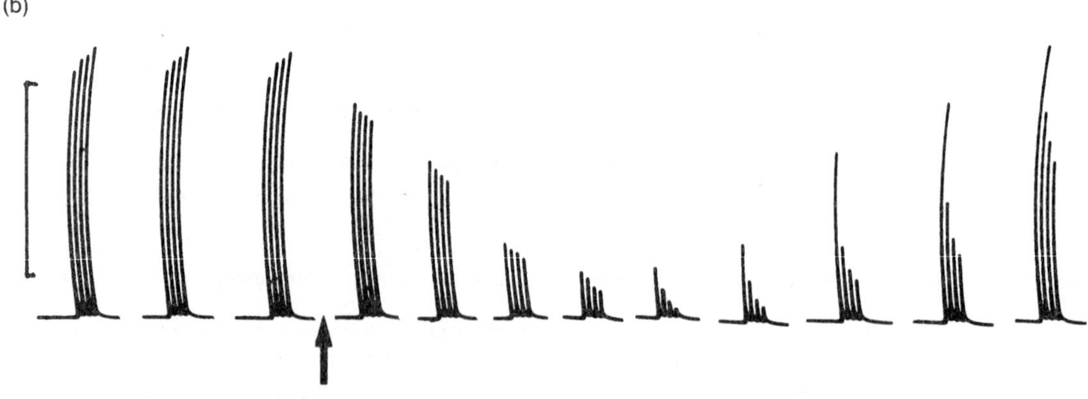

FIGURE 12.4 (a) Diagram illustrating the proposed actions of released acetylcholine on prejunctional and postjunctional nicotinic acetylcholine receptors. Mobilization (mob) should be taken to include all those processes that serve to place acetylcholine in a readily releasable situation between nerve impulses, and not merely the movement of vesicles towards the terminal membrane as suggested by the diagram. (b) Cat, chloralose anaesthesia. Maximal twitches of a tibialis muscle were evoked by stimulation of the motor nerve with train-of-four stimulation (2 Hz for 2s) applied every 20 s. Vecuronium (30 μg/kg) was injected intravenously at the arrow. Selected groups of stimuli are illustrated during the onset of and the recovery from the block. Groups were selected in pairs to show matching degrees of block of the first twitches in each pair of groups during onset and recovery. Note that fade of trains is much more marked during recovery than during onset; that is, fade has a slower onset than has initial twitch depression. Depression of T_1 amplitude is a consequence of postjunctional receptor block whereas fade is regarded as mainly a consequence of prejunctional receptor block. (Reproduced with permission from the International Anesthesia Research Society from Bowman WÇ. *Anesthesia and Analgesia* 1980; 59: 935–43.)

type in the electric organs of the electric eel and the electric rays, and the ability of α-toxins from certain elapid snakes, notably cobra toxin from the Thailand cobra and α-bungarotoxin from the Malaysian or Taiwanese banded krait, to bind selectively and virtually irreversibly to this type of receptor. The powerful binding properties of these α-toxins have permitted the isolation, purification and chemical characterization of the receptors. The receptors are protein, or glycoprotein, in nature and for many species the complete amino-acid sequence is known. Figure 12.5 gives a diagrammatic representation of nicotinic acetylcholine receptors inserted in the lipid membrane of the motor endplate. The receptors are anchored to the cytoskeleton on the inside and they extend right through the membrane and project into the extracellular fluid. Each receptor is composed of five protein subunits or protomers. Two are identical in composition and are designed the α (alpha)-subunits; the others, in electric fish and fetal mammalian receptors, being the β (beta)-, γ (gamma)- and δ (delta)-subunits. In the adult mammalian receptor, the subunit corresponding to the γ-subunit differs in composition and is designated the ϵ (epsilon)-subunit. The two α-subunits contain the binding sites for acetylcholine, one on each. The same binding sites combine with snake α-toxins and with neuromuscular-blocking agents. The five subunits are arranged around a central pore which is the ion channel. In the resting state, this ion channel is in the closed conformation and therefore impermeable to ions.

Much is known, or has been deduced, about the structure of the proteins that comprise the subunits. The polypeptide chain of each subunit crosses the membrane four times, the four transmembrane stretches being designated M1, M2, M3 and M4 (Fig. 12.5(b)). Both the NH_2 end and the COOH end of the chain are on the outside. The ion channel is lined by the five M2-spanning regions, one contributed by each subunit. The M2, and probably the M4, regions are twisted into α-helices, whereas the other two transmembrane spanning regions are probably β-pleated sheets. The acetylcholine binding site, that is, the recognition site of the receptor on each of the two α-protomers, is in a pocket of the protein 2–3 nm above the lipid membrane surface, and involves the amino acids Tyr-93, Trp-149, Tyr-190, Cys-192 and Cys-193 of the N-terminal hydrophilic domain. On the cytoplasm side is the region where the proteins of the cytoskeleton and certain protein kinases interact. Phosphorylation of a site on the cytoplasmic side causes desensitization of the receptor. One especially important protein is that designated 43K protein, which serves to anchor the receptors to the underlying cytoskeleton, thereby restricting their lateral movement.

Acetylcholine released from the nerve terminals traverses the hurdle of the acetylcholinesterase of the basement membrane, and much of it (though not all) reaches the acetylcholine receptors on the shoulders of the junctional folds. There is a large excess of spare receptors so that the safety factor in transmission is high.

Binding of an acetylcholine molecule at its binding site on one α-subunit facilitates the binding of a second acetylcholine molecule at the other α-subunit. That is to say that binding exhibits positive co-operativity (cf. the binding of oxygen with haemoglobin). When both binding sites at the receptor complex are occupied by acetylcholine, and only when both are occupied, a conformational change is induced in the protein of the α-subunit which is then transmitted throughout the complex. The change takes the form of opening of the ion channel through the receptor complex. The open ion channel is selective for cations (Na^+, K^+, Ca^{2+}, Mg^{2+}, NH_4^+) which then passively flow through the membrane in accordance with their concentration and electrical gradients. At the neuromuscular junction, the cations in greatest concentration are Na^+ and K^+. The concentration gradient for Na^+ is inwards whereas that for K^+ is outwards. However, the electrical gradients for both cations are inwards. Hence, the electrical gradient sums with the concentration gradient for Na^+ but opposes that for K^+. The net result is that when the ion channel opens, the main change is an influx of Na^+ ions; that is, there is an inward flowing electric current carried by sodium ions. Figure 12.6(a) illustrates activation of a receptor complex by acetylcholine.

The inward Na^+ current occurs through a large number of receptor channels and constitutes the miniature endplate current (MEPC) or the full sized endplate current (EPC) depending upon the amount of acetylcholine released and the number of receptors activated (about 1700 receptors in a MEPC and about 340 000 in an EPC). Flow of current through a membrane changes the potential differences across it, and so the endplate current lowers the membrane potential at the endplate (i.e. depolarizes the endplate) to produce a MEPP or a full-sized endplate potential (EPP). A full-sized EPP in a focally innervated muscle fibre triggers off a propagating action potential that passes around the muscle fibre membrane and along the transverse tubules to initiate contraction. In a multiply innervated muscle fibre, depolarization by released acetylcholine, of the large number of endplates all over the muscle fibre surface may make the propagating action potential unnecessary. The acetylcholine-induced depolarization may therefore directly activate the contractile mechanism so that a *contracture* results. A contracture is defined as a contraction during which propagating action potentials are absent.

Patch clamp

The so-called patch clamp technique allows measurement of the current that flows through a single activated ion channel. The highly polished tip of a glass micropipette (1–2 μm tip diameter) is pressed against

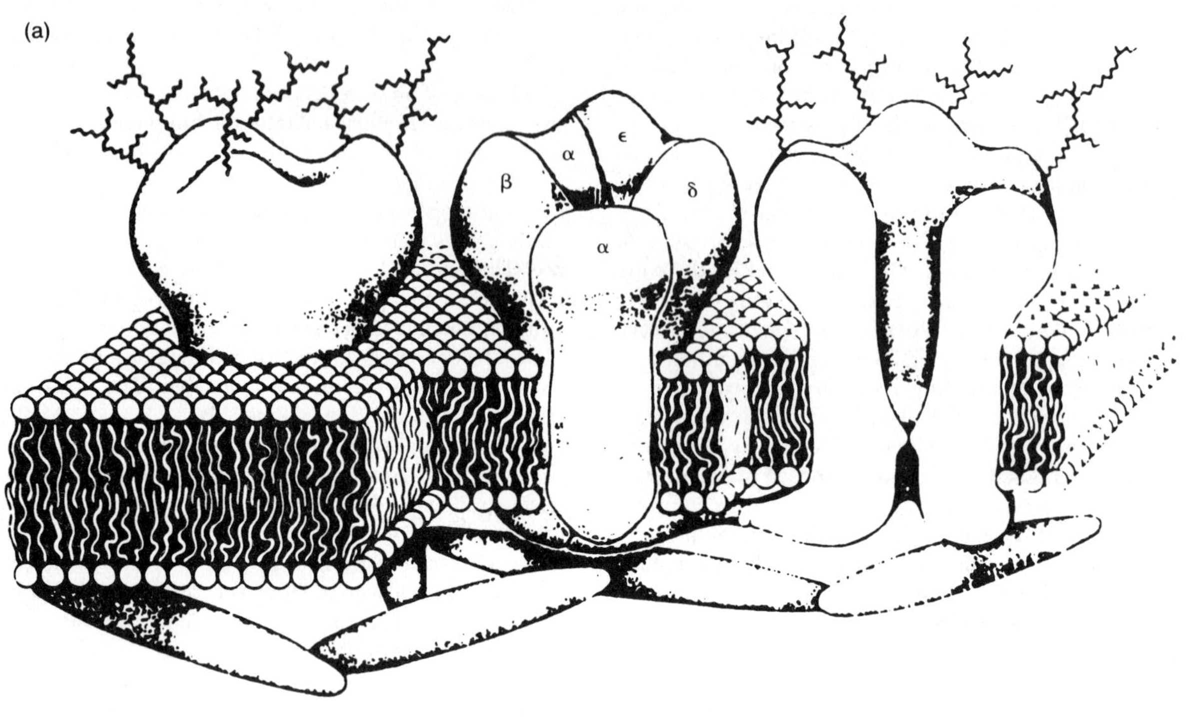

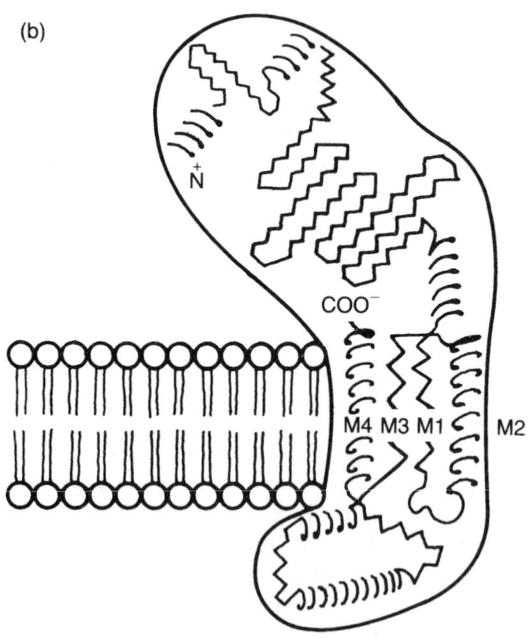

FIGURE 12.5 Nicotinic acetylcholine receptors embedded in the lipid membrane of the motor endplate. Three receptors are shown, the centre one having its protein subunits labelled ($\alpha_2\beta\delta\epsilon$), and the one on the right being sectioned to show the ion channel. Carbohydrate moieties project like antennae from the upper (outer) surface. At the lower (inner) surface, the receptors are anchored to the cytoskeleton. The two α-subunits possess the binding sites for acetylcholine molecules, one on each of the outer surfaces. The receptors were originally drawn on the basis of electron microscopy and neutron scattering data from Torpedo electric organ membranes, but mammalian receptors are similar in appearance. In the Torpedo receptor, the subunit corresponding to the ϵ-subunit is called the γ-subunit. (Reproduced with permission from Lindstrom J, Schoepfer R, Whiting P. *Cold Spring Harbor Symposia on Quantitative Biology* 1983; **XLVII**: 89–99.) (b) A proposed model for the transmembrane arrangement of the polypeptide chain in a protomer.

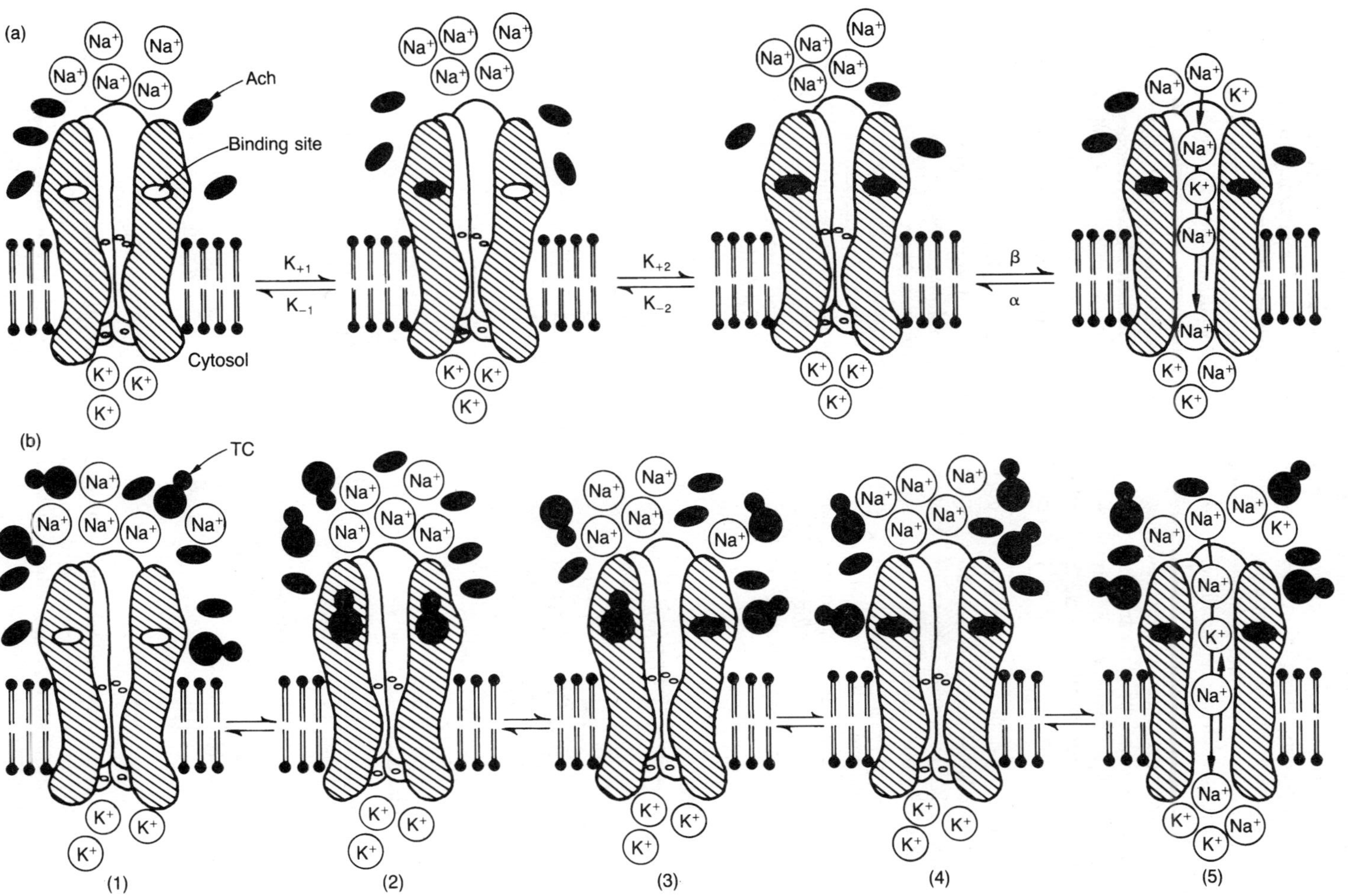

FIGURE 12.6 Diagram of the interaction of acetylcholine (Ach) with endplate acetylcholine receptors. Two acetylcholine molecules combine with the recognition sites of the receptor and induce a conformational change that results in the opening of a cation channel allowing the diffusion of sodium and potassium ions. The combination of the first Ach molecule facilitates combination with the second (positive co-operativity). (b) The interaction of acetylcholine molecules and molecules of a reversible blocking drug (e.g. tubocurarine) with endplate acetylcholine receptors. (1) An unblocked, non-activated receptor complex; (2) a receptor complex with both binding sites occupied by antagonist molecules; (3) a receptor complex with one binding site occupied by an antagonist molecule and the other by an acetylcholine molecule; (4) a receptor complex with both binding sites occupied by acetylcholine molecules but before the ion channel has opened; and (5) a receptor complex in which the ion channel has been opened by acetylcholine molecules. Note that the blocking drug does not prevent the acetylcholine–receptor interaction but merely reduces its probability.

the membrane and suction is applied to form an electric seal of high leak resistance. The patch of membrane containing one or perhaps up to three receptors may be broken away from the cell as illustrated in Fig. 12.7. Techniques are available for inverting the membrane so that the receptor recognition sites are towards the outside. However, in the diagram of Fig. 12.7, the receptor recognition sites would be inside the pipette, and therefore drugs, such as acetylcholine, must be dissolved in the fluid inside the pipette, which acts both as a means of applying drugs and as a recording electrode. The resistance between the glass and the membrane surface is so high ($10^9\Omega$) that the only way that current can flow into or out of the pipette is through an open ion channel. Currents as small as 1 pA can be resolved.

Acetylcholine dissolved in the fluid inside the pipette causes the ion channel to open and close repeatedly so that small rectangular pulses of current of constant amplitude (a few pA) but variable duration are recorded. The mean duration, that is the mean open time of the channel, is constant (a few ms) for a particular nicotinic agonist. For example, it is shorter for nicotine than for acetylcholine, and longer for certain synthetic esters of choline (e.g. suberylcholine). If the concentration of acetylcholine (or other agonist) is increased, the only change is an increase in the frequency of channel openings. The amplitude of the current pulses and the mean open time remain constant. These observations are important in that they demonstrate the properties of the channel, and the fact that agonists in the biophase around the receptors interact in a dynamic way, repeatedly and transiently combining with and dissociating from their binding sites. The situation for transmitter acetylcholine in the intact neuromuscular system is, however, slightly different because of the presence of acetylcholinesterase. This enzyme is so efficient that acetylcholine molecules released from the nerve, and that reach the postjunctional membrane intact, on the whole last long enough to activate only one receptor and only once. Hence the EPC, and consequently the EPP, are the summated result of thousands of single receptor activations. If cholinesterase is inhibited by an anticholinesterase agent, then a situation more similar to that in the patch clamp electrode is produced. More of the released acetylcholine then reaches the receptor sites, and the molecules may activate the same and different receptors repeatedly as they bounce their way across the endplate membrane while escaping by diffusion

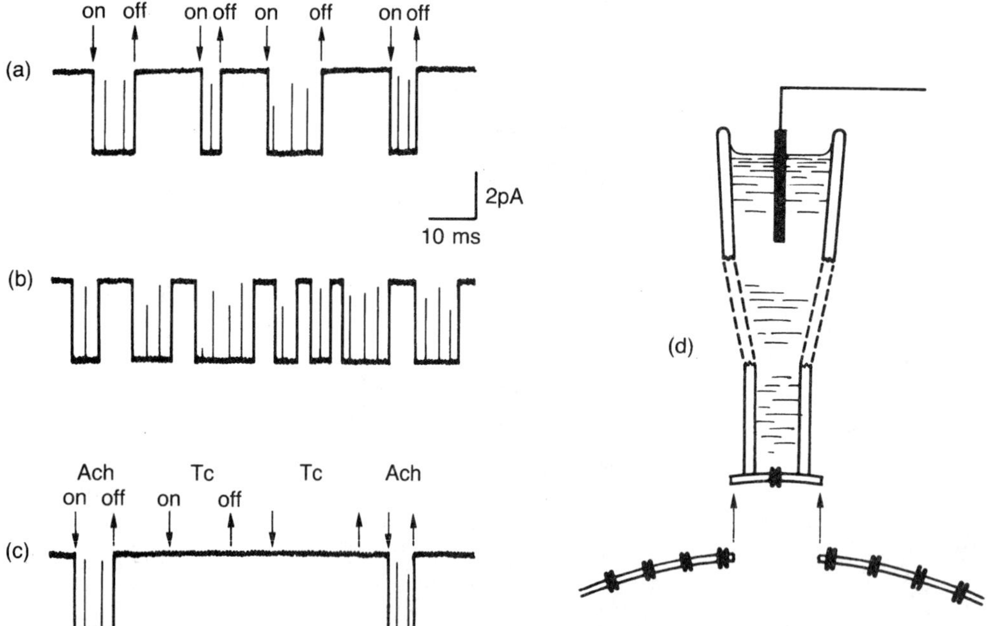

FIGURE 12.7 Three facsimile records of acetylcholine (Ach) currents through a single receptor channel made with a patch clamp electrode are shown on the left. Current flow is represented by downward deflections. (a) Four openings (or rather four bursts of openings) with a given concentration of acetylcholine in the pipette. (b) Seven openings (bursts) in an equivalent oscilloscope sweep when the acetylcholine concentration is increased. (c) The response when the acetylcholine concentration in (b) is mixed with tubocurarine (Tc); the frequency of openings or bursts is reduced to two in the oscilloscope sweep. Association with and dissociation from the receptor by acetylcholine or tubocurarine are indicated by 'on' and 'off'. (d) Diagram (not to scale) of a patch clamp pipette with a trapped patch of membrane containing a single receptor. The highly polished tip of a glass micropipette (1–2 μm tip diameter) is pressed against the membrane, and suction is applied to form an electric seal with a leak resistance of more than 10^9 Ω. The patch of membrane may be broken away as illustrated. Electric currents flowing from the pipette can do so only through the open receptor channel. In this arrangement, drugs are added to the fluid inside the pipette, which also serves as the recording electrode. (Reproduced with permission from Bowman WC. In: Bowman WC, Denissen PAF, Feldman S eds. *Neuromuscular blocking agents, past, present and future.* Amsterdam: Excerpta Medica, 1990: 20–35.)

from the junctional cleft. Hence, in the presence of an anticholinesterase agent, the EPC and EPP become larger in amplitude and longer in duration.

Variations in receptor number

Prolonged application of excess acetylcholine, as occurs for example through prolonged use of an anticholinesterase drug, causes a reduction in the number of receptors (i.e. the receptors are down-regulated) because the rate at which they are taken back into the cell by endocytosis and destroyed in the lysosomes is increased, and the insertion of newly synthesized ones into the membrane is slowed. The opposite occurs (i.e. the receptors are up-regulated) if receptor activation is reduced, for example, by the prolonged application of a neuromuscular-blocking agent.

When the motor nerve to a skeletal muscle is severed and chronic denervation occurs, receptors begin to appear outside the endplate region and eventually spread to cover the whole surface of the muscle fibre membrane to a density of about $1000/\mu m^2$. The density at the crests of the junctional folds of an innervated endplate is about ten times greater but outside the endplate region of an innervated muscle the receptor density is generally less than $10/\mu m^2$. The increase in extrajunctional receptor density following denervation arises because the motor nerve can no longer exert its, as yet mysterious, depressant effect on extrajunctional receptor synthesis and insertion.

The disease myasthenia gravis is associated with the presence of circulating antibodies to the α-subunits of muscle nicotinic receptors. The receptors became cross-linked in pairs by the antibodies, and this triggers endocytosis and internal destruction of the receptors. From 70 to 90% of the receptors may be lost.

MECHANISMS OF ACTION OF NEUROMUSCULAR-BLOCKING AGENTS

There are two main and fundamentally different mechanisms through which drugs may produce neuromuscular block by acting on postjunctional nicotinic acetylcholine receptors. The drugs are therefore broadly divided into two classes, the non-depolarizing and the depolarizing blocking agents, depending upon their mechanism of action.

Non-depolarizing blocking agents

Tubocurarine is the prototype drug of this class, and most experiments concerned with mechanism of action have been carried out with it. There is, however, sufficient evidence to indicate that the other members of this class act in essentially the same way. Snake α-toxins are also included under this heading, although their action is largely irreversible and they are not used clinically. Their main importance lies in their toxicology and in their use as tools to count and study receptors.

Tubocurarine combines with the same binding sites as does acetylcholine on the α-subunits of the receptor complex. However, it differs from acetylcholine in that it does not induce a conformational change in the proteins and therefore does not open the ion channel; that is, it has *affinity* for the receptors but lacks the property called *efficacy* or *intrinsic activity*. The effect of tubocurarine is therefore to prevent the access of acetylcholine to its binding sites and thereby to block the receptor. This is the classical action of a receptor antagonist. Since the binding sites on both α-subunits must be occupied by acetylcholine in order to activate the receptor, block of only one of the binding sites by a tubocurarine molecule is sufficient to prevent that activation. Although both α-subunits are identical in their amino-acid composition, their binding properties with respect to neuromuscular-blocking agents differ, possibly because their environments differ. Thus, one α-subunit and its surroundings might be defined as δ-α-β, whereas the other might be defined as β-α-ϵ. Some neuromuscular-blocking agents (e.g. aminosteroids) appear to have more affinity for one of the α-subunits, whereas other agents (e.g. benzyl tetrahydroisoquinoliniums) may have more affinity for the other α-subunit. This preferential affinity may be the basis of the observations that pairs of drugs from the same chemical class are simply additive in their actions, whereas pairs made up of one from each class produce a block that is greater than the sum of their separate effects, i.e. true potentiation occurs. The snake α-toxins appear not to exhibit a preferential affinity for one binding site over the other.

When tubocurarine is present in a patch clamp pipette, along with acetylcholine, in an arrangement of the type illustrated in Fig. 12.7, the frequency of channel opening produced by the acetylcholine is reduced but the channel is not totally inactivated (Fig. 12.7). There is no change in the channel's mean open time, nor in the shape and size of the elementary currents. This type of experiment confirmed what had been long supposed; that is, that the tubocurarine, while present in the biophase, does not combine and remain combined with the receptor, but rather repeatedly associates with and dissociates from it with a submillisecond time course (see Fig. 12.6(b)). In this way, it reduces the probability that acetylcholine can combine with the receptor but does not totally prevent that combination. If the concentration of acetylcholine is increased while maintaining the concentration of tubocurarine, then the dice are loaded in favour of the acetylcholine, and the frequency of channel openings increases toward or beyond the original frequency again. This is the basis of reversible block by competition and is the basic reason why a tubocurarine block is reversible by an anticholinesterase agent.

Theoretically, with a reversible competitive blocking agent, oscillation between depressing and restoring the frequency would go on indefinitely as the concentrations of the antagonist and then the agonist were successively increased. However, with higher concentrations of tubocurarine, an additional action comes into play that prevents the restoration of the frequency of receptor activation by acetylcholine. At higher concentrations, tubocurarine begins to produce receptor-operated ion channel block. The dimensions of the molecule are such that it can enter and occlude an ion channel that has been opened by acetylcholine (i.e. like a cork in a bottle). When the appropriate concentration of tubocurarine is reached, additional acetylcholine then begins to facilitate its ability to enter and occlude the channels, and can therefore no longer reverse the block, which at this stage, can no longer be described as competitive. It is doubtful whether, under normal conditions of anaesthetic practice, the concentration of tubocurarine in the junctional clefts reaches that necessary to produce ion channel occlusion. Even so, the phenomenon should be borne in mind in the event that high doses of tubocurarine are administered. At the stage of ion channel occlusion, anticholinesterase agents can no longer reverse the block, but may even enhance it by causing more channels to open and become occluded.

The situation in the intact neuromuscular junction differs from the equilibrium conditions that prevail in a patch clamp pipette. In the intact junction, the concentration of tubocurarine in the cleft builds up to a maximum and then declines, and the acetylcholine released by the nerve impulse is present for only about a millisecond, so that equilibrium conditions cannot be reached. An acetylcholine molecule that reaches the receptor region will either bind with a binding site or will find that binding site already occupied by tubocurarine. It will probably not survive long enough for that receptor to become free from tubocurarine, or to diffuse to another receptor, and hence the true equilibrium conditions for block by competition do not hold for the situation *in vivo*. The reduced probability that acetylcholine molecules combine with free receptors means that the EPC and therefore the EPP are reduced. When the latter is reduced below the critical threshold that triggers a propagating action potential, the muscle fibre fails to contract. If cholinesterase is inhibited, a situation closer to that in the patch clamp pipette comes into play. Not only does more acetylcholine survive to reach the receptor region, but it now survives long enough to make repeated approaches to its binding sites. The EPC and EPP therefore increase and the latter may reach the threshold necessary to trigger the action potential and the contraction.

If an effective concentration of a snake α-toxin, such as α-bungarotoxin, is placed in the patch clamp pipette in place of tubocurarine, its interaction with the receptor is not a dynamic one; it combines with and remains combined with the binding site. Hence the effect of acetylcholine is totally abolished and no amount of excess can restore activity. The molecules of the polypeptide toxins are too large to enter and occlude the ion channels. In the intact neuromuscular system, a limited reversal of an α-toxin block can be achieved by an anticholinesterase agent. This is because there is a large surplus of spare receptors, and the preserved transmitter acetylcholine may then survive to reach those that are less accessible.

This large safety factor in transmission has already been referred to and should be borne in mind. The number of receptors present is considerably in excess of those necessary to produce the critical degree of EPP necessary to trigger-off the propagating action potential and the contractile sequence. It has been estimated that about 70% of the receptors have to be blocked before contraction fails. Hence, restoration of a normal contraction is not evidence of fully restored normal transmission.

The role of autoreceptors at synapses and neuroeffector junctions, including the neuromuscular junction, has been briefly referred to. There is both electrophysiological evidence and evidence from experiments in which released transmitter was collected and assayed, that the nerve endings possess nicotinic receptors that function in a positive feedback mechanism. The evidence for the presence of such receptors is less convincing than that for postjunctional receptors, mainly because prejunctional receptors are relatively few and there is as yet no irreversible ligand, analogous to α-bungarotoxin at postjunctional receptors, for visualizing, counting and extracting them. Although the postulated nerve terminal receptors appear to be of the nicotinic type, they differ in some respects both from the postjunctional motor endplate receptors and from autonomic ganglionic receptors. They may therefore constitute a separate subtype of nicotinic acetylcholine receptors, possibly similar to some of those in the central nervous system. The evidence suggests that activation of these prejunctional receptors enhances the rate of mobilization of stored transmitter into the readily releasable immediately available situation. Hence, they play an essential role in maintaining transmitter output when the traffic of nerve impulses is high (i.e. 2 Hz and above). When these receptors are blocked, the muscle responses rapidly wane in amplitude during bursts of nerve stimulation at frequencies of 2 Hz and above. Consequently, during brief trains of EPCs or EPPs, successive responses rapidly run down to a plateau. Similarly, tetanic tension rapidly fades, often to an undetectable level, during continuous stimulation at say 50 or 100 Hz.

Monitoring degree of block

Anaesthetists commonly monitor depth of neuromuscular block by stimulating the ulnar nerve through the skin and recording the compound EMG or the contractions (or some derivative of the latter) of the adductor pollicis muscle. A common pattern of stimulation is the so-called train-of-four in which the nerve is stimulated every 20 s with a group of four stimuli delivered at a frequency of 2 Hz (see p. 166). Tubocurarine not only depresses the amplitude of the initial response in each group (attributed to postjunctional receptor block) but also causes successive run down or fade of the remaining three responses in each group (attributed to prejunctional block). Figure 12.4 illustrates the concept of pre- and post-junctional receptors and the pattern of responses when these are blocked by a clinically-used non-depolarizing blocking drug. α-Bungarotoxin blocks only the postjunctional receptors, and therefore depresses amplitude in a uniform fashion; there is no fade.

Depolarizing blocking agents

Although acetylcholine is the transmitter at the neuromuscular junction, paradoxically, in large doses injected into the arterial supply, it is capable of blocking transmission. Its effect is transient because of the highly efficient action of cholinesterase, but a longer-lasting block may be produced if an anticholinesterase agent is first administered. The block is a consequence of prolonged endplate depolarization and is known as depolarization block. The explanation lies in the fact that depolarization of many electrically excitable membranes, including that of skeletal muscle fibres, has two consecutive effects on sodium channels. The initial effect is that the sodium channels open and there is an influx of Na^+ which, if abrupt enough, excites the tissue by giving rise to a propagated action potential. The secondary effect is that the membrane depolarization induces a conformational change in the proteins of the sodium channels that prevents them from permitting any more Na^+ influx. The channels are said to be inactivated. In response to a transient depolarization, inactivation is transient and accounts for the refractory period of the membrane. However, in response to a prolonged depolarization, although the initial opening of the Na^+ channels remains brief, inactivation persists until the depolarization terminates. The depolarized endplate is an island of external negativity in the centre of a normal membrane. It acts like a cathodal electrode causing persistent local currents to flow through the surrounding membrane. The local currents initially excite, but their persistent effect is to cause inactivation of the Na^+ channels in the region of membrane surrounding the endplate. Hence there is a zone of inexcitability around the endplate that resembles a prolonged refractory period, and this prevents the generation of action potentials so that flaccid paralysis of the muscle results. Figure 12.8 is an attempt to represent a depolarization block diagrammatically. The flaccid block is a consequence of the focal innervation of the muscle fibre. In a multiply innervated fibre, islands of depolarization occur all over the membrane and these activate the contractile mechanism directly so that contracture results.

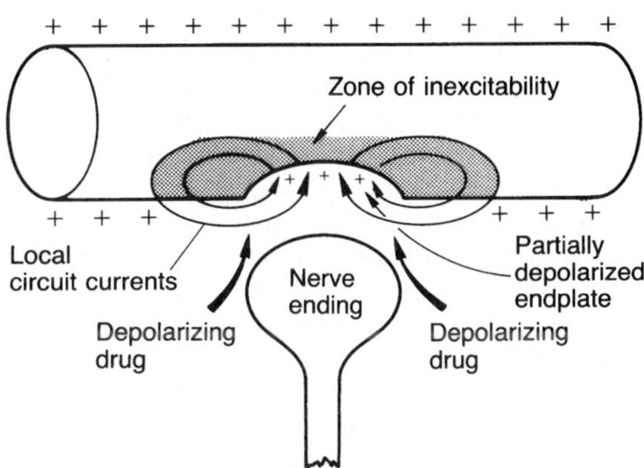

FIGURE 12.8 Probable mechanism underlying block by depolarization. The depolarizing drug, injected intravenously, reaches the endplates relatively gradually so that the endplate depolarization is slow to develop. Consequently, the opening of potassium channels in the surrounding membrane keeps pace with the opening of sodium channels and the depolarization does not therefore give rise to a propagating action potential. The continuous flow of local circuit currents into the depolarized endplate region causes inactivation of sodium permeability and increased potassium permeability in the surrounding membrane, thereby giving rise to a zone of inexcitability through which an action potential cannot propagate. (Reproduced with permission from Bowman WC *Pharmacology of neuromuscular function.* Wright-Butterworth Scientific, London, 1990.)

Any nicotinic agonist, including nicotine itself, is capable of producing depolarization block but for clinical use the drug must be free from pronounced effects on other types of acetylcholine receptor.

In the late 1940s and early 50s, Barlow and Ing, and Paton and Zaimis synthesized a series of compounds known as the methonium compounds with the general formula:

$$(CH_3)_3{}^+N - (CH_2)_n - N^+(CH_3)_3.$$

The two most interesting compounds were hexamethonium (in which $n = 6$) and decamethonium (in which $n = 10$). Hexamethonium is now a virtually obsolete ganglion-blocking drug, but was the first of its kind. Decamethonium is a neuromuscular-blocking drug which Paton and Zaimis showed to be of the depolarizing type. It was the first clinically useful drug of this class, but it is also now obsolete, largely because it has no special advantages and it has the disadvantage that there is no suitable antagonist. Other neuromuscular-blocking agents of the depolarizing type that have been developed since decamethonium are suxamethonium (succinyldicholine, Fig. 12.1), suxethonium, carbolonium, and dioxonium. Of these, only suxamethonium continues to be commonly used in anaesthetic practice, because of its short duration of action and rapid onset of effect. The latter makes suxamethonium especially useful for rapid intubation.

Prolonged endplate depolarization by a nicotonic agonist arises from the inflow of Na^+ current through the receptor-operated cation channels at the endplate. There are two interacting components to the effect seen when studying the endplate response at molecular level. The channels open, and they open repetitively. Different agonists cause the channels to open for different mean open times; for example, as already mentioned, mean open time is longer with suberylcholine than with acetylcholine, and is shorter with decamethonium than with acetylcholine. However, a shorter open time may be compensated for by a higher frequency of opening at maximum effect. This is in fact the case with these three drugs. Decamethonium produces the highest and suberylcholine the lowest frequency so that, at maximum effect, the amount of Na^+ current and therefore the degree of endplate depolarization is the same for all three drugs.

An additional problem with depolarizing blocking drugs is that the type of block produced does not always remain the same throughout the effect, especially if large doses are given or the block is maintained for a long time. Some anaesthetic agents, especially halogenated inhalational anaesthetics, may hasten the change from one type of block to another. The first phase of block (Phase I block) is a consequence of endplate depolarization as described. However, this may gradually merge into a second phase (Phase II block) that exhibits different characteristics, superficially bearing some resemblance to block produced by an acetylcholine antagonist such as tubocurarine. There is no convincing evidence that Phase II block is in fact a non-depolarizing block of the type produced by tubocurarine.

Despite much work, the change remains a pharmacological mystery. There are a number of possibilities as detailed below.

Receptor desensitization

In isolated muscles bathed in an artificial medium, prolonged application of a nicotinic agonist causes activation of a protein kinase that phosphorylates the receptor protein causing a conformational change that results in them becoming non-functional. The receptors are said to be desensitized. There is no convincing evidence that receptor desensitization occurs in the intact organism with normal clinical doses of depolarizing drugs, but if it does, it may contribute to Phase II block.

Ion-channel occlusion

Just as non-depolarizing acetylcholine antagonists, such as tubocurarine, can enter and occlude the already opened ion channels, so also can the depolarizing drugs. The difference with the latter is that they both cause the opening and then occlude the ion channels. It is not known whether this effect occurs *in vivo* with the doses used in anaesthetic practice.

Nerve terminal depolarization

Many non-myelinated nerve fibre membranes are depolarized by large concentrations of nicotinic agonists, including acetylcholine. Motor nerve terminals are apparently no exception. It remains a pharmacological mystery as to why such membranes possess receptors that mediate this effect, since endogenous acetylcholine does not appear to have access to them under physiological conditions. At the neuromuscular junction, these prejunctional receptors (which appear to be a different population from those mediating the feedback control of transmitter mobilization described above) are normally protected from transmitter acetylcholine by the junctional cholinesterase. It is possible that prolonged application of a depolarizing drug produces nerve terminal depolarization to the extent that conduction of the nerve impulse is blocked before it can evoke transmitter release. The characteristics of Phase II block are compatible with such a mechanism.

Hemicholinium-like action

High doses of depolarizing drugs might impair acetylcholine synthesis in a manner resembling the effect of hemicholinium (Table 12.1). Depolarizing drugs have in fact been shown capable of inhibiting acetylcholine synthesis *in vitro*.

Stimulation of electrogenic sodium pump

Under the prolonged influence of a depolarizing drug, the excessive Na^+ entry at the endplate stimulates the activity of a metabolic sodium pump which drives sodium ions out of the cell in exchange for potassium ions. The exchange is on the basis of 2 Na^+ for 1 K^+, and so the endplate repolarizes despite the continued presence of the depolarizing drug. Presumably the drug molecules continue to interact with the receptors, yet their normal effect – depolarization – is prevented. Hence, they may merely act to impede the access of acetylcholine to the receptors.

All of the above five mechanisms can be shown to occur in *in vitro* experiments set up to detect such actions. The problem lies in determining which, if any, contribute to Phase II block in human patients, for the nature of the tests needed to make the assessment are impossible to carry out in an intact individual.

NEUROMUSCULAR-BLOCKING AGENTS IN CURRENT USE

The main drugs in current use (Table 12.2) are the non-depolarizing agents, tubocurarine, its trimethyl analogue (called metocurine in the USA), alcuronium, gallamine (now almost obsolete), pancuronium,

TABLE 12.2 **Currently used neuromuscular-blocking drugs**

DRUG	APPROX. RELATIVE POTENCY BY WEIGHT IN MAN (TUBOCURARINE = 1)	APPROX. RELATIVE DURATION IN MAN (TUBOCURARINE = 1)	DISTRIBUTION, METABOLISM AND EXCRETION IN MAN
Tubocurarine	1 (0.25 mg/kg produces 50% twitch block at 0.15 Hz)	1 (About 80 min from injection to 25% recovery after dose to produce 98% twitch block)	Rapid fall in plasma concentration (15 min) is followed by a slower fall over many hours; 16% is bound to plasma albumin and 24% to gammaglobulin. Tubocurarine also binds to cartilage, chondroitin sulphate and basement membrane. Some tubocurarine may be metabolized; 30–40% is excreted via the kidneys and most of the remainder in the bile
Metocurine	2 (i.e. twice as potent)	1	Although metocurine appears to have certain advantages, it has not been widely used in anaesthetic practice. It undergoes little or no metabolic change. Up to 58% is excreted in the urine within 48 h, but only about 2% in the bile. About 35% is bound to plasma protein. Like tubocurarine, it is bound to cartilage and mucopolysaccharides
Alcuronium	1.5	1	Alcuronium is probably not metabolized. Most is excreted unchanged in the urine although a minor secondary pathway via the bile exists. About 75% is bound to plasma albumin
Gallamine	0.2	0.6	Rapid fall in plasma concentration to 25% of initial dose in 5 min, followed by slower second and third phases. First phase due to redistribution to organs with high blood flow: second phase to organs with less abundant blood flow, and final phase to gradual elimination from a large hypothetical volume of distribution. Partially bound to β and γ-globulin. Not metabolized. Excreted almost entirely by kidneys.
Pancuronium	5.7	0.8	Rapid fall in plasma concentration in first 5 min followed by slower fall; 60–80% eliminated in urine; some is eliminated in bile. Theoretically, pancuronium may be deacetylated to the 3-OH, the 17-OH or the 3,17-diOH derivatives but only the 3-OH has been detected in man. The 3-OH derivative is about half as potent as the parent drug. The other possible metabolites have only about 2% of the potency of the parent drug. About 34% of pancuronium is bound to albumin and about 53% to gammaglobulin.
Pipecuronium	6.5	1.2	Largely eliminated via the kidneys. Theoretically may be metabolized in an analogous way to pancuronium. About 75% is bound to albumin
Vecuronium	6	0.25	Plasma clearance 2–3 times faster than for pancuronium. Theoretically metabolized to the 3-OH, the 17-OH and the 3,17-diOH derivatives but the quantities produced in man are uncertain. The 3-OH derivative has 60% of the potency of vecuronium. The others are only weakly active. About 70% is bound to plasma proteins. Binds to cartilage and mucopolysaccharides. Mainly eliminated in the bile. The kidneys are a secondary minor route of elimination. Repeated doses only mildly cumulative. Unstable in solution.
Rocuronium	1	0.25	Important property is its rapid onset of action allowing fast intubation at 1 min. Otherwise similar to vecuronium in time course of action. About 33% excreted in urine in 24 h. Plasma clearance mainly due to liver uptake and biliary excretion
Atracurium	2	0.25	Rapidly broken down in plasma and tissue fluid by Hofmann elimination and to some extent by ester hydrolysis. Liver and kidneys unimportant in removal. Block slightly enhanced by mild acidosis and decreased by alkalosis (these changes decrease and increase Hofmann elimination respectively). Cumulation with repeated doses is minimal. About 80% is bound to plasma proteins

TABLE 12.2 (continued)

DRUG	APPROX. RELATIVE POTENCY BY WEIGHT IN MAN (TUBOCURARINE = 1)	APPROX. RELATIVE DURATION IN MAN (TUBOCURARINE = 1)	DISTRIBUTION, METABOLISM AND EXCRETION IN MAN
Mivacurium	6	0.15	Rapidly hydrolysed by plasma cholinesterase to products inactive at the neuromuscular junction. Rate of hydrolysis is about 80% that of suxamethonium. Onset of block about the same as that of atracurium after 1 ED_{95} dose (i.e. 3–4 min)
Doxacurium	20	1.5	Little or no metabolism. Mainly excreted in urine with a minor secondary biliary excretion
Suxamethonium	3*	0.075	Rapidly hydrolysed (70% within 1 min) by plasma cholinesterase to succinylmonocholine which has only very weak neuromuscular-blocking potency. Then 6–7 times more slowly to inactive succinate and choline. This is the only currently used depolarizing blocking drug. Use virtually restricted to rapid intubation, which is possible within 1 min

*Relative potency with tubocurarine has rarely been determined with accuracy because suxamethonium is usually deliberately used in a large dose (1 mg/kg) to produce rapid and complete block for intubation.

pipecuronium, vecuronium, rocuronium, mivacurium and doxacurium, and the depolarizing agent suxamethonium (succinylcholine). All are quaternary ammonium compounds (Figs 12.1, 12.9 and 12.10) and, in solution, are therefore highly ionized and consequently poorly absorbed after oral ingestion, and do not penetrate the blood–brain barrier. They are injected intravenously. With four exceptions (tubocurarine, vecuronium, rocuronium and gallamine) they are bisquaternary compounds. Gallamine has three quaternary ammonium groups, and tubocurarine, vecuronium and rocuronium each have only one. However, these last three contain a second nitrogen which is tertiary, and which at body pH is strongly protonated so that they each contain two charged nitrogen centres. In accordance with structure : activity data that have been worked out over many years, the distance between the two charged centres in the molecules of all of the above named drugs (in the case of gallamine, between the two at the greatest distance) lies in the optimal range, a little above 1 nm.

Thin flexible molecules with methyl groups attached to the quaternary nitrogens are of the depolarizing type, and this is characteristic of suxamethonium. The molecules of non-depolarizing agents are generally bulkier (Fig. 12.9).

The potencies and time courses of action of the main neuromuscular-blocking agents are given in Table 12.2. Because of its rapid onset of action and brief duration, suxamethonium is usually used when rapid intubation is desired, and this is its main use. Rocuronium has a rapid onset of action approaching that of suxamethonium, and may be used for intubation. Its duration of action is similar to that of vecuronium. Mivacurium has a brief duration of action, although its onset of action is not very rapid. All of the non-depolarizing drugs are used, more or less interchangeably, to produce muscle relaxation during surgery, the individual choice being much dependent on the personal preference of the anaesthetist, although certain side-effects specific to some of the drugs (histamine release, ganglion block, tachycardia) or their route or mechanism of elimination (kidneys, liver, enzymatic or other breakdown) may dictate choice for some patients. At the end of surgery, neuromuscular block produced by the non-depolarizing agents may be readily reversed by an anticholinesterase drug (neostigmine, pyridostigmine, or occasionally edrophonium). Atropine or glycopyrronium (glycopyrrolate in USA) is necessary to prevent the muscarinic effects of the anticholinesterase drug.

Distribution, metabolism and excretion

Details relating to the individual drugs are given in Table 12.2. Highly ionized drugs, such as neuromuscular-blocking agents, that do not penetrate cell membranes, might be expected to have a volume of distribution that is similar to the extracellular fluid volume. This is essentially the case with most neuromuscular-blocking drugs which have a volume of distribution in the range of 0.2–0.3 l/kg. Tubocurarine and metocurine have volumes of distribution that are a little greater (*c.* 0.4 l/kg) probably because they are more extensively bound to mucopolysaccharides in cartilage and basement membrane than are the other agents. Neuromuscular-blocking agents are bound both to mucopolysaccharides and to plasma proteins, but the latter binding does not much affect their volume of distribution.

Elimination occurs via the kidneys and the liver, or by breakdown. The longer-acting drugs (tubocurarine, metocurine, gallamine, alcuronium, pipecuronium, pancuronium, doxacurium) have similar

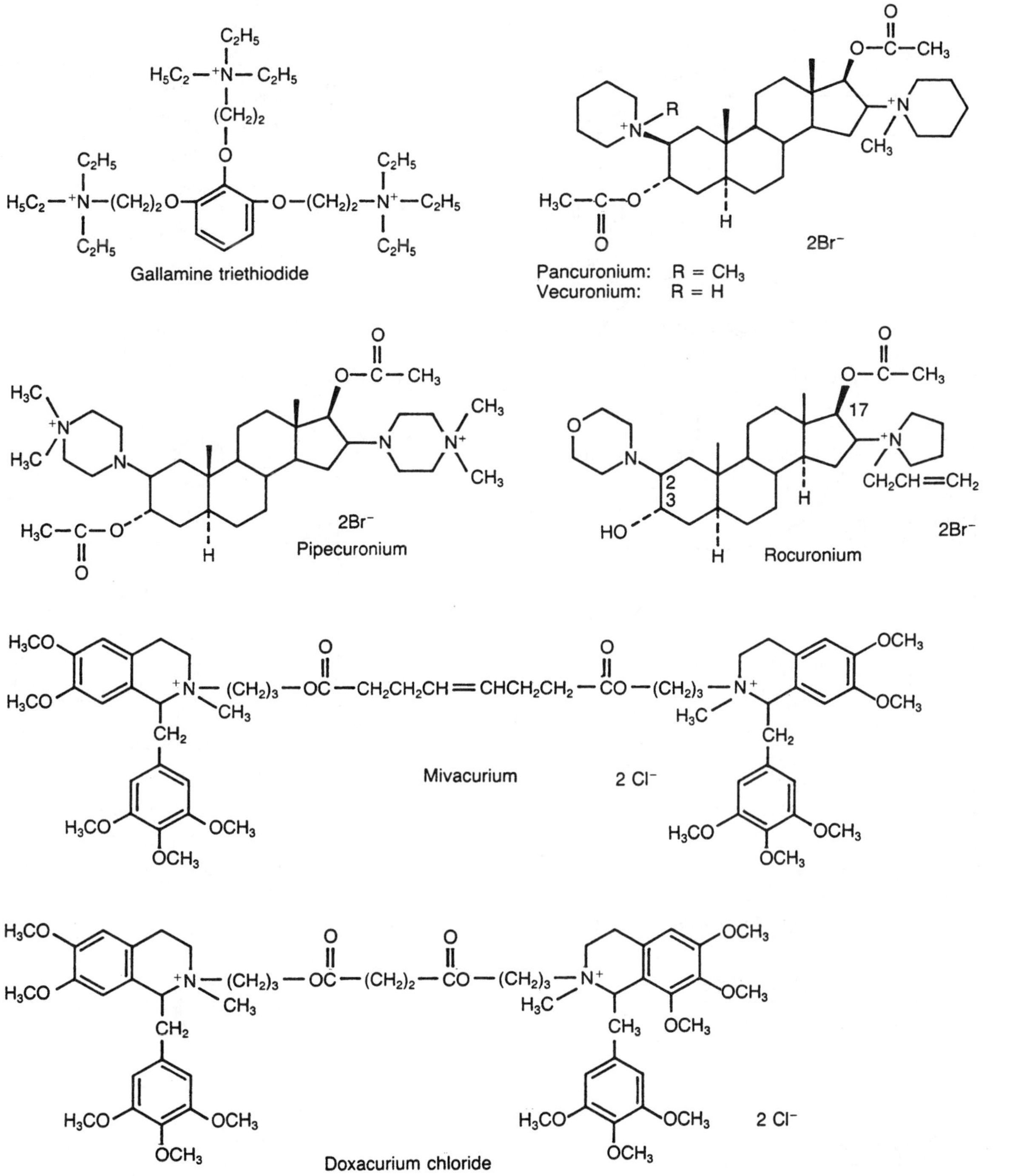

Gallamine triethiodide

Pancuronium: R = CH_3
Vecuronium: R = H

$2Br^-$

Pipecuronium

Rocuronium

Mivacurium $2\ Cl^-$

Doxacurium chloride $2\ Cl^-$

FIGURE 12.9 The chemical structures of synthetic non-depolarizing blocking drugs, other than atracurium which is given in Fig. 12.10. Note that the ester groups in mivacurium and doxacurium are the other way around from those in atracurium making the first two incapable of Hofmann elimination. Mivacurium, but not doxacurium, is rapidly hydrolysed by plasma cholinesterase.

elimination half-lives (about 150 min), similar volumes of distribution (0.2–0.3 l/kg), and similar clearances (1–2 ml/kg/min), the last being approximately equal to the normal glomerular filtration rate. Shorter-acting drugs are cleared faster than can be accounted for by the glomerular filtration rate. Vecuronium and rocuronium with a clearance rate of 4.6 ml/kg/min are taken up by the liver and eliminated in the bile. Atracurium with a clearance rate of 5.5 ml/kg/min depends on spontaneous and enzymatic breakdown, as described below. Mivacurium and suxamethonium are rapidly hydrolysed by plasma cholinesterase.

Atracurium is spontaneously broken down at body pH and temperature by a process known as Hofmann elimination (Fig. 12.10), after the German chemist who

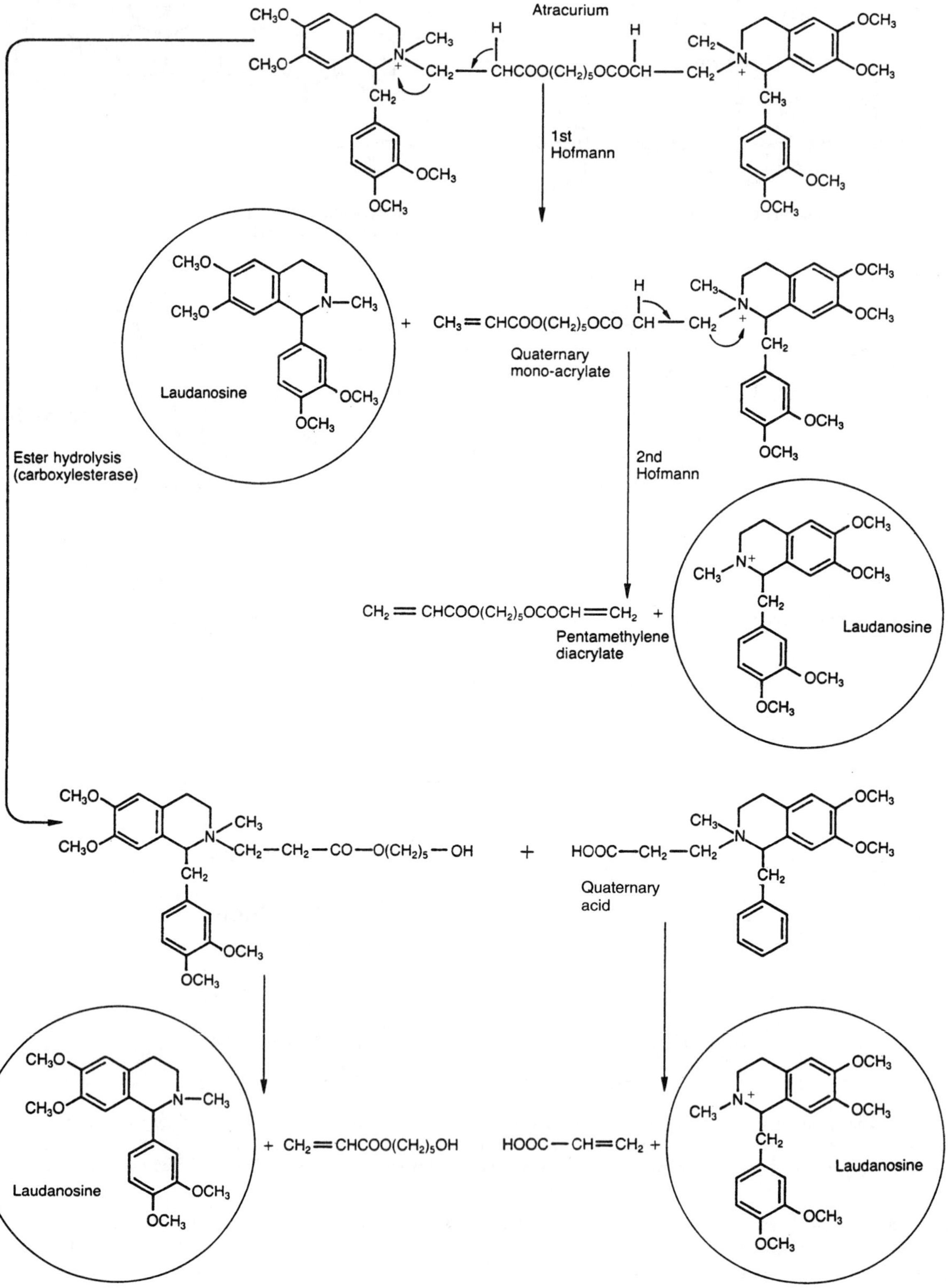

Atracurium

1st Hofmann

Laudanosine

+ $CH_2{=}CHCOO(CH_2)_5OCO\ CH{-}CH_2$

Quaternary mono-acrylate

Ester hydrolysis (carboxylesterase)

2nd Hofmann

$CH_2{=}CHCOO(CH_2)_5OCOCH{=}CH_2$ +

Pentamethylene diacrylate

Laudanosine

$-CH_2{-}CH_2{-}CO{-}O(CH_2)_5{-}OH$ + $HOOC{-}CH_2{-}CH_2-$

Quaternary acid

Laudanosine

+ $CH_2{=}CHCOO(CH_2)_5OH$

$HOOC{-}CH{=}CH_2$ +

Laudanosine

FIGURE 12.10 Atracurium and its breakdown by Hofmann elimination (the principal route in man) and by ester hydrolysis. Laudanosine (circled) is a product of four reactions.

first described the reaction in 1851. In this reaction, a quaternary ammonium group is converted into a tertiary amine which is eliminated from the molecule by the breaking of a carbon–nitrogen bond. The tertiary amine released from atracurium is laudanosine, which is an alkaloid of opium that possesses a weak stimulant action on the central nervous system.

Atracurium is an ester, although the carbonyl group and the ether oxygen are in the reverse order from those in acetylcholine, suxamethonium and mivacurium. This means that atracurium is not a substrate for cholinesterase. However, it is a substrate for another esterase called carboxylesterase (Fig. 12.10). In man, the activity of this enzyme is low so that the main route of breakdown is by Hofmann elimination. The spontaneous breakdown of atracurium means that it is not dependent on liver or kidneys for its removal, and this may be an important attribute in some patients.

Unwanted effects

Neuromuscular-blocking agents are designed to interact with nicotinic acetylcholine receptors on the motor endplate, so it would not be surprising if they were also found to interact to some extent with other peripheral acetylcholine-binding sites, on cholinesterase, in autonomic ganglia, and at muscarinic receptors. In searching for new agents, chemists and pharmacologists therefore carry out tests to ensure that such activity is as low as possible.

Pancuronium inhibits plasma cholinesterase in concentrations that may be achieved in patients during surgical anaesthesia. None of the other non-depolarizing agents is active against any form of the enzyme in concentrations that could be achieved clinically. Suxamethonium and mivacurium are substrates for plasma cholinesterase and this accounts for the brevity of their effects. Interaction between pancuronium on the one hand and suxamethonium and mivacurium on the other in relation to plasma cholinesterase, is theoretically possible, but of little importance.

Tubocurarine blocks nicotinic receptors in autonomic ganglia in neuromuscular-blocking doses. A number of autonomic reflexes may be abolished by this action, which also contributes to the hypotension produced by tubocurarine. Ganglion block is unimportant with the other neuromuscular-blocking drugs used in anaesthetic practice. Suxamethonium possesses a weak stimulant action on ganglionic nicotinic receptors, although this is generally unimportant.

Gallamine, pancuronium, alcuronium and, to a small extent, rocuronium block a particular subtype of muscarinic receptors, the M_2 subtype (p. 130). M_2 receptors in the SA node mediate vagal inhibition of the heart, and the main consequence of M_2 receptor block produced by gallamine, pancuronium, alcuronium and, to a small extent, rocuronium is tachycardia through preventing vagal inhibition. Muscarinic receptor block is unimportant with the other agents in current use; vecuronium, especially, possesses a very wide margin of safety between its neuromuscular blocking and M_2-receptor blocking doses. Suxamethonium has a weak stimulant action on muscarinic receptors which may give rise to bradycardia.

Some agents exert complex actions on the sympathetic nervous system, including block of noradrenaline reuptake (Uptake 1). These effects are important probably only with pancuronium and gallamine. Their actions in this respect may enhance the tachycardia arising from their muscarinic M_2-receptor blocking action.

The main remaining unwanted effects are consequences of hypersensitivity reactions and release of mediators from mast cells. Life-threatening hypersensitivity reactions to neuromuscular-blocking drugs are rare, but do occasionally occur during the induction stage of anaesthesia. They include cardiovascular collapse, bronchospasm, angioneurotic oedema and occasionally pulmonary oedema. The patients are often young women with a history of allergy to cosmetics, shampoos or penicillin. The reactions generally belong to the Type I (immediate) allergic reactions. Most hypersensitivity reactions involve suxamethonium, followed by alcuronium and tubocurarine. Reactions to the other drugs are very rare, especially to the steroidal agents.

Many basic compounds can liberate histamine and other mediators from mast cells by a different mechanism that does not involve IgE antibody and antigen interactions. In fact they interact directly with binding sites on the mast cell. Through an unknown mechanism this leads to a rise in intracellular Ca^{2+} and release of histamine. Among the neuromuscular-blocking agents, tubocurarine is the most powerful direct histamine liberator of this type, whereas pancuronium and vecuronium are the least effective. The other agents fall between these extremes.

Unwanted drug interactions

The main unwanted interactions with neuromuscular-blocking agents are with certain general anaesthetics, some local anaesthetics and some antibacterial agents. They all lead to enhanced paralysis which is sometimes not reversible by anticholinesterase agents. Potentiation of tubocurarine by ether was observed soon after the introduction of tubocurarine into anaesthetic practice. Of the commonly used anaesthetic agents, isoflurane and enflurane are the most effective in potentiating non-depolarizing blocking drugs. Halothane is the next most effective, whereas nitrous oxide, barbiturates and other intravenous anaesthetics are the least effective.

The main action of the anaesthetic agents in potentiating non-depolarizing blocking drugs is exerted on the postjunctional endplate membrane where they interfere with acetylcholine receptor-operated ion channel function. Minor actions to impair acetylcholine release may be exerted on the nerve endings, and there may also be minor effects through modification of distribution or elimination. For example, halothane may reduce renal excretion by reducing kidney blood flow, and isoflurane may increase the fraction of neuromuscular-blocking drug that reaches the neuromuscular junction by increasing muscle blood flow.

Antibiotics that potentiate non-depolarizing neuromuscular-blocking drugs generally do so by one of two main mechanisms. Either they act on the nerve endings to reduce acetylcholine release (aminoglycosides, spectinomycin and tetracyclines act in this way), or they act on the postjunctional membrane to interfere with the function of the ion channels opened by acetylcholine (polymyxins, lincomycin and clindamycin act in this way).

Penicillins, cephalosporins and chloramphenicol have negligible effects at the neuromuscular junction, and do not interact with blocking agents at normal clinical dose levels.

Several drugs whose mechanisms of action depend upon blocking ion channels at other sites (local anaesthetic agents, anti-arrhythmic drugs of the quinidine or disopyramide types, calcium-channel blocking drugs) may exert a similar action on the acetylcholine receptor-operated channels in the postjunctional endplate membrane. This action is not detectable when the transmission process is normal because of the substantial safety margin in transmission that exists. However, it is reflected in enhanced neuromuscular block when transmission is impaired by non-depolarizing neuromuscular-blocking drugs.

New neuromuscular-blocking drugs

There is a continuing search for improved agents, and especially for a non-depolarizing equivalent of suxamethonium. Suxamethonium has a number of disadvantages, and its continued widespread use for rapid intubation is a consequence only of its rapid onset of action. In general, rapid onset requires a large dose in order that the drugs may reach the biophase quickly and flood the receptive area. This is possible with suxamethonium because of its rapid rate of inactivation, which prevents what would otherwise be a long-lasting block. In addition, rapid onset is more likely with a depolarizing agent because the drug begins to act as soon as interaction with the receptors commences. Because of the large number of spare receptors at the motor endplate, a large proportion of the receptors must be blocked by a non-depolarizing agent before interference with the contractile sequence begins. Hence, it may not be possible to achieve with a non-polarizing agent, the rapidity of onset that is characteristic of suxamethonium. Even so, considerable improvement over the current situation should be possible, and so the search continues.

Over the past 100 years or so, since the work of Crum Brown and Fraser in Edinburgh, the search for new neuromuscular-blocking drugs has largely been confined to bis onium compounds of one kind or another. However, we have long known of the virtually irreversible acetylcholine receptor block produced by certain polypeptide snake toxins of the Elapidae and Hypdrophiidae families, showing that acetylcholine antagonism, albeit non-competitive, may be found among different chemical species. More recently it has been shown that certain shorter polypeptides (α-conotoxins G1 and M1), originally obtained from the marine cone snails (*Conus geographus* and *C. magnus*) but which may be synthesized in the laboratory, have reversible neuromuscular-blocking properties in anaesthetized animals that seem to exhibit the main properties desirable in a clinically useful muscle relaxant. It might be therefore that such polypeptides could act as starter compounds for the synthesis of new drugs for use in anaesthetic practice.

FURTHER READING

Agoston S, Bowman WC eds. *Muscle relaxants. Monographs in Anaesthesiology* 1990; **19**. Amsterdam: Elsevier.

Bevan DR, Bevan, JC, Donati F. *Muscle relaxants in clinical anaesthesia.* Chicago: Year Book Medical Publishers, 1988.

Bowman WC. *Pharmacology of neuromuscular function.* London: Wright-Butterworth Scientific, 1990.

Clementi F, Meldolesi J eds. *Neurotransmitter release: the neuromuscular junction.* London: Academic Press, 1990.

Hull CJ. *Pharmacokinetics for anaesthesia.* Oxford: Butterworth-Heinemann, 1991.

Feldman S A ed. Introduction to *Anaesthetic Pharmacology Review* 1993; **1** (1): 1–92.

Kharkevich DA ed. *New neuromuscular blocking drugs. Handbook of Experimental Pharmacology* **79**. Berlin: Springer-Verlag, 1986.

Martyn JAJ, White DA, Gronert GA, Jaffe RS, Ward JM. Up- and down-regulation of skeletal muscle acetylcholine receptors. *Anesthesiology* 1992; **76**: 822–43.

McGuinness TL, Greengard P. Protein phosphorylation and synaptic transmission. In: Sellin LC, Libelius R, Thesleff S eds. *Neuromuscular junction.* Amsterdam: Elsevier, 1988: 111–124.

Unwin N. Neurotransmitter action: opening of ligand-gated ion channels. *Cell* **72** and *Neuron* **10**: Supplement: 1993; 31–41.

Vincent A, Wray D eds. *Neuromuscular transmission, basic and applied aspects.* Manchester: Manchester University Press, 1990.

PART II CLINICAL PHARMACOLOGY OF NEUROMUSCULAR-BLOCKING AGENTS

B Astley

Neuromuscular-blocking drugs are traditionally classified into two broad groups, the depolarizing agents, typified by suxamethonium, and the non-depolarizing (or competitive acetylcholine antagonists) typified by tubocurarine. However, in many series of closely related compounds that interact with endplate cholinoceptors, it is possible to pass from substances that mimic acetylcholine (i.e. full agonists) through substances that have different degrees of both agonist and antagonist activity (i.e. partial agonists) to substances devoid of agonist activity although they combine with cholinoceptors (antagonists). Not only do different compounds in the same series exhibit this range of properties but the same compounds in different species, or even in the same muscle under different conditions, might also do so. The situation is therefore not as clear cut as the classification into two broad groups might imply even though the classification remains useful.

DEPOLARIZING AGENTS

After inhibition of acetylcholinesterase by an anticholinesterase drug, acetylcholine may produce blocks of twitches evoked at a frequency of 0.1 Hz.[1] Even in the presence of functional acetylcholinesterase a large dose of acetylcholine injected directly into the arterial supply to a muscle produces a transient neuromuscular block. Since such a block lasts for less than 10 s it is necessary to stimulate the motor nerve at a higher frequency than 0.1 Hz to demonstrate it.[2] Thus acetylcholine may stimulate the muscles to contract, or may block contractions according to the concentration present and the length of time for which it persists. Burns and Paton[3] showed convincingly that the block in transmission was a consequence of its depolarizing action, for when an anodal (hyperpolarizing) electrode was placed on the endplate region neuromuscular transmission was restored. They went on to show that the depolarized endplate region and its immediate surroundings become a zone of inexcitability through which a muscle action potential evoked by direct stimulation could not propagate. The persistent endplate depolarization itself failed to excite the muscle for the same reason. This type of block is a consequence of the fact that the muscle fibres are focally innervated. Where this is not so, as in multiply innervated fibres, the widespread acetylcholine induced depolarization itself can activate the contractile process resulting in contracture accompanying the sustained depolarization.

The characteristic features of depolarizing neuromuscular block are as follows:

- Depression of twitches preceded by muscle fasciculations and by an increase in the amplitude of evoked contractions. This is an initial acetylcholine-like effect.
- During subsequent depression of twitches there is no tetanic fade.
- The block is followed by a secondary augmentation of twitches which may be the result of increased contractility arising either from secondary membrane hyperpolarization[4] or increased availability of calcium to the contractile mechanism.
- Anticholinesterase drugs do not reverse the block.
- A small dose of an acetylcholine antagonist, for example tubocurarine reverses the block.
- Tachyphylaxis occurs with decamethonium. Burns and Paton[3] explained this by postulating that membrane penetration by the agonist was an essential part of the depolarization. In the case of acetylcholine, molecules that enter the sarcoplasm are rapidly destroyed by cholinesterase, but with a stable agonist such as decamethonium repeated application would result in a gradually diminishing concentration gradient across the endplate membrane and diminishing responsiveness would thereby result. This limited its use clinically and decamethonium is now obsolete.

Suxamethonium

Succinyldicholine (suxamethonium) is the only depolarizing agent now available. It was first synthesized by Hunt and Taveau in 1906 and a full account of its history and development is provided by Dorkins.[5] It was introduced into Great Britain in 1951 by Scurr.

The drug has a rapid onset of action (one circulation time) and so is ideally suited for intubation of the trachea, particularly in the emergency situation where it remains the drug of choice for rapid sequence induction. Its duration of action is brief, about 3–5 min because of its rapid hydrolysis to the relatively inactive succinylmonocholine by plasma pseudocholinesterase. Succinylmonocholine is itself hydrolysed to succinate and choline. Structurally suxamethonium consists of two acetylcholine molecules linked by a carbon chain.

After administration of a single bolus dose of suxamethonium the tetanic and train of four responses diminish without fade. This is called phase I block. If suxamethonium is then given repeatedly or by infusion (a technique no longer used) fade, post-tetanic potentiation and tachyphylaxis gradually appear on repeated stimulation. This is called phase II block. This change in the nature of the block may be due to the inclusion of halogenated anaesthetics[6] either changing the postjunctional endplate membrane or acting prejunctionally to reduce the output of transmitter. This is not the 'dual block' first described by Zaimis in which certain laboratory animals developed both types of block after the first dose.

Suxamethonium has a number of disadvantages that have led to numerous but as yet unsuccessful attempts by medicinal chemists to design a non-depolarizing or competitive type of muscle relaxant, free from side-effects and with an equally rapid onset of action.

Side-effects of suxamethonium

Fasciculations

These have been linked with the postoperative muscle pains associated with suxamethonium but the relationship is not straightforward. A patient may show few fasciculations and yet develop severe pain and vice versa. Prior administration of a small dose of a competitive agent, for example tubocurarine 3 mg or gallamine 10 mg will reduce the incidence of fasciculations but not necessarily abolish them. Following this pretreatment a larger dose of suxamethonium is then needed to produce the same degree of neuromuscular block. Fasciculations and myalgia (see below) probably arise from stimulation of motor nerve endings, motor endplates and muscles spindles.[7] Plasma creatine phosphokinase levels are increased reflecting possible muscle damage.

Muscle pains – myalgia

The incidence of muscle pains following the use of suxamethonium is very variable making techniques for elimination difficult. Studies have reported up to 90% incidence of pains, particularly in young fit ambulant patients, especially female. Pain is experienced in the diaphragm, between the scapulae and over the back. The muscle ache may last up to 4 days[8] and can be worse than the discomfort from the surgical procedure! Other workers[9] observed no difference in the incidence of myalgia when vecuronium was substituted for suxamethonium and Trepanier *et al.*[10] found 20% incidence of myalgia postoperatively when no relaxant had been given. Pretreatment with competitive muscle relaxants, dantrolene, aspirin, lignocaine, benzodiazepines, magnesium sulphate and preoperative exercise have all been tried in the hope of reducing the incidence of both fasciculations and myalgia and although the incidence can be reduced it cannot be reliably eliminated. Jones[11] reviews the subject with respect to its occurrence in outpatient surgery and advocates the prior administration of gallamine 15 mg. Care is necessary after the administration of even a small dose of competitive agent for the reason that response to relaxants is very variable.

Hyperkalaemia

In the course of a depolarizing block, sodium channels close and the potassium channels remain open resulting in a leak of potassium ions into the circulation which under normal conditions raises the serum potassium by 0.5 mmol/l. In patients suffering from soft tissue trauma, burns or neurological injuries suxamethonium may, several weeks after the time of injury, produce an exaggerated rise in serum potassium which has caused cardiac arrest.[12] Following the administration of suxamethonium to patients with severe burns the serum potassium may rise to 13 meq/l. This susceptibility exists between 10 and 60 days post-burn so that suxamethonium should be avoided during this time. In all these patients the area of chemosensitive muscle fibre membrane spreads as a result of chronic denervation. Consequently, there is a more widespread depolarization and greater loss of muscle potassium. This rise in serum potassium is not abolished by precurarization.

Increased intraocular pressure

Suxamethonium produces a rise in intraocular pressure,[13] which may be of importance in a patient with a penetrating eye injury when the contents may be extruded. The effect appears to be due to the contracture produced in the multiply innervated fibres of the extraocular muscles, and to rises in intravascular pressure in the eye. This effect is not abolished by precurarization. This rise in pressure is manifested 1 min after the administration of suxamethonium and subsides within 6–8 min. The pressure rise after suxamethonium is in the order of 7 mmHg[13] whereas intubation performed on a patient who is not paralysed can produce rises in pressure of up to 30 mmHg. It is obvious therefore that to minimize the rise in intraocular pressure intubation must be performed on a fully anaesthetized and paralysed patient.

Suxamethonium is the only relaxant that provides reliably favourable intubating conditions within 60 s. Thiopentone lowers intraocular pressure both by lowering the central venous pressure and by abolishing the tonic contracture produced by suxamethonium in the extraocular muscles.[14] Thiopentone given prior to suxamethonium as part of a rapid sequence induction results in intraocular pressure not altering significantly from baseline values.[15] Edmonson *et al.* recommend its use in the emergency patient with a penetrating eye injury.[15] Alfentanil, fentanyl and sufentanil also attenuate the haemodynamic responses to laryngoscopy and tracheal intubation and have been recommended for use in this situation.[16,17] Debate continues regarding the use of suxamethonium in the emergency patient with a penetrating eye injury. Libonati, Leahy and Ellison[18] describe the management of seventy-three cases of penetrating eye injuries given suxamethonium with no loss of global contents. Perhaps despite the theoretical disadvantages of suxamethonium causing a rise in intraocular pressure this is not a problem in clinical practice.

Increased intracranial pressure

Although suxamethonium does cause a small rise in intracranial pressure it is felt that the reliable paralysis and therefore good intubating conditions provided outweigh any risk.

Increased intragastric pressure

This is related to the incidence of fasciculations. If there are no fasciculations there is no rise in intragastric pressure. The incidence of both is less in children. As the intragastric pressure rises so does lower oesophageal pressure (in the anatomically normal patient) and hence the important 'barrier' pressure does not alter significantly.

Bradycardia

Repeated injections of suxamethonium may cause this, and occasionally nodal rhythm and more usually ventricular arrhythmias which are further encouraged by the release of potassium from skeletal muscle. This bradycardia occurs more often in children in whom resting vagal tone is higher. This is presumably due to a muscarinic action of suxamethonium and it is wise to have an antimuscarinic agent to hand under these circumstances. In children anticholinergic premedication is advisable prior to suxamethonium administration but in adults anticholinergic premedication as a routine with its association of a dry and sore throat postoperatively is not necessary.[19] Suxamethonium may produce an elevation in heart rate and arterial pressure secondary to ganglionic stimulation.[20] For a full view of cardiovascular effects of suxamethonium see Miller and Savarese.[21]

Myotonia

Suxamethonium results in a spastic paralysis in patients with dystrophia myotonica.

Malignant hyperpyrexia

Suxamethonium acts as a trigger for the muscle rigidity and metabolic derangement characteristic of this rare but potentially fatal complication.

Masseter spasm

After the administration of suxamethonium there is an increase in masseter muscle tone, especially in children,[22] which is not necessarily followed by malignant hyperpyrexia. Leary and Ellis[23] measured the myotonic response of the masseteric muscles following suxamethonium with a myotonometer in fifty patients. In the majority the rise in tone lasted less than 100 s and seventeen developed tensions large enough to be termed masseteric spasm. Therefore they too questioned the value of this spasm as a predictor of malignant hyperpyrexia.

Anaphylaxis

Suxamethonium is considered to be the muscle relaxant most frequently implicated in allergic reactions.[24]

Prolonged duration of action

Plasma pseudocholinesterase is synthesized in the liver and deficiency of it may accompany various forms of liver disease. Diminished activity of the enzyme may arise from the use of drugs that inhibit plasma cholinesterase, for example anticholinesterase drugs, metoclopramide,[25] ester-type local anaesthetics, for example procaine, amethocaine, which are themselves substrates for the enzyme and the competitive muscle relaxants pancuronium and mivacurium, and from ecothiopate, phenothiazines and cyclophosphamide. Clinically, low pseudocholinesterase levels do not give rise to problems as the duration of neuromuscular blockade is only moderately increased by low levels of normal enzyme.[26]

However, a suxamethonium neuromuscular blockade can be prolonged if the patient has an abnormal, genetically derived variant of the enzyme. An excellent review by Pantuck and Pantuck[27] details the subject. Abnormal variants of the enzyme exist in about 4% of the population. The four main variants of the enzyme are normal, atypical, fluoride resistant and silent. Normal plasma cholinesterase is inhibited by more than 70% by cinchocaine (also known as dibucaine in the USA) whereas the atypical enzyme is inhibited by less than 30%. In the rare individuals with no enzyme activity, that is homozygous SS variant (1 : 3000) suxamethonium may produce neuromuscular block for up to 2–4 h during which time the drug is eliminated by glomerular filtration. In a heterozygote (1 in 25) this may only take 10–30 min. The picture clinically is not always clear cut in that affected patients may breathe and move initially, later to become unresponsive and apnoeic. Cholinesterase activity in suspected cases can be assayed by the laboratory for future records and in the meantime intermittent positive pressure ventilation with sedation is the appropriate treatment. Fresh frozen plasma does contain the enzyme and may be given.

NON-DEPOLARIZING (COMPETITIVE) MUSCLE RELAXANTS

These drugs work by true competitive antagonism at the receptor (see p. 145), which is discussed in depth by

Ginsborg and Jenkinson[28] and in addition produce a membrane-potential dependent block of open ion channels.[29]

Characteristics of competitive neuromuscular blockade

- There is depression of twitches not preceded by muscle fasciculations so that there is generally no increase in the amplitude of the maximal twitch. However, Payne[30] and Blaber[31] noted an initial increase in twitch height, albeit transient, after sub-paralysing doses. Blaber found that the quantal content of the first endplate potential rose to 170% of control due to an increase in the fractional release of acetylcholine. When larger doses are given there is no change in the quantal content. Hence there is some overlap in depolarizing and non-depolarizing relaxant behaviour.
- During the depression of twitches the tension of an interposed tetanus is reduced and rapidly wanes (tetanic fade) during the period of stimulation. After the tetanus in the partially blocked muscle the twitches and compound action potentials are strikingly increased in amplitude for a short time (anticurare effect of a tetanus). This effect is the result of an increased output of acetylcholine by each post-tetanic impulse.
- The block can be antagonized by the injection of a stable depolarizing drug.
- The block is antagonized by anticholinesterase drugs.

A full history of the discovery of tubocurarine and the subsequent development of synthetic competitive relaxants is given by Bowman.[32] Tubocurarine was first used in anaesthesia in 1942 by Griffiths and Johnson in Montreal. Despite the introduction of a number of competitive neuromuscular-blocking drugs into everyday use following the discovery of curare there were still sufficient deficiencies among these drugs to prompt Savarese and Kitz to define the profile of an ideal neuromuscular blocking drug.[33]

Features of such an ideal drug included:

- competitive mechanism of action
- rapid onset of action
- short duration of action
- non-cumulative and independent of renal or hepatic elimination
- non-toxic
- free from cardiovascular side-effects
- no histamine release

To quite a large extent these criteria were fulfilled by the introduction of atracurium and vecuronium in the early 1980s. Prior to the introduction of these drugs the relaxants in common use included tubocurarine, pancuronium, alcuronium, gallamine and fazadinium. The principal deficiencies of these agents were as follows:

- Ganglion blockade. This occurred with tubocurarine[34] so that hypotension occurred which was potentiated by associated histamine release.
- Atropine-like block of cardiac muscarinic receptors or block of noradrenaline uptake. Gallamine and pancuronium block the actions of acetylcholine released from the cardiac vagus, facilitate release of noradrenaline from cardiac sympathetics and facilitate transmission through sympathetic ganglia. Pancuronium and fazadinium block the uptake of noradrenaline into sympathetic nerve endings.[7] These effects result in tachycardia and hypertension when the agents are used injudiciously.
- Histamine release. Although all basic compounds may disrupt mast cells and release histamine if the dose is large enough the effect is most pronounced with tubocurarine. The problem has been fully discussed by MacLagen.[35]
- Anticholinesterase activity. Since acetylcholine combines with both, there must be some resemblance between cholinoceptors and the active sites of cholinesterases. The neuromuscular-blocking drug benzoquinonium which would otherwise have been a useful relaxant has powerful acetylcholinesterase-inhibiting actions which limited its ease of reversibility.
- Recovery unduly dependent upon renal and hepatobiliary mechanisms so that there is prolongation of neuromuscular block in patients with impaired renal function or diminished drug metabolism.

Tubocurarine

This is the relaxant taken as the standard by which others are compared.

Minimal metabolism of curare occurs in the body. Within 24 h of a bolus dose 12% will be extracted in the bile (this percentage is increased in patients with renal failure) and 44% appears in the urine. A percentage (35–60%) of the drug is protein bound, although the clinical significance of protein binding is unclear. Furthermore, binding of muscle relaxants with other sites, for example cartilage, may be as important as that to plasma proteins. It would appear that the protein binding of tubocurarine is not altered in patients with renal and hepatic disease.

The intubating dose of tubocurarine is 0.5 mg/kg and maximum block occurs in 220 s. Time to 10% recovery of the twitch response occurs in 48 min.[36] The drug causes hypotension by a combination of ganglion blockade and histamine release and possibly by inhibiting calcium ion transport in heart cells.[37] The ganglion-blocking effects of tubocurarine and fazadinium occur closer to their neuromuscular-blocking dose range than in the case of other muscle relaxants. The amount of histamine released is related to the dose and the speed of injection.

Pancuronium

Pancuronium was introduced into anaesthetic practice in Britain in 1967.[38] It has a steroid nucleus and 15–40% of an injected dose is deacetylated in the liver to the 3-OH, 17-OH and 3,17-OH pancuronium derivatives. Of these, the 3-OH is the most potent in neuromuscular-blocking terms with 50% of the potency of pancuronium.[39] Eighty per cent of the drug is eliminated in the urine and the 3-OH metabolite is cleared poorly in renal failure patients and very high levels appear in patients with renal failure in the intensive care units (ICU) who have received infusions of pancuronium.[40] Therefore the drug should be avoided in patients with renal disease. Somogyi *et al.*[41] found that the duration was also prolonged in patients with biliary obstruction.

The intubating dose is 0.1 mg/kg and the onset time is long. Time to recover to 90% of the control twitch response is 90 min. Pancuronium has a sympathomimetic action (see above) resulting in tachycardia and hypertension. It does not release histamine.

Alcuronium

Alcuronium is derived from toxiferin. The drug is minimally metabolized and excreted unchanged in the urine and hence care is required with infusions in patients with renal failure. Intubating dose is 0.2–0.25 mg/kg. It was introduced as a medium-duration relaxant but in fact has a similar duration of action to tubocurarine (long acting) with an elimination half-life of 200 min. Thus, alcuronium cannot be considered a medium-duration non-depolarizing muscle relaxant.[42]

*Alcuronium does produce a degree of vagal blockade but has little sympathomimetic effect. This vagolytic effect is not as marked as with gallamine and pancuronium and there is no net effect on blood pressure.[43,44] It has very weak ganglion-blocking properties. Alcuronium does not release histamine but anaphylactoid reactions are recorded more commonly following its use than with any other non-depolarizing agent.[24]

Gallamine

Gallamine was the first widely used synthetic neuromuscular-blocking drug introduced in 1950. It is not a potent drug and the intubating dose is 160 mg. It is not metabolized but excreted almost entirely by the kidney and its use should be avoided in patients with renal failure.[45] It is suitable for patients with liver failure because there is minimal excretion in bile. The duration of action of gallamine is about 0.6 that of tubocurarine. Gallamine causes a tachycardia by both vagolysis and sympathetic stimulation. It releases less histamine than tubocurarine and allergic reactions are rare. It readily crosses the placental barrier and is therefore contraindicated in obstetric practice.

Fazadinium

Fazadinium is excreted mainly unchanged in urine. The intubating dose is 1–1.5 mg/kg and the duration of action is slightly shorter than that of tubocurarine. It is strongly vagolytic and always causes a tachycardia since dose–response curves for vagal and neuromuscular block overlap.[46] It causes ganglion blockade with occasional hypotension. It is not a potent releaser of histamine. The combination of tachycardia and occasional hypotension rendered it unpopular and it was withdrawn in 1984.

Newer muscular blocking agents

During the 1970s research continued for agents that would more closely approximate to the ideal competitive agent described by Savarese and Kitz.[33] This research resulted in the introduction of atracurium and vecuronium which come some way towards fulfilling these criteria.

Atracurium

This drug was designed and synthesized by a university pharmaceutical chemist, JB Stenlake, who commenced work on the project in 1970. He had long been interested in the possibility of utilizing the classical method of degrading quaternary ammonium compounds, the Hofmann elimination reaction, so that the molecule would possess a built-in 'self-destruct' mechanism. In this way elimination of the molecule would be independent of enzyme reactions and hepatobiliary or renal excretion. This he successfully achieved in the form of atracurium besylate. The first clinical report of its uses in patients was published in 1980.[47]

Atracurium is chemically related to some of the curare alkaloids. It is formulated as an aqueous injection with a pH 3.5 which is stable under refrigeration to 5°C for up to 2 years. (Degradation will occur at room temperature albeit at a slower rate than at body temperature.) Atracurium undergoes non-enzymatic Hofmann degradation to produce laudanosine and the quaternary monoacrylate. It also undergoes enzyme-catalysed ester hydrolysis at a lower pH to yield the quaternary acid and alcohol (see Fig. 12.10). The degree to which these occur is species dependent and is uncertain in humans. There is some recent evidence to suggest that this second pathway of ester hydrolysis may be of more importance than originally thought.[48] To emphasize the fact that the metabolism of atracurium is complicated and not completely resolved, Nigrovic and Smith[49] suggested that there may yet be other additional routes of metabolism. The ED_{90} dose is 0.1–0.25 mg/kg and atracurium is eliminated independently of the kidney[50] and liver.[51] Atracurium is non-cumulative. This was demonstrated by Payne and Hughes[52] who found that repeated doses of 0.1 mg/kg of atracurium produced less than a 5% increase in duration of action following the fourth dose compared with the first dose. The rate constant for recovery after atracurium infusion is the same as that following a bolus dose, implying lack of cumulation.[53]

The product of Hofmann degradation, laudanosine, is known to produce cerebral irritation in animals and seizure activity in dogs[54] at blood levels of 14 mg/ml. After hours of continuous infusions in the ICU the highest level recorded in humans was 5.1 mg/ml by Yate *et al.*[55] It is impossible to evaluate the toxic level in humans but this level may be exceeded if used in ill patients long term. Laudanosine crosses the blood–brain barrier and unlike atracurium is almost totally metabolized in the liver and has a long elimination half-life. Delayed clearance therefore occurs in patients with obstructed liver disease[56] and laudanosine levels are higher in patients with renal failure than in normal subjects.[57] Further studies on these central effects are warranted.

Atracurium has a wide autonomic margin of safety with little effect on the heart rate. However atracurium may release histamine at three times the dose producing muscle relaxation.[58] There is clinical evidence that atracurium releases histamine at a dose of 0.5 mg/kg. Atracurium has a 0.1% incidence of possible adverse reactions including flushing.[59] The incidence of anaphylaxis and histamine release is reduced by decreasing the dose and speed of injection and possibly with histamine antagonists.[60]

Neonates are more sensitive than adults to atracurium although this phenomenon is not as marked as following the use of tubocurarine or pancuronium.[61] Its profile of action is unchanged in elderly patients.

Following a dose of 0.6 mg/kg of atracurium, 20% recovery of T_1 (first twitch in the train of four) occurs within 40 min. Atracurium has an intermediate duration of action. Because of its shorter half-life reversal may not be necessary if neuromuscular monitoring indicates good recovery of neuromuscular function. Because of its short elimination half-life (20 min) is it used successfully in patients with neuromuscular disorders, for example myasthenia gravis and myotonic dystrophy. It is also an ideal drug for administration by infusion as the offset is rapid. Hutton[62] and Eger *et al.*[63] have reviewed and investigated respectively the use of atracurium given by infusion. Even when given to patients on the ICU with respiratory and renal failure, the mean time from cessation of infusion to recovery to T_1 without reversal was 60 min.[64]

Vecuronium

Vecuronium was synthesized in 1980 after preliminary work on a large number of diesters. It has a steroid nucleus and is related to pancuronium. Vecuronium is liable to conversion by deacetylation after only 30 min.[65] A ready-for-use aqueous preparation is therefore not practicable. Hence a buffered lyophilized product that is stable was developed which is easily constituted with sterile water for use. The additional lipophilicity of vecuronium compared with pancuronium means that its distribution and elimination differ from those of pancuronium and although they are equipotent in their actions the duration of action of vecuronium is much shorter than that of pancuronium.

The main metabolite of vecuronium is 2% as potent as the parent drug in terms of neuromuscular blockade. This contrasts with one of the main metabolites of pancuronium which has 50% of the neuromuscular-blocking activity of pancuronium. Rapid total plasma clearance of vecuronium is mainly due to hepatic uptake.[66] The proportion of free drug excreted in the urine is much smaller than in the case of other conventional neuromuscular-blocking agents.[67] Patients with liver disease demonstrate a prolonged duration of action of vecuronium.[68] Repeated doses of vecuronium in healthy patients without liver dysfunction are cumulative. Fahey *et al.*[69] showed that when repeating small doses (0.04 mg/kg) of vecuronium there was a 40% increase in duration of the fourth dose compared with the duration of the first dose. While the early pharmacokinetic data on vecuronium justify the conclusion that there is a rapid diminution of blood levels following injection, there is really no justification for referring to it as non-cumulative. Indeed, following prolonged infusion or repeated injection the recovery characteristics for vecuronium may not be significantly better than most of the older compounds.[70] Vecuronium has an elimination half-life of 70 min[71] compared with 20 min for atracurium.[72] Hence the two agents have a very similar duration of action after a single dose but not after repeated doses or infusion. Feldman[73] found that following an infusion of vecuronium which lasted for >90 min the recovery index was prolonged compared with a single bolus dose technique. Smith *et al.*[74] investigated the duration of vecuronium infusions in patients with renal and respiratory disease and found very variable results. The range of time for T_1 to recover to control from a level 20% of control was 6–37 h!

Vecuronium is 5–20 times more potent in studies in man than atracurium, and the ED_{90} value varies between studies and depends upon several factors, for example anaesthetic used and methods of peripheral nerve stimulation. ED_{90} for vecuronium ranges from 0.02 to 0.04 mg/kg and for atracurium 0.1–0.25 mg/kg.

Like pancuronium, vecuronium does not release histamine in clinically effective doses.[75] It has a wide autonomic margin of safety and does not cause tachycardia. Occasional reports of bradycardia and asystole have appeared in the literature after vecuronium.[76] This is generally thought to be associated with narcotic administration and not due to the vecuronium itself.[77]

Mivacurium (BW1090u)

Mivacurium is a short-acting competitive muscle relaxant. Although the speed of onset of action is longer than atracurium, its recovery is rapid and non-cumulative.[78] Its duration of action is approximately twice that of suxamethonium (or 33–50% that of atracurium). About 70% of a dose is broken down by plasma cholinesterase.[79] Ninety-five per cent recovery after 0.25 mg/kg occurs within 30 min. It is suitable for infusion. Brandon *et al.*[80] compared suxamethonium and mivacurium administered by bolus dose and infusion and confirmed that suxamethonium has a faster onset and shorter duration of action. It is reversible by neostigmine.

Mivacurium is structurally similar to atracurium and like atracurium has minimal cardiovascular side-effects. It releases rather less histamine than atracurium. Histamine release is not a problem within the normal clinical dose range but may occur at high doses (Savarese *et al.*[81]). The authors marked relaxants according to the likelihood of histamine release; tubocurarine > metocurine > mivacurium > doxacurium. There is no evidence that mivacurium has vagal-blocking properties.

Doxacurium (BWA93U)

This is a long-acting competitive neuromuscular blocker. It is minimally hydrolysed by plasma cholinesterase and largely excreted unchanged by the kidney.[82] The duration of action is similar to that of pancuronium. Onset of block takes about 3 min, and maximum block is slow to develop (10–12 min). It is the most potent relaxant ever studied in man. It exhibits cardiovascular stability and does not release histamine in the clinical dose range. Cashman *et al.*[83] studied the effects in patients with renal failure and found recovery to be prolonged.

Pipecuronium

Pipecuronium is an analogue of pancuronium developed in Hungary in 1980. Onset and recovery from neuromuscular block are similar to those of pancuronium. Between 40 and 80% of a bolus dose is excreted through the kidney unchanged and its effect is prolonged in renal failure patients.[84] The remainder of the drug is slowly deacetylated in the liver. It exhibits cardiovascular stability (unlike pancuronium) and does not release histamine.

Org 7617, Org 9616, Org 9426 (Rocuronium)

These steroidal compounds have been investigated in animal studies. Org 9616 and Org 7617 were found to produce very short-lasting neuromuscular blockades (comparable to suxamethonium) with only minor autonomic and cardiovascular side-effects.[85] Neither drug is potent and Org 9616 lacks potency to a degree that may make commercial development unlikely. It is, however, the only non-depolarizing relaxant with an onset time that approaches that of suxamethonium. Org 9426 has a duration of action similar to that of vecuronium but its onset of action, although not as fast as suxamethonium, is faster.[86] Org 9426 was developed and became available for use in this country under its generic name rocuronium.

Potent reversible neuromuscular activity is also attributable to molecules other than the traditional quaternary compounds (e.g. peptides). Perhaps future developments may lie in this direction.[87] Anaphylactoid reactions continue to occur to drugs which contain quaternary nitrogen groups so that the search for new relaxants continues.

Onset of action of non-depolarizing muscle relaxants

The search for a non-depolarizing relaxant with an onset of action comparable to that of suxamethonium continues. Why is the onset of a non-depolarizing block slower than that with suxamethonium? Scott and Marman[88] postulated that due to the naturally large margin of safety of neuromuscular transmission, competitive blockers need to block all the spare receptors to produce complete block. Depolarizing agents on the other hand only need to produce depolarization via 20–30% receptors to render the junctional insensitive. Second, because of the short half-life of suxamethonium it can be given in a relative overdose thus increasing the concentration gradient. If this is indeed the case then a depolarizing block will always develop faster than a non-depolarizing one.

The time taken to produce satisfactory intubating conditions is often equated with the onset of action. However, criteria for suitability for intubation are multifactorial and include anatomy of the larynx, skill of the operator and individual patient response to the relaxant. Payne[89] concluded that smooth intubation after 0.5 mg/kg of atracurium should be possible within 2 min. Agoston *et al.*[90] reported good intubating conditions after 0.08 mg/kg of vecuronium within 100 s.

These findings are very similar and it has been claimed that the onset times (time from injection of drug to maximum effect) are similar for all non-depolarizing relaxants at equivalent dosage.[91] Increasing the dose has been tried in order to improve the speed of onset but results are unconvincing and increasing the dose may render reversal difficult. Harrison and Feldman[92] tried increasing the dose of vecuronium to 0.15 mg/kg and found minimal improvement in intubating conditions at 1 min. Scott and Goat[93] repeated the experiment with atracurium and came to the same conclusion; that is, despite increasing the dose of relaxant, the onset of action after atracurium or vecuronium is not as fast as after suxamethonium.

Intubation can be carried out faster if the muscle relaxants are given in divided doses. The first dose should block about 75% of the receptors and the second dose about 90%. If the doses are given 6 min apart, intubation can be achieved as rapidly as following suxamethonium with vecuronium[94] or atracurium.[95] However, care should be exercised with the divided dose technique. Owing to the very wide variation in patient response to muscle relaxants, some will experience weakness after the first dose. This is unacceptable in the unanaesthetized patient and Jones[96] believes that the disadvantages outweigh the advantages. However, Miller and Savarese[21] argue that this technique is fast enough for a rapid sequence induction and should be used when there is a valid contraindication to the use of suxamethonium.

Finally, Bowman *et al.*[97] have demonstrated that for steroidal relaxants a faster onset and shorter duration of action is correlated with lower potency (see above for Org 9616).

FACTORS THAT INFLUENCE THE ACTION OF NEUROMUSCULAR-BLOCKING AGENTS

The subject is reviewed by Payne and Hughes[52] and factors include route of administration, variations in sensitivity of different muscle groups, rate of stimulation, acid–base balance, drug interactions, temperature and age of the patient.

Route and method of administration

Muscle relaxants are all administered by the intravenous route in order to obtain the levels of necessary for neuromuscular blockade rapidly. The pharmacodynamic and pharmacokinetic variability of competitive neuromuscular-blocking agents makes it impossible to predict accurately in an individual patient the magnitude of block at completion of surgery when simple criteria, for example dose, duration and body weight are used. One must titrate drug administration against effect by way of monitoring neuromuscular function. The administration of frequent small doses allows some control but is difficult and inconvenient.

The continuous infusion of a muscle relaxant provides a flexible and accurate method for maintaining a precise degree of muscle relaxation during surgery. The advantages of the technique are most pronounced where shorter-acting agents are used. The offset of these is relatively fast so that termination of their action, either by spontaneous recovery or by reversal with an anticholinesterase drug, is more reliable than that following the longer-acting agents. Indeed from the safety aspect one wonders if there is a future for new long-acting relaxants. The infusion rate necessary to maintain a stable neuromuscular blockade quickly becomes constant because of the short duration of action and lack of cumulative effects of these agents.

Systems for infusion vary from simple systems that are manually altered according to the number of twitches felt during a train of four stimulation[98] to more complex computer-assisted closed loop systems. Atracurium is very suitable for infusion as dose requirements are relatively unaffected by age and an infusion rate of 0.4–0.5 mg/kg/h maintains adequate surgical relaxation in the majority of patients.[99]

Acid–base balance

There seems to be general agreement that respiratory acidosis enhances and respiratory alkalosis reduces the potency of tubocurarine and pancuronium. The reverse is true for gallamine[7] and atracurium, although affected *in vitro*, is probably not affected *in vivo*.[52]

General anaesthetics

General anaesthetic agents have a depressant effect on neuromuscular transmission such that the effect of non-depolarizing muscle relaxants is potentiated. Gissen *et al.*[100] attribute this to an effect on the postjunctional membrane. The twitch response to indirect stimulation is unaffected[101] but fade on high frequency tetanic stimulation occurs. Recent studies have shown that isoflurane reduces the average duration of opening of acetylcholine receptor channels, impairing neuromuscular transmission.[102] In addition, general anaesthetics can produce muscle relaxation through their central CNS actions.[103]

Inhalation anaesthetics augment relaxants in the decreasing order: isoflurane > desflurane, enflurane > halothane > N_2O-barbiturate-narcotic anaesthesia.[21] Atracurium and vecuronium appear to be less affected by the choice of anaesthetic than are tubocurarine and pancuronium.[104]

Temperature

The degree of block produced by non-depolarizing agents is reduced by moderate hypothermia (owing to reduction in acetylcholinesterase activity) but the duration is prolonged because of delayed urinary and biliary excretion at low temperatures.[105]

Age

Much has been written about the action of non-depolarizing muscle relaxants at the extremes of life. It is generally accepted that neonates (and in particular premature babies) are more sensitive to their effects than adults. Stead[106] suggested that neonates are ‘miniature myasthenics' since tetanus was not sustained in this age group in the absence of relaxants. Certainly it is true to say that the neuromuscular junction is not fully developed at birth and that maturation of neuromuscular transmission occurs within the first few months of life.[107] Also babies have a higher percentage of body water than adults, which presumably affects the volume of distribution of drugs. Meretoja[108] found that infants up to 1 year were more sensitive to the effects of vecuronium than adults. This has not been demonstrated with atracurium.

Do elderly patients respond differently? Separating the influence of age from disease is difficult. However, it is probable that in healthy elderly patients the pharmacokinetic and pharmacodynamic response to muscle relaxants is similar to that of younger patients.[109]

REVERSAL OF NEUROMUSCULAR BLOCKADE/ANTICHOLINESTERASES

If the response to the administration of muscle relaxants was uniform, that is, there was no variation in individual response, then the whole problem of reversal of neuromuscular blockade would be very much simpler. However, in clinical practice the response to competitive neuromuscular-blocking agents has been found to be highly variable. Katz[110] found that 0.1 mg/kg of tubocurarine caused no neuromuscular block in 6% of patients and 100% depression of the twitch response in 7%, with a range of neuromuscular block in between. The factors that cause the variability can be analysed in terms of pharmacodynamics and pharmacokinetics, and then the effect of other drugs, for example, general anaesthetics, can be taken into consideration.

In the absence of monitoring neuromuscular function, residual curarization in the recovery room remains a problem. In a study at three Copenhagen University Hospitals, Viby-Mogensen[111] found that 42% of patients who had received a muscle relaxant had evidence of incomplete reversal of neuromuscular blockade on arrival in the recovery room. Subsequent studies in Sweden[112] and Australia[113] have supported this. The most serious consequence of residual curarization is postoperative respiratory failure and a marked increase in the incidence of this potentially lethal complication was noted soon after the introduction of relaxants into clinical practice.[114] Even now postoperative respiratory failure is still an important cause of anaesthetic mortality. Lunn *et al.* attribute 19% of anaesthetic deaths to postoperative respiratory failure following residual paralysis[115].

The findings of Viby-Mogensen[111] may be explained by the observation that most attempts to antagonize a competitive block occur when there is greater than 90% depression of the twitch height compared with control. Antagonism of this degree of neuromuscular blockade with an anticholinesterase may take 30 min or more.[116] Rapid and reliable antagonism of a competitive neuromuscular blockade will only occur if the block has spontaneously recovered to a sufficient degree by the time of reversal.

Following the recent introduction of atracurium and vecuronium, antagonism of neuromuscular blockade can be achieved more quickly and reliably than following block achieved with drugs with a longer duration of action.[117] Many of the above studies refer to such drugs. However, the duration of action of $3 \times ED_{95}$ of both drugs is approximately 1 h[118,119] and therefore after short surgical procedures reversal is advisable, especially if there is no recovery area. This situation regrettably exists today in many hospitals.[120] Reversal is also advised after the use of longer-acting agents. It has been argued that even in the presence of an adequate train of four response (i.e. with evidence of adequate neuromuscular function), reversal should be given as the risks of administering reversal agents do not outweigh the risks of residual paralysis.[121] The opposite viewpoint has also been put forward.[122] It is now appreciated that if neostigmine is given to a patient who has recovered his or her neuromuscular function, then clinically significant neuromuscular blockade can be caused by the anticholinesterase itself. This appears not to be such a problem after edrophonium. Thus Jones[123] suggests that if recovery is adequate (assessed by neuromuscular monitoring) then no anticholinesterase need be given at the end of surgery or, if in doubt, edrophonium should be used rather than neostigmine (see later).

The most important factors that influence the ability to antagonize residual paralysis reliably are:

- Density of block at the point reversal is attempted. Unless the concentration of relaxant present at the neuromuscular junction has decreased to a critical level, the administration of an anticholinesterase drug cannot re-establish neuromuscular transmission. For prompt reversal the twitch height should be 20% of control or have three twitches present on train of four stimulation.[116,123]
- Specific relaxant used. It is easier to antagonize atracurium and vecuronium than longer-acting agents.
- Presence of drugs potentiating relaxants (or antagonizing). Aminoglycoside antibiotics and calcium antagonists potentiate relaxants.
- Age of patient. It has been suggested that children up to 8 years of age require 33–50% less neostigmine than adults.[124]
- Acid–base status of patient. Respiratory acidosis potentiates competitive relaxants.

Administration of anticholinesterases remains the principal method of antagonizing residual neuromuscular blockade. Anticholinesterases are quaternary ammonium compounds with a structural similarity to acetylcholine. They act either by reversible occupation of the active site of the acetylcholinesterase enzyme, for example edrophonium, or by acylation of the esteratic site, for example carbamates (physostigmine, pyridostigmine and neostigmine) and organophosphates.

Whereas edrophonium has a brief duration of action presumably due to its reversible attachment and subsequent rapid renal clearance, deacylation of carbamylated and phosphorylated acetylcholinesterase takes longer and until this has taken place the enzyme remains inhibited. Both neostigmine and pyridostigmine form the same carbamylated enzyme and so the duration of enzyme inhibition produced by these drugs is similar and exceeds that produced by edrophonium.

There is still uncertainty as to whether their effect on neuromuscular transmission is due entirely to inhibition of acetycholinesterase.[125,126] The anticholinesterases used for their anticurare (nicotinic) action are neostigmine, edrophonium and pyridostigmine. An antimuscarinic agent must be given at the same time to counteract the unpleasant muscarinic side-effects also produced such as salivation, excessive bronchial secretions, colic and bradycardia. Atropine and glycopyrronium are the commonly used antimuscarinic agents. Atropine produces a vagolytic effect much more rapidly than glycopyrronium and, in theory, to minimize any cardiovascular changes atropine is better suited for use with edrophonium, which has a fast onset of action, and glycopyrronium is better suited for use with neostigmine, which has a slower onset of action. Glycopyrronium offers some advantages over atropine in terms of stability of heart rate and a lower incidence of dysrhythmias, and lack of central antimuscarinic actions.[127] However, glycopyrronium was less effective than atropine on inhibiting the action of neostigmine on the bowel.[128]

The main effect of anticholinesterases on normal unblocked muscle is to cause paralysis partly by producing a depolarizing block from a postsynaptic action of acetylcholine and perhaps by a reduction in acetylcholine release.[7,129,130] It is only when neuromuscular transmission is impaired by drugs such as tubocurarine or in myasthenia gravis that anticholinesterases lead to facilitation.

Physostigmine

Physostigmine antagonizes non-depolarizing neuromuscular block in animals but the results are disappointing in humans.[131] Its lipid solubility and consequent ability to cross the blood–brain barrier causing excitement is the reason for its application in the reversal of general anaesthesia. It is not used clinically to reverse the actions of non-depolarizing drugs.

Neostigmine

Neostigmine is the most widely used agent in the UK for reversal of neuromuscular blockade at present. It is used in a dose range 2.5–5.0 mg. A number of isolated cases of cardiac arrest occurred after its introduction[132,133] attributable to the bradycardia associated with its muscarinic action. These reports led to the practice of giving atropine prior to neostigmine to counteract this but Kemp and Morton[134] showed that if atropine and neostigmine were mixed together this did not happen as atropine worked within 30 s and neostigmine after this in 100 s. As mentioned above, glycopyrronium mixed with neostigmine is gaining popularity as dysrhythmias are less common. Neostigmine should be used with caution in operations involving bowel anastomosis as it causes increased gastrointestinal motility. It has also been implicated in postoperative nausea. King *et al.* noted an incidence of postoperative vomiting of 68% compared with 32% in the control group after lower limb prosthetic surgery.[135]

The neuromuscular-blocking properties of neostigmine have been known for many years.[136,137] The author has seen tetanic fade which lasted for 20 min following the administration of neostigmine to a fully recovered patient.[138] This may be clinically significant and is in contrast with edrophonium, which only caused a very transient block under the same circumstances (3 min). Goldhill *et al.*[139] also noted fade of the train of four response which lasted for 10 min after neostigmine was given to a patient who had not received muscle relaxants. This was associated with muscle fasciculations. It would seem prudent therefore to give edrophonium to a patient who already has a significant degree of spontaneous recovery of neuromuscular function.

However, when reversing patients with little or no apparent recovery of neuromuscular function the outcome, as has already been discussed, is often protracted and unsatisfactory. Neostigmine is preferable to edrophonium under these circumstances. Katz[110] noticed that neostigmine could reverse patients with no twitch response when this was not possible following edrophonium. This finding has been confirmed by Rupp *et al.*[140] The author has shown that while the twitch response was facilitated under these circumstances following edrophonium, the tetanic response was not. Perhaps edrophonium depletes acetylcholine stores as a result of its presynaptic action (see below) and at high frequencies of stimulation cannot cope with mobilization.

The facilitatory drug 4-aminopyridine potentiates the effects of neostigmine[141] so that the dose of neostigmine may be reduced (and hence the muscarinic side-effects). However 4-aminopyridine cannot be used as the sole antagonist because of the central nervous system stimulation that it causes.

Edrophonium

Edrophonium has not been widely used as an anticurare agent in this country because of the apparently short duration of action, unreliable antagonism and the possibility of recurarization.[110,142–147]

Some of these reports of unsustained and unreliable reversal were due to inadequate dosage (10–20 mg), imprecise (or lack of) monitoring of neuromuscular function, or trying to antagonize a very dense neuromuscular blockade. Recent studies measuring the twitch response suggest that when used in higher doses (0.5–1.0 mg/kg) the duration of action of edrophonium is almost the same as neostigmine. In equiantagonistic doses the duration of antagonism during steady-state 90% block of the twitch response produced by tubocurarine was 66 min for edrophonium (0.5 mg/kg) and 76 min for neostigmine (0.04 mg/kg).[127] The pharmacokinetic profile of the two drugs has been shown to be very similar.[148] There has therefore been a revival of interest in edrophonium as a reversal agent.

The importance of cholinesterase inhibition in the mechanism of action of edrophonium is unclear. It has been shown to be less than that of neostigmine[149,150] and muscarinic side-effects of edrophonium are less obvious, which supports this finding;[127] that is, edrophonium possesses a greater selectivity for the nicotinic receptor although it does produce muscarinic side-effects. It requires a smaller dose of an anticholinergic agent to be used with it and it has been suggested that atropine is a suitable anticholinergic as both drugs have a quick onset of action. Part of the anticurare action of edrophonium may involve an increase in the quantal release of acetylcholine. Blaber[31,151,152] showed that tubocurarine reduced the rate of refilling of the acetylcholine store in nerve terminals and demonstrated that edrophonium could reverse this. Donati *et al.*[153] examined the fade of the train of four response after antagonism of a pancuronium blockade with neostigmine, pyridostigmine or edrophonium and found the highest train of four ratios after reversal with edrophonium. They concluded that it was a more effective antagonist at the presynaptic receptor, a view shared by Jones *et al.*[154]

Large doses of edrophonium (0.5–1.4 mg/kg) produce adequate and sustained reversal of neuromuscular blockade provided that some spontaneous recovery of neuromuscular function has occurred.[155–159]

As a reversal agent edrophonium has a quicker onset of action than neostigmine and pyridostigmine.[127,154,159,160] This may be due to the initial rapid release of acetylcholine from the motor nerve terminal or it may be related to the size of the molecule. The molecular weight of edrophonium is 166 compared with 223 for neostigmine and it may diffuse more rapidly to its site of action.

Its efficacy in reversing dense neuromuscular blockade is not as great as neostigmine (see above).

Pyridostigmine

Pyridostigmine is an analogue of neostigmine with one-quarter of its potency so that 10 mg of pyridostigmine are equivalent to 2.5 mg of neostigmine. Katz[161] concluded that it exhibited fewer muscarinic effects on the bowel and myocardium than neostigmine although Fogdall and Miller[162] found no difference. It has been shown to have a slower onset of action and longer duration of action than neostigmine.[163]

The liver is the major site of metabolism for anticholinesterase drugs, which are then excreted by the kidney. Renal excretion accounts for 75% of the clearance of pyridostigmine, 70% of edrophonium and 50% of neostigmine.[164] The effects of anticholinesterases are prolonged in patients with renal failure.[165]

ASSESSMENT OF NEUROMUSCULAR FUNCTION

In the absence of neuromuscular monitoring the anaesthetist equates neuromuscular function with tests of muscle strength such as head raising, handgrip strength, eye opening or with respiratory measurements, for example tidal volume, vital capacity and inspiratory and expiratory airway pressures. Unfortunately tidal volume and vital capacity are influenced by a number of factors unrelated to neuromuscular function and the presence of respiration is in itself no guarantee of adequate recovery from neuromuscular blockade.[166] Competitive neuromuscular-blocking agents have been shown to have a 'sparing' effect on the muscles of respiration compared with peripheral muscles[167–170] so that spontaneous breathing can occur in the presence of marked peripheral neuromuscular blockade. Although gas exchange may be satisfactory in a patient whose airway is safeguarded by an endotracheal tube, this degree of recovery may not leave enough margin of safety for a patient to overcome airway obstruction or vomiting.

Various studies have highlighted the inadequacy of the anaesthetists' clinical judgement as to the adequacy of recovery of neuromuscular function after the use of muscle relaxants. Harrison[171] carried out a retrospective survey of deaths in South Africa and discovered that ten out of fifty-three were due to inadequate respiration following neuromuscular blockade. Viby-Mogensen *et al.*[111] found in Sweden that 42% of patients in the recovery room had inadequate muscle strength when precise neuromuscular monitoring was applied and they concluded that residual paralysis remained a problem in unmonitored patients. Lunn *et al.*[115] attributed 19% of anaesthetic deaths in the UK in a retrospective survey to postoperative respiratory failure from residual curarization. Of the clinical tests that require co-operation and therefore an awake subject (impossible when in the operating theatre) probably head lift for 5 s is the most sensitive. This requires sustained tetanic effort. In an excellent study by Pavlin *et al.*[172] awake volunteers were given tubocurarine until the mean inspiratory pressure fell from –90 cmH_2O to –20 cmH_2O. As they recovered, patients who could sustain head lift for 5 s (mean inspiratory pressure –53 cmH_2O) could perform all airway protective manoeuvres, for example Valsalva, swallow and maintain a patent airway. Those who could not sustain head lift could not do this. Also, Engbaek *et al.*[173] have shown that head lift could not be sustained for 5 s in any patient with a train of four ratio (see later) of 0.5 or less during recovery from atracurium. This ratio had to recover to 0.8 for this to be achieved in all patients.

As most patients are too drowsy at the end of surgery to perform such co-operative tests the need has evolved for precise monitoring during routine anaesthesia. This is more important as the response to muscle relaxants in individuals is so variable[110] and in order for anticholinesterases to be successful there must be some degree of spontaneous recovery present. Precise neuromuscular monitoring involves stimulating a peripheral nerve with a nerve stimulator and quantifying the evoked muscle response. An early report of this being performed in clinical anaesthesia comes from Christie and Churchill-Davidson[174] at St Thomas' Hospital. The nerve must always be stimulated supramaximally to ensure recruitment of all fibres, and because different muscle groups can exhibit different sensitivities to relaxants it follows that the same one should always be compared.

The ulnar nerve at the wrist is most often chosen because of the ease of access, and the response of the adductor pollicis muscle measured. The responses to twitch, train of four and tetanic stimulation can be examined.

The single twitch response

Performed at a frequency of 0.1 Hz, this is a relatively insensitive test as 75–80% of receptors have to be occupied before there is any diminution of control height.[175] Observation of the single twitch is not particularly useful as observer memory of the control (which must be performed as a baseline measurement) is unreliable. Most workers agree that recovery of the simple twitch to its control value does not indicate satisfactory recovery of neuromuscular function. The sensitivity of testing can be increased by increasing the stimulation frequency as in the train of four at 2 Hz[176] or by using tetanic stimulation at 50 Hz.[177]

Train of four response

This is performed at 2 Hz. Under conditions of partial neuromuscular blockade as the rate of stimulation of the single twitch is increased, a reduction in twitch height is seen.[176] This phenomenon was first used clinically by Roberts and Wilson[178] who utilized a train at 4 Hz in the diagnosis and treatment of myasthenia gravis. It was then adapted by Ali *et al.*[176] and introduced for the assessment of neuromuscular blockade. The first twitch in the train is unconditioned and the extent of diminution of subsequent twitches is proportional to magnitude of block present; that is, the fade of the train or the ratio of the fourth twitch to the first twitch is proportional to the degree of block. Therefore, since a ratio can be examined, no control measurement is necessary. However, evaluation of the ratio by inspection or palpation following stimulation with a nerve stimulation even in expert hands is poor.[179,180] A more precise evaluation can be obtained using a force transducer with recording apparatus which provides both a record for the control single twitch and allows detailed analysis of fade. Alternatively, the EMG can be recorded and simple EMG devices are now available that provide an analogue reading of the compound electromyogram with a meter display of the degree of block.[181] Close correlation between this EMG measurement and that of the force transducer has been confirmed for single twitch and train of four modes of stimulation.[182] The EMG measurement has some advantages over tension measurement for any mode of stimulation. It is free from errors of change in position and the patient need not be immobilized. It can be used on small infants where a force transducer would be too heavy. It has been shown that the best readings are obtained if the active electrode is placed over the adductor pollicis for hypothenar muscles and the indifferent over the second or fifth finger.[183]

It would appear that the train of four ratio need not return to unity for recovery of neuromuscular function to be judged adequate (see below). It is therefore a much more sensitive index than the single twitch response.

Tetanic stimulation

This is normally performed at 50 Hz, the stimulation frequency which Merton[184] equated with maximum volitional effort. After administration of a competitive relaxant there is a fall in the amplitude of the response (postjunctional receptor block) and fade of the response (due to prejunctional receptor block) which is analogous to train of four fade. The degree of fade is dependent upon the degree of block, the frequency and duration of stimulation and how often it is applied.[177] The use of high-frequency stimulation may reveal effects at presynaptic sites not apparent from single twitch stimulation and therefore it is a more sensitive test than the single twitch. A disadvantage of tetanic stimulation is that it is painful and under certain circumstances can itself influence the course of neuromuscular block with a decurarizing effect.[185] Thus while the tetanic response may recover to be fully sustained, in the same patient the ratio of the train of four may be less than one (see below). It seems curious that fade of the train of four at 2 Hz should be greater than when tetanic stimulation is performed at 50 Hz. One would imagine that tetanic stimulation would stress the neuromuscular junction at this high frequency of traffic impulses far more and reveal more fade. Studies by Wali and Payne[186] throw some light on this problem. They suggested that the output of acetylcholine from the nerve ending at 2 Hz was greater than at 50 Hz and furthermore in the presence of atracurium the decline in acetylcholine output was greater at 2 Hz than at 50 Hz.

CORRELATION OF TESTS OF NEUROMUSCULAR FUNCTION WITH ADEQUACY OF VENTILATION AND SIGNS OF RECOVERY

Walts *et al.*[187] found that sustained muscle contraction in response to tetanic stimulation at 30 Hz was a useful end-point as it correlated with 90% recovery of vital capacity in human volunteers. In their study, the ability to raise the head did not return to control and this was probably because head raising is a more sensitive test than sustained tetanus performed at 30 Hz. That head lift is a sensitive test is supported by the study of Johansen, Jorgensen *et al.*[168] who found that head lift was 38% of control when inspiratory and expiratory flow rates were > 90% of control. Ali and Kitz[188] found that when vital capacity was recovered to >90%, tetanus at 50 Hz was fully sustained and that the train of four ratio was 0.75 following the administration of tubocurarine to anaesthetized patients. A similar study performed on conscious volunteers found that at a train of four ratio 0.6, tetanus was fully sustained.[166]

Thus the train of four appears to be a more sensitive test of neuromuscular function than the tetanus and the ratio need not recover to unity for antagonism to be judged adequate. Miller[189] collected data from several studies and suggested that the sensitivities of test of neuromuscular function were head lift > inspiratory force > train of four > sustained tetanus at 30 Hz and normal vital capacity > normal tidal volume and twitch height. He concluded that even when the test is normal one cannot assume all receptors are free of relaxant.

RECENT DEVELOPMENTS

Double burst stimulation (DBS)

To overcome the difficulties in manual estimation of the fade of the train of four response, a new pattern of stimulation, double burst stimulation, has been introduced.[190] The rationale behind this is that it is easier to compare two movements rather than four in the accurate estimation of a ratio. It consists of two 50 Hz tetanic stimuli separated by a 750-ms interval, and these are compared to give a fade ratio. Drenck *et al.*[191] detected fade in response to DBS at a higher ratio than train of four stimulation and concluded that manual evaluation of the response to DBS was more sensitive than that to train of four. This has been confirmed by Gill *et al.*[192] Brull *et al.*[193] found a high degree of correlation of train of four and DBS ratios over a wide range of stimulating currents and varying degrees of neuromuscular block.

Acceleration

Instead of measuring the force of muscle contraction, acceleration is measured. This eliminates the need for immobilization. Viby-Mogensen *et al.*[194] found good correlation between acceleration and force measurements for the train of four response during recovery from vecuronium blockade using the 'accelograph', but that the control readings varied.

Post-tetanic count

Non-depolarizing block is characterized by the occurrence of post-tetanic facilitation. This phenomenon is used in the post-tetanic count to estimate when spontaneous recovery from a very deep neuromuscular block can be anticipated.[195] A 50-Hz tetanic stimulus is applied for 5 s (for longer than is physiological) and the number of single twitches at 0.1 Hz elicited after a 3-s interval are counted.

Also, Stanec *et al.*[196] have used the phenomenon of post-tetanic facilitation to define an end-point for adequate recovery in day case patients. If standard train of four stimuli at 2 Hz are interrupted for tetanic stimulation at 50 Hz for 10 s, the ensuing train of four response is enhanced in the presence of residual block. They maintain that disappearance of this enhancement is a useful sign of recovery.

Perhaps the introduction of muscle relaxants with an intermediate duration of action are as important in the fight against residual curarization as neuromuscular monitoring. It must be obvious from the constant introduction of new techniques and methods in monitoring that the subject is complex and yet unresolved.

REFERENCES

1 Bacq ZM, Brown GL. Pharmacological experiments on mammalian voluntary muscle in relation to the theory of chemical transmission. *Journal of Physiology* 1937; **89**: 45–60.

2 Riker WF. Actions of acetylcholine on the mammalian motor nerve terminal. *Journal of Experimental Therapeutics* 1966; **152**: 397–416.

3 Burns BD, Paton, WDM. Depolarisation of the motor end-plate by decamethonium and acetylcholine. *Journal of Physiology* 1951; **115**: 41–73.

4 MacLagan J, Vrbova G. A study of the increased sensitivity of denervated and reinervated muscle to depolarising drugs. *Journal of Physiology* 1966; **182**: 131–43.

5 Dorkins HR. Suxamethonium – the development of a modern drug from 1906 to the present day. *Medical History* 1982; **26**: 145.

6 Zaimis E. The neuromuscular junction: areas of uncertainty. In: Zaimis E, ed. *Neuromuscular junction. Handbook of experimental pharmacology*, Vol 42. Berlin: Springer-Verlag, 1976: 1–21.

7 Bowman WC. *Pharmacology of neuromuscular function.* Bristol: John Wright, 1980.

8 Urbach CM, Edelist G. An evaluation of the anaesthetic used in an outpatient unit. *Canadian Anaesthetists Society Journal* 1977; **24**: 401–7.

9 Zahl K, Apfelbaum JL. Muscle pain occurs after outpatient laparoscopy despite the substitution of vecuronium for succinylcholine. *Anesthesiology* 1989; **70**: 408–11.

10 Trepanier CA, Brousseau C, Lacerte L. Myalgia in outpatient surgery: comparison of atracurium and succinylcholine. *Canadian Journal of Anaesthesia* 1989; **35**: 255–9.

11 Jones RM. Muscle relaxants for day stay surgery. In: Healy TJ ed. *Anaesthesia for day case surgery. Clinical Anaesthesiology*, **4**(3). London: Bailliere Tindall, 1990: 679–89.

12 Smith SE. Neuromuscular blocking drugs in man. In: Zaimis E, ed. *Neuromuscular junction. Handbook of experimental pharmacology*, Vol 42. Berlin: Springer-Verlag, 1976: 593–660.

13 Cook JH. The effects of suxamethonium on intraocular pressure. *Anaesthesia* 1981; **36**: 354–5.

14 Mirakhur RK, Shepherd WFI, Darrah WC. Propofol or thiopentone: effects on intraocular pressure associated with induction of anaesthesia and tracheal intubation (facilitated with suxamethonium). *British Journal of Anaesthesia* 1987; **59**: 431–6.

15 Edmonson L, Lindsay SL, Lanigan LP, Woods M, Chew HER. Intra-ocular pressure changes during rapid sequence induction of anaesthesia. *Anaesthesia* 1988; **43**: 1005–10.

16 Sweeney J, Underhilll S, Dowd T, Mostafa SM. Modification by fentanyl and alfentanil of the intraocular pressure response to suxamethonium and tracheal intubation. *British Journal of Anaesthesia* 1989; **63**: 688–91.

17 Stirt JA, Chin GJ. Intraocular pressure during rapid sequence induction: use of moderate doses of sufentanil or fentanil and vecuronium or atracurium. *Anaesthesia and Intensive Care* 1990; **18**: 390–4.

18 Libonati MM, Leahy JJ, Ellison N. The use of succinylcholine in penetrating eye injuries. *Anesthesiology* 1985; **62**: 637.

19 Valentine S, McVey FK, Coe A. Postoperative sore throat. *Anaesthesia* 1990; **45**: 306–8.

20 Goat VA, Feldman SA. The dual action of suxamethonium on the isolated rabbit heart. *Anaesthesia* 1972; **27**: 149.

21 Miller RD, Savarese JJ. Pharmacology of muscle relaxants and their antagonists. In: Miller RD, ed. *Anaesthesia*, 3rd edn. New York: Churchill Livingstone, 1990: 389–435.

22 Van der Spek AF, Reynolds PI, Fang WB, Ashton Miller JA, Stohler CB, Schork MA. Changes in resistance to mouth opening induced by depolarising and non-depolarising neuromuscular relaxants. *British Journal of Anaesthesia* 1990; **64**: 21–7.

23 Leary NP, Ellis RF. Masseteric muscle spasm as a normal response to suxamethonium. *British Journal of Anaesthesia* 1990; **64**: 488–92.

24 Watkins J. Adverse anaesthetic reactions. An update from a proposed national reporting and advisory service. *Anaesthesia* 1985; **40**: 797–800.

25 Kao JY, Yurner DR. Prolongation of succinylcholine block by metoclopramide. *Anesthesiology* 1989; **70**: 905–8.

26 Viby Mogensen J. Correlation of succinylcholine duration of action with plasma cholinesterase activity in subjects with genotypically normal enzyme. *Anesthesiology* 1980; **53**: 517.

27 Pantuck EJ, Pantuck CB. Cholinesterases and anticholinesterases. In: Katz RL, ed. *Muscle relaxants.* Amsterdam: Excerpta Medica, 1975.

28 Ginsborg BL, Jenkinson DH. Transmission of impulses from nerve to muscle. In: Zaimis E, ed. *Handbook of experimental pharmacology*, Vol 42. Berlin: Springer-Verlag, 1976; 229.

29 Colquhoun D, Dreyer, F, Sheridan RE. The action of tubocurarine at the frog neuromuscular junction. *Journal of Physiology* 1979; **293**: 247.

30 Payne JP. The initial transient stimulating action of neuromuscular blocking agents in the cat. *British Journal of Anaesthesia* 1961; **33**: 285.

31 Blaber LC. The prejunctional actions of some non-depolarising blocking drugs. *British Journal of Pharmacology* 1973; **47**: 109–16.

32 Bowman WC. Discoveries in pharmacology. In: Parnham, Brunivels, eds. *Psycho and neuropharmacology*, Vol 1. Amsterdam: Elsevier Science Publishers, 1983; 135.

33 Savarese JJ, Kitz RJ. The guest for a short-acting non-depolarising neuromuscular blocking agent. *Acta Anaesthesiologica Scandinavica* 1973; **53** (Suppl): 43.

34 Bowman WC, Webb SN. Neuromuscular blocking and ganglion blocking activities of some acetylcholine antagonists in the cat. *Journal of Pharmacy and Pharmacology* 1972; **24**: 762–72.

35 MacLargen J. Competitive neuromuscular blocking drugs. In: Zaimis E, ed. *Neuromuscular junction. Handbook of experimental pharmacology*, Vol 42. Berlin: Springer-Verlag, 1976: 421–86.

36 Hunter JM, Jones RS, Utting JC. Comparison of vecuronium, atracurium and tubocurarine in normal patients and in patients with no renal function. *British Journal of Anaesthesia* 1984; **56**: 941–51.

37 Johnstone M, Mahmoud AA, Mrozinski RA. Cardiovascular effects of tubocurarine in man. *Anaesthesia* 1978; **33**: 587–93.

38 Baird WLM, Reid AM. The neuromuscular blocking properties of a new steroid compound, pancuronium bromide (a pilot study in man). *British Journal of Anaesthesia* 1967; **39**: 775–80.

39 Miller RD, Agoston S, Booij LHDJ, Kersten UW, Crul JF, Ham J. The comparative potency and pharmacokinetics of pancuronium and its metabolites in anaesthetised man. *Journal of Pharmacology and Experimental Therapeutics* 1978; **207**: 539.

40 Segredo V, Matthay MA, Sharma ML. Prolonged neuromuscular blockade after long-term administration of vecuronium in two critically ill patients. *Anesthesiology* 1990; **72**: 566–70.

41 Somogyi AA, Shanks CA, Triggs EJ. Disposition kinetics of pancuronium bromide in patients with total biliary obstruction. *British Journal of Anaesthesia* 1975; **49**: 1103.

42 Astley BA, Hughes R, Payne JP. Recovery of respiration after neuromuscular blockade with alcuronium. *British Journal of Anaesthesia* 1987; **59**: 206.
43 Hunter JM. Muscle relaxants. *Current Anaesthesia and Critical Care* 1989; 38–46.
44 Tamisto T, Welling I. The effect of alcuronium and tubocurarine on blood pressure and heart rate. A clinical comparison. *British Journal of Anaesthesia* 1969; **41**: 317.
45 Hunter JM. Adverse effects of neuromuscular blocking drugs. *British Journal of Anaesthesia* 1987; **59**: 46–60.
46 Savage TM, Blogg CE, Ross L. The cardiovascular effects of AH 8165. *Anaesthesia* 1973; **28**: 253.
47 Hunt TM, Hughes R, Payne JP. Preliminary studies with atracurium in anaesthetised man. *British Journal of Anaesthesia* 1980; **52**: 238P.
48 Stiller RL, Cook DR, Chakravorti S. *In vitro* degradation of atracurium in human plasma. *Anesthesia and Analgesia* 1985; **64**: 289.
49 Nigrovic V, Smith MA. In activation of atracurium evidence of an additional route. *Anesthesia and Analgesia* 1987; **66**: S129.
50 Hughes R, Chapple DJ. The pharmacology of atracurium: A new competitive neuromuscular blocking agent. *British Journal of Anaesthesia* 1981; **53**: 31.
51 Hunter JM, Jones RS, Utting JE. Use of atracurium in patients with no renal function. *British Journal of Anaesthesia* 1982; **54**: 1251.
52 Payne JP, Hughes R. Evaluation of atracurium in anaesthetised man. *British Journal of Anaesthesia* 1981; **53**: 45–54.
53 Madden AP, Hughes R, Payne JP. Recovery from neuromuscular blockade after infusion of atracurium. *British Journal of Anaesthesia* 1982; **54**: 226.
54 Hennis PJ, Fahey MR, Miller RD, Canfell D, Ski W-Z. Pharmacology of laudanosine in dogs. *Anesthesiology* 1984; **61**: A305.
55 Yate PM, Flynn PJ, Arnold RW, Weatherley BC, Simmonds RJ, Dopson J. Clinical experience and plasma laudanosine concentrations during atracurium infusions in the intensive therapy unit. *British Journal of Anaesthesia* 1987; **59**: 211–17.
56 Vine P, Boheimer N, Ward S, Weatherley B, Buick A, Smith I. Laudanosine pharmacokinetics after bolus atracurium in patients with hepatobiliary dysfunction. *British Journal of Anaesthesia* 1986; **58**: 1327.
57 Fahey MR, Rupp SM, Canfell C, Fisher DM, Miller RD, Sharma M, Castagnoli K, Hennis PJ. Effect of renal failure on laudanosine excretion in man. *British Journal of Anaesthesia* 1985; **57**: 1049–51.
58 Basta SJ, Savarese JJ, Ali HH, Moss J, Gionfriddo M. Histamine releasing properties of atracurium besylate (BW33A), metocurine and *d*-tubocurarine. *Anesthesiology* 1982; **57**: A201.
59 Hughes R. Atracurium – a year on. *Postgraduate Medical Digest*. Wellcome Foundation Limited, 1984.
60 Scott RPF, Savarese JJ, Basta SJ, Sunder N, Ali HH, Gargarian M, Gionfriddo M, Batson AG. Atracurium: Clinical strategies for preventing histamine release and attenuating the haemodynamic response. *British Journal of Anaesthesia* 1985; **57**: 550–3.
61 Nightingale DA, Bush GH. Atracurium in paediatric anaesthesia. *British Journal of Anaesthesia* 1983; **55**: 115S.
62 Hutton P. Atracurium: Automatic or manual. In: Jones RM, Payne JP, eds. *Recent developments in muscle relaxation; atracurium in perspective*. RSM Services International Congress and Symposium Series No 131. Published by RSM Services Ltd, 1988.
63 Eger BM, Flynn PJ, Hughes R. Infusion of atracurium for long surgical procedures. *British Journal of Anaesthesia* 1984; **56**: 447–52.
64 Griffiths RB, Hunter JM, Jones RS. Atracurium infusions in patients with renal failure on an ITU. *Anaesthesia* 1986; **41**: 375–81.
65 Savage DS, Sleigh T, Carlyle I. The emergence of Org NC45 from the pancuronium series. *British Journal of Anaesthesia* 1980; **52**: 3S.
66 Bencini A, Scaff AHJ, Sohn YJ, Kersten U, Agoston S. Clinical pharmacokinetics of vecuronium. In: Agoston S, ed. *Experiences with norcuron*. Symposium. Amsterdam: Excerpta Medica, 1983: 115.
67 Upton RA, Nguyen TL, Miller RD, Castaguoli NL. Renal and biliary elimination of vecuronium (Org NC45) and pancuronium in rats. *Anesthesiology and Analgesia* 1982; **61**: 313.
68 Hunter JM, Parker CJR, Jones RS *et al.* The use of different doses of vecuronium in patients with liver dysfunction. *British Journal of Anaesthesia* 1985; **57**: 758.
69 Fahey MR, Morris RB, Miller RD, Sony YJ, Cronelly R, Gencarelli P. Clinical Pharmacology of Org NC45 (Norcuron). *Anesthesiology* 1981; **55**: 6.
70 Spence A. Forward. In: Agoston S, ed. *Clinical experiences with norcuron*. Symposium. Amsterdam; Excerpta Medica, 1983.
71 Cronelly R, Fisher DM, Miller RD, Gencarelli P, Nguyen GN. Pharmacokinetics and pharmacodynamics of vecuronium (Org NC45) and pancuronium in anaesthetised humans. *Anesthesiology* 1983; **58**: 405.
72 Ward S, Meill EAM, Weatherley BC, Corrall IM. Pharmacokinetics of atracurium besylate in healthy patients (after a single intravenous bolus dose). *British Journal of Anaesthesia* 1983; **55**: 113S.
73 Feldman SA. The new muscle relaxants. In: Kaufman L, ed. *Anaesthesia review* 3. London: Churchill Livingstone, 1985; 64.
74 Smith CL, Hunter JM, Jones RS. Vecuronium infusions in patients with renal failure in an ITU. *Anaesthesia* 1987; **42**: 387–93.
75 Basta SJ, Savarese JJ, Ali HH, Sunder N, Moss J, Gionfriddo M, Embree P. Vecuronium does not alter serum histamine within the clinical dose range. *Anesthesiology* 1983; **59**: A273.
76 Clayton D. Asystole associated with vecuronium. *British Journal of Anaesthesia* 1986; **58**: 937.
77 Cozanitis DA, Erkola O. A clinical study into the possible intrinsic bradycardic activity of vecuronium. *Anaesthesia* 1989; **44**: 648.
78 Savarese JJ, Ali HH, Basta SJ, Embree PB, Scott RPF, Sunder N, Weakly JN, Wasula WB, El-Sayad HA. The clinical neuromuscular pharmacology of mivacurium chloride. A short-acting non-depolarising ester neuromuscular blocking drug. *Anesthesiology* 1988; **68**: 723–32.
79 Cook DR, Stiller RL, Weakly NZ. *In vitro* metabolism of mivacurium chloride (BE1090) and succinylcholine. *Anesthesia and Analgesia* 1989; **68**: 452.
80 Brandon BW, Woelfel SK, Cook DR, Weber S, Powers DM, Weakly JN. Comparison of mivacurium and suxamethonium administered by bolus and infusion. *British Journal of Anaesthesia* 1989; **62**: 493.

81 Savarese JJ, Ali HH, Basta SJ, Scott RPF, Embree PB, Wastila WB, Abu-Doria MM, Celb C. The cardiovascular effects of mivacurium chloride (BW1090U) in patients receiving nitrous-oxide–opiate–barbiturate anaesthesia. *Anesthesiology* 1989; **70**: 368–94.

82 Basta SJ, Savarese JJ, Ali HH, Embree PB, Schwartz AF, Rudd D, Wastila WB. Clinical pharmacology of doxacurium chloride. A new long-acting non-depolarising muscle relaxant. *Anesthesiology* 1988; **69**: 478–86.

83 Cashman JN, Luke JJ, Jones RM. Neuromuscular block with doxacurium (BWA938U) in patients with normal or absent renal function. *British Journal of Anaesthesia* 1990; **64**: 186–92.

84 Caldwell JE, Castagnoli KP, Canfell PC, Fahey MR, Lynham DP, Fisher DM, Miller RD. Pipecuronium and pancuronium: comparison of pharmacokinetics and duration of action. *British Journal of Anaesthesia* 1988; **61**: 693–7.

85 Muir AW, Houston J, Marshall RJ, Bowman WC, Marshall IG. Comparison of the neuromuscular blocking and autonomic effects of two short-acting muscle relaxants with those of succinylcholine in the anesthetised cat and pig. *Anesthesiology* 1989; **70**: 533–40.

86 Wierda JMKH, De Wit APM, Kuikenga K, Agoston S. Clinical observations on the neuromuscular blocking action of Org 9462, a new steroidal non-depolarising agent. *British Journal of Anaesthesia* 1990; **64**: 521–3.

87 Marshall IG, Harvey AL. Selective neuromuscular blocking properties of alpha-conotoxins *in vitro*. *Toxicon* 1990; **28**: 231–4.

88 Scott RPF, Marman J. Editorial III. Do we need more muscle relaxants? *British Journal of Anaesthesia*, 1988; **61**: 528–31.

89 Payne JP. Atracurium. In: Katz RL, ed. *Seminars in anesthesia* 3. Orlando: Grune & Stratton, 1984: 303.

90 Agoston S, Salt P, Newton D, Bencini A, Broomsma P, Ermann W. The neuromuscular blocking action of Org NC45 (norcuron): A new pancuronium derivative in anaesthetised patients. A pilot study. *British Journal of Anaesthesia* 1980; **52**: 53S.

91 Basta SJ, Ali HH, Savarese JF, Sunder N, Gionfriddo M, Gloutier G, Lineberry C, Cato EAE. Clinical pharmacology of atracurium besylate (BW33A). A new non-polarising muscle relaxant. *Anesthesia and Analgesia* 1982; **61**: 723.

92 Harrison P, Feldman SA. Intubating conditions with Org NC45. A preliminary study. *Anaesthesia* 1981; **36**: 874.

93 Scott RPF, Goat VA. Atracurium: its speed of onset. A comparison with suxamethonium. *British Journal of Anaesthesia* 1982; **54**: 909.

94 Foldes FF, Schwartz S, Ilias W, Lackner F, Nagashima H, Mayrhofer O. Rapid tracheal intubation with vecuronium: the priming principle. *Anesthesiology* 1984; **61**: A294.

95 Nagashima H, Nguyer HD, Lee S, Kaplan R, Duncalf D, Foldes FF. Facilitation of rapid endotracheal intubation with atracurium. *Anesthesiology* 1984; **61**: A289.

96 Jones RM. The priming principle. How does it work and how should we be using it? *British Journal of Anaesthesia* 1989; **61**: 1.

97 Bowman WC, Rodger IW, Houston J, Marshall RJ, McIndewar I. Structure : action relationships among some desacetoxy analogues of pancuronium and vecuronium in the anaesthetised cat. *Anesthesiology* 1988; **69**: 57–62.

98 Thisted B, Howardy P, Administration of atracurium using a simple infusion set. *Insights into Anaesthesia* 1987; **1**: 5–7.

99 Ewen A, Casson WR, Havitt PB, Adams AP. Atracurium infusions during neurosurgery. *Insights into Anaesthesia* 1987; **1**: 9–12.

100 Gissen AJ, Karis JG, Nastuk WL. Effect of halothane on neuromuscular transmission. *Journal of the American Medical Association* 1966; **197**: 770–4.

101 Hughes R, Payne JP. Interaction of halothane with non-depolarising neuromuscular blocking drugs in man. *British Journal of Clinical Pharmacology* 1979; **7**: 485.

102 Brett RS, Dilger JP, Yland KF *et al*. Isoflurane causes 'flickering' of the acetylcholine receptor channel: observations using the patch clamp. *Anesthesiology* 1988; **69**: 161.

103 Ngai SH. Action of general anaesthetics in producing muscle relaxation: interaction of anaesthetics with relaxants. In: Katz R L, ed. *Muscle relaxants*. Amsterdam: Excerpta Medica, 1975: 279.

104 Miller RD, Rupp SM, Fisher DM *et al*. Clinical Pharmacology of vecuronium and atracurium. *Anesthesiology* 1984; **61**: 444.

105 Buzello W, Schluermann D, Pollmaecher T, Spillner G. Unequal effects of cardiopulmonary bypass-induced hypothermia on neuromuscular blockade from constant infusion of alcuronium, *d*-tubocurarine, pancuronium and vecuronium. *Anesthesiology* 1987; **66**: 842.

106 Stead AL. The response of newborn infants to muscle relaxants. *British Journal of Anaesthesia* 1955; **27**: 124.

107 Goudsounzian NG. Maturation of neuromuscular transmission in the infant. *British Journal of Anaesthesia* 1980; **52**: 205.

108 Meretoja DA. Is vecuronium a long acting neuromuscular blocking agent in neonates and infants? *British Journal of Anaesthesia* 1989; **62**: 184.

109 Rupp SM, Castagnoli KP, Fisher DM, Miller RD. Pancuronium and vecuronium pharmacokinetics and pharmacodynamics in younger and elderly adults. *Anesthesiology* 1987; **67**: 45.

110 Katz RL. Neuromuscular effects of *d*-tubocurarine, edrophonium and neostigmine in man. *Anesthesiology* 1967; **28**: 327–36.

111 Viby-Mogensen J, Jorgensen BC, Ording H. Residual curarisation in the recovery room. *Anesthesiology* 1979: **50**: 539–41.

112 Lenmarken C, Lofstrom JB. Partial curarisation in the postoperative period. *Acta Anaesthesiologica Scandinavica* 1984; **28**: 260–2.

113 Beemer GH, Rozental P. Postoperative neuromuscular function. *Anaesthesia Intensive Care* 1986; **14**: 41–5.

114 Breecher HI, Todd DP. A study of deaths associated with anaesthesia and surgery based on a study of 599 548 anaesthetics in 10 institutions. 1948–1953 inclusive. *Annals of Surgery* 1954; **50**: 2–34.

115 Lunn JN, Hunter AR, Scott DB. Anaesthesia related surgical mortality. *Anaesthesia* 1983; **38**: 1090–6.

116 Katz R. Clinical neuromuscular pharmacology of pancuronium. *Anesthesiology* 1971; **34**: 550–6.

117 Cashman JN, Jones RM, Adams AP. Atracurium recovery; prediction of safe reversal times with edrophonium. *Anaesthesia* 1989; **44**: 805–7.

118 Payne JP, Hughes R. Clinical assessment of neuromuscular transmission. *British Journal of Clinical Pharmacology* 1981; **11**: 537.

119 Fragen RJ, Robertson EN, Booij LHD, Crul JF. A comparison of vecuronium and atracurium in man. *Anesthesiology* 1982; 57: A253.

120 Lunn J, Mushin W. Mortality associated with anaesthesia. Nuffield Provincial Hospitals Trust, 1982.

121 Cronelly R. Reversal, metabolism and elimination of neuromuscular blocking agents. *ASA Annual Refresher Course Lectures* 1987; 122.

122 Sneyd JR. Recovery after atracurium. *British Journal of Anaesthesia* 1987; **59**: 1477–8.

123 Jones RM. Reversal of residual neuromuscular blockade. In: Jones RM, Payne JP, eds. *Recent developments in muscle relaxants*. London: Royal Society of Medicine, 1988: 31–8.

124 Fisher DM, Cronelly R, Miller RD, Sharma M. Neuromuscular pharmacology of neostigmine in infants and children. *Anesthesiology* 1983; **59**: 220–5.

125 Hobbiger F. Pharmacology of anticholinesterase drugs. In: Zaimis E, ed. *Handbook of experimental pharmacology*, Vol 42. Berlin: Springer-Verlag, 1976; 487.

126 Astley BA. Recovery from neuromuscular blockade. In: Kaufman L, ed. *Anaesthesia review* **4**. London: Churchill Livingstone, 1987: 180–93.

127 Cronelly R, Morris RB, Miller RD. Edrophonium: duration of action and atropine requirement in humans during halothane anaesthesia. *Anesthesiology* 1982; **57**: 261–6.

128 Childs CS. Glycopyrrolate and the bowel. *Anaesthesia* 1984; **39**: 495.

129 Barnes JM, Duff JI. The role of cholinesterase at the myoneural junction. *British Journal of Pharmacology* 1953; **8**: 334–9.

130 Blaber LC, Bowman WC. Studies on the repetitive discharges evoked in motor nerve and skeletal muscle after injections of anticholinesterase drugs. *British Journal of Pharmacology* 1963; **20**: 326–44.

131 Baraka A. Antagonism of neuromuscular block by physostigmine in man. *British Journal of Anaesthesia* 1978; **50**: 1075–6.

132 Clutton M, Brock J. Death following neostigmine. *British Medical Journal* 1949; 1: 1007.

133 Mackintosh RR. Death following injection of neostigmine. *British Medical Journal* 1949; **1**: 852.

134 Kemp SW, Morton HJV. The effect of atropine and neostigmine on the pulse rate of anaesthetised patients. *Anaesthesia* 1962; **17**: 170–5.

135 King MJ, Milazkiewicz R, Carli F, Deacock AR. Influence of neostigmine on postoperative vomiting. *British Journal of Anaesthesia* 1988; **61**: 403–6.

136 Briscoe G. Shift in optimum rate of stimulation due to prostigmin. *Journal of Physiology* 1936; **86**: 48P.

137 Payne JP, Hughes R, Al-Azawi S. Neuromuscular blockade by neostigmine in anaesthetised man. *British Journal of Anaesthesia* 1980; **52**: 69–76.

138 Astley BA, Katz RL, Payne JP. Electrical and mechanical responses after neuromuscular blockade with vecuronium and subsequent antagonism with neostigmine and edrophonium. *British Journal of Anaesthesia* 1987; **59**: **983–8**.

139 Godhill DR, Wainwright AP, Stuart CS, Flynn PJ. Neostigmine after spontaneous recovery from neuromuscular blockade. Effect on depth of blockade monitored with train of four and tetanic stimuli. *Anaesthesia* 1989; **44**: 293–9.

140 Rupp SM, McChristian JW, Miller RD. Neostigmine antagonises a profound neuromuscular block more rapidly than edrophonium. *Anesthesiology* 1984; **61**: A297.

141 Booij LHDJ, Miller RD, Crul JF. Neostigmine and 4-aminopyridine antagonism of lincomycin and pancuronium neuromuscular blockade. *Anesthesia and Analgesia* 1978; **57**: 316–21.

142 Artusio JF, Riker WF, Wescoe WC. Studies on the interrelationship of certain cholinergic compounds. *Journal of Pharmacology and Experimental Therapeutics* 1952; **100**: 227–36.

143 MacFarlane DW, Pelikan EW, Unna KR. Evaluation of curarising drugs in man. *Journal of Pharmacology and Experimental Therapeutics* 1950; **100**: 382–92.

144 Doughty AG, Wylie WD. Antidotes to true curarising agents. *British Journal of Anaesthesia* 1952; **24**: 175–86.

145 Hunter A. Tensilon: a new anticurare agent. *British Journal of Anaesthesia* 1952; **24**: 175–86.

146 Nastuk WL, Alexander JT. The action of 3-hydroxyphenyldimethyl-ethylammonium (Tensilon) on neuromuscular transmission in the frog. *Journal of Pharmacology and Experimental Therapeutics* 1954; **111**: 302–28.

147 Sugai N, Payne JP. The skeletal muscle response to edrophonium during neuromuscular blockade by tubocurarine in anaesthetised man. *British Journal of Anaesthesia* 1975; **47**: 1087–92.

148 Morris RB, Cronelly R, Miller RD, Stanski DR, Rahey MR. Pharmacokinetics of edrophonium and neostigmine when antagonising tubocurarine neuromuscular blockade in man. *Anesthesiology* 1981; **54**: 399–402.

149 Randall LO, Lehman G. Pharmacological properties of some neostigmine analogues. *Journal of Pharmacology and Experimental Therapeutics* 1950; **99**: 16–32.

150 Smith CM, Mead JC, Unna KR. Antagonism of tubocurarine. Time course of action of pyridostigmine, neostigmine and edrophonium in vivo and in vitro. *Journal of Pharmacology and Experimental Therapeutics* 1957; **120**: 215–28.

151 Blaber LC. The effect of facilitatory concentrations of decamethonium on the storage and release of transmitter at the neuromuscular junction in the cat. *Journal of Pharmacology and Experimental Therapeutics* 1970; **175**: 664–72.

152 Blaber LC. The mechanism of the facilitatory action of edrophonium in the cat. *British Journal of Pharmacology* 1972; **46**: 498–507.

153 Donati F, Ferguson A, Bevan DR. Twitch depression and train of four ratio alter antagonism of pancuronium with edrophonium, pyridostigmine or neostigmine. *Anesthesia and Analgesia* 1983; **62**: 314–16.

154 Jones RM, Pearce AC, Williams JP. Recovery characteristics following antagonism of atracurium with neostigmine or edrophonium. *British Journal of Anaesthesia* 1984: **56**: 453–7.

155 Baird WLM, Bowman WC, Kerr WJ. Some actions of Org MC45 and of edrophonium in the anaesthetised cat and in man. *British Journal of Anaesthesia* 1982; **54**: 375–84.

156 Baird WLM, Kerr WJ. Reversal of atracurium with edrophonium. A pilot study in man. *British Journal of Anaesthesia* 1983; **55**: 635.

157 Bevan DR. Reversal of pancuronium with edrophonium. *Anaesthesia* 1979; **34**: 614–19.

158 Kopman A. Edrophonium antagonism of pancuronium induced neuromuscular blockade in man. *Anaesthesia* 1979; **51**: 139–42.

159 Ferguson A, Egerszegi P, Bevan DR. Neostigmine, pyridostigmine and edrophonium as antagonists of pancuronium. *Anesthesiology* 1980; **53**: 390–4.

160 Astley BA, Hughes R, Payne JP. Antagonism of atracurium induced neuromuscular blockade by neostigmine or edrophonium. *British Journal of Anaesthesia* 1986; **58**: 1290–5.

161 Katz RL. Pyridostigmine (Mestinon) as an antagonist of tubocurarine. *Anesthesiology* 1967; **28**: 528–34.

162 Fogdall RP, Miller RD. Antagonism of tubocurarine and pancuronium induced neuromuscular blockades by pyridostigmine in man. *Anesthesiology* 1973; **39**: 504–9.

163 Miller RD, Van Nyhuis LS, Eger EI, Vitez TS, Way WL. Comparative times to peak effect and duration of action of neostigmine and pyridostigmine. *Anesthesiology* 1974; **41**: 27–33.

164 Cronelly R, Stanski DR, Miller RD, Sheiner LB, Sohn YJ. Renal function and the pharmacokinetics of neostigmine in anaesthetised man. *Anesthesiology* 1979; **51**: 222–6.

165 Morris RB, Cronelly R, Miller RD, Stanski DR, Fahey MR. Pharmacokinetics of edrophonium in anephric and renal transplant patients. *British Journal of Anaesthesia* 1981; **53**: 1311–13.

166 Ali HH, Wilson RS, Savarese JJ, Kitz RJ. The effect of tubocurarine on the indirectly elicited train of four muscle response and respiratory measurement in humans. *British Journal of Anaesthesia* 1975; **47**: 570–3.

167 Foldes FF, Monte AP, Brunn HM, Wolfson B. Studies with muscle relaxants in unanaesthetised subjects. *Anesthesiology* 1961; **22**: 230–6.

168 Johansen SH, Jorgensen M, Molbech S. Effect of tubocurarine on respiratory and non-respiratory muscle power in man. *Journal of Applied Physiology* 1964; **19**: 990–4.

169 Gal TJ, Smith TC. Partial paralysis with tubocurarine and the ventilatory response to carbon dioxide. *Anesthesiology* 1976; **45**: 22–8.

170 Wymore ML and Eisele JH. Differential effects of tubocurarine on inspiratory muscles and two peripheral muscle groups in anaesthetised man. *Anesthesiology* 1978; **48**: 360–2.

171 Harrison GG. Death attributable to anaesthesia. A 10 year survey (1967–1976). *British Journal of Anaesthesia* 1978; **50**: 1041–6.

172 Pavlin EG, Holle R, Schoene RB. Recovery of airway protection compared with ventilation in humans after paralysis with tubocurarine. *Anesthesiology* 1989; **70**: 381–5.

173 Engbaek J, Ostergaard D, Viby Mogensen J, Svovgaard LT. Clinical recovery and train of four ratio measured mechanically and electromyographically following atracurium. *Anesthesiology* 1989; **71**: 391–5.

174 Christie TH, Churchill-Davidson HC. The St Thomas' Hospital Nerve Stimulator in the diagnosis of prolonged apnoea. *Lancet* 1958; **i**: 776.

175 Paton WDM, Waud DR. The margin of safety of neuromuscular transmission. *Journal of Physiology* 1967; **191**: 59–90.

176 Ali HH, Utting JE, Gray C. Stimulus frequency in the detection of neuromuscular block in human. *British Journal of Anaesthesia* 1970; **40**: 967–77.

177 Gissen AJ, Katz RL. Twitch, tetanus and post-tetanic potentiation as indices of nerve muscle block in man. *Anesthesiology* 1969; **30**: 481–7.

178 Roberts DV, Wilson A. Physiology of neuromuscular transmission. In: Green R, ed. *Electromyography in diagnosis and treatment of myasthenia gravis*. London: Heinemann, 1969: 14.

179 Savarese JJ, Ali HH. Accurate prediction of individual metocurine dosage by clinical observation of the threshold of fade on train of four stimulation. Meeting of the American Society of Anaesthetists. New Orleans (Abstract). 1977.

180 Viby-Mogensen J, Engbaek J, Jensen NH, Jorgensen BC, Ording H. New developments in clinical monitoring of neuromuscular transmission: monitoring without equipment. Clinical experiences with novocuron. Symposium. Geneva, 1983: 66–71.

181 Lam HS, Cass NM, Ng KC. Electromyographic monitoring of neuromuscular block. *British Journal of Anaesthesia* 1981; **53**: 1351–6.

182 Windsor JPW, Sebel PS, Flynn PJ. The neuromuscular transmission monitor. *Anaesthesia* 1985; **40**: 146–51.

183 Kalli I. The effect of surface electrode positioning on the compound action potential evoked by ulnar nerve stimulation in anaesthetised infants and children. *British Journal of Anaesthesia* 1989; **62**: 188–93.

184 Merton PA. Voluntary strength and fatigue. *Journal of Physiology* 1954; **123**: 553.

185 Feldman SA, Tyrell MF. A new theory of the termination of muscle relaxants. *Proceedings of the Royal Society of Medicine* 1970; **63**: 692.

186 Wali FA, Payne JP. Effect of atracurium on release of acetylcholine at the vertebrate neuromuscular junction in response to nerve stimulation at 2 Hz and at 50 Hz. *British Journal of Anaesthesia* 1983; **55**: 911–12.

187 Walts LF, Levin N, Dillon JB. Assessment of recovery from tubarine. *Journal of the American Association* 1970; **213**: 1894–6.

188 Ali HH, Kitz RJ. Evaluation of recovery from non-depolarising neuromuscular block using a digital neuromuscular transmission analyser. *Anesthesia and Analgesia* 1973; **52**: 740–3.

189 Miller RD. Antagonism of neuromuscular blockade. *Anesthesiology* 1976; **44**: 318–30.

190 Engbaek J, Ostergaard D, Viby Mogensen J. Double burst stimulation (DBS): A new pattern of nerve stimulation to identify residual neuromuscular blockade. *British Journal of Anaesthesia* 1989; **62**: 274–8.

191 Drenck ME, Ueda M, Olsen NV, Engbaek J, Jensen E, Skovgaard LT, Strat, C, Viby Mogensen J. Manual evaluation of residual curarisation using double burst stimulation: A comparison with train of four. *Anesthesiology* 1989; **70**: 578–81.

192 Gill SS, Donati F, Bevan DR. Clinical evaluation of double burst stimulation. Its relationship to train of four stimulation. *Anaesthesia* 1990; **45**: 543–8.

193 Brull SJ, Cronelly NR, Silverman DG. Correlation of train of four and double burst stimulation ratios at varying amperages. *Anesthesia and Analgesia* 1990; **71**: 489–92.

194 Viby-Mogensen J, Jensen E, Werner MN, Kirkegaardnielsen HK. Measurement of acceleration: a new method of monitoring neuromuscular function. *Acta Anaesthesiologica Scandinavica* 1988; **32**: 45–8.

195 Viby-Mogensen J, Howardy-Hansen P, Chraemmer-Jorgensen B. Post-tetanic count (PTC): a new method of evaluating an intense non-depolarising neuromuscular blockade. *Anesthesiology* 1981; **55**: 458–61.

196 Stanec A, Conelly T, Lobel E, Monzon R, Baker T. The recovery from residual neuromuscular blockade in surgical outpatients. *Anesthesia and Analgesia* 1990; **70**: S390.

13

The Adrenergic Nervous System—Adrenoceptor Agonists

AG Ramage, AD Scott, RO Feneck, NH Kellow

INTRODUCTION

Oliver and Schafer first reported the pressor effects of extracts of suprarenal gland on various animal tissues in their classical experiments of 1895, and since then the sympathetic nervous system has been the focus of considerable interest. The term 'sympathomimetic', which relates the action of a specific agent to innervation by the sympathetic nervous system, was described by Barger and Dale in 1911. Subsequently, the structure and function of the naturally occurring catecholamines adrenaline, noradrenaline and dopamine have been characterized together with those of the directly and indirectly acting synthetic agents. Furthermore, drugs antagonizing the effects of sympathetic stimulation have been investigated, and their actions described at all levels of the sympathetic axis, from the cerebral cortex to the adrenergic receptor where they either augment or antagonize sympathetic stimulation. Clearly, it is necessary to have a broad understanding of the sympathetic pathways involved if a consideration of the pharmacology of drugs affecting adrenergic transmission is to be undertaken.

TYPES OF ADRENOCEPTOR

The catecholamines noradrenaline, adrenaline and dopamine are remarkable biological agents which, despite their structural simplicity, can induce responses as diverse as glycogenolysis, aggregation of platelets, contraction of the myometrium, increased contractility of the heart and lipolysis of adipose tissue. Earlier in this century, Dale observed that ergot alkaloids could inhibit some of the physiological responses caused by catecholamines. In addition, the pressor action of adrenaline was reversed to a depressor action after treatment with ergotoxine (the name given to the first alkaloid fraction isolated from ergot). It had also been observed by Cannon that the physiological actions of stress that are mediated by the sympathetic nervous system (tachycardia and inhibition of gut motility) were similar to the actions of adrenaline. The ability of the sympathetic portion of the autonomic nervous system and adrenaline to cause both inhibitory and excitatory effects was clarified by Ahlquist with the development of the concept that the sympathetic nervous system and adrenaline act via at least two different types of receptor.

The method proposed by Ahlquist in 1948, which is still one of the major ways used to identify receptors today, involves the relative potency of agonists in eliciting a tissue response and of blocking that response with a particular antagonist. Ahlquist carried out a study to identify drugs that would cause uterine relaxation in order to develop a treatment for dysmenorrhoea. He used a series of catecholamines including noradrenaline, adrenaline and isoprenaline and found that the rank order of potency of these drugs on organ responses could be placed in two distinct groups:

Adrenaline > noradrenaline ≫ isoprenaline (α)
Isoprenaline > adrenaline ≥ noradrenaline (β)

indicating two types of catecholamine receptor which he termed 'α' and 'β'. Furthermore, he found that all α responses were excitatory, except for that on the gut which caused intestinal relaxation, while all β responses were inhibitory, except for that on the heart. The demonstration by Powell and Slater that dichloroisoproterenol (dichloroisoprenaline) was selective in blocking the inhibitory effects of catecholamines, and by Moran and Perkins that this drug also blocked the excitatory effects of catecholamines on the heart, led to acceptance of Ahlquist's theory of two types of adrenoceptor.

Subdivision of β-adrenoceptors

Land, again comparing the potency of various catecholamine derivatives on various tissues containing β-adrenoceptors, concluded in 1967 that there must be two types of β-adrenoceptor (β_1 and β_2). Noradrenaline and adrenaline were found to be equipotent on β_1-adrenoceptors while adrenaline is a 100 times more potent on β_2-adrenoceptors than noradrenaline. This probably reflects the role of adrenaline as a circulating hormone. Innervated β-adrenoceptors are of the β_1 subtype; that is, heart (positive chronotropy and inotropy), kidney (renin secretion) and adipose tissue (lipolysis).

However, it should be noted that tissues do not always contain a homogeneous population of β-adrenoceptors; for instance, the heart has also been shown to contain β_2-adrenoceptors while the lungs (bronchial smooth muscle) also contain β_1-adrenoceptors. Further, it has been suggested that adipocytes contain an atypical β-adrenoceptor termed β_3. The existence of three types of β-adrenoceptor is supported by the identification of three different genes for this receptor.

Subdivision of α-adrenoceptors

It had been observed in the late 1930s that contraction caused by adrenergic transmission could be potentiated by α-adrenoceptor antagonists. However, it was the attempts to interpret Brown and Gillespie's observation that α-adrenoceptor antagonists could increase the release of noradrenaline from the cat spleen, that led to the subdivision of the α-adrenoceptor, although the increase in noradrenaline could have been due to blockade of neuronal uptake by the antagonist used. It was only when Starke and Langer in the early 1970s moved to studying a sympathetic response mediated by β-adrenoceptors and also used an α-adrenoceptor antagonist that did not interfere with uptake of transmitter, that the correct interpretation was made. This was that α-adrenoceptors are involved in controlling, by negative feedback, the release of noradrenaline. These receptors were termed presynaptic α_2-adrenoceptors (receptors with this function are also known as autoreceptors): the postsynaptic receptors were termed α_1-adrenoceptors (heteroreceptors). However, it is now known that α_2-adrenoceptors exist postsynaptically as well as presynaptically. Evidence indicates that noradrenaline released from sympathetic nerves acts on postsynaptic α_1-adrenoceptors while circulating catecholamines act preferentially on postsynaptic α_2-adrenoceptors.

It should be noted that β_2-autoreceptors are involved in the positive feedback control of noradrenaline release from sympathetic nerve endings.

More recently α_1-adrenoceptors have been divided into α_{1A}-, α_{1B}- and α_{1D}- adrenoceptors, while α_2-adrenoceptors have been divided into α_{2A}-, α_{2B}- and α_{2C}-adrenoceptors.

DISTRIBUTION AND FUNCTION OF ADRENOCEPTORS

The distribution of α- and β-adrenergic receptors in various tissues in man is shown in Table 13.1. In common with the diversity of action of the sympathetic nervous system, the effects of the α and β adrenoceptor activation are wide ranging and consequent on these effects is a correspondingly large spectrum of clinical applications. However, their principal uses are directed towards the manipulation of function of smooth and cardiac muscle. The β_2-agonists remain in the forefront of the acute and chronic treatment of asthma. Adrenaline remains the first-line treatment of life-threatening anaphylaxis, having favourable actions on inflammatory cells and mediator release together with the advantageous circulatory effects, and the catecholamines remain first-line treatment for the management of the failing circulation in a number of settings. The β-blockers are widely used in the therapy of cardiac disease, and are currently one of the most prescribed group of drugs with a large range of clinical applications for the anaesthetist.

A knowledge of the distribution and function (Table 13.1) of the various adrenoceptors is essential for the understanding of the pharmacology of the agonist and antagonist agents. The mechanism of action of this class of drugs on end-organs is related not only to the type but also to the relative density of receptors present in different tissues. These factors and the responsiveness of the particular receptor are not constant but exist in a continuous state of flux, with modulation occurring as a result of pathophysiological states.

Age is now known to alter the response of effector organs to sympathomimetics. There appears to be a down-regulation of β-activated inotropic and chronotropic responses with variable alteration of α-mediated vascular effects. This phenomena is thought to be brought about by excessive production of noradrena-

TABLE 13.1 Distribution and function of adrenoceptors

EFFECTOR ORGAN	RECEPTOR	RESPONSE
CVS		
Central vasomotor	β_2	Hypotension
Vasculature		
All blood vessels	α_1/α_2	Constriction
Skeletal vessels	β_2	Dilatation
EDRF	α_2	Release (vasodilatation)
Heart		
SA node	β_1	Increase in HR
Atria	β_1	Increase in contractility & conduction velocity
A-V node & conducting system	β_1	Increase in conduction velocity
Ventricles	β_1	Increase in conduction velocity & contractility
Respiratory system		
Central	α_2	Decrease in ventilation
Smooth muscle	β_2	Dilatation
Platelets	α_2	Aggregation, granule release
Eye		
Radial muscle of iris	α_1	Contraction (mydriasis)
Ciliary muscle	β_2	Relaxation
Gastrointestinal tract		
Motility/tone	α_2 & $\beta_{1\&3}$	Decrease (inhibition of ACh release)
Sphincter	α_1	Contraction
Salivary glands	α_2	Inhibition of ACh release (reduction)
Urinary bladder		
Detrusor	β_2	Relaxation
Trigone & sphincter	α_1	Contraction
Kidney		
Juxtaglomerular	β_1	Renin release
	α_2	Inhibition of ADH release/block ADH action
		Increase GFR/inhibition renin release, all mediating *diuresis*
Sex organs		
Vas deferens/prostate	α_1	Contraction (ejaculation)
Uterine smooth muscle	α_1	Contraction
	β_2	Relaxation
Liver	β_2/α	Glycogenolysis
	α	Gluconeogenesis
Pancreas	β_2	Increase insulin/glucagon release
	α_2	Decreased insulin release (B cells)
Adipose tissue	β_1/β_3	Lipolysis
Mast cells	β_2	Inhibition of mediator release
Skeletal muscle		
Membrane Na^+-K^+ ATPase	β_2	Stimulation (hypokalaemia)
	β_2	Tremor
	β_2	Glycogenolysis and lactate production

ADH, antidiuretic hormone; GFR, glomerular filtration rate.

line attendant on the gradual increase in sympathetic tone that occurs with advancing age.

α-Adrenoceptors

Although many sympathomimetics are α-agonists it was not understood until the 1970s that the α-adrenoceptor population was heterogeneous. In addition to the proposed postjunctional receptors, α-adrenoceptors are also located on presynaptic and prejunctional adrenergic nerve endings. Activation of these receptors inhibits the release of noradrenaline. This confers a system of negative feedback as the release of noradrenaline is modulated. Agonist drugs possess a spectrum of selectivity for the two subclasses of receptor. Methoxamine and phenylephrine are moderately selective for α_1-receptors with dexmedetomidine being the most selective α_2 agonist. It has an

TABLE 13.2 Selectivity of various α-adrenergic agonists. Reproduced and adapted from Maze M, Tranquilli W. *Anesthesiology* 1991; 74(3): 581–605.

$\alpha_1 > \alpha_2$	$\alpha_1 = \alpha_2$	$\alpha_2 > \alpha_1$	$\alpha_2 \gg \alpha_1$
Methoxamine	Adrenaline	Clonidine	Azepexole
Phenylephrine	Noradrenaline	α-methylnoradrenaline	Medetomidine
		Xylazine	Dexmedetomidine

$>$ indicates 100 times more selective
$\gg$ indicates 1000 times more selective

α_2/α_1 selectivity ratio of approximately 2000:1. Clonidine has a ratio of 220:1 with important α_1 effects appearing at relatively low doses. Noradrenaline and adrenaline demonstrate equal affinity for both receptors (Table 13.2).

α_1-Adrenoceptors (postjunctional) are responsible for vasoconstriction mediated by the classical α_1 agonists (e.g. phenylephrine). In addition postjunctional α_1-receptors mediate positive inotropism thought until recently to be an exclusively β-adrenoceptor-mediated activity. Phenylephrine has been shown to double contractility in comparison to a seven-fold increase demonstrated by isoprenaline. It has been proposed that a degree of co-operation exists between α_1- and β-adrenoceptor-mediated cardiac inotropy.

Using selective α- and β-blockade, the contribution of pure alpha-1 inotropy is 30–50% in the absence of β-mediated effects. When α- and β-effects occur concurrently this contribution falls to 20–30%. Controversy exists over the role of vasoconstrictors in the maintenance of arterial blood pressure. Recent studies have demonstrated the benefits of the use of infusions of noradrenaline in vasodilated septicaemic patients who have remained hypotensive despite adequate volume loading and the use of inotropic agents (see Chapter 17). The use of vasoconstrictors where there is inappropriate and potentially deleterious vasodilation such as that occurring following the institution of local anaesthetic subarachnoid or epidural blockade, is also widespread. However, there may be adverse effects on myocardial oxygen balance in patients with coronary artery disease. Clearly the maintenance of an adequate perfusion pressure in the presence of a critical coronary artery stenosis is vital, but an increased afterload and hence cardiac work and myocardial oxygen consumption may be deleterious.

The management of patients with critical coronary stenoses undergoing the stress of anaesthesia and both cardiac and non-cardiac surgery presents a dilemma. The controversy exists as to whether α-mediated vasoconstriction may be beneficial by preventing steal from 'at-risk' areas, or deleterious by reducing flow to already underperfused areas of myocardium. In the presence of a critical epicardial stenosis, coronary vasoconstriction in the transmural coronary vasculature may protect the vulnerable subendocardium from 'steal' under conditions where flow is critical for example during tachycardia. The distribution of α_1- and α_2-receptors in the coronary circulation has not yet been fully evaluated but it would appear that α-receptor-mediated coronary vasoconstriction is protective against the 'steal' phenomenon in patients with coronary artery disease.

α-Adrenoceptors are also implicated in the production of ischaemia-induced arrhythmias. Animal work has shown a proliferation of α-receptors on the surface of myocytes in response to ischaemia. The stimulus is as yet unknown but a link to acyl-carnitines is proposed, and antagonism of acyl carnitine transferase or prazosin-mediated α-blockade reduces the incidence of such arrhythmias. Independent workers have demonstrated the protective effect of α_1 blockade with prazosin in this setting, although this effect is limited by the vasodilatation produced by prazocin.

Prejunctional α_2-adrenoceptors act as a negative feedback mechanism reducing the release of noradrenaline from adrenergic neurones. In the CNS, activation of this receptor subpopulation results in a general reduction in central sympathetic activity. Clonidine, a pure agonist at the α_2-adrenoceptor, produces sedation and reduces anaesthetic requirements. Its use is discussed later.

β-Adrenoceptors

Cardiac β-adrenoceptors were defined as the β_1 subtype, with the bronchiolar and smooth muscle types classified as β_2-adrenoceptors. However, with the discovery that both types co-existed in the heart, the anatomical classification was discontinued. Functional studies have demonstrated that both subtypes are functionally coupled to adenylate cyclase and contribute to the positive inotropic response to both endogenous and exogenous β-agonists. It is now agreed that activation of adenylate cyclase in β_1- and β_2-adrenoceptors leads to the accumulation of 3, 5 cyclic adenosine monophosphate (cAMP) and that this is responsible for the observed effects. The concentration of cAMP is determined by the relative activity of adenyl cyclase and the phosphodiesterase enzymes. Intracellular cAMP is responsible for the activation of certain protein kinases, which in the case of bronchial and vascular smooth muscle leads to the reduction of phosphorylation of the myosin light chain, causing a reduction of calcium-dependent coupling of actin and myosin leading to smooth muscle relaxation.

The explanation for differing effects of the sympathomimetic agents on different organs and smooth muscle groups is complex. The effect of β-adrenoceptor agonists on smooth muscle is one of relaxation. This is in contrast to its effect on other tissues, for example the pancreas, where they stimulate the secretion of insulin from islet cells.

A third receptor subtype (β_3) is now known to be present in a number of peripheral tissues, notably on brown adipose tissue and on certain smooth muscles of the large intestine. The action of sympathomimetic drugs to stimulate adipocyte lipolysis and heat production (thermogenesis) is now thought to be mediated through this receptor subtype. The effects of β_3-adrenoceptor stimulation by selective β_3-adrenoceptor agonists in patients have suggested a possible role in the treatment of obesity (see Chapter 33). Non-selective β-agonists tend to have unacceptable side-effects from their stimulant actions on cardiovascular β_1-adrenoceptors and β_2-receptors on skeletal muscle which lead to tremor.

It was shown over 10 years ago that the total population of cardiac β-adrenoceptors, and more recently that the β_1 subpopulation in particular, are down-regulated in patients with chronic heart failure. The β_2 population remains unaltered (although they are numerically proportionately increased) and appears to retain a near full inotropic response to selective β_2-agonists. The chronic elevated levels of circulating noradrenaline found in patients with heart failure is a likely explanation for this down-regulation given that noradrenaline has a 10-fold increase in affinity for β_1-adrenoceptors. The discovery of this change in receptor density clearly has implications for the therapeutic use of β-agonists in such patients.

The presence of β-adrenoceptors in bronchial smooth muscle mediating relaxation and hence bronchodilatation has been known for some time. The receptors on airway and vascular smooth muscle and on airway epithelium appear to be exclusively of the β_2 type. Those present on submucosal glands and alveolar walls are of mixed type. *In vitro*, β-agonists have a direct relaxant effect on preconstricted or spontaneously contracting bronchiolar smooth muscle. In this setting they are extremely potent. *In vivo*, they are less effective at relaxing preconstricted muscle in human bronchioles. Salbutamol is a partial agonist compared with isoprenaline. The relaxant effect seen with the β-agonists is physiological, since it seems to occur regardless of the stimulus.

As long ago as 1936 adrenaline was shown to inhibit the release of histamine, and all the β-agonists are potent inhibitors of histamine release in a variety of settings. The receptors on mast cells are of the β_2 type as are those present on lymphocytes and leukocytes. It is difficult to separate the actions of this class of drugs when considering their ability to reduce the response to inhaled antigen and exercise. Some of the effects may be due to reduction of mediator release whereas others are probably due to a reduction in the response of the airway to the stimulus. The β- adrenoceptor agonists tend to reduce the degree of mucosal oedema associated with asthma but this is probably secondary to the suppression of mediator release rather than a direct effect on capillaries. Work performed on the actions of sympathomimetics in the presence of acid-induced pulmonary injury has shown an increased capillary leak. They have been shown to enhance mucociliary clearance and stimulate the production of mucus. The use of β_2-agonists in the treatment of reversible airways obstruction is widespread.

SYMPATHOMIMETICS

All the sympathomimetic amines are based on a skeleton formed by the β-phenylethylamine molecule. The term 'catecholamine' is derived from the name given to the nucleus of such agents as dopamine, adrenaline, dobutamine, isoprenaline and noradrenaline (Fig 13.1). This 'catechol' nucleus is formed by the hydroxyl substitution of the 3- and 4-positions on the benzene ring. The presence of no more than two carbon atoms separating the benzene ring and the amino group confers maximal sympathomimetic activity on the molecule. Further substitutions at these carbon atoms and at the terminal amino group allow almost limitless variation in structure and function (Fig. 13.1).

The sympathomimetics all have activity at both α- and β-adrenoceptors, each agent possessing differing affinity for each receptor. Thus this class of drugs exhibits a spectrum of activity at adrenoceptors.

In general, β-activity is enhanced by increasing the size of the radical on the amino group and α-activity enhanced by reducing it. An inspection of the structures of isoprenaline, adrenaline and noradrenaline possessing $-CH(CH_3)_2$, $-CH_3$, and $-H$ respectively bears this out.

Substitution at the benzene ring has important implications for activity. 3-, 4-Hydroxylation confers maximal α- and β-activity and the absence of one of these groups reduces potency. 3-, 5-Hydroxylation produces enhanced β_2-specificity seen in the case of terbutaline, a drug used in the treatment of bronchospasm.

The indirectly acting agents such as ephedrine, which release noradrenaline from sympathetic nerves, tend to lack the hydroxylation of the benzene ring or side-chain, and the lipophilicity of a given molecule will affect its ability to cross the blood–brain barrier and produce central effects.

Directly acting sympathomimetics

Noradrenaline

Noradrenaline activates both types of α-adrenoceptor and the β_1-adrenoceptor and therefore would be expected to cause all the effects described for the acti-

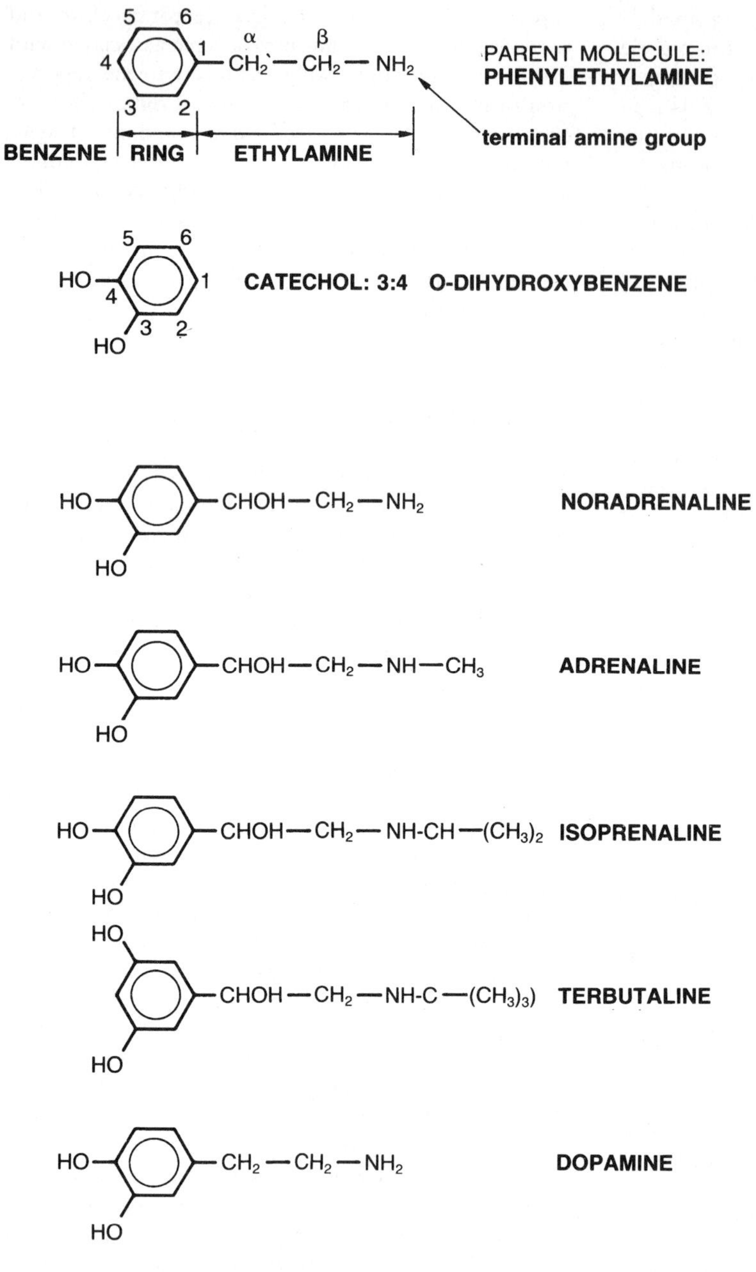

CH_2—CH_2—NH_2 PARENT MOLECULE: **PHENYLETHYLAMINE**

BENZENE RING **ETHYLAMINE** **terminal amine group**

CATECHOL: 3:4 O-DIHYDROXYBENZENE

CHOH—CH_2—NH_2 **NORADRENALINE**

CHOH—CH_2—NH—CH_3 **ADRENALINE**

CHOH—CH_2—NH-CH—$(CH_3)_2$ **ISOPRENALINE**

CHOH—CH_2—NH-C—$(CH_3)_3$) **TERBUTALINE**

CH_2—CH_2—NH_2 **DOPAMINE**

FIGURE 13.1 Structures of some of the commonly used sympathomimetics.

vation of these receptors. However, it would be incorrect to list these as effects caused by noradrenaline when it is given iv or subcutaneously, as the effects observed would depend on the ability of noradrenaline to gain access to these receptor sites. The most obvious effect of noradrenaline will be vasoconstriction through activation of α-adrenoceptors causing a rise in blood pressure. However, the increase in heart rate and circulating renin caused by activation of β_1-adrenoceptors will be masked by a baroreceptor reflex elicited by the rise in blood pressure causing a withdrawal of sympathetic drive to these receptors and, in the case of the heart, an increase in vagal drive combining to cause a reflex bradycardia. High doses will also cause glucose to be liberated from the liver and, interestingly enough, contractions of the pregnant uterus.

Subcutaneous noradrenaline and adrenaline in very low doses will cause local sweating by acting on α-adrenoceptors on apocrine sweat glands. These are non-thermoregulatory. The eccrine glands are involved in thermoregulation and are activated through muscarinic receptors; this cholinergic innervation is part of the sympathetic nervous system.

Adrenaline

Adrenaline differs from noradrenaline in that it has a more marked effect on β-adrenoceptors. In this respect bronchodilatation will be observed with adrenaline. It should be noted that adrenaline will also cause inhibition of mediator release from mast cells; that is, 'stabilization' of mast cells. Furthermore, adrenaline can enter the CNS causing symptoms of fear, anxiety and restlessness. Adrenaline's action on the cardiovascular system depends on dose. Low doses cause tachycardia and an increase in the force of contraction of the heart, which will cause an increase in systolic blood pressure. However, diastolic blood pressure will be reduced, because of the fall in peripheral resistance due to adrenaline causing the skeletal muscle vasculature to dilate. As there will be no overall change in mean blood pressure, a baroreceptor reflex will not be activated. Higher doses will begin to activate vascular α-adrenoceptors causing vasoconstriction and therefore an increase in total peripheral resistance so that diastolic pressure will rise and mean blood pressure will increase causing activation of the baroreceptor reflex. Another important action of adrenaline will be to increase skeletal muscle tremor by activation of β_2-adrenoceptors.

Adrenaline also causes relaxation of uterine smooth muscle by inhibiting tone and contraction, especially in the last trimester, and causes relaxation of gastrointestinal muscle. The overall action of adrenaline on the bladder results in hesitancy which may contribute to urinary retention by relaxing the detrusor muscle, through activation of β_2-adrenoceptors, and contracting the trigone and sphincter muscles, through activation of α-adrenoceptors.

In the eye, activation of α_1-adrenoceptors by adrenaline will cause dilation of the pupil (mydriasis). However, adrenaline can also cause a decrease in intraocular pressure by increasing outflow of aqueous humour through the trabecular meshwork and may reduce the production of aqueous humour. In this respect it is interesting that the non-selective β-adrenoceptor antagonist timolol can also reduce intraocular pressure.

Metabolic effects

Adrenaline elevates blood glucose (hyperglycaemia) and lactic acid (hyperlactacidaemia) by activation of β_2-adrenoceptors causing a rise in cAMP by increasing the activity of adenylate cyclase. This will cause glycogen to be broken down in the liver and muscle, first to glucose-1-phosphate and then to glucose in the liver cells and to lactic acid in the muscle cells. Adrenaline also initially inhibits insulin release by activation of α_2-adrenoceptors and then increases insulin release by activation of β_2-adrenoceptors. A similar biphasic effect is seen with serum potassium activation of α-adrenoceptors (subtype unknown) causing release of potassium from the liver (hyperkalaemia) and then activation of β_2-adrenoceptors on skeletal muscle causing increased uptake of potassium by stimulation of Na^+-K^+ ATPase causing hypokalaemia. Adrenaline also raises plasma free fatty acid levels by inducing lipolysis at adipocytes by activation of triglyceride lipase which accelerates the breakdown of triglycerides to form free fatty acids and glycerol. The receptor involved is thought to be an atypical β-adrenoceptor which has been termed a β_3-adrenoceptor.

Absorption and fate

Neither adrenaline nor noradrenaline can be orally absorbed as they are rapidly conjugated and oxidized in the gastrointestinal mucosa and by first-pass metabolism by the liver. Adrenaline or noradrenaline when given subcutaneously will be absorbed slowly due to the vasoconstriction that they cause. However, absorption is more rapid when given intramuscularly. In the blood, both adrenaline and noradrenaline are rapidly removed by neuronal uptake (uptake 1) and extraneuronal uptake (uptake 2) and then metabolized by either monoamine oxidase (MAO-A) found in mitochondria or catechol-O-methyltransferase (COMT). Drugs that interfere with these processes, such as antidepressants, will prolong the actions of adrenaline and noradrenaline.

Ephedrine

Ephedrine is both an α- and β-adrenoceptor agonist. It is not metabolized by MAO-A and is therefore active orally (see below).

β-Adrenoceptor agonists – isoprenaline and salbutamol

Isoprenaline (Fig. 13.1) differs from adrenaline in that it does not activate α-adrenoceptors. Thus isoprenaline causes a fall in blood pressure associated with a large tachycardia. Part of this tachycardia will be due to a baroreceptor-mediated increase in sympathetic drive as well as a withdrawal of any vagal tone. As salbutamol (Fig. 13.2), which is not a catecholamine, activates

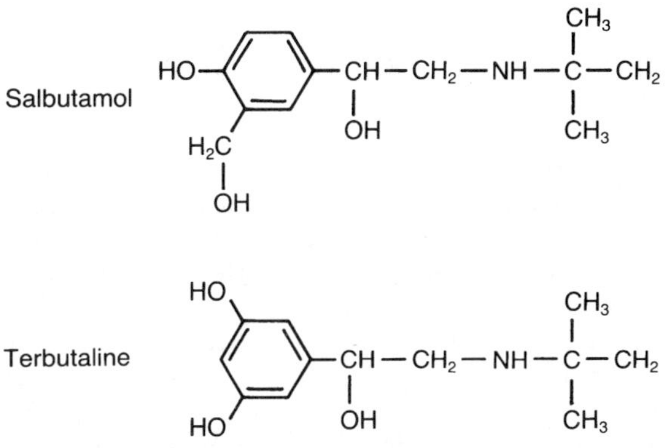

Salbutamol

Terbutaline

FIGURE 13.2 Structure of β_2-adrenoceptor agonists.

only β_2-adrenoceptors the fall in blood pressure will be associated with a smaller tachycardia as this is indirectly due to the fall in blood pressure activating the baroreceptor reflex. Both drugs will cause tremor through activation of β_2-adrenoceptors on skeletal muscle plus bronchodilation as well as 'stabilizing' mast cells. Isoprenaline also stimulates the CNS whereas salbutamol seems weaker in this action. Uterine smooth muscle relaxation can be induced by both drugs.

Metabolic effects

Both isoprenaline and salbutamol will cause hyperglycaemia. This will be less than that observed with adrenaline. However, both isoprenaline and salbutamol are just as effective in increasing free fatty acid concentrations and inducing hypokalaemia as adrenaline.

Absorption and fate

Both drugs can be orally absorbed although, as a result of sulphate conjugation in the gut, considerably less is available than when given parenterally. Isoprenaline is, however, absorbed through the oral mucosa so it can be given sublingually. Removal of isoprenaline from the blood differs from adrenaline in that it is not removed by neuronal uptake and is resistant to metabolism by MAO-A although it is metabolized by COMT. Salbutamol is subject to first-pass metabolism in the liver so when given orally about half is excreted as the sulphate conjugate, while the remaining half is excreted unchanged via the urine.

Terbutaline is a β_2 selective bronchodilator and is not affected by COMT. It has a long duration of action and has a place in the management, not only of obstructive airways disease, but also status asthmaticus.

α-Adrenoceptor agonists

There are two groups of agonists, those related to the catecholamines, phenylephrine and methoxamine, which are selective for the α_1-adrenoceptor and the imadazolines, clonidine, naphazoline and oxymetazoline, which are selective for α_2-adrenoceptors.

Phenylephrine and methoxamine (α_1-adrenoceptor agonists)

Phenylephrine differs from adrenaline in that it lacks a hydroxyl group on the benzene ring in the para (C4) position and has little or no effect on β-adrenoceptors (Fig. 13.3). The actions of phenylephrine are similar to those of noradrenaline although it is less potent in raising blood pressure than noradrenaline and has a longer duration of action. Methoxamine is similar to and has a more prolonged action than phenylephrine (Fig. 13.3). Interestingly, methoxamine has been reported to cause piloerection (goose pimples) and a desire to micturate. Neither drug has been reported to have central actions.

Absorption and fate

Phenylephrine is only metabolized by MAO-A whereas methoxamine is unaffected by either MAO-A or COMT, explaining the longer duration of action of these compounds when compared with noradrenaline.

α_2-Adrenoceptor agonists

The substances naphazoline and oxymetazoline as well as clonidine are vasoconstrictor agents (Fig. 13.4), although surprisingly clonidine is not used as a vasoconstrictor, for which it was originally developed, but is used as an antihypertensive. In fact all of these compounds can cause a fall in blood pressure associated with a bradycardia. The ability of these drugs to induce hypotension varies and is due to an action on central α_2-adrenoceptors which causes sympathoinhibition and sedation. Another feature that these drugs have in common is the ability to cause a rebound effect when administration is stopped. In the case of naphazoline and oxymetazoline, which are used as nasal decongestants, a rebound vasodilatation, that is, drug-induced rhinitis, is caused. Clonidine, used as a hypotensive agent, causes rebound hypertension. This rebound effect is believed to be related to the ability of these drugs to interfere with the negative feedback control of noradrenaline release from sympathetic nerve endings.

All these drugs can cause dry mouth, dizziness and headache. Fluid retention is also observed with clonidine although this is difficult to explain as a consequence of activation of α_2-adrenoceptors, as activation of renal α_2-adrenoceptors causes a reduction in renin release. Whether this effect is presynaptic or postsynaptic remains to be determined. Clonidine can also cause constipation, presumably by acting on α_2-adrenoceptors which reduce the release of acetylcholine from parasympathetic nerve endings in the gut. High doses of clonidine can also cause hyperglycaemia,

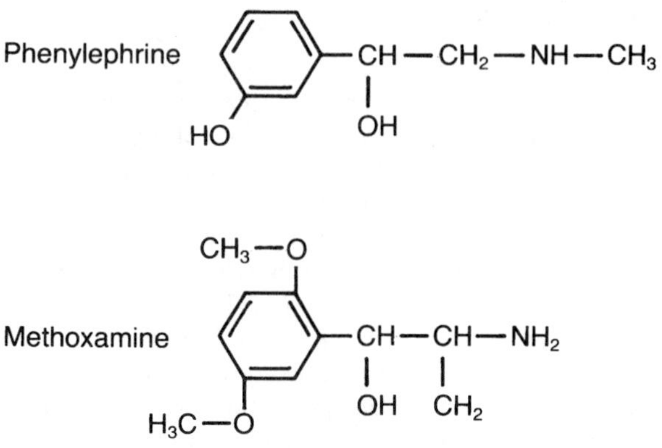

Phenylephrine: (HO-substituted benzene ring)—CH(OH)—CH_2—NH—CH_3

Methoxamine: (CH_3—O and H_3C—O substituted benzene ring)—CH(OH)—CH(CH_2)—NH_2

FIGURE 13.3 Structure of α_1-adrenoceptor agonists.

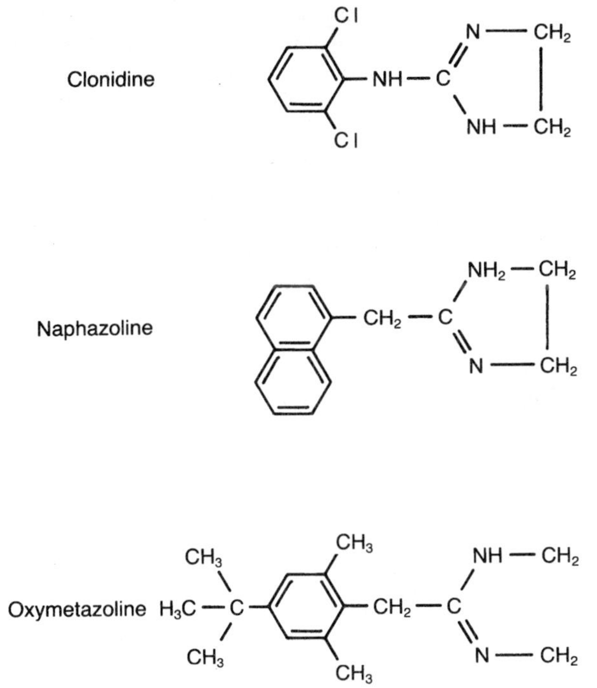

Clonidine

Naphazoline

Oxymetazoline

FIGURE 13.4 Structure of α_2-adrenoceptor agonists.

again due to a reduction in insulin release through activation of α_2-adrenoceptors.

Absorption and fate

As these compounds are lipid soluble they are easily absorbed by any route and broken down by the liver.

Indirectly acting sympathomimetics

Compounds that are classified as indirectly acting sympathomimetics are compounds that depend for their action on an intact existence of intraneuronal noradrenaline stores. These compounds are tyramine, ephedrine and amphetamine (Fig. 13.5). The action of these compounds is further complicated by varying direct effects as well as varying abilities to stimulate α- and β-adrenoceptors. Further responses of these drugs decline with repetitive use (tachyphylaxis).

Indirect sympathomimetics act by entering the nerve terminal via neuronal uptake, although they can diffuse in and, once inside the nerve terminal, displace noradrenaline from vesicular stores causing a flooding of the neuroeffector junction with noradrenaline. Administration of tyramine can be considered as a way of chemically stimulating the sympathetic nervous system. It has very weak direct sympathomimetic actions. Its effects are only seen clinically when patients are undergoing MAO inhibitor therapy for depression since it is a good substrate for MAO. Large amounts are found in a variety of foods such as cheese, Chianti wine, etc. In patients on MAO inhibitors the sympathomimetic response observed is known as the 'cheese' reaction. Tyramine does not cross the blood–brain barrier, so its actions are restricted to the periphery.

Ephedrine is orally active and causes a rise in blood pressure through α-adrenoceptor activation although it can excite β-adrenoceptors as indicated by a bronchodilator action. It produces tachycardia, although this can sometimes be masked, presumably due to a baroreceptor-induced bradycardia. It also causes a reduction in intestinal motility and relaxation of uterine smooth muscle. Ephedrine will also cause dilation of the pupil. It also has a central stimulatory action including that on the respiratory centre.

Ephedrine is largely excreted unchanged in the urine ($t_{1/2}$ = 3–6 h); however, the rate of excretion is increased if the urine is acidified.

Amphetamine differs from ephedrine in one major respect in that it has a very potent central stimulant action.

SITE OF ACTION OF DRUGS THAT AFFECT ADRENERGIC TRANSMISSION

There are many sites at which adrenergic transmission can be affected. Alteration of input from higher centres with tranquillizers and sedatives will have effects on the peripheral elements of the CNS. The mechanism for these phenomena remains obscure but it is clear that cortical functions (mood, emotion, etc.) exert an effect on sympathetic outflow. More specifically, drugs acting on adrenergic neurones, either centrally or peripherally, autonomic ganglia or at the pre- or post-synaptically situated adrenergic receptors have important actions on the various functions of the sympathetic nervous system.

Tyramine

Ephedrine

Amphetamine

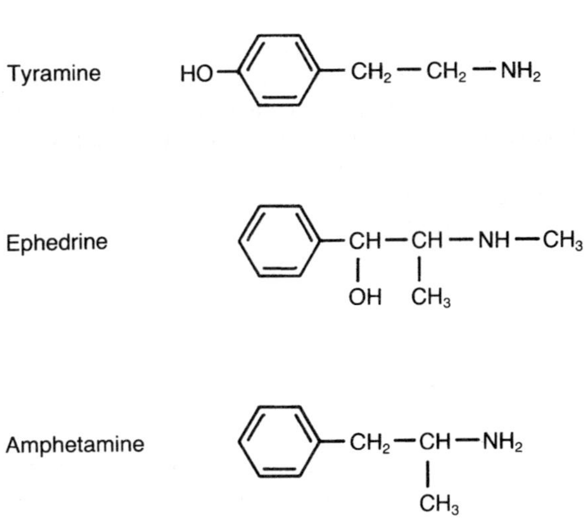

FIGURE 13.5 Structure of indirect acting sympathomimetics.

The cerebral cortex

Major and minor tranquillizers, independent of any peripheral effects, reduce the level of sympathetic outflow, as is the case with anaesthetic and analgesic drugs. The magnitude of the effect on sympathetic outflow is variable and governed by the prevailing level of sympathetic activity. Conversely, CNS stimulants will increase the level of sympathetic activity.

The midbrain and brain stem

A number of agents influence sympathetic activity by their actions on preganglionic neurones in the midbrain. Reserpine, formerly used in the treatment of hypertension exerts its action by depletion of noradrenaline and serotonin in neurones situated mainly in the brain but also in the adrenal medulla. It achieves this by irreversibly preventing the uptake of noradrenaline into chromaffin granules in adrenergic neurones. Normal function is only restored by the provision of new granules. There is an initial-sympathomimetic effect following administration of reserpine as the level of free noradrenaline transiently rises, but the subsequent production of noradrenaline is reduced as free catecholamine exerts a negative feedback on tyrosine hydroxylase.

Agonist activity at central α_2-receptors situated postsynaptically in the brain stem is responsible for reductions in sympathetic activity. The α_2-agonist clonidine was originally developed for the central control of blood pressure. Together with an increasing number of related substances, clonidine is thought to exert its action on central α_2-adrenoceptors although the precise site of action remains obscure. At lower doses the central α_2-adrenoceptor agonist effects predominate over the peripheral vasoconstrictor actions and mediate reductions in sympathetic outflow, probably via actions on receptors situated in the lateral reticular nucleus and the locus coeruleus which normally mediates a pressor response. This reduction in outflow is essential to the hypotensive action of these agents since it is not seen in tetraplegic patients receiving clonidine. The agent methyldopa uses the potent action of its metabolite α-methylnoradrenaline on central α_2-adrenoceptors and was formerly a first-line drug used in the treatment of hypertension. The β-adrenoceptor antagonists are thought in part to exert their actions via an, as yet unidentified, central mechanism.

Sympathetic ganglia

Blockade of sympathetic ganglia will reduce the rate of depolarization and thus the release of noradrenaline from postsynaptic adrenergic neurones. Alteration of ganglionic transmission will affect both the sympathetic and parasympathetic nervous systems, and the response of a particular target organ will depend on the ambient predominance of sympathetic or parasympathetic tone. There are few uses for drugs altering ganglionic transmission in clinical practice since the unwanted parasympathetic effects limit their acceptability. Trimetaphan, a short-acting agent used in the production of controlled hypotension, is the only agent used in this context. Its hypotensive action is achieved by a combination of ganglionic blockade and histamine release.

Post-ganglionic neurones

The release of stored noradrenaline from adrenergic nerves can be either enhanced in the case of the indirectly acting sympathomimetics (e.g. amphetamines) or inhibited in the case of the adrenergic neurone-blocking drugs. This latter mechanism has been an important method for inhibiting noradrenergic transmission. The guanidine derivative guanethidine is the best known drug of this class (which also includes bethanidine and debrisoquine) and is taken up by adrenergic nerves and stored in intraneuronal granules where it displaces noradrenaline (see also Chapter 14). The method of uptake is similar to that applied to endogenous catecholamines (uptake 1) and is blocked by the tricyclic antidepressants (e.g. imipramine). There is an initial hypertensive response following guanethidine administration as existing noradrenaline is displaced from stores. Thereafter, stimulation of the nerve is associated with release of guanethidine. Following establishment of treatment, denervation supersensitivity develops in the effector receptors. In contrast tyramine, ephedrine and amphetamine cause a short-lived release of noradrenaline producing a transient sympathomimetic effect.

Another method of interfering with noradrenergic transmission at this level is by the inhibition of reuptake of noradrenaline into the postganglionic nerve endings leaving released noradrenaline open to enzymatic degradation and diffusion away from the synaptic cleft. The rauwolfia alkaloids (reserpine) exert their effect partly by this mechanism.

DOPAMINE RECEPTORS

There are known to be at least two types of dopamine receptor in the periphery; those that cause renal and mesenteric vasodilatation being known as D_1 receptors, and those that inhibit the release of noradrenaline from sympathetic nerves known as D_2. Dopamine, when given iv, causes mesenteric and renal vasodilatation and increases urine output. Dopamine also stimulates β_1-adrenoceptors on the heart, causing mainly a positive inotropic response. At high doses some α-adrenoceptor agonist actions will be observed, resulting in vasoconstriction.

Dopamine is the immediate precursor of noradrenaline. It is produced by the action of aromatic amino acid decarboxylase (DOPA decarboxylase) and metabolized by dopamine β-hydroxylase (to noradrenaline) or by MAO. Dopmaine is preferentially oxidized by an isozyme of MAO known as MAO-B. The selective MAO-B inhibitor selegiline can therefore be used to restore dopamine levels in the brain without affecting the metabolism of the other monoamines. Until recently, dopamine agonists and antagonists have been employed mainly for CNS disorders including Parkinsonism (see Chapter 23) and schizophrenia (see p. 337).

Role of dopamine receptors

Classification of dopaminergic receptors into D_1 and D_2 occurred over 10 years ago. More recently they have been subdivided into D_1, D_2, D_3 and D_4 receptors. Those in the D_1 subtype are situated on the smooth muscle of the blood vessels supplying the kidney, the mesentary and the myocardium. Activation leads to vasodilatation of these vascular beds with resulting increases in blood flow. The potential usefulness of dopaminergic stimulation in conditions where there is borderline tissue perfusion is evident. In addition D_1 receptors situated on the renal tubules mediate promotion of natriuresis and diuresis. Further receptors situated on the juxtaglomerular apparatus mediate an increase in renin secretion tending to antagonize these effects. However, the overall result of stimulation of D_1 receptors is a promotion of sodium and water excretion.

D_2 receptors were first discovered on postganglionic sympathetic nerve terminals. These prejunctional receptors mediate inhibition of noradrenaline release causing hypotension and bradycardia. The effects are complex and depend on the prevailing level of sympathetic tone. In general, the higher the level of sympathetic tone the greater the effects of D_2 receptors agonism. Inhibition of aldosterone release is brought about by activation of D_2 receptors situated on the zona glomerulosa. This further promotes sodium and water excretion. The action of sympathomimetic agents on β_1-adrenoceptors situated on the juxtaglomerular apparatus will tend to oppose these effects by promoting renin release.

The use of dopaminergic stimulation with the endogenous catecholamine dopamine to increase organ perfusion is widespread and newer agents such as dopexamine, fenoldopam and ibopamine are rising to prominence in the treatment of cardiac failure and situations of compromised organ perfusion.

Dopamine

Dopamine is 3-hydroxytyramine and is the precursor of noradrenaline. Many of the actions of dopamine result from the release of endogenous noradrenaline and at higher rates of infusion its pharmacological effects are similar to, although less potent than, noradrenaline. Combined with these α- and β-effects are those resulting from activation of specific dopamine D_1 receptors (qv). At lower doses (< 2 μg/kg/min) the dopaminergic actions predominate, producing hypotension and renal, coronary and mesenteric vasodilatation. Increasing the dose (2–5 μg/kg/min) produces β-mediated cardiac effects, and α-mediated vasoconstriction occurs when the dose exceeds 10 μg/kg/min. It is these vasoconstrictor actions, together with the production of arrhythmias, that limit the usefulness of dopamine in the support of the failing circulation. The effectiveness of dopamine at these moderate doses in improving cardiac function has led to the development of drugs that combine the dopaminergic and β-effects while lacking the α-mediated vasoconstriction.

Dopexamine

Dopexamine is a relatively new compound that is structurally related to dopamine. Like dopamine, it can only be given intravenously. It has been shown to activate postjunctional dopamine receptors equipotently with dopamine, and possesses substantial β_2 activity, has no β_1 activity and unlike dopamine has no activity at α-receptors. However, at higher doses it has been reported to inhibit the neuronal reuptake of noradrenaline and therefore mimics the action of dopamine at these doses. The actions of the drug have been studied in patients with congestive cardiac failure in whom it induces beneficial effects on stroke volume, cardiac output and systemic vascular resistance. It also produces renal vasodilatation. Dopexamine appears to be effective in the treatment of such patients and its natriuretic effects may offer an added bonus.

The potential usefulness of dopamine receptor stimulation is evident in situations of borderline organ perfusion. However, there are few reports identifying actual benefit in terms of the preservation of organ function, particularly renal. Numerous studies have failed to demonstrate reductions in the incidence of renal impairment in various high-risk settings such as following cardiac surgery.

Fenoldopam

This benzazepine compound is the only orally active dopaminergic agonist available. However, bioavailability is poor. It is also available in the intravenous form. Specific fenoldopam receptors have been characterized on renal tubules and studies have shown functional similarity to dopaminergic receptors. Fenoldopam produces hypotension, renal vasodilatation, natriuresis and diuresis. The latter two actions are produced without significant haemodynamic effects indicating a tubular site of action. It has been shown to be effective in reducing blood pressure while enhancing renal flow.

Ibopamine

This is an orally active prodrug. Ibopamine is a butyric acid ester of the active *n*-methyldopamine. Once absorbed, it is converted by non-specific plasma esterases to the active form epinine, which has pharmacological properties similar to those of dopamine. It exhibits a favourable haemodynamic profile with a fall in systemic vascular resistance, a modest inotropic effect and almost no effect on the heart rate. Its diuretic effect mediated via its action on D_1 receptors is another potential benefit.

Dobutamine

Dobutamine, a synthetic analogue of dopamine (Fig. 13.6), was introduced in 1975 and was synthesized in order to reduce the potentially deleterious chronotropic effects of isoprenaline. It possesses minimal α- and β_2-activity and thus exerts its effects through β_1-activity. The resulting increases in cardiac output are reputedly achieved in the absence of significant tachycardia and the resulting vasodilatation optimizes ventricular–vascular coupling whereby improvements in cardiac function are combined with afterload reduction. This minimizes the increase in myocardial oxygen consumption seen with other sympathomimetics. In practice, however, tachyarrhythmias, particularly sinus tachycardia, are fairly frequent with its use at higher doses. Dobutamine has been shown to be clinically useful in the support of the failing circulation in a wide range of settings including following acute myocardial infarction, cardiac surgery and in a variety of intensive care settings, and is regarded by many to be the drug of choice in such settings.

The ability of dobutamine to produce vasodilatation probably occurs as a result of direct action on the vasculature coupled with a reduction in sympathetic activity attendant on the alleviation of cardiac failure. Cardiac filling pressures are reduced by dobutamine to a greater degree compared with dopamine and greater increases in cardiac output seen, largely due to the absence of α-adrenoceptor activity.

CLINICAL ASPECTS OF SYMPATHOMIMETIC DRUGS

Introduction

The sympathomimetic agents have actions on a wide variety of tissues. The majority of their use in clinical practice is directed towards harnessing their actions on the heart and smooth muscle, both vascular and bronchial. This group of drugs remains the mainstay of acute positive inotropic intervention as well as in the field of resuscitation. Reasons for this dominance include favourable pharmacological profiles, predictable pharmacological responses including adverse reactions and a wide range of haemodynamic responses. This also applies to their use as bronchodilators. The use of α_2-adrenoceptor agonists, for example clonidine, originally licensed for use as antihypertensive agents is increasing. This group of drugs, most notably medetomidine and xylazine, has been used extensively in veterinary practice as an adjunct to general anaesthesia or as sole sedative–analgesic agents, and is currently undergoing intensive clinical research for potential use in human anaesthetic practice. The ability of these compounds to reduce anaesthetic and opioid requirements when administered intravenously or into the epidural or subarachnoid space has been the main feature accounting for this interest. A detailed consideration of their use appears below under α_2-Adrenoceptor agonists.

Pharmacology

The catecholamines are ineffective when taken orally, being inactivated in the gut mucosa and by first-pass metabolism in the liver. They are, however, well absorbed from the buccal mucosa and lung. Once ingested catecholamines are rapidly removed from

Dobutamine (slight β_2)

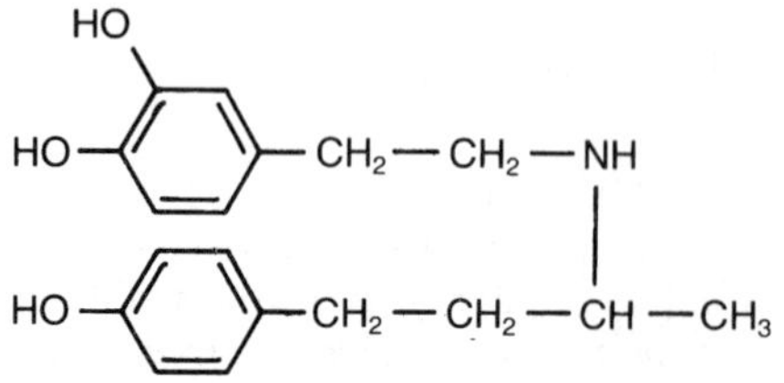

HO, HO–(ring)–CH_2—CH_2—NH
HO–(ring)–CH_2—CH_2—CH—CH_3

Prenalterol

HO–(ring)–O—CH_2—CH(OH)—CH_2—NH—CH(CH_3)$_2$

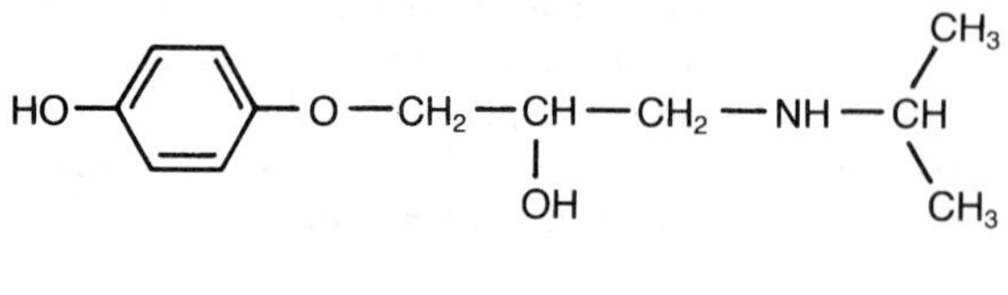

FIGURE 13.6 Structure of β_1-adrenoceptor agonists.

the circulation either by active uptake mechanisms or via metabolism by COMT or MAO.

There are two active processes by which catecholamines are removed from the synaptic cleft: uptake 1 and uptake 2. In uptake 1 catecholamines are actively taken up into the sympathetic nerve terminal itself where they can be re-incorporated into vesicles. This is an important method of termination of the actions of adrenaline and noradrenaline but not of isoprenaline. This process is inhibited by agents such as cocaine and the tricyclic antidepressant imipramine. Uptake 2 involves the uptake of catecholamines including isoprenaline into non-neuronal tissue such as smooth muscle where enzymatic degradation occurs. COMT substitutes a methyl group at the 3-position on the catechol nucleus and MAO cleaves the molecule between the α C-atom and the amine group. The catecholamines are largely excreted either unchanged or as metabolites in the urine.

The non-catecholamines in contrast are effective when given orally and frequently have longer durations of action. This is due to a relative resistance to the inactivating effects of the liver enzymes and also to the fact that larger doses are commonly given. Following ingestion they are partially conjugated during first-pass metabolism. In the case of salbutamol, about 95% is absorbed, of which half is conjugated with sulphate. Reductions in water solubility will increase absorption following oral administration. Non-catecholamines are not affected by uptake 1 or 2, and molecules lacking one or both of the hydroxyl groups at the 3- or 4-positions are resistant to the action of COMT. The non-catecholamines, in addition, tend to have relatively large substitutions at the amine group rendering them less amenable to degradation by MAO. They tend to be excreted in the urine either unchanged or as conjugates and rely on the existence of an intact adrenergic nerve terminal for their actions. They enter the nerve terminal by diffusion or by neuronal uptake where they then displace noradrenaline from storage vesicles, for example phenylethylamines such as octopamine. In addition, some have direct agonist activity on adrenergic receptors, and others are taken up into storage vesicles at the expense of noradrenaline and, having much less agonist activity on adrenoceptors than noradrenaline, cause a greatly diminished response to neuronal depolarization. This constitutes the 'false transmitter' concept.

The half-life of the sympathomimetics commonly used, particularly in the acute setting of cardiovascular support, is short, being of the order of 2–3 min. Steady-state blood levels are thus achieved in 10–15 min. This removes the requirement for a loading dose which may be undesirable in unstable situations. Furthermore, on discontinuation of the infusion, drug is removed from the circulation rapidly with the corresponding rapid disappearance of any unpleasant cardiovascular effects. In addition, the correct administration of this class of drug is rarely associated with any 'surprises' – be these idiosyncratic reactions or other unexpected effects. There is a degree of tachyphylaxis associated with their use and the changes in pharmacodynamics referred to earlier will affect their efficacy. They have, on the whole, a predictable pharmacological profile. An important drug interaction occurs when there is concomitant administration of antipsychotic drugs such as the monoamine oxidase inhibitors (MAOIs). In the adrenergic nerve terminal noradrenaline is accumulated in two forms. The stable pool contains noradrenaline combined with adenosine triphosphate, and the labile pool contains noradrenaline ready for immediate release. There is constant exchange between the two stores, with MAO as the mediator. Inhibition increases the size of the stable and hence the labile pool. Administration of the indirectly acting drugs, such as ephedrine, will result in unpredictable and sometimes dangerous levels of hypertension as the larger stores are released. Denervation supersensitivity will augment the effects of exogenous directly acting agents, and these effects will be prolonged. Caution is advised when used with MAOIs. Since the reaction between MAO and MAOI is largely irreversible, noradrenaline stores are likely to be prolonged for several weeks following discontinuation of the drug while synthesis of fresh enzyme occurs.

Chronic therapy with other antidepressant agents such as reserpine, which depletes adrenergic neurones of noradrenaline, and imipramine, which prevents uptake 2, will increase the likelihood of the necessity of careful dosage administration.

CATECHOLAMINES

Adrenaline

The use of adrenaline as a combined vasopressor and inotropic agent is now well established in clinical practice. It remains in the front line of agents for use in cardiopulmonary resuscitation, supporting the failing circulation, and in the treatment of anaphylaxis.

Adrenaline acts on both α- and β-adrenoceptors and actions on target organs are complex. It elevates arterial blood pressure by increasing myocardial contractility, increasing heart rate and producing peripheral vasoconstriction. It produces coronary vasodilatation not only secondary to increased myocardial oxygen consumption, but also due to a direct vasodilator action. Indeed, at low doses adrenaline has a predominantly vasodilator action. it is less chronotropic than isoprenaline and considered by some to be suitable for the treatment of low cardiac states when combined with vasodilators such as glyceryl trinitrate. The dose of adrenaline required to produce useful increases in cardiac output may vary widely. Adrenoceptor downgrading referred to earlier, together with a degree of tachyphylaxis attendant on the use of all the catecholamines in this setting, will lead to a degree of dosage unpredictability.

Adrenaline has an important role in the treatment of patients with septic shock. In such patients, despite significant vasodilatation leading to increases in cardiac output, myocardial depression is evident. The mechanism remains controversial but the presence of a number of myocardial depressant factors is proposed. This, combined with the vasodilator effects of endotoxins, alters the response to infused catecholamines and dosage requirements are much higher. The drawbacks of vasoconstriction with potential organ hypoperfusion found with adrenaline have to be balanced against the increased inotropy produced. In addition, at high doses the production of arrhythmias may limit the usefulness of adrenaline.

Adrenaline remains the most useful drug in cardiopulmonary resuscitation. The α-mediated vasoconstriction maintains perfusion pressure to the benefit of the cerebral and coronary circulations. The β-effect may prove successful in restarting an asystolic heart but may increase the myocardial oxygen consumption in ventricular fibrillation. However, the assessment of pure α-adrenoceptor agonists in this setting has failed to reveal any improvement in outcome. The dose of adrenaline used in the CPR setting has been the subject of a recent review. Current guidelines suggest that adrenaline be administered in increments of 1 mg for the treatment of asystole. However, recent animal work has suggested that this may be insufficient with larger doses increasing coronary perfusion pressure, myocardial blood flow and resuscitation success. Human studies comparing 1 and 5 mg showed a significantly improved success rate but hospital discharge rate was not improved. Administration of resuscitation drugs by the tracheal route is sometimes necessary owing to the problem of intravenous access. Satisfactory blood levels of lignocaine and atropine can be achieved by this route but, possibly due to pulmonary capillary vasoconstriction, this route has not proved reliable for adrenaline in the doses normally used. For optimal levels the dose should be nebulized into the distal trachea in a large volume of diluent.

The metablic effects of adrenaline have been described above (p. 179).

Noradrenaline

This endogenous catecholamine is synthesized and stored in granules in the adrenergic neurones. It has effects on both α- and β-receptors and therefore its haemodynamic effects are dependent on the particular clinical scenario in which it is used. Its predominant action is one of vasoconstriction, which is more intense than that seen with adrenaline. The rise in blood pressure elicits a baroreceptor-mediated reflex bradycardia. The powerful vasoconstrictor activity raising arterial blood pressure has been used to raise perfusion pressure in shocked patients, theoretically to shunt blood from skin and muscle to the more vital cerebral, myocardial and renal vascular beds. In the setting of sepsis syndrome, where there is profound arterial hypotension with an inappropriately low systemic vascular resistance, the use of a vasoconstrictor is logical and there are several reports that carefully titrating an infusion of noradrenaline to achieve vasoconstriction and raise perfusion pressure is clinically beneficial. Clearly, this should only be undertaken while employing invasive haemodynamic monitoring. Certain assumptions are made – namely that the vasoconstrictors act on the 'overdilated' vessels shunting blood to the hypoperfused regions and not those supplying already underperfused tissues. However, despite the fact that noradrenaline has been shown to cause reductions in renal blood flow, its use in this setting has repeatedly been shown to improve arterial blood pressure and urine flow using relatively high doses (0.5–1 μg/kg). In the management of certain patients requiring therapy with noradrenaline, the addition of low-dose dopamine may prevent excessive renal vasoconstriction thereby reducing the risk of renal dysfunction.

Like adrenaline, noradrenaline is rapidly removed by neuronal and extraneuronal uptake. They are metabolized by either mitochondrial MAO or COMT. The inactive metabolite vanillyl mandelic acid is excreted in the urine.

Isoprenaline

Isoprenaline is a potent non-selective β-adrenoceptor agonist causing increased myocardial contractility and heart rate. There is often a significant fall in systemic vascular resistance mediated by the predominantly β-effect. It is of use in the management of bradydysrhythmias including those due to excessive β-adrenoceptor blockade and complete heart block. There is little evidence to support its use as a sole inotropic agent, for example following myocardial infarction, since its chronotropic effects tend to affect adversely myocardial oxygen balance. There is concern that the coronary vasodilator action may actually induce a degree of steal. Isoprenaline has been shown to increase infarct size experimentally. It is, however, used to support the failing circulation following cardiac surgery in both adults and children.

β_2-Adrenoceptor agonists

The non-catecholamine analogue salbutamol acts purely on β_2-adrenoceptors and is used widely in the treatment of bronchoconstriction. This and terbutaline are the most widely used sympathomimetics used in the treatment of asthma. Using the inhaled route of administration, the documented side-effects of tachycardia and tremor are minimized since efficacy is improved with delivery directly into the bronchi allowing a reduction of the dose.

There are minor differences between the various other β_2-agonists available in this setting. Rimiterol, being a catecholamine, is shorter acting than the other agents which commonly last for between 3 and 5 h. Salmeterol has recently been introduced. Its longer duration of action allows twice-daily administration. Unlike the shorter-acting agents, it is not suitable for the treatment of the acute attack. The dose of all the β_2-agonists can be reduced by the concomitant administration of inhaled corticosteroids with which they have an additive bronchodilator effect.

The phosphodiesterase inhibition seen *in vitro* with theophylline suggested that this class of agents might produce a synergistic effect on the airways when combined with β-agonists. This has not proved to be the case in the clinical setting, with theophylline producing a mere 5–10% increase over that seen with β-agonists alone. One study showed that aminophylline, when added to inhaled β-agonists for the treatment of acute asthma, contributed nothing more than an increase in side-effects. The use of ipratropium bromide similarly increases the FEV_1 by a further 5–10% over the increase seen with β-agonists alone. Both isoprenaline and salbutamol have similar metabolic effects to adrenaline and in particular can cause hypokalaemia although this is not usually a problem when using the correct dose of a metered inhaler. Reductions in serum potassium concentration of the order of 0.4–0.9 mmol/l have been recorded in the acute situation and these changes are not sustained with chronic therapy. Diabetic ketoacidosis has been triggered in diabetic patients by β-agonists.

These agents are absorbed following oral administration although extensive sulphate conjugation in the gut limits bioavailability. Isoprenaline is effective if taken sublingually. Salbutamol is subject to extensive first-pass metabolism in the liver with about half excreted as the sulphate conjugate and half excreted unchanged in the urine.

The duration of action of the inhaled β-agonists is very dependent on the dose. Increasing the delivered dose increases the effective half-life and, despite the fact that a mere 10% of the metered dose enters the lungs, this would seem to be adequate to achieve near maximal bronchodilatation in most patients. Inadequate dosage is most often caused by faulty technique in operating the inhaler, in which case an alternative device should be sought. Inhaled catecholamines have a rapid onset of action producing their effect within 5 min. Their duration of action is correspondingly short, being of the order of 30 min–2 h.

α_2-Adrenoceptor agonists

The use of α_2-adrenoceptor agonists in anaesthetic practice in patients remains limited despite an increasing body of evidence promoting their usefulness. This is in sharp contrast to the situation in veterinary anaesthetic practice, where their use has been widespread for nearly two decades. The agent, xylazine, has been used since the 1970s as an adjunct to anaesthetic agents such as ketamine but its link to the stimulation of α_2-receptors was not established until 1980. When used with ketamine, the hypotensive and bradycardiac effects seen on intravenous administration were moderated by the cardiostimulant effects of ketamine. Xylazine has also been administered epidurally where it produced longer-acting analgesia than lignocaine at equipotent doses, while demonstrating less motor paralysis. The cardiodepressant effects of epidurally administered xylazine could be effectively reversed with tolazoline without the loss of the sedative and analgesic effects.

The α_2-adrenoceptor agonist clonidine has been used for 30 years as a centrally acting antihypertensive agent. This site of action has also been harnessed by the use of methyl dopa, which is metabolized to methyl noradrenaline; a full agonist at the α_2-adrenoceptor having a relative affinity of 10:1. Biotransformation to the active compound is slow and unpredictable and this limits its use.

Clonidine only has a licence for use as an antihypertensive agent but is gaining popularity for the beneficial effects it exerts over a number of organ systems. It is structurally related to naphazoline, a nasal decongestant, and in the 1960s underwent clinical trials in this regard. The first volunteer to receive intranasal clonidine subsided into a prolonged but rousable sleep. The absence of a perceived niche as a sedative agent at the time prevented its development as an adjunct to anaesthetic agents.

Medetomidine, a more selective agonist at the α_2-receptor, has been in use in veterinary anaesthetic practice for some time. Dexmedetomidine, the most selective agent isolated to date, is the subject of much animal work.

The actions of clonidine and allied compounds relate to their ability to reduce the sympathetic outflow and enhance the parasympathetic outflow from the CNS. The activation of α_2-adrenoceptors in the 'medullary vasomotor centre' resets the gain of the system so that blood pressure is maintained at a lower level. In contrast to the more peripherally acting agents, this does not mediate a reflex response from the unblocked portion of the control loop and results in a more integrated mechanism of blood pressure control. The exact site of action is unknown but clonidine is ineffective in controlling the blood pressure of tetraplegic hypertensive patients in whom the central control of sympathetic system is lacking.

Postural hypotension is a recognized feature of their use and there is an enhanced bradycardiac response to increases in systolic blood pressure and the valsalva manoeuvre. Slowing of conduction through the A-V node occurs at higher doses and may lead to prolongation of the P-R interval. This is thought to be a result of the central vagomimetic actions.

Following abrupt withdrawal of clonidine after a prolonged period of use there is a sometimes a rebound phenomenon mimicking the signs of phaeochromocytoma. This is variable in nature and severity but may comprise hypertension, anxiety, insomnia, restlessness, tremor, nausea and vomiting. There have been reports of angina pectoris, myocardial infarction, ventricular fibrillation and even death. The incidence and severity of these effects is related to the dose and duration of use and is not seen following short-term use in the anaesthetic setting.

There are few data on the effects of α_2-agonists on the respiratory system. Animal work has demonstrated a reduction in the response to CO_2 which is less than that seen with morphine. Clonidine has been demonstrated to reduce bronchospasm in asthmatics.

The α_2-adrenoceptor agonists produce an increase in urine flow. Several mechanisms are proposed mostly relating to the release and action of antidiuretic hormone (ADH). The renal tubular action of ADH is inhibited by α_2-agonist and a reduction in the release of ADH was seen in dogs receiving clonidine.

Following oral dosing, the bioavailability of clonidine is good. Peak serum concentrations are reached after 1.5–2 h following administration. The half-life varies between 6 and 24 h with a mean of 10 h. Clonidine is excreted largely unchanged in the urine.

There is a fine dividing line between the doses required to produce the α_2- and α_1-effects. Excessive dosing with clonidine causes the peripheral α_1-hypertensive effects to predominate.

In addition to its use in the treatment of hypertension, including that of renal origin, clonidine has been shown to have beneficial effects in patients with ischaemic heart disease. Improvements in myocardial oxygen balance, reductions in the frequency of anginal attacks and limitations in infarct size have been reported. Beneficial alterations in afterload and preload leading to improvements in cardiac function have been demonstrated in patients with chronic congestive cardiac failure who received 150 μg of intravenous clonidine.

Studies of the effects of clonidine in the perioperative period were carried out as long ago as 1976. A 'smoothing out' of the haemodynamic profile was seen in addition to the sedative effect that was already recognized. Subsequently, there have been numerous reports of reduction in requirements for volatile agents and opioids in patients undergoing a variety of procedures. Initially, the inhibition of central noradrenergic neurotransmission was proposed as the mechanism for these findings. However, it is now thought that the α_2-agonists has anaesthetic properties. In animal studies, the new agent dexmedetomidine has reduced mean alveolar concentration (MAC) values for halothane by more than 90%.

Clonidine has been shown to confer a greater degree of cardiovascular stability as judged by a number of variables including the haemodynamic response to intubation, incision, and sternotomy, thus maintaining favourable myocardial oxygen balance in patients undergoing cardiac surgery. It has also been shown to reduce the levels of circulating catecholamines during major vascular surgery as well as incidence and severity of postanaesthetic shivering.

The mechanism of analgesic action of clonidine has been thought to be the same as that mediating the spinal analgesic action of the opioids since specific opioid antagonists (naloxone) have antagonized α_2-mediated analgesia. Subsequent work has suggested the presence of α_2-adrenoceptors in the dorsal horn of the spinal cord which inhibit the release of substance P. There is substantial evidence to support the synergism of α_2-agonists and opioids in the spinal cord and the efficacy of spinal and epidurally administered clonidine in the treatment of postoperative or chronic pain.

The rebound hypertension seen after withdrawal of clonidine has been mentioned earlier. Other undesirable effects of clonidine include bradycardia and hypotension seen after intravenous administration. The removal of sympathetic tone from certain patients may be deleterious, particularly if they are relying on this to maintain an adequate circulation, as is the case in acute left ventricular failure or hypovolaemic shock. These adverse effects can be overcome easily with the administration of vagolytic and vasoconstrictor drugs.

The administration of α_2-agonists with selective antagonists has been the subject of considerable interest in the field of veterinary anaesthetic practice. Yohimbine has been extensively investigated and has been granted a licence for the reversal of the sedative effects of xylazine in dogs. For some time it has been used for rousing wild animals anaesthetized with 'Imobilon', a mixture of α_2-adrenoceptor agonists and opioids. The use of these antagonists is not without hazard. In particular, hypotension and bradycardia have been reported, albeit rarely, and the use of a carefully titrated dose prevents such sequelae.

NON-CATECHOLAMINES

Ephedrine

This is one of the most commonly used indirect-acting sympathomimetic amines in anaesthetic practice which also has direct actions on adrenoceptors. It occurs naturally, being found in several plant species, and has been used for centuries in Chinese medicine. Unlike the catecholamines, it is active after oral administration and has a much longer duration of action.

Its actions are similar to those of adrenaline but last many times longer. When administered intravenously it causes a rapid rise in systolic and diastolic blood pressure. Owing to a direct action on β-adrenoceptors it also causes bronchodilatation and an increase in heart rate and contractility, which differentiates it from the purely indirect agents which, lacking any direct stimulatory action on β-adrenoceptors, lead to a reflex baroreceptor-mediated bradycardia which can often offset the desired increase in blood pressure. The rise in blood pressure caused by one incremental dose of intravenous ephedrine may last up to 1 h. However, if repeated doses are required the clinical effect diminishes as the number of repeated administrations increases. This tachyphylaxis is a phenomenon shared by all the indirect-acting sympathomimetics and is due to the progressive depletion of neuronal stores of noradrenaline with repeated depolarization due to the displacement of noradrenaline from storage vesicles.

It is the most widely used vasoconstrictor in routine anaesthetic practice due to its effects on increasing vascular tone and on stimulating the heart, and thus avoiding the problems of bradycardia which may occur with pure α-adrenoceptor agonists. Another point of note is that it does not have a significant effect on placental blood vessels, and is thus the vasoconstrictor of choice in obstetric regional anaesthesia. It may be given orally but is usually given intramuscularly or intravenously, as either an infusion or as a carefully administered bolus.

It is available in 1-ml ampoules containing 30 mg ephedrine sulphate as the *l*-isomer. For hypotension following spinal anaesthesia, it is usually administered in aliquots of 3 mg intravenously which will cause a sustained increase in blood pressure of around 20% within 1 min. The heart rate will also increase by a similar amount. Larger doses need to be given intramuscularly whereupon the latency to clinical effect is naturally prolonged.

Metaraminol

Metaraminol is 3-hydroxyphenylisopropanolamine. It is like ephedrine in that it has both direct and indirect actions, but its actions are predominantly those of α-adrenoceptor agonist and it does not have a central effect. The lack of effect on β-adrenoceptors means that the unopposed vasoconstriction will lead to a baroreceptor-mediated reflex bradycardia unless vagal activity is blocked by the prior administration of an anticholinergic agent. This is a real phenomenon with important clinical implications and should be borne in mind whenever pure vasoconstrictors are used in anaesthetic practice. It constricts placental vessels and should thus not be used in obstetric practice.

It causes a sustained increase in both systolic and diastolic blood pressure and also constricts venous capacitance vessels leading to an increase in central venous pressure. It causes a reduction in renal and splanchnic blood flow and disrupts autoregulation of cerebral blood flow. In the absence of a change in heart rate, cardiac output remains either unchanged or falls, although if atropine has been administered the cardiac output in those with normal myocardial function tends to rise substantially.

It is available in 1-ml ampoules containing 10 mg metaraminol tartrate BP with methylparaben, propylparaben and sodium bisulphite as preservatives. The solution is rendered isotonic by the addition of normal saline. It is usually given in doses of 0.5–1.0 mg, which cause a prompt increase in blood pressure by 20–30%. It is used in regional anaesthetic practice to counteract the hypotension produced by paralysis of the spinal sympathetics, and it is also used in cardiac anaesthesia to maintain perfusion pressure during cardiopulmonary bypass. Associated bradycardia may be sudden and dramatic and may be treated with atropine, but is best avoided altogether by the prophylactic administration of an anticholinergic if there is the possibility of bradycardia developing.

Phenylephrine

Phenylephrine is the drug resulting from the removal of the hydroxyl group from the 4-position on the benzene ring of the adrenaline molecule. It is an extremely potent α-adrenoreceptor agonist with minimal β-activity and acts predominantly by direct stimulation of postsynaptic α-receptors. Its actions are mediated predominantly by constriction of peripheral arterioles leading to an increase in systemic vascular resistance. It also constricts renal, splanchnic and cerebral blood vessels, and causes a sustained rise in pulmonary artery pressure due to its actions on the pulmonary vasculature. Unlike metaraminol it has little effect on venous tone.

It is available in 1-ml ampoules containing phenylephrine 10 mg as the *l*-isomer. For anaesthetic use it can be administered as either an intramuscular depot of 5 mg, by slow intravenous infusion or by careful administration of a bolus of up to 0.5 mg as a dilute solution. It has a prompt vasoconstricting effect which persists for about 30 min after intravenous administration. Its uses are similar to those of metaraminol.

Methoxamine

Methoxamine is similar to phenylephrine in that it is almost exclusively a directly acting α-adrenoceptor agonist with little effect on release of stored noradrenaline. It causes a sustained increase in systolic and diastolic blood pressure with an associated baroreceptor-mediated reflex bradycardia. It has no β-actions so cardiac output falls or remains unchanged and it has no central effects. Renal and splanchnic blood flow are affected in a similar manner as following administration of other vasoconstrictors.

It is prepared as methoxamine hydrochloride BP 20 mg in 1 ml. Its hypertensive effect tends to occur slightly more gently than with phenylephrine but is similar quantitatively after the administration of an intravenous bolus of 2 mg with a duration of action of around 20 min. Pure vasoconstrictors have been used for the treatment of supraventricular tachydysrhythmias by attempting to invoke the baroreceptor-mediated slowing of heart rate that is characteristic of this group of agents, but they are little used for this purpose today.

Amphetamine

Amphetamine is racemic β-phenylisopropylamine and is active after oral administration. It has substantial stimulatory effects on central sympathetic function which last for several hours in addition to the peripheral effects which are common to other indirectly acting sympathomimetics. After oral administration, systolic and diastolic blood pressure rise and heart rate tends to fall. Cardiac arrhythmias may occur with large dosages.

It causes contraction of the sphincter of the urinary bladder predisposing to urinary retention. It may indeed be used to treat enuresis but is rarely done so today. It has unpredictable effects on gastrointestinal tone and motility and may produce either constipation or diarrhoea.

Its effects on the CNS are, however, pronounced and merit particular attention. Owing to its ability to stimulate central adrenergic function it causes an increase in arousal and general CNS activity due to stimulation of the reticular activating system and cerebral cortex. This leads to an increase in alertness and wakefulness, elevation of mood, and increased ability to concentrate. Appetite is also suppressed by a central action which has led to its use as an aid to weight loss in obese individuals. This practice is not to be recommended as any weight lost is due to decreased food intake rather than an increase in metabolism. There may be an associated increase in physical activity due to the generalized central arousal but this effect tends to be subject to dependence and should not be relied upon as a means of losing weight without dietary restriction.

It can enhance physical performance and has thus been subject to abuse by athletes although it is now banned. With continued use or overdosage it may lead to fatigue or depression, in addition to dizziness, headache, palpitations or vasomotor disturbances. It is likely to cause psychological dependence with prolonged use and substantially disrupted sleep pattern. Indeed, following abrupt discontinuation, normal sleep and dietary patterns may not resume for several months. It is unlikely that an anaesthetist will encounter a patient taking prescribed amphetamine but it should be remembered that it is a sympathomimetic amine with peripheral circulatory effects in addition to the better-known psychological effects.

Cocaine

Benzoylmethylecgonine (cocaine) is an ester of benzoic acid and ecgonine, an amino alcohol that closely resembles tropine, the amino alcohol in atropine. It is a powerful local anaesthetic drug whose actions on nerve conduction are discussed elsewhere in this book. In the context of sympathetic nervous system activity it causes stimulation of adrenergic function by inhibiting uptake-1, the process whereby released noradrenaline is actively collected and re-stored in the nerve ending from where it was released. As has been already discussed, this is the major means of termination of the actions of released noradrenaline. It is thus an indirectly acting non-catecholamine.

It is absorbed into the CNS where it causes arousal, euphoria, agitation and other symptoms characteristic of central sympathetic stimulation. It causes intense psychological addiction and has been a substance of abuse for many centuries.

It is absorbed through intact mucosal surfaces as well as after oral administration. Once in the blood it is broken down by plasma esterases with a half-life of approximately 1 h. It is not available for internal use or injection and its only clinical use nowadays is as a topical vasoconstrictor when used as a 1% or 4% paste (or a 10% or 20% solution), predominantly for preventing bleeding during operations in the nasal cavity.

Tyramine

Tyramine is not a drug that is available for clinical use but it is nevertheless an important non-catecholamine. It closely resembles the parent molecule phenylethylamine, the only difference being the addition of an hydroxyl group at the 4-position on the aromatic ring. Its importance stems from its relationship with the MAOIs. MAO is an enzyme found in mitochondrial membranes of a wide range of tissues, particularly adrenergic nerve endings and hepatocytes, and plays an important part in the inactivation of released noradrenaline. MAOIs thus tend to lead to an increase in local noradrenaline concentrations around noradrenergic nerve terminals, particularly within the brain with associated elevation of mood and lifting of depression. They are starting to be used again with increasing frequency.

The effects of exogenously administered sympathomimetic amines are prolonged and exaggerated in patients receiving MAOI treatment, more so with the indirectly acting agents such as amphetamine and ephedrine. Tyramine is another example of such an indirect acting sympathomimetic amine which is found in high concentrations in certain food substances. True catecholamines are affected to a lesser extent as these are largely inactivated by COMT and are not so dependent on MAO for termination of their effects.

The dose of tyramine or other monoamines which may be contained in an average portion of certain foodstuffs may be enough to provoke a dramatic rise in blood pressure or even a hypertensive crisis. The most dangerous products are matured cheeses such as cheddar or stilton, yeast products or cheap red wines. Other products include coffee, broad beans, canned figs and citrus fruits. These hypertensive episodes are commonly associated with headaches, and intracranial bleeding sometimes resulting in death has been reported. The administration of pethidine to patients taking MAOIs may lead to the development of a serious hyperpyrexic reaction which is thought to be due to the release of 5-hydroxytryptamine (5-HT) and is not related to the actions of tyramine.

MAOIs can also potentiate the respiratory-depressant effects of pethidine but not other opioids.

FURTHER READING

Barnes PJ, Chung KF. Questions about inhaled β_2-adrenoceptor agonists in asthma. *Trends in Pharmacological Sciences* 1992, **13**: 20–3.

Chernow B, Roth BL. Pharmacologic manipulation of the peripheral vasculature in shock: clinical and experimental approaches. *Circulatory Shock* 1986, **18**: 141–55.

Maze M, Tranquilli DVM. (1991) Alpha$_2$ adrenoceptor agonists: defining the role in clinical anaesthesia. *Anesthesiology* 1991; **74**: 581–605.

Maze M, *et al.* Clonidine and other alpha$_2$-adrenergic agonists: strategies for the rational use of these novel anaesthetic agents. *Journal of Clinical Anesthetics* 1988; **1**: 146–57.

Molinoff PB. α- and β-adrenergic receptor subtypes; properties, distribution and regulation. *Drugs* 1984; **28** (Suppl 2): 1–15.

Potter, DE. Adrenergic pharmacology of aqueous humor dynamics. *Pharmacology Review* 1981; **33**: 133–53.

Ruffolo RR. Review: the pharmacology of dobutamine. *American Journal of Medical Science* 1987; **294**: 244–8.

Seiden LS, *et al.* Amphetamine: effects on catecholamine systems and behaviour. *Annual Review of Pharmacology and Toxicology* 1993; **32**: 639–77.

Stjarne L. Basic mechanisms and local modulation of nerve-impulse induced secretion of neurotransmitters from individual sympathetic nerve varicosities. *Physiology, Biochemistry and Pharmacology* 1989; **112**: 1–137.

14

The Adrenergic Nervous System—Adrenoceptor Antagonists

AG Ramage, NH Kellow, AD Scott, RO Feneck

INTRODUCTION

There are many sites at which a drug can act to interfere with adrenergic transmission. Drugs can act within the CNS to reduce central sympathetic drive, thus causing a reduction in noradrenaline released from postganglionic sympathetic nerve terminals. They can also act on afferent inputs and reduce central sympathetic drive by increasing baroreceptor input for a given blood pressure by sensitizing baroreceptor nerve endings, for example veratridine. Blockade of sympathetic ganglia would also reduce release of noradrenaline from sympathetic nerve terminals. However, ganglion-blocking drugs also block parasympathetic ganglia causing a number of unwanted effects such as diminished movement of the gastrointestinal tract and bladder, reduced gastric and salivary secretion and blurred vision. These drugs are now obsolete, except for the short-acting ganglion-blocking drug trimetaphan. Drugs can also act at sympathetic nerve terminals to reduce the release of noradrenaline and finally drugs can act on the postsynaptic receptors to block the effects of noradrenaline and adrenaline.

DRUGS THAT AFFECT THE STORAGE AND RELEASE OF NORADRENALINE

Reserpine (Fig. 14.1) causes depletion of the sympathetic nerve endings of noradrenaline. It will also deplete other stores of catecholamines and tryptamines in nerve endings in the CNS and peripheral tissues. It does this by irreversibly blocking the uptake of amines into the storage granules thus increasing the level of the plasma concentrations of amines which are quickly removed by monoamine oxidase (MAO). The rate and extent of catecholamine depletion mainly depends on the rate of turnover of catecholamines in that particular tissue. Recovery from depletion is slow and can only occur by transport of fresh storage granules down the axons from the cell bodies. Reserpine is lipid soluble and easily absorbed from the gastrointestinal tract and can enter the CNS. Depletion of central monoamines causes sedation and depression.

The adrenergic neuron-blocking drugs guanethidine, bethanidine, debrisoquin (Fig. 14.1) and bretylium are very polar substances which contain a basic guanidinium group or a quaternary N^+ and therefore do not cross into the CNS. Guanethidine and bretylium are poorly absorbed orally, while bethanidine and debrisoquin are readily absorbed. Guanethidine differs from the other compounds in that it causes depletion in noradrenergic nerves and can act initially as an indirect sympathomimetic. Before these compounds can exert their pharmacological action they must be taken up by sympathetic nerve terminals by neuronal uptake. These drugs then accumulate in the varicosities of sympathetic nerve terminals to prevent exocytosis. The accumulation of these drugs is thought to produce a local anaesthetic action (blockade of Na^+ channels) preventing invasion of the action potential into the varicosity thus preventing exocytosis. These drugs are thought to have little or no effect on the release of adrenaline from the adrenal medulla. Drugs that block neuronal uptake

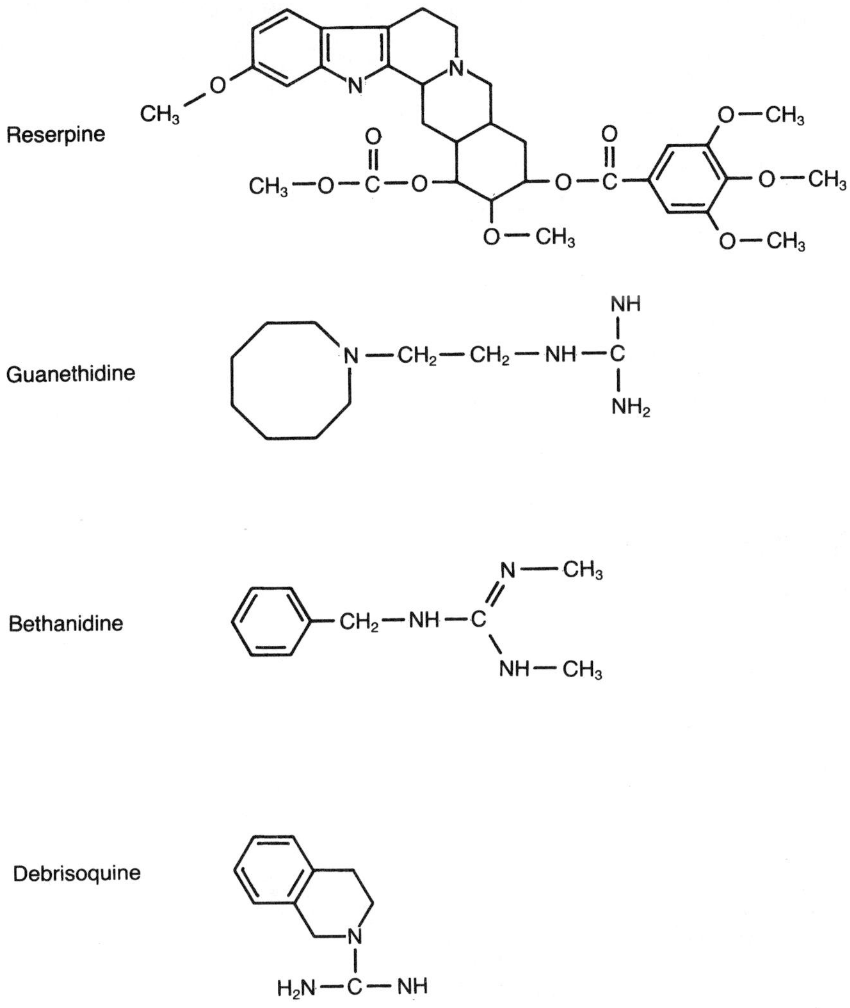

Reserpine

Guanethidine

Bethanidine

Debrisoquine

FIGURE 14.1 Structure of drugs that interfere with release of noradrenaline from sympathetic varicosities.

will attenuate the action of noradrenergic neurone-blocking drugs.

As these compounds inhibit α-adrenoceptor-mediated sympathetic vasoconstrictor drive, their major effects will be to cause vasodilatation which causes a lowering of blood pressure and nasal congestion. The fall in blood pressure will be associated with postural hypotension as the subject will be unable to venoconstrict on standing up as there is a sharp pooling of blood in the legs causing a reduction in venous return and therefore cardiac output. The reduction in cardiac output will often produce fainting due to cerebral ischaemia. Another major effect of these compounds is to cause blockade of the sympathetic nerve supply to the gastrointestinal tract while leaving the parasympathetic drive unopposed, causing diarrhoea. These drugs inhibit ejaculation. They will also cause fluid retention due to stimulation of renin release. The mechanism for this is complex and is related to the fall in blood pressure. As these drugs prevent transmitter release they also cause postsynaptic supersensitivity; that is, circulating catecholamines have a more potent effect when activating adrenoceptors.

Guanethidine will also cause a reduction in intraocular pressure when applied to the eye. Interestingly, this is the same effect as produced by sympathomimetics. There may also be a tendency to cause miosis due to blockade of sympathetic drive to the pupil.

Adrenoceptor antagonists

α-Receptor antagonists occur naturally (ergot alkaloids and yohimbine) but the majority of therapeutically useful drugs are synthetic. These include the imidazolines (tolazoline and phentolamine) and the β-haloalkylamines (phenoxybenzamine) (Fig. 14.2). The imidazolines demonstrate simple competitive inhibition at the α-receptor with no significant β-effects. Presynaptic α_2-adrenoceptors are also blocked thus

Non-selective

Phentolamine

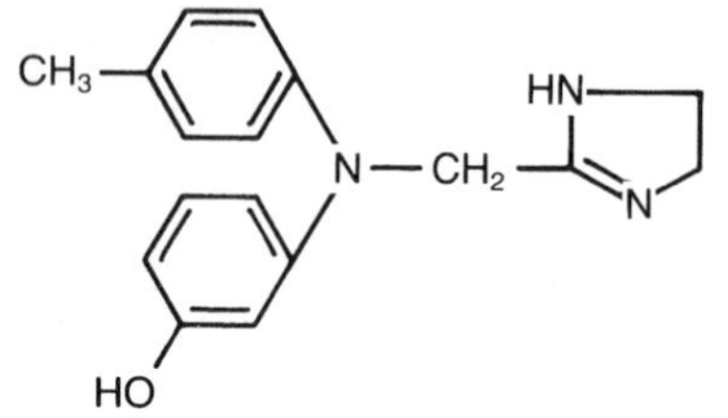

Phenoxybenzamine

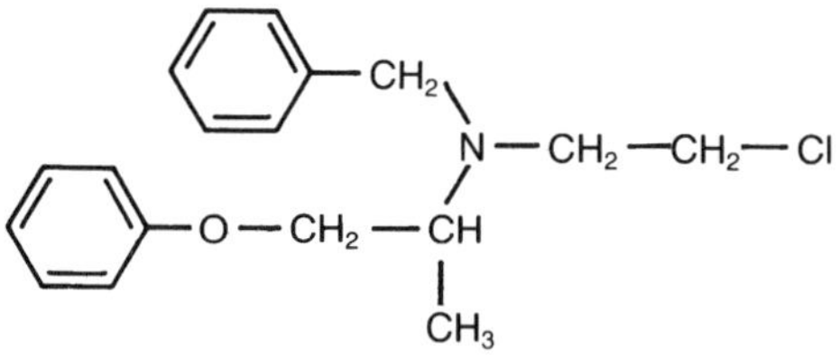

α_1 *Selective*

Prazosin

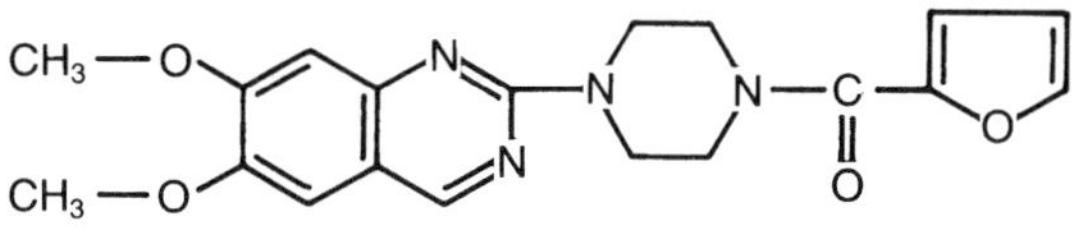

Doxazosin

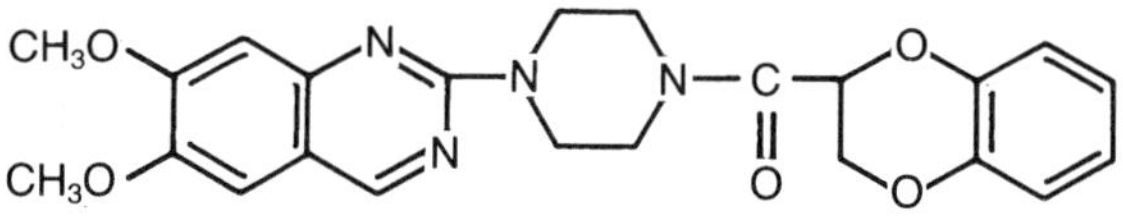

α_2*-Selective*

Yohimbine

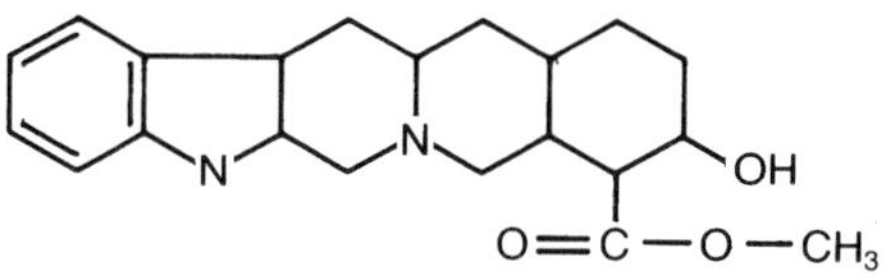

Idazoxan

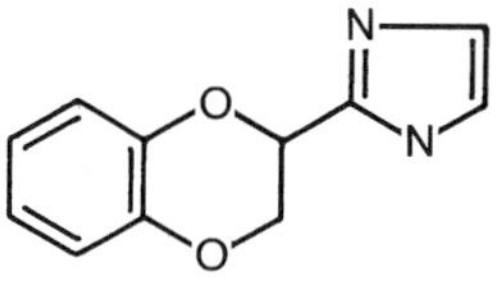

FIGURE 14.2 Structure of α-adrenoceptor antagonists.

interfering with the negative feedback control of noradrenaline release. Phenoxybenzamine also produces a reversible competitive antagonism at low doses, but at higher doses a covalent bond is formed resulting in non-competitive and irreversible antagonism.

The first α-adrenoceptor antagonists to be described, the ergot alkaloids, still have therapeutic applications. Briefly, ergotamine is a partial agonist used mainly for its vasoconstrictor action in acute migraine attacks and dihydroergotamine is nearly a full antagonist and has non-clinical uses. It should be mentioned that these drugs also have what is called an oxytocic-like action, although this is very weak for both ergotamine and dihydroergotamine. However, ergometrine, which has very weak effects on α-adrenoceptors, has a very potent oxytocic effect and is used for the treatment of postpartum haemorrhage.

Other non-selective α-adrenoceptor antagonists are phenoxybenzamine, a haloalkylamine, and tolazoline and phentolamine, which are imidazolines. These drugs cause a similar action to adrenergic neurone-blocking drugs (see above); however, they differ in that they do not interfere with innervated β_1-adrenoceptor-mediated actions. Thus, the fall in blood pressure caused by blockade of α-adrenoceptor-mediated vasoconstrictor tone causes a reflex tachycardia and stimulates the renin–angiotensin system again through reflex activation of β_1-adrenoceptors. The increase in angiotensin levels causes vasoconstriction and increased aldosterone synthesis causing sodium and water retention. These combined effects will obviously tend to reduce the blood pressure lowering action of these drugs. The reflex effects will be even more pronounced as presynaptic α_2-adrenoceptors are blocked, thus interfering in the negative feedback control of noradrenaline release. These antagonists differ in their duration and onset of action. Phenoxybenzamine is a non-competitive or irreversible antagonist that forms a covalent bond with α-adrenoceptors and is very long-acting with a slow onset of action. Phentolamine is poorly absorbed when given orally and so is usually given intramuscularly or intravenously.

All non-selective α-adrenoceptor antagonists can cause miosis; however, this is more often seen with phenoxybenzamine.

α_1-Adrenoceptor antagonists

Prazosin, doxazosin (Fig. 14.2) and terazosin are highly selective for the α_1-adrenoceptor subtype. These drugs all cause a fall in blood pressure by blocking α_1-adrenoceptor-mediated vasoconstrictor tone. The fall in blood pressure is associated with little or no increase in heart rate or renin levels due to the lack of α_2-adrenoceptor blockade. Further, these agents cause only slight postural hypotension and no diarrhoea. These effects obviously indicate a difference between the location of α_1- and α_2-adrenoceptors. As these drugs do not block presynaptic α_2-adrenoceptors, negative feedback control of noradrenaline release is not interfered with and so these drugs should cause less tachycardia and a smaller increase in renin levels when compared with non-selective α-adrenoceptor antagonists for the same fall in blood pressure. However, little change is seen in these variables and these drugs must modulate the baroreceptor-induced reflex increase in sympathetic drive. These compounds can cause slight sedation, indicating that they enter the CNS. (Table 14.1.)

It is well known that both types of α-adrenoceptor are found in central pathways involved in the control of blood pressure and it has been shown that these compounds can cause sympathoinhibition, suggesting that central α_1-adrenoceptors have a sympathoexcitatory role. In this respect it should be pointed out that activation of central α_2-adrenoceptors causes sympathoinhibition. Therefore, it is blockade of central α_1-adrenoceptors that is responsible for the failure to see a reflex tachycardia and also the expected reflex increase in renin release through activation of β_1-adrenoceptors. Interestingly, the baroreceptor reflex does not seem to be impaired centrally or peripherally. The reason for reduced postural hypotension is that venoconstriction is only slightly impaired by prazosin as it is mainly mediated by postsynaptic α_2-adrenoceptors. Furthermore, sympathetic inhibition of the gastrointestinal tract is mediated primarily through α_2-adrenoceptors found on parasympathetic nerve endings which reduce the release of acetylcholine. Thus if these receptors were blocked there would be an increase in parasympathetic drive to the gut causing diarrhoea; however, they are not blocked by prazosin.

TABLE 14.1 Consequence of non-selective α-adrenoceptor blockade

Reflex tachycardia
Reflex activation of renin/angiotensin system
Hypotension
Postural hypotension
Nasal stuffiness
Diarrhoea
Failure to ejaculate
Miosis

α_2-Adrenoceptor antagonists

Yohimbine is the classical drug in this group (Fig. 14.2). There are a large number of these drugs under development; idazoxan being one of the newer α_2-adrenoceptor antagonists (Fig. 14.2). Interestingly, yohimbine is a very weak hypotensive agent; in fact it can produce hypertension and tachycardia. These latter effects are not simply due to blockade of presynaptic α_2-adrenoceptors but are also due to a central sympathoexcitatory action. Again central noradrenergic sympathetic pathways are sympathoinhibitory and are tonically active, thus blockade of central α_2-adrenoceptors will cause central sympathoexcitation. It should be mentioned that these central α_2-adrenoceptors are located postsynaptically. It has been proposed that the α_1-adrenoceptors are located presynaptically in this pathway. Yohimbine also causes postural hypotension which could be simply explained by a peripheral action but again may involve a central one as well. α_2-Adrenoceptors will also cause an increase in insulin release. Interestingly, yohimbine has been reported to be an aphrodisiac through its effects on the penile vasculature. Its central actions include anxiogenesis.

β-Adrenoceptor antagonists

As is evident from the distribution of β-receptors shown in Table 13.1, the effects of β-adrenoceptor agonism and blockade can be simply identified (Table 14.2). The chemical structures of the β-receptor antagonists are much more closely related to the structure of the agonists than is the case with the α-receptor antagonists. In particular, this structural similarity holds true for three characteristics: (1) alkyl or aralkyl substitution on the terminal amine radical is associated with an increased β-receptor affinity; (2) steric configuration of the OH-bearing β-carbon atom in the side-chain confers specific β-receptor affinity; and (3)

TABLE 14.2 Consequence of β-adrenoceptor blockade

Reduced exercise tolerance
Breathlessness
Bradycardia
Hypotension
Cold extremities
Fatigue
Vivid dreams

methyl substitution on the α-carbon atom increases the duration of action.

In addition to a variation in receptor selectivity, β-adrenoceptor antagonists may also demonstrate intrinsic sympathomimetic actions (or partial agonism) and local anaesthetic (membrane stabilizing) effects. The relative prevalence of these additional features is shown in Table 14.3.

Propranolol can be considered to be the classical non-selective β-adrenoceptor antagonist. Other β-adrenoceptor antagonists which are termed cardio-selective, for example atenolol, vary in their ability to block β_2-adrenoceptors, in their ability to enter the CNS, to have intrinsic sympathomimetic activity or membrane-stabilizing action. Labetalol is a mixed α_1- and non-selective β-adrenoceptor antagonist and is used as an antihypertensive. It is seven times more potent at β- than α-adrenoceptors. It is also used in hypotensive anaesthesia and here its action is potentiated by halothane (see Table 14.4 for the various properties of a range of β-adrenoceptor antagonists).

TABLE 14.3 Additional features of β-adrenoceptor antagonists

	β_1	β_2	ISA	LA	POTENCY	$T_{1/2}$ (h)
Dichloroisoprenaline	+	++	++	–	–	–
Propranolol	+	++	–	++	1	3–6
Oxprenolol	+	++	++	++	1	2–3
Pindolol	+	++	++	+	20	3–4
Sotalol	+	++	–	–	0.1	2–3
Metoprolol	++	–	–	–	3	3–4
Atenolol	++	–	–	–	1	6–9
Timolol	+	+	–	–	10	4–6
Labetalol	++	+/–	–	++	0.25	4–6
Esmolol	++	–	–	–	0.02	9 min

β_1, cardioselective; β_2, non-cardioselective; ISA, intrinsic sympathomimetic effect; LA, membrane-stabilizing (local anaesthetic) effects; potency, relative to propranolol.

TABLE 14.4 Properties of β-adrenoceptor antagonists

NAME	β_1 (CARDIAC) SELECTIVE	ISA	CNS Pen	LA	5-HT_1
Propranolol	No	No	+++	+++	++
Atenolol	Yes	No			No
Acebutolol	Yes	Yes	+	++	?
Betaxolol	Yes	No	++		No
Bisoprolol	Yes	No	++		?
Carteolol	No	Yes	++		?
Metoprolol	Yes	No	++		?
Nadolol	No	No	++		?
Oxprenolol	No	Yes	++	+	++
Penbutolol	No	No	++		?
Pindolol	No	Yes	++	+	+++
Sotalol	No	No			?
Timolol	No	No	+		?

ISA, intrinsic sympathomimetic action.
LA, local anaesthetic action, i.e. membrane-stabilizing action.

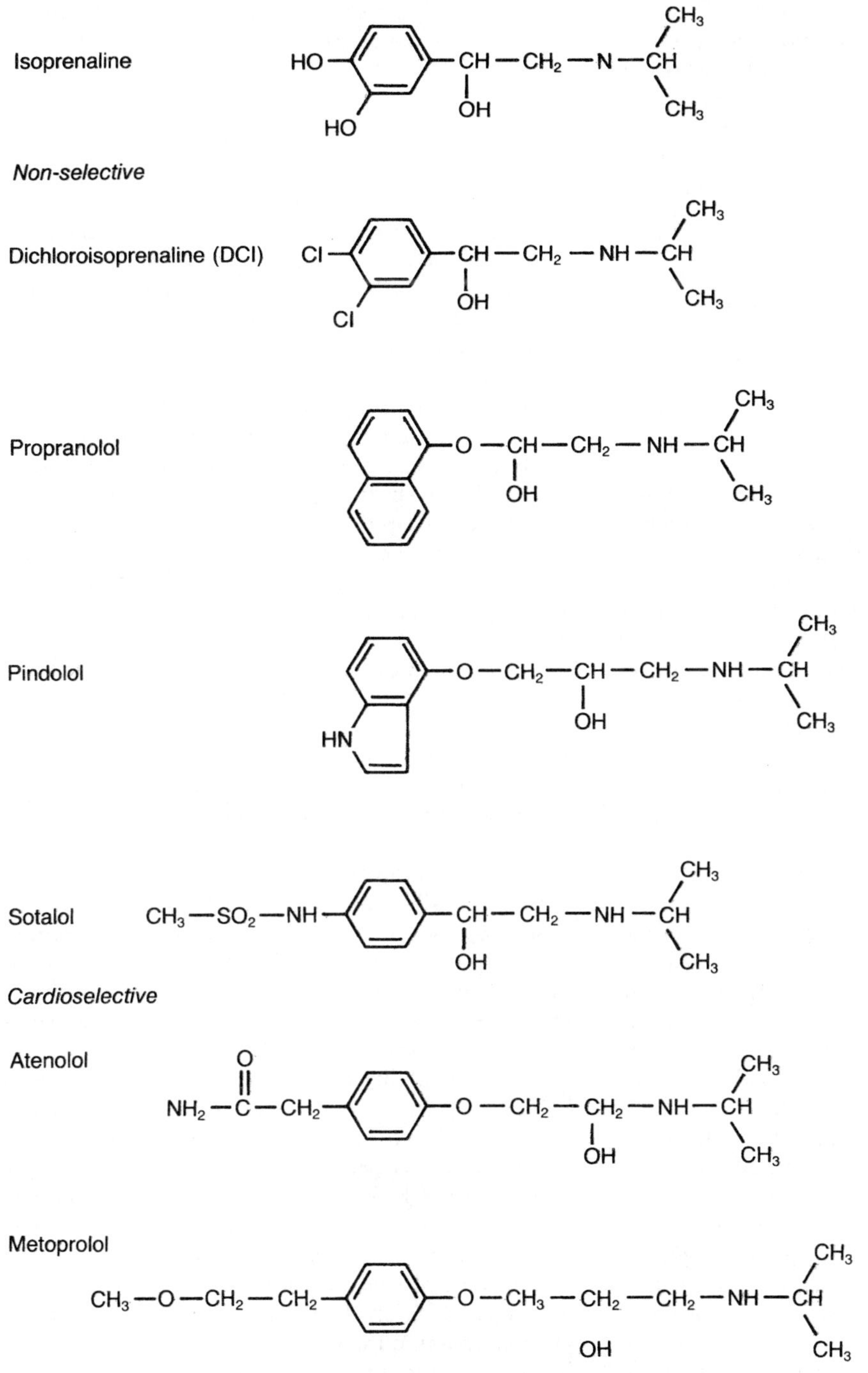

Isoprenaline

Non-selective

Dichloroisoprenaline (DCI)

Propranolol

Pindolol

Sotalol

Cardioselective

Atenolol

Metoprolol

FIGURE 14.3 Structure of some β-adrenoceptor antagonists.

Receptor selectivity

The structural similarity of isoprenaline and a number of the modern β-receptor antagonists is shown in Fig. 14.3. Cardioselectivity (i.e. β_1-effect) is conferred by substitution of a side-chain in the *para*-position on the benzene ring. The stereoisomerism of the compounds is most important, since activity is strongly influenced by the isomeric position of the β-carbon atom in the ethanolamine side-chain bearing the hydroxyl group.

Clearly, the original concept that β-receptors were distributed such that β_1- or β_2-receptors were present in any specific tissue has been shown to be somewhat simplistic. It is now understood that both β_1- and β_2-receptors are present, but the proportions in any given tissue may vary. Thus the heart and adipose tissue contain a greater proportion of β_1- than β_2-receptors, and bronchial, uterine and vascular smooth muscle contain the reverse. It should also be remembered that potency and selectivity may vary. Thus while propranolol is five times more potent at blocking β_1-receptors than practolol, it is 100 times more effective than practolol in blocking β_2-bronchial smooth muscle receptors. Selective affinity is a relative phenomenon that reflects the observed rank order of potency of a given antagonist at different receptor sites and in response to a given agonist.

Intrinsic sympathomimetic activity

Dichloroisoprenaline, a supposed β-adrenoceptor antagonist, was found to demonstrate effects compatible with a partial agonist effect, and since that time other β-adrenoceptor antagonists (practolol, oxprenolol, pindolol) have also been shown to be partial agonists, or have intrinsic sympathomimetic activity (ISA). There have been a number of attempts made to exploit this effect, particularly in patients with mild heart failure following acute myocardial infarction. In this setting, β-adrenoceptor antagonists are usually contraindicated since they may significantly worsen the severity of heart failure, and yet some degree of myocardial protection conferred by β-adrenoceptor blockade may be advisable to prevent extension of the myocardial infarction. Furthermore, the antiarrhythmic effect of β-adrenoceptor blockade may be useful and lead to an increase in cardiac output if the reduction in cardiac output is in part due to arrhythmia. Despite studies with newer compounds, there is currently no β-adrenoceptor antagonist with ISA licensed for clinical use in the UK that has proven safety and efficacy in acute heart failure. Some authors have suggested that, in contrast to other β-adrenoceptor antagonists, β-adrenoceptor antagonists with ISA may be used with a greater margin of safety during anaesthesia, particularly if volatile anaesthetics are used. In fact a variety of β-adrenoceptor atagonists have been safely used in the perioperative period, and safety is best enhanced by close attention to every aspect of the anaesthetic rather than reliance on the properties of a single drug (Table 14.3).

Local anaesthetic activity

Many β-adrenoceptor antagonists demonstrate local anaesthetic activity when applied to surface mucous membranes, and this effect is not dependent on their β-antagonism. For example, both the *d*- and *l*-isomers of propranolol demonstrate local anaesthetic properties, but only the *l*-isomer acts as a clinically useful β-adrenoceptor antagonist. Experimental work in normal and catecholamine-depleted animals has shown that the membrane-stabilizing effect is not responsible for direct myocardial depression, except when massive doses are used.

Cardiovascular effects of β-adrenoceptor blockade

Propranolol will cause a decrease in heart rate. This decrease in heart rate will be dependent on the level of sympathetic drive to the heart and will thus depend on whether the subject is resting and supine or active and upright. The rise in heart rate during exercise will be severely blunted. This will cause a considerable reduction in exercise tolerance as the reduction in heart rate will be related to a reduction in cardiac output. The blunting of the sympathetic response to the heart reduces the oxygen consumption of heart muscle. It has been suggested that the blunting of the β_2-adrenoceptor-induced vasodilatation in the skeletal muscle bed may contribute to reduced exercise tolerance; however, this is doubtful as autoregulation will occur quickly once skeletal muscle begins to contract.

β-Adrenoceptor antagonists were unexpectedly found to lower blood pressure. Although a reduction in cardiac output would be expected to cause a fall in blood pressure (blood pressure is the product of cardiac output and peripheral resistance) the initial fall in blood pressure should induce a baroreceptor-mediated reflex rise in total peripheral resistance. This reflex rise in peripheral resistance is suggested to be responsible for the cold extremities reported in some subjects. Further, it may be expected that blockade of β_2-adrenoceptor-mediated vasodilatation in the skeletal muscle beds adds to this rise in peripheral resistance; however, there seems to be little background drive in this system. The fall in blood pressure is due to the ability of β-adrenoceptor antagonists to 'switch off' this reflex rise in peripheral resistance. The mechanism for this is not completely understood. The fall in blood pressure caused by propranolol has been shown to be slow in onset. However, propranolol, although well absorbed orally, is subject to extensive hepatic tissue binding and first-pass metabolism and thus the plasma concentration varies greatly from individual to individual. Therefore there can be a great variation in the time indicated for the maximum hypotensive effect to be seen of between 24 h and 2 weeks. This delay led to the suggestion that the hypotensive effect of propranolol was due to a resetting of baroreceptors, presumably by a central action. Such a resetting would cause a 'switch off' of the reflex rise in peripheral resistance. More recently, the 'switch off' of the reflex rise in peripheral resistance has been shown to occur within 4 h. Other theories have also been proposed to explain the 'switch off' of this reflex rise in peripheral resistance. The theories are:

- Baroreceptor resetting, as already mentioned.
- Central inhibition of sympathetic drive.

- Reduction in renin release.
- Autoregulatory response to the decrease in cardiac output.
- Blockade of presynaptic β-adrenoceptors preventing positive feedback. An intriguing suggestion involving this mechanism is that in hypertension there is a high degree of circulating adrenaline that accumulates in sympathetic nerve terminals and when released has a preferential action on presynaptic β-adrenoceptors causing a potentiation of the overall release of transmitter and thus a rise in total peripheral resistance, which causes hypertension. Blockade of these presynaptic β-adrenoceptors will reverse this process.
- An adrenergic neurone-blocking action.

It should be stressed that it may be a combination of these effects that causes the 'switch off'.

Recent evidence from hypertensive patients using the selective β_2-adrenoceptor antagonist ICI 118,551 indicates that β_1-adrenoceptor blockade is crucial for the antihypertensive action of β-adrenoceptor antagonists, as the selective β_2-adrenoceptor antagonist ICI 118,551 failed to lower blood pressure.

Antiarrhythmic effects

β-Receptor blockers are Class II antiarrhythmic drugs, based on the Vaughan–Williams classification (see Chapter 15). They act as antagonists to the arrhythmogenic effects of sympatho-adrenal stimulation, but their effectiveness is influenced by the other factors already discussed – receptor selectivity, intrinsic sympathomimetic activity and membrane-stabilizing activity.

Respiratory function

Blockade of β_2-adrenoceptors causes exacerbation of bronchospasm in asthmatic patients. Interestingly, there is only a slight difference between cardioselective and non-selective β-adrenoceptor antagonists in causing this effect. Breathlessness is in fact a common problem, even with non-asthmatic patients treated with β-adrenoceptor antagonists. The precise mechanism for this action of β-adrenoceptor antagonists other than that of blockade of the β_2-adrenoceptors on bronchial smooth muscle remains to be determined.

Skeletal muscle tremor

This arises from the stimulation of β_2-adrenoceptors and is therefore reduced more effectively by non-selective β-adrenoceptor antagonists. It is occasionally observed following excessive doses of β_2 agonists such as salbutamol in asthmatic patients.

Metabolic effects

Catecholamine-induced hyperglycaemia is blocked by β_2-adrenoceptor antagonists. Blockade of β_2-adrenoceptors on the pancreas causes a decrease in the release of insulin. Therefore, non-selective β-adrenoceptor antagonists might impair glucose tolerance. However, this effect seems to be very minor and there is little difference between non-selective and cardioselective β-adrenoceptors. Non-selective β-adrenoceptor antagonists delay the recovery of normal blood glucose levels in insulin-induced hypoglycaemia. In diabetic patients these drugs will increase the likelihood of exercise-induced hypoglycaemia. A cardioselective β-adrenoceptor antagonist should have little effect on the rate of recovery from insulin-induced hypoglycaemia as the adrenaline released in response to hypoglycaemia can activate the β_2-adrenoceptors in the liver to cause glycogenolysis.

Another possibility is that the delay in recovery from hyperglycaemia caused by non-selective β-adrenoceptor antagonists may be related to the greater peripheral uptake of glucose, as the ability of adrenaline to cause lipolysis and raise the free fatty acid levels in the plasma is diminished due to blockade of β_1-adrenoceptors on adipocytes. In this respect, both non-selective and β_1-adrenoceptor antagonists reduce the resting level of free fatty acids. Further, propranolol has a greater lipid-lowering effect than cardioselective drugs during exercise and hypoglycaemia. The reason for this discrepancy may be the existence of an atypical β-adrenoceptor – a β_3-adrenoceptor. A new drug, BRL 26,830A, has been shown to have a selective action on these receptors (see Chapter 33).

It should be noted that in diabetics the contribution of adrenaline to recovery from hypoglycaemia is heightened because glucagon release is impaired, thus making this compensation mechanism more important. The ability of adrenaline to cause anxiety, sweating, palpitations and tremor is also important. These are the premonitory signals that a diabetic patient is hypoglycaemic and will be masked to varying degrees by β-adrenoceptor blockade. Propranolol has greater masking effects than the cardioselective drugs. Interestingly, none of the β-adrenoceptor antagonists interferes with sweating induced by hypoglycaemia. Another problem of non-selective β-adrenoceptor antagonists is that the adrenaline released by hypoglycaemia causes a rise in blood pressure as the dilator effects caused by activation of β_2-adrenoceptors on the vasculature of skeletal muscles will be blocked. Normally, when no drug is present hypoglycaemia causes tachycardia. In this respect other drugs that cause release of adrenaline, such as caffeine and nicotine, will cause a rise in blood pressure in subjects receiving non-selective β-adrenoceptor antagonists.

Fatigue

Fatigue is another effect of β-adrenoceptor blockade. This is due to the diminished cardiac output and also to the above metabolic effects.

DRUGS THAT ACT ON PRESYNAPTIC RECEPTORS TO BLOCK NORADRENALINE RELEASE

Drugs acting on presynaptic α_2-adrenoceptors

The principal drug that has this action is clonidine. However, as discussed in the previous chapter, its antihypertensive action is due mainly to a central action causing a reduction in central sympathetic drive.

Another substance that has this action is α-methylnoradrenaline, produced by the action of dopa decarboxylase on methyl dopa, which is a very widely used antihypertensive agent. α-Methylnoradrenaline is known as a 'false transmitter' as it accumulates in sympathetic nerve terminals, is not metabolized by MAO, and displaces noradrenaline from the vesicles. Thus, being released instead of noradrenaline, α-methylnoradrenaline is much less effective than noradrenaline on postsynaptic α_1-adrenoceptors. However, this does not explain fully its hypotensive action nor its presynaptic action. Again, as for clonidine, a central site of action is important. The major unwanted actions of α-methyl dopa are mild sedation and drowsiness. Other unwanted actions are postural hypotension, flushing of the skin and failure of ejaculation, which are consistent with peripheral sympathetic blockade.

Less common but nevertheless serious side-effects necessitating discontinuation of the drug include haemolytic anaemia (less than 1%) and a hepatitis that resembles viral hepatitis and is characterized by fatigue and anorexia.

FURTHER READING

Berlan M. *et al.* Pharmacological prospects for α_2-adrenoceptor antagonist therapy. *Trends in Pharmacological Sciences* 1992; **13**: 277–81.

Brodde OE. The functional importance of beta$_1$ and beta$_2$ adrenoceptors in the human heart. *American Journal of Cardiology* 1988; **62**: 24C–29C.

Cruickshank JM. The clinical importance of cardioselectivity and lipophilicity in beta blockers. *American Heart Journal* 1980; **100**: 160–78.

Cubeddu LX. New alpha$_1$-adrenergic receptor antagonists for the treatment of hypertension: role of vascular alpha receptors in the control of peripheral resistance. *American Heart Journal* 1988; **116**: 133–62.

Feely J, Peden N. Use of beta blockers in hyperthyroidism. *Drugs* 1984; **27**: 425–46.

Gengo FM *et al.* Lipid soluble and water soluble beta-blockers: comparison of the central nervous system depressant effect. *Archives of Internal Medicine* 1987; **147**: 39–43.

McDevitt DG. Comparison of pharmacokinetic properties of beta-adrenoceptor blocking drugs. *European Heart Journal* 1987; **8** (Suppl M): 9–14.

Ruffalo RR. Pharmacologic and therapeutic application of α_2-adrenoceptor subtypes. *Annual Review of Pharmacology and Toxicology* 1993; **32**: 243–79.

SECTION FOUR

Drugs Affecting the Cardiovascular System

15

Pharmacology of Drugs Affecting the Heart

RO Feneck

NORMAL CARDIAC FUNCTION AND THE PATHOPHYSIOLOGY OF HEART FAILURE

Normal cardiac function is dependent on a number of interlinking processes. An adequate supply of energy substrate and oxygenated blood to the myocardium is essential for the maintenance of normal contractile function. In addition, the contractile function of the myofibril will be enhanced by an optimum resting length of the constituent sarcomeres.

The myocardial cell consists of a number of components. The sarcolemma or plasma membrane surrounds the cell, and the intracellular components consist of a nucleus and other organelles including the sarcoplasmic reticulum and mitochondria, which in turn are enclosed by the sarcoplasmic reticular and mitochondrial membranes, and the contractile proteins.

The myocardial cells are arranged into structures known as myofibrils, which are themselves arranged in a syncytial formation, with the sarcolemma apparently differentiated in intercalated discs which separate the cells. Each myofibril is composed of the structural contractile proteins actin and myosin. The thin actin filaments surround the thicker myosin filaments, and the actin filaments are attached at one end to the Z line. The areas where the actin and myosin overlap can be seen under the light microscope as the characteristic dark A bands, and the actin filaments identified as the lighter I bands (Fig. 15.1). The thin actin filament is in fact a twin chain of actin monomer arranged in a double helix with the polypeptide tropomyosin aligned in the groove of the double helix, and with the troponin

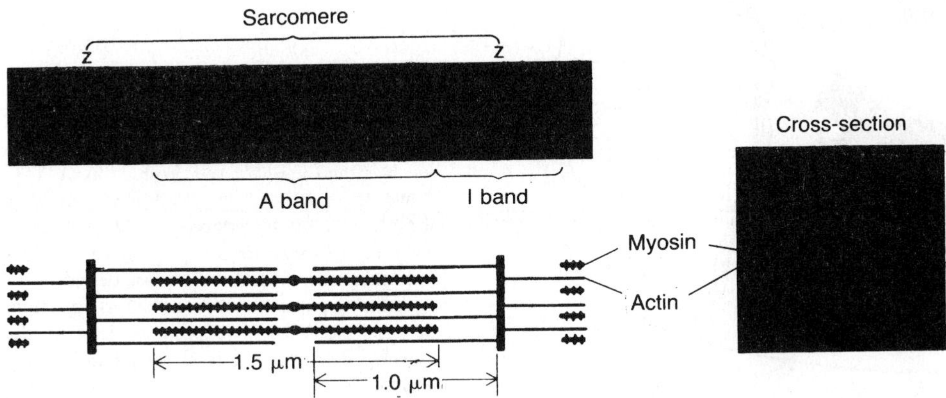

FIGURE 15.1 Morphology of the myofibril, showing the relation of actin and myosin fibres.

complex bound to the tropomyosin and located at regular intervals in the chain at every seventh actin monomer. Troponin is a complex of three subunits; C, which contains the calcium binding site; I, which inhibits cross-bridge formation with myosin; and T, which binds troponin to tropomyosin. The myosin filaments contain thick heads that protrude to close proximity with the actin helix, and whose actions are central to the function of the contractile unit.

The contractile process

In order to initiate the contractile process, the myosin head is associated with ATP, and hydrolysis of that ATP leads to the formation of ADP and P, which are transiently stored on the myosin head. Critically, the myosin head, previously angulated, now becomes realigned but completion of the cross-bridging process with the actin helix is prevented by troponin-I. However, calcium ions are released from intracellular stores following membrane depolarization and are bound to troponin C, which induces a protein interaction and releases the troponin-I induced inhibition of actin–myosin interaction, probably through a process of reconfiguration of the troponin–tropomyosin complex which exposes the actin-binding sites. The myosin head, still containing the stores of ADP and P, becomes aligned to the actin-binding site as a result of flexion of the tail of the myosin, and thus activated myosin and actin are attached and the cross-bridge formed. The next step is the force-generating step, in which the myosin head, still attached to the actin in the form of the cross-bridge, flexes thereby moving the actin relative to the myosin molecule and initiating the sliding filament process resulting in contraction of the myofibril without the change in actual length of the actinomyosin filaments. With this step, energy is consumed leaving the cross-bridge flexed and the actinomyosin complex deactivated. Further ATP combines with the myosin head and the cross-bridge is broken, leaving the myosin–ATP complex ready for the next cycle.

From the above it can be seen that normal contractile processes are heavily dependent on calcium and high-energy phosphates for their normal function. The invaginations of the sarcolemma in the myocardial cell (the T tubules) are broader than in skeletal muscle cells, thus allowing extracellular or sarcolemmal calcium to be more rapidly transported into the cell. The sarcoplasmic reticulum is a major intracellular storage site of calcium and may account for the clearance of calcium from the sarcoplasm during diastole, but the exact role of the sarcoplasmic reticulum during the phase of rapid release of calcium is not fully understood. The mitochondria, whose primary role is the intracellular production of energy, may also be implicated in calcium storage and transport, but more probably in the regulation of calcium deficiency or excess rather than in the beat-to-beat regulation of intracellular calcium.

The energy source from which the contractile proteins form actinomyosin cross-bridges and then angulate and perform the work of shortening and tension development is ATP. The release of energy from ATP is controlled by the activity of ATPase, located in the head of the myosin filament. This enzyme is sensitive to both calcium and magnesium. The supply of ATP is regulated through the metabolic utilization of many substrates including glucose, free fatty acids, pyruvate and even lactate. Normal cardiac metabolism is strictly aerobic in contrast to skeletal muscle which has to utilize anaerobic metabolic mechanisms in order to provide adequate energy for bursts of activity. The heart is very sensitive to relative hypoxia, which will lead to normal metabolic processes being rapidly disrupted. Lactate, which under circumstances of normal aerobic metabolism is consumed as a fuel, may then be produced as a product of anaerobic metabolism (Fig. 15.2). Although capable of using many fuel sources, non-esterified free fatty acids are the preferred substrate.

The strength and duration of the interactions of contractile proteins are therefore dependent on a number of factors. The number of actinomyosin cross-bridge interactions is dependent on the degree of overlap between thick and thin filaments, which means that the force of contraction of the myofibril will be dependent on the resting length of the sarcomeres. Intracellular calcium ions will affect the number

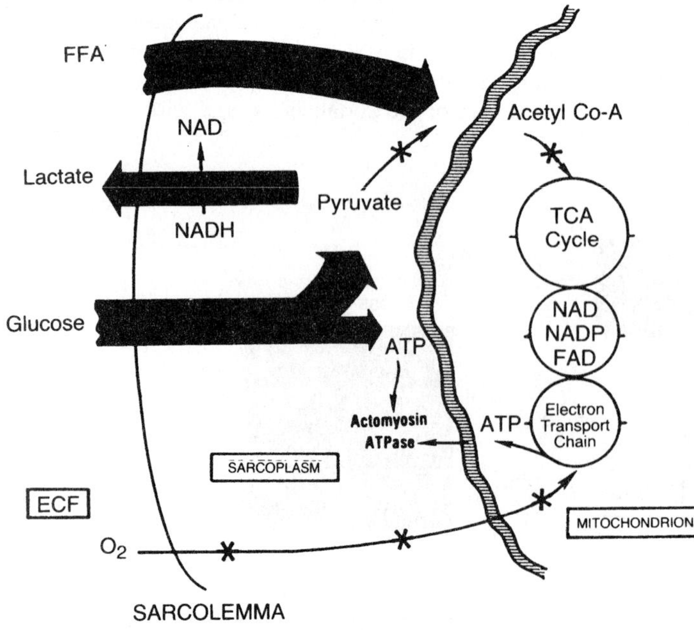

FIGURE 15.2 During normal aerobic cardiac metabolism, pyruvate is continuously transformed by pyruvate dehydrogenase into Acetyl Co-A, which is then used for the production of ATP. However, under hypoxic conditions, oxidative phosphorylation is reduced and Acetyl Co-A levels in the mitochondria are increased. This and other factors inhibit pyruvate dehydrogenase, causing pyruvate levels in the sarcoplasm to increase. Increased H^+ production leads to the conversion of pyruvate to lactate. Thus, during aerobic metabolism the heart *extracts* lactate, during anaerobic metabolism the heart *produces* lactate.

of actinomyosin cross-bridges and their formation rate. Finally, changes in the morphology of the contractile proteins themselves may affect contractile performance. In physiological terms, resting sarcomere length, the rate of stimulation, and the hormonal effects, in particular of β-adrenergic stimulation, are the most important factors affecting contractile performance of the myofibril.

It is not surprising that as such a number of factors are involved in affecting normal contractile function, that the pathophysiology of the failing heart may involve the disruption of a number of normal processes.

Cardiac failure

Cardiac failure is most simply defined as the inability of the heart to pump blood at a flow rate commensurate with the requirements of the metabolizing tissues, despite an elevated filling pressure. Failure may occur as a result of myocardial failure (i.e. as a result of failure of the normal contractile processes) or as heart failure resulting from a profoundly increased volume load (i.e. acute aortic regurgitation) or inadequate filling (constrictive pericarditis) or as circulatory failure in which cardiac function may be initially unimpaired, as in the early stages of septic shock.

Hypoxia and ischaemia are processes that are commonly involved in the development of myocardial failure. Both of these will lead to a substantial disruption of energy production and utilization within the myocardial cell, leading to reduced pumping performance. One of the first adaptive mechanisms in response to this deficit is to retain sodium and water, thus increasing blood volume and thereby increasing the sarcomere length (preload) to provide the optimum overlap between thick and thin filaments to enhance contraction. This is followed by hypertrophy of the muscle mass with eventual chamber enlargement, and a substantial enhancement of catecholamine release both by cardiac adrenergic nerve endings and the adrenal medulla, in addition to activation of the renin–angiotensin–aldosterone and other neurohumoral systems. This enhanced sympathoadrenal state serves initially to restore cardiac output and later to preserve systemic blood pressure. However, prolonged exposure to elevated catecholamine levels leads to a reduction in density and down-regulation of cardiac β-adrenoceptors. Other adaptive mechanisms include alterations in the density of the mitochondria and sarcoplasmic reticulum, alterations in action potential propagation and the appearance of slow myosin and increased collagen. The short-term consequences of these adaptations are not severe but in the longer term they may be deleterious to cardiac function.

THEORETICAL FACTORS IN THE TREATMENT OF CARDIAC FAILURE

One of the earliest adaptive mechanisms in heart failure is to retain fluid thereby increasing preload and restoring cardiac output by the Frank–Starling mechanism. Furthermore, vasoconstriction induced by enhanced release of adrenergic transmitters and activation of other mechanisms as part of another adaptive mechanism may increase the impedance to left ventricular ejection (afterload) thereby causing an increased level of cardiac work in order to maintain cardiac output and eventually a reduced level of output for the same work. It is not surprising, therefore, that considerable benefit may be gained in both acute and chronic heart failure by factors that optimize the state of the peripheral circulation. Drug therapy that causes arteriolar vasodilatation will reduce ventricular afterload and therefore lead to an enhancement of ventricular emptying, thereby increasing stroke volume, ejection fraction and cardiac output. This is true of both ventricles, although in the case of the right ventricle improving stroke volume simply by afterload reduction may be a more difficult therapeutic manoeuvre.

Reduction in preload may have beneficial cardiac effects in the overdistended and acutely failing heart, but in general venodilatation resulting in a reduction in preload will serve to reduce cardiac output by the Frank–Starling mechanism. However, reduction in preload may be necessary in the chronic failing heart in order to reduce pulmonary venous pressure and lessen pulmonary congestion and oedema. Both venodilatation and reduction in extracellular fluid following diuretic therapy may be beneficial. Although markedly elevated pulmonary venous pressure will eventually cause pulmonary oedema, in the patient with chronic heart failure adaptive changes in the pulmonary capillary bed will protect against the early formation of oedema.

Improvements in myocardial contractility may be brought about by a wide range of positively inotropic drugs. Both systolic contraction and diastolic relaxation are active energy-consuming processes that can be impaired by disease and may respond to appropriate pharmacologic therapy. Systolic failure is manifest by a shift to the right of the left ventricular pressure/volume loop and an increase in left ventricular end-systolic volume, with a reduction in stroke volume. End-diastolic volume, and hence end-diastolic pressure are both increased. In contrast, in diastolic failure the left ventricular pressure volume loop is shifted upwards, and an increased end-diastolic pressure required to achieve the same level of end-diastolic volume, denoting a reduction in left ventricular diastolic compliance (Fig. 15.3).

Improvements in cardiac output may be brought about by altering preload and afterload, without any direct effect whatsoever on myocardial contractility. It may be difficult therefore to identify whether drug treatment leading to an improvement in cardiac output is having an effect on contractility, since the effects seen may be due to peripheral circulatory effects rather than cardiac effects. A number of indices have been used as assessments of contractility. The rate of rise of left ventricular pressure (LV dP/dT max) and the maximum rate of shortening of ventricular muscle (V max) have been used as indices of contractility, and the rate of fall of left ventricular pressure (negative LV dP/dT max) has been used as an assessment of diastolic relaxation. However, as discussed in the previous section, both force of contraction and maximum rate of shortening are dependent on initial sarcomere length, and therefore both positive and negative LV dP/dT max are influenced by preload. Further, since end-systolic volume is increased in systolic failure, a reduction in end-systolic volume could be the result of an inotropic effect. However, end-systolic volume is also influenced by the impedance to ventricular ejection, and therefore

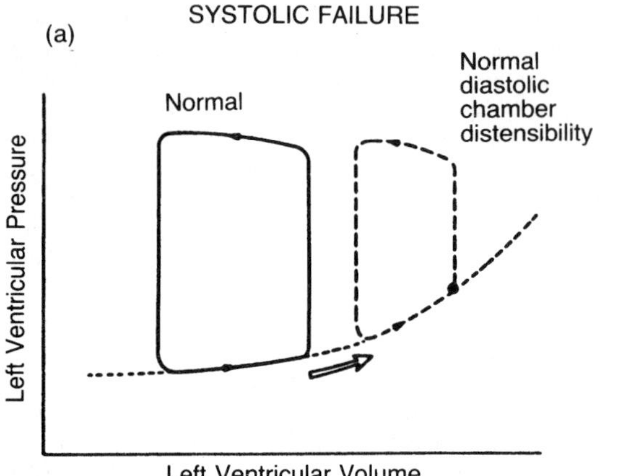

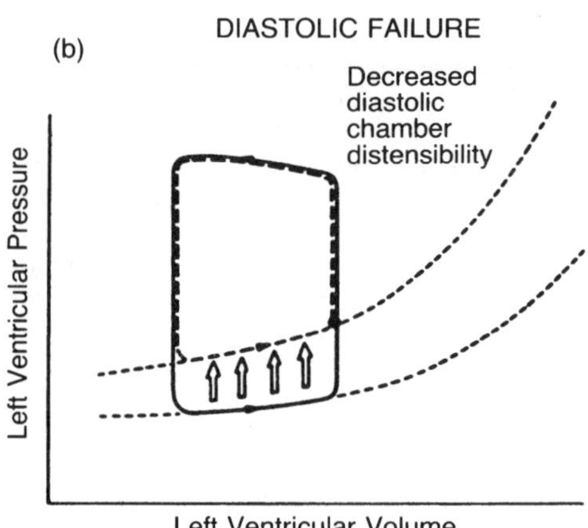

FIGURE 15.3 The differences between systolic and diastolic failure. In systolic failure (a), the failing LV pressure/volume curve is displaced to the right (dotted line). The main features are an increase in left ventricular end-diastolic pressure associated with an increase in left ventricular end-diastolic volume, and a reduction in stroke volume. In diastolic failure (b) there is an increase in left ventricular pressure for any given left ventricular volume, denoting a reduction in distensibility. An increased left ventricular end-diastolic pressure is therefore needed to maintain the left ventricular end-diastolic volume.

a reduction in end-systolic volume and increase in ejection fraction could simply occur as a result of afterload reduction. Thus isovolumic contraction phase indices such as LV dP/dT max and ejection phase indices such as end-systolic volume and ejection fraction are load-dependent indices of contractility, and may not be a true indicator of an enhanced contractile state.

Load-independent indices of contractility are complex. The most accurate technique is to construct a series of ventricular pressure/volume loops at differing preload, identify the end-systolic point in each loop and link them with a straight line, thereby constructing the end-systolic pressure volume relationship (ESPVR). An increase in contractility will increase the slope of the ESPVR, and a negative inotropic effect will result in a flattening of the slope (Fig. 15.4)

However, in the therapeutic context of the treatment of cardiac failure it may not be necessary or even desirable for a drug to have effects only on myocardial contractility and many of the drugs used have direct effects on both cardiac and vascular muscle.

DRUGS THAT IMPROVE CARDIAC PERFORMANCE

From the above discussion, it is clear that drugs may improve cardiac performance by increasing the amount of intracellular calcium available for contractile processes, and by increasing the generation of energy. These may be identified as the final pathway common to many of the drugs that have positive inotropic effects. However, there are a number of mechanisms whereby drugs may improve cardiac performance by a positive inotropic effect, and these are considered in detail below.

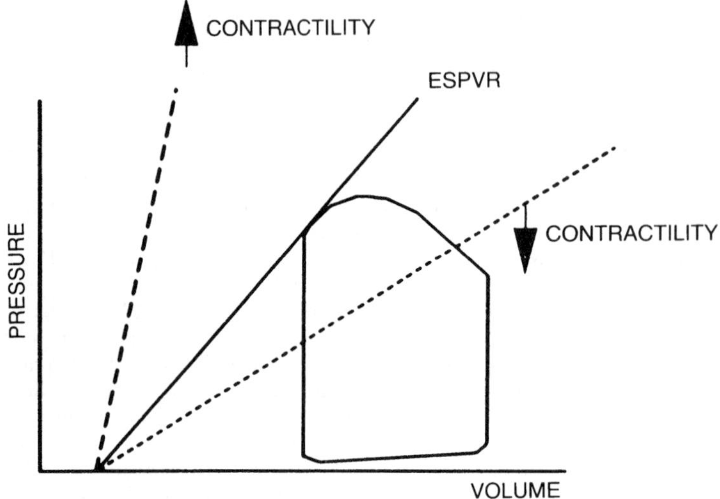

FIGURE 15.4 The slope of the end-systolic pressure volume relationship (ESPVR) is proportional to contractility.

Forskolin

Forskolin acts by direct activation of adenyl cyclase thereby increasing accumulation of 3′5 cAMP within the cell and thus increasing the concentration of calcium available for contractile processes. It is not available for use in humans.

Adrenergic β-receptor agonists

The general pharmacology of these compounds is dealt with more extensively in Chapter 13. In this section, the effects of β-agonists on cardiac function and on the peripheral circulation as it relates to cardiac function, are considered.

Adrenergic β-agonists enhance cardiac function by a positive inotropic effect mediated by adrenergic β_1-receptors. By this mechanism, adenyl cyclase is activated promoting an increase in 3′5 cAMP and hence in available calcium, as discussed earlier. The effect of catecholamines on α- and β-receptors is shown in Table 15.1 and, as can be seen, none of the compounds shown has a dose-independent specificity for β_1-receptors. The consequence of this is that, as the dosage is increased, other α- and other non-β_1-effects are increasingly seen which are both variable and may not be desirable or effective in improving cardiac function. Furthermore, as discussed earlier, the efficacy of adrenergic agonists will in part be dependent on the density and sensitivity of the adrenergic receptor population in a specified tissue. In patients with chronic heart failure, plasma catecholamine levels are raised initially as part of the adaptive process, but eventually this results in a marked reduction in the density and specificity of cardiac β-receptors. In this patient group, catecholamines are much less effective in normal dosage than in patients with a normal β-receptor density.[1]

Activation of β_1-receptors by any of the agonists shown will result in an increase in isovolumic contraction phase indices (LV d*P*/d*T* max) and in ejection phase indices (increase in ejection fraction, decrease in end-systolic volume) and in load-independent indices (ESPVR). There is also an increase in negative LV d*P*/d*T* max suggesting an enhancement in the rate of ventricular relaxation. *In vivo*, the increase in cardiac contractility will cause an increase in cardiac output and a reflex vasodilatation, resulting in a marked fall in systemic vascular resistance. The actual change in systemic blood pressure is more variable and partly dependent on the pretreatment level. Activation of cardiac β-receptors also causes a positive chronotropic effect resulting in a tachycardia.

The interaction between the β_1-effects and other adrenergic receptor effects seen with catecholamines will produce a range of haemodynamic effects that are markedly influenced by the pre-existing state of the myocardium. Activation of peripheral α-receptors via noradrenaline, or following high dose infusions of adrenaline, dopamine or possibly dobutamine, will lead to systemic and pulmonary vasoconstriction and an increase in pulmonary and systemic arterial pressures and vascular resistances. The increase in impedance to ventricular ejection may result in a reduction in cardiac output, particularly in the failing heart. However, in the situation of profound systemic hypotension, an increase in aortic diastolic blood pressure may serve to improve coronary perfusion pressure and hence to enhance coronary blood flow and myocardial oxygen delivery resulting in improved contractile function. Activation of peripheral β_2-receptors following isoprenaline may result in active vasodilatation, particularly in skeletal muscle and the pulmonary vascular bed. The reduction in preload may result in little or no change in stroke output, and any enhancement in overall cardiac output is often achieved only as a result of the developing tachycardia. This tachycardia may serve to shorten diastolic coronary filling time and thereby reduce coronary perfusion thus potentially worsening myocardial oxygen balance. However, the vasodilator effects may offset this by reducing other factors (LV systolic wall stress, left ventricular end-diastolic pressure (LVEDP) or preload) known to

TABLE 15.1 Features of the phosphodiesterase isoenzymes. (Km, Michaelis constant; cGMP, cyclic guanosine monophosphate; cAMP, cyclic adenosine monophosphate)

ISOENZYME FAMILY	SUBSTRATE CHARACTERISTIC	ISOENZYME SELECTIVE INHIBITORS	FUNCTIONAL EFFECT OF INHIBITION
I	Ca^{2+} and calmodulin-dependent	Vinpocetine	Smooth muscle relaxation
II	cGMP stimulated	No selective inhibitor	Unknown
III	cGMP inhibits the cAMP hydrolytic action. Low K_m for cAMP and cGMP	Milrinone, enoximone, piroximone, amrinone	Positive inotrope; vascular and airway smooth muscle relaxation Platelet aggregation inhibition
		Pimobendan, imadazodan	Ca^{2+} sensitization
IV	cAMP specific. Low K_m only for cAMP	Rolipram, denbufylline	Airway, smooth muscle relaxation; inhibition of inflammatory mediators
V	cGMP specific. Isoenzymes with high and low K_m for cGMP	Zaprinast, dipyridamole	Platelet aggregation inhibition

increase myocardial oxygen consumption. The overall effects on combined β_1- and β_2-stimulation on the peripheral circulation are to reduce systemic and pulmonary vascular resistances. It is for this latter effect in particular, as well as the chronotropic effects, that isoprenaline is used therapeutically.

Phosphodiesterase inhibitors

The phosphodiesterase isoenzyme is present in a wide range of tissue, including vascular and bronchial smooth muscle, cardiac muscle, platelets, lung and liver. The phosphodiesterase inhibitors are a heterogeneous group of drugs whose effects are to inhibit the enzymatic degradation of 3′5 cAMP and cGMP in various tissues. In cardiac tissue this leads to an increase in 3′5 cAMP and the consequent improvement in contractility outlined above.

The various isoenzymes of phosphodiesterase and the consequent effects of inhibition are shown in Table 15.1. Inhibition of isoenzyme III is associated with cardiovascular effects, and the drugs used currently to treat heart failure are PDE III inhibitors. The different classes of drugs that are able to inhibit phosphodiesterase are also shown in Table 15.1. The drugs currently available are enoximone (imidazolone derivative) and the bipyridine derivatives amrinone and milrinone. Although these are all described as selective for isoenzyme PDE III, inhibition of other PDE isoenzymes is likely. Both amrinone and milrinone have shown the ability to inhibit platelet aggregation,[2] which is a functional effect of inhibiting isoenzyme V. Drugs that inhibit all PDE isoenzymes may theoretically be used for their cardiovascular effects. In practice, the alkylxanthines demonstrate an unacceptably high level of unwanted effects (nausea, cerebral irritability, arrhythmia) to be clinically useful. Papaverine is used predominantly for its peripheral vascular effects.

The effect of increasing the intracellular concentration of cAMP is to enhance myocardial contractility, although there would appear to be a time lag effect between the onset of maximum contractility and the peak concentration of cAMP following PDE III therapy, which is similar to the effects seen with catecholamines. The explanation for this is not clear, but it may be that cAMP and PDE isoenzymes are compartmentalized within cells and that these compartments have different sensitivities to PDE inhibition. Furthermore, the ability of some PDE inhibitors to directly sensitize the myofibrils to calcium may be more important in determining an inotropic effect than the effect of increased cAMP. However, with currently available compounds it is likely that the cAMP-related effects are the most important.

In addition to the cardiac effects, PDE III inhibitors have direct effects on vascular smooth muscle. The increase in cAMP in vascular smooth muscle causes a liberation of calcium which is rapidly taken up by the sarcoplasmic reticulum thereby reducing the amount of calcium available for contractile processes. The vasodilatation seen with PDE III inhibitors is an active process, in contrast to that seen with the β_1-agonist catecholamines where much of the vasodilator response may be a reflex response to an increased cardiac output.

The therapeutic effects of PDE III inhibitors are therefore to improve contractile performance and to cause a reduction in vascular tone, but the detailed haemodynamic responses seen may be more dependent on the pre-existing state of the circulation. Intravenous studies in patients with chronic heart failure show that PDE III inhibitors are able to increase cardiac output and reduce systemic and pulmonary vascular resistance.[3] The vasodilator effects result in a reflex tachycardia. Studies of myocardial energetics in these patients suggest that the increase in oxygen consumption that would be consequent on an inotropic effect are offset by a reduction in LV wall stress, such that overall myocardial oxygen balance is not affected, although it should be said that there is considerable variation between individual patients.[4] The intravenous studies of patients with acute low output syndrome, usually following cardiac surgery, mirror the intravenous chronic heart failure studies almost exactly.[5] Cardiac output is increased with a small reflex tachycardia, pre- and afterloading conditions are reduced and systemic and pulmonary vascular resistances are also reduced, particularly where they are markedly elevated before treatment. Similarly, systemic and pulmonary arterial pressures are reduced, and myocardial energetics are not disturbed. There are data to suggest an antischaemic effect, which is not surprising since the effects on LV relaxation, end-systolic and end-diastolic volumes and wall stress are similar to those seen following nitroglycerine. Furthermore, the effects on inhibition of platelet aggregation may be important in inhibiting thrombus formation and propagation.[6]

Oral studies

Oral studies with PDE III inhibitors were encouraging initially, but the long-term results have proved disappointing. It is salutary to recall that the development of PDE III inhibitors was stimulated in part by a search for alternatives to digoxin in chronic heart failure patients, and that efficacy and safety must equal or exceed digoxin. The oral preparation of amrinone has been withdrawn due to thrombocytopenia, and oral milrinone was withdrawn following an unfavourable outcome in a large placebo-controlled trial in chronic heart failure patients.[7] Oral enoximone has also been withdrawn for safety reasons and thus there are no oral PDE III inhibitors currently available in Europe or the USA. However, the use of intravenous PDE III inhibitors in the hospital setting is widespread and increasing. The effects of bipyridine and imidazolone compounds are terminated by renal excretion either of the drug or of active metabolites. Milrinone has a terminal half-life of approximately 1 h in normals, increased to 2.3 h in patients with chronic heart failure. Eighty per cent of the drug is excreted unchanged via the kidneys, and the dosage should be substantially reduced in renal failure. By contrast, enoximone is metabolized mainly by the liver, and has a long-acting active sulphoxide metabolite with approximately one-seventh of the activity of the parent compound. The metabolite is also excreted renally and therefore the dosage of enoximone will need to be reduced in renal failure also.

The adverse effects of treatment with PDE III inhibitors are predictable from their known pharmacological profile. The main circulatory problems are hypotension and arrhythmia, but these can be minimized by careful attention to dosage. The arrhythmogenic effects of intravenous PDE III inhibitors in patients recovering from major cardiovascular surgery have not been marked, in contrast to the arrhythmogenic effects of the oral preparation in chronic heart failure patients. The inhibitory effects on platelet aggregation may cause postoperative bleeding, and nausea and vomiting have been reported.

Direct calcium-channel activators

Studies of the pharmacology of the dihydropyridine compounds have revealed that these compounds possess calcium agonist effects as well as calcium antagonistic, or calcium-channel blocking effects. Although there are no compounds available for clinical use, a number of drugs have been studied experimentally, including BAY k8644, CGP 28-392, H 160/51, YC 170 and 202-791. These studies have revealed not only a potential new class of inotropic drugs but also new information about the nature of the calcium channels and calcium physiology.

The dihydropyridine (DHP) calcium agonists exist in two enantiomers, but only one enantiomer has calcium agonist properties, the other possessing calcium-channel blocking effects. Clearly, the overall effect of the drug will depend on the relative potencies and preponderance of the two enantiomers. In all compounds but 202-791 the relative preponderance of enantiomers is firmly in favour of the Ca agonist moiety. In that sense, the drugs prescribed are partial agonists, and indeed the effects of the drugs may differ at different concentrations, with higher concentrations revealing a more effective calcium-channel blocking effect.

The relative potency of the inotropic versus vasoconstrictor effects may also be variable between compounds. Whereas BAY k8644 and CGP 28-392 exhibit almost identical inotropic and vasoconstrictor potencies, YC 170 exhibits only vasoconstrictive effects.

The mechanism of action of calcium agonists is complex and reflects current understanding of the calcium channel. This channel is supposed to exist in three different states (resting, inactivated, open) and the DHPs have a state-dependent action on the channel, increasing the open probability by binding to the open channel and stabilizing this state. Although the positive inotropic effects of calcium agonists are well reported, it should also be said that studies are by no means exhaustive, and an improvement in isovolumic contraction phase indices has largely been taken to indicate a positive inotropic effect.

Changes in the left ventricular function curve suggest vasoconstriction +/– inotropy (shift upwards to the right), but simultaneous treatment with sodium nitroprusside to remove the vasoconstrictor effects reveals LV function curve changes more in keeping with classic positive inotropy. These effects may make the calcium agonists more appropriate therapy for patients with acute heart failure and severe hypotension, rather than chronic congestive heart failure, although the partial agonist properties of the DHPs may facilitate the development of more appropriate compounds in the future.

Drugs that act on Na/K membrane-bound ATPase

DPI 201-106

DPI 201-106 is a piperazinyl-indole derivative. The effect of the drug is to maintain the open state of sodium channels during the action potential which transiently loads the cell with sodium, which in turn increases intracellular free calcium via stimulation of the sodium/calcium exchange mechanism. In addition, DPI 201-106 may increase the sensitivity of contractile proteins in cardiac muscle to calcium, and these combined effects may result in an inotropic effect. DPI 201-106 has shown potential as a positive inotropic agent in patients with congestive cardiomyopathy and chronic heart failure, although studies in patients following cardiac surgery were not as encouraging. Furthermore, electrophysiologic changes including QTc prolongation, ST segment elevation and T wave changes have all been described which are similar to those changes seen during myocardial ischaemia but which do not appear to be related to active ischaemia as identified by studies of cardiac metabolism.[8] DPI 201-106 has been shown to have other haemodynamic effects including a negative chronotropic effect and vasodilator effects, possibly related to inhibition of slow calcium channels, and antiarrhythmic effects have been produced experimentally.

Digitalis and the cardiac glycosides

Although a large number of plant extracts containing cardiac glycosides have been used therapeutically since Roman times, the therapeutic value of digitalis came to be more widely recognized after William Withering published *An account of the foxglove and some of its medical uses: with practical remarks on dropsy and other diseases* in 1785.[9] However, it is John Ferriar in 1799 who is credited with ascribing to digitalis a primary effect on the heart, in contrast to the diuretic effect which he felt was of secondary importance. In the early 20th century the value of the drug in the treatment of atrial fibrillation was gradually established, and since that time digoxin has been used both for its positive inotropic effects in the treatment of congestive heart failure and as an antiarrhythmic, particularly in the treatment of atrial fibrillation.

The chemical structure of the cardiac glycosides is such that they combine an aglycone with between one and four sugar molecules. The pharmacological activity is determined by the aglycone whereas the sugar molecules determine lipid and water solubility and affect potency. The pharmacology of the cardiac glycosides is complex. They have direct effects on force of contraction and on electrophysiology; in addition there are a number of important secondary cardiovascular effects to consider.

Hydrolysis of ATP by Na/K-bound ATPase provides the energy for the mechanism whereby Na is actively extruded and K imported into the sarcolemma of cardiac fibres. Cardiac glycosides bind to Na/K ATPase and inhibit its activity thereby impairing the active transport of Na and K ions. There is, therefore, a gradual increase in intracellular sodium. However, the resultant effect is that the exchange of intracellular Ca for extracellular Na is diminished, leading to an increase in intracellular calcium ions. The consequence of this is that calcium stores in the sarcoplasmic reticulum are increased, and more calcium is available for enhancement of contractility. In addition, the increase in intracellular calcium leads to an increase in the slow inward current during the action potential. This slow inward current is the result of calcium ions moving intracellularly and contributes to the plateau phase (phase 2) of the action potential. Furthermore, other modes of action of the inotropic properties of cardiac glycosides have been proposed, including stimulation of the Na/K pump and alterations in calcium binding by sarcolemmal phospholipids. However, it does appear that an effective inotropic action is dependent on some degree of inhibition of active transport of Na and K ions.

The electrical effects of cardiac glycosides are complex and should be differentiated into direct and indirect effects. These are dealt with later in this chapter under the heading of antiarrhythmics.

ANTI-ISCHAEMIC DRUGS

Ischaemic heart disease is the largest single cause of mortality in the UK and accounts for approximately 150 000 deaths per year in England and Wales.[10] This represents a massive morbidity and mortality in the adult population overall, and the treatment of patients with ischaemic heart disease is therefore a vitally important topic.

General principles of therapy

There are a number of rare causes of coronary artery occlusion, but the most common and hence the most important is the build up of atheroma in larger coronary arteries. The aetiology for the development of atheroma in the general population is not clear, but there do appear to be a number of factors that may be significantly contributive – that is, lack of exercise and heavy cigarette smoking. In certain individuals, familial predisposition to hyperlipidaemia and hypercholesterolaemia may be associated with a high incidence of early severe ischaemic heart disease and a family history of early cardiac infarction. Modifying the serum lipid profile in an attempt to reduce the development of early atheroma is important in these individuals. However, the value of reducing the serum lipids and serum cholesterol in otherwise normal patients as a means of protecting against ischaemic heart disease has been questioned. Thus the first line of the therapeutic strategy lies in lifestyle modification and, where appropriate, lipid-lowering drugs in an attempt to prevent the onset of coronary atheroma.

The second line of the therapeutic strategy is to prevent the development of myocardial oxygen imbalance once significant coronary atheroma has developed thus producing symptoms of ischaemic heart disease. A number of haemodynamic factors have been identified which will have effects on myocardial oxygen balance, and these are shown in Fig. 15.5. Some haemodynamic changes, most notably tachycardia, may be particularly troublesome, but it should be noted that overall there is a poor correlation between the development of intraoperative ischaemia and notable haemodynamic abnormality. This would suggest that there are other factors involved in the generation of perioperative ischaemia, and attention is now being directed to areas such as the stability of coronary vascular tone.

The management of patients with proven significant coronary artery disease entails the use of drugs to maximize coronary vasodilatation and reduce systemic vasoconstriction (calcium-channel blockers), to reduce heart rate and myocardial work and hence oxygen consumption (adrenergic β-blockers) and to reduce preload and hence left ventricular end-diastolic pressure, redistribute intramyocardial blood flow from the epicardial to the endocardial layers and also dilate large epicardial coronary vessels (i.e. nitrates). In the

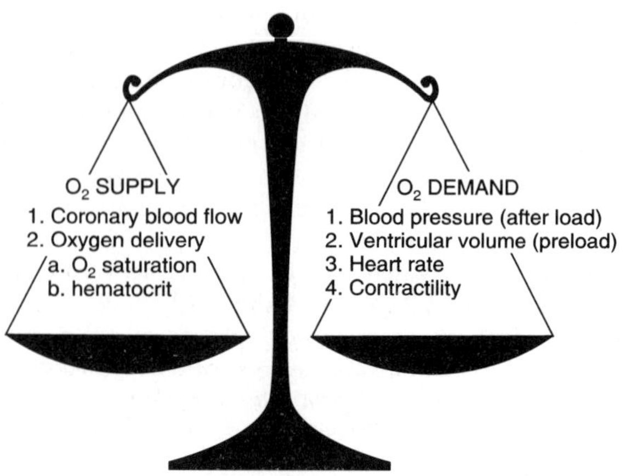

FIGURE 15.5 Haemodynamic factors affecting myocardial oxygen balance.

setting of chronic stable angina, calcium-channel blockers, β-blockers and nitrates are taken orally, and sublingual nitrates are used to treat an acute anginal attack. The pharmacology of the relevant drugs is described in Chapters 14 and 16.

The third line of therapeutic strategy lies in the treatment of acute myocardial infarction. There are variants in the aetiology of acute infarction, but one common mechanism involves the rupture of an atheromatous plaque in a coronary artery. This leads to the acute generation of thrombus to repair the ruptured plaque, with the consequence that the thrombus so generated may lead to a substantial or total occlusion of the coronary artery. Debris from the ruptured plaque may further complicate the picture. Myocardial tissue distal to the acute occlusion may become acutely ischaemic and infarct unless flow through adequate collateral channels is maintained.

Treatment is directed toward two goals. The first is the removal of any blood clots by thrombolytic therapy. A number of drugs have been developed for this purpose, including streptokinase and related compounds, and recent data suggest that they may reduce mortality from myocardial infarction when given early.[11] These drugs are discussed in detail in Chapter 27.

The second goal is to improve collateral flow and the intramyocardial distribution of blood flow, usually with conventional antischaemic drugs such as intravenous nitrates or, more rarely, calcium-channel blockers. The detailed pharmacology is discussed in the relevant sections on adrenergic β-receptor antagonists, nitrovasodilators and calcium-channel blocking agents.

NORMAL CARDIAC ELECTROPHYSIOLOGY

The aetiology and treatment of arrhythmias is a large and controversial subject. Many aspects are currently topical, particularly in the field of prophylaxis in patients with cardiac failure or suffering recent myocardial infarction. For anaesthetists, arrhythmias have always been a subject of great relevance. The use of ECG monitoring during anaesthesia began in the 1930s, and it immediately became apparent that the incidence of intraoperative arrhythmias was high.[11] Perioperative arrhythmias are common, but fortunately since generally patients undergoing surgery do well, the overwhelming majority of intraoperative arrhythmias must be benign. However, whatever the clinical context, it is necessary to identify the mechanisms for arrhythmia generation if we are to understand the therapeutic potential of the different drugs available for treatment.

Cellular basis of rhythmicity

The schematic representation of a cardiac cell action potential is shown in Fig. 15.6. After rapid depolarization (phase 0) there is a short period of rapid repolarization (phase 1) followed by a plateau (phase 2) and then another rapid phase completing repolarization (phase 3). Slow diastolic depolarization occurs (phase 4) until a critical threshold is reached, whereupon rapid phase 0 depolarization commences and the cycle is repeated. During phase 0 depolarization, the opening of fast response sodium channels is responsible for the massive influx of Na^+ ions which increase transmembrane potential from –90 to +20 mV, and the terminal notch (phase 1) is caused by deactivation of the Na^+ current and an inward Cl^- current. Slow Ca channels open during phase 0 depolarization at about –40 mV and these remain open for between 30 and 300 ms and thus are responsible for the phase 2 plateau. This slow inward Ca current is inactivated during phase 3, and the outward K^+ current is activated, thus causing a reduction in transmembrane potential. During phases 3–4 the Na/K pump re-establishes the baseline concentration gradient of the relative cations with 2 K^+ ions moving into the cell for every 3 Na^+ ions moving out.

Pacemaker cells have a much less negative resting membrane potential (–50 to –60 mV) and at this level fast Na channels are refractory. Thus slow Ca channels are responsible for depolarization resulting in a slow rising action potential. At –40 mV a secondary phase of rapid depolarization

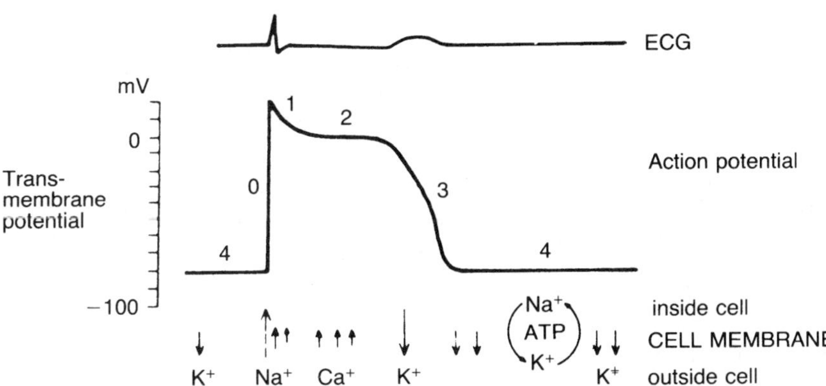

FIGURE 15.6 Schematic representation of an action potential in a myocardial cell, correlated with the ECG and the major ionic movements.

occurs associated with inward Na^+ currents. The prolonged repolarization phase is associated with termination of inward cation movement and the efflux of K^+ ions.

Cardiac fibres have the characteristic of refractoriness. The refractory period may be absolute, during which period no stimulus, no matter how large, will generate a further action potential, or relative, during which time a larger than normal stimulus may generate an action potential, although this action potential may be smaller than normal and fail to propagate fully. Temporally, the absolute refractory period occurs during phase 2, and the relative refractory period starts midway through phase 3.

Cardiac pacemaker tissue will also demonstrate automaticity, classically seen as a gradual upward (less negative, more positive) trend in phase 4 depolarization toward the threshold potential. Alterations in threshold potential and maximum diastolic potential will also influence automaticity.

Once initiated, propagation of an action potential will depend on the 'strength' of the action potential, and on the 'resistance' to propagation through surrounding tissue. Excitation of nearby fast response fibres is more likely to result in successful impulse propagation than excitation of slow response fibres, and the excess of activation current over the minimum that is required to ensure successful impulse propagation may be considered as the safety factor of conduction. Fast response fibres have a higher conduction safety factor than slow response fibres.

CELLULAR MECHANISMS OF ARRHYTHMOGENESIS

The main cellular mechanisms responsible for arrhythmogenesis include: conduction of the depressed fast response; abnormal automaticity; triggered automaticity; triggered activity; and the re-entry of excitation. Many provoking factors have been implicated including drugs, local hypoxia or ischaemia, and abnormal biochemical or physiological states.

In many of these situations, loss of membrane potential in fast-response fibres may be influential. This results in slowed conduction, but this slowed conduction is not likely to be uniform throughout the conducting system with the result of uneven conduction and refractoriness. Either re-entry or heart block could occur as a result.

Abnormal automaticity (usually enhanced automaticity) has been demonstrated in experimental ischaemia. It differs from triggered automaticity, which is dependent on a prior trigger stimulus for the initiation of the arrhythmia. This latter phenomenon may occur during phases 2–3 of the action potential, and may be due to oscillations in the transmembrane potential, called early afterdepolarizations (EAD), or early potentials. Different types of EAD have been described, no doubt associated with different ionic mechanisms, but EAD-triggered arrhythmic activity is more likely to occur at slow heart rates.

Triggered activity occurs in association with delayed afterdepolarizations, or late potentials, which are oscillations in the transmembrane potential that occur during phase 4 repolarization, often preceded by hyperpolarization of the membrane which may occur due to calcium overload. In contrast to EADs, late potentials tend to be dependent on fast heart rates.

Following the original criteria for re-entry arrhythmia,[12] the possible scenarios for generation of re-entry arrhythmias have expanded substantially. None the less, the simplest variant of re-entry is easily understood. It relies on an impulse being conducted to a circuit in which there is a unidirectional conduction block. The impulse is then conducted in a circular fashion and be seen to re-enter the conducting pathway, and interruption of the circus pathway would terminate the arrhythmia. This original concept of circus re-entry was thought to be due to an anatomical block, but other mechanisms including electrophysiological states have since been proposed.

Overview of arrhythmogenic mechanisms

Whatever cellular mechanisms are involved, it is clear that the clinical environment that may be considered to be arrhythmogenic is widely diverse. However, in surgical patients it is clear that both pathophysiological and pharmacological factors combine to produce a very high possibility of arrhythmogenesis. For example, preoperative anxiety and/or pain, the premedicant drugs used to alleviate it, the anaesthetic agents and muscle relaxants used and the neuroendocrine responses and biochemical alterations during and after surgery all have the potential to be considered arrhythmogenic (Table 15.2). Given that arrhythmias are common, and that almost everything about anaesthetic practice can be considered to be potentially arrhythmogenic, it is clear that many perioperative arrhythmias carry little relevance to the fit individual, although to the patient with concomitant cardiac disease a new arrhythmia may have a very poor effect on outcome.

TABLE 15.2 Perioperative arrhythmogenic factors

Pain, anxiety, agitation
Pre-existing cardiac disease
Pre-existing arrhythmia, including anti-arrhythmic drugs
Endocrine disorders, especially thyroid
Blood gas and acid–base disturbance
Electrolyte imbalance, especially K, Ca, Mg
Anaesthetic premedicants with autonomic NS effects
Anaesthetic drugs, especially volatile agents
Neuromuscular relaxants (pancuronium, suxamethonium)
Local anaesthetics with vasoconstrictors (adrenaline)
Temperature changes
Sympatho-adrenal activation due to surgical stress
Parasympathetic activation due to surgical traction (peritoneum, extraocular muscles)
Changes in haemoglobin and circulating volume
Causes of prolonged QT interval

Classification of arrhythmias

There have been a number of different methods for classifying arrhythmias. From the discussion of cellular mechanisms, it would appear that a subdivision into disorders of impulse formation, and disorders of impulse conduction or propagation would be an appropriate classification. Attempts have been made to classify arrhythmias based on anatomical site (supraventricular and ventricular), heart rate (bradyarrhythmias and tachyarrhythmias), the effective drug treatment and other criteria. The following is a method of classification that has the advantage of combining practicality with theory:

- arrhythmias of sinus origin
- ectopic rhythms
- conduction blocks
- pre-excitation syndromes.

Arrhythmias of sinus origin

The electrical activity follows the usual conduction pathways but is either too fast, too slow or irregular. Apart from sinus tachycardia and bradycardia, sinus arrest or exit block is the other notable arrhythmia.

Ectopic rhythms

These are usually due to either abnormal automaticity or re-entry. In the former setting, a single focus or multiple foci take over as the driving pacemaker. Since the ectopic focus may occur within either the atria or ventricles, it is important to be able to distinguish between atrial and ventricular ectopic rhythms. This will be aided by observing the presence of p waves, the width of the QRS complex, the regularity of the rhythm and the relationship between the p wave and the QRS complex.

The cellular mechanism of re-entry has already been described, but the consequence of the re-entry mechanism is to create a focus of abnormal electrical activity. Re-entry mechanisms appear to be important in the generation of a number of arrhythmias, including atrial flutter, paroxysmal supraventricular tachycardia and ventricular tachycardia.

Conduction blocks

Conduction block may occur at the level of the SA node, the AV node, and within the His–Purkinje system. The degree of AV block (first degree, second degree Mobitz type I and II, third degree or complete) is determined by the relationship of the p waves to the QRS complexes. The nature of bundle branch block (right or left, or left anterior or posterior hemiblock) is determined by the width and configuration of the QRS complexes, and the ECG axis.

Pre-excitation syndromes

In this situation, the normal delay between atrial and ventricular depolarization is bypassed by an accessory pathway, resulting in premature ventricular depolarization. Although a number of accessory pathways have been identified they are not common, occurring in less than 1% of individuals, usually in males. The two most common pre-excitation syndromes are Wolff–Parkinson–White and Lown–Ganong–Levine. Pre-excitation circuits may act as an effective substrate for re-entry tachycardia, which may be particularly severe.

ANTIARRHYTHMIC DRUGS

The usual contemporary classification of antiarrhythmic drugs is the Vaughan–Williams classification, shown in Table 15.3. This classification, although useful, is not infallible. In particular, the association between the clinical antiarrhythmic effect of different drugs and the electrophysiological effect is often weak, and there is often both considerable variation between differing subgroups of drugs in the same class and distinct similarities between drugs in supposedly different classes. In addition, digoxin, a drug with potent antiarrhythmic effects, is not easily classified and therefore either ignored or given its own class. None the less, no other classification combines accuracy and simplicity as effectively.

TABLE 15.3 Vaughan–Williams classification

Class I	Membrane-stabilizing drugs
Ia	Quinidine, disopyramide, procainamide
Ib	Lignocaine, mexiletine
Ic	Flecainide, encainide
Class II	β-Adrenergic receptor antagonists, i.e. propranolol, metoprolol, esmolol
Class III	Drugs that increase action potential refractory period (antifibrillatory drugs), i.e. amiodarone, bretylium
Class IV	Calcium-channel blockers i.e. verapamil, diltiazem
Others	Cardiac glycosides (class V)
	Adenosine

Class I

Class I drugs are membrane stabilizers, resulting in the inhibition of fast-channel depolarization due to the blockade of sodium channels. However, these are a pharmacologically diverse group of compounds and they have been further classified into class Ia, Ib, and Ic. The differing electrophysiological effects seen within each class are shown in Table 15.4.

Although depression of fast sodium channels may be the primary antiarrhythmic mechanism, a number of other mechanisms may be involved – the most important of which involve abolishing re-entry.

Class Ia

Quinidine has classic class Ia effects and depresses cardiac excitability by raising the threshold potential level, decreasing both fast and slow depolarization, prolonging duration of the action potential and the effective refractory period and slowing intra-atrial, atrioventricular and intraventricular conduction.

Quinidine has anticholinergic effects that may be responsible for a variety of cardiac and non-cardiac effects. Gastrointestinal irritation, tinnitus and visual disturbances, and eventually severe CNS symptoms including confusion and psychosis may be seen in overdosage. The cardiac effects include an increase in sinus rate and a variable effect on AV nodal conduction which may be enhanced or depressed, depending on the balance between the direct depressive effect and the anticholinergic enhancement. Infranodal conduction is slowed and in overdosage intraventricular conduction block, including complete heart block, may occur. The QT interval on the ECG may be prolonged, and monitoring the QT interval may provide a useful guide to dosage. Prolongation of the QT interval with quinidine therapy has been associated with severe tachyarrhythmias.

Quinidine is usually administered orally, partly as a precaution against the adverse haemodynamic consequences of parenteral administration and partly because absorption from the gastrointestinal tract is rapid and effective. Peak plasma levels are reached 1–2 h after oral dosing, and the elimination half-life is such that the drug should be administered three or four times daily. In non-responders, increasing the frequency may be more effective than increasing the dosage.

Quinidine is used to treat atrial and ventricular arrhythmias. The ventricular response in atrial fibrillation may, however, be accelerated with quinidine therapy, due to the combination of a reduction in atrial rate and enhancement of AV nodal conduction. Thus more impulses are conducted effectively through the AV node. In this respect it differs in its effects from digoxin, and quinidine is often combined with β-blockade or digoxin for this reason. Indeed, quinidine may interact with digoxin since both drugs are protein bound and quinidine may displace digoxin from plasma proteins thereby increasing serum digoxin levels. Quinidine is partially excreted unchanged by the kidneys (20%); the remainder undergoes hepatic metabolism.

Procainamide decreases the rate of rise of depolarization (V max) during phase 0 and decreases the rate of phase 4 depolarization in a similar fashion to quinidine. Anticholinergic effects may also be seen, but there is less prolongation of the QT interval than with quinidine. Procainamide is even more likely than quinidine to increase the ventricular response in patients with atrial fibrillation, and therefore although it may be used for supraventricular arrhythmias its use is usually confined to ventricular arrhythmias. In this regard it is usually used as a second line drug after lignocaine, and may be used for either multiple VEs, R on T phenomenon or ventricular tachycardia. Slow intravenous administration of 1.5 mg/kg may be repeated up to a total dose of 15 mg/kg, and the drug may also be given by continuous infusion. However, the total dose should be reduced markedly in patients with hepatic or renal impairment. Procainamide is cleared by the kidneys (50%) and the remainder undergoes hepatic metabolism.

Adverse cardiac effects may be seen in overdosage, and ventricular tachycardia associated with QT prolongation is a feature although it is less likely with procainamide than with quinidine.

TABLE 15.4 Electrophysiology of class I drugs

ELECTROPHYSIOLOGICAL ACTIVITY	Ia	Ib	Ic
Phase 0	Depressed	Slight effect	Depressed^{++}
Depolarization	Prolonged	Slight effect	Slight effect
Conduction	Decreased	Slight effect	V max reduced
ERP	Increased	Slight effect	Slight effect
APD	Increased	Decreased	Slight effect
ERP : ADP ratio	Increased	Decreased	Slight effect
QRS duration	Increased	No effect	Increased^{++}

ERP, effective refractory period; ADP, action potential duration.

Disopyramide also possesses anticholinergic effects which may facilitate AV nodal conduction. It may be used for both ventricular and supraventricular tachyarrhythmias, although it too may cause ventricular tachycardia in association with a prolonged QT interval. It has marked negative inotropic effects; elimination is via both the hepatic and renal routes equally.

Class Ib

Class Ib drugs have no autonomic effects and therefore the antiarrhythmic effects seen are due solely to the electrophysiological effects. The rate of rapid (phase 0) depolarization may be reduced and the slope of slow (phase 4) depolarization may also be depressed in Purkinje fibres. The action potential and the effective refractory period are shortened.

Of the drugs available, lignocaine is clearly the most widely used, but its lack of bioavailability when given orally has led to the development of other compounds, notably mexiletine.

Lignocaine has been used for all forms of ventricular arrhythmia with the exception of those precipitated by a prolonged QT interval. It is ineffective in treating supraventricular arrhythmias. Lignocaine increases the threshold for VF, and its effects on fast sodium channels and the linkage between Na^+ and K^+ current effects may make lignocaine ineffective in hypokalaemic patients. The reduction in action potential duration may make lignocaine effective in combating re-entry arrhythmias in ventricular tissue although this is controversial.[14]

The distribution of lignocaine within the myocardium has been shown to have an important bearing on its antiarrhythmic effect. The concentration within the ischaemic arrhythmogenic areas of myocardium is the important factor determining efficacy, not blood levels.

Lignocaine has a short elimination half-life (100 min) and is extensively metabolized by the liver. Active metabolites are produced that are excreted renally.

Therapeutic plasma levels lie in the range of 1.5–5 μg/ml. Toxicity is usual over 10 μg/ml. Whatever the therapeutic regimen used, it should aim to achieve and maintain effective plasma levels without risk of overdosage. Thus, a 100-mg bolus followed by a 2 mg/min infusion in a 70-kg adult may be effective, although the dose should be reduced in patients with severe heart failure.

The major toxic effects of lignocaine are CNS effects, including drowsiness and disorientation, progressing to agitation, twitching, tinnitus and other auditory manifestations, and finally convulsions. Profound and sudden overdosage, such as may occur with tourniquet failure during a Biers block, will produce convulsions with very little warning. However, provided that respiratory and cardiovascular problems are dealt with appropriately, lignocaine-induced convulsions have no permanently damaging effects.

Mexiletine but not lignocaine may be given orally, although mexiletine has also been used intravenously. The mechanism of action is similar to that of lignocaine, and the profile of use is also similar although there is some suggestion that mexiletine may be effective intravenously where lignocaine has failed. Mexiletine undergoes hepatic metabolism and may therefore be affected by hepatic microsomal induction and by liver failure.

Class Ic

Class Ic drugs are highly effective in suppressing phase 0 activity thereby causing a marked reduction in conduction velocity. However, in recent years class 1c drugs have become notorious for their ability to be pro-arrhythmic, a phenomenon identified as arrhythmia precipitated or exacerbated by antiarrhythmic drug therapy. Both flecainide and encainide have been implicated in pro-arrhythmic effects, and a trial involving both drugs in the setting of ventricular ectopic activity following acute myocardial infarction had to be discontinued due to excess mortality in the patients receiving flecainide and encainide compared with those patients taking a placebo (Chronic Arrhythmia Suppression Trial – CAST). The exact mechanism of pro-arrhythmia in Ic drugs is not fully clear, but it may be related to decreased conduction in abnormal areas of myocardium which may actually favour re-entry.

Flecainide suppresses phase 0 activity but also increases the action potential duration. It is well absorbed after oral administration and has a plasma half-life of 20 h. Normal dose ranges from 50 mg orally bd to a maximum of 300 mg daily for supraventricular arrhythmias, and 100 mg bd to a maximum of 400 mg daily for ventricular arrhythmias. The results of the CAST trial have led to flecainide being withdrawn in some countries,[15] but in the UK the drug is available chiefly for the treatment of AV nodal reciprocating tachycardia, paroxysmal atrial fibrillation and ventricular arrhythmias unresponsive to other therapy.

Class II – β-adrenergic receptor antagonists

The pharmacology of the β-blockers is dealt with at length in Chapter 17. In this section the antiarrhythmic effects of the drugs are discussed.

In addition to the direct electrophysiological effects of β-receptor antagonism, the β-blockers may affect cardiac conduction by other mechanisms including the membrane stabilizing or local anaesthetic effect, the partial agonist or intrinsic sympathomimetic effect and the relative affinity for β_1- and β_2- or indeed α_1-receptors.

The electrophysiologic effects of β-blockade are:

- a reduction in automaticity
- an increase in the action potential duration, particularly in the ventricles
- an increase in the effective refractory period in the AV node.

The latter effect may be the most important anti-arrhythmic effect. Automaticity is reduced at the SA and AV nodes as well as elsewhere in the conducting system. Although the heart rate is reduced, this effect is overshadowed by the potent inhibition of catecholamine-induced tachycardia induced either by exercise, emotion, or drug-induced hypotension.

Some β-adrenergic blocking drugs have direct effects causing a reduction in potassium efflux and, at higher concentrations, a reduction in inward sodium current. This effect, similar to class I activity, is the membrane stabilizing (or quinidine-like or local anaesthetic) effect, and is seen with propranolol at high concentrations. Although effective β-blockade is achieved with propranolol at a concentration of 1–300 ng/ml, a plasma concentration 3–5 times higher may be necessary to produce a membrane stabilizing effect.

Propranolol is well absorbed from the gastrointestinal tract, but hepatic first-pass metabolism may account for two-thirds of the administered dose, although this will be reduced with chronic therapy. The elimination half-life is 3–4 h, although this may be increased with chronic therapy also. Propranolol is 90% protein bound, and is metabolized before excretion. At least one metabolic product, 4-hydroxypropranolol, is active although it has a short half-life.

The simultaneous administration of heparin may increase the free plasma concentration of propranolol since heparin may increase free fatty acid levels which in turn inhibited the protein binding. This process is reversible with protamine.

Anti-arrhythmic therapy may be continued in the fasting patient, and propranolol may be given intravenously by bolus injection or by continuous infusion. Repeat boluses of 0.5–1.0 mg may be given up to a total of 0.15 mg/kg, or an infusion of 2–4 mg/h for a 70-kg adult.

Propranolol may be particularly useful for treating AV nodal re-entry tachycardia and some catecholamine-induced ventricular arrhythmias. Overdosage will produce signs of excessive β-blockade, chiefly cardiac failure, hypotension, and evidence of depressed intracardiac conduction including complete heart block and asystole. Furthermore, since propranolol has β_1- and β_2-effects, overdosage may increase the tone in bronchial smooth muscle and produce an increase in airways resistance, and may inhibit the sympathomimetic response to hypoglycaemia in diabetic patients. However, sudden withdrawal of propranolol may be inadvisable in surgical patients and may provoke hypertension, myocardial ischaemia and arrhythmia, dependent on the underlying pathology.

Metoprolol differs from propranolol in that it is much more highly selective for β_1-receptors. Metoprolol has only 2% of the activity of propranolol at the β_2-receptor site, and is not devoid of any membrane-stabilizing effect.

Metoprolol is also well absorbed orally but less drug undergoes first-pass hepatic metabolism. The plasma half-life of approximately 3 h is similar to propranolol, but it may be considerably longer in certain individuals. The drug is 90% metabolized and there are no active metabolites.

Despite its relative β_1-specificity, metoprolol may reduce the FEV_1 in asthmatic patients, and will also inhibit the sympathomimetic response to hypoglycaemia. As with propranolol, the main effects of overdosage are the consequences of excessive β-blockade on the myocardium.

Esmolol is an ultra-short-acting β-adrenergic blocker with a high specificity for β_1-receptors, and no demonstrable effect on α-receptors. The electrophysiological effects are similar to those of other class II drugs, namely, an increase in SA nodal recovery time and a prolongation of the effective refractory period in the AV node.

The short duration of action of esmolol is due to its rapid metabolism in the blood by hydrolysis of its methyl ester linkage. The esterase responsible is located in red cells, however, and is not inhibited by cholinesterase inhibitors such as neostigmine or physostigmine. There is no metabolic interaction between esmolol and other ester molecules and esmolol does not modify the neuromuscular effects of suxamethonium.

In asthmatic patients, esmolol causes a mild increase in airways resistance. The other cardiac effects are those of β-blockade (reductions in contractility) but again this effect is short lived following termination of the drug.

Class III

The class III drugs primarily exert an antifibrillatory effect by increasing electrical stability, rather than an anti-ectopic effect. The most frequently used compound in this class is the benzofuran derivative, amiodarone.

Amiodarone

Although developed as an anti-anginal agent, the anti-arrhythmic potential of amiodarone soon became clear, and it is used to treat supraventricular arrhythmias including pre-excitation syndromes such as Wolf–Parkinson–White, and ventricular arrhythmias including ventricular tachycardia and fibrillation.

The electrophysiological effects of amiodarone are complex. Experimentally, it has been shown to increase action potential duration and to reduce the slope of phase 4 depolarization and SA node automaticity. Phase 0 depolarization is depressed, repolarization and the effective and absolute refractory period are prolonged. There are clear differences in electrophysiology when the drug is given acutely compared with chronic oral therapy. Following acute administration, the effective refractory period is prolonged particularly in ventricular muscle and conduction tissue and there is no prolongation of the QTc. This is in contrast with chronic administration in which the effective refractory period is prolonged chiefly in AV nodal tissue, and the QTc interval is prolonged also. The effects of chronic therapy have been described as similar to thyroid ablation, and some of the effects of amiodarone are reversed by T3. It may be that the slow onset of action is explained by the development of a blockade of the cardiac effects of T3. Amiodarone increases the threshold for ventricular fibrillation, and is effective against refractory ventricular tachycardia when given acutely. It appears to have a selective activity in diseased tissue in a manner similar to lignocaine. Amiodarone also has some α- and β-adrenergic blocking effects but the importance of this is not clear.

When given intravenously, amiodarone causes a reduction in LV dP/dT, mean aortic pressure, peak LV pressure and heart rate. Left ventricular afterload is reduced, and hence cardiac output may increase or remain the same apart from those patients with severe LV failure in whom cardiac function may be further impaired.

When given orally, the drug is characterized by a profoundly slow onset of action. Peak plasma levels may occur 3–7 h after ingestion, but the bioavailability of the ingested dose is low, probably due to poor absorption. The drug has a large volume of distribution and a half-life following chronic oral therapy of 14–107 days. Because of these factors, it may be better to combine oral and intravenous loading rather than to rely on the oral route alone. A suggested regime would be to give 5 mg/kg intravenously over 30 min, followed by 800 mg/day orally for 7 days followed by 600 mg/day orally for 3 days. In fasting patients, the intravenous loading dose may be followed by an intravenous infusion of similar dosage.

The use of chronic amiodarone therapy is limited by a number of untoward effects, some of them severe.

Untoward effects of amiodarone

Skin manifestations include photosensitivity, pigmentation and rashes, and corneal deposits may occur. A pulmonary syndrome similar radiologically to cryptogenic fibrosing alveolitis may occur, with cough, dyspnoea, hypoxia and a reduction in diffusion lung function tests (e.g. carbon monoxide transfer) and a reduction in total lung capacity as features. Pulmonary manifestations occur in approximately 6% of patients but often resolve on discontinuation of the drug. They may be caused by the production of an abnormal phospholipid.

Both hyper- and hypothyroidism may occur with chronic amiodarone therapy. These thyroid effects are not wholly explained by the content of iodine in the amiodarone molecule, since the amount of iodine ingested during chronic amiodarone therapy is not enough to cause adverse thyroid effects.

In contrast to the hazards of chronic oral therapy, acute intravenous therapy appears relatively free of adverse effects and this fact coupled with its effective action in treating supraventricular and ventricular arrhythmias has led to an increase in the use of amiodarone in the perioperative period. However, hypotension, bradycardia and severe resistance to vasopressors have been described in anaesthetized patients. Adrenaline may be required to reverse these effects.

Bretylium

Bretylium is a quaternary ammonium compound that produces a biphasic response after acute intravenous administration. Initially, there is displacement of noradrenaline from nerve endings thereby giving rise to sympathomimetic effects, which is rapidly followed by adrenergic blockade.

Bretylium prolongs the effective refractory period, and may delay the conduction of premature impulses in normal and diseased myocardium. It may effectively convert ventricular fibrillation to sinus rhythm and has been recommended for refractory ventricular tachycardia (VT) or ventricular fibrillation (VF), when 5–10 mg/kg may be given as an intravenous bolus, repeatable up to 30 mg/kg. The antiarrhythmic effect of bretylium has been shown to occur in the presence of cardiac denervation and therefore cannot be said to be a simple anti-adrenergic effect. However, the onset of action may be relatively slow and, in patients with VF, resuscitative efforts should be continued for 20–30 min after administration. In patients with VT, an intravenous infusion of 2 mg/min may be used to maintain plasma levels.

The efficacy of bretylium in the setting of ventricular arrhythmia is controversial, and this coupled with the slow onset of action still places it as a second-line drug for VT/VF after intravenous lignocaine.

Adverse reactions include nausea and vomiting.

Class IV – calcium-channel antagonists

Calcium-channel blockers inhibit the inward flow of calcium ions during depolarization, particularly late phase 0 depolarization through to the phase 2 plateau, which is primarily calcium dependent. The nature and mechanism of activation of calcium channels is discussed more fully in Chapter 16, Part II. The WHO classification of calcium-channel antagonists divides the drugs into the papaverine derivatives (verapamil), the dihydropyridines (nifedipine, etc.) and the benzothiazepines (diltiazem). Although drugs in each subclass have activity in cardiac and vascular smooth muscle, the dihydropyridines and the benzothiazepine drug, diltiazem, have a profile of activity that renders them useless practically as antiarrhythmic drugs. The main anti-arrhythmic drug in this class is the papaverine derivative, verapamil.

Verapamil

The electrophysiological effects of verapamil are seen predominantly in SA and AV nodal tissue, since these are largely calcium dependent for phase 0 and phase 4 depolarization. The rate of discharge in the SA node is reduced and recovery is prolonged. These effects may be seen with other calcium channel blockers. Verapamil slows AV conduction and prolongs the effective refractory period, but the QRS duration and QTc interval are not significantly affected. Transatrial conduction is more likely to be slowed than intraventricular conduction.

After oral administration, substantial hepatic extraction occurs such that bioavailability is reduced, although this may be increased significantly in patients with hepatic disease. Verapamil is metabolized and excreted via the kidneys, but the principal metabolite, norverapamil, is active and may accumulate to therapeutic concentrations.

When given intravenously, verapamil is cleared from the plasma at a rate equivalent to splanchnic blood flow. For the treatment of supraventricular tachycardias (SVTs), 0.07–0.15 mg/kg may be given over 1 min, and repeated up to a maximum of approximately 10 mg.

There is no doubt that verapamil may have negative inotropic effects, and it appears that this effect may be synergistic with the cardiac effects of volatile anaesthetics, such that profound cardiovascular depression and conduction disorders may occur. Also, verapamil has been shown experimentally to potentiate neuromuscular blockade, and this possibility must be taken into account in patients receiving muscle relaxants.

Verapamil is useful therapeutically in the treatment of supraventricular tachycardias including PSVT, atrial fibrillation and atrial flutter. AV node conduction is delayed or blocked and refractoriness is prolonged, which may be useful in preventing re-entry. The reduction in AV nodal conduction is useful in treating patients with atrial flutter and/or fibrillation, but the therapeutic effect is usually a reduction in the ventricular response rather than a return to sinus rhythm. In this respect its therapeutic effect is similar to digoxin, but the more rapid onset of effect may make verapamil preferable in the acute setting.

One area where verapamil may be inadvisable is in the treatment of PSVT associated with WPW syndrome. Verapamil is successful in treating PSVT when conduction is anterograde through the AV node and retrograde through the accessory pathway. However, when conduction is anterograde through the accessory pathway and retrograde (or re-entering the circuit) through the AV node, verapamil will be ineffective. Furthermore, in patients with atrial fibrillation, if the effective refractory period in the AV node is reduced by treatment with verapamil or digoxin, the ventricular response may be increased and VF may ensue. Class I (procainamide) or class III drugs (amiodarone), or adenosine may be more successful.

Class V – digoxin

The failure of Vaughan–Williams classification to categorize the cardiac glycosides adequately has led to their identification as class V compounds. The effects of digoxin and the cardiac glycosides on the force of contraction in the myocardium and their role in the treatment of heart failure has been dealt with earlier in this chapter. In this section the electrophysiological effects of digoxin and related compounds and their role in the treatment of arrhythmias are described.

The antiarrhythmic effects of digoxin are due to both direct and indirect effects. The primary direct effect is the inhibition of Na/K-dependent ATPase. In Purkinje fibres, digoxin increases the slope of phase 4 depolarization and reduces the resting potential such that phase 0 depolarization begins at a higher (less negative) resting potential, thereby inhibiting conduction velocity of the action potential. The phase 4 effect is inversely proportional to the extracellular K^+ concentration; thus under conditions of hypokalaemia, phase 4 depolarization and automaticity may be increased, which may explain the potential arrhythmogenic effect of digoxin and low serum K^+. At toxic levels, digoxin induces delayed after-depolarizations (DADs) which may trigger depolarization and produce ectopic beats. The main consequence of the direct effect of digoxin is to reduce conduction velocity, and this may occur in SA node and AV node tissue and myocardial tissue as well as in Purkinje fibres. However, other indirect effects occur involving the autonomic nervous system, and these may predominate. The indirect effects of digoxin are in part due to the inhibition of the pathophysiological responses to congestive heart failure following an increase in inotropic state. Vagal activity may be increased, and the SA node sensitivity to acetylcholine enhanced. In high concentrations, digoxin may reduce the sensitivity of the SA and AV nodes to catecholamines, although it is not clear if this is due to a CNS medullary or peripheral neuronal effect. The reduction in heart rate may therefore occur as a result of both increased vagal tone and reduced sympathetic tone.

The AV node is particularly sensitive to both the direct and indirect effects of digoxin. The effective refractory period is lengthened and conduction through the AV node is slowed. At high concentrations, transnodal conduction may be blocked entirely. This effect is important, since the rate of atrial contraction may actually increase with digoxin, and it is the effect of the drug at the AV node that effectively controls the ventricular response.

Although other cardiac glycosides are available, digoxin is the most commonly used compound, both for intravenous and oral therapy. In adults, 0.5 mg iv may be given slowly, followed by further increments as necessary. Digoxin is approximately 25% protein bound, and a significant clinical effect should be seen within 5–30 min of intravenous administration. Digoxin is excreted renally, and the dose should be adjusted in renal insufficiency. Oral digitalizing regimes should aim to provide between 125–750 μg daily in adults, with the dose reduced by half in the elderly. Side-effects and toxic effects are not uncommon and include gastrointestinal and visual disturbances, as well as the more important disorders of cardiac conduction including heart block and severe bradycardia. It may be necessary to check plasma levels regularly.

Digoxin is a useful drug for controlling atrial fibrillation, and for converting atrial flutter to fibrillation by increasing the atrial rate as described above. The resting ventricular response is well controlled, but the response to exercise may be poorly controlled. Thus sympathoadrenal activity may well produce a severe tachycardia, which may occur in the awake patient under conditions of exercise or in the anaesthetized patient during the stress of surgery. This potential drawback has to be balanced against the fact that digoxin is the only available antiarrhythmic drug for treating atrial fibrillation that does not have negative inotropic or vasodilator effects, a factor that may be very important in the anaesthetized patient.

Adenosine

Adenosine is an endogenous molecule produced as an intermediate metabolite of adenosine monophosphate. It has been shown to have effects on cardiac conduction and on coronary vasomotor tone. Adenosine is a highly potent coronary vasodilator and has been shown to abolish effectively the autoregulation of coronary flow over a wide perfusion pressure, resulting instead on coronary flow being directly proportional to coronary perfusion pressure.

The electrophysiological effects of adenosine are mediated by the A_1 receptor, which is linked to the ionic channel for K^+ and Ca^{2+}. The effects seen may be related to an increase in K^+ conductance, since activation of the α_1-receptor at the SA and AV node activates the outward adenosine-regulated potassium current. In ventricular myocardium, adenosine may lead to a depression of calcium-mediated slow channel conductance which in effect antagonizes the effect of catecholamines.

Adenosine has been shown to link with specific adenosine receptors linked to G proteins (guanine nucleotide binding proteins), which are responsible for cardiac and vascular effects, including negative inotropic and chronotropic effects. SA nodal activity and AV nodal conductivity are reduced, as is ventricular automaticity.

The serum half-life of adenosine is less than 10 s and it is totally cleared from the plasma in less than 30 s, thereby necessitating rapid intravenous administration by bolus injection. The effect of adenosine may be potentiated by dipyridamole and antagonized by theophylline, but there appears no contraindication to adenosine in patients currently taking calcium-channel or β-blockers, ACE inhibitors or quinidine. In adults, an initial dose of 200 μg/kg should be given by rapid iv injection, and followed by a second dose of up to 400 μg/kg if required. The effects at the AV node are particularly impressive, and adenosine has been used to treat re-entry SVT and to aid in the diagnosis of a broad complex tachycardia, since a reduction in the atrial rate may make atrial activity more easily recognizable. Adenosine will not convert VT.

Adenosine may be preferable to verapamil as an antiarrhythmic, since the onset of action is faster, the duration of action shorter and the incidence of adverse effects smaller.

PERIOPERATIVE ANTIARRHYTHMIA THERAPY

Since so many aspects of anaesthesia and surgery may be considered to be arrhythmogenic (see Table 15.2), it is clear that high-quality anaesthesia is the most effective method of both preventing and treating perioperative arrhythmias. In fact, the general conduct of anaesthesia is of paramount importance in that regard, but where perioperative arrhythmias do not respond to other non-specific measures, therapy with antiarrhythmic drugs should be considered.

One common scenario may involve the patient who has a pre-existing arrhythmia (e.g. atrial fibrillation) and in whom the ventricular response is now suboptimal, in that it may be either too fast or too slow. Such an example is useful because it involves two of the major mechanisms that produce significant perioperative arrhythmias. The first is an additive effect between antiarrhythmic therapy and anaesthesia. We have seen that digoxin may increase AV nodal block and reduce the ventricular rate. AV nodal block may be further produced by high concentrations of volatile anaesthetics (e.g. halothane, enflurane) and thus these two effects may combine to produce a high level of AV blockade and a severe reduction in the ventricular rate. Alternatively, the sympatho-adrenal stimulation following surgery and perioperative pain, and the lack of antiarrhythmic therapy consequent on perioperative fasting may reduce effective digoxin levels significantly while at the same time increasing SA node activity, transatrial and AV conduction and intraventricular conduction and automaticity such that a severe tachycardia may ensue.

In such patients it is important to tailor the anaesthetic to the patient and their antiarrhythmic drug therapy, while at the same time ensuring that the dose and route of adminstration of drug therapy is appropriate for the perioperative period.

REFERENCES

1 Goldsmith SR, Francis GS, Cohn JN. Norepinephrine infusions in congestive heart failure. *American Journal of Cardiology* 1985; **56**: 802

2 Weishaar RE, Burroes SD, Kobylarz DC, *et al.* Multiple molecular forms of cyclic nucleotide phosphodiesterase in cardiac and smooth muscle and in platelets. Isolation characterization and effects of various reference phosphodiesterase inhibitors and cardiotonic agents. *Biochemical Pharmacology* 1986; **35**: 787.

3 Anderson JL, Hemodynamic and clinical benefits with intravenous milrinone in servere chronic heart failure; results of a multicentre study in the United States. *American Heart Journal* 1990; **21**: 1956.

4 Monrad ES, Baim DS, Smith HS, *et al.* Effects of milrinone on coronary hemodynamics and myocardial energetics in patients with congestive heart failure. *Circulation* 1985; **71**: 972.

5 Feneck RO and the European Milrinone Multicentre Trial Group. Intravenous milrinone following cardiac surgery. Effect of bolus infusion followed by variable dose maintenance infusion. *Journal of Cardiothoracic and Vascular Anesthesia* 1992; **6**: 554.

6 Feneck RO. Milrinone and Postoperative pulmonary hypertension *Journal of Cardiothoracic and Vascular Anesthesia* 1993; **7**: 21.

7 Skoyles JR, Sherry KM. Mechanisms of action and uses of selective phosphodiesterase inhibitors. *British Journal of Anaesthesia* 1992; **68**: 2937.

8 Davis ME, Jones C, Walesby RK, Feneck RO, Assessment of the effects of DPI 201-106 on cardiac performance and metabolism following CABG surgery. *International Journal of Cardiology* 1990; **7**: 332.

9 Withering W. An account of the foxglove. London: Robinson, 1785.

10 Office of Population Censuses and Surveys. Mortality Statistics; cause. London: HMSO. 1992.

11 Gruppo Italiano per lo Studio della Streptochinasi nell'infarcto miocardico (GISSI) Effectiveness of intravenous thrombolytic in acute myocardial infarction. *Lancet* 1986; **i**: 397.

12 Kurtz CM, Bennett JH, Shapiro HH. ECG studies during surgical anaesthesia. *Journal of the American Medical Association* 1936; **106**: 434.

13 Mines GR. On circulating excitations in heart muscles and their possible relation to tachycardia and fibrillation. *Transcripts of Royal Society of Canada* (Section IV) 1914; 43–52.

14 El-Sherif N, Scherlag BJ, Lazzara R, *et al.* Reentrant ventricular arrhythmias in the late myocardial infarction period. 4: Mechanism of action of lidocaine. *Circulation* 1977; **56**: 395.

15 Echt DS, Liebsan PR, Mitchell B, *et al.* Mortality and morbidity in patients receiving encainide, flecainide or placebo. *New England Journal of Medicine* 1991; **324**: 781.

16

Drugs Affecting Vascular Tone, Function and Vasodilatation

PART I DRUGS AFFECTING VASCULAR TONE AND FUNCTION

NH Kellow, RO Feneck

INTRODUCTION

The cardiovascular effects of the autonomic nervous system and drugs affecting it are covered in Chapters 13 and 14. The aim of this chapter is to concentrate on the specific pharmacology of vascular smooth muscle and its associated endothelium, incorporating recent developments in the understanding of vascular structure and function and thus of the pharmacological control of vascular smooth muscle. The realization of the importance of the vascular endothelium in overall vascular function, and the identification of nitric oxide as the endothelium-derived relaxing factor (EDRF) have been recent developments of great impact. Also, the ultrastructure of vascular smooth muscle has been further elucidated, and important discoveries have been made regarding the biochemical processes underlying its contractile mechanism and the development of vascular tone.

Thus we are now aware of the extremely complex nature of vascular structure and function and are better able to understand the mechanisms of action of the majority of pharmacological agents used to affect it. Several alternative pathways have been identified for the processes of both vasoconstriction and vasodilatation, and it has been suggested that nitric oxide (NO) is the final result of several pharmacological pathways aimed at producing a reduction in vascular tone.

This new understanding has already led to the development of new pharmacological interventions designed to influence vascular tone and to attempt to reduce the secondary effects of its derangements. For example, potassium channel activators such as nicorandil have been developed for the treatment of angina and inhaled NO is being used experimentally to reduce elevated pulmonary arterial pressures.

VASCULAR STRUCTURE

The parent of the arterial system is the aorta, a thick elastic structure with a diameter of about 2.5 cm in the adult and a thickness of about 1.5 mm. This divides into numerous generations of smaller diameter arteries whose proportions of elastic tissue become progressively less while the proportion of smooth muscle becomes proportionally greater as the overall calibre of the vessel reduces (Fig. 16.1).

The most muscular vessels are the small diameter arteries and arterioles that lead into the capillary network which itself is composed of a single layer of endothelium. The total cross-sectional area of the arterial system multiplies many times in these smaller divisions and it is these that control total vascular resistance largely by virtue of their muscular content.

Three distinct layers can be identified following examination of the cross-sectional appearance of arteries and veins. Named from within to without these are the tunica intima, tunica media and tunica adventitia. Each has a characteristic appearance which, although somewhat variable, none the less remains identifiable throughout the vascular system.

For example, the tunica intima generally consists of a single layer of endothelium supported by a delicate layer of subendothelial connective tissue, usually arranged longitudinally. The tunica media extends from the internal to the external elastic lamina and is organized circumferentially. This has a highly variable structure that is predominantly elastic tissue in large arteries which are designed to absorb and dissipate the considerable circumferential and longitudinal wall stresses imposed on them by left ventricular contraction with the associated addition of 60–80 ml of blood to the aorta with each systole. The tunica adventitia surrounds the external elastic lamina and is a layer of longitudinally arranged connective tissue which merges with the surrounding fibro-areolar tissue.

A single layer of longitudinally arranged endothelial cells is a feature found throughout the vascular system, in the chambers of the heart, in the pulmonary circulation and throughout the systemic circulation including the capillaries and veins. This plays a vital role in controlling vascular function in a multitude of ways and these will be considered below.

In large arteries, the tunica media is composed almost exclusively of concentrically arranged fenestrated elastic lamellae, up to forty layers thick in a normal adult aorta, which are separated by fibrous tissue and in which are embedded smooth muscle cells. These cells are responsible for the synthesis and deposition of the elastic tissue and also the collagen and glycoproteins between them. Elastic tissue is almost absent in the neonatal aorta, which is a largely muscular conduit, but its relative amount is considerably increased in elderly patients and in those with hypertension.

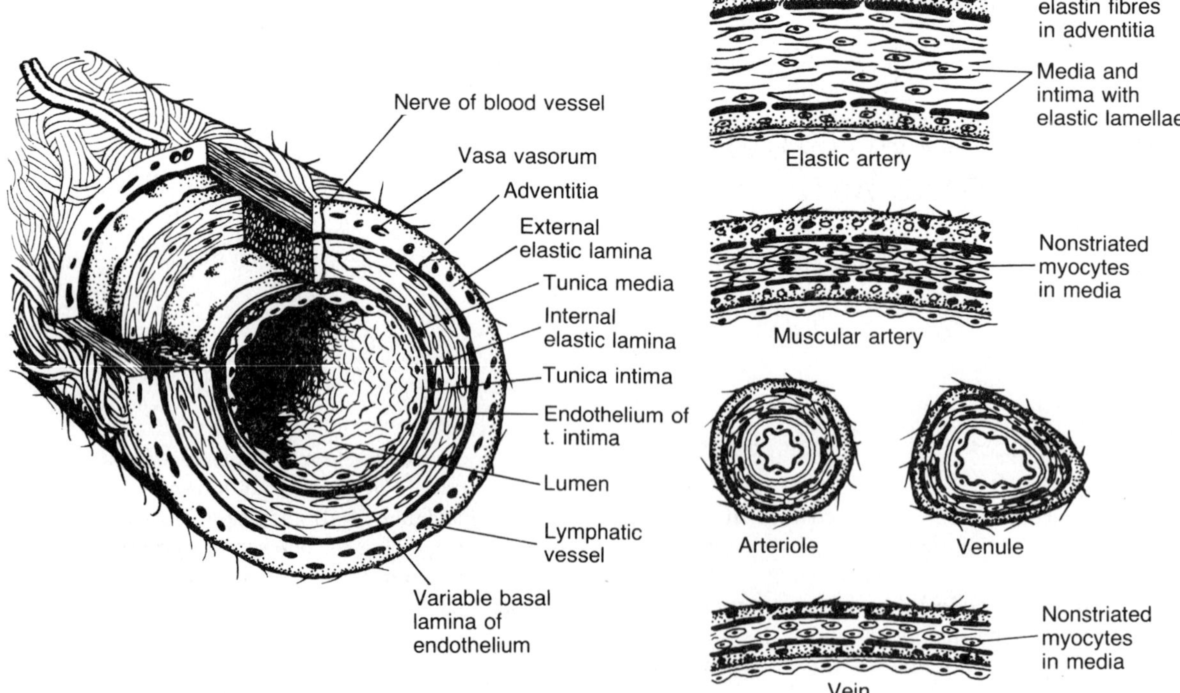

FIGURE 16.1 A diagram showing the principal architectural features of the larger blood vessels. On the left the major layers and associated structures are depicted. On the right the particular features of an elastic artery, muscular artery, arteriole, venule and vein are shown.

In smaller arteries, the tunica media is composed predominantly of circumferentially arranged smooth muscle cells with a much smaller proportion of elastic tissue. Arteries of this size are extensively innervated and an intimate relationship exists between their endothelium and the underlying smooth muscle cells. Indeed, it is now apparent that endothelial function in small arteries and arterioles is one of the most important determinants of vascular smooth muscle tone and hence vascular resistance and blood pressure.

ENDOTHELIAL PHYSIOLOGY AND FUNCTION

In simple terms, the endothelium represents a barrier preventing the particulate components of blood including blood cells, platelets and large molecules, from leaving the circulation. It is not a passive barrier; for example, from the parent molecule arachidonic acid it manufactures and secretes prostaglandin I_2 (PGI_2 or prostacyclin). This is released towards the luminal surface of the blood vessel and prevents the aggregation of platelets on the collagen and smooth muscle of the vessel wall. It may also be responsible for inactivating serotonin released by aggregating platelets and thus preventing this from reaching vascular smooth muscle cells. Endoperoxides released by platelets may also be taken up into endothelial cells and converted to prostacyclin which will inhibit further platelet aggregation. Endothelial cells represent an important transducer of vasoactive substance signals released from platelets and hence influence the contractile state of the underlying muscle. This can obviously have important implications for such conditions as angina, myocardial infarction, stroke and hypertension.

Endogenous mediators of vascular smooth muscle tone

The first evidence of the obligatory role of the endothelium in the control of vascular smooth muscle tone was provided by Furchgott and Zawadski[1] who showed that if intact isolated arteries were exposed to acetylcholine they relaxed. However, if their endothelium was removed this relaxation no longer took place. This led them to suppose that an intact endothelium somehow translated the acetylcholine signal, which in itself is not directly vasodilatory to smooth muscle cells, into a vasodilatory messenger which exerted a paracrine effect on the neighbouring smooth muscle cells thus causing relaxation.

Other substances have since been shown also to cause relaxation of vascular smooth muscle only via an intact endothelium. Such substances include arachidonic acid, thrombin, α_2-adrenoceptor agonists, histamine, bradykinin and substance P, as well as ADP and ATP. As stated above, endothelial cells convert arachidonic acid to prostacyclin, which is then secreted by endothelial cells and itself mediates vasodilatation. However, smooth muscle cell relaxation is mediated for the other agents by EDRF.

Nitric oxide (NO)

EDRF is highly unstable with a half-life of only a few seconds. Its action is destroyed by oxyhaemoglobin and preserved by superoxide dismutase (thus demonstrating that superoxide anions could inactivate it). Its identity was discovered in 1987 when Furchgott[2] and Ignarro[3] independently pointed out that EDRF shared very similar properties to NO. Soon after, Moncada and his coworkers[4] showed that NO accounted for the biological activity of EDRF and that L-arginine was its precursor.

It has been known for some time that the nitrovasodilators are metabolized in target cells to a nitrosothiol compound and/or nitric oxide. However, recent developments have identified that the final common pathway in a number of therapeutic avenues aiming to produce vasodilatation is the release of NO which then exerts a paracrine hormonal influence on the underlying smooth muscle to cause relaxation of vascular smooth muscle tone.

Nitric oxide is formed from the precursor molecule L-arginine. Cultured endothelial cells deprived of L-arginine are incapable of synthesizing NO whilst the addition of L-arginine restores this capacity. If an analogue of L-arginine such as L-N-monomethyl arginine (L-NMMA) is added to isolated intact arteries they are rendered unable to relax in response to the addition of acetylcholine. This can be reversed by the addition of L-arginine. Neurohumoral mediators stimulate the formation of NO by combining with luminal endothelial surface receptors.

NO enters the vascular myocytes by diffusion where it stimulates soluble guanylate cyclase (Fig. 16.2) which increases intracellular levels of cyclic guanosine monophosphate (cGMP) which in turn mediates smooth muscle relaxation. There is a basal level of release of NO from vascular endothelium which rises in response to various stimuli such as certain hormones, platelet-derived vasoactive substances and stretching of the endothelial cell itself. Although the formation of NO is the final common pathway of a number of vasodilator drugs, the actual mechanism for its formation varies according to the drug in question. For example, the organic nitrates such as glyceryl trinitrate (GTN) only form NO if thiol-containing compounds such as cysteine are present, when they will act as cofactors for the formation of NO. Meanwhile, the syndonimine derivatives such as molsidomine and sodium nitroprusside (SNP) release NO spontaneously. A third group, the nitrosothiols, also release NO directly and appears also to have the ability to directly activate guanylate cyclase.

Arteries with an intact endothelium have a reduced responsiveness to exogenously administered NO

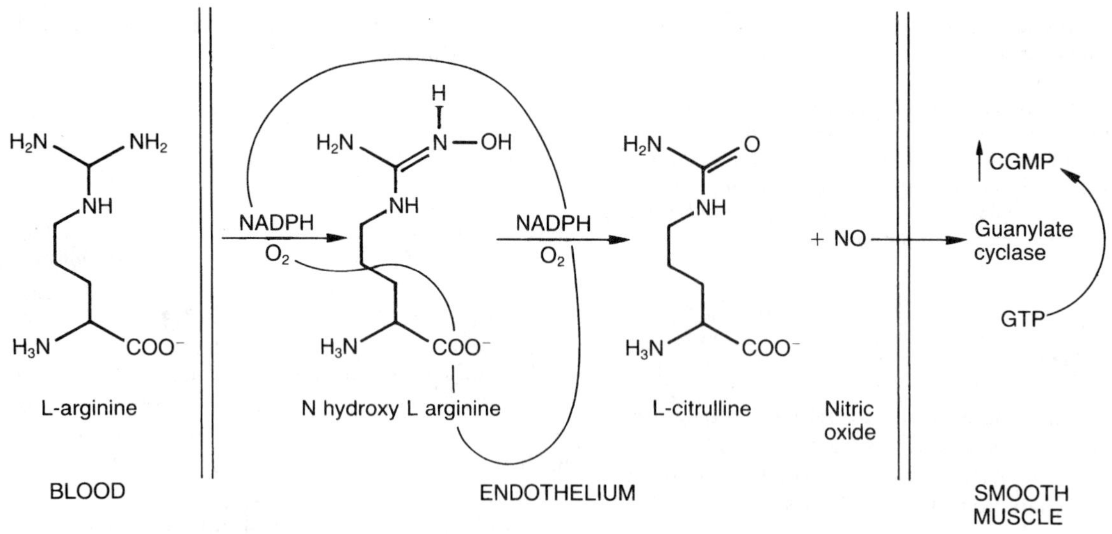

FIGURE 16.2 Nitric oxide production by endothelium and its effect on vascular smooth muscle. GTP, guanosine triphosphate: NADPH, reduced nicotinamide adenine dinucleotide phosphate: cGMP, cyclic guanosine monophosphate.

precursors such as nitrates or SNP due to their basal formation of NO. Veins, conversely, have a lower basal rate of NO formation and this is reflected in their increased responsiveness to such agents. Of course, the nitrovasodilators do not require the presence of intact functioning endothelium in order to produce vasodilatation as they all produce NO independently of it. It is also released towards the luminal surface of the vessel where it has certain important action on platelet function. It stimulates guanylate cyclase within platelets which effects a reduction in platelet intracellular calcium concentration. This reduces platelet adhesiveness and aggregation and potentiates prostacyclin-induced increased in cAMP. It also inhibits the release of platelet-derived growth factor and may inhibit smooth muscle cell proliferation.

5-Hydroxytryptamine (5HT) (serotonin)

Serotonin is released by activated platelets and it has different effects on endothelium and on the underlying smooth muscle cells. In the presence of an intact endothelium, serotonin interacts with a specific receptor in the luminal surface of the endothelial cell which stimulates the cell to produce NO and this causes vascular relaxation in the usual way. However, the direct application of serotonin on to the underlying smooth muscle causes vasoconstriction mediated by specific 5-HT_2 serotonergic receptors located in the myocyte cell membrane. Similarly, the application of serotonin to the outer surface of the vessel wall also causes vasoconstriction. Thus it seems that serotonin only causes vasodilatation if it is placed in contact with the endothelial surface of an intact blood vessel. The relaxation caused by aggregating platelets and by exogenous serotonin is antagonized by methysergide but not by ketanserin. This would suggest that the endothelial serotonin receptors are different from the myocyte serotonin receptors.

It therefore appears that NO is a classical paracrine hormone. If released into the bloodstream, it is immediately inactivated by oxyhaemoglobin and converted to nitrate. However, it does have important actions on its luminal surface particularly with regard to modulating platelet function. When released abluminally it mediates vasodilatation. It shares a different but complementary action with prostacyclin; while NO mediates vasodilatation via cGMP, prostacyclin acts via cAMP.

Endothelins

Vascular endothelium also synthesises and secretes a family of three, similar, 21-amino acid sequence polypeptides known as endothelin-1, endothelin-2, and endothelin-3 (ET-1, 2, and 3 respectively). All are released as pre-proendothelin, with 200 amino acid residues; this is cleaved to proendothelin (38 residues), which is further cleaved by an endothelin converting (ET-converting) enzyme to the endothelins. These act upon specific receptors of which two sub-types, ET-A and ET-B, have so far been identified. Both receptor sub-types are coupled to G-proteins. ET-A seems to be specific for ET-1, whilst ET-B is coupled through another G protein to phospholipase C, mediating an increase in intracellular calcium. The ET-A receptor seems to mediate vasoconstriction, whilst the function of the ET-B receptor remains unknown.

Endothelins are the most potent vasoconstrictors yet identified, ET-1 being about 10 times as potent as angiotensin II. An intravenous injection of ET-1 produces a substantial and sustained increase in blood pressure.

Tolerance to vasodilators

The phenomenon of tolerance to exogenously administered nitrates has long been recognized but the mechanisms have only recently been identified. Tolerance predominantly develops when dosing strategies are designed to give therapeutic effects throughout the 24-h period. It cannot be circumvented by a change of route of administration or by changing the nitrate used. It may develop within hours in a patient given continuous nitrates for severe angina pectoris. In practice, its effects can be minimized by allowing a nitrate-free period every day, which is usually aimed to be overnight when myocardial oxygen demands are likely to be at their lowest.

A number of mechanisms have been proposed to account for the phenomenon such as desensitization of guanylate cyclase, depletion of pools of reduced sulphydryl groups, counterregulatory neurohormonal activation and plasma shifts. The most widely accepted theory is that of the depletion of reduced sulphydryl groups in vascular smooth muscle cells. The presence of reduced sulphydryl groups is necessary for the conversion of organic nitrates to NO and also for the formation of nitrosothiol compounds. It has been shown that the administration of sulphydryl groups in the form of N-acetylcysteine can partly reverse nitrate tolerance although this has not been shown to occur in patients chronically treated with oral slow-release preparations. Meanwhile, only slight tolerance has been reported to SNP or to molsidomine, presumably because these increase NO directly. Molsidomine has been used as an adjunct to nitrate interval treatment in an alternative attempt to circumvent the tolerance problem.

VASCULAR SMOOTH MUSCLE PHYSIOLOGY

Vascular smooth muscle cell structure

Smooth muscle cells are fusiform or branched cells, approximately 100–500 μm in length and about 3–6 μm in diameter. They have a very large surface area to volume ratio due predominantly to the presence of large numbers of invaginations of the cell membrane known as caveolae, which can increase the surface area by as much as 75%. Vascular smooth muscle cells synthesize collagen, elastin, glycoproteins and proteoglycans, which are used to produce the extracellular matrix in which the cells lie and which also determine the functional characteristics of the tissue. The extracellular secretion of these substances can be regulated by agents such as heparin and growth factors. Smooth muscle cells can also undergo both hypertrophy and hyperplasia; mitotic figures can commonly be seen in hypertensive and atherosclerotic blood vessels and are believed to contribute to their development.

Gap junctions are found between smooth muscle cells, formed in areas where there is direct contact between the cell membranes of two neighbouring cells. They are regions where there is facilitated transmission of electrical and hormonal messages. They are dynamic in nature and number, their electrical resistance being able to change with fluctuations in ionic concentration and pH. They are extensive in number in vascular smooth muscle allowing the rapid transmission of electrical signals between large numbers of cells, producing a functional syncytium. They also allow the passage of small molecules between neighbouring cells thus producing metabolic as well as electrical communication within an area of smooth muscle cells. Such small molecules would be of the order of size of amino acids, sugars or nucleotides.

The cell membrane of vascular myocytes can be divided into three structural regions: the caveolae, the area of cell membrane attached to underlying junctional sarcoplasmic reticulum (SR), which forms areas of surface coupling, and the remainder of the cell membrane which is not associated with either of these. The caveolae are flask-shaped invaginations of the cell membrane about 50–80 nm in diameter which are arranged in longitudinal groups along the cell surface. They do not undergo pinocytosis and their function is still unknown. The areas of surface coupling are believed to be important sites of signal transduction. A major part of the remainder is accounted for by intercellular contacts and dense bodies which are sites of insertion of actin filaments.

The smooth muscle SR, like its counterpart in striated muscle, is the main source of intracellular Ca^{2+}. It is an apparently continuous system of intracellular tubules that occupies between 1–7% of the cellular volume. It seems to possess functionally independent units that respond to different stimuli. It forms surface couplings with the cell membrane through a space about 12–18 nm wide which is traversed by ‘bridging structures’. These ‘feet’ are partially composed of the ryanodine-binding protein which is thought to be, at least in striated muscle, the Ca^{2+} channel of the SR through which Ca^{2+} ions are released during excitation–contraction coupling.

In common with striated muscle, the main contractile elements of vascular smooth muscle are actin and myosin. The myosin molecules are bundled together to form thick filaments with their heads pointing outwards. They undergo a cycle of high- and low-affinity binding to actin in a process driven by the consumption of ATP, the formation of each cross-bridge requiring the consumption of one molecule of ATP. Tension is generated as a result of the change in orientation of the myosin heads from 90° to 45° with respect to the long axis of the actin/myosin complex. The direction of development of tension is determined by the orientation of the contractile elements. While in skeletal muscle, the myofilaments are all orientated in the same direction so that the entire muscle exerts its tension in unison; in smooth muscles they are arranged in a large number of different directions so that the overall result depends on the predominant direction of orientation of myofilaments. Vascular smooth muscle cells tend to be somewhat elongated in shape and lie in a circumferential manner around the wall of a blood vessel. The effect of both single myocyte contraction and that of overall contraction of myocytes in a blood vessel is to reduce the diameter of that vessel.

In vascular smooth muscle, thin filaments which comprise actin, tropomyosin and other binding proteins are attached to the internal surface of the myocyte cell membrane by means of specialized areas known as ‘membrane plaques’.

The molecular basis of vascular smooth muscle contraction and relaxation

There are three second messenger systems which are widely encountered in cardiovascular pharmacolgy: the cGMP system which has already been mentioned, the inositol 1,4,5 tri-phosphate (IP_3) system, and the cyclic AMP (cAMP) system. In the IP_3 system the binding of a ligand to its receptor activates phospholipase C on the inner surface of the membrane via a specific G protein (Fig. 16.3). The phospholipase C thus activated catalyses the hydrolysis of phosphatidylinositol 4,5 diphosphate to IP_3 and diacylglycerol (DAG). The IP_3 diffuses to the sarcoplasmic reticulum where it triggers the release of calcium (Ca^{2+}) ions, which initiates the contractile process. However the increase in intracellular Ca^{2+} is short-lived for two reasons. First, Ca^{2+} ions are actively pumped out of the cytoplasm into the extracellular space, and back into the sarcoplasmic reticulum, and secondly because IP_3 production is rapidly switched off because of receptor desensitisation.

In the cAMP system, when an appropriate ligand binds to a stimulatory receptor, adenylyl cyclase is activated via another specific G protein (Fig. 16.4). Conversely, when a ligand binds to an inhibitory receptor, adenylyl cyclase is inhibited through another G protein.

Calcium-channel blockers

Calcium ions are essential for the activation of contractile proteins in vascular smooth muscle as well as in striated muscle and cardiac muscle. As discussed above the sustained contraction of vascular smooth muscle occurs due to the inward flux of extracellular Ca^{2+} ions after the Ca^{2+} stores in the SR are used to initiate contraction. The slow inward calcium current is also particularly important in the maintenance of cardiac function, and it may be increased by other drugs (adrenergic agonists) and pathophysiological states such as ischaemia and hypoxia. Calcium channels may therefore be influenced by a variety of factors, and channels may be voltage operated (i.e. activated by depolarization) or receptor operated, and non-selective channels may allow the passage of other ions including sodium.

There are three subtypes of voltage operated channel. These are L (large conductance and long lifetime), N (intermediate channels) and T (short mean lifetime and low conductance carrying transient currents). Although L channels appear to be most important in cardiac muscle, both L and T channels, as well as receptor-operated channels, appear to be implicated in the regulation of vascular muscle tone. The intracellular movement of calcium ions can be blocked at the L-type Ca^{2+} channel by a number of different classes of drug. This chemical heterogeneity suggests that calcium-channel blockers contain chemical moieties that bind to receptors. These receptors are functionally linked to calcium channels, and indeed there is evidence that this drug–receptor interaction may be reversed following the administration of calcium-channel agonists.

The current classification of calcium-channel blockers is shown below:

- Selective for slow calcium channels:
  Class 1 – papaverine derivatives (e.g. verapamil)

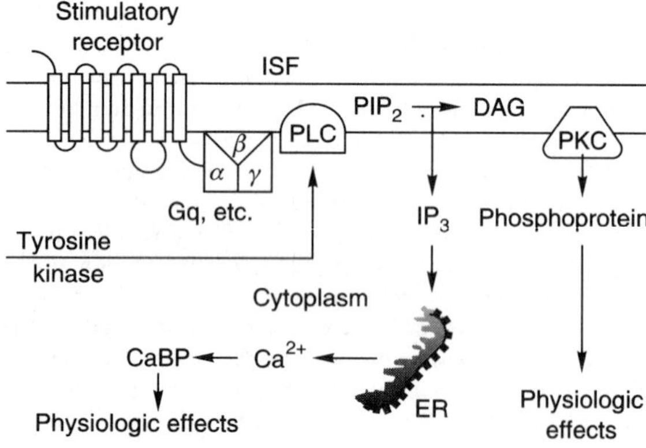

FIGURE 16.3 Diagrammatic representation of release of inositol triphosphate (IP_3) and diacylglycerol (DAG) as second messengers. Binding of ligand to G protein-coupled receptor activiates phospholipase C (PLC) β, or β2. Alternatively, activation of receptors with intracellular tyrosine kinase domains can activate $PLC_{\gamma 1}$. The resulting hydrolysis of PIP_2 produces IP_3, which releases Ca^{2+} from the endoplasmic reticulum (ER), and DAG, which activates protein kinase C (PKC). CaBP, Ca^{2+}-binding proteins. ISF, interstitial fluid.

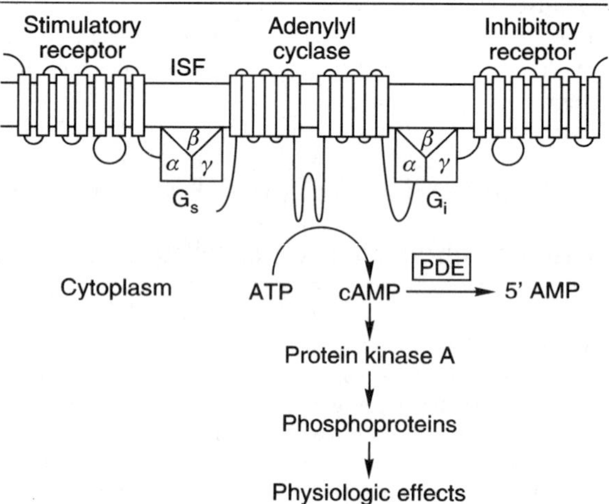

FIGURE 16.4 The cyclic AMP system. Activation of adenylyl cyclase catalyzes the conversion of ATP to cyclic AMP. Cyclic AMP activates protein kinase A, which phosphorylates proteins, producing physiologic effects. Stimulatory ligands bind to stimulatory receptors and activate adenylyl cyclase via G_s. Inhibitory ligands inhibit adenylyl cyclase via inhibitory receptors. ISF, interstitial fluid.

Class 2 – the dihydropyridines (e.g. nifedipine, nicardipine, isradipine, nisoldipine, nimodipine, amlodipine, etc.)
Class 3 – the benzothiazepines (e.g. diltiazem)

- Non-selective for slow calcium channels:
  Diphenylpiperazines (e.g. cinnarizine)

Class 1 – papaverine derivatives

Verapamil is the only Class 1 calcium-channel blocker in current use. Verapamil is effective at reducing systemic vascular resistance and left ventricular afterload by calcium-channel blocking effects on vascular smooth muscle, and it has therefore been used in the treatment of hypertension and angina. However, verapamil also possesses highly significant effects on myocardial contractility and conduction. Sinus node automaticity and atrioventricular nodal conduction are both reduced, and myocardial contractility is reduced as a direct result of a negative inotropic effect. These effects may be problematic in patients with angina and in some patients with hypertension also, and as a result verapamil has been largely superseded by other drugs for these indications. However, verapamil is a highly effective anti-arrhythmic agent and it is largely used for this purpose. The effects of verapamil on myocardial contractility, resting vascular tone and intracardiac conduction may be enhanced by concomitant therapy with other drugs. Verapamil in combination with β-blockers may cause bradyarrhythmias and conduction defects and, in exceptional cases, congestive heart failure. ACE inhibitors and other vasodilators given in combination with verapamil may cause severe hypotension. The combination of verapamil with potent inhalational agents such as halothane, enflurane and isoflurane, may also cause an enhanced reduction in myocardial contractility, and produce arrhythmias and hypotension.

Class 2 – dihydropyridine derivatives

The introduction of the parent compound, nifedipine, has proved to be a substantial therapeutic success with the result that the development of other dihydropyridine derivatives has proceeded apace and these compounds threaten to be as prolific as adrenergic β-blockers. Nifedipine and related compounds are effective in the treatment of systemic hypertension and angina. Indeed, their haemodynamic effects may be seen to be beneficial to both pathophysiological states.

Nifedipine will cause a direct reduction in vascular tone, systemic vascular resistance and arterial blood pressure. Coronary vasodilatation is induced, thereby maximizing coronary perfusion, and by preventing calcium overload nifedipine may cause an enhanced relaxation in myocardial diastolic wall tension thus improving diastolic relaxation and diastolic function. These effects are particularly prominent in patients given intravenous Class 2 calcium-channel blockers for the treatment of perioperative hypertension. The prominent chronotropic and intracardiac conduction effects seen with verapamil are not seen with Class 2 drugs, in particular with nicardipine and isradipine. Studies have shown that the maximum rate of rise in left ventricular systolic pressure (LV dP/dT max) is actually enhanced *in vivo* with isradipine. However, this is likely to be due to baroreceptor-mediated sympathoadrenergic activation in response to the vasodilatation rather than as a result of a direct effect. More detailed studies of the effects of nicardipine on myocardial contractility using end systolic pressure volume relationship (ESPVR) as an index of contractile state have suggested that nicardipine does produce a mild negative inotropic effect, and the same is probably true for other Class 2 drugs. This effect is therapeutically irrelevant unless other negatively inotropic drugs are used concomitantly, including β-blockers and volatile anaesthetics.

There is a mild inhibition of sinoatrial node activity, which serves to reduce the chronotropic response to vasodilatation, and cardiac output and stroke volume may be substantially increased, particularly in those patients with a high baseline level of left ventricular afterload. This is further enhanced by the fact that venodilatation is minimally affected, and so pulmonary capillary wedge pressure and left ventricular filling is maintained.

The effects of Class 2 drugs on the coronary circulation are particularly important. Coronary vascular resistance is reduced and coronary blood flow is increased. Nifedipine has been used as a treatment for coronary vasospasm by direct intracoronary injection, and isradipine has been recommended for prophylaxis or treatment of internal mammary graft spasm following coronary bypass graft surgery. However, rapid coronary vasodilatation may produce a redistribution of coronary blood flow such that non-ischaemic areas receive luxury perfusion and ischaemic areas may be underperfused, resulting in worsening ischaemia via an intracoronary steal mechanism. Nifedipine and other Class 2 drugs have been associated with a sudden worsening of anginal symptoms and treatment may need to be stopped for this reason.

The effects of Class 2 drugs on other vascular beds appears variable. Many have reported an increase in urine output following intravenous therapy but this could be due to the increase in cardiac output rather than as a result of renal vasodilatation. There is some evidence that nifedipine may be effective in pulmonary hypertension, but in general this is a weak effect. Pulmonary vasodilatation with Class 2 calcium blockers is less potent than that seen following nitrates, sodium nitroprusside, prostacyclin, inhaled nitric oxide or phosphodiesterase inhibitors. Significant pulmonary vasodilatation is not seen when nicardipine or isradipine are given acutely to control perioperative blood pressure, and this may have important implications in preventing an increase in intrapulmonary shunting and hypoxaemia.

Finally, the effects on the cerebral circulation have been investigated. There are data to suggest that both Class 1 and 2 drugs are effective in reducing experimental vasospasm, and much experimental evidence to suggest that the area of cerebral infarction may be reduced. Nimodipine may improve the prognosis after intracranial aneurysm rupture. Calcium-channel blockers may have beneficial cerebrovascular antispasmodic effects, but their vasodilator effects may lead to increase in cerebral blood flow and hence rises in intracranial pressure.

Class 3 – benzothiazepines

Diltiazem is the only Class 3 calcium-channel blocker in clinical use, and the drug is used almost exclusively in the treatment of angina and ischaemic heart disease. Diltiazem causes a small reduction in sinoatrial node automaticity and hence in heart rate. Coronary vasodilatation is a prominent feature, but systemic vasodilatation is minimal and therefore the effects on blood pressure and systemic vascular resistance seen with Class 2 drugs are not seen with diltiazem. The effects on cardiac output are variable, and there is a reduction in myocardial contractility. The effects of coronary vasodilatation, reduction in myocardial work and control of heart rate have identified diltiazem as being more effective than nifedipine as monotherapy in the treatment of angina. Diltiazem alone or in combination with a nitrate is frequently used to control chronic stable angina in patients who are intolerant to β-blockers. Calcium-channel blockers have been shown to be less effective than β-blockers at preventing perioperative ischaemia in patients undergoing coronary artery bypass graft surgery. However, recent data have called into question these findings, since the plasma levels of diltiazem following cardiopulmonary bypass were shown to be subtherapeutic despite supposedly adequate oral dosing on the morning of surgery. Thus it may have been the dosage and route of administration rather than the drug itself that was in fact ineffective.

In combination with the calcium-binding protein calmodulin, Ca^{2+} ions are responsible for the activation of the enzyme myosin light chain kinase (MLCK). Vascular myocyte myosin is composed of two heavy chains and two sets of light chain subunits. MLCK phosphorylates one of the residues of a light chain (the regulatory 20 000 Da light chain, or LC_{20}). This phosphorylation is the trigger that sets in motion the cycling of cross-bridging and hence contraction, by increasing 1000 times the speed of inorganic phosphate release, which is the rate-limiting step in the actin–myosin–ATPase cycle.

During the contraction of vascular smooth muscle the increases in cytosolic Ca^{2+} levels and myosin light chain phosphorylation are transient; they return to little above resting levels while tension is maintained in the actin–myosin complexes probably by means of non-phosphorylated and slowly cycling cross-bridges – a phenomenon known as 'latch state'. This is an energy-efficient condition as ATP is consumed much more slowly than it is during the process of tension development. This is a 'dynamic steady state' whose mechanism is poorly understood. The latches do break and need to be reformed with the associated consumption of ATP, Ca^{2+} ions and myosin light chain phosphorylation also being required.

In most vascular smooth muscle preparations, the addition of phorbol esters will lead to the production of slowly developing and sustained contractions. Phorbol esters are well known to be activators of protein kinase C. It has been suggested that the diacylglycerol produced in the generation of IP_3 activates protein kinase C and that this may be responsible for the generation of tonic contraction.

Potassium channels

Potassium channels of several types have been identified in vascular smooth muscle. If these are activated an increase in membrane K^+ conductance leads to an influx of K^+ ions into the intracellular compartment which produces a hyperpolarization of the cell membrane, with subsequent inactivation of voltage-sensitive Ca^{2+} channels and enhanced Ca^{2+} extrusion via Na^+–Ca^{2+} exchange. Both lead to a reduction in developed tension in the contractile elements resulting in vasodilatation. ATP-sensitive K^+ channels can be activated by agents such as nicorandil, pinacidil, minoxidil or diazoxide, and inactivated by sulphonylureas such as glibenclamide.

Potassium-channel openers

The main effect of these agents is to open potassium channels in the membranes of vascular smooth muscle cells leading to an efflux of potassium channels from within the cell to the extracellular space which hyperpolarizes the cell membrane and produces relaxation of the vascular myocyte.

This class of drugs is typified by the compounds nicorandil, pinacidil and cromakalin, all of which predominantly open potassium channels in smooth muscle. Minoxidil and diazoxide also act via this mechanism. It is thought that they open a potassium channel that is regulated by the intracellular concentration of ATP.

Nicorandil dilates arterial muscle by means of its activity as a potassium-channel opener. It also has a nitrate group that confers nitrate-like activity on it. In the treatment of angina pectoris it has been shown in clinical studies to be as effective as isosorbide dinitrate, β-blockers and calcium antagonists. It dilates large coronary arteries by 10–20% and decreases coronary vascular resistance via potassium-channel activation by between 25 and 50% resulting in a significant increase in coronary blood flow. It decreases systemic vascular resistance and blood pressure in addition to pulmonary capillary wedge pressure and left ventricular end-diastolic presure. This can be associated with a moderate rise in heart rate.

Its haemodynamic effects reach a peak within 1–2 min of intravenous injection or within 1 h of a single oral dosage, and last for up to 8 h. In contrast to the nitrovasodilators, these agents are not associated with the phenomenon of tolerance. It appears to be an effective anti-anginal agent through a combination of coronary vasodilatation and a decrease in cardiac preload and afterload. Its main adverse effects seem to be a relatively high incidence of headache and dizziness.

Pinacidil has been mainly investigated as an antihypertensive agent, for which indication it has been shown to be effective. It is frequently associated with the development of fluid retention, necessitating concomitant treatment with a thiazide diuretic. When given alone, it has a favourable effect on plasma lipid profiles but this effect is lost when a thiazide is coprescribed. In contrast, cromakalim does not seem to be associated with fluid retention which may be due to its effect on increasing renal blood flow and glomerular filtration.

These drugs have also been investigated for use in the treatment and prophylaxis of asthma and peripheral vascular disease with promising results.

Vasodilatation can also be produced by phosphodiesterase inhibitors which increase intracellular levels of 3′5 cAMP by inhibiting the enzyme phosphodiesterase which converts it to the inactive 5′-AMP, and also by activating cAMP-dependent protein kinase. The phosphorylation of MLCK reduces its affinity for the Ca^{2+}–calmodulin complex resulting in the dephosphorylation of myosin light chains and a cessation of tension development. Another means of producing vasodilatation is by means of increasing intracellular levels of cGMP as has been discussed above.

DRUGS AFFECTING ENDOTHELIAL AND VASCULAR SMOOTH MUSCLE FUNCTION

Drugs affecting predominantly endothelial function

Nitric oxide (NO)

The cellular effects of NO have already been discussed in the preceding sections. This section deals with its potential therapeutic role and does not discuss the role of the nitrodilators such as glyceryl trinitrates and associated compounds, which all work via NO.

The main area of therapeutic interest with direct NO therapy is in the management of right heart failure and pulmonary hypertension. There are, unfortunately, no available agents that selectively dilate the pulmonary vascular bed or increase right ventricular inotropy. The right heart and its associated pulmonary circulation are designed to be a high flow–low resistance circuit. The right ventricle is an appropriately thin-walled structure which, under normal circumstances, is incapable of generating pressures of the same order of magnitude as are found in the systemic circulation.

Some conditions are associated with the development of increased resistance in the pulmonary vascular bed. Examples include long-standing chronic lung disease such as cystic fibrosis, or chronic mitral valve disease due to the development of back pressure from the left atrium. The right ventricle will hypertrophy to a certain extent in order to generate a higher pressure to overcome the increased resistance but it will eventually dilate and fail. The treatment of pulmonary hypertension and right ventricular failure is notoriously difficult. The newer phosphodiesterase inhibitors, such as enoximone, amrinone or milrinone, are often used in an attempt to treat it. However, although these agents improve contractility and dilate the pulmonary vascular bed, they do not do so selectively and systemic hypotension may ensue which limits their usefulness.

Recently, inhaled NO has been tried as a selective pulmonary vasodilator. However, this is also not without problems. NO is an effective pulmonary vasodilator in a narrow range of concentrations. Its administration requires special equipment including the ability to monitor its concentration and that of its main metabolite nitrogen dioxide. NO strongly binds to oxyhaemoglobin leading to the conversion of the latter to methaemoglobin. Although this normally remains within safe limits, its levels should be measured. In the presence of oxygen, NO is rapidly oxidized to nitrogen dioxide. This can then be converted into nitrous acid and nitric acid, producing considerable acid-induced pulmonary damage, leading to pulmonary oedema and even death.

The risks of intrapulmonary acid formation can be minimized by keeping NO concentrations to the minimum that are clinically effective, by maintaining the lowest possible inspired oxygen concentration and by minimizing the contact time between NO and oxygen.

Nitrovasodilators

The nitrovasodilators such as glyceryl trinitrate (GTN), and isosorbide mononitrate and dinitrate spontaneously generate nitric oxide in blood vessel walls. The NO thus produced stimulates soluble guanylyl cyclase within vascular smooth cells resulting in the generation of cGMP. This inhibits the formation of cross-bridges between actin and myosin by causing the dephosphorylation of the myosin light chain leading to relaxation of developed tension. This process does not depend on the integrity of the endothelium as NO is released directly from the vasodilator molecules themselves and does not rely on the endothelial pathway of NO generation from its precursor L-arginine.

This group of compounds causes the relaxation of almost all types of smooth muscle. They cause bronchodilatation by relaxing bronchial smooth muscle tone. They also cause relaxation of the gastrointestinal tract and both tone and motility can be affected, but it is in the treatment of angina pectoris that they have been used extensively since the latter half of the 19th century.

They relax the vascular smooth muscle in both arteries and veins, although at low concentrations venodilatation tends to predominate. This apparent selectivity may be due to different bioavailabilities between arterial and venous muscular tissue, or different cellular metabolism of the drugs to NO. It may also be due to the different levels of basal formation of NO between the two types of tissue as discussed earlier. The venodilatation results in reductions in end-diastolic pressures of the right and left ventricles and a fall in cardiac preload. This fall in preload is proportionately greater than the fall in afterload associated with a reduction in systemic and pulmonary arterial pressures. Heart rate tends to increase slightly due to a baroreceptor-mediated increase in central sympathetic discharge and reduction in vagal tone. In the normal patient, cardiac output remains the same or falls slightly.

The mechanism whereby nitrovasodilators relieve attacks of angina pectoris has been considerably debated. Typical anginal pain is caused by myocardial ischaemia, which is the manifestation of an imbalance between the demand and supply of oxygen to the myocardium. This imbalance can be redressed by either increasing the supply of oxygen to the myocardial areas where it is deficient or by reducing its demand. It must be remembered that in most cases there is a regional rather than global supply/demand imbalance and this can be confined to the territory of branches of the coronary arteries. Furthermore, subendocardial tissue is particularly susceptible to ischaemia due to the forces to which it is subjected during ventricular systole.

Nitrovasodilators increase regional myocardial blood flow including that to the subendocardium. They selectively dilate large epicardial vessels including submaximal epicardial stenoses and the resultant increase in regional blood flow is preferentially distributed to ischaemic areas which have dilated in response to normal autoregulation. They increase subendocardial flow by reducing intracavitary pressures, creating a more favourable pressure gradient for flow to these regions.

Global myocardial oxygen consumption is also reduced by a combination of a reduction in preload and afterload, and it is believed that this constitutes the main means whereby anginal attacks are relieved. GTN and isosorbide dinitrate (but not isosorbide mononitrate) are subject to extensive hepatic first-pass metabolism. Nitrates are inactivated by the enzyme glutathione-organic nitrate reductase, which converts the lipid-soluble nitrates into water-soluble denitrated metabolites and inorganic nitrite. These metabolites are substantially less active than the parent compounds.

GTN has a plasma half-life of about 2 min and its plasma concentration peaks less than 4 min after sublingual administration. Isosorbide dinitrate plasma concentrations peak about 6 min after sublingual administration and it has a plasma half-life of 45 min. Its main metabolites are isosorbide mononitrates which have prolonged half-lives and favourable bioavailability in addition to reduced, although still significant, therapeutic activity.

Because of the extensive first-pass hepatic metabolism of GTN it is not given orally. Its main routes of administration are sublingual, transdermal, buccal and intravenous. Isosorbide dinitrate is given orally in large doses in order to saturate the routes of hepatic metabolism. This results in delayed onset of action due to initial effective clearance followed by prolonged duration of action due to delayed further inactivation and activity of the mononitrate metabolites. Isosorbide 5-mononitrate has been available for several years as a sustained-release preparation which is not subject to substantial first-pass metabolism.

Tolerance can develop to long-term exposure to organic nitrates and is thought to be due to the reduced availability of reduced sulphydryl groups which are essential for the conversion of nitrate to NO. It is currently recommended that to minimize tolerance a nitrate-free period of several hours duration should be provided each day in order to allow sulphydryl stores to be replenished. GTN dosages of 0.3 mg sublingually are usually employed as required to relieve acute anginal episodes. This is normally effective in 1–3 min and lasts up to 1 h. It should preferably be taken before activity that is known to precipitate an anginal episode. Isosorbide mononitrate is given in daily divided doses of between 30 and 120 mg for the prophylaxis of angina.

In anaesthetic usage GTN is used by the intravenous route whereby it acts as a reliable hypotensive agent, reducing first central venous pressure and pulmonary capillary wedge pressure, and systemic arterial pressure at higher doses. It also reduces pulmonary arterial pressure and can be used as part of the intraoperative management of patients with pulmonary hypertension. It can also be used intravenously in patients with coronary artery disease undergoing surgery, when it can be effective at reversing ischaemic changes on electrocardiogram. It is usually prepared as a solution of 1 mg/ml and is given as a bolus dose of 0.25–1 mg or as an infusion of 0.5–2 μg/kg/min.

Prostacyclin (PGI_2)

Prostaglandin I_2, PGI_2, or prostacyclin is produced in both endothelial cells and in vascular myocytes.

While the endothelium synthesizes greater amounts of PGI_2, the muscle mass in the blood vessel wall is greater, so the overall production is evenly divided. As discussed previously, it is a vasodilator and inhibitor of platelet aggregation, acting through the stimulation of adenylate cyclase to produce cAMP. In common with other prostaglandins it causes vasodilatation and hypotension but, unlike other members of the group, it is not metabolized on passage through the lungs endowing it with a potential therapeutic role.

An infusion of PGI_2 into healthy volunteers has no effect on reducing blood pressure until the dosages are increased to such a level that unacceptable side-effects occur, such as nausea, vomiting, flushing and agitation. It seems likely, therefore, that rather than acting like a true hormone it acts in an autocrine or paracrine manner. However, if the synthesis of prostaglandins is inhibited or prevented by the inhibition of cyclo-oxygenase (e.g. by non-steroidal anti-flammatory agents) their antihypertensive actions do not occur.

Although most blood vessels react in a predictable manner to PGI_2 by dilating, some vessels exhibit unusual responses; for example, it causes relaxation of the human umbilical artery at low doses but constriction at high doses. There are also interspecies differences; it causes either coronary artery constriction or dilatation depending on the species studied.

Although it is believed that the main mechanism responsible for the vasodilatation seen with PGI_2 is the intracellular increase in cAMP, it has recently been shown that the PGI_2 analogue, iloprost, mediates vasodilatation by membrane hyperpolarization through stimulation of potassium channels. Although this has not yet been demonstrated with PGI_2 the possibility exists that this mechanism may at least be partly responsible for the vasodilatation seen with this agent.

Prostacyclin has been evaluated for use in a number of therapeutic fields. It has been tried in both moderate and malignant hypertension. It was hoped that its effect on inhibiting platelet aggregation would enhance its therapeutic benefits in the latter, but it was poorly tolerated by infusion for either indication. Its overall haemodynamic effects were to produce a fall in systemic vascular resistance, manifested by an initial fall in diastolic blood pressure, followed at higher infusion rates by a fall in systolic blood pressure. These were accompanied by a reflex increase in heart rate, the overall effect producing an increase in cardiac index.

It also produces a fall in pulmonary arterial blood pressure and vascular resistance which has led to its investigation as an agent with potential usefulness in the management of pulmonary hypertension. Although it does improve cardiac performance and reduce pulmonary arterial pressure it is accompanied by unpleasant side-effects which preclude its routine use in adults.

It is useful, however, in the short-term management of neonates with congenital heart defects associated with a reduction in pulmonary blood flow. In these cases an infusion of PGI_2 may be used to maintain patency of the ductus arteriosus and hence permit the passage of blood into the pulmonary circulation, until corrective surgery can be undertaken.

It has also been used in recent years in patients requiring continuous anticoagulation, such as those undergoing renal haemofiltration or cardiopulmonary bypass. These patients are particularly susceptible to platelet activation, damage and consumption leading to a qualitative defect in platelet activity, even if the laboratory-measured platelet count is not remarkably abnormal. This platelet defect can cause substantial bleeding and further platelet loss.

It may also be of use in patients who have heparin-induced thrombocytopenia (HIT). In this condition, complement-mediated IgG antiplatelet antibodies are produced following exposure to heparin. The condition usually manifests itself as thrombocytopenia, and tachyphylaxis to heparin with thrombotic complications commonly about 7–10 days after the initial exposure to heparin. Subsequent exposure may lead to extensive thrombosis formation, bleeding due to thrombocytopenia and even death from thrombus formation in the coronary or cerebral circulation. Prostacyclin has been effectively used in these patients to deactivate platelets prior to heparin exposure for cardiopulmonary bypass. Although other agents such as ancrod may be used in these patients, an infusion of prostacyclin is probably the method of choice.

Hydralazine

This was one of the first antihypertensive agents in clinical practice but its use was associated with a high incidence of unacceptable adverse effects, particularly fluid retention and tachycardia. It causes direct relaxation of arteriolar smooth muscle by a mechanism that is not entirely understood but which is thought to involve NO. Some of its activity relies on the presence of the endothelium. In addition hydralazine can generate NO *in vitro*. It can also cause hyperpolarization of isolated arteries, which may be a reflection of potassium-channel activation.

Angiotensin II

Angiotensin II is an eight-residue peptide formed by the removal of the two terminal amino acids from the carboxyl terminal of angiotensin I by ACE. It exists in two types: circulating and endogenous. Circulating angiotensin II is produced by the action of endothelial-bound ACE found in large quantities in the pulmonary circulation. The precursor, angiotensin I, has in turn been cleaved from angiotensinogen by renin released from the juxtaglomerular apparatus of the kidney.

Angiotensin II binds to specific receptors on cell membranes whereupon membrane-bound guanine nucleotide binding proteins (G-proteins) are activated. IP_3 is produced by activated phospholipase C leading to the flooding of the cytoplasm by Ca^{2+} ions.

In the heart, this Ca^{2+} influx leads to prolongation of the action potential and an increase in contractility which is augmented by indirect activation of the sympathetic nervous system. It is not associated with a change in heart rate, presumably due to a baroreceptor-mediated reduction in central sympathetic tone in response to the increased contractility. It predisposes to arrhythmias and prolonged exposure results in ventricular hypertrophy.

Angiotensin II is an extremely potent constrictor of vascular smooth muscle, both arterial and venous, and it also constricts coronary arteries. Overall, it tends to cause an increase in arterial blood pressure with a modest rise in venous pressure and predisposes towards myocardial ischaemia.

In addition to enhancing central sympathetic outflow it also facilitates peripheral synaptic transmission by both increasing noradrenaline release from postganglionic nerve endings and by increasing end-organ response.

In the kidney, angiotensin II produces generalized contraction of the glomerular arterioles and mesangium affecting the efferent proportionately more than the afferent arteriole. This tends to cause an increase in filtration pressure although there is an associated global reduction in permeability of the glomerular apparatus leading to a reduction in effective renal plasma flow and glomerular filtration.

Angiotensin II also stimulates the zona glomerulosa of the adrenal cortex to release aldosterone which acts on the distal convoluted tubule and collecting duct to promote retention of Na^+ ions and excretion of K^+/H^+ ions.

Although angiotensin II is not commercially available in the UK, it is undergoing clinical evaluation. It has been shown to be of value in the management of patients with catastrophic hypotension secondary to systemic inflammatory response syndrome (SIRS) who have not responded to noradrenaline. It has also been used to manage hypotension during cardiopulmonary bypass and for the management of patients with severe hypotension directly attributable to ACE inhibition.

Vasopressin and its analogues

Vasopressin (AVP) is a ring-shaped peptide containing nine amino-acid residues. Currently two subtypes of surface-bound AVP receptor have been identified based on ligand characteristics and intracellular messengers. Stimulation of V_1 receptors leads to an increase in intracellular calcium ion concentrations via stimulation of membrane-bound G-proteins and IP_3 generation.

Stimulation of V_2 receptors leads to an increase in intracellular cAMP concentrations via activation of adenylate cyclase. While V_1 receptors in vascular smooth muscle membranes mediate an increase in vascular tone with resulting vasoconstriction, V_2 receptors in the renal medulla mediate water reabsorption. V_1-type AVP receptors have also been found in the membranes of platelets, where they mediate platelet aggregation in the presence of extracellular calcium.

The potential applications of AVP receptor agonists and antagonists are numerous, and much effort has been directed towards identifying suitable compounds. AVP itself is the most potent agonist yet identified at the vascular V_1 receptor. Although the potential uses of such a powerful vasoconstrictor are limited, it could, for example, be used in patients with pathological vasodilatation due to SIRS. Another potential use is in the management of massive upper gastrointestinal bleeding, particularly from oesophageal varices. Specific V_1 antagonists may be useful in the management of patients with elevated vascular resistances such as systemic hypertension, and in the inhibition of platelet aggregation in high-risk groups such as smokers and surgical patients.

V_2 agonists can be used in conditions of excessive water loss. Deaminated (D-Arg8) AVP or (or dDAVP) is used in the management of central diabetes insipidus. V_2 antagonists may be useful in the management of patients with hepatic cirrhosis or congestive heart failure.

Most of the agents discovered experimentally have mixed actions at both V_1 and V_2 receptors, and a drug that reduces excessive vascular tone and inhibits platelet aggregation (V_1 antagonism) while inhibiting water retention (V_2 antagonism) may have many uses in cardiovascular medicine.

Sodium nitroprusside

Sodium nitroprusside acts via the spontaneous release of NO in vascular tissue itself. It acts on both arteries and veins to effect a reduction in both preload and afterload. It reliably reduces systemic arterial blood pressure and usually pulmonary arterial pressure, and its use is associated with a baroreceptor-mediated increase in heart rate and stimulation of the renin–angiotensin system producing a rise in plasma renin activity. It reduces cardiac work and myocardial oxygen consumption. Cardiac output is usually maintained at pretreatment levels or is slightly increased, as are renal and cerebral blood flow. Hepatic blood flow is not greatly affected. It is available as a freeze-dried powder, usually as 50 mg to be reconstituted with 2–3 ml of 5% glucose. This concentrated solution is noticeably pink in colour and should be further diluted in at least 50 ml of 5% glucose. The pink coloration should still be slightly detectable. If the solution is tainted blue it should be discarded as this suggests some deterioration and breakdown of the nitroprusside. It decomposes spontaneously on exposure to light and should be appropriately protected. However, the spontaneous decomposition is relatively slow: it loses 10% of its activity in 3 h and still has over 50% of its original activity after 2 days of exposure to bright light.

It must only be given intravenously, and its highly potent effect dictates that invasive blood pressure monitoring is appropriate. The usual dose range is 0.5–10 μg/kg/min. It has a very rapid onset and offset of action and blood pressure can be controlled quite satisfactorily. Blood pressure will be seen to rise starting about 1 min after discontinuation of an infusion. It is rapidly broken down in contact with erythrocytes with the production of NO and hydrocyanic acid. The production of cyanomethaemoglobin may lead to the appearance of cyanosis even in the absence of cyanide poisoning at a cellular level. Cyanide ions formed by the dissociation of hydrocyanic acid mainly remain in the red blood cells, and they do not substantially alter red cell function. This is termed 'bound' cyanide and is only slowly released into the plasma as 'free' cyanide. The latter is metabolized in the liver by combining with thiosulphate in the presence of the enzyme rhodanase to produce the non-toxic thiocyanate.

Thiocyanate is subject to enterohepatic circulation and has a biological half-life of several days before undergoing eventual renal excretion. In the presence of renal impairment, thiocyanate can accumulate. In prolonged administration to patients with or without impaired renal function it may reach toxic levels (1.7 mmol/l serum). Toxicity associated with nitroprusside treatment is almost exclusively due to overdosage. However, the administration of large doses over a prolonged period may be associated with either cyanide poisoning or accumulation of thiocyanate as described above. Cyanide ions inhibit oxidative phosphorylation by binding to cytochrome oxidase leading to the interruption of cellular oxidative respiration and the development of metabolic acidosis by the replacement of aerobic respiration with obligatory anaerobic cellular respiration. An unexplained metabolic acidosis shown on arterial blood sampling should be considered as a sign of developing toxicity due to cyanide accumulation in a patient receiving nitroprusside therapy. Clinical manifestations include tachycardia, sweating, hyperventilation and cardiac arrhythmias. Plasma cyanide levels may be measured and should be considered toxic when in excess of 3 μg/l. Another possible cause of cyanide poisoning is a deficiency in thiosulphate groups, necessary for the inactivation of the cyanide ions.

If cyanide toxicity is suspected the following treatment should be instituted:

- Discontinue the nitroprusside infusion, and moderately hyperventilate the patient (if anaesthetized) with 100% oxygen. Support the circulation and treat arrhythmias as appropriate. Plus, either
- Administer sodium thiosulphate 12.5 mg in 50 ml 5% glucose over 5–10 min. This may be repeated. Or,
- Administer dicobalt edentate 300 mg in 20 ml over about 1 min. This too, may be repeated. This chelates the cyanide ions forming a stable compound with it, thus inactivating it.

The sudden increase in production of thiocyanate ions that will occur following treatment of cyanide poisoning with thiosulphate may result in the plasma levels of the former becoming toxic. Excess thiocyanate ions may be removed by haemodialysis.

It is recommended that no patient should receive nitroprusside at a rate greater than 4 μg/kg/min under any circumstance and that to those under anaesthesia it should be limited to a maximum of 1.5 μg/kg/min due to the synergistic effect it has with anaesthetic agents. Acid/base status should be frequently measured during therapy to exclude the development of a metabolic acidosis. It is suggested that thiocyanate levels be measured if treatment is continued for more than 3 days, that plasma or blood cyanide levels should also be measured during prolonged infusion or if there is a metabolic acidosis, and that the total dose in any 14-day period should not exceed 70 mg/kg body weight.

Despite the above, sodium nitroprusside remains a highly effective agent for the emergency treatment of severe hypertension and has a place in the management of pulmonary hypertension and severe congestive heart failure. It is widely used to control blood pressure in the perioperative period and is still the 'gold standard' against which other agents are compared.

REFERENCES

1 Furchgott RF, Zawadski JV. The obligatory role of endothelial cells in the relaxation of arterial smooth muscle by acetyl choline. *Nature* 1980; **288**: 373–6.

2 Khan MT, Furchgott RF. Similarities of behaviour of nitric oxide (NO) and endothelium derived relaxing factor in a perfusion cascade bioassay system. *Federation Proceedings* 1987; **46**: 385.

3 Ignarro LJ, Byrns RE, Buga GM, Woods KS. Endothelium derived relaxing factor (EDRF) released from artery and vein appears to be nitric oxide or a closely related radical species. *Federation Proceedings* 1987; **46**: 644.

4 Palmer RM, Ferrige AG, Moncada S, Nitric oxide release accounts for the biological activity of endothelium derived relaxing factor. *Nature* 1987; **327**: 524–6.

5 Silke B, Tennet H, Fischer-Hansen J, Keller N, Heikkila J, Salminen K. A double-blind, parallel group comparison of flosequinan and enalapril in the treatment of chronic heart failure. *European Heart Journal* 1992; **13**: 1092-1100.

Part II Vasodilator drugs used in the management of cardiovascular diseases

CJC Roberts

Four major groups of drugs produce vasodilatation by separate pharmacological mechanisms. They are the nitrates, the α-adrenoceptor-blocking agents, the calcium-channel blocking agents and the angiotensin-converting enzyme (ACE) inhibitors. There are three categories of cardiovascular disease in which vascular dilatation provides an important therapeutic approach – angina pectoris, cardiac failure and hypertension. However, not every vasodilator drug group has found an indication in every clinical entity. Thus the nitrates are not used in hypertension, the ACE inhibitors are not used in angina and some of the calcium antagonists have found indication in the treatment of arrhythmias and one in the management of cerebral vascular pathology (Table 16.1). The usage of vasodilators is dictated by differences in their other pharmacological actions, pharmacokinetic properties and dose–response relationship and consequent ease of dosing and risk of tolerance. The aim here is to explore these aspects for each group.

CALCIUM-CHANNEL BLOCKERS

The rapid expansion in the number of these drugs becoming available is a reflection of the recognition of their usefulness in angina and hypertension. Other indications are emerging and the need for a calcium antagonist with an ideal pharmacological profile increases.

Cellular mechanism of action

The cross-linking of actin and myosin filaments in the contractile unit of cardiac, striated and smooth muscle requires the ready availability of calcium ions. In striated muscle there is a well-developed mechanism for recycling calcium from intracellular stores in the sarcoplasmic reticulum. In smooth muscle the availability of calcium is dependent on entry of the ion into the cell through voltage-dependent and receptor-operated channels on the cell surface (Fig. 16.5). Cardiac muscle cells are also dependent on inward movement of calcium but to a much lesser extent. Thus it can be predicted that any drug blocking the entry of calcium through the surface channels will have its greatest effect on smooth muscle, some effect in the heart and minimal effect in skeletal muscle. The voltage-dependent channels open in response to depolarization initiated by rapid influx of sodium ions during the rapid upstroke of the action potential. Inward flow of calcium is slower, and more sustained and accounts for the plateau of the action potential (Fig. 16.6). Receptor-operated calcium channels are sensitive to the presence of catecholamines which enhance calcium entry. The available calcium-channel blockers all bind stereoselective receptors in the voltage-dependent channels. The reduction in calcium entry in response to excitation accounts for the muscle relaxation.

Calcium flux is of importance in the pacemaker and conducting system in the heart. Resting potential in the sinoatrial and atrioventricular nodes is less negative than elsewhere in the heart. Consequently, the voltage-dependent calcium channels are more readily opened and the action potential is slower in onset and largely attributable to calcium inward movement. At these sites the pacemaking capacity of the heart is determined by slow depolarization in phase 4 of the action potential which is also caused by inward calcium ion movement. Clearly, therefore, blockade of calcium channels will result in reduced myocardial excitability and automaticity.

There are fundamental differences in the cellular pharmacodynamics of the available calcium blockers.

TABLE 16.1 Clinical indications for pharmacological drug groups

HEART FAILURE	ANGINA	HYPERTENSION	ARRHYTHMIAS
Diuretics	β-Blockers	β-Blockers	Sodium-channel blockers
Digoxin	Calcium blockers	Calcium blockers	β-Blockers
Nitrates	Nitrates	ACE inhibitors	Amiodarone
ACE inhibitors		α-Blockers	Some calcium blockers
α-Blockers		(Nitrates)	Digoxin

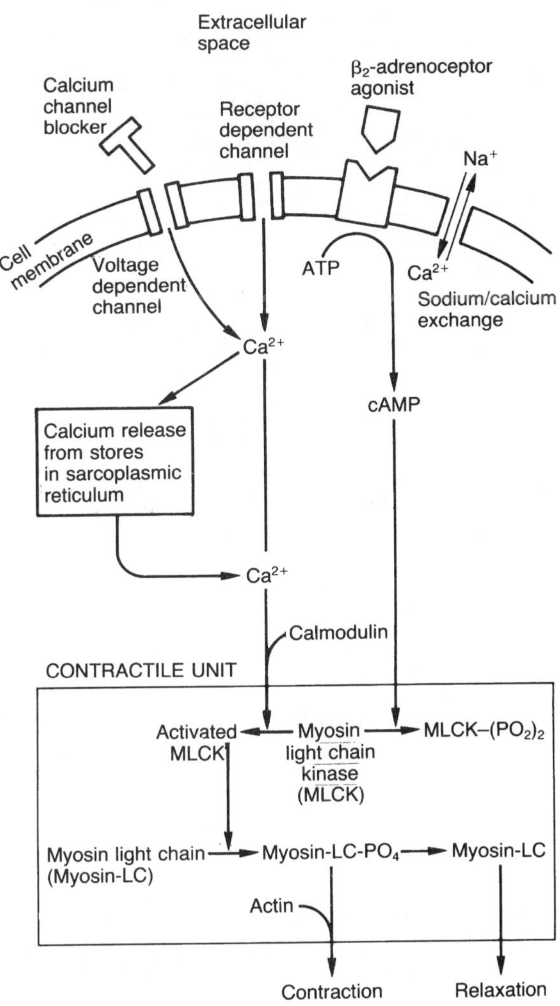

FIGURE 16.5 Role of calcium in facilitating muscle wall contraction.

There is more than one receptor at the calcium channel and it is probable that the distribution of these receptors varies with the tissues. This may account for verapamil's profound effect within the heart in contrast to nifedipine's small effect at therapeutic doses. Diltiazem's effect on the heart is intermediate and the newer dihydropyridine calcium blockers have less effect on the heart than nifedipine.

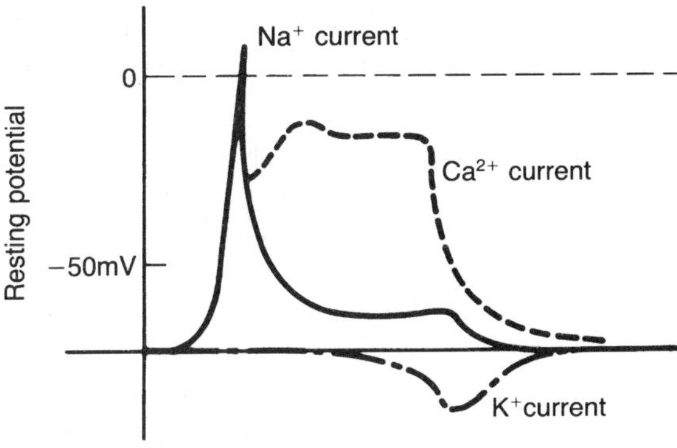

FIGURE 16.6 Contributions of ionic movements to action potential.

Mechanism of clinical effects

These derive from the three major pharmacological actions – generalized arteriolar dilatation, decreased myocardial contractility, decreased myocardial excitability and automaticity (Fig. 16.7).

Following the use of calcium blockers for angina, there is reduced myocardial contractility which decreases the oxygen requirement of the heart. The vasodilatation results in reduced afterload with reduced myocardial tension in systole. This results in reduced work and further reduction in myocardial oxygen requirement and also tends to improve flow of blood within the myocardium. Coronary artery vasodilatation may also occur, especially where spasm is a precipitant of the angina attack. There is a view that the anti-anginal efficacy is partly offset by the tendency to cause reflex tachycardia following the fall in peripheral resistance and that those drugs with more pronounced action in the myocardium that suppress such tachycardia may be more effective. Indeed nifedipine has been reported to increase angina, possibly by diverting blood flow away from ischaemic areas or by causing coronary underperfusion secondary to a fall in blood pressure. The dihydropyridines can be expected to reduce the frequency of angina attacks by about 50% and they increase exercise capacity and time to angina in formal testing.

In hypertension the reduction in peripheral resistance is the basis of the antihypertensive effect. Large artery compliance is increased and wall tension reduced. In addition most, if not all, have a diuretic action which may contribute. In contrast to diuretics at high dose and β-adrenoceptor blockers, the calcium blockers have no discernible adverse effect on patients' lipid profiles – a factor that has to be weighed in making a choice for long-term therapy. When used alone, the degree of antihypertensive effect achieved is similar to that with β-blockade or diuretic treatment. Their effect is additive not only to that of diuretics and β-blockers but also to that of ACE inhibitors and other vasodilators.

The vasodilatory and smooth muscle relaxant effects have provided the basis for studies in peripheral vascular disease, migraine, irritable bowel syndrome, oesophageal spasm, etc. Beneficial effects in Raynaud's phenomenon have been documented with nifedipine.

Because of their powerful afterload-reducing effect and minimal negative inotropic effect, the dihydropyridines have been assessed in heart failure. While immediate improvements in haemodynamic parameters have been measured, these drugs have been disappointing in controlled long-term studies and this is

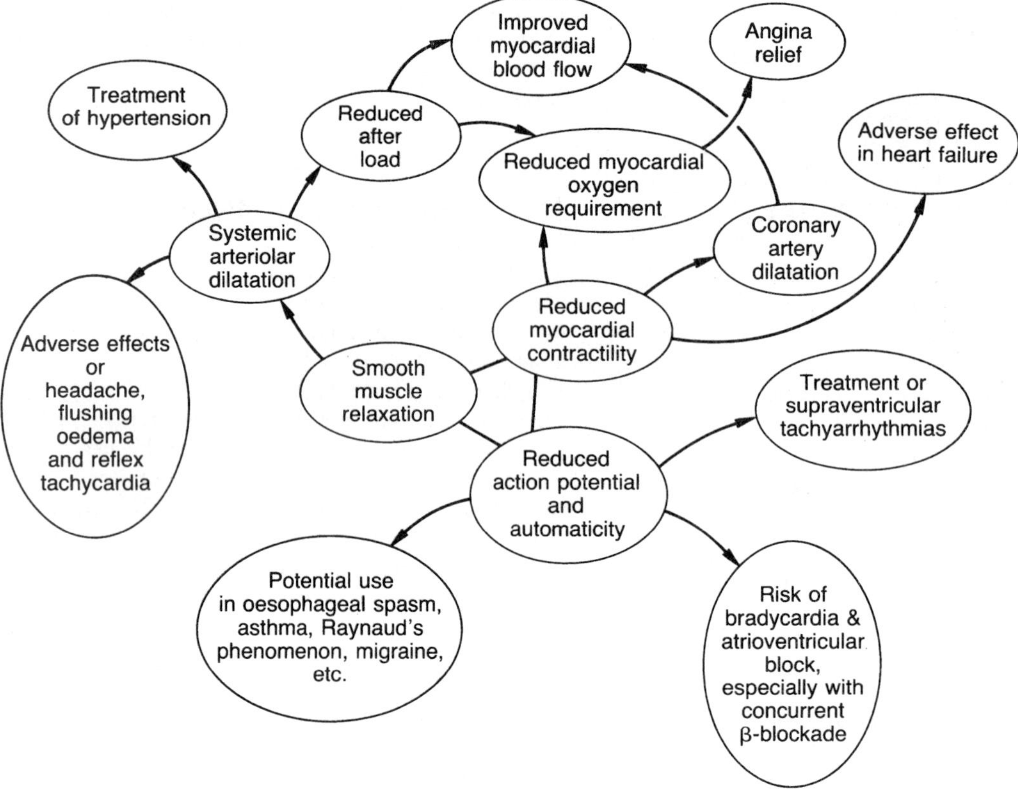

FIGURE 16.7 Mechanisms of the effects of calcium channel blockers.

not regarded as a valid approach. Studies of the use of calcium-channel blockers after myocardial infarction have suggested deterioration in patients with left ventricular dysfunction.

Calcium blockers are cerebral vasodilators but at present only nimodipine has been shown to be an important treatment in the prevention of cerebral spasm associated with subarachnoid haemorrhage. Hopes that they might be of benefit in patients with cerebral infarction seem unlikely to be realized.

Classification of calcium blockers

Three groups can be distinguished based upon chemical structure and this classification coincides with the qualitative differences in actions (Table 16.2). While verapamil and diltiazem stand alone in their groupings, the dihydropyridine group contains all the recently marketed drugs as well as several still under development or in use outside the UK. The important ones are nifedipine, nicardipine, isradipine, amlodipine, felodipine and nimodipine. Of these neither isradipine nor felodipine is yet licensed for angina and nimodipine is only used in subarachnoid haemorrhage. Nitrendipine is not available in the UK.

TABLE 16.2 Classification of calcium blockers

CLASS	DIHYDROPYRIDINES	VERAPAMIL	DILTIAZEM
Sinus node activity	0	++	++
A-V node conduction	0	++	++
Myocardial contractility	+	+++	+
Arterial vasodilatation	+++	++	++
Coronary vasodilatation	+++	++	++

0, no effect; +, marginal effect; ++, important effect; +++, major effect.

Pharmacokinetic aspects

As with the β-blockers and the ACE inhibitors, there are differences in the kinetic profiles of the calcium blockers (Table 16.3). They are all cleared by the

TABLE 16.3 Pharmacokinetics of calcium blockers

DRUG	BIOAVAILABILITY %	PLASMA HALF-LIFE (h)
Verapamil	10–35	3–7
Diltiazem	30–60	3–6
Nifedipine	30–60	2–6
Nicardipine	15–45	3–8
Isradipine	15–25	2–8
Amlodipine	50–90	35–50

liver and most suffer considerable presystemic metabolism, low bioavailability and short elimination half-life. However, amlodipine has a low clearance profile and an extensive apparent volume of distribution. This accounts for its relatively high bioavailability, its slow rise to peak concentration and its long duration of action. Most of the metabolic products have little or no pharmacological activity and are rapidly excreted in the urine. As can be predicted, markedly increased bioavailability of the highly cleared agents has been shown in liver disease and when enzymes have been inhibited, such as by cimetidine. The whole group is susceptible to interaction from drugs affecting hepatic drug-metabolizing capacity, either enzyme inducers or inhibitors, and the wide interpatient variability is increased by ageing. Because of the need for repeated dosing within each day for all except amlodipine some have been reformulated in slow-release preparations and these are used to reduce the peak plasma concentrations that are associated with adverse effects as well as to improve compliance.

Adverse effects and interactions

Considering that these agents interfere with a basic physiological mechanism, they are remarkably safe. Most of the adverse effects experienced are a direct consequence of the arteriolar vasodilatation. However, risks associated with the negative inotropic effect are being increasingly realized. Facial flushing, headache and palpitation may be experienced in as many as half the patients. Peripheral oedema is common. It is not amenable to diuretic treatment and is thought to be due to increased capillary permeability secondary to the vasodilatation. The reflex tachycardia together with a degree of hypotension accounts for the occasional precipitation of angina when the dihydropyridines are started. Effects on other smooth muscle are less obvious but constipation is a common complaint of patients taking verapamil.

Because of verapamil's potent effect on the sinus node, A-V conducting system and myocardial contractility great care must be exercised when prescribing this drug. Clearly, it is contraindicated in patients with actual cardiac failure or when cardiac decompensation seems possible. It should not be given in the presence of cardiac conduction abnormalities. There is considerable controversy over the use of verapamil with β-blockers. There is no doubt that the two groups potentiate each other's cardiac depressant effects and that verapamil should not be given intravenously to patients who have received β-blockers within 24 h and vice versa. Heart block, pronounced hypotension and death have resulted. Symptomatic bradycardia and heart failure may also follow oral combination therapy. While verapamil may be used orally with β-blockers in the management of hypertension in selected cases and in experienced hands with careful monitoring, this combination is not recommended for routine work.

Evidence is accumulating that the dihydropyridine calcium blockers and diltiazem should not be used where there is compromised myocardial function. They are not suitable vasodilators for the management of heart failure and there is some evidence that they may increase the risk of late heart failure after myocardial infarction. It seems that the negative inotropic effects of these agents is enough to precipitate cardiac failure despite initial improvements in haemodynamic measurements.

Verapamil increases the steady-state levels of digoxin by about 70% by interfering with both its renal and non-renal routes of elimination. Digoxin toxicity may be provoked in as many as 15% of patients and deaths have been attributed to this interaction. A 50% reduction in digoxin dose is required if the two groups are used together.

Verapamil impairs the metabolism of quinidine and theophylline and both verapamil and diltiazem impair the metabolism of carbamazepine. Significant elevations in the blood concentrations of the drugs may be expected with the predictable consequences. Particular caution is needed if either calcium blocker is stopped in patients whose epilepsy is stabilized on carbamazepine as fits may be precipitated.

Levels of cyclosporin are also elevated by some of the calcium blockers.

The calcium blockers are not recommended for use in pregnancy as some have been teratogenic in animal models.

Potassium-channel openers

Diazoxide and minoxidil were formerly classified as 'direct-acting' vasodilators. It is now known that these drugs act by opening potassium channels in the smooth muscle cell of the arteriolar wall. The resulting hyperpolarization impedes the calcium channel and contraction is prevented. Both these drugs are virtually obsolete because of adverse effects – hirsutism with minoxidil and fluid retention and diabetes with diazoxide. However, pinacidil is a drug available with this mode of action and appears to be free of unpredictable adverse effects. It is a powerful vasodilator that has been shown to be an effective antihypertensive agent. The drug has a high bioavailability but short half-life (about 2 h) being extensively metabolized to an oxidative product which retains pharmacological activity. Experience with pinacidil is limited. Whether it heralds a new group of important therapeutic agents remains to be seen.

Nicorandil has recently become available for the management of angina. It acts primarily by opening ATP-sensitive potassium channels but also has some nitrate-like action. The drug causes a high incidence of symptomatic adverse effects but may be useful in some patients where other therapies have failed.

ANGIOTENSIN-CONVERTING ENZYME (ACE) INHIBITORS

Nine drugs that inhibit ACE can now be prescribed in the UK. They are the most recent addition to the treatment of hypertension and cardiac failure and represent a major advance. Despite the undisputed benefits to patients that can be obtained from these drugs, their history has been far from smooth.

Captopril was launched in 1981 for the management of severe hypertension and when renin might perpetuate the high blood pressure. However, a catalogue of major adverse effects marred the drug's early reputation. Of these, the development of nephrotic syndrome and bone-marrow depression were the most worrying. These problems are now explained by the use of too high a dose in patients with multisystem disease whose kidneys and bone marrows were at risk and who were liable to drug accumulation. Experience has dictated a maximum daily dose below which serious adverse effects are rare.

The dose recommendation for enalapril also had to be amended months after the drug had been released. The starting dose was found to be too high – causing profound hypotension and transient renal impairment in a significant proportion of patients. As a result strict guidelines on starting ACE inhibitors have been drawn up.

The reputations of the newer agents are unscathed but experience with the group is still accumulating and so policies and guidance need constant updating.

Mechanism of action

The renin–angiotension system provides the mechanism whereby renal perfusion and glomerular filtration are maintained in the face of physiological variations such as those due to dehydration, posture, vasodilatation, blood loss, etc. (Fig. 16.8). Renin output from the juxtaglomerular apparatus of the nephron is stimulated by a fall in perfusion detected by stretch receptors in the afferent arteriole and juxtaglomerular cells and by activation of the sympathetic nervous system following a fall in systemic blood pressure. Circulating angiotensinogen is converted to angiotensin I and this to angiotensin II catalysed by ACE. The latter causes systemic arteriolar constriction both directly and by augmenting the activity of the sympathetic nervous system. Angiotensin II stimulates the release of aldosterone which acts at the distal part of the renal tubule to promote sodium retention and potassium excretion. Angiotensin II stimulates thirst by increasing the synthesis of antidiuretic hormone and within the kidney causes a redistribution of blood flow towards the medullary nephrons, which causes further volume retention. The volume expansion, together with the increased peripheral resistance, improve flow to the kidney and the fraction of blood flow that is filtered by the glomeruli is increased as a result of efferent arteriolar constriction in the nephron.

The system serves the kidney well but can have a damaging effect elsewhere. When activated by stenosis of a renal artery or because of renal parenchymatous disease it may create and perpetuate hypertension. The accelerated phase of idiopathic hypertension is usually associated with hyper-reninaemia. When the reduction in renal perfusion is caused by a low cardiac output because of cardiac muscle disease the increase in peripheral resistance puts an excessive afterload on the heart. This not only physically impairs its capacity to eject an adequate stroke volume but increases the oxygen requirement of the heart muscle while decreasing coronary perfusion. The volume retention contributes to cardiac dilatation and congestive symptoms as well as oedema (Fig. 16.9).

It follows that to block the renin–angiotensin system provides a valid line of therapy in hypertension and cardiac failure accepting a risk to renal function. In practice, renal function in most patients improves either because of reduction in the damaging effect of uncontrolled hypertension or in cardiac failure because of an overall improvement in cardiac output.

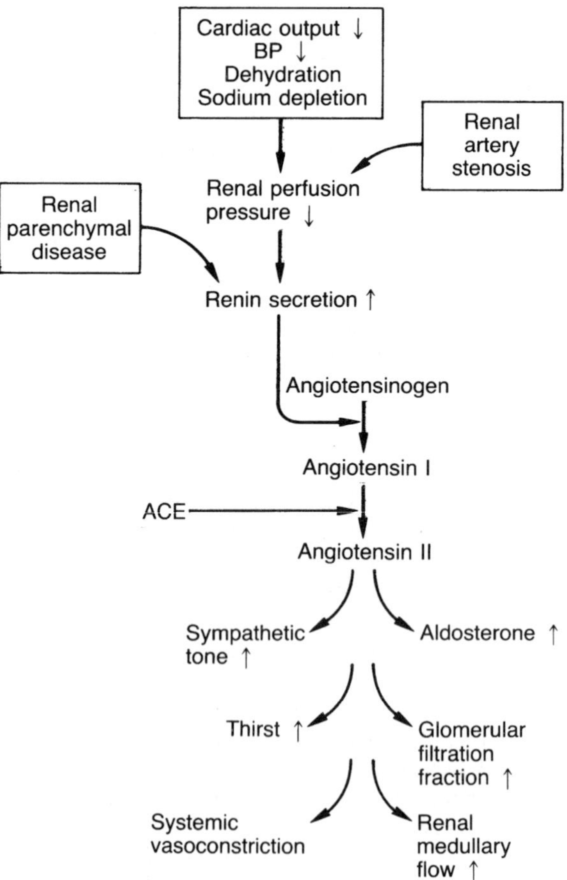

FIGURE 16.8 Stimulants and effects of the renin-angiotensin system.

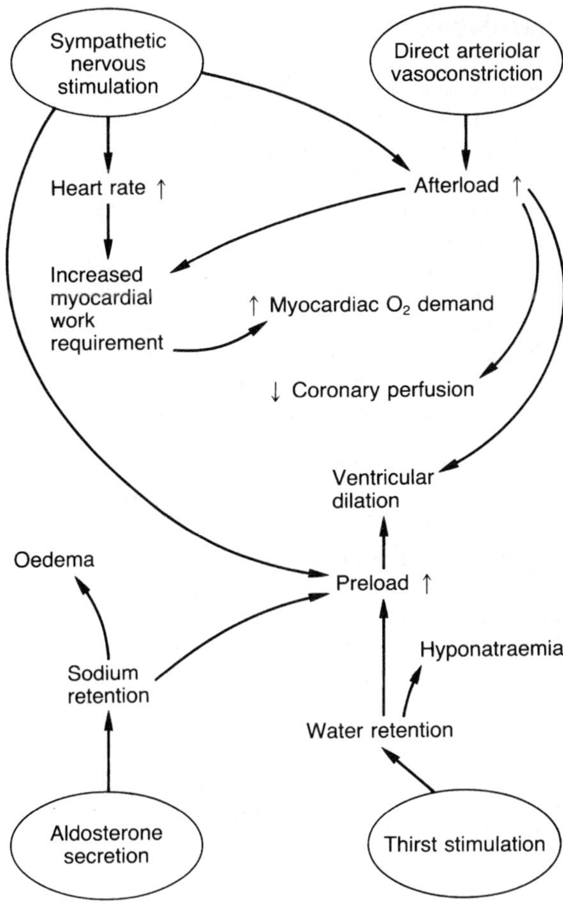

FIGURE 16.9 Adverse effects of the renin–angiotensin system in heart failure.

It should be remembered that ACE is also kinase II – the enzyme responsible for the breakdown of the circulating vasodilatory kinins such as bradykinin. Kinins produce marked vasodilatation in several vascular beds including heart, kidney and skeletal muscle either by direct action or by the release of arteriolar vasodilatory prostaglandins PGE_2 and PGI_2. In the veins they cause constriction probably via the release of $PGF_{2\alpha}$. The relevance of promoting these substances to the therapeutic action of ACE inhibitors continues to be debated.

Indications

Hypertension

Each of the ACE inhibitors has been shown to be effective in reducing blood pressure in all forms of hypertension – whether or not mediated by the renin–angiotensin system. In combination with loop diuretics they are particularly useful in the accelerated phase of hypertension. However, if there is bilateral stenosis of the renal arteries – a situation increasingly recognized – when blood pressure is critically dependent on angiotensin disastrous falls in blood pressure may occur. The place of these drugs in the management of mild to moderate hypertension remains uncertain. Most patients tolerate them well and they are as effective as β-blockers and have been shown to complement their action. Many use them as first-line agents arguing that the quality of life is better on these agents than on diuretics or β-blockers. Others await more definitive evidence that they have material advantages which justify their cost and use them only when patients are intolerant of the older drugs or have specific contraindications.

ACE inhibitors have become popular in the first-line management of hypertension associated with diabetes because they have been shown to slow down the progression of microalbuminuria to overt diabetic nephropathy and to reduce the rate of fall of renal function. This probably relates to the changes in glomerular capillary hydraulic pressure. Apart from this, diuretics and β-blockers have specific adverse effects in diabetes.

Heart failure

ACE inhibitors relieve shortness of breath in heart failure and increase exercise and functional capacity. The improvement in haemodynamics remains for longer than during treatment with conventional vasodilators such as prazosin, probably because volume expansion is prevented. Enalapril has been shown to reduce cardiovascular mortality by 40% after 6 months' treatment in severe heart failure apparently by reducing the risk of progression to intractable congestion. It has been shown that ACE inhibitors delay the onset of severe symptoms if used much earlier in patients with cardiac muscle disease and left ventricular hypertrophy regresses in some patients with ACE inhibitors. They are superior to conventional vasodilators in reducing cardiac failure mortality.

After myocardial infarction administration of ACE inhibitors can prevent progressive ventricular dilatation and dysfunction. They reduce the mortality when given to patients in the postmyocardial infarction period who are identified as having left ventricular dysfunction but are not appropriate in the immediate management of all patients with infarction. They are no substitute for diuretics in symptomatic patients. ACE inhibitors should be used in all patients with proven cardiac failure in the absence of contraindications. Elderly patients are likely to respond well despite evidence that the renin–angiotensin system's activity is reduced.

Contraindications and precautions

Every attempt must be made to avoid hypotension and renal impairment. Renal function should be assessed in all patients in whom ACE inhibition is being considered by measurement at least of serum creatinine. Where this is elevated, the dose should be reduced and renal function carefully monitored during the first few days of treatment and at intervals subsequently. Great care is required in using these drugs to control the hypertension of renal artery stenosis and hospitalization is advisable. Otherwise in the management of hypertension it is acceptable to start treatment in the community. A low dose as recommended by the manufacturer should be given on retiring especially if the patient is also taking a diuretic drug. Maintenance therapy can then be started but it is advisable to monitor plasma potassium and urea regularly.

In heart failure, patients with valvular stenosis or who are severely hypotensive are unsuitable and the response in patients with cor pulmonale may be disappointing. The risk of hypotension following the first administration is greater than in hypertensive patients. Who will develop this reaction cannot be predicted but hyponatraemic patients, those with renal insufficiency, the elderly and those who have been receiving large doses of diuretics are particularly liable. Initiation of treatment should be followed by blood-pressure monitoring for several hours. That usually means admission to hospital but is not mandatory. If a small test dose is tolerated, regular therapy can be instituted and the dose increased according to response ensuring that the systolic blood pressure does not fall below 100 mmHg and that the serum creatinine does not rise unduly.

Differences between the drugs

No significant differences in effectiveness have been shown between the available ACE inhibitors either in hypertension or cardiac failure. However, the pharmacokinetic properties, duration of action and adverse effect profile are not the same and there is a small cost difference (Table 16.4). Choice of drug depends on these.

TABLE 16.4 Characteristics of the ACE inhibitors

DRUG	SH GROUP PRESENT	PRODRUG	APPROX EFFECTIVE HALF-LIFE (h)
Captopril	+	–	2
Enalapril	–	+	11
Lisinopril	–	–	13
Quinapril	–	+	3*
Perindopril	–	+	25
Ramipril	–	+	11

*Duration of action in hypertension greater than that implied by half-life.

Pharmacokinetics

Captopril is rapidly absorbed and active but has a short half-life and should be given three times per day. The rapidity in the onset of action has advantages when starting patients on treatment as early hypotensive reactions can be readily detected and are of short duration. Enalapril requires conversion in the liver to enalaprilat for activity. The maximum effect of a single dose is delayed therefore for some hours. Enalaprilat has a long half-life and enalapril is suitable for once-daily administration. Quinapril, ramipril and perindoril have similar profiles. Lisinopril is active, slowly and poorly absorbed from the gastrointestinal tract and has a slow elimination so that it also can be given once daily (Table 16.4).

It has been suggested that the drugs with the longer duration of action are more liable to cause long-term hypotension and secondary elevations in serum creatinine in patients with heart failure. It may be then that captopril should be considered first in this condition. Conversely, in hypertension once-daily treatment is clearly an advantage and so enalapril, lisinopril or one of the other agents have kinetic profiles more suited.

Adverse effects and interactions

Some adverse effects are attributable to the action of ACE inhibition and are common to the group. However, captopril at the high doses previously used caused an unacceptable incidence of specific adverse effects – neutropenia, nephropathy and skin rashes. This toxicity may well have been related to the sulphydryl group in its molecules. At currently used doses the problems have virtually disappeared. Disturbance of taste is an effect unique to captopril and occurs at a rate about two times that in a control population.

Predictable adverse effects from ACE inhibition are hypotension and hyperkalaemia. The latter is not usually clinically significant, except in renal insufficiency, but ACE inhibitors should not be administered with potassium supplements or potassium-retaining diuretics without careful monitoring. Angioedema, which may come on within days of starting treatment and may be severe, should be watched out for. Dry irritating cough coming on weeks after starting treatment is now well recognized with these drugs and may have an incidence as high as 20%. It occurs more frequently in women and is unrelated to initial diagnosis. These effects are probably due to inhibition of the breakdown of bradykinin and substance P by kininase II and possibly the build up of certain prostaglandins. Interestingly non-steroidal anti-inflammatory agents have been shown to suppress the cough but this is not a recommended therapeutic manoeuvre. Disodium cromoglycate may ameliorate it. Diarrhoea also occurs and this may have a similar pharmacological basis.

Few drug interactions that could not be predicted have been reported. Captopril may reduce the clearance of digoxin and it is thought that renal function might be particularly susceptible to the combination of non-steroidal anti-inflammatory agents and ACE inhibitors.

Lozarten is the first angiotension II receptor antagonist to be introduced into clinical practice. The adverse effect of cough is eliminated by the use of this drug but its place in the treatment of hypertension has still to be established.

NITRATES

While the organic nitrates can be regarded as old drugs, having been introduced into medicine in the 19th century, our understanding of their mode of action and pharmacokinetics is relatively recent. This improved understanding has not only optimized the way in which they are used in angina but has widened the indications for their use to include heart failure.

Cellular mechanism of action

All of this group achieve relaxation of smooth muscle throughout the body and have virtually no other pharmacological actions. While smooth muscle in bronchi, gastrointestinal tract and genitourinary systems is demonstrably relaxed, these actions are rarely of clinical value because of their short duration and their importance is minimal compared with the overwhelming vasodilatation. All segments of the vascular system relax in response to nitrates but arterioles and precapillary sphincters are dilated less than the veins at therapeutic doses. The result is a greatly increased venous capacitance and decreased ventricular preload.

Glyceryl trinitrate (nitroglycerin) is the prototype of the group. It and its analogues are denitrated in the smooth muscle cell in a process requiring sulphydryl groups and catalysed by organic nitrate ester reductase. The nitric oxide released is thought to activate guanylate cyclase by combining with a further sulphydryl-containing receptor. Production of cGMP is promoted and subsequent dephosphorylation of phosphorylated myosin light chains results in smooth muscle relaxation (Fig. 16.10). While there is some evidence that prostacyclin may also be produced and involved, the effect is completely independent of autonomic receptors. Indeed, autonomic reflexes may be invoked to counter the hypotensive effect of the drugs.

Mechanism of clinical effects

Nitrates are used in the management of myocardial ischaemia – both acute coronary insufficiency and in the relief of anginal symptoms – and they are used to

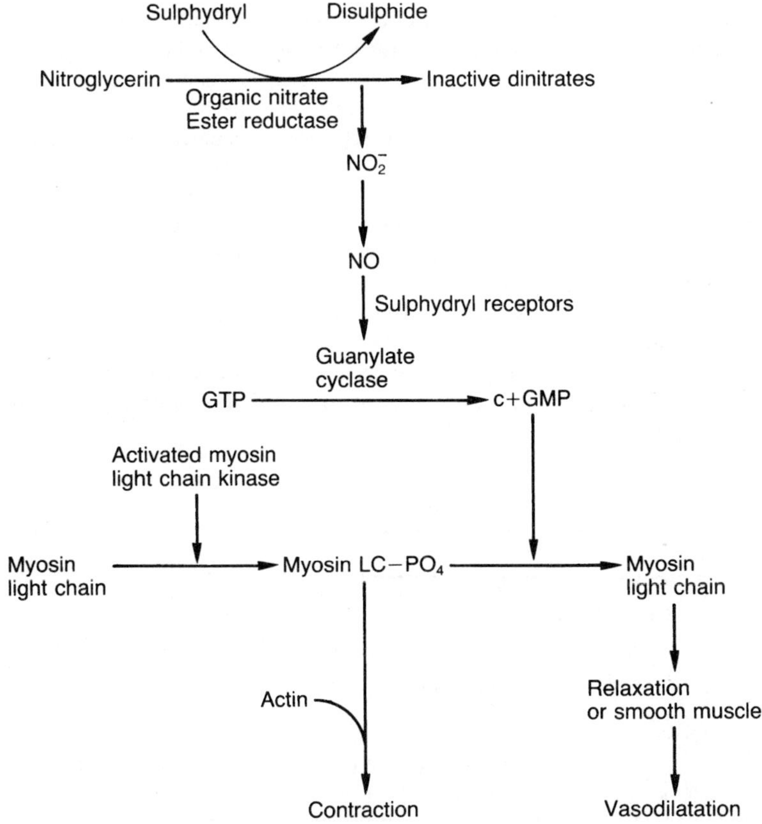

FIGURE 16.10 Cellular mechanism of nitrate action.

treat heart failure, predominantly left ventricular failure.

Relief of myocardial ischaemia

Myocardial blood flow is limited by coronary artery dimension, intramyocardial tension during diastole (particularly through subendocardial vessels) and perfusion pressure. Myocardial oxygen requirement increases with heart rate and with intramyocardial tension during systole (afterload). The possible beneficial effects of nitrates in myocardial ischaemia are therefore firstly coronary vasodilatation. This certainly seems to be an important factor in variant angina which is mediated by coronary spasm and may be a contributing factor where atheroma is the cause by opening collateral channels allowing perfusion of ischaemic areas. Second, by reducing the venous return, end-diastolic pressure falls and intramyocardial tension is reduced. Third, by decreasing peripheral resistance and afterload, work requirement and oxygen demand is reduced. These beneficial effects may be countered if the vasodilatation is so great as to cause significant hypotension as heart rate will increase by baroreceptor reflexes and time for perfusion as well as perfusion pressure in the coronary artery system falls (Table 16.5).

The predominant role of systemic vasodilatation is supported by the finding that the intracoronary administration of small amounts of nitroglycerin which improves overall coronary flow does not relieve pacing-induced angina, whereas systemic administration can stop angina despite a small reduction in total coronary blood flow.

Heart failure

Many patients with left ventricular dysfunction are able to maintain a reasonable cardiac output but only at the expense of a greatly increased left ventricular end-diastolic pressure and volume. Once filling pressure exceeds the oncotic pressure on the venous side of the pulmonary capillary bed, pulmonary oedema will develop. This is followed by decreased blood oxygenation and a deteriorating situation. Drugs that either reduce volume (such as diuretics) or increase capacitance vessels (the nitrates), thereby decreasing venous return and preload, can reverse the situation. Too drastic a reduction in venous return will, however, adversely affect cardiac output. The arteriolar vasodilating effect of the nitrates will cause further improvement by afterload reduction.

Pharmacokinetic aspects

The nitrates are a pharmacokinetically awkward group of compounds. Amyl nitrite is a volatile substance which can only be administered by inhalation. It provided the only effective treatment for angina in the early part of this century but is now obsolete. Attempts to produce nitrates with a prolonged duration of action resulted in drugs such as pentaerythritol tetranitrate whose efficacy remains uncertain. Three compounds are of importance in cardiovascular therapeutics – glyceryl trinitrate, isosorbide dinitrate and isosorbide mononitrate. Glyceryl trinitrate is relatively volatile and begins to be significantly lost from tablets once unsealed after about 2 months. Glyceryl trinitrate undergoes such extensive presystemic metabolism in the liver if swallowed that its bioavailability reduces to less than 10% – inadequate for any therapeutic effect. This is because of a high capacity enzyme system – glutathione-dependent organic nitrate reductase. This enzyme system also accounts for its rapid clearance from the circulation with a half-life of 2–3 min. Consequently, it must be administered buccally by conventional tablet, slow release tablet or spray, intravenously or percutaneously via one of the commercially available transdermal release preparations. The onset of action is within 2–4 min of buccal administration and because some of the metabolites are active, its duration of action is about 8 min. Isosorbide dinitrate also achieves much higher blood concentrations if given buccally but some preparations are available to be swallowed. The onset of action is slower than that of glyceryl trinitrate. This drug also undergoes extensive, rapid and variable metabolism to isosorbide-2-mononitrate and isosorbide-5-mononitrate, both of

TABLE 16.5 Effects of nitrates in myocardial ischaemia

Beneficial:	
Decreased systolic ventricular volume and tension	Decreased myocardial oxygen requirement
Dilatation of epicardial coronary arteries	Relief of coronary artery spasm
Increased collateral flow	Improved perfusion of ischaemic myocardium
Decreased LV diastolic pressure	Improved subendocardial perfusion
Potentially adverse:	
Reflex tachycardia	Increased myocardial oxygen requirement and decreased diastolic perfusion time
Hypotension	Decreased coronary perfusion

which are active. The half-life of the parent drug is about 30 min, while that of the 2- and 5-mononitrates is 1.8 and 5 h respectively. The latter is popular in the UK as the drug isosorbide mononitrate because of its high bioavailability and long duration of action.

Clinical indications

These are listed in Table 16.6. Sublingual glyceryl trinitrate remains the most widely used drug for treatment of and prophylaxis against acute episodes of angina. The rapid onset of absorption from the buccal mucosa either from tablets or the increasingly popular spray causes immediate off-loading of the heart and reduction in symptoms. The drug is very safe for self-administration and patients should be encouraged to use it when exercise is anticipated.

Intravenous nitrate therapy is valuable in the management of patients with unstable angina and is sometimes used after thrombolytic therapy for myocardial infarction. The aim of therapy is to maintain coronary artery flow and patency and to limit ischaemic damage. Intravenous preparations are expensive and many physicians believe that buccal, transdermal or high dose oral therapy can achieve as much. The administration of nitrates after myocardial infarction requires careful monitoring of heart rate and blood pressure. Myocardial ischaemia may worsen if central aortic blood pressure falls excessively, resulting in hypotension and reflex tachycardia. Occasionally a paradoxical bradycardia occurs. This is thought to be due to a vagal reflex stimulated by volume receptors in the atria which sense a markedly reduced venous return. The resultant syncope can only harm the critical intramyocardial situation.

Success in the use of these agents in the management of both biventricular and left ventricular failure also depends on careful monitoring. If preload is reduced excessively, cardiac output will fall.

The nitrates are useful if not essential drugs in the anaesthetic management of cardiac surgery, particularly coronary bypass. A primary concern during such surgery is myocardial infarction subsequent to disturbance of the balance between myocardial oxygen supply and demand. Intraoperative hypertension will clearly adversely affect that balance and intravenous glyceryl trinitrate is effective in its prevention and control.

Nitrate tolerance

A major problem when using these drugs discovered in recent years is the rapid development of tolerance. It is well known that the headache associated with their therapeutic use can be short-lived when long-acting agents are used. Workers in explosive factories who may be exposed to high levels of volatile organic nitrate compounds have reported headache and dizziness on starting work on Mondays and reduction in the symptoms during the week, only for them to restart after the weekend break. There is now good evidence that tolerance to the therapeutic effects of nitrates may occur within 24 h of continuous use. Blood vessels become hypo- or non-reactive to nitrate administration, resulting in a decrease in the duration of anti-anginal effect or loss of the beneficial actions in preventing or limiting myocardial ischaemia. In congestive cardiac failure it has been shown that there is attenuation of the pulmonary capillary wedge pressure response. Pharmacokinetic mechanisms are not responsible for the effect as vascular nitrate metabolism is decreased as is systemic clearance. Tolerance is associated with high levels of circulating nitrate and metabolites. Tolerance is a particular problem when large doses, frequent dosing regimes and long-acting formulations are used. It has been reported particularly with some transdermal glyceryl trinitrate preparations whose effect may be reduced by 18–24 h after application and whose anti-anginal effect is completely lost after 1–2 weeks' continuous use. Tolerance also develops to continuous intravenous infusion. Normal compensatory mechanisms such as volume expansion in response to the vasodilatation account for only a minor part of the tolerance as evidenced by its reversal

TABLE 16.6 Uses of nitrate therapy

Ischaemic heart disease
Relief of angina
Prophylaxis against angina
Treatment of unstable angina
After thrombolytic therapy for myocardial infarction
Cardiac failure
Long-term management of biventricular failure
Emergency management of left ventricular failure
Blood pressure control
Control of hypertension associated with left ventricular failure
Hypertensive emergency
Intra- and postoperative blood pressure control, e.g. coronary bypass surgery, neurosurgical and orthopaedic procedures

by the administration of drugs that provide sulphydryl groups such as N-acetylcysteine. The present theory is that the smooth muscle cell becomes depleted of sulphydryl groups essential for the chain of metabolism and action of the nitrates. This finding does not provide a suitable therapeutic approach and so nitrates are best used intermittently allowing a period of a few hours without nitrate administration in each 24 h. Thus slow release preparations should not provide 24-h therapeutic blood levels, transdermal applications should be stopped at night and intravenous infusions should be discontinued for a few hours each day.

Adverse effects

Hypotension is a predictable adverse effect which accounts for the palpitations and tachycardia commonly experienced. Severe hypotension must be avoided when the drugs are used intravenously and syncope may occur when the drugs are self-administered. The vagally mediated effect mentioned above may be precipitated if venous pooling is exacerbated by the patient remaining still and standing.

Headache is common and is due to meningeal artery dilatation. Susceptible patients may develop a full migraine attack. Care with dosage can minimize this symptom.

Although amyl nitrite readily induces methaemoglobinaemia, this is extremely rare with the therapeutic uses of the other nitrates.

α-BLOCKERS

α-Adrenoceptor blockers have been available for many years. Phentolamine and phenoxybenzamine lost their place in routine management of hypertension rapidly because of the reflex tachycardia and flushing commonly experienced. Prazosin was originally thought to be a 'direct-acting' vasodilator but it soon became clear that it was actually an α_1-receptor antagonist. The presynaptic α_2-receptors located in the adrenergic neurone terminals are unaffected by prazosin. This receptor sensitivity accounted for its hypotensive effect without undue tachycardia. Noradrenaline may continue to exert unopposed negative feedback on its own release. In contrast, phentolamine which blocks both types of receptor causes reflex stimulation of sympathetic neurons and greater release of transmitter onto the cardiac β-receptors and correspondingly greater cardioacceleration. Recently two further α_1-blockers have been developed for the management of hypertension but their role remains uncertain.

Prazosin has been used in both hypertension and in heart failure. It is an effective antihypertensive but lost favour because of the development of profound hypotension in some patients on commencing therapy ('first-dose effect'). This effect is particularly likely to occur in patients taking diuretics or sodium deplete for some other reason. It is mandatory to advise patients to start treatment last thing at night before retiring to bed. In the management of heart failure, immediate haemodynamic improvement can be demonstrated but over the course of weeks tachyphylaxis develops to the drug and improvement in exercise tolerance is lost. This appears to be partly explained by a degree of fluid retention which, however, can be reversed by concurrent diuretic treatment. A further suggestion for the tolerance is that there is increased noradrenaline release from the neuronal terminal. The long-term effect of prazosin on mortality in heart failure has been studied with disappointing outcome. Prazosin is well absorbed from the gastrointestinal tract with a bioavailability of about 50%. It undergoes extensive hepatic metabolism which accounts for its low bioavailability. It has an elimination half-life of 2.5 h which may be prolonged up to about 7 h in heart failure, reflecting the sensitivity of its clearance to the effect of changes in liver blood flow. There is also prolongation of its elimination in renal failure. Under normal circumstances it must be given in divided doses. Prazosin is relatively free of serious side-effects although some patients develop positive antinuclear factor and acute polyarthropathy has been rarely reported. Gastrointestinal symptoms, headache, palpitations, drowsiness, depression and sexual dysfunction occur infrequently. Prazosin and the other α_1-blockers do not adversely and may even beneficially affect lipid profiles. They cause an approximate 2% reduction in total cholesterol and a rise in HDL-C.

Because diuretics and β-blockers have been shown to increase serum lipids there is a trend for these drugs to be demoted to second-line therapy. Arguments in favour of such a major change in therapeutic policy ignore the fact that the low doses of diuretic drugs now in use have no important effect on lipids and that in the long term the effect of β-blockers is indiscernible. However, it has reawakened the development of vasodilator agents which have no effect on lipids. Two α_1-blockers – terazosin and doxazosin – are now available. They differ from prazosin only in their pharmacokinetic profile being longer acting, allowing once-daily dosing. Neither are licensed for use in the treatment of heart failure. Experience with them is limited but apart from the improved dosing regime they appear to offer little advantage over prazosin.

CONCLUSIONS

The groups of drugs described in this chapter have had a dramatic impact on the treatment of common cardiovascular diseases carrying a high mortality. They all have great potential to save life but carry significant hazard if used unwisely. The prescriber who ignores the guidelines for when and how to use them may magnify the risk to the extent that it outweighs the benefit.

FURTHER READING

Abrams J. Glyceryl trinitrate (nitroglycerin) and the organic nitrates: choosing the method of administration. *Drugs* 1987; **34**: 391–403.

Brogden RA, Todd PA, Sorkin EM. Captopril: an update of its pharmacodynamic and pharmacokinetic properties and therapeutic use in hypertension and congestive heart failure. *Drugs* 1988; **36**: 540–600.

Cohn JN. The prevention of heart failure – A new agenda. *New England Journal of Medicine* 1992; **327**: 725–7.

Editorial. Calcium antagonists caution. *Lancet* 1991; **337**: 885–6.

Flaherty JT. Nitrate tolerance: a review of the evidence. *Drugs* 1989; **37**: 523–50.

Freedman DD, Waters DD. 'Second generation' dihydropyridine calcium antagonists: greater vascular selectivity and some unique applications. *Drugs* 1987; **34**: 578–96.

Johnston CI, Arnolda L, Hiwatari M. Angiotensin-converting inhibitors in the treatment of hypertension. *Drugs* 1984; **27**: 271–7.

Lancaster SG, Todd PA. Lisinopril: a preliminary review of its pharmacodynamic and pharmacokinetic properties and therapeutic use in hypertension and congestive heart failure. *Drugs* 1988; **35**: 646–69.

McTavish D, Sorkin EM. Verapamil: an updated review of its pharmacodynamic and pharmacokinetic properties and therapeutic use in hypertension. *Drugs* 1989; **38**: 19–76.

Roberts CJC. Role of angiotensin converting enzyme inhibitors in the management of hypertension and of heart failure. In: Rowlands DJ ed. *Recent advances in cardiology* **10**. London: Churchill Livingstone, 1987: 175–200.

Roberts CJC. Therapy: angiotensin converting enzyme (ACE) inhibitors and vasodilators. *Current Opinion in Cardiology* 1988; **3**: 344–56.

Sharpe, N, Smith H, Murphy J, Greaves S, Hart H, Gamble G. Early prevention of left ventricular dysfunction after myocardial infarction with angiotensin converting enzyme inhibition. *Lancet* 1991; **337**: 872–6.

Sorkin EM, Brogden RN, Romankiewicz JA. Intravenous glyceryl trinitrate (nitroglycerin): a review of its pharmacological properties and therapeutic efficacy. *Drugs* 1984; **27**: 45–80.

The CONSENSUS trial study group. Effects of enalapril on mortality in severe congestive heart failure: results of the cooperative North Scandinavian enalapril survival study. *New England Journal of Medicine* 1987; **316**: 1429–34.

Todd P, Goa KL. Enalapril: an update of its pharmacological properties and therapeutic use in congestive heart failure. *Drugs* 1989; **37**: 141–61.

17

Control of Blood Pressure by Drugs

PART I DRUG TREATMENT OF HYPERTENSION

NH Kellow, RO Feneck

EPIDEMIOLOGY OF ESSENTIAL HYPERTENSION

Hypertension affects about one-fifth of the adult population in industrialized countries and is a major contributor to mortality, sufferers having a substantially greater risk of dying from myocardial infarction, stroke, congestive heart failure and renal failure. Its incidence is also higher among certain populations, particularly the elderly, diabetics and blacks.

While reducing blood pressure in hypertensive patients has been consistently shown to reduce substantially overall mortality, and particularly mortality from strokes, there has always been a confusing paradox. More than three times as many hypertensive patients die from myocardial infarctions as from strokes, yet antihypertensive treatment has had a singularly minimal effect in reducing coronary artery disease related deaths. There have been many theories put forward to explain this phenomenon but it seems most likely that coronary artery disease has a multifactorial aetiology with several factors such as obesity, lipid and thrombotic disturbances, and insulin resistance acting in parallel with hypertension rather than in series with it to create atheroma within the coronary vessels. It thus follows that a reduction in coronary artery disease related deaths in hypertensive patients will only ensue when simultaneous attempts are undertaken to tackle the other factors leading to its formation in addition to measures aimed specifically at reducing elevated blood pressure.

TABLE 17.1 Classification of hypertension by blood pressure

CLASSIFICATION	SYSTOLIC BLOOD PRESSURE (mm Hg)		DIASTOLIC BLOOD PRESSURE (mm Hg)
Normal	< 140	and	<90
Mild hypertension	140-180	and/or	90-105
Subgroup: borderline hypertension	140-160	and/or	90-95
Moderate and severe hypertension*	⩾ 180	and/or	⩾ 105
Isolated systolic hypertension	⩾ 140	and	<90
subgroup: borderline isolated systolic hypertension	140-160	and	<90

* Risk to be indicated by reporting actual values of systolic and diastolic blood pressure

DIAGNOSIS AND CRITERIA FOR TREATMENT

Before one embarks on treating a patient for probably the rest of his or her life it is important to establish criteria for the diagnosis of what value of blood pressure constitutes an elevation that should be treated. Arterial blood pressure exhibits a unimodal normal distribution within populations and numerous epidemiological studies over several decades have shown reliably that those patients with blood pressures in the upper end of the range are subject to a significantly greater risk of cardiovascular morbidity and mortality. The decision whether to treat a given value of blood pressure in the upper end of this range must be taken after careful consideration of the potential prognostic benefit that could be expected from commencing drug treatment aimed at reducing this elevation compared with the potential adverse effects of any such therapy.

Since the early days of the relatively toxic antihypertensives, such as reserpine and the ganglion blockers, newer drugs have been developed with much enhanced tolerability that have led to a steady fall in the threshold for treating elevated blood pressure. It can be stated reasonably safely that patients with a blood pressure of less than 140/85 fall within the normal range and are not subject to greater cardiovascular risk related to their blood pressure. Above this value there are several categories of elevated blood pressure with different recommendations for the management of each (Table 17.1).

However, blood pressure is an extremely labile measurement and the decision over the value that is representative of the patient's characteristic blood pressure should be reached very carefully. For example, the diagnosis of hypertension should not be made after one isolated elevated value. Initial elevated readings should be confirmed on at least two subsequent occasions. Furthermore, because blood pressure can be affected by many extraneous factors it should be measured in a standardized and repeatable way. The following procedure should be followed:

1 Patients should be seated with their arm bared and supported. They should not have smoked or ingested caffeine within the 30-min period prior to the measurement.
2 Measurements should be made after 5 min of seated rest.
3 The appropriate cuff size should be chosen. The rubber bladder should encircle at least two-thirds of the upper arm. A cuff that is too large will lead to under-reading of the patient's blood pressure.
4 Measurements may be taken with a mercury sphygmomanometer, a recently calibrated aneroid device or a validated electronic device.
5 The appearance (Korotkoff phase I) of sounds should be taken as the value of systolic pressure and the disappearance (Korotkoff phase V) should be taken as the diastolic value.
6 Two or more readings should be averaged at each sitting.

If there is still doubt about the patient's normal blood pressure after several visits to the clinic, then 24-h ambulatory measurement should be considered. It has long been recognized that blood pressure exhibits a diurnal pattern, being lowest during sleep and highest on waking. Hypertensive patients maintain this diurnal pattern but there is sustained elevation throughout the 24-h period. Nevertheless, suspicion should be aroused in a patient whose blood pressure is consistently elevated in clinic visits, regardless of any apparent patient anxiety that appears to be related to the clinic environment. These patients often have an exaggerated and sustained pressor response to stress and treatment should be considered, even if their blood pressure is shown to be predominantly within the normal range during 24-h measurement.

Before considering treatment, other factors should be carefully evaluated. A careful history should be taken, paying particular attention to other cardiovascular risk factors such as positive family history, smoking, obesity, excessive alcohol consumption, diabetes, and psychosocial circumstances. A physical examination should include height and weight and a painstaking examination of the cardiovascular system, not forgetting the optic fundi and major arteries for evidence of aneurysm, bruits or other manifestation of arterial disease. The presence of an enlarged thyroid gland should also be excluded as should evidence of enlarged kidneys, suggesting polycystic disease. Truncal obesity with abdominal striae and muscle wasting may suggest Cushing's syndrome. Although in 95% of hypertensive patients no cause is found (essential hypertension), it is important to exclude secondary hypertension with a treatable primary cause.

The aim of therapy is to reduce the patient's blood pressure into the range that is not associated with a significantly greater risk of cardiovascular morbidity. It may be possible to achieve this by considering first non-pharmacological approaches, such as weight reduction, reduction in dietary salt intake, cessation of smoking, reduction in alcohol consumption and the adoption of favourable lifestyle changes.

There is a clear correlation between obesity and hypertension. If individuals gain weight, there is a concomitant increase in arterial pressure. Weight reduction in obese individuals is associated with a fall in blood pressure and all such patients should be encouraged to remain within 115% of their ideal body weight.

There is much argument about whether excessive sodium intake leads to hypertension, but there is little doubt that in patients who have already been diagnosed as hypertensive reduction in sodium intake may lead to a fall in blood pressure such that antihypertensive medication may no longer be necessary. Furthermore, a high sodium intake may lead to relative resistance to treatment by antihypertensive medication.

Smokers have a considerably increased risk for lung cancer and pulmonary disease and twice the risk of non-smokers for coronary artery disease and sudden death. Smoking is associated with an acute rise in blood pressure due to circulating nicotine, although prolonged tobacco usage has not been associated with an increased prevalence of hypertension. However, smoking is the single most preventable worldwide cause of death and every effort should be made to encourage patients to stop.

Small amounts of alcohol taken daily are known to have a high-density lipoprotein (HDL)-related cardioprotective effect but excessive alcohol intake may lead to hypertension. Furthermore, the patient who drinks too much alcohol is at considerably greater risk for the development of non-cardiovascular disease and he or she should be encouraged to reduce alcohol consumption to no more than 30 ml of ethanol daily.

Finally, hypertensive patients should also be encouraged to take regular, moderate amounts of aerobic exercise which will serve both to aid weight reduction and may also reduce blood pressure. The patient's intake of dietary fats, particularly of the saturated variety, should also be reduced.

CURRENT TREATMENT GUIDELINES

Large-scale studies have shown a clear association between a reduction in blood pressure in patients with mild to moderate hypertension and a reduced incidence of morbidity and mortality from cardiovascular disease. However, it is believed that the benefits that have been demonstrated in randomised studies have actually underestimated the actual benefits that long-term anti-hypertensive treatment may confer on appropriate patients. This is at least partly because most studies were of a relatively short duration (three to five years) and the full benefits of a reduction in elevated blood pressure may take more than ten years to realise. In addition, the initial goal in young hypertensive patients is not so much to reduce the incidence of cardiovascular events, which in this population is low, but rather to prevent the progression of the disease process, such as the development of atherosclerosis and left ventricular hypertrophy.

It should be emphasised that levels of both systolic and diastolic blood pressure are important in deciding whether to treat a patient with elevated blood pressure (Fig. 17.1). However, other factors may influence the decision to start treatment early. For example, men generally and post-menopausal women in particular should have treatment started early. Evidence of existing cardiovascular or renal disease, or diabetes should also encourage early treatment. The reduction of blood pressure (even from normal) in patients with diabetes reduces microalbuminuria and delays the development of diabetic nephropathy. Treatment should be started early in patients with cardiovascular risk factors, such as continued smoking, dyslipidaemias, and elevated blood glucose.

The elderly population derive particular benefit from the treatment of elevated blood pressure. The ten-year risk of a major cardiovascular event amongst Western populations with mild hypertension ranges from less than 1% in those aged 25–34 to more than 30% in those aged 65–74 years.

What level of blood pressure should be aimed for? The simple answer is the lowest tolerated. There is a continuous relation between blood pressure and cardiovascular risk, which even extends to subjects with blood pressures in the normal range. Even in specific populations, such as patients with coronary artery disease, there are no proven adverse consequences of reducing blood prepssure to the low part of the normal range.

There are several non-pharmacological steps that should be taken before starting drug therapy in patients with mild hypertension. These include losing weight in obese patients, stopping smoking, reducing alcohol intake to less then 30g per day, the taking of regular moderate aerobic exercise, and the reduction of salt intake. These efforts will frequently reduce blood pressure into the normal range, although there is not

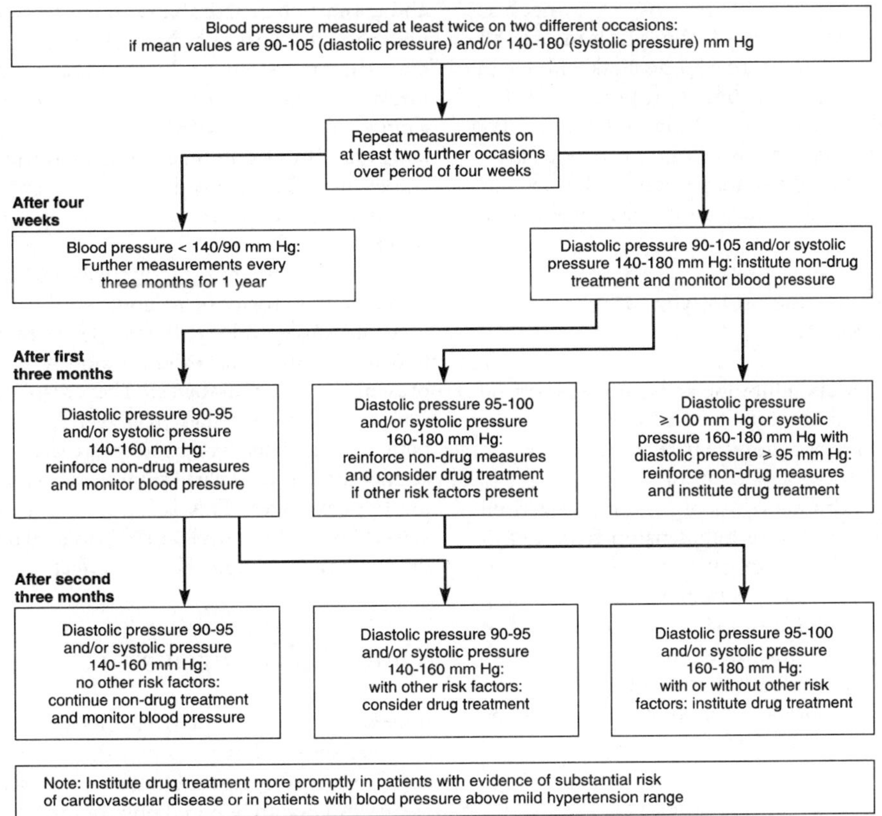

FIGURE 17.1 Management of mild hypertension (diastolic blood pressure 90–105 mm Hg or systolic blood pressure 140–180 mm Hg, or both)

yet any evidence that they are associated with a reduction in cardiovascular events in susceptible patients.

When starting drug therapy current guidelines favour an individualised approach. The majority of large-scale prognostic studies have been undertaken using diuretics and beta-blockers, so these are still favoured as first-line agents. However, there are also provisions for starting newly diagnosed hypertensive patients on angiotensin-converting enzyme inhibitors, calcium-channel blockers or α-adrenoceptor antagonists, depending on the particular profile of the patient in question. It must be emphasised that there is no proven benefit associated with one particular class of drugs, neither is one class more effective at lowering blood pressure than another. If treatment with one class of compound on its own has been ineffective then a drug from another class may be added.

DRUGS USED TO TREAT ESSENTIAL HYPERTENSION

Diuretics

This group of compounds has formed the mainstay of antihypertensive therapy for almost 40 years. When given either alone or in combination with other agents they produce a sustained and reliable reduction in blood pressure. Three types of diuretics which act via different mechanisms are used (thiazides, potassium-sparing diuretics and loop diuretics) but it is the thiazides and related compounds that have proved to be most clinically useful as blood-pressure lowering agents due to their effective antihypertensive action, which is not accompanied by polyuria following the first few days of treatment.

Even after such a wealth of clinical experience the exact mechanism of antihypertensive action of these agents is not precisely known. Upon starting treatment there is an abrupt urinary loss of sodium and water leading to a fall in extracellular volume, cardiac filling pressures and cardiac output that is accompanied by a fall in blood pressure. After a few days, however, the sodium loss ceases and sodium balance becomes more positive. This pushes extracellular volume towards pre-treatment levels although it remains about 5% lower, and cardiac output returns to normal. However, whereas systemic vascular resistance remains unchanged during initial therapy, it tends to fall after a few days and it is this modest but sustained reduction that accounts for the long-term antihypertensive effect of diuretics.

They are ineffective as antihypertensives in anephric patients and a high intake of sodium leads to an increase of extracellular volume to normal and a loss of antihypertensive effect. It has been postulated that the sustained fall in systemic vascular resistance may be due to an alteration in transmembrane smooth muscle sodium balance, which may reduce intracellular calcium ion concentrations to reduce tonic contraction.

Loop diuretics (frusemide, ethacrynic acid, bumetanide, piretanide)

These agents all act via inhibiting sodium reabsorption from the ascending limb of the loop of Henlé. They are potent and cause a brisk diuresis that starts within 1 h of oral administration and continues for about 6 h. They can lead to a dramatic loss of sodium, potassium and water, producing severe hypotension from extracellular volume depletion. In general, the milder thiazides are preferable as antihypertensive agents but loop diuretics retain a useful position for the treatment of patients with impaired renal function where the former group of compounds is relatively ineffective. There are, however, other non-diuretic compounds that should be preferentially considered for these patients.

Potassium-sparing diuretics (amiloride, triamterene, spironolactone, potassium canrenoate)

These are weak diuretics that are rarely effective as antihypertensives on their own. They are normally used in conjunction with thiazides or loop diuretics to reduce the potassium loss that occurs with these agents.

Thiazides and related compounds (hydrochlorothiazide, bendrofluazide, chlorthiazide, chlorthalidone, benthiazide, clopamide, cyclopenthiazide, hydroflumethazide, mefruside, methyclothiazide, polythiazide, indapamide, metolazone, xipamide)

These are a closely related group of diuretic compounds that are most frequently used for the treatment of essential hypertension. They act by inhibiting sodium reabsorption at the start of the distal convoluted tubule and are less potent than loop diuretics. They act within 2 h of oral administration, have a duration of action of 12–24 h and are normally taken in the morning so that the diuresis does not affect sleep. They are more effective with moderate dietary sodium restriction and there is normally no advantage in blood-pressure control by increasing the dose. They have a high incidence of adverse effects.

Hypokalaemia may be associated with muscle weakness and fatigue although previous worries about ventricular irritability in moderately hypokalaemic patients, particularly those undergoing non-cardiac surgery, seem to be unfounded. As previously mentioned, the concurrent administration of a potassium-sparing agent with a thiazide may prevent hypokalaemia. If this combination is prescribed, the patient should not also be given potassium supplements as an excessive and dangerous rise in serum potassium may occur.

They are known to increase plasma uric acid levels, which may predispose to gout, so they should not be used in susceptible patients. They may also cause hypercalcaemia and raised blood sugar which may present as overt diabetes. They also cause elevated serum cholesterol and triglyceride levels in some patients and this has been postulated as a possible contributor to coronary atherogenesis in diuretic-treated hypertensives. This is an area of current research activity with the newer antihypertensive agents which do not have this lipid-altering effect.

Sympatholytic agents

Interference with the pharmacology of the sympathetic nervous system has provided the other main limb of antihypertensive treatment since its inception. These agents can act anywhere between the origins of central adrenergic neurones in the brain which form the central sympathetic outflow, via paravertebral sympathetic ganglia, through to adrenergic nerve endings where they can act on either pre- or postsynaptic adrenoceptors or on the mechanisms of noradrenaline storage, release and reuptake.

Centrally acting antihypertensive agents

Centrally acting antihypertensive agents such as methyldopa, clonidine and guanbenz share a similar mechanism of action: they are all false agonists (methyldopa via its active metabolites methyladrenaline and methylnoradrenaline) at α_2 adrenoceptors in the pons and medulla. They inhibit central sympathetic outflow, which leads to a fall in plasma noradrenaline concentrations, systemic vascular resistance and blood pressure while heart rate and cardiac output are reduced to a lesser extent.

Methyldopa is associated with a positive direct Coomb's test in up to 20% of patients in which autoantibodies are produced that are directed against the Rhesus (Rh) component of red cell membranes. The positive Coomb's test may lead to interference with some laboratory tests, including cross-matching of blood, but in a small number of individuals it may lead to overt haemolytic anaemia that requires prompt drug discontinuation.

Hepatic dysfunction related to methyldopa may occur that is characterized by elevated transaminases and a systemic flu-like illness. The changes are usually reversible although fulminant hepatic failure has been reported. It should not be prescribed to patients with active liver disease.

All these agents tend to cause modest fluid accumulation which may lead to a loss of antihypertensive effect 'pseudotolerance' which may be successfully treated by the concurrent administration of a diuretic. A secondary central effect is a relatively high incidence of drowsiness and sedation which may limit their usefulness as long-term oral antihypertensive agents but which has led to the investigation of their use, particularly that of clonidine, in anaesthesia where they have been shown to reduce anaesthetic requirements and also to have potentially useful antiemetic, sedative and analgesic effects.

An undesirable feature of this group of drugs is the unusual but well recognized syndrome of rebound hypertension on following abrupt withdrawal. This is usually heralded by feelings of anxiety, apprehension and headaches and is characterized by a dramatic rise in blood pressure which parallels an increase in plasma noradrenaline levels within 24 hours of discontinuing the drug to values substantially greater than pretreatment levels. It can be readily treated by restarting therapy or by the administration of intravenous phentolamine or hydralazine.

Ganglion-blocking drugs

Ganglion-blocking drugs are no longer available for the long-term control of blood pressure. Indeed trimetaphan is the only such drug that is available for any indication in the UK and is licensed only for the intraoperative control of blood pressure when given by intravenous infusion. The onset of action is within 5 min of starting therapy and offset occurs in 15 min from the discontinuation of an infusion. It can produce respiratory arrest when given at high dosage and other features related to blockade of autonomic ganglia frequently occur: bladder dysfunction, dry mouth and eyes, disturbance of heat regulation, tachycardia and paralytic ileus. It is also subject to tachyphylaxis after prolonged use (24–48 h). It is rarely used today, even in the operating theatre environment.

Pentolinium, hexamethonium and pentamethonium are no longer commercially available in this country and they are only of historical interest as being members of a group of drugs whose importance to pharmacology examiners has far exceeded the lifespan of their clinical usefulness.

Adrenergic neurone-blocking drugs

Adrenergic neurone-blocking drugs such as guanethidine, guanadrel, bethanidine, debrisoquine and the rawolfa alkaloids including reserpine are also of largely historic interest and they are mentioned primarily because they illustrate some important pharmacological principles. Only guanethidine, bethanidine and debrisoquine are still available in this country, but it will be rare to encounter a patient who is taking one of these drugs.

They are actively transported into the endings of postganglionic adrenergic nerves by the same mechanisms that are responsible for the reuptake of noradrenaline. Here they combine with the storage vesicles and lead initially to a failure of release of catecholamines into the synaptic cleft following depolarization of the nerve terminal by an action potential, followed by destruction of the storage vesicles, the released catecholamines being degraded by monoamine oxidase in the cytoplasm of the nerve terminal.

Because of the lack of release of noradrenaline from patients tested with these compounds, effector cells such as vascular smooth muscle become exquisitely sensitive to adrenoceptor agonists. The antihypertensive response may take weeks to disappear as adrenergic neuronal competence requires the synthesis of new vesicles, which is a slow process. A serious adverse effect of reserpine is its ability to deplete central stores of noradrenaline, which may lead to severe and sometimes suicidal depression. It should not be prescribed to patients with a history of depression and should be promptly discontinued in patients who exhibit signs of affective disorder.

The particular historical importance of reserpine is that it was one of the drugs used in the first study to show a reduction in mortality from antihypertensive treatment. These agents are associated with a high incidence of adverse effects and, with the current availability of clinically superior and better-tolerated drugs, there are few indications for their continued use.

α-Adrenoceptor antagonists

α-Adrenoceptor antagonists used today for the oral treatment of hypertension are mainly the newer agents such as prazosin, doxazosin, trimazosin and terazosin.

Phenoxybenzamine remains available, but is now only used in conjunction with β-blockers in the preoperative control of blood pressure in patients with a phaeochromocytoma. It binds irreversibly to α_1-receptors by a strong covalent bond leading to prolonged hypotension, even after discontinuation of medication. It is associated with profound postural hypotension and a tachycardia that is mediated by reflex vagal inhibition. Furthermore, the pressor response to exogenous or endogenous catecholamines is significantly obtunded.

Phentolamine is a short-acting competitive antagonist at α_1-receptors that is only available as a preparation for intravenous administration. It retains a useful role in the treatment of hypertensive emergencies, particularly those occurring in relation to phaeochromocytoma, withdrawal of monoamine oxidase inhibitors and during surgery, and it is probably most often used today to control blood pressure of patients undergoing cardiac surgery, particularly during cardiopulmonary bypass.

Prazosin is a selective α_1-adrenoceptor antagonist that exerts little effect on α_2-receptors. Thus, the α_2-mediated effect of negative feedback control on noradrenaline release remains competent and noradrenaline release is not increased. It is by this mechanism that a tachycardia is not apparent during treatment with these agents. They are, however, commonly associated with a profound fall in blood pressure, particularly following the first dose. This may be linked to extracellular fluid depletion, particularly in patients who have been treated with diuretics, and caution should be exercised when starting treatment with these compounds.

β-Adrenoceptor antagonists

Although β-blockers have been in use for 30 years, there is still debate over the exact mechanism of their antihypertensive action, but it seems likely to be due to a combination of the following: reduction of cardiac output, central-adrenoceptor blocking effect, baroreceptor sensitization and by interference with prostaglandin synthesis. This subject is examined in greater depth in Chapter 14.

There are currently fourteen β-blockers licensed for use in the UK. Their differing properties can largely be accounted for by differences in lipid solubility, partial agonist (intrinsic sympathomimetic) action, membrane-stabilizing ability and selectivity for the myocardial β_1-adrenoceptor, in addition to such factors as hepatic first-pass metabolism and mode of excretion.

β-Adrenoceptor blockade leads to a fall in heart rate and myocardial contractility due to β_1-antagonism. This combination causes a fall in cardiac output and secondarily in blood pressure that is detected by the arterial baroreceptors located primarily in the carotid sinus and aortic arch. The increased activity in these receptors leads to a reflex central efferent effect to try to increase blood pressure towards normal by increasing central sympathetic outflow. It is this which may account for the phenomenon of cold peripheries that is experienced by some patients treated with β-blockers. In most instances, however, vascular resistance will return to normal within a few days and the persistent reduction in cardiac output in conjunction with a normal vascular resistance accounts for the fall in blood pressure that occurs with these agents. The fall in cardiac output is normally associated with a reduction in effective renal plasma flow but this is not normally reflected by a deterioration in renal function.

Intrinsic sympathomimetic activity or partial agonist activity is an important pharmacological property shared by a number of compounds with β-adrenoceptor antagonist properties such as practolol, acebutolol, pindolol and oxprenolol. Agents with this characteristic tend to produce less myocardial depression, bradycardia and reduction in cardiac output. Their hypotensive effect is thought to be due to the stimulation of vascular β_2-receptors mediating vasodilatation, as resting heart rate and cardiac output are little affected.

When prescribing β-blockers to diabetics, it should be borne in mind that they can interfere with carbohydrate and fat metabolism in a complex manner and that they can lead to persistent hypoglycaemia largely by inhibiting β_2-receptor-mediated glycogenolysis. In addition, the clinical signs of hypoglycaemia such as sweating, anxiety and tachycardia, which are largely mediated via increased sympathetic discharge and an increase in circulating catecholamines, will be reduced due to β-adrenoceptor blockade. For these reasons, caution should be exercised when considering β-blockers as potential antihypertensive treatment for diabetics.

Propranolol is a lipid-soluble agent that readily crosses the blood–brain barrier. It has been associated with CNS disturbances such as fatigue, depression and disturbances of sleep but it is unlikely that these are due to a central β-adrenoceptor effect as these adverse effects are also associated with water-soluble agents, such as atenolol, which do not cross into the brain. However, propranolol does have a significant membrane-stabilizing ability and is almost as potent a local anaesthetic as lignocaine. This phenomenon may contribute to its antiarrhythmic effect, but the majority of its cardiovascular properties are likely to be due to blockade of β-adrenoceptors.

Several drugs in this class also exhibit relative specificity for the myocardial β_1-receptor. Avoidance of blockade of β_2-receptors will theoretically reduce the incidence of peripheral vascular constriction and cooling, bronchospasm in those with reactive airways disease, and metabolic disturbances. Metoprolol, atenolol, bisoprolol, acebutolol and betaxolol are the cardioselective agents available in the UK and, of these drugs, atenolol and metoprolol are the most widely used. They are about 3 and 100 times more specific respectively for β_1-receptors as propranolol but both agents have been associated with a deterioration in pulmonary function in some asthmatics. It is for this reason that the Committee on Safety of Medicines has recommended that all β-blockers, even the supposedly cardioselective agents, should be avoided in patients with reactive airways disease if there are other suitable agents available.

Labetalol is a unique drug that is of particular interest to the anaesthetist in the operating theatre. It has both non-selective β-receptor or antagonist properties and selective α_1-antagonism. It also inhibits the reuptake of noradrenaline into nerve terminals and has some intrinsic sympathomimetic activity. After intravenous administration the ratio of α- to β-blockade is roughly 1 to 7. It can be used orally for the long-term control of blood pressure but its main interest to anaesthetists is as an agent to control hypertension during surgery and to contribute to controlled intraoperative hypotension. As such, it is dealt with in greater detail later in this chapter.

Vasodilators

These direct-acting arterial vasodilators are little used today for the treatment of essential hypertension due to their high incidence of adverse effects, poor tolerance and the availability of superior drugs. Diazoxide is only available as a parenteral formulation for the treatment of hypertensive emergencies. It is diabetogenic and causes significant fluid retention. Hydralazine is still available as an oral preparation although it is usually used parenterally in anaesthesia and intensive care for the emergency control of blood pressure. It causes fluid retention and a reflex tachycardia and should not be used without concomitant β-blockade or diuretic therapy for oral treatment. It may also cause a systemic lupus erythematosus-like syndrome when given in large doses for long periods. Minoxidil is a potent but toxic vasodilator that also causes fluid retention and tachycardia and should not be used alone. Its most notable side-effect is an increase in body hair growth, which further restricts its use in women.

Calcium-channel blockers

An increased availability of intracellular calcium ions leads to a greater interaction of muscular contractile elements and thereby to an increase in vascular smooth muscle tone and an increase in myocardial contractility. Some workers believe that hypertensive patients have a disturbance of transmembrane calcium homeostasis that leads to an increase in intracellular calcium ion concentration and thus to an increased vascular contractile state. The agents available for clinical use in the UK are as follows: verapamil, nifedipine, nicardipine, amlodipine, nimodipine, diltiazem and isradipine. Their pharmacology is described in Chapter 16.

Verapamil was the first available agent in this class and is used for the treatment of arrhythmias (particularly supraventricular) and angina in addition to the treatment of hypertension. It is chemically a phenylalkylamine and affects myocardial tissue relatively more than vascular tissue. It is negatively inotropic and chronotropic and indeed the reflex tachycardia that is observed with the other less cardioselective calcium-channel blockers is less evident with verapamil owing to its negative chronotropic effect. Caution should be exercised if verapamil is administered to patients with congestive heart failure. The decrease in myocardial contractility may quantitatively exceed in importance the vasodilatation, thus dangerously increasing myocardial work which may precipitate acute left ventricular failure.

The dihydropyridines, such as nifedipine, nicardipine and nimodipine, are potent coronary and systemic vasodilators and lead to a significant increase in coronary and forearm blood flow. They tend to cause little venous pooling and their antihypertensive effect is caused mainly by arterial vasodilatation. This leads to a reflex sympathetic tachycardia and an attempt to increase myocardial contractility. Overall, blood pressure falls and heart rate, contractility and cardiac output increase modestly while myocardial work is reduced. They should be avoided in patients with overt congestive heart failure and in those with SA and AV nodal problems, but they are particularly useful for patients with reactive airways disease, peripheral vascular disease, diabetes, hyperlipidaemia and renal dysfunction. Furthermore, they are not associated with a rise in serum lipids which has been implicated as one of the potential reasons why otherwise successful antihypertensive treatment with diuretics has not led to a fall in the incidence of coronary artery disease related morbidity.

Angiotensin-converting enzyme (ACE) inhibitors

The renin–angiotensin system (RAS) is one of the many intricately interwoven mechanisms that contribute to circulatory control and to the regulation of sodium and water balance. Patients with essential hypertension do not normally exhibit increased activity of plasma renin, which is normally used as the marker to indicate the degree of activity of the RAS, and this was partly at fault for the delay in the investigation of this group of compounds as potential cardiovascular therapeutic agents. However, with the discovery of agents that selectively inhibit ACE, it became apparent due to parallel research that there is a wide distribution in levels of plasma renin activity and that ACE inhibitors are effective at lowering blood pressure in patients with normal or even low plasma renin activity.

Further investigation and large-scale clinical studies showed this to be a group of drugs with enormous clinical potential. For example, they are the only single group of compounds that has been shown to improve survival in patients with degrees of left ventricular dysfunction ranging from asymptomatic systolic impairment to severe overt congestive heart failure. They have also been shown to reduce left ventricular dilatation and to improve survival following myocardial infarction and have favourable myocardial protective properties following periods of ischaemia. They decrease myocardial oxygen consumption by reducing afterload while heart rate remains little changed and they have also been shown to cause regression of vascular and left ventricular hypertrophy in hypertensive patients.

It is also well established that they are effective at controlling blood pressure throughout the 24-h period, but their main attraction is their low incidence of adverse effects and impressive tolerance coupled with clinical efficacy that has led to the consistent demonstration of improved quality of life on ACE-inhibitor treatment when compared with other antihypertensives. Finally, they have not been shown to have adverse metabolic effects on either lipid or glucose homeostasis.

Captopril was the first available agent in this class and was launched in the early 1980s as a treatment for hypertension that was refractory to other available therapy. When prescribed for this indication, it was usually given in large doses to achieve a rapid response and was associated with a high incidence of adverse clinical events, which led to some initial bad press for this class of drugs. With subsequent research it became apparent that an adequate antihypertensive response may be achieved with a much lower dosage and that the majority of side-effects could thus be avoided.

It is important that ACE inhibitors should not be prescribed to patients with bilateral renal artery stenosis or with a stenosis of the artery to a single functioning kidney. Kidneys with such a reduced blood flow rely on high levels of circulating angiotensin II to produce sufficient efferent glomerular arteriolar constriction to allow adequate glomerular filtration and if these levels are reduced, as they would be by inhibition of ACE, sudden acute renal failure may occur. In patients other than these, there is conflicting evidence about ACE inhibitors' effect on renal function in those in whom it is already impaired – although there is, however, convincing evidence that they have the ability to preserve renal function in diabetics with or without hypertension.

Caution should be exercised when initiating therapy in patients who may be fluid depleted from any cause, but particularly in those who have been treated with diuretics. Sudden and severe hypotension may occur in response to the ACE-inhibitor-mediated arterial vasodilatation, which may necessitate urgent intravenous fluid resuscitation. Treatment should therefore be started at night in these patients and it is preferable that previous diuretic therapy should be stopped several days before it is planned to commence ACE inhibitor treatment.

A common side-effect with ACE inhibitor therapy is a persistent dry cough. This is due to the local accummulation in the lungs of bradykinin which is also broken down by ACE. Cessation of therapy leads to a disappearance of the cough, which may not recur on recommencement of the same therapy. Angioedema has also been reported which is readily reversible on discontinuation of therapy.

Finally, in the early days of ACE inhibitors it was thought that the sulphydryl group of the captopril molecule was responsible for the high incidence of adverse effects that were seen. Therefore, newer agents were developed without this moiety before it was shown that the excessive dosages used were responsible for the majority of adverse events. Indeed, it has been an area of recent speculation that the —SH group may in fact confer desirable properties on the molecule due to its action as a scavenger of oxygen-derived free radicals. It has also been shown that —SH-containing ACE inhibitors can produce faster and greater improvement in coronary artery blood flow than those agents that do not.

More recently has been the introduction of specific angiotensin II receptor antagonists. On the evidence of early studies these seem to have a more favourable side-effect profile than ACE inhibitors, and they do not seem to be associated with the development of a cough. This is presumably due to the lack of interference with the breakdown of bradykinin that is seen with ACE inhibitors.

HYPERTENSIVE PATIENTS, SURGERY AND ANAESTHESIA

Untreated hypertensive patients undergoing anaesthesia and surgery exhibit extremely labile changes in haemodynamics. Almost all anaesthetic agents cause profound hypotension following their introduction to hypertensive patients due to a combination of systemic vasodilatation and direct myocardial depression. However, during laryngoscopy there is an exaggerated pressor response and during surgery patients tend to have greater peroperative anaesthetic and analgesic requirements to obtund the stress response related to surgical stimulation.

It has been shown that this group of patients is at greater risk of perioperative myocardial ischaemia and arrhythmias than treated hypertensives, although there is still debate over whether hypertensive patients *per se* are at greater risk of suffering perioperative myocardial infarction than normotensive individuals. However, it is accepted that patients with elevated blood pressure presenting for non-emergency surgery should have their surgery postponed pending investigation of possible hypertension. They should then be started and stabilized on appropriate therapy whose efficacy should be confirmed before rescheduling surgery.

Hypertensive patients who are well controlled on therapy may safely undergo surgery but it should nevertheless be borne in mind that these patients have demonstrated cardiovascular disease and they should have a detailed history taken and an examination performed by the anaesthetist at the preoperative visit. As at the presentation of a newly diagnosed hypertensive patient to the general physician, before the commencement of antihypertensive therapy particular attention should be paid at the visit to symptoms or signs suggestive of coronary artery disease, impaired cardiac function including overt heart failure, occlusive and aneurysmal arterial disease, renal impairment, endocrine disease and possible causes of secondary hypertension.

A preoperative chest radiograph is mandatory. This will show signs of longstanding untreated hypertension: left ventricular enlargement, unfolded aortic arch, or overt cardiac failure: generalized cardiac enlargement, pleural effusions, increased pulmonary vascular markings or overt pulmonary oedema. Rarely, rib notching will be seen which is caused by hypertrophy of the intercostal vessels in patients with aortic coarctation and a retrosternal goitre may occasionally be seen in thyrotoxic patients.

Coronary artery disease is the main cause of death in hypertensive patients and every effort should be made to exclude this in the hypertensive patient scheduled for surgery. It must be remembered that resting ECGs are usually of little use in demonstrating significant coronary artery disease, even in patients with severe angina requiring multiple therapy. They are, however, useful for diagnosing old transmural myocardial infarctions where pathological Q waves can be seen for some time following the infarction. They are also sensitive indicators of longstanding left ventricular hypertrophy with or without strain, and other abnormalities such as P-wave changes, conduction abnormalities, rhythm disturbances and repolarization abnormalities are useful indicators of cardiac disease. However, if coronary artery disease is strongly suspected then an exercise ECG should be performed proceeding to coronary angiography and further intervention if this is indicated.

If there is any doubt about the patient's overall cardiac function this should be investigated. Echocardiography is now widely available and can readily provide a relatively accurate, albeit subjective, indication of cardiac performance both non-invasively and at the bedside. Should more objective assessments be required, other more accurate methods using radionuclide imaging or ventriculography could be employed.

Hypertensive patients are at greater risk of impaired renal function secondary to hypertension-induced nephron loss. This can have a substantial effect on the clearance of drugs used in the perioperative period and may also lead to further renal deterioration following surgery. It is therefore vital that the renal function of a hypertensive surgical patient should be established before surgery and that appropriate measures be taken to avoid drugs that accumulate in renal impairment and to try to prevent further renal impairment during or after surgery.

It is now accepted practice that hypertensive patients who are established on therapy should have their normal therapy continued up to and including the operative day and that it should be restarted as soon as is practicable following surgery. In patients who are unable to take their normal oral medication on the day after surgery an appropriate parenteral substitute should be given and continued until normal therapy can be recommenced.

FURTHER READING

Joint National Committee on Detection, Evaluation and Treatment of High Blood Pressure. The fifth report of the Joint National Committee on detection, evaluation and treatment of high blood pressure (JNC-V), *Archives of Internal Medicine* 1993; **153**: 154–83.

Sever P, Beevers G, Bulpitt C, *et al.* Management guidelines in essential hypertension: report of the Second Working Party of the British Hypertension Society. *British Medical Journal* 1993; **306**: 983–7

Subcommittee of WHO–ISH Mild Hypertension Liaison Committee. Summary of 1993 World Health Organisation–International Society of Hypertension guidelines for the management of mild hypertension. *British Medical Journal* 1993; 307: 1541–6.

PART II PHARMACOLOGY OF DRUGS USED TO PRODUCE HYPOTENSION IN ANAESTHESIA

R Langford, K Bakhshi

The use of elective hypotension in anaesthesia is still a controversial subject. Many anaesthetists feel that the risks of reducing systemic arterial pressure in order to reduce bleeding and facilitate surgery outweigh the benefits. However, others justify its use with modern monitoring techniques and in the hands of experienced anaesthetists in many situations. They argue that a mean arterial blood pressure as low as 50–60 mmHg appears to be well tolerated in healthy patients.[1] Also, improved visibility with decreased blood loss improves the surgical field and therefore benefits the patient.

Simpson[2] has classified its use as applicable to situations in which the operation would otherwise be impossible (e.g. cerebrovascular surgery), situations in which excessive blood loss might be detrimental (e.g. orthopaedic spinal and maxillofacial operations) and situations where blood loss interferes with surgical visibility or technique (e.g. middle ear surgery). Particular areas of controversy include its use for cosmetic surgery and to preserve blood loss in situations where transfusion is undesirable or when the patient has a low preoperative haemoglobin.

CARDIOVASCULAR PHYSIOLOGY

The mean arterial pressure is the most important factor in determining the extent of perioperative haemorrhage.

Mean arterial pressure = Cardiac output × Total peripheral resistance.

Cardiac output is dependent on stroke volume and heart rate; peripheral resistance depends on peripheral vasodilatation.

Arterial bleeding is considerably reduced by a reduction in mean arterial pressure and heart rate. Drugs that cause vasodilatation will produce a reduction in mean arterial pressure. These may act centrally, such as volatile anaesthetic agents on the vasomotor centre, or by interruption of peripheral sympathetic pathways (e.g. at the sympathetic ganglia or postganglionic noradrenergic terminals). They may also act directly on blood vessels.

Capillary bleeding is dependent on local flow in the capillary bed and is reduced by elective hypotension, local vasoconstriction (e.g. infiltration with adrenaline) and good venous drainage of the area.

Venous bleeding is related to venous return and venous tone and therefore depends on posture. Spinal and extradural anaesthesia, as well as directly acting vasodilators, will reduce venous tone. The consequent venous pooling will reduce venous return and cardiac output leading to reduction in mean arterial pressure.

ADJUVANTS TO INDUCED HYPOTENSION

Anaesthetic technique and anaesthetic drugs may be used as adjuvants to specific hypotensive drugs. Posture has already been mentioned. In addition, good anaesthesia will prevent the response to surgical stimulation. The use of intermittent positive pressure ventilation (IPPV) will reduce venous return by raising mean intrathoracic pressure (especially with the addition of positive end expiratory pressure). The reduction in P_{CO_2} during controlled ventilation will reduce circulating endogenous catecholamines. Hypocapnia also produces vasoconstriction, which further reduces blood loss.

GENERAL ANAESTHETIC AGENTS

The inhalational anaesthetic agents may be used to produce hypotension (either on their own or as an adjuvant to other treatments). These drugs depress the cardiovascular control centres within the CNS. They also directly depress vascular smooth muscle and myocardium.

Halothane decreases peripheral resistance by reducing efferent sympathetic activity. (Total peripheral resistance is reduced by approximately 15–18% and this is mainly due to vasodilatation in the skin and splanchnic vascular beds. There is, however, vasoconstriction in skeletal muscle.) It causes bradycardia due to increased vagal stimulation as well as a direct effect on the SA node. This together with direct myocardial depression causes a fall in cardiac output. Enflurane acts similarly; however at equal MAC concentrations it causes greater depression of myocardial contractility and cardiac output. It also causes a reflex tachycardia (unlike halothane).

Isoflurane does not significantly depress myocardial contractility at low inspired concentrations. It causes arteriolar vasodilatation and a reduction in systemic vascular resistance and this is readily adjusted by alterations in inspired concentration. CNS depression prevents compensatory tachycardia and vasoconstriction. It does not raise intracranial pressure as much as halothane or enflurane in patients with normal preoperative values.[3] Much has been written in the literature about 'coronary steal' with isoflurane due to a greater reduction in peripheral resistance than cardiac output in patients with ischaemic heart disease. However, this has not been associated with any increase in morbidity or mortality.[4] When a moderate reduction in pressure is required, this may act as a good hypotensive agent.

SPINAL AND EPIDURAL ANAESTHESIA

Local anaesthetics inserted in the subarachnoid or epidural space will block sympathetic outflow and produce arteriolar vasodilatation together with loss of venomotor tone. The former produces a fall in peripheral resistance, the latter results in venous pooling producing a decreased venous return and consequently cardiac output. The net result is hypotension. If the cardiac sympathetic nerves (T_1–T_4) are involved, reflex tachycardia will not occur.

NEUROMUSCULAR-BLOCKING DRUGS

When used as part of the general anaesthetic technique both tubocurarine and alcuronium will produce histamine release and consequent vasodilatation. They also have a mild ganglion-blocking effect (see below). However, they should be avoided in patients with a history of atopy.[5]

HYPOTENSIVE DRUGS

Pentolinium and hexamethonium

The manufacture of these drugs has now been discontinued. However, they have been widely used in the past for hypotensive anaesthesia.[6] They are autonomic ganglion-blocking agents that act by competitive inhibition of acetylcholine. When used to produce hypotension during anaesthesia, they gave good operating conditions. However, the variability in the initial dose required meant that fine control of blood pressure was difficult. Pentolinium also had a long duration of action which made it less appropriate for shorter cases.[7]

Trimetaphan

Trimetaphan produces hypotension by blocking sympathetic ganglia. In addition, it has a direct effect on the vessel wall and some of its action is thought to be mediated through histamine release.[8] The drug is usually given by infusion and although it produces rapid onset of hypotension, its dose response is variable (younger patients generally require more than older to produce the same effect). As with other ganglion-blocking drugs, patients may develop tachycardia following hypotension. Tachyphylaxis (the need for increasing doses) is particularly marked with trimetaphan. In addition, return to normotension may be prolonged following cessation of treatment. It has been suggested that it should not be used in asthmatic patients; however, MacRae[7] has used the drug over many years in patients with allergic diathesis undergoing ENT surgery and has not found any clinical problems (although many patients will have a weal and flare response around the infusion site).

Sodium nitroprusside

Sodium nitroprusside was first described by Jonson in 1929 and was used as an oral hypotensive in the 1950s.[9] However, its use was abandoned as its action by this route was too short lived. It was reintroduced into clinical practice in the late 1960s as an intravenous hypotensive agent[10,11] and its use by this route has been evaluated fully.

Sodium nitroprusside acts directly on smooth muscle of blood vessels to produce relaxation and hence vasodilatation. The mode of action probably involves sulphydryl (SH) groups bound to smooth muscle membrane.[12] It exerts its effect mainly on arterial vessels and both cardiac output and tissue perfusion are usually well maintained. There is often a reflex tachycardia due to baroreceptor stimulation.

The commercial preparation (Nipride) is a freeze-dried powder and must be dissolved in 500 ml of 5% dextrose for clinical use (100–200 μg/ml). The solution must be protected from light as there is a 10% decrease in potency in 3 h if exposed (50% decrease in bright light).

Sodium nitroprusside is a good hypotensive agent with rapid onset and return to normotension on cessation; however, its main disadvantage is toxicity. It is rapidly metabolized in the bloodstream (both in plasma and red blood cells) producing nitric oxide (NO) and hydrocyanic acid which conjugates with thiosulphate to produce thiocyanate. Overdosage leads to accumulation of free cyanide ions.[13] It is also thought that cyanide is produced by photodegradation in solution before administration to the patient.[14]

The risk of toxicity is greatly decreased by restricting the amount of sodium nitroprusside administered. Opinions differ on the maximum dose for short-term administration, but levels of up to 1.5 mg/kg in such cases have not proved clinically to produce complications.[15] For longer term administration (hours or days), thiocyanate levels can be measured and a maximum rate in the order of 10 μg/kg/min has been suggested.[16] The drug should be avoided when normal cyanide metabolism is inhibited (e.g. liver and renal failure). The development of a metabolic acidosis as indicated by a low standard bicarbonate on blood gas measurement is an early sign of cyanide accumulation. If cyanide toxicity develops, the infusion must be discontinued. Sodium thiosulphate may be administered intravenously.[17] This will combine with cyanide to produce hydroxocobalamin (a relatively inert substance). In severe cases intravenous sodium bicarbonate may also be necessary.

The decrease in peripheral resistance and consequent drop in blood pressure produced by sodium nitroprusside gives rise to a compensatory physiological response the extent of which depends on the particular patient and the attenuating effect of anaesthetic and other drugs being used. Catecholamines are released through the action of the baroreceptors and these produce both α- and β-stimulatory effects. This will particularly manifest itself as a rise in pulse rate. The renin–angiotensin system will also be activated but at a slower rate (15–30 min). Angiotensin II produced by this system is a potent vasoconstrictor. At the end of the operation, when the sodium nitroprusside is switched off, its effects wear off rapidly and accumulation of both catecholamines and angiotensin II may produce rebound hypertension.

Sodium nitroprusside and trimetaphan combined

MacRae[7] has used this combination to offset the toxic effects of nitroprusside and to create a manageable hypotensive infusion. A modest fall in blood pressure is first achieved with the trimetaphan and this is decreased further with a small amount of sodium nitroprusside thus avoiding the unpredictable hypotension caused by trimetaphan and the toxic effects of large doses of sodium nitroprusside. Maximal synergism of the combination occurs when the drugs are infused together in the ratio 4 trimetaphan to 1 sodium nitroprusside. Previous studies in which the drugs were infused separately produced an unreliable and poorly controlled fall in blood pressure.

Nitroglycerine

This is the raw material of dynamite and was first used in the treatment of angina in 1879 by William Murrell.[18] Its use as an intravenous hypotensive agent compares favourably with sodium nitroprusside and it is claimed that the course of hypotension is smoother with fewer peaks and troughs of arterial pressure.[19]

It relaxes smooth muscle in the vessel wall and acts mainly on venous capacitance. It also improves coronary perfusion and can cause a rise in intracranial pressure. Lack of toxicity is a particular advantage, making it a drug of choice in situations where hypotension is required over many hours or days (e.g. postcardiac surgery). However, it is not as good at the low levels of blood pressure sometimes required in hypotensive anaesthesia to produce a good operative field.[20]

Nitroglycerine solutions are absorbed by polyvinyl chloride containers and tubing so that polythene or glass must be used.

α-ADRENOCEPTOR-BLOCKING DRUGS

These act on sympathetic postsynaptic α-adrenergic receptors to produce vasodilatation. Phentolamine, a short-acting α-blocker with rapid reversal, is used when rapid induction of vasodilatation is required (e.g. to control blood pressure on cardiopulmonary bypass). Phenoxybenzamine has a longer duration of action as it forms an irreversible receptor complex. It is used in the preparation of patients for surgical removal of phaeochromocytoma.

β-ADRENOCEPTOR-BLOCKING DRUGS

Propranolol and oxprenolol

These drugs reduce both heart rate and cardiac output. Many anaesthetists believe that a slow heart rate considerably reduces operative bleeding. Unselective blockade of β-receptors at sites outside the heart may lead to bronchospasm in asthmatic patients and an increase in peripheral vascular resistance due to paralysis of dilator fibres in the smooth muscle of blood vessels. The negative chronotrophic effects of propranolol and oxprenolol are used to prevent or treat the tachycardia produced by ganglion-blocking drugs or sodium nitroprusside. These drugs may precipitate cardiac failure when a diminished functional capacity is being countered by enhanced sympathetic activity. Also the removal of sympathetic discharge to the heart may unmask the direct depression by potent anaesthetic agents and lead to a further fall in cardiac output.

Esmolol

Esmolol is a relatively new β_1-selective adrenergic blocker with a rapid onset and a half-life of approximately 9 min. It is used in the treatment of supraventricular tachycardia and is also effective in the treatment of perioperative hypertension and to minimize β-sympathetic autonomic responses to noxious stimuli with minimal side-effects and no known toxicity.[21] Recent studies have demonstrated its efficacy as an adjunct to sodium nitroprusside and as a primary drug for controlled hypotension.[22,23]

Labetalol

This drug was first used in anaesthesia by Scott *et al.*[24] in 1976 and is a popular drug used quite widely by many anaesthetists.[25] It has a combination of α- and β-blocking effects. The ratio of α- to β-blockade varies depending on the dose and may be as much as 1 to 7. Also it is not possible to increase the α-effect (drop in peripheral resistance) without significantly increasing β-blockade (bradycardia which may be undesirable).The half-life of labetalol given intravenously is between 3.5 and 6.3 h, depending on the dose administered and other drugs being used. Should marked bradycardia occur, atropine may be given; however, this may produce a rise in arterial pressure. When used with care and with an appreciation of its shortcomings, it is a very useful agent in young and fit patients.

Adenosine and adenosine triphosphate

Until recently, there has been little use of these drugs in the western world.[7] Their use, however, has long been advocated in Japanese literature. Pulse rates are thought to remain stable when these drugs are used for elective hypotension. Owall *et al.*[26] studied forty-seven patients undergoing cerebral aneurysm surgery under neurolept analgesia in whom hypotension was induced using adenosine triphosphate. Stable, easily controlled hypotension was produced without tachycardia, tachyphylaxis or rebound hypertension. There is much interest in its use in neurosurgical practice and one study in cats has shown a much lower increase in intracranial pressure (when either normal or artificially induced) using adenosine triphosphate compared with sodium nitroprusside.[27] Adenosine triphosphate may cause increases in serum uric acid concentrations and further studies of the pathological effects of long-term administration are required.[28]

COMPLICATIONS OF INDUCED HYPOTENSION

If arterial pressure is reduced excessively and autoregulation fails, tissue oxygenation of vital organs will be impaired.

Brain

Cerebral blood flow remains constant over a wide range of perfusion pressures (60–130 mmHg). The autoregulation curve is shifted to the right in hypertensive patients and to the left when vasodilators such as sodium nitroprusside and nitroglycerine are used. Autoregulation may be lost completely during a period of marked hypotension. The reduction in supply of oxygenated blood may cause severe ischaemic damage as the brain has high energy requirements and little reserve (a reduction in cerebral blood flow by 50% will produce ischaemic signs and damage may be permanent). The risk is increased in patients with pre-existing cerebral disease; however, anaesthetic agents that reduce cerebral metabolism (e.g. thiopentone) may give some degree of brain protection during hypotensive anaesthesia. Also sodium nitroprusside and nitroglycerine are potent cerebral vasodilators and preserve cerebral blood flow at lower levels of arterial pressure (although the vasodilator effect will also increase intracranial pressure).

Methods of monitoring cerebral perfusion (e.g. cerebral function monitor, jugular venous oxygen content) are only able to demonstrate more severe global ischaemia.

Heart

A reduction in arterial pressure reduces myocardial work. However, a reduction in systolic pressure below 60 mmHg (higher in hypertensive subjects) will reduce coronary artery perfusion pressure and a compensatory tachycardia will reduce perfusion time. This may produce myocardial ischaemia. Monitoring ST segment depression would appear to be the most reliable way of detecting myocardial ischaemia from induced hypotension.

Kidney

A reduction of systolic arterial pressure below 80 mmHg will reduce renal perfusion and glomerular filtration. This may produce oliguria.

Lungs

A reduction in arterial pressure and the effect of gravity will reduce blood flow to the upper parts of the lungs. This produces ventilation perfusion mismatch and an increase in physiological dead space (which may be up to 80% of the tidal volume).[2] The use of controlled ventilation and increasing the inspired oxygen concentration will counter this physiological imbalance.

Despite these possible complications associated with hypotensive anaesthesia, several large series have found a very low mortality and morbidity with induced hypotension in experienced hands.

CONCLUSION

Hypotensive drugs may be used in combination with anaesthetic drugs and technique to reduce blood pressure and control bleeding during surgery. These drugs were first introduced into anaesthetic practice in the 1940s when hypertensive episodes during surgery were a problem. Improvements in anaesthesia and technique have led many to question their role and safety in reducing bleeding in modern-day anaesthesia. However, in experienced hands and with adequate monitoring, these drugs still appear to have an important role in situations where hypotension is essential as well as in reducing bleeding and improving the operative field.

REFERENCES

1 Prys-Roberts C. Induced hypotension, overview. *Current Opinions in Anaesthesiology* 1988; **1**: 81–2.

2 Simpson P. Peri-operative blood loss and its reduction: the role of the anaesthetist. *British Journal of Anaesthesiology* 1992; **69**: 498–507.

3 Michenfelder JD. Does isoflurane aggravate regional cerebral ischaemia? Editorial. *Anesthesiology* 1987; **66**: 451–2.

4 Slogoff S, Keats AS, Dear WE, Abadia A, Lawyer JT, Moulds JP, Williams TM. Steal-prone coronary anatomy and myocardial ischaemia associated with four primary anaesthetic agents in humans. *Anesthesia and Analgesia* 1991; **72**: 22–7.

5 Coleman AJ, Downing JW, Leary WP *et al.* The immediate cardiovascular effects of pancuronium, alcuronium and tubocurarine in man. *Anaesthesia* 1972; **27**: 415.

6 Enderby GEH. Pentolinium tartrate in controlled hypotension. *Lancet* 1954; **ii**: 1097–8.

7 MacRae WR. Induced hypotension. In: MacRae WR, Wildsmith JAW eds. *Monographs in anaesthesiology* 1991.

8 Fahmy NR, Soter NA. Effects of trimetaphan on arterial blood histamine and systemic haemodynamics in humans. *Anesthesiology* 1985; **62**: 562–6.

9 Page IH, Corcoran AC, Dustan HP, Koppanyi T. Cardiovascular actions of sodium nitroprusside in animals and in hypertensive patients. *Circulation* 1955; **11**: 188.

10 Jones GOM, Cole P. Sodium nitroprusside as a hypotensive agent. *British Journal of Anaesthesiology* 1968; **40**: 804.

11 Taylor TH, Styles M, Lamming AJ. Sodium nitroprusside as a hypotensive agent in general anaesthesia. *British Journal of Anaesthesiology* 1970; **42**: 859.

12 Cole PV. In: Hewer CL, Atkinson RS eds. *Recent advances in anaesthesia and analgesia* **13**. Edinburgh: Churchill Livingstone, 1979.

13 Vesy CJ, Simpson PJ, Adams L, Cole PV. Metabolism of sodium nitroprusside and cyanide in the dog. *British Journal of Anaesthesiology* 1979; **51**: 89–97.

14 Bisset WIK, *et al.* Photochemistry of the nitroprusside ion and the consequences for the detection of cyanide in mixtures of nitroprusside and blood: use of sodium nitroprusside as a hypotensive agent. *Journal of Chemical Research* **299**: 3501.

15 Cole PV. The safe use of sodium nitroprusside. *Anaesthesia* 1978; **33**: 473.

16 Editorial. Controlled intra-vascular sodium nitroprusside treatment. *British Medical Journal* 1978; **2**: 784.

17 Cole PV, Vesey CJ. Sodium thiosulphate decreases blood cyanide concentrations after the infusion of sodium nitroprusside. *British Journal of Anaesthesiology* **59**: 531–5.

18 Murrell W. Nitroglycerin as a remedy for angina pectoris. *Lancet* 1879; **ii**: 80–1.

19 Atkinson RS, Rushman GB, Lee JA. *Synopsis of anaesthesia*, 10th edn. Oxford: Butterworth-Heinemann, 1987.

20 Maktabi M, Warner D, Sokoll M, Boarini D, Adolphoson A, Speed T, Kassell N. Comparison of nitroprusside, nitroglycerine and deep isoflurane anaesthesia for induced hypotension. *Neurosurgery* **19**: 350–5.

21 Gorczynski RJ. Basic pharmacology of esmolol. *American Journal of Cardiology* 1986; **56**: 3F–13F.

22 Edmondson R, Del Valle O, Shah N, *et al.* Esmolol for potentiation of nitroprusside induced hypotension. Impact on the cardiovascular adrenergic and renin–angiotensin systems in man. *Anesthesia and Analgesia* 1989; **69**: 202–6.

23 Blair JL, McGuire R, Killian J, Amundson G. Esmolol as primary agent for controlled hypotension (abstract). *Anesthesia and Analgesia* 1989; **68**: S31.

24 Scott DB, Buckley FP, Drummond GB, Littlewood DG, Macrae WR. Cardiovascular effects of labetalol during halothane anaesthesia. *British Journal of Clinical Pharmacology* 1976; (suppl) 817–21.

25 Mcnulty S, Sharifi Azad S, Farole A. Induced hypotension with labetalol for orthagnathic surgery. *Journal of Oral and Maxillofacial Surgery*; **45**: 309–11.

26 Wall A, Gordon E, Lagerkranser M, Lindquist C, Rudehill A, Sollevi A. Clinical experience with adenosine for controlled hypotension during cerebral aneurysm surgery. *Anesthesia and Analgesia* 1987; **66**: 229–34.

27 Thiagarajah S, Azar I, Lear E, Machetnis EM. Intracranial pressure changes during infusions of adenosine triphosphate and sodium nitroprusside. *Bulletin of the New York Academy Medicine* 1987; **63**: 186–92.

28 Wildsmith JAW, MacRae WR. Intravenous agents for induced hypotension. *Current Opinions in Anaesthesiology* 1988; **1**: 83–7.

PART III DRUGS IN THE TREATMENT OF SHOCK AND HYPOTENSION

RF Armstrong

INTRODUCTION

The popularity and long-practised measurement of blood pressure as an expression of circulatory function has led to a traditional therapeutic approach to the hypotensive patient based on the maintenance of this pressure above certain limits. While these limits will, to some extent, depend upon pre-illness levels, it is generally agreed that a mean arterial pressure $(2D + S)/3$ below 60 mmHg is insufficient to guarantee essential organ perfusion. More recently, this pressure-driven approach has been challenged by those who favour attention to blood flow with the objective of maximizing transport of oxygen to the tissues. Noble[1] points out that the purpose of manipulating the circulation in intensive care should be to optimize stroke volume not arterial pressure, and Shoemaker[2] in his studies draws attention to the basic physiological problem in acute circulatory crisis being the disparity between the supply and demand for oxygen by the tissues.

Before considering the use of drugs to improve circulatory function, it is necessary to review briefly the physiology and terminology of this supply and demand system.

CARDIAC FUNCTION

Central to the supply side of the circulation is the heart and its stroke volume regulated by preload, afterload and myocardial contractility. Not all the ventricular contents are ejected at each contraction. The ejection fraction in man is normally between 0.5 and 0.75, increasing with exercise and inotropic stimulation.

As the heart fails, ejection fractions of less than 0.5 are seen with rising end-systolic volumes. Using angiography or echocardiography, ejection fraction may be calculated from the formula:

$$EF = \frac{SV}{LVEDV}$$

where EF is ejection fraction; SV is stroke volume; and LVEDV is left ventricular end-diastolic volume.

Preload

Preload or venous return refers to a property of cardiac muscle fibres, that of increasing contractile power occurring with increasing fibre length. The effects of ventricular filling on stroke volume were originally described by Otto Frank and Ernest Starling. Since then many variants of this curve have been used with other indices of contractile energy on the Y axis (stroke volume, stroke work, systolic muscle tension) and of filling pressure (right ventricular end-diastolic pressure, CVP, left ventricular end-diastolic pressure and volume, and left atrial pressure) on the X axis. These ventricular function curves underline the fundamental point that the stretching of cardiac muscle cells produces an increase in their contractile energy and provides the basis for optimal filling of the vascular system during resuscitation. Because of the ease of measurement of central venous pressure (CVP) and pulmonary artery wedge pressure (PAWP), these filling pressures are widely used as indices of preload. While there is no denying the value of pressure measurements, it has to be borne in mind that the relationship between end-diastolic pressure and volume is not linear. In the case of a stiff and uncompliant ventricular wall, filling pressures may be misleadingly high in the presence of low stroke volumes (Fig. 17.2).

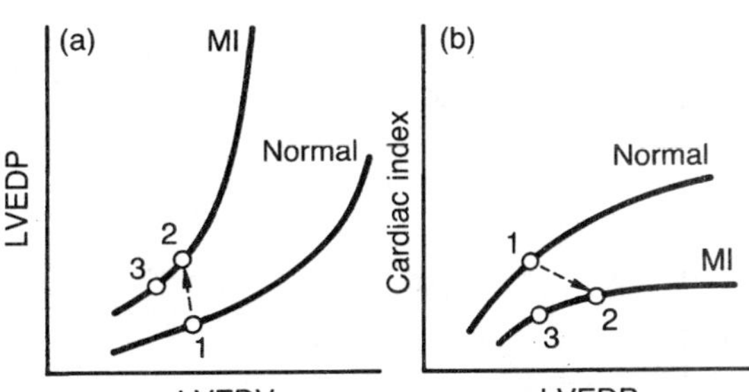

FIGURE 17.2 End-diastolic pressure/volume relationship. Changes in left ventricular compliance (a) and performance curves (b) following acute myocardial infarction (MI) complicated by heart failure. At point 1, the patient has a normal left ventricular end-diastolic volume and pressure (LVEDV and LVEDP respectively). Cardiac index is also normal. Following myocardial infarction, LVEDP rises without a significant change in LVEDV (point 2) and a reduction in cardiac index. Diuretics move the patient to point 3 where LVEDP is reduced to normal levels but cardiac index is further reduced. (From Chattejee K. *Dobutamine. A ten year review.* NCM, 1989, with permission of Eli Lilly and Company, Indiana, USA).

Afterload

This is the force required by the myocardium to eject a stroke volume and depends upon aortic pressure and the peripheral resistance presented by the size and compliance of the vascular bed.

Contractility

Contractility is defined by Levick as a change in contractile energy not related to alterations in the length of the cardiac fibres.[3] It can be improved by inotropic agents and sympathetic nervous system stimulation acting probably by increasing calcium influx into the myocardial cells. Increasing contractility results in a more forceful contraction with shorter systole and an increased ejection fraction.

Sarnoff curves demonstrate the beneficial effects of sympathetic stimulation. In this 'family' of curves, stroke work is plotted against mean left atrial pressure for different degrees of sympathetic stimulation. Figure 17.3 describes several such curves showing the effects of sympathetic stimulation, myocardial failure and adrenaline on cardiac function in the open chest dog preparation. Individual curves represent the increase in contractile energy generated by increasing filling pressures. Increases in contractility, on the other hand, are seen by moving upwards from one curve to the next at a constant filling pressure.

From these studies, it is clear that stroke volume can be increased up to a point by increasing filling pressure or by increasing contractility. It is also important to note that the ejection of blood is opposed by the arterial pressure and the total peripheral resistance. As afterload increases, the stroke volume initially decreases and then recovers as end-diastolic fibre length increases. Contraction of cardiac muscle in these circumstances is achieved at the price of higher energy consumption and will therefore demand a satisfactory flow of energy substrates from the coronary circulation. Furthermore, as the size of the ventricular chambers increases, there is a decrease in efficiency of the ventricular expulsive effort. This mechanical effect is described by Laplace's law which states that the pressure developed within a sphere is proportional to wall tension and inversely proportional to radius. Thus as the failing heart dilates, its increasing chamber radius will result in a decrease in the pressure generated by the contracting ventricle.

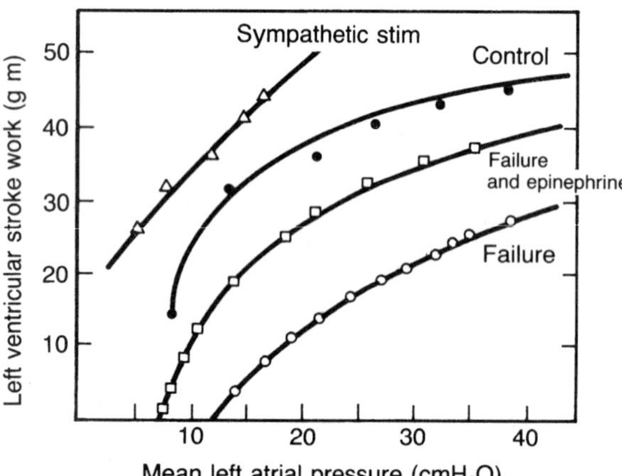

FIGURE 17.3 The effects of sympathetic stimulation, myocardial failure, and adrenaline on cardiac function in the open chest dog preparation. (From Little RC, Little WC. *Physiology of the heart and circulation*, 4th Edition. Chicago: Year book Med Publications. Modified from Sarnoff, SJ. *Physiological Reviews* 1955 and *Circulation Research* 1960. Reproduced by permission of Mosby Year Book, St Louis USA.)

Effects of afterload and preload changes

The importance of the interaction between arterial pressure and stroke volume can be appreciated by a study of pressure volume loops. These are described in more detail in the referenced texts by Noble,[1] Levick[3] and Little and Little.[8]

Figure 17.4 shows three pressure loops occurring within the ventricle during a normal cardiac cycle (1), with increased preload (2) and afterload (3).

With the aid of the pressure volume loop it is now possible to visualize the effects of increasing preload and afterload. As preload increases, the end-diastolic volume rises but the ventricle contracts down to the same end-systolic point and stroke volume increases. With increase in afterload, higher intraventricular pressures are developed in order to overcome the higher aortic diastolic pressure and allow ejection. Because of the slope of the isovolumetric systolic curve the stroke volume will be reduced and more energy will be

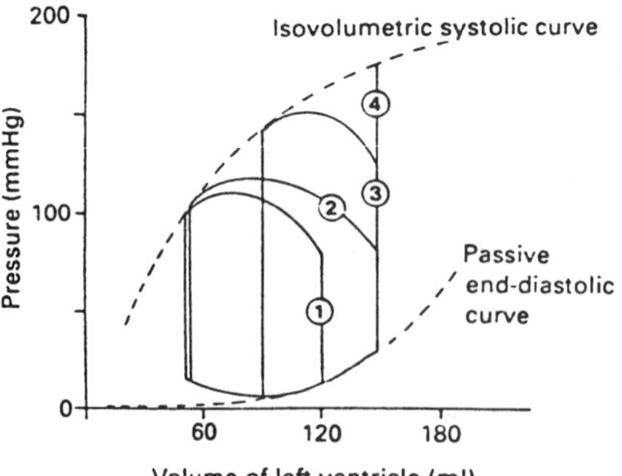

FIGURE 17.4 Effect of increased preload and afterload on the normal pressure loop (1) during a normal cardiac cycle; (2) with increased preload; and (3) with increased afterload. (From Levick JR. *An introduction to cardiovascular physiology*. Oxford: Butterworths, 1991, with permission.)

expended overcoming pressure rather than in myocardial fibre shortening. In this situation pressure work will result in significantly higher myocardial oxygen consumption than for the same volume work.

The clinical relevance of this lies in the recognition that achieving an improved arterial blood pressure by vasoconstriction may reduce stroke volume and increase myocardial work. Vasodilators act by reducing afterload and allowing the heart to increase stroke volume with less work done overcoming pressure.

Oxygen flows and uptake

Efforts to improve stroke volume and cardiac index (CI) are of limited value if consideration is not given to oxygen content (Cao_2) and therefore haemoglobin and arterial oxygen saturation. Oxygen delivery (Do_2) can be calculated from the product of arterial oxygen content and cardiac index according to the formula:

$$\underset{\text{ml/min/m}^2}{Do_2I} = \underset{\text{ml}}{Cao_2} \times \underset{\text{l/min/m}^2}{\frac{CO}{BSA}} \times 10$$

where BSA = body surface area.

This index of oxygen flow to the tissues is referred to as oxygen delivery though, as Bihari[4] points out, this implies an arrival and acceptance at the target site which is not necessarily the case.

If oxygen delivery represents the supply side of the circulatory system, then oxygen uptake (Vo_2) can be measured to indicate demand. This is now routinely calculated from measurements of cardiac output and arterial to mixed venous oxygen (CVo_2) content difference.

$$Vo_2I = (Cao_2 - CVo_2 \times \frac{CO}{BSA} \times 10\ (\text{ml/min/m}^2))$$

The relationship between oxygen delivery and uptake in normal and disease states is shown in Fig. 17.5.

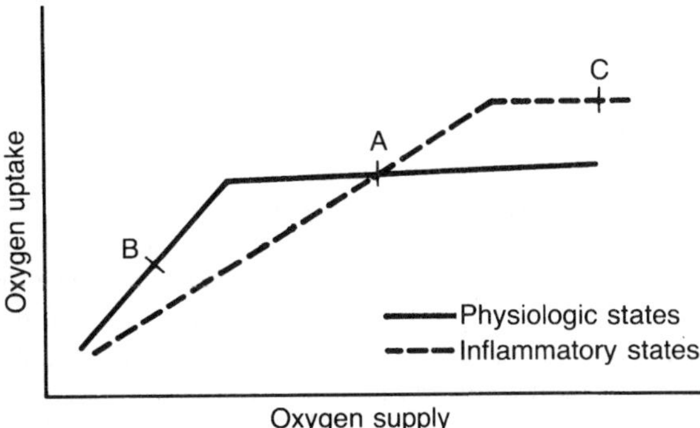

FIGURE 17.5 The relationship between oxygen supply and oxygen uptake. (From Chatterjee K. *Dobutamine. A ten year review*. NCM, 1989, with permission of Eli Lilly and Company, Indiana, USA.

Following Cain's work in 1977,[5] it seems that as oxygen supply decreases, oxygen uptake is maintained until a critical point is reached. At this point increasing tissue oxygen extraction fails to compensate for the decreasing supply and oxygen uptake falls. In the septicaemic patient, this point may be considerably higher. The change from supply independency to supply dependency corresponds to the development of anaerobic metabolism, lactate production and circulatory shock. This concept has led to efforts to increase oxygen delivery with the use of inotropes and fluid. Although studies[6,7] have shown that increasing oxygen delivery in certain patient groups is associated with improved survival, supranormal goals of oxygen delivery and uptake in critically ill patients remains a controversial issue.

DRUGS IN THE MANAGEMENT OF SHOCK

From the above, it is clear that the objectives in shock management are to fill the intravascular space, raise cardiac output and direct high oxygen flow to the tissues. Once proper vascular filling is achieved[7] further benefits may be obtained with the use of inotropic drugs and in particular the catecholamines.

Pharmacology of the catecholamines

This most important group of drugs used to treat hypotension is based on a catechol nucleus consisting of benzene ring, hydroxyl groups and an ethylamine side-chain (Fig. 17.6).

The sympathomimetic actions of these drugs are produced by interaction with receptors at pre- and postsynaptic sympathetic nerve terminals situated in the heart, and the smooth muscle of blood vessels, bronchi and uterus. Activation of the receptors in the heart produces inotropic responses, increasing myocardial contractility by altering intracellular AMP and calcium concentrations (see Chapter 13).

These receptors, first described by Ahlquist in 1948, are labelled α- and β- according to their response to sympathetic agonists and antagonists. Since then further subdivisions of receptors have been described, including: α_1 (cardiac inotropy and peripheral vasoconstriction), β_1 (cardiac chronotropic and inotropic effects), β_2 (vasodilatation and bronchodilatation), and the dopaminergic receptors DA_1 (vasodilatation of renal and splanchnic blood vessels).

In the critically ill patient the effects of catecholamines will depend upon the extent to which the receptors are stimulated (Table 17.2) as well as dosage.

In addition, their effects may be modified by such factors as altered receptor sensitivity, presence of other agonists or antagonists, alteration in second and third messenger activity as well as homeostatic reflexes responding to a particular change – that is, pressure

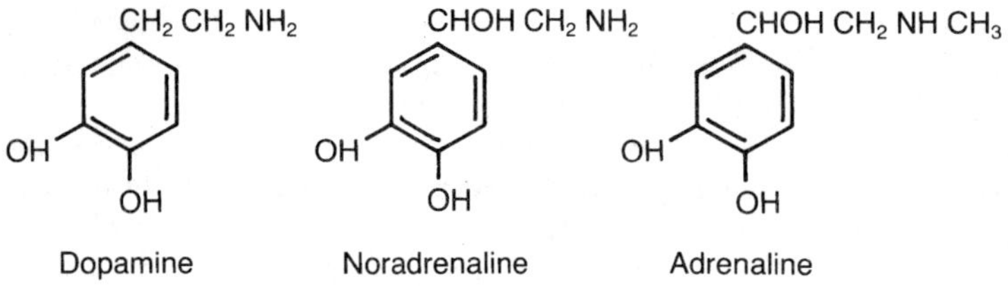

$CH_2\,CH_2\,NH_2$	$CHOH\,CH_2\,NH_2$	$CHOH\,CH_2\,NH\,CH_3$
OH, OH	OH, OH	OH, OH
Dopamine	Noradrenaline	Adrenaline

FIGURE 17.6 Chemical structure of the common inotropic drugs.

TABLE 17.2 Adrenergic receptor activity of commonly used catecholamines. (From Lollgren H, Drexler H. *Critical Care Medicine* **18**. Williams & Wilkins, 1990.)

DRUG	α PERIPHERAL	β_1 CARDIAC	β_2 PERIPHERAL	DA_1 PERIPHERAL	DA_2 PERIPHERAL
Noradrenaline	++++	++++	0	0	0
Adrenaline	++++	++++	++	0	0
Dopamine	++++	++++	++	++++	++++
Dobutamine	+	++++	++	0	0

and heart rate. As a result, dosage has to be determined by clinical response to a trial and error approach.

Receptor behaviour

A feature common to many drugs is a reduction in response, or tachyphylaxis, developing after prolonged exposure of a receptor to an agonist. This phenomenon has been extensively studied in β-receptors which show a reduction in surface density and numbers (down-regulation) after long-term stimulation. Patients with congestive cardiac failure have been reported[9] to show marked reduction in β-receptor density related to the severity of heart failure and associated with resistance to the effects of β-agonists. It is interesting to note in this context that down-regulation affects β_1-receptors to a greater extent than β_2-receptors.

Drugs

Adrenaline

Adrenaline is a naturally occurring catecholamine and is the main hormone liberated from the adrenal medulla. It stimulates both α- and β-receptors to varying degrees depending on dose. Its cardiac effects are to increase heart rate and contractility with an increase in cardiac output. Myocardial oxygen consumption is increased. On the peripheral vasculature it has mainly β-effects at low dose (1–2 μg/min), with mixed α- and β-effects at moderate doses (2–10 μg/min). At high dosage rates (10–20 μg/min), peripheral vasoconstriction occurs as a result of the predominantly α-effects. This causes a rise in total peripheral resistance and blood pressure. At high doses, adrenaline is arrhythmogenic, producing ventricular tachycardia and fibrillation by its action on conducting tissues. Although it has a half-life of about 2 min, β-effects may persist longer than α- at termination of an infusion causing hypotension. It has a place in the treatment of low cardiac output states (below 2.0 l/min), cardiac arrest, anaphylaxis and resistant bronchospasm. Its effects on preload and afterload are dose dependent but tend to be unpredictable.

A useful way of calculating inotrope dosage has been described at the Freeman and Royal Victoria Hospitals in Newcastle:[10]

For adrenaline, noradrenaline, and isoprenaline:
(BW in kg × 3)/100 = mg to add to 50 ml of solution
Then 1 ml/h = 0.01 μg/kg/min

For dopamine and dobutamine:
(BW in kg × 3) = mg to add to 50 ml of solution
Then 1 ml/h = 1 μg/kg/min

Dopamine

This is a precursor of noradrenaline with moderate α-effects, strong β-effects and also specific effects on dopaminergic receptors in the vascular smooth muscle of kidneys, heart, brain and gut. It releases noradrenaline from stores, so it may also act indirectly. The effects of dopamine administration depend on dosage. At low dosage rates (0.1–2.0 μg/kg/min) there is increased renal blood flow, a rise in glomerular filtration rate and natriuresis. As the dose increases (2.0–5.0 μg/kg/min) β-effects predominate with an increase in myocardial contractility and cardiac output. At high rates of infusion, peripheral vasoconstriction occurs due to intense α-stimulation with increasing peripheral vascular resistance and reduction in renal blood flow. Filling pressures may increase due to increased venous tone. In the blood, dopamine is broken down rapidly by dopamine hydroxylase and monoamine oxidase. Because extravasation will cause sloughing (treat with phentolamine) it should be administered via a wide bore central line. Mixing with alkaline solutions should be avoided. Currently, the most common use of dopamine is in promoting renal blood flow and diuresis, though it can be useful in patients who require an increase in cardiac output and a pressor effect.

Noradrenaline

Noradrenaline is a naturally occurring sympathomimetic amine acting as a transmitter at adrenergic nerve endings. It has marked α-effects and mild β_1-activity. As a result of widespread vasoconstriction total peripheral resistance increases. Systolic and diastolic pressures rise and cardiac output may fall. Reflex slowing of the heart is caused by the rise in blood pressure. Extravasation at drip site will cause necrosis. Dosage is from 1 to 10 μg/min. Noradrenaline has a half-life of approximately 3 min. It is useful, though controversial, in septic shock states but should be avoided in late pregnancy and myocardial ischaemia.

Isoprenaline

A synthetic catecholamine acting on β_1- and β_2-receptors only, isoprenaline increases cardiac contractility and heart rate via the β_1-receptors. β_2-Stimulation causes vasodilatation in vascular beds of skeletal muscle, kidney and gut causing a fall in TPR and diastolic blood pressure. Systolic blood pressure may also fall. Although it has very potent bronchodilator effects, its propensity for causing tachycardia and arrhythmia has led to the use of more selective β_2-agonists in asthma. Rare indications for its use now include the emergency treatment of heart block or possibly pulmonary embolism associated with severe bronchoconstriction. The fall in mean arterial pressure and tachycardia occurring after use means that intravenous administration should be undertaken with caution and adequate monitoring. Dosage is from 0.5 to 5.0 μg/min.

Dobutamine

This synthetic catecholamine has mainly inotropic effects on the heart acting on β_1-receptors and possibly cardiac α_1 receptors. As a result, there is an increase in myocardial contractility and cardiac output. Peripheral effects include β_2-stimulation and some minimal α_1-instigated vasoconstriction, producing an overall slight reduction in systemic vascular resistance (SVR). At low to moderate doses (2.5–10 μg/kg/min), dobutamine does not adversely affect the myocardial oxygen supply and demand ratio nor provoke tachycardia. However, in the hypovolaemic patient and at high doses, there may be an increase in heart rate. Its half-life is 1.5–2.5 min due to rapid metabolism by catechol-*o*-methyl transferase to inactive breakdown products. Dosage starts at 2.5–1.0 μg/kg/min up to 40 μg/kg/min. Because it has such mild α-effects, dobutamine extravasation does not cause tissue necrosis and may be given peripherally. Mixing with alkaline solutions should be avoided.

Dopexamine hydrochloride

This is a synthetic compound designed for use in low cardiac output states. It has powerful β_2-adrenergic effects as well as activity at DA_1 and DA_2 receptors producing vasodilatation and an increase in blood flow in the renal and peripheral vascular bed. It has no α-vasoconstrictor activity and improves cardiac output by combined chronotropic and inotropic effects. Overall it reduces afterload and increases cardiac output and urine flow. A summary of its effects relative to dopamine is seen in Table 17.3

Administration

Dopexamine has a short half-life of approximately 7 min, being metabolized in the liver to inactive breakdown products excreted in the urine. Dosage is 0.5–6.0 μg/kg/min but clinical experience is limited. Tachycardia may prove a problem at higher dosage and as with all vasodilators careful monitoring is mandatory.

Phosphodiesterase inhibitors

Inhibition of phosphodiesterases in the myocardial cell and vascular smooth muscle will produce elevated cAMP concentrations and a resulting increase in calcium influx. This is the basis of the inotropic effects of amrinone, milrinone and enoximone whose peripheral

TABLE 17.3 The pharmacological properties of dopexamine hydrochloride relative to dopamine and dobutamine. (From Smith GW, O'Connor SE. *Americal Journal of Cardiology* 1988; **62**: 9C–17C.)

	DA_1	DA_2	β_1	β_2	α	UPTAKE-1 INHIBITION
Dopexamine hydrochloride	++	+	(+)	+++	0	+++
Dopamine	+++	++	++	(+)	+++	++
Dobutamine	0	0	+++	++	++	+

arterial and venous vasodilatating effects have led to their designation as inodilators.[11]

So far, clinical studies with these agents have been restricted to patients with congestive cardiac failure. In these cases the effects have been to increase cardiac index, lower peripheral resistance and reduce filling pressures without increasing myocardial oxygen consumption. Because of their relatively long elimination time and their vasodilatatory properties, particular care must be exercised with their use and full cardiovascular monitoring employed. In heart failure, as well as hepatic and renal malfunction, marked persistence of their effects has been reported.

Vasodilators

This group of drugs is dominated by the nitrates and in particular nitroglycerine, isosorbide dinitrate and sodium nitroprusside. Their main effect is to produce relaxation of vascular smooth muscle by nitric oxide released in the vessel walls. The resulting vasodilatation in the arteriolar (good) and venous beds (better) produces significant reduction in afterload and especially preload. Tolerance is a significant problem.

Sodium nitroprusside (SNP)

This vasodilator acts on both arteriolar and venous beds. It has a rapid onset and brief duration (1–3 min) giving minute by minute control of haemodynamic effects. It is converted to cyanmethaemoglobin, cyanide and thiocyanate and excreted by the kidneys. When therapy is continued for more than 12 h cyanide levels should be checked. Invasive monitoring is required because of the danger of sudden hypotension. Solutions are prepared by adding 50 mg of SNP to 2 ml 5% glucose and diluting to 50 ml. Infusion can start at 10 μg/min up to 300 μg/min but should not exceed 4 μg/kg/min. Nitroprusside solutions should be protected from light and discarded after 4 h. It is particularly useful in low output cardiac failure where arterial pressure is satisfactory.

Glyceryl trinitrate (GTN)

Nitroglycerine produces dilatation of arterial and venous beds but is predominantly a venodilator. As a result there is a fall in venous return with reduction of right atrial and pulmonary artery wedge pressure (PAWP). For this reason it can be most effective in relieving acute pulmonary oedema. By its arteriolar dilating effects ventricular wall tension diminishes and myocardial oxygen demands may decrease. Solutions are prepared by adding 50 mg GTN in 50 ml 5% glucose in a polycarbonate syringe (not PVC infusion bags). The infusion is started at 5 μg/min and increased slowly up to 200 μg/min.

Isosorbide dinitrate (ISDN)

Like nitroglycerine, isosorbide dinitrate has arteriolar and venodilator effects reducing preload and afterload by vasodilatation. It has, however, a longer terminal half-life than nitroglycerine, being broken down by the liver to mono-nitrates which also have active vasodilatory properties. It is more stable in solution than nitroglycerine. Normally 50 ml ISDN 0.1% (50 mg) are added to 50 ml solution This is infused at 1.25–5 mg/h.

MANAGEMENT OF HYPOTENSION AND SHOCK

Acute heart failure in myocardial infarction

Following acute ischaemic changes in the myocardium there is a sharp deterioration in both systolic and diastolic function of the heart. Myocardial contractility is reduced and the end-systolic volume line moves downwards and to the right. At the same time, the ventricular wall becomes stiffer and less compliant and the ventricular end-diastolic pressure volume curve moves upwards and to the left. These changes[12] result in a fall in stroke work and a reduction in ejection fraction with a rise in left ventricular end-diastolic pressure (LVEDP). Coincident with these mechanical changes is an alteration in the balance between myocardial oxygen supply and demand (Fig. 17.7).

Several factors conspire to upset this balance. Tachycardia brought about by increased sympathetic activity increases myocardial oxygen demands as does any increase in myocardial wall tension. Concurrent reductions in coronary perfusion caused by shortened diastole, lowered aortic pressure and compression of the myocardial microcirculation by high end-diastolic pressures compound the problem.

Under these circumstances clinical objectives are clear cut. Myocardial oxygen demands should be reduced by bed rest and attention to the relief of pain and anxiety. Oxygen therapy improves arterial oxygen content and lowers pulse rates and should be monitored by pulse oximetry, keeping oxygen saturation above 95% whenever possible.

In the presence of heart failure, vasodilator therapy with nitroglycerine or isosorbide dinitrate may bring about improvement. The consequent reduction in afterload increases stroke volume and reduces myocardial wall tension allowing the ventricle to perform more volume and less pressure work at lower oxygen consumption rates.

With effective venodilatation, a fall in venous return reduces ventricular end-diastolic pressure, thereby lowering pulmonary venous pressures and improving dyspnoea and pulmonary function. Any fall in diastolic

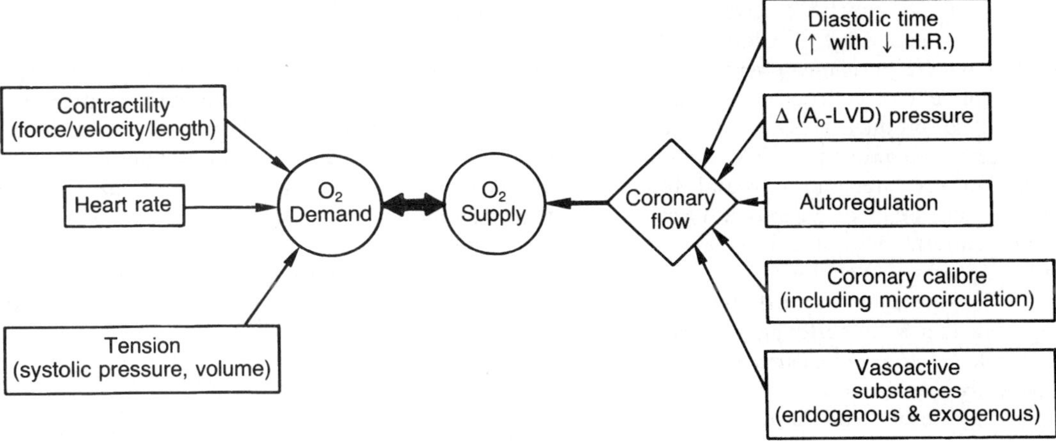

FIGURE 17.7 Myocardial energetics. (Reproduced with permission from Ferlinz J. Nifedipine in myocardial ischaemia, systemic hypertension and other cardiovascular disorders. *Annals of Internal Medicine* 1986; **105** 714–29. H.R., heart rate; (A_0-LVD), aortic–left ventricular diastolic pressure.

pressure within the heart also enhances blood flow through the microcirculation of the ventricular wall.

Although vasodilator therapy has beneficial actions, it is clear that its administration is capable of producing unwanted effects. In particular, vasodilators should be avoided in hypotension or obstructive valvular heart disease.[13] The presence of hypovolaemia may be unmasked by vasodilator therapy causing sharp falls in ventricular end-diastolic pressure sufficient to lower stroke volume and cardiac output. Excessive afterload reduction may allow aortic diastolic pressure to fall below the level necessary to perfuse the coronary circulation. For this reason invasive monitoring may be necessary in certain subsets of this group of patients. Insertion of a flow-guided pulmonary artery catheter with the facility for thermodilution cardiac output estimation allows repeated measurement of both filling pressures and stroke volume so that therapy can be more accurately directed. Pulmonary artery wedge pressures in the region of 18–22 mmHg are recommended[12] but it should be remembered that changes in the compliance of the ventricular wall may give rise to high filling pressures even though stroke volume is not optimal. Although the value of pulmonary artery catheters in this situation is controversial[14] Raper makes the point 'that the principles of treatment applied to patients by clinicians who do not use this device are in large measure dependent upon the understanding derived from its widespread use'.[15]

With the use of the catheter, stroke volume and the cardiac output can be repeatedly assessed. If venous oximetry is available then continuous mixed venous oxygen measurement[16,17] can be displayed and maintained above tensions of 30 mmHg or saturation of 60%.

The place of frusemide in cardiac failure management is contentious. Although it may reduce pulmonary venous pressure and thus relieve dyspnoea by its vasodilatory action, excessive diuresis can bring about uncontrolled reduction in filling pressure with impairment of cardiac function. Intravenous doses should therefore be kept low (5–10 mg) and as with all aspects of critical care their effects monitored with frequent reassessment of circulating volume, blood pressure and stroke volume.

If there is hypotension, or evidence of a low cardiac output or if symptoms of heart failure intensify, consideration should be given to the use of inotropes. At present, dobutamine is a common choice after myocardial infarction, because of its useful effects on contractility without increasing heart rate or enzymatically estimated infarct size.[18] Because of its short half-life (several minutes) an infusion can be easily managed starting at a dose of 2.5 μg/kg/min and increasing to 10 μg/kg/min.

Cardiogenic shock

After infarction of a significant volume of cardiac muscle has occurred, cardiogenic shock may develop. This is characterized by hypotension (mean arterial pressure (MAP) < 60 mmHg) and a low cardiac index (< 2.0 l/min/m^2). In these circumstances hypovolaemia, due to fluid restriction, diuretic therapy and fluid redistribution, may be present, as well as regional underperfusion, impairment of renal function, confusion and early hepatic insufficiency. High left atrial pressures may have induced pulmonary oedema with a rising respiratory rate and arterial hypoxaemia and acidosis produced by poor tissue perfusion may further impair cardiac function.

In these circumstances inotropic support is clearly required, though not before correction of any hypovolaemia. Colloid challenges[7] may have advantages over crystalloids in this situation and need to be guided by reference to stroke volume, cardiac output or filling pressures in order of preference. Oxygen therapy using the high flow oxygen enrichment venturi masks ensures known inspired oxygen concentrations and should be selected to produce oxygen saturations over 95%. Appropriate monitoring of ECG, pulmonary artery occlusion pressures, intra-arterial blood pressure, cardiac output and mixed venous and arterial oxygen saturation should be instituted according to local skills and equipment availability.

Several studies have suggested that dobutamine is superior to dopamine in patients suffering from cardiogenic shock. Fowler[19] reported beneficial haemodynamic effects with rises in cardiac index, falls in SVR and pulmonary artery end-diastolic pressure. No hypotension was noted, though heart rate increases were seen. Comparisons of dobutamine and dopamine,[20] showed both agents were capable of increasing cardiac index but that dopamine in doses >5 μg/kg/min increased pulmonary artery wedge pressure. An increase in filling pressure caused by dopamine has also been reported by other workers[21] and has been ascribed to its vasoconstrictive effects on venous tone.

Because of the slight fall in SVR produced by dobutamine, several workers suggest dopamine should be used in very low cardiac output states or when dobutamine fails to raise MAP above the level needed to guarantee good coronary perfusion. However, the main value of dopamine in shock management relies on its effects at low dosage (0.5–2.5 μg/kg/min) on the DA_1 receptors of renal tubular cells causing an increase in renal blood flow and sodium excretion.

Where severe hypotensive and low cardiac output states persist there is a place for adrenaline infusion (Fig. 17.8) though increasing afterload is obviously a major problem. At this stage options become limited. Continuous positive airway pressure (CPAP) by mask, or endotracheal intubation and intermittent positive pressure ventilation are useful techniques, particularly when respiratory function is poor and oxygen saturations fall below 90%. Both these techniques reduce the respiratory workload, thus sparing oxygen for other sites. Finally, intra-aortic balloon pumping may be considered if surgical treatment or angioplasty is considered a possibility.

SHOCK IN THE HIGH-RISK SURGICAL PATIENT

Attitudes to the management of the shocked surgical patient were changed by a series of articles by WC Shoemaker from the UCLA School of Medicine at Los Angeles. He pointed out that the clinical measurements traditionally used as descriptions of the shock state such as blood pressure, heart rate, CVP and urine output correlated poorly with outcome. Furthermore, restoration of these indices to normal using vasopressors, crystalloids and diuretics did not affect survival rates. Investigation of the oxygen transport variables, CI, oxygen delivery (Do_2) and oxygen consumption (Vo_2) demonstrated marked differences between survivors and non-survivors. Essentially the survivors exhibited better myocardial performance (increased CI and flow related variables), better oxygen transport and lower oxygen extraction rates. Reduced Vo_2 was considered to be the fundamental pathogenic characteristic of non-survivors. As a result of these studies efforts were made to increase Do_2 and Vo_2 in shocked patients by fluid therapy, inotropes and/or vasodilators. The supranormal goals of therapy were defined as follows:[22]

- CI 50% above normal (4.5 l/min/m^2)
- Do_2 greater than normal (>600 ml/min/m^2)
- Vo_2 30% above normal (>170 ml/min/m^2)
- Blood volume 500 ml above normal (3.2 l/m^2 for males, 2.8 l/m^2 for females)

Although fluid therapy with colloid is the cornerstone of this approach, drugs play a significant role. Colloid infusion is used to bring filling pressures to appropriate levels (wedge pressure 18 mmHg). If an adequate Do_2, CI and Vo_2 have not been reached, dobutamine is commenced starting at 2 μg/kg/min and increased until the optimal goals are reached. Comparisons of dobutamine and dopamine in 25 critically ill postoperative general surgical patients demonstrated superior results with dobutamine producing greater rises in HR, CI, stroke work, Do_2 and Vo_2 as well as falls in wedge pressure.[23] Vasodilators including prostacycline have also been recommended for subsets of patients with high MAP and SVR. Correct doses are achieved by titration while monitoring CI, Do_2 and Vo_2 and avoiding hypotension.

SEPTIC SHOCK

Most cases of septic shock originate from Gram-negative infections, though Gram-positive organisms also have a role.[24] In particular, *E. coli*, *Klebsiella* and *Staphylococci* have been found to be common causative organisms in these highly dangerous (40–60% mortality) infections. Following bacteraemia, a variety of mediators are described. These are released into the blood initiating cascades of reactions involving the complement system, coagulation and the release of various cytokines culminating in the familiar clinical picture of septic shock. Fever, tachycardia, tachypnoea, systemic organ hypoperfusion and hypotension with warm vasodilated peripheries are common clinical findings. Investigations reveal leucocytosis, thrombocytopaenia, lactic acidosis and hypoxaemia. In this situation the sequential development of multiple system organ failure must be avoided if mortality rates are to be lowered. Drainage of infected fluid collections and removal of necrotic tissue is of elementary importance in association with correct antibiotic therapy. Failure to improve in these circumstances mandates repeated searches utilizing ultrasound, CT scans and

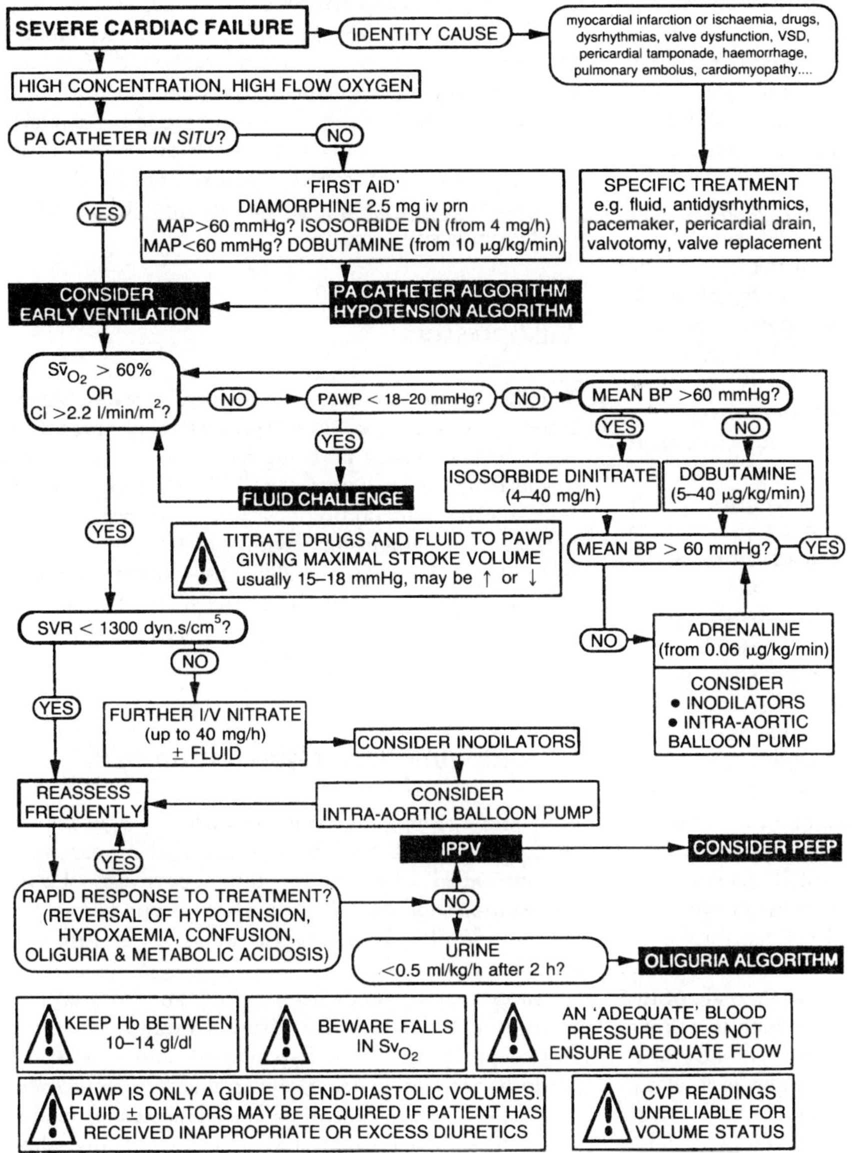

FIGURE 17.8 Management algorithm for severe cardiac failure. (From Armstrong RF, Bullen C. Cohen SL, Singer M, Webb AR. *Critical care algorithms.* Oxford: Oxford University Press; 1991, with permission.) VSD, ventricular septal defect; PA, pulmonary artery; MAP, mean arterial pressure; SV_{O_2}, mixed venous oxygen saturation; CI, cardiac index; PAWP, pulmonary artery wedge pressure; BP, blood pressure; SVR, systemic vascular resistance; IPPV, intermittent positive pressure ventilation; PEEP, positive end expiratory pressure; CVP, central venous pressure.

even laparotomy, if necessary, in an effort to identify the sources of the infection.

THERAPEUTIC OBJECTIVES

Although sepsis may ultimately affect all organs it is disorders of the heart and peripheral circulation that dominate the early clinical picture. Cardiac dysfunction is now well documented[25] though the causes of this are not yet clear. While there is wide support for the presence of a circulating myocardial depressant substance (MDS), there is no consensus as to its identity. Endotoxin, a lipopolysaccharide released from the outer membrane of Gram-negative bacilli, produces a similar clinical picture to septic shock but does not explain the myocardial depression seen after Gram-positive infections. The proposal that other mediators such as tumour necrosis factor (TNF) or interleukin 2 cause myocardial depression revives the possibility of pharmacological mediator blockade as a potential treatment option. In this context it is interesting that ibuprofen has been demonstrated to block the cardiovascular response to interleukin 1 and TNF.[26] Other developments in treatment include the use of immunological therapy and, in particular, antibodies to the core lipid A component of the endotoxin molecule. Although monoclonal antibodies to endotoxin[27] and TNF antibodies have been used in clinical and experimental situations, there is, as yet, no clear evidence of benefit.

Whatever the circulating mediators of sepsis are, there is no doubt that both right- and left-sided myocardial dysfunction exists in sepsis. In the case of the right ventricle the problem is made worse by the development of pulmonary hypertension occurring in association with acute respiratory failure. This increase in afterload provides a major obstruction to the thin-walled right ventricle, causing a reduction in ventricular ejection fraction. To this difficulty in ejection is added poor ventricular wall perfusion due to the low aortic diastolic pressure experienced in sepsis. Efforts to lower pulmonary artery pressure by prostacyclin infusion (epoprostenol) are usually made in these circumstances though the resulting vasodilatation may critically reduce perfusion pressures to the point where vasopressors (noradrenaline) are needed.

Although cardiac malfunction can be a problem in sepsis, cardiac output is usually high. It is peripheral vasomotor failure that is the primary mechanism bringing about circulatory collapse. Release of vasodilatory mediators causes marked falls in SVR and filling pressures such that there is a reduction in the effective circulating blood volume and hypotension. Increases in capillary permeability cause interstitial oedema and extend diffusion distances for the transportation of oxygen to target cells. Widespread maldistribution in the microcirculation, though unproven, may cause the fall in oxygen extraction that is so characteristic of the septic state and that results in areas of high metabolic demand receiving inappropriately low blood flow. Against this background of poor oxygen extraction, there is a generalized increase in metabolic activity. The consequence of this imbalance is anaerobic cellular respiration and the production of lactic acid. Ischaemic changes in the intestinal mucosa impair the barrier effect of the gut wall, possibly allowing bacterial translocation[28] and thus contributing to the sequential pattern of multiple organ failure.

Treatment

Correcting the cause is the most important therapy in the treatment of septic shock. Next is the administration of an adequate volume of intravenous fluid. Colloids are more effective at restoring plasma volume than crystalloids but concern persists at their potential for increasing extravascular lung water. Blood transfusion should be considered whenever reduction in haematocrit occurs and insertion of a pulmonary artery catheter will facilitate fluid management as well as allowing measurement of cardiac output and mixed venous oxygen. Respiratory and renal support is commonly needed. Because of peripheral vasomotor failure the use of vasopressors is often necessary.[29] Cardiac output is usually high but if mean arterial pressures fall below 60 mmHg either dopamine or noradrenaline is indicated. Commonly a combination of low dose dopamine and noradrenaline is used. Finally the use of steroids is restricted to those situations where adrenal failure is suspected.

Vasopressors

Whether or not to use vasopressors in severe shock states is a vexed question. Misgivings about precipitating ischaemic bowel are being reinforced by studies of mucosal pH using tonometry.[30] Nevertheless, if after fluid replacement, antibiotics and inotropes there is persistent hypotension with MAPs less than 60 mmHg there is really no other option. Noradrenaline infusion is often successful in the severely hypotensive patient and can be weaned down at the earliest opportunity.

Cardiopulmonary resuscitation (CPR)

Adrenaline (1 mg) has been the vasopressor of choice in cardiac arrest for many years and is currently recommended by both the American Heart Association and the British Heart Foundation for resumption of spontaneous circulation in all forms of cardiac arrest.

Several factors influence recovery and hospital discharge rates after cardiac arrest. Duration of arrest, degree of hypoxia and hypercapnia and severity of acidosis are clearly major determinants of outcome. If these factors are controlled and minimized as in animal studies there is evidence that the dose of adrenaline necessary to maintain minimal cerebral and myocardial blood flow requirements may be higher than currently recommended.[31] Lindner[32] showed that high dose adrenaline (5 mg) was associated with higher initial resuscitation success in adults suffering asystole or electromechanical dissociation than the normal dose of 1 mg. However, a large multicentre trial showed no advantage of 0.2 mg/kg adrenaline over the standard dose in out of hospital arrests[33] nor of high doses (7.0 mg) in inpatients.[34] Evidence that noradrenaline may have advantages over adrenaline has also been proposed,[35] demonstrating better results in terms of overall oxygen balance and shorter resuscitation times. However, optimal dosage has yet to be determined. Of the other drugs used in CPR, sodium bicarbonate has historically had an important role in the treatment of the associated metabolic acidosis. Recent work, however, has failed to show any improvement in outcome in animal models after bicarbonate administration.[36] The reason for this is thought to be the interaction of bicarbonate with hydrogen ions to produce CO_2. In the presence of inadequate ventilation this may worsen intracellular acidosis. The hypertonicity produced by the administration of bicarbonate solution adds further insult by decreasing aortic pressure and thus myocardial perfusion. A recent review concludes that the early or late use of buffering agents is of no proven value.[37] Finally calcium chloride is also currently out of fashion in CPR, though levels of ionized calcium have been shown to decrease during prolonged resuscitation.

CONCLUSION

The last decade has seen new emphasis in the management of shock and hypotension. Volume correction, maintenance of high blood flow and repeated measurement and support of stroke volumes and oxygen delivery have received massive attention in medical literature with some evidence of improved results. Peripheral vasomotor failure remains a topic clouded in uncertainty as do the regional effects of vasopressors. Efforts to prevent the lethal cascades of multiple organ failure have received new support from the field of immunology and searches continue for a pharmacological mediator blocker. As in all other areas of medicine, prevention or early intervention in the course of severe illness has a major impact on both outcome and cost of therapy.

REFERENCES

1 Noble MM. Inappropriateness of inotropic support with epinephrine. In: Vincent JL ed. *Update in intensive care and emergency medicine*. Berlin: Springer-Verlag, 1988; 81–9.

2 Shoemaker WC, Appel PL, Waxman K., Schwartz S. Chang P. Clinical trial of survivors cardiorespiratory patterns as therapeutic goals in critically ill postoperative patients. *Critical Care Medicine* 1982; **10**: 398.

3 Levick JR. *An introduction to cardiovascular physiology*. Oxford: Butterworths, 1988.

4 Kox W, Bihari D eds. *Shock and the adult respiratory distress syndrome*. Berlin: Springer-Verlag.

5 Cain MC. Oxygen delivery and uptake in dogs during anaemic and hypoxic hypoxia. *Journal of Applied Physiology* 1977; **42**: 228–34.

6 Shoemaker WC, Appel PL, Kram HB. Prospective trial of supra normal values of survivors as therapeutic goals in high risk surgical patients. *Chest* 1988; **94**: 1176.

7 Boyd O, Grounds RM, Bennett ED. A randomised clinical trial of the effect of deliberate perioperative increase of oxygen delivery on mortality in high risk surgical patients. *Journal of the American Medical Association* 1993; **270**: 2699–2707.

8 Little RC, Little WC. *Physiology of the heart and circulation*, 4th edn. Chicago: Mosby Year Book, 1988.

9 Bristow MR, Ginsburg R, Minobe W, Cubicciotti RS, Sageman WS, Lurie K, Billingham ME, Harrison DC, Stinson EB. Decreased catecholamine sensitivity and beta adrenergic receptor density in failing human hearts. *New England Journal of Medicine* 1982; **302**: 205–11.

10 Guzman M, Hedley Brown A, Been M, Cook S, Wren C, Richens D. *Manual of cardiorespiratory critical care*. Oxford: Butterworths, 1989.

11 Mason DT ed. Review. Intravenous milrinone. Therapeutic responses in heart failure. *American Heart Journal* (Suppl) 1991; **121**: 1937–2000.

12 Perret C. Acute heart failure in myocardial infarction. Principles of treatment. *Critical Care Medicine* 1990; **18**: 526.

13 Opie LH. *Drugs for the heart*, 3rd edn. Philadelphia: W.B. Saunders, 1991.

14 Robin ED. The cult of the Swan–Ganz catheter. *Annals of Internal Medicine* 1985; **103**: 445–9.

15 Raper RF, Fisher M McD. The heart and circulation in sepsis. *Baillière's Clinical Anaesthesiology* 1990; **4**: (2).

16 Armstrong RF, Secker-Walker J, Cobbe S, St Andrew D, Lincoln JCR, Cohen S. Continuous monitoring of MVo_2 tension in cardio-respiratory disorders. *Lancet* 1978; **i** (8064): 632–4.

17 Baele PL, McMichan JC, Marsh HM, Sill JC, Southorne PA. Continuous monitoring of mixed venous oxygen saturation in critically ill patients. *Anesthesia and Analgesia* 1982; **61**: 513–17.

18 Gillespie TA, Ambos HD, Sobel BE, Roberts R. Effects of dobutamine in patients with acute myocardial infarction. *American Journal of Cardiology* 1977; **39**: 588–94.

19 Fowler MB, Timmis AD, Crick JP, Vincent R, Chamberlain DA. Comparison of haemodynamic responses to dobutamine and salbutamol in cardiogenic shock after acute myocardial infarction. *British Medical Journal* (Clinical Research) 1982; **284**: 73–6.

20 Frances GS, Sharma B, Hodges M. Comparative haemodynamic effects of dopamine and dobutamine in patients with acute cardiogenic circulatory collapse. *American Heart Journal* 1982; **103**: 995–1000.

21 Lang RM, Carroll JD, Nakamura S, Itoh H, Rajfer SI. Role of adrenoceptors and dopamine receptors in modulating left ventricular diastolic function. *Circulation Research* 1988; **63**: 126–34.

22 Shoemaker WC, Appel PL, Kram HB, Waxman K, Lee TS. Prospective trial of supra normal values of survivors as therapeutic goals in high risk surgical patients. *Chest* 1988; **94**: 1176–86.

23 Shoemaker WC, Appel PL, Kram HB. Comparison of haemodynamic and oxygen transport effects of dobutamine and dopamine in critically ill surgical patients. *Chest* 1988; **96**: 120–4.

24 Rackow EC, Astiz ME. Pathophysiology and treatment of septic shock. *Journal of the American Medical Association*. 1991; **266**: 548–54.

25 Parker MM, Shelhamer JH, Bacharach SL, Green MV, Natanson C, Frederick TM, Damske BA, Parillo JE. Profound but reversible myocardial depression in patients with septic shock. *Annals of Internal Medicine* 1984; **100**: 483–90.

26 Okusawa S, Gelfaud J, Ikejma T, Connolly R, Dinarello C. Interleukin-1 induces a shock-like state in rabbits: synergism with tumour necrosis factor and the effect of cyclo-oxygenase inhibition. *Journal of Clinical Investigation*. 1988; **81**: 1162–72.

27 Ziegler E, HA-IA. Sepsis Study Group. Treatment of Gram-negative bacteraemia and septic shock with

HA-1A human monoclonal antibody against endotoxin. *New England Journal of Medicine* 1991; **324**: 429–36.

28 Marston A, Buckley GB, Fiddian-Green RG, Haglund UH. *Splanchnic ischaemic and multiple organ failure.* London: Edward Arnold, 1989, Chapter 17.

29 Snell RJ, Parillo JE. Cardiovascular dysfunction in septic shock. *Chest* 1991; **99**: 1000–9.

30 Fiddian-Green RG. Should measurements of tissue pH and P_{O_2} be included in the routine monitoring of ICU patients? *Critical Care Medicine* 1991; **19**: 141–3.

31 Brown CG, Werman WA, Davies EA, Hobson J, Hamlin RL. The effects of graded doses of epinephrine on regional myocardial blood flow during cardiopulmonary resuscitation in swine. *Circulation* 1987; **75**: 491–7.

32 Lindner KH, Ahnefeld FW, Prengel AW. Comparison of standard and high dose adrenaline in the resuscitation of asystole and electro-mechanical dissociation. *Acta Anaesthesia Scandinavica* 1991; **35**: 253–6.

33 Brown CG, Martin DR, Pepe PE, Stueven H, Cummins RO, Gonzalez E, Jastremski M. A comparison of standard dose and high dose epinephrine in cardiac arrest outside hospital. *New England Journal of Medicine* 1992; **327**: 1051–5.

34 Sherman BW, Munger MA, Panacek EA, Foulke GE, Rutherford WF. High dose epinephrine in patients failing pre-hospital resuscitation. *Annals of Emergency Medicine* 1991; **20**: 949 (Abstract).

35 Lindner KH, Ahnefeld FW, Schurmann W, Bowdler IM. Epinephrine and norepinephrine in cardiopulmonary resuscitation. Effects on myocardial oxygen delivery and consumption. *Chest* 1990; **97**: 1458–62.

36 Kette F, Weil MH, Gazmuri RJ. Buffer solutions may compromise cardiac resuscitation by reducing coronary perfusion pressure. *Journal of the American Medcical Association* 1991; **266**: 2121–6.

37 Niemann JT. Cardiopulmonary resuscitation. *New England Journal of Medicine* 1992; **327**(15): 1075–9.

SECTION FIVE

Drugs Affecting the Respiratory System

18

Neurohumoral Control of Respiration

IP Hall

INTRODUCTION

This chapter is concerned with the mechanisms underlying the neurohumoral control of respiration and the ways in which these mechanisms are altered by drug administration or disease. The inherent rhythmicity of respiration is dependent on the generation of spontaneous inspiratory and expiratory impulses which originate from the respiratory centre in the brain stem. The exact anatomical localization of the respiratory centre and its connections remain to be precisely defined but it is essentially localized to the reticular formation. The majority of upper motor neurones originate from the lower end in the floor of the 4th ventricle and descend the spinal cord in the ventral and lateral columns. The main muscles of respiration are supplied by lower motor neurones in the phrenic nerve (to the diaphragm, arising from roots C 3, 4, 5), and the intercostal nerves (to the intercostal muscles, arising from roots T 1–12).

Many inputs can potentially vary respiration and ventilation. These are considered in the next two sections, and are summarized in Fig. 18.1.

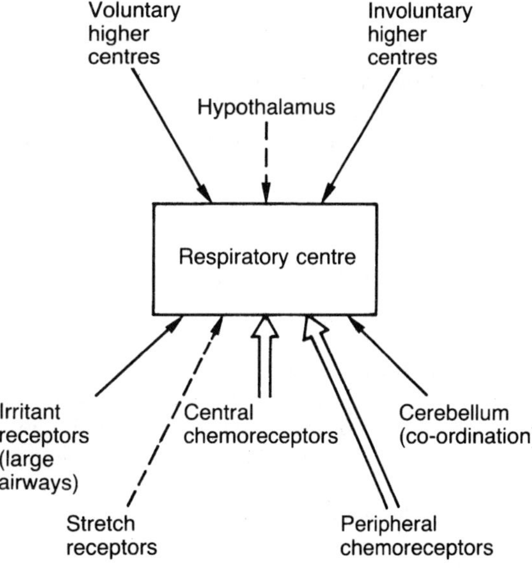

FIGURE 18.1 Inputs to the respiratory centre. Major inputs are shown by broad arrows. The contribution of inputs indicated by dotted arrows is controversial in normal adults.

CONTROL OF RESPIRATION: INPUTS

Higher centres

Voluntary control of respiration is dependent upon pathways from the pyramidal and extrapyramidal systems to the respiratory centre. However, other involuntary higher inputs also exist. The co-ordination of respiration movements during speech is believed to depend upon input from the cerebellum. It is well recognized that anxiety produces hyperventilation. The precise mechanism whereby the hyperventilation induced by anxiety occurs is unclear, but it is presumably mediated through the pyramidal or extrapyramidal systems. There are additional inputs from the hypothalamus that are believed to be involved in the control of body temperature. However, although a rise in body temperature causes hyperventilation this is not entirely due to direct links between the hypothalamus and the reticular formation; in pyrexial patients, the increased metabolic rate results in the production of greater amounts of CO_2 which itself stimulates ventilation (qv).

Control of respiration by pulmonary reflexes

In animals and babies a forced maintained lung inflation results in a delay in the onset of the following spontaneous inspiratory effort and a forced maintained deflation increases the spontaneous inspiratory rate. These effects are mediated through vagal efferents and collectively are known as the Herring–Brauer reflex. However, it is uncertain how important this reflex is in normal adults, although pulmonary stretch reflexes may become more important in patients with abnormal lung compliance due to interstitial lung disease (see p. 278).

The other major reflex initiated through pulmonary afferent input is the cough reflex which can be induced by mechanical irritation of the lower trachea or through stimulation of irritant receptors in the lower airways. This reflex is discussed in more detail in Chapter 19.

As well as the above reflexes, there may be an additional proprioreceptive input to the respiratory centre from the diaphragm and intercostal muscles. The importance of this potential input is unclear, but it may be involved in the appreciation of respiratory workload.

Control of respiration: chemoreceptors

Physiological control of ventilation in normal individuals and in disease states is dependent on changes in $Paco_2$, pH and Pao_2. The effects of alteration of these inputs are mediated through peripheral and central chemoreceptors. The central chemoreceptors lie in the area close to the nuclei of the 8th, 9th and 10th cranial nerves near the lateral recesses of the 4th ventricle. Peripheral chemoreceptors are in the carotid body (supplied with afferent fibres in the glossopharyngeal nerve) and aortic bodies (supplied via the vagus nerve). Although present during infancy, aortic bodies subsequently regress and are not believed to be of functional importance in adults. The carotid bodies are situated at the bifurcation of the common carotid artery, and receive their blood supply from branches of the occipital or ascending pharyngeal arteries. Efferent nerve fibres from the carotid bodies travel via the cervical sympathetic system. The chemoreceptors in the carotid body are sensitive to changes in Pao_2, this effect being potentiated by accompanying acidosis. In addition, the carotid bodies are thought to play a role in the increased sensitivity to CO_2 seen in patients with hypoxia. Studies on individuals in whom the carotid bodies have been removed have shown no real alteration in ventilation in otherwise healthy individuals at rest. Approximately 70% of the CO_2 drive persists, lending support to the idea that the majority of CO_2 drive to ventilation arises from the central chemoreceptors. If Pao_2 remains above about 6 kPa, hypoxic drive remains relatively unimportant. However, when Pao_2 falls below this value chronically (e.g. at high altitude, or in patients with chronic lung disease), patients in whom the carotid bodies have been removed demonstrate severe blunting of their ventilatory responses to hypoxia.

CONTROL OF RESPIRATION BY $Paco_2$, pH AND Pao_2

The regulation of respiration by changes in $Paco_2$, pH or Pao_2 is a classical example of homeostatic control, with negative feedback responses designed to counteract change predominating.

Effect of changing $Paco_2$

The most important chemoreceptor input comes from the central chemoreceptors which are sensitive to changes in the partial pressure of CO_2. The Pco_2 of cerebrospinal fluid is similar to the venous Pco_2 ($Pvco_2$); hence changes in ventilation tend to follow changes in $Pvco_2$. The basic relationship of changing Pco_2 on ventilation is shown in Fig. 18.2, from which it can be seen that large changes in ventilation occur with relatively small alterations in inspired Pco_2. Concentrations of inspired CO_2 above 11 kPa result in decreased respiratory effort, probably due to central nervous system depression. Although the majority of the CO_2 drive originates from the central chemorceptors, as discussed above, a variable amount also arises from the peripheral chemoreceptors in the carotid bodies.

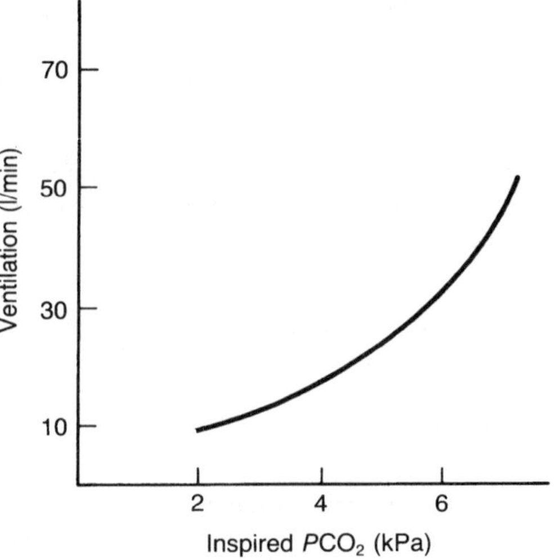

FIGURE 18.2 The effect of alteration in inspired Pco_2 on ventilation.

Effect of changing inspired O_2

In order to show the effect of changing inspired O_2 on ventilation, it is useful to examine ventilation in relation to alveolar P_{CO_2} at different inspired levels of CO_2. A series of relationships for ventilation and alveolar CO_2 can be constructed (see Fig. 18.3). The effect of altering inspired O_2 levels is to increase the sensitivity of the respiratory centre to elevation of CO_2, but not to alter the threshold of the system (Fig. 18.3). Using this approach to quantify changes in ventilation, it can be shown that increasing inspired O_2 above the level in room air produces a less steep linear relationship, implying that a small degree of hypoxic stimulation occurs in normal respiration. The effect of altering P_{O_2} is maximal between inspired P_{O_2} values of 5–9 kPa. It should be noted that the effects of chronic hypoxia are more complex (see below).

Increased hypoxic drive can be demonstrated in normal individuals during exercise or hyperthermia, and in patients with hyperthyroidism.

Effects of changing pH

Using the relationships shown in Fig. 18.3, changes in ventilation at different pH values can be described. For a given P_{O_2}, the effect of acidosis is to reduce the threshold without altering the sensitivity to P_{CO_2}.

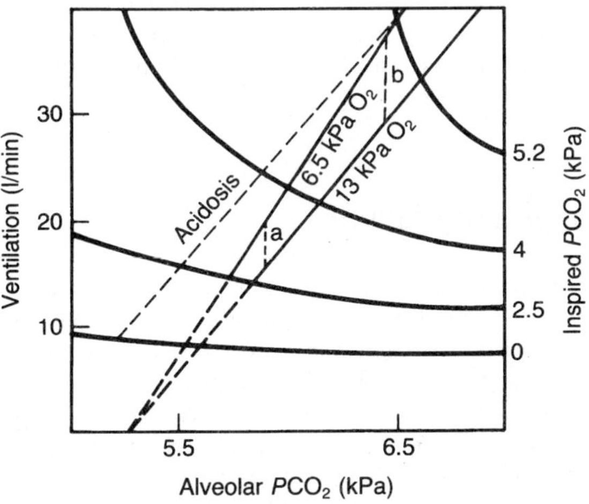

FIGURE 18.3 Changes in ventilation in relation to alveolar P_{CO_2} at different inspired P_{CO_2} values. Note that as inspired P_{CO_2} rises, marked increases in ventilation are required to reduce alveolar P_{CO_2}. The effect of hypoxia is to alter the sensitivity to P_{CO_2} without altering threshold. The effect of reducing inspired P_{O_2} from 13 kPa to 6.5 kPa is shown. Note the much larger increase in ventilation observed with hypoxia at higher inspired P_{CO_2} values (b compared with a). The effect of acidosis is to shift the relationship to the left (i.e. to alter the threshold for stimulation of ventilation by CO_2 but not to alter the sensitivity to CO_2) (dotted line).

This results in a parallel shift of the linear relationship shown for a given P_{O_2} to the left (Fig. 18.3). Alkalosis produces, as would be predicted, a parallel shift to the right of this relationship – that is, an increased threshold to changes in P_{CO_2}.

The above relationships only hold for an ideal system over short time periods, and *in vivo* the effects of changes in P_{CO_2}, P_{O_2} or pH cannot be considered in isolation. The longer term effects of alterations in acid–base balance are more complex. For example, metabolic acidosis initially increases ventilation as would be predicted from the above model, but the increase in ventilation results in a lower P_{aCO_2}, which in turn will increase cerebrospinal fluid (CSF) pH, offsetting the increase in ventilation. Finally, over a period of hours, CSF $[HCO_3]$ will fall (because the blood–brain barrier is less permeable to HCO_3 than to CO_2, so $[HCO_3]$ alters more slowly), and ventilation will again increase.

FACTORS AFFECTING CONTROL OF RESPIRATION

A number of physiological alterations occur in normal individuals which affect control of respiration. Both exercise and sleep produce effects upon respiratory control mechanisms. In addition, respiratory control is altered during exposure to abnormal environmental conditions, of which the best documented situation is exposure to high altitude.

Exercise

The hyperventilation associated with exercise arises as a result of several factors. There is an initial neural stimulus, which is believed to be transmitted through the corticospinal pathways, and acts to produce the early hyperventilation of exercise in conjunction with stimulation from the higher centres. With higher levels of exercise there is a significant CO_2 stimulus and the lactic acidosis of exercise provides a further input. With very high levels of exercise, hypoxia can occur even in normal individuals. In addition to the above, the rise in body temperature occurring on exercise may contribute to hyperventilation.

Sleep

The major change in respiration which occurs during sleep in normal individuals is a reduction in ventilation during rapid eye movement (REM) sleep probably due to reduced hypercapnic drive. The breathing pattern may become erratic. In non-REM sleep chemical drive to respiration is well maintained.

Altitude

A large volume of data exists regarding the physiological response of the body to high altitude. Symptoms of exposure to high altitude occur in most individuals at heights above about 3000 m, and initially consist of headache and nausea with mild breathlessness on exertion due to increased hypoxic drive. With time, CSF $[HCO_3]$ falls in response to the fall in P_{CO_2} caused by hyperventilation. This in turn results in a rise in CSF pH with a subsequent further increase in ventilation, which again causes P_{CO_2} to fall and reduces ventilation. Eventually, acclimatization occurs and a new equilibrium is attained. At very high altitudes (>6500 m), as experienced by Himalayan mountaineers, acclimatization is only partial. Two severe complications of high altitude exposure occur in some individuals, namely high-altitude pulmonary and cerebral oedema, although the mechanisms underlying the aetiology of these conditions remain controversial. The carbonic anhydrase inhibitor, acetazolamide, has been shown to reduce symptoms of acute mountain sickness, although whether it is effective in preventing the life-threatening complications of high altitude exposure remains to be ascertained. Altitude exposure also results in abnormal breathing patterns, with Cheyne–Stokes respiration frequently occurring. This condition also occurs in people with left ventricular failure or bilateral cerebral hemisphere lesions, and is believed to be due to an exaggerated response to hypercapnia; the increase in ventilation lowers P_{CO_2}, which then reduces ventilation, P_{CO_2} rises, and ventilation again increases.

DISEASES AFFECTING RESPIRATORY CONTROL

Hypoventilation and hyperventilation

Hypoventilation can occur due to abnormal respiratory drive, neurological disease affecting the afferent nerve supply to the respiratory muscles, abnormal respiratory muscle function, an abnormal chest wall, or abnormal lungs. In isolated pulmonary disease, the respiratory drive will usually be normal, but the ventilatory response may be reduced. However, in interstitial lung disease (e.g. cryptogenic fibrosing alveolitis), hyperventilation may be a marked feature. Although this in part is due to increased hypoxic drive due to ventilation perfusion mismatch, some of the drive to respiration may come from stimulation of pulmonary stretch receptors. As mentioned above, these receptors are not believed to play a role in the control of respiration in healthy individuals, but when lung compliance is altered by interstitial lung disease, they may become more important. Some of the causes of hypoventilation are given in Table 18.1.

TABLE 18.1 Conditions causing hypoventilation

Central nervous system abnormalities
Cerebrovascular accidents
Arnold–Chiari malformation
Syringomyelia
Viral encephalitis
Other neurological conditions
Cervical cord transection
Guillan–Barré syndrome
Myasthenia gravis
Primary muscle disease
Diaphragmatic paralysis
Myopathies
Other conditions
Primary alveolar hypoventilation
Obesity-hypoventilation (Pickwickian syndrome)
Kyphoscoliosis and other chest-wall deformities

Hyperventilation attacks, characterized by presyncope, numbness, paraesthesia and tetany due to the ensuing respiratory alkalosis, occur in individuals with otherwise normal lung function, and may be a particularly difficult clinical problem. Classically, these attacks may be aborted in some individuals by rebreathing using, for example, a paper bag, which prevents the fall in Pa_{CO_2} which hyperventilation otherwise induces.

Respiratory failure

Respiratory text books tend to recognize two distinct kinds of respiratory failure, with hypoxic respiratory drive being maintained in type I but lost in type II respiratory failure. This distinction has given rise to the description of two kinds of patients, the so-called 'pink puffer' and 'blue bloater'. In reality, there is a continuum within these two extremes. In the patient with maintained hypoxic drive, chronic lung disease (usually due to airflow obstruction) results in a thin, breathless patient who maintains their arterial oxygen saturation well. The patient with type II respiratory failure, on the other hand, is often overweight, cyanosed but not particularly breathless, and has evidence of right heart failure with marked peripheral oedema. The explanation for the loss of hypoxic drive in some individuals with chronic lung disease is unclear, although genetic factors may play a role. Treatment should be aimed at correcting reversible causes of hypoxia (e.g.

reversible airflow obstruction with β_2-adrenoceptor agonists, anticholinergic agents, and, in responsive individuals, steroids), and treating right heart failure if present with diuretics. Trials of long-term domiciliary oxygen (16 h/day) have demonstrated improved survival in patients with cor pulmonale who demonstrate improvement in their hypoxia on oxygen therapy.

Sleep apnoea

Abnormal breathing patterns during sleep may result in significant falls in arterial Po_2. Two major forms of sleep apnoea are recognized, central and obstructive. In the former, periods of apnoea resulting in arterial oxygen desaturation are due to reduced respiratory drive. The aetiology is unclear, but it is presumably due to primary abnormalities of control of the medullary respiratory centre. In contrast, obstructive sleep apnoea is due to intermittent closure of the upper airways by the soft tissues of the pharynx. This condition is commoner in obese individuals and is exacerbated by a high alcohol intake. Nocturnal nasal CPAP can be effective in preventing dips in oxygen saturation during sleep. If left untreated, right heart failure may develop in individuals with frequent episodes of desaturation.

DRUGS AFFECTING RESPIRATORY DRIVE

Respiratory depressants

A number of classes of drugs depress respiratory drive due to their direct central nervous system depressant effects. In addition, agents that act as muscle relaxants will also reduce ventilation, without affecting respiratory drive. These drugs are summarized in Table 18.2.

TABLE 18.2 Drugs causing respiratory depression

General anaesthetics
Narcotic analgesics
Barbiturates
Alcohol
Muscle relaxants

The effects of opiate agents upon respiration can be reversed using naloxone, and the effects of benzodiazepines reversed with flumezanil.

Respiratory stimulants

Central nervous system stimulants increase ventilation by increasing respiratory drive. Agents such as doxapram have been used to some effect in patients with type II respiratory failure, but unfortunately the use of these agents is sometimes limited by poor efficacy or side-effects, the most frequent of which is agitation. In some individuals, convulsions may occur with the use of such agents. Theophyllines produce only small effects on ventilation through their central actions, but have other potential beneficial effects such as bronchodilatation. Progesterone produces a small increase in ventilation and may be responsible for the increased ventilation seen during pregnancy. These agents are summarized in Table 18.3. It should be noted that the use of respiratory stimulants is potentially dangerous in the management of respiratory depression due to overdoses or poisoning.

TABLE 18.3 Drugs stimulating respiration

Theophyllines
Progesterone
Nikethamide
Doxepram
Ethamivan

SUMMARY

This chapter has summarized the factors controlling respiratory drive, and the alterations of respiratory drive control in disease states and by drugs.

FURTHER READING

Kryger MH ed. *Pathophysiology of respiration.* New York: John Wiley, 1981.

19

Pharmacology and Therapeutics

PART I PHARMACOLOGY OF THE AIRWAYS

IP Hall, SJ Hill

INTRODUCTION

The lungs are composed of a variety of tissue types including airway smooth muscle, vascular smooth muscle, inflammatory cells, glandular tissue, secretory epithelial surfaces and the specialized pneumocytes of the alveoli. The majority of the information regarding the effect of drugs on the lungs concerns interactions of these drugs with airway smooth muscle and inflammatory cells. However, it is important to note that the net effect of any agent on the respiratory system as a whole depends upon the balance of the agent's effect on all the tissue types upon which the agent acts within the lungs. This chapter summarizes the effects of a range of drugs important in respiratory pharmacology on airway tone and airway reflexes and in addition covers some aspects of the pharmacology of asthma.

CONTROL OF AIRWAY TONE

The major physiological factor controlling airway tone is the input from the vagus nerve. Postganglionic fibres from the vagus supply all of the airways down to the level of the terminal bronchioles. The stimulation of these fibres results in the release of acetylcholine which contracts the airway smooth muscle via an action at muscarinic receptors. Recently, it has become apparent that several different muscarinic receptor subtypes exist and a range of selective agonists and antagonists have been developed for these receptor subtypes. Airway smooth muscle contains all three muscarinic receptors, the contractile response being mediated through the M_3 subtype.

The initiation of the contractile response of airway smooth muscle in response to spasmogens such as acetylcholine is believed to be mediated through the production of the intracellular second messengers inositol 1,4,5 trisphosphate and diacylglycerol. Inositol 1,4,5 trisphosphate is able to release calcium from intracellular stores, while diacylglycerol can activate protein kinase C and hence alter the sensitivity of the contractile apparatus to changes in intracellular calcium content (Fig. 19.1). The inositol phosphate response to muscarinic stimulation of airway smooth muscle is, like the contractile response, mediated through the M_3 subtype, further supporting a role for the inositol phospholipid signalling system in pharmacomechanical coupling in airway smooth muscle. Following the initiation of the contractile response, calcium may additionally enter the cell from the extracellular stores, either through voltage-dependent channels, or possibly through putative receptor operated (voltage independent) channels.

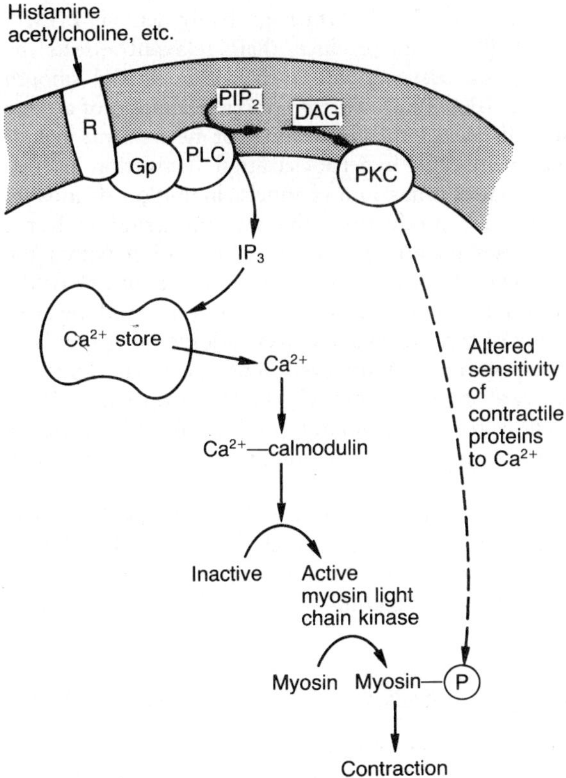

FIGURE 19.1 Inositol phospholipid hydrolysis and contraction of airway smooth muscle. Activation of membrane receptors (R) activates phospholipase C (PLC) via the intermediacy of a GTP-binding protein (G_P) leading to the hydrolysis of a membrane phospholipid (phosphatidylinositol-4,5-bisphosphate; PIP_2) located on the inner leaflet of the cell membrane to form inositol-1,4,5-trisphosphate (IP_3; which is released into the cytosol) and diacylglycerol (DAG; which remains within the membrane environment). IP_3 mobilizes intracellular calcium while DAG activates protein kinase C (PKC) which appears to alter the sensitivity of the contractile proteins to Ca^{2+} ions. Raised intracellular levels of free Ca^{2+} ions lead to the activation of myosin light chain kinase, the phosphorylation of myosin and actin–myosin cross-bridge formation.

In addition to acetylcholine, a wide range of other agents have also been demonstrated to contract airway smooth muscle. The relative importance of these agents in the physiological control of airway tone remains to be determined; however, it is clear that many of them act as mediators of inflammatory and immediate hypersensitivity responses. These agents include histamine, 5-hydroxytryptamine, products of arachidonic acid metabolism such as the leukotriene LTD_4, and a group of agents collectively known as tachykinins, which includes substance P, neurokinin A and neurokinin B. Some of these mediators can be readily demonstrated to be released by inflammatory cells within the airway such as the mast cell in response to a range of stimuli. Others have a potential role as neurotransmitters (including a range of neuropeptides) since they have been identified in nerve endings using immunohistochemical techniques in human airway tissue. Of these neuropeptides some, for example substance P, are potent spasmogens of airway smooth muscle.

Bronchoconstrictor responses can also be elicited by irritant stimuli which are not spasmogens in their own right. This mechanism accounts for the increase in airway resistance seen following provocation with cold air or sulphur dioxide. Stimulation of irritant receptors in the bronchial walls leads via C-fibre afferents to vagally mediated bronchoconstriction. There is some evidence to suggest that, in addition, a local axon reflex may exist in the airways (Fig. 19.2). The afferent input to this reflex again is believed to originate from the stimulation of irritant receptors in the bronchial wall. This is proposed to result in the release of potent bronchoconstrictor neuropeptides such as substance P and neurokinin A from the nerve endings of axon collaterals in the submucosa and underlying airway smooth muscle. Because the neurotransmitters involved are not acetylcholine or noradrenaline, this pathway is known as an excitatory nonadrenergic noncholinergic (e-NANC) system.

As mentioned above, a major source of bronchoconstrictor agents within the airways is inflammatory cells within the bronchi. Both mast cells and eosinophils are likely to be the important sources of histamine and constrictor arachidonic acid metabolites, and can be stimulated to release a range of mediators by a variety of stimuli including allergen. Some of these mediators (e.g. histamine) are spasmogens *per se*, while others are able to influence airway responsiveness by initiating inflammatory response in the bronchial wall resulting in the migration of other inflammatory cells into the lungs. Platelet activating factor (PAF) has attracted attention as a potentially important mediator, but many other pro-inflammatory mediators are formed in inflammatory cells including a group of compounds collectively called cytokines. The cytokines include a range of interleukins which are able to initiate both chemotactic responses and proliferative responses among other inflammatory cell types. In asthmatic airways, interleukins 4 and 5 may play a

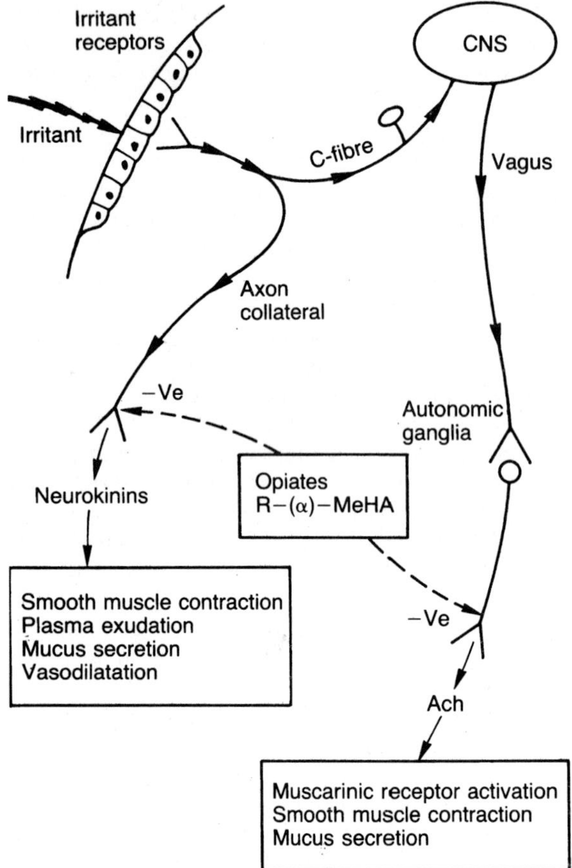

FIGURE 19.2 Neural control of smooth muscle contraction in airways. Stimulation of irritant receptors in the walls of the airways leads via C-fibre activation to vagally mediated smooth muscle contraction. Nerve impulses in the C fibres can also travel along axon collaterals to release neurokinins from the peripheral ends of these bipolar nerve cells leading to smooth muscle contraction, vasodilatation etc. Releases of both acetylcholine (ACh) and neurokinins from vagal or axon collateral nerve endings can be inhibited by opiates or the histamine H_3 receptor agonist R-(α)-methylhistamine (R-(α)-MeHA).

particularly important role. The importance of other inflammatory cell types present in the airway such as alveolar macrophages and neutrophils to the control of airway tone in normal airways is uncertain, but both cell types are potential sources of these inflammatory mediators and may be relevant to the pathogenesis of a range of disease states in which these cells are activated.

BRONCHODILATOR MECHANISMS

Although in some species of animal a functional sympathetic innervation to the airways has been identified, this appears to be absent in man. Hence circulating catecholamines are thought to be the major endogenous source of agents which relax airway smooth muscle by interaction with the β_2-adrenoceptor present on this tissue. There is, however, evidence that an additional mechanism exists for reducing airway smooth muscle tone by stimulation of an inhibitory non-adrenergic, non-cholinergic (i-NANC) pathway. The relevant neurotransmitter remains to be firmly identified in human airways although it may well be vasoactive intestinal peptide (VIP) which is a potent relaxant agent of airway smooth muscle, presumably through its ability to elevate tissue cAMP content through stimulation of adenylate cyclase. There is also increasing evidence that airway epithelium can release a relaxant factor analogous to endothelial derived relaxant factor (EDRF; nitric oxide) which has been labelled epithelial-derived relaxant factor. Finally some products or arachidonic acid metabolism (e.g. PGE_2) are able to relax airway smooth muscle and may play a role in the regulation of airway tone.

All of the above relaxant agents, with the possible exception of EDRF (which probably acts via cGMP) are believed to produce their relaxant effects by increasing tissue cAMP levels within airway smooth muscle (Fig. 19.3). This produces relaxation of airway smooth muscle through a range of mechanisms including membrane hyperpolarization, activation of calcium-gated potassium channels, inhibition of inositol phosphate production (thereby interfering with the processes governing calcium mobilization within the cell; Fig. 19.1), and alteration in the sensitivity of the contractile apparatus to changes in calcium. However, many of these agents may have additional effects (as a result of raised cAMP levels in other cell types) that are relevant to their bronchodilator properties. These include reduced mediator production and release by inflammatory cells and inhibition of the changes in vascular permeability.

In addition to agents elevating cAMP, some agents (e.g. nitric oxide, nitroprusside and probably EDRF) can elevate cGMP within airway smooth muscle leading to tissue relaxation.

BRONCHOSECRETION IN THE AIRWAYS

The airways are capable of secreting both water and mucus. Mucus hypersecretion is a feature of some inflammatory diseases affecting the airways, such as chronic bronchitis. Relatively little is known about the mechanisms underlying these responses *in vivo*. The major controlling influence on mucus secretion appears to be the vagus nerve. The receptor involved in this response is a muscarinic receptor. Histamine is also capable of simulating mucus secretion and both the muscarinic and histaminergic secretory responses can be inhibited by corticosteroids in *in vitro* systems. Recently, mucus secretion has been demonstrated in response to e-NANC stimulation, suggesting the involvement of neuropeptides such as substance P in the control of mucus secretion. This response can be inhibited by opioid agonists (see also p. 284).

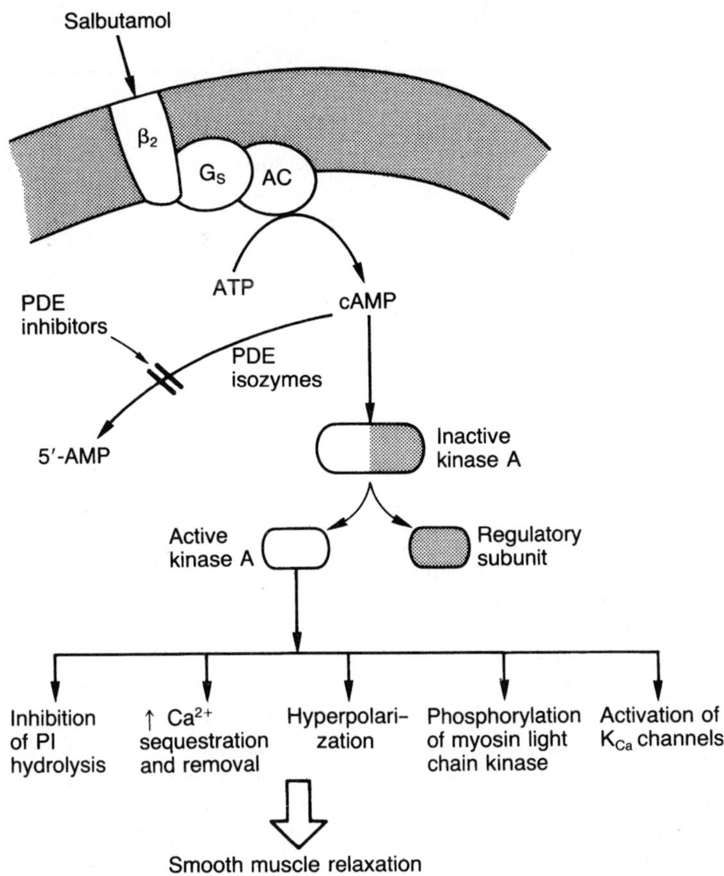

FIGURE 19.3 Accumulation of cyclic AMP (cAMP) and relaxation of airway smooth muscle. Activation of β_2-adrenoceptors leads to the formation of intracellular cyclic AMP from ATP via the enzyme adenylate cyclase (AC). The GTP-binding protein G_S acts as the interface between the extracellular receptor and the catalytic unit of adenylate cyclase. Cyclic AMP then binds to the regulatory unit of protein kinase A to release the active enzyme which produces a number of effects on cell function by phosphorylating a variety of target proteins leading to smooth muscle relaxation. Cyclic AMP is broken down by phosphodiesterases within the cell (see Table 19.1).

BRONCHODILATOR AGENTS

The various agents used as bronchodilators are briefly surveyed below; their detailed clinical pharmacology is given below (p. 287ff).

β-Agonists

β_2-Adrenoceptor agonists are the mainstay bronchodilator agents in clinical use. The most widely used agents are salbutamol and terbutaline (see p. 287). Recently, long-acting inhaled β_2-adrenoceptor agonists, such as salmeterol have been increasingly used. Such agents have the advantage that they can be delivered locally in high dose via inhalers or nebulizers. Cardiac side-effects are kept to a minimum by the use of β_2-selective agents. Although tachyphylaxis to some of the metabolic effects of β-agonists has been reported, there is no evidence to suggest that tachyphylaxis occurs to the bronchodilator effects of these agents.

Muscarinic receptor antagonists

The only muscarinic antagonists in regular clinical usage as a bronchodilator are ipratropium bromide and oxitropium. These are poorly absorbed from the airways and thus side-effects due to muscarinic receptor blockade in other parts of the body can be kept to a minimum following local application (see p. 291). As discussed above, the muscarinic receptor involved in the airway smooth muscle contractile response appears to be the M_3 receptor. Ipratropium bromide is relatively non-selective with regard to muscarinic receptor subtypes and there is clear potential for development of an M_3 antagonist which should have selective effects upon the airway. Ipratropium bromide can be delivered by inhaler or nebulizer.

Phosphodiesterase (PDE) inhibitors

Non-selective phosphodiesterase inhibitors such as the methylxanthine theophylline, often used clinically as theophylline-ethylenediamine (aminophylline), are effective bronchodilator agents given via the intravenous or oral route but have little effect given by nebulizer due to poor local bioavailability. It has become clear that many tissues contain a range of distinct phosphodiesterase isozymes with different selectivity for cAMP, cGMP and differing Michaelis constants (Km) values for their respective substrates (Table 19.1). These individual isozymes are likely to have

TABLE 19.1 Selective inhibitors of phosphodiesterase isozymes. Adapted from Beavo JA, Reifsnyder DH. *Trends in Pharmacological Science* 1990; **11:** 150–5.

ISOZYME FAMILY	SELECTIVITY	SELECTIVE INHIBITORS
PDE_1 Ca^{2+}-calmodulin stimulated	cAMP = cGMP	Trofluoperazine Vinpocetine
PDE_2 cGMP-stimulated	cAMP = cGMP (high concentrations)	None known
PDE_3 cGMP-inhibited	cAMP > cGMP	Milrinone Cilostamide Imazodan
PDE_4 cAMP-specific	cAMP ≫ cGMP	Rolipram
PDE_5 cGMP-specific	cGMP ≫ cAMP	Dipyridamole Zaprinast

Non-selective inhibitors include theophylline, isobutyl-methylxanthine, papaverine and enprophylline.

important regulatory roles within each tissue type. The development of a range of selective inhibitors of the different phosphodiesterase isozymes (Table 19.1) raises the possibility of selectively inhibiting an individual isozyme in a given tissue, and hence improving the therapeutic value of phosphodiesterase inhibitors. Most of the available agents are currently only available as research drugs but there is potential for the development of isozyme selective phosphodiesterase inhibitors for clinical use. Airway smooth muscle cAMP content can be elevated by inhibitors of the type IV isozyme and to a lesser extent in some species by inhibitors of the type III isozyme. Hence, selective inhibitors of these phosphodiesterase isozymes may prove to be useful bronchodilator agents.

There is debate regarding the mode of action of theophylline in the airways. This stems from the observation that theophylline can act as an antagonist at adenosine receptors. However, enprophylline, a related compound which is a PDE inhibitor devoid of adenosine receptor antagonist properties, is also an effective bronchodilator. This suggests that the mechanism of action of theophylline is more likely to be linked to its properties as a non-selective phosphodiesterase inhibitor.

Other agents

A range of other agents have been used as potential bronchodilators. H_1 receptor antagonists would be expected to act as bronchodilators in situations where histamine is being released (e.g. by degranulation of mast cells) but classical H_1 antihistamines are clinically of limited value, although they do provide some protection against the late response to antigen in antigen challenge tests. Recent interest has focused on the efficacy of a number of H_1 antagonists that do not cross the blood–brain barrier (the so-called non-sedating H_1 antihistamines e.g. terfenadine and astemizole). However, the multitude of mediators released in inflammatory reactions makes it unlikely that antagonism of the action of one particular mediator will be an effective strategy. Despite this reservation, 5-lipooxyenase inhibitors and LTD_4 antagonists have shown some potential in initial studies.

Airway smooth muscle contains both calcium-sensitive and ATP-sensitive K^+ channels in common with vascular smooth muscle. Recently, a range of agents capable of activating the ATP-sensitive K^+ channel have been developed. Of these, cromakalim has been the most extensively studied in airway smooth muscle and produces smooth muscle hyperpolarization and relaxation *in vitro*. This and similar compounds (e.g. pinacidil and nicorandil) may have potential as bronchodilator drugs.

A number of agents have been identified that act on presynaptic receptors located on vagal or e-NANC nerve terminals to inhibit neurotransmitter release and hence smooth muscle contraction. These include μ-opiate receptor agonists (e.g. morphine) and histamine H_3-receptor agonists (e.g. R-(α)-methylhistamine) (Fig. 19.2). However, their clinical efficacy remains to be established.

Prophylaxis against bronchoconstriction

Many clinically useful agents for the treatment of asthma depend for their effect not on a bronchodilator action *per se* but upon the ability to reduce the bronchoconstrictor response to subsequent challenge. These agents include corticosteroids, which probably act mainly by inhibiting the synthesis of potential bronchoconstrictor mediators (e.g. PAF and leukotrienes) within airway cells. Although corticosteroids such as hydrocortisone and prednisolone can be administered parenterally or orally, the development of inhaled corticosteroids such as beclomethasone, fluticasone and budesonide has reduced the likelihood of steroid-related side-effects when these agents are used prophylactically in the treatment of asthma. In addition, disodium cromoglycate and nedocromil belong to the category of drugs that act as prophylactic agents in the therapy of asthma. Their mechanism of action *in vivo* remains uncertain although *in vitro* they are both capable of inhibiting mast cell degranulation.

ASTHMA

Asthma can be defined as reversible airflow obstruction resulting in clinical symptoms such as wheeze, cough and breathlessness. The pathological features of asthma include epithelial damage, mucosal oedema and mucus plugging of airways leading to the hypothesis that a chronic inflammatory response is occurring in the airways. It is associated with an increase in non-specific bronchial reactivity to a range of irritant stimuli such as inhaled histamine, methacholine and cold air. Airway reactivity may be measured by determining the dose of an agent such as histamine causing a 20% fall in FEV_1 compared with baseline. This is known as the PD_{20}, and is a useful measurement to enable comparisons of airway reactivity to be made before and after treatment with a given drug. Drugs that act purely as bronchodilators (e.g. ipratropium bromide) have relatively little effect on PD_{20} whereas anti-inflammatory drugs, such as inhaled steroids, can produce marked alterations in PD_{20} when used in subjects with asthma. Many clinical studies of potential anti-asthmatic drugs use change in PD_{20} as an indication of potential therapeutic value. However, although this is a valuable technique, it should be emphasized that not all patients with asthma have demonstrable bronchial hyperresponsiveness and, in addition, increased bronchial reactivity can be demonstrated in a range of other clinical conditions as diverse as cystic fibrosis and heart failure.

Whereas measurement of change in bronchial responsiveness is of potential value in helping to evaluate new anti-asthmatic agents, drugs that act specifically as bronchodilators are best assessed by examining their effects on spirometry alone, or if small changes are being examined, by measuring changes in specific airway conductance (sGAW) using plethysmography in a 'body box'.

Another method of assessing potential anti-asthmatic agents is to examine the effect of the agent upon the airway response to antigen. Sensitive individuals may display a typically biphasic response to antigen challenge, with an early, acute bronchoconstrictor response that resolves relatively rapidly but is then followed several hours later by a late response that resolves more slowly over a period of hours. Agents which have anti-inflammatory properties may attenuate the late response without having an effect upon the early response, whereas agents acting predominantly as bronchodilators will attenuate the early response but will have little effect upon the development of a subsequent late response (Fig. 19.4).

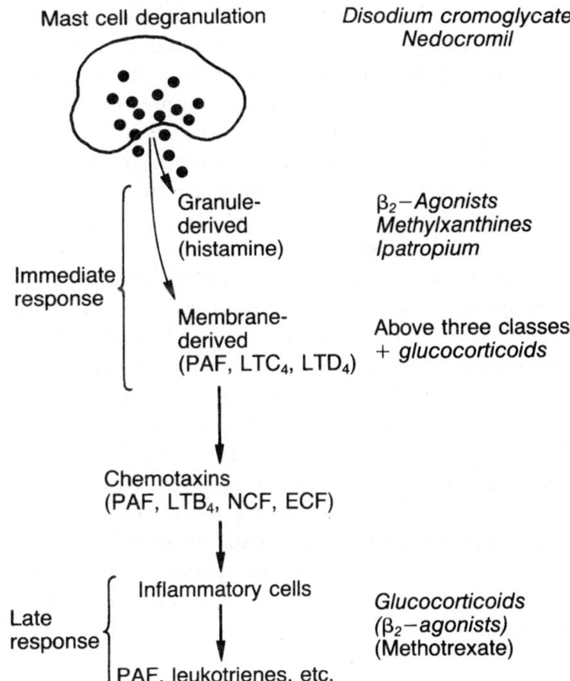

FIGURE 19.4 Treatment of asthma. The rationale behind the use of different agents in the treatment of asthma is partly governed by their underlying mechanism of action. Disodium cromoglycate and nedocramil are used prophylactically because they act to prevent mast cell degranulation. Similarly glucocorticoids are prophylactic because they rely on *de novo* protein synthesis to mediate their inhibitor effects on phospholipase A_2 activity leading to inhibition of leukotriene (LTC_4, LTD_4 and LTB_4) and platelet activating factor (PAF) formation from membrane phospholipids. The direct bronchodilator properties of β_2-agonists, methylxanthines and ipratropium are particularly effective against the immediate bronchoconstrictor responses to both membrane- and granule-derived mediators. Late responses are a consequence of chemotaxin release (e.g. PAF; NCF, neutrophil chemotactic factor; ECF, eosinophil chemotactic factor) and the infiltration of a range of inflammatory cells. These effects can be controlled by corticosteroids and the resulting bronchoconstriction can also be relieved by bronchodilators.

Treatment of asthma

Agents used in the treatment of asthma fall into two categories: (1) bronchodilators, and (2) anti-inflammatory agents. Whereas mild asthmatics will only require occasional doses of inhaled β-agonists, moderately severe asthmatic patients are best controlled on a combination of an inhaled steroid (e.g. beclomethasone or budesonide) and an inhaled β_2-agonist. Some patients obtain additional benefit with inhaled ipratropium bromide or oral theophylline, both of which act predominantly as bronchodilators. Patients with severe symptoms may require long-term oral steroid treatment or frequent short courses of reducing dose steroids. Some of these patients can reduce their steroid intake with the use of disodium cromoglycate or nedocromil, the former being particularly useful in children. Recent studies have suggested that steroid-dependent asthmatics can also reduce their steroid requirement by taking immunosuppressive agents such as methotrexate and cyclosporine.

There has been considerable concern about potential side-effects of the treatment of asthma. The major problems encountered with oral steroids are weight gain, adrenal suppression and osteoporosis. In many patients these effects can be avoided by the use of appropriate doses of inhaled steroids instead of oral prednisolone. Theophylline has a relatively narrow therapeutic window, the therapeutic range being below 20 μg/l. At higher plasma levels, toxic effects may occur such as tachyarrhythmias and convulsions. For this reason intravenous aminophylline should probably be avoided in the emergency treatment of asthma unless the patient is not taking an oral theophylline preparation or the plasma theophylline level is already known. Within the therapeutic range, gastrointestinal side-efects have proved the major therapeutic problem.

Cough reflex and antitussives

Stimulation of irritant receptors in the airway submucosa and epithelial layers results in a forced expiratory manoeuvre against the closed glottis – that is, the cough reflex. The efferent part of this pathway is carried by the vagus. Afferent input is mainly from irritant receptors in the walls of the airways. There is, in addition, evidence that a local axon reflex can result in release of neuropeptides from e-NANC nerve endings which causes further airway narrowing and inflammation, which may in turn exacerbate cough. This is the mechanism whereby capsaicin, an extract from peppers, is believed to produce cough, and this property of capsaicin has been used in clinical studies of cough. Cough can be a major problem clinically, both from a diagnostic point of view and in terms of appropriate treatment. Patients with intractable cough due to local pressure effects from, for example, tumours may respond to radiotherapy or chemotherapy. Antitussives are contraindicated in conditions where cough is appropriate due to increased production of secretions as in pneumonia. The cough reflex can be inhibited by local anaesthetics instilled locally in the airways (e.g. at bronchoscopy), by anticholinergics interfering with vagal efferents and by central suppression with opiates. There are also peripheral μ-opioid receptors present within the airways which may be inhibitory on the local axon reflex although whether this mechanism is relevant to regulation of the cough reflex in healthy human airways remains to be determined. Cough may be a symptom of inadequately controlled asthma, and may then respond to increased anti-asthmatic medication. Finally, in patients with no obvious airway disease, it is worth remembering that cough may be produced by gastro-oesophageal reflux and then may respond to treatment with antacids and/or H_2 antagonists or omeprazole. Cough is also a side-effect of angiotensin-converting enzyme (ACE) inhibitors such as captopril.

FURTHER READING

Beavo JA, Reifsnyder DH. Primary sequence of cyclic nucleotide phosphodiesterase isozymes and the design of selective inhibitors. *Trends in Pharmacological Science* 1990; **11**: 150–5.

British Thoracic Society. Guidelines for management of asthma in adults: 1. Chronic persistent asthma. *British Medical Journal* 1990; **301**: 651–4.

British Thoracic Society. Guidelines for management of asthma in adults: 2. Acute severe asthma. *British Medical Journal* 1990; **301**: 797–800.

Chung KF, Barnes PJ ed. *Pharmacology of the respiratory tract: Experimental and clinical research.* New York: Dekker, 1993.

Coburn RF, Baron CB. Coupling mechanisms in airway smooth muscle. *American Journal of Physiology* 1990; **258**: L119–L133.

Hall IP, Chilvers ER. Inositol phosphates and airway smooth muscle. *Pulmonary Pharmacology* 1989; **2**: 113–20.

PART II THERAPEUTICS IN RESPIRATORY MEDICINE

V Mak, SG Spiro

INTRODUCTION

This part will deal with drugs that are used commonly in respiratory care. Medications such as cytotoxics and immunosuppressive agents, other than inhaled corticosteroids used in the treatment of asthma, will not be discussed.

β_2-ADRENOCEPTOR AGONISTS

β_2-Adrenoceptor agonists are probably the commonest prescribed medication in respiratory practice. They are used in the treatment of asthma and the reversible element of airways obstruction commonly found in chronic obstructive airways disease (COAD). Although there are several different types of β_2-agonist, most are pharmacologically similar and all are used in a similar fashion. The group will therefore be discussed as a whole with individual differences highlighted.

The two commonest β_2-agonists prescribed in the UK are salbutamol (Ventolin^R, Ventodisk^R) and terbutaline sulphate (Bricanyl^R). Other less common drugs include fenoterol hydrobromide (Berotec^R), rimiterol hydrobromide (Pulmadil^R), pirbuterol (Exirel^R), reproterol hydrochloride (Bronchodil^R) and tulobuterol hydrochloride (Brelomax^R). There is no place for the use of orciprenaline and isoprenaline in current practice as they are not β_2-selective and therefore they will not be discussed.

Pharmacology

Salbutamol, terbutaline and fenoterol have a similar molecular structure based on the isoprenaline molecule, but rimiterol has not.

All four agents are selective β_2-adrenoceptor agonists with effects on smooth and skeletal muscle, which include bronchodilatation, relaxation of the uterus and tremor. Both salbutamol and terbutaline are highly β_2-receptor selective, fenoterol less so and rimiterol twenty times less than fenoterol. Therefore, both fenoterol and rimiterol may stimulate the β_1-receptors as well, causing an increase in heart rate and myocardial contractility. Both salbutamol and terbutaline will also increase the heart rate, but this may be due to a reflex response following relaxation of vascular smooth muscle resulting in vasodilatation rather than stimulation of β_1-receptors.

Smooth muscle relaxation is thought to occur following stimulation of the β_2-receptor in the cell membrane causing conversion of ATP to cAMP, which then activates protein kinase. This leads to phosphorylation of proteins which then bind intracellular calcium, reducing its availability for actin–myosin cross-linkage and therefore relaxation of the muscle.

β_2-Agonists also have mild anti-inflammatory activity because they have been shown to inhibit the release of bronchoconstrictor mediators from mast cells *in vitro* and the release of mediators into the circulation following provocation challenge testing *in vivo*. β_2-Agonists have also been shown to enhance mucociliary clearance and have metabolic effects such as raising free fatty acid, glucose and insulin concentrations. Hypokalaemia also occurs commonly, especially following intravenous administration, and is thought to be related to linkage of β_2-receptors to Na^+/K^+-ATPase.

Pharmacokinetics

All β_2-agonists are commonly administered by inhalation of the drug as an aerosol (either from a metered dose inhaler (MDI) or a nebulizer) or as a powder. Salbutamol and terbutaline are also available as oral slow-release tablets, syrups and intravenous preparations. MDIs deliver an aerosol containing particles of drug with a mean median aerodynamic diameter of 2–3 μm which should reach the peripheral airways of the lung. Using direct labelling techniques, it was previously thought that only about 10% of the inhaled aerosol dose actually entered the lungs, the remainder being swallowed. However, recent studies using directly labelled drugs suggest a much higher percentage deposition in the region of 20% in both normal subjects and patients with asthma, and the percentage distribution to the periphery of the lungs can be improved by use of a large volume spacer device (Volumatic^R or Nebuhaler^R), which also greatly reduces the swallowed dose. The maximal therapeutic effect is seen within 15 min of inhalation, which suggests a local action within the lungs as the peak plasma concentration of the drug occurs about 3 h after inhalation. When given as a nebulized solution, an initial peak plasma concentration is seen within 30 min, which is probably due to absorption from the lungs.

Oral preparations of salbutamol are well absorbed (approximately 85%), and terbutaline slightly less so (25–80%), both probably being affected by food in the gastrointestinal tract, and both undergoing significant first-pass metabolism. Oral salbutamol is now only available as Volmax[R], a specially designed capsule that osmotically controls release of the drug by holding it within a core surrounded by a semipermeable membrane with a single pore 250 μm in diameter and produces peak plasma levels 5–6 h after ingestion. The plasma half-life of both drugs is about 2.5–5 h although the terminal half-life of terbutaline is much longer being 14–18 h. When administered intravenously, because of the avoidance of first-pass metabolism, both salbutamol and terbutaline circulate mostly as unchanged drug.

Because of their local effect within the lungs, none of the currently available β_2-agonists shows any relation between plasma concentrations and efficacy when inhaled. However, there is a dose-dependent response when salbutamol or terbutaline are administered orally or intravenously, although assay of levels is not relevant in clinical respiratory practice.

Salbutamol, terbutaline and fenoterol, unlike isoprenaline and rimiterol, are not substrates for metabolism by catechol-O-methyl-transferase (COMT), and are metabolized by conjugation to the sulphate, although some terbutaline is also conjugated as the glucuronide. The main route of excretion is by the kidneys. Rimiterol is metabolized by COMT and the product conjugated by the liver, and as a consequence, has the shortest duration of action of the four agents.

Therapeutic use

These agents are used for their bronchodilator properties in the management of asthma and the reversible airflow element of chronic obstructive bronchitis. Salbutamol and terbutaline are also used in obstetric practice for their tocolytic properties in the management of premature labour.

In the treatment of mild asthma, the agents are given by inhalation as the aerosol or powder for the relief of symptoms or prior to exercise to prevent exercise induced asthma. Recent studies suggest that better control of symptoms may be obtained by 'as required' rather than regular dosing. If symptoms dictate the use of the inhaler more than twice a day, then prophylactic therapy in the form of an inhaled corticosteroid or mast cell stabilizing agent should be considered. Oral preparations of β_2-agonists are useful in patients unable to use the inhaled forms of therapy, although with the introduction of spacer devices and easy-to-use powder delivery systems, this is uncommon. Oral therapy is also useful for the control of troublesome nocturnal symptoms and also daytime symptoms not controlled by high dose inhaled corticosteroid therapy.

In the management of acute severe asthma, the nebulized route is preferred because there are fewer systemic side-effects and a more prolonged effect than when β_2-agonists are given parenterally. Nebulizers can deliver an aerosol with the particle size range of 2–5 μm, similar to the MDI. The nebulized dose of both salbutamol (2.5–5 mg) and terbutaline (5–10 mg) is equivalent to 25–50 puffs of the equivalent MDI and some studies have shown that 25 puffs from an MDI given via a spacer device has an equivalent clinical effect in acute severe asthma. Nebulizers can be driven by oxygen for patients with asthma or air for patients with chronic bronchitis and suspected carbon dioxide retention. Nebulized doses can be given safely every 2–4 h and in very severe cases, even hourly doses can be used, although in this situation the patient may have too small a tidal volume and assisted ventilation should be considered. In ventilated patients, nebulized drug can be given via the ventilator circuit and may be especially useful prior to physiotherapy.

Both salbutamol and terbutaline may be administered intravenously in acute severe asthma, but this has no significant advantages over the inhaled route. Salbutamol can be given as a slow bolus of 250 μg initially followed by an infusion of 5–20 μg/min according to response. Terbutaline is given as a slow bolus of 250–500 μg followed by an infusion 1.5–5 μg/min. The most common side-effects of intravenous therapy are tachycardia and tremor, which may limit the dosage given. Hypokalaemia is also more common during intravenous therapy.

Some patients with chronic bronchitis respond only to very large doses of bronchodilator and in this group, home nebulization using an air compressor has been useful and may replace the MDI. Continuous subcutaneous infusion of terbutaline or salbutamol has also been used in some patients with very variable ('brittle') asthma. In emergencies, both salbutamol and terbutaline can be given as subcutaneous injection, and some patients with a history of sudden catastrophic attacks of asthma may carry preloaded syringes.

Recent surveys into the high mortality rate among asthmatics in New Zealand may have found links with the use of fenoterol. It is now recommended that patients presently using fenoterol should use an alternative β_2-agonist until the matter has been clarified.

Side-effects and overdosage

β_2-agonists have proved extremely safe and free from serious toxic effects. The main side-effect that may limit usage is fine tremor although switching to an alternative agent usually works. Other side-effects include muscle cramps, anxiety and headache. Both tremor and palpitations are more commonly seen when oral dosing or high dose nebulizers are used. Theoretically, care should be taken in patients with ischaemic heart disease or a history of cardiac dysrhythmias when high doses or parenteral treatment are used. Significant hypokalaemia may be seen, especially when parenteral therapy is used, although whether this is clinically significant has not been determined. No fatalities have been reported with overdosage, the main effects being tremor, anxiety, tachycardia, flushing and hypokalaemia and the treatment is mainly supportive.

SALMETEROL

Recently, a new class of long-acting β_2-agonist, salmeterol xinafoate (Serevent[R]) has been introduced. Although undoubtedly a very effective drug, its role in the management of asthma has yet to be determined.

Pharmacology

Salmeterol is similar in structure to salbutamol except that it has the addition of a long non-polar side-chain. Salmeterol is a highly selective β_2-adrenoreceptor agonist, being at least as equipotent as isoprenaline as a bronchodilator. It is fifteen times more potent than salbutamol at the β_2-receptor, but at the cardiac β_1-receptor, it is four times less potent than salbutamol and 10 000 times less potent than isoprenaline. Salmeterol has been shown to protect against bronchoconstriction caused by histamine, methacholine and exercise, and in suppressing late phase bronchoconstriction suggesting that it has some degree of anti-inflammatory activity in addition to its bronchodilator role. It has been shown to suppress the release of inflammatory mediators in the lung and the migration of inflammatory cells.

It is postulated that the prolonged duration of action of salmeterol is due to the long side-chain that may attach itself on to an exoreceptor site near to or within the β_2-receptor. This may allow the active phenylethanolamine head of salmeterol to oscillate in and out of the β_2-receptor site, repeatedly stimulating it. The action of salmeterol can be competitively reversed by β_2-antagonists, but when the antagonist is removed, the muscle-relaxant activity returns without further dosing with salmeterol, suggesting that it may be permanently anchored near the β_2-receptor site.

Pharmacokinetics

Salmeterol can be administered as an aerosol or inhaled as a powder. Its onset of action is slightly slower than that of other inhaled β_2-agonists and, therefore, should not be used as an as-required (reliever) drug. Its duration of action is up to 12 h so that twice-daily dosing is sufficient to control the symptoms of mild asthma. Salmeterol is rapidly absorbed from the lung and is rapidly eliminated, with a plasma half-life of between 2 and 8 h. Salmeterol is extensively metabolized.

Therapeutic use

Because of the slower onset of action of salmeterol compared with other β_2-agonists, it is recommended to be used as a prophylactic agent rather than in the relief of acute symptoms. Because of its long duration of action, salmeterol can control the symptoms of asthma for up to 12 h after dosing, with little evidence of tachyphylaxis to its effects. However, there is concern that this prolonged bronchodilatation may mask underlying inflammation in the lung, the consequence of which in the long term is unknown. For this reason, the use of salmeterol is at present only recommended in those patients whose asthma symptoms are poorly controlled on moderate or high doses of inhaled steroids. However, the addition of salmeterol is complementary to, rather than instead of, inhaled steroids. Whether salmeterol has an effect on the underlying disease process remains to be determined, and until then, its sole use in the management of asthma cannot be recommended.

Side-effects and overdosage

The side-effect profile is similar to that of other β_2-agonists with tremor and palpitations being the most prominent, and there is a risk of hypokalaemia in overdosage. The incidence of side-effects is dose related, and patients seem to develop tachyphylaxis to the unwanted side-effects with time with no reduction in bronchodilator properties. It has been reported to cause anginal-type pain.

THEOPHYLLINE

Theophylline has bronchodilator properties and is used in the treatment of asthma and COAD. Despite theophylline being widely available in a large number of proprietary preparations, its precise mode of action is still unclear (see p. 284). Theophyllines are very popular in the USA and on the continent, but some respiratory physicians in the UK still have reservations about its use, mainly because of the high incidence of side-effects, particularly at the upper limit of its therapeutic range, and the availability of more potent and less toxic alternatives. However, it still retains an important role in the treatment of acute severe asthma.

Pharmacology

Theophylline is a naturally occurring alkaloid found in tea and is a methylxanthine similar to caffeine. It is available as a number of different salts, the most common of which are aminophylline (the ethylenediamine) and choline theophyllinate. All three behave similarly and are considered together.

Theophylline works as a bronchodilator by the relaxation of bronchial smooth muscle. Several mechanisms have been proposed, which include the inhibition of phosphodiesterase to increase intracellular cAMP levels. However, the concentrations of theophylline required to produce measurable increases in cAMP are far outside the levels at which there is a clinical effect. Theophylline is an antagonist of adenosine at pharmacological doses, but a theophylline analogue, enprofylline, does not antagonize adenosine yet still retains potent bronchodilator activity. Recently, theophylline has also been shown to have some anti-inflammatory activity, inhibiting the activity of CD_4 lymphocytes *in vitro* and mediator release from mast cells, and can inhibit bronchoconstriction produced by exercise and challenge testing. Theophylline has also been shown to increase the force of contraction of the diaphragm in patients with COAD although this mechanism of action, and any clinical value of this function, is still disputed.

Theophylline produces bronchodilatation in a concentration-dependent manner and continuous therapy can reduce the symptoms of chronic asthma, reduce the dosage of oral corticosteroids in steroid-dependent asthma, and reduce the requirement for symptomatic use of β_2-agonists. However, theophylline also reduces dyspnoea in patients with COAD without alteration of their lung function which could be due to a central, cardiovascular or diaphragmatic effect. Theophylline is a central nervous system stimulant and can increase minute ventilation in man by stimulation of the medullary respiratory centres. This is thought to be mediated by augmentation of hypoxic ventilatory drive and could account for its effectiveness in reducing apnoeic episodes in premature infants and reducing Cheyne–Stokes respiration. Other effects of theophylline include peripheral and coronary vasodilatation, but in the central nervous system, cerebrovascular vasoconstriction and reduced cerebral blood flow. Theophylline also increases catecholamine release from the adrenal medulla, and as a consequence increases heart rate, force of contraction, cardiac output and blood pressure, and also has mild diuretic properties. Clinically, tolerance develops rapidly to the cardiac, diuretic and central stimulant effects of theophylline but not its bronchodilator properties.

Pharmacokinetics

Theophylline is well absorbed from the gastrointestinal tract with up to 90–100% bioavailability. Peak levels are achieved within 1–2 h following ingestion, but this is slowed by the presence of food. Theophylline is approximately 60% plasma-protein bound and has a mean volume of distribution of 0.5 l/kg. Plasma-protein binding is reduced in infants and in patients with liver cirrhosis. The mean plasma half-life of theophylline is about 8 h in adults although there is large intra- and interindividual variation. It also varies greatly with age, being approximately 30 h in premature neonates, 12 h within the first 6 months, 5 h up to the first year of life and approximately 3.5 h up to the age of 20 years gradually increasing again thereafter.

Because of the relatively short plasma half-life of theophylline, there are many sustained-release preparations available commercially. These all vary as to their bioavailability and the time to peak plasma concentrations. Therefore, once stabilized on one sustained release preparation, patients should not be changed to another without monitoring of plasma levels.

Theophylline is mainly metabolized in the liver by demethylation or oxidation using the cytochrome P-450 system. Only small amounts are excreted by the kidney unchanged, and dosage adjustments in renal failure are unnecessary. However, caution needs to be exercised when using other drugs that are also metabolized by the cytochrome system when dosage adjustments need to be made in conjunction with the measurement of plasma levels.

Many drugs may interfere with the metabolism of theophylline. Special care should be taken with certain antibiotics as patients with acute infective exacerbations of their airways obstruction may be inadvertently put on them without consideration of the effects on theophylline metabolism. These include the macrolide (e.g. erythromycin) and quinolone (e.g. ciprofloxacin) families of antibiotics which both reduce theophylline clearance to varying degrees. Other drugs that reduce theophylline clearance include cimetidine, allopurinol and propanolol (although this would be a rather unusual therapeutic combination). Drugs that increase theophylline metabolism include rifampicin, phenobarbitone and particularly phenytoin and carbamazepine but not the oral contraceptive pill.

The rate of metabolism of theophylline is increased substantially in cigarette smokers (the half-life can be halved), although may not be significant in those who smoke less than 10/day. Smoking marijuana has a similar effect, as can eating a high protein diet. Hepatic dysfunction, heart failure and cor pulmonale all reduce the elimination of theophylline, and low albumin states reduce the amount of protein-bound drug in the blood, thus results of plasma levels need to be interpreted with caution. Therefore, as the clinical state of the patient with heart failure or respiratory failure with cor pulmonale improves, the clearance of theophylline alters, and dosage adjustments may be necessary.

Therapeutic use

Theophylline is used both in the prophylaxis of chronic asthma and COAD, and as emergency treatment in acute severe asthma. Generally theophyllines are used as third- or fourth-line drugs in the control of troublesome asthma. If patients are still symptomatic whilst taking high doses of inhaled corticosteroids and requiring frequent 'rescue' doses of β_2-agonists, especially if they have nocturnal or early morning symptoms, the addition of an oral theophylline preparation may be useful. Sustained release preparations (e.g. Theo-dur, Phyllocontin, Uniphyllin) are preferred because they produce smoother plasma levels throughout a 24-h period and have better patient compliance. Alternatively, if nocturnal and morning symptoms are the most prominent problem with good control during the day, a single bedtime dose of a sustained-release preparation, tailored to give peak levels during the most troublesome hours, may be sufficient.

If theophyllines are required for both day and night time control, plasma levels should be measured to ensure that the patients are within the therapeutic range. Although a rough guide to total daily dosage is 10–15 mg/kg in adults (higher in children) in two divided doses for sustained-release preparations, the interindividual variation in metabolism of theophylline and the effect of smoking, drugs and other factors, can make the initial estimate of dosage requirements in an individual patient a hit and miss affair. It is best to start at a low end of the scale and measure levels after at least 48 h at the same dosage and adjust accordingly.

In acute severe asthma, intravenous theophylline (in the form of aminophylline) is used only when patients fail to respond to the initial treatment of repeated high doses of nebulized β_2-agonists and ipratropium bromide with intravenous corticosteroids. Aminophylline should be given initially as a loading dose of 5–6 mg/kg (in patients not already on oral theophylline) as an intravenous infusion over 15–30 min, followed by a continuous maintenance infusion (see below). In patients that are taking oral theophylline, the use of intravenous theophylline can cause problems as the plasma level will not be known. The measurement of plasma theophylline levels is seldom available in an emergency, and the patient may be uncertain as to when or if they took their last dose (the compliance with oral theophylline can be very poor because of the high incidence of side-effects) or may have taken more than the prescribed dose because of their deteriorating control. Therefore, the administration of a loading dose in this situation may be dangerous as toxic levels may be achieved. In this situation, it is best not to give a loading dose, but to take blood for a theophylline level and just start a maintenance-dose infusion until the result is known and give a loading dose if the result is very low.

The calculation of the maintenance infusion dosage needs to take into account the age of the patient, their smoking history, any concurrent disease and medication. As a rough guide, adult non-smokers should be given 0.4–0.5 mg/kg/h, adult smokers 0.6–0.7 mg/kg/h, and patients with liver dysfunction, heart failure or cor pulmonale 0.2–0.3 mg/kg/h. Adolescents and young children may require higher dosages. Plasma levels should be measured within 24 h of starting the maintenance infusion and the infusion rate adjusted accordingly. There are now several computer programs that can predict plasma levels given certain details of the patient and advise on adjustments in dosage.

Side-effects and overdosage

One of the factors that limits the usefulness of theophylline is the high incidence of side-effects within the therapeutic range and the narrow therapeutic index. As plasma levels exceed 15 mg/l (normal therapeutic range 10–20 mg/l), the frequency of side-effects increases, the most common being a sinus tachycardia, nausea, tremor and indigestion. Indigestion is probably due to theophylline increasing gastric secretion and relaxing the gastro-oesophageal sphincter causing gastro-oesophageal reflux. Patients may also complain of central stimulatory effects such as anxiety, nervousness and insomnia.

Deaths associated with theophylline toxicity have been reported. These may be due to cardiac toxicity leading to life-threatening dysrhythmias, especially in association with anaesthetic agents such as pancuronium and halothane and sympathomimetics. Most deaths are associated with neurotoxicity, and the mortality from theophylline related seizures approaches 30%. These seizures are often initially focal progressing to generalized tonic–clonic convulsions and an encephalopathic picture. There is no close relationship between the plasma level of theophylline and the onset of seizures as this may be also influenced by the presence of hypoxia, hypercapnia and acidosis.

Other clinical features of acute theophylline overdosage include nausea, vomiting, metabolic acidosis, hypokalaemia, gastrointestinal bleeding and rhabdomyolysis. There is no specific treatment, but general measures such as gastric lavage and oral activated charcoal may help reduce plasma levels. With life-threatening levels, haemoperfusion is the most effective form of clearance.

IPRATROPIUM BROMIDE

Ipratropium bromide (Atrovent^{R}) is an anticholinergic agent that is used in the treatment of asthma and the reversible element of chronic obstructive airways disease.

Pharmacology

Ipratropium is a competitive muscarinic acetylcholine receptor antagonist. When given intravenously, it is most potent at inhibition of bronchial receptors, less so of salivary receptors, and has minimal effects on cardiac and urinary bladder receptors. When given by the inhaled route, even in high dosage, the systemic effects are negligible. It produces a dose-related inhibition of bronchoconstriction to a variety of inhaled bronchoconstrictors, including methacholine, and also to exercise-induced asthma. Its effects are dose related but it is a less potent bronchodilator than the β_2-agonists in asthma although it may be equipotent in patients with COAD and in the elderly. In patients with asthma, the combination of ipratropium and a β_2-agonist may be synergistic.

Pharmacokinetics

The onset of action of ipratropium when given by the inhaled route is slower than that of the β_2-agonists, being in the region of 30–60 min and its effects last up to 4 h. Very little of the drug is absorbed following inhalation or ingestion so hepatic or renal impairment has little effect on its therapeutic use.

Therapeutic use

Ipratropium is used in the management of patients with asthma whose symptoms are poorly controlled on prophylactic therapy with high-dose inhaled corticosteroids and regular β_2-agonists. It may be used before or after the addition of theophylline, but because of its slower onset of action, it is not recommended to be used as a first-line therapy in the management of mild asthma.

In acute severe asthma, nebulized ipratropium (250–500 μg 2–4 hourly) in conjunction with nebulized β_2-agonists can be used when patients fail to respond satisfactorily to initial treatment with high doses of nebulized β_2-agonists and intravenous corticosteroids.

Ipratropium is more commonly used in the management of COAD, especially in those who respond poorly to inhaled β_2-agonists alone. Ideally, a demonstrable improvement in an index of lung function following inhalation of ipratropium should be sought before commencing a patient on treatment with the drug, although in practice this is rarely done. The use of nebulized ipratropium (250–500 μg 4–6 hour) in combination with a nebulized β_2-agonist is common in patients with severe COAD using home nebulizer therapy.

Care should be taken with treatment with nebulized ipratropium as paradoxical bronchoconstriction has been reported. Initially, this was thought to be due to the preservatives used (benzalkonium chloride and EDTA) or the hypotonic nature of the nebulizer solution, but there have been similar reports with the unpreserved isotonic preparation.

Side-effects and overdosage

These are rare as there is little systemic absorption. Some patients may report a dry mouth due to effects on the salivary glands. Drying of bronchial secretions with difficulty with expectoration, glaucoma and acute urinary retention are theoretically possible. However, systemic effects are rarely seen, even with high-dose nebulized therapy.

INHALED CORTICOSTEROIDS

Inhaled corticosteroids are now widely used in the management of asthma. Their proven efficacy and safety has led them to be regarded as the mainstay of therapy in the prophylaxis of asthma. The two drugs available are beclomethasone dipropionate (Becotide[R], Becloforte[R]) and budesonide (Pulmicort[R]). Bextasol is now no longer available.

Pharmacology

Both beclomethasone dipropionate (BDP) and budesonide (BUD) are topically active glucocorticoids that have both anti-inflammatory and immunosuppressive activity. Both have glucocorticoid effects when given systemically in that they bind to the glucocorticoid receptor and have the usual effects on protein and carbohydrate metabolism as hydrocortisone and prednisolone. When inhaled, both drugs inhibit phospholipase A_2 locally, thereby reducing the formation of prostaglandins and leucotrienes, and they also inhibit neutrophil and macrophage adherence in the capillaries of inflamed tissues, reducing the inflammatory response.

Both drugs reduce bronchial hyperresponsiveness in asthmatics and a single dose can modify the late-phase response to inhaled allergens. When taken over a period of several days, both drugs may also prevent the early-phase response to inhaled allergens and exercise. Clinically, both drugs when taken regularly reduce the frequency of asthma symptoms and 'rescue' bronchodilator requirements, and for patients on long-term oral corticosteroid therapy, may allow a reduction in dose or complete withdrawal of oral steroids.

Pharmacokinetics

Both drugs can be inhaled either as an aerosol from a MDI or nebulizer, or as a powder. Although both drugs rely on their topical activity, there may be significant systemic absorption from the lungs. Also, because a large proportion of the inhaled dose impacts in the oropharynx, they are absorbed from the gastrointestinal tract, but undergo significant first-pass hepatic metabolism. The plasma half-life of BUD is 90–120 min in adults and is metabolized in the liver to inactive metabolites. BDP, however, as well as hepatic metabolism to inactive metabolites, also undergoes metabolism the lung to beclomethasone monopropionate which is pharmacologically active (although less potent than BDP) and cleared four times slower than BUD.

Therapeutic use

Both drugs are used in the control of asthma (and also rhinitis). It is now recommended that any asthmatic patient that needs to use a bronchodilator more than once or twice a day on a regular basis should be treated with a prophylactic anti-inflammatory agent such as an inhaled corticosteroid. It should be stressed to patients that an inhaled corticosteroid will have no effect when taken for acute symptoms as this misunderstanding can lead to poor compliance with these agents. Also, if a patient is just starting on inhaled corticosteroids, they should also be warned that it may take a week or two before they see an improvement in their symptoms. Inhaled corticosteroids are now preferred to oral steroids because of the reduced incidence of glucocorticoid side-effects for the equivalent clinical effect.

The usual dose for maintenance treatment is in the range 200–800μg/day for both BDP and BUD, usually in 2–4 divided doses. BUD is clinically slightly more potent than BDP. For patients who are still poorly controlled, dosages can be increased up to 2000μg/day for BDP and 1600μg/day for BUD, but it is thought that dosages above this level convey no further advantages, and oral steroid therapy should be added if control is still poor. Also, in patients poorly controlled on high doses of inhaled corticosteroids, four times a day dosing is thought to be more effective than twice daily. For BDP, the dose using a powder delivery system for the same clinical effect is usually double that of aerosol, but for BUD, the dose of the powder is equivalent to that of the aerosol.

It is now recommended that patients increase the dosage of their inhaled corticosteroids whenever they detect a deterioration in their asthma control (by home peak flow monitoring). They can be given a set of written instructions as to how much to increase the dosage by according to their peak flow, and at what stage to seek further medical advice. By this means, early intervention may avoid further deterioration requiring a course of oral steroids.

Side-effects and overdosage

The side-effects of the two drugs can be divided into those caused by local deposition in the oropharynx, and those caused by systemic absorption. Patients may complain of a sore or dry throat, and occasionally, oropharyngeal candidiasis may occur. This can be prevented to some extent by gargling and rinsing of the mouth after inhaling the drug and the use of a large volume spacer device (Volumatic^{R}, Nebuhaler^{R}) to reduce oropharyngeal deposition. Severe cases may need treatment with antifungal lozenges. Hoarseness and dysphonia may occur, and this may be due to atrophy of vocal cord tissues or a localized myopathy of the vocal cord musculature. This is reversible on reducing the dose, using a spacer device or withdrawal of treatment.

Systemic side-effects are seen in high dosage. Both drugs can cause suppression of the hypothalamic–pituitary–adrenal (HPA) axis (usually at dosages >1500μg/day for BDP and >1600μg/day for BUD in adults). Suppression of the HPA axis has been seen in children taking 800μg/day of BDP but there has been no convincing evidence of growth suppression. Although HPA axis is known to occur, no serious effects due to acute glucocorticoid deficiency have been reported in patients taking these drugs. Because most of the systemic activity is due to absorption via the lungs, the use of spacer devices may not prevent this, and may actually increase delivery to the lungs.

Recently, there have been reports of increased bone turnover in normal subjects taking BDP but not BUD, which may lead to osteoporosis in long-term use. Other systemic effects that have been reported include increased easy bruising and dermal thinning and possibly cataract formation. It should be noted that systemic effects may be common with BDP rather than BUD because of the faster systemic clearance of BUD with the formation of inactive metabolites.

OTHER ANTI-ALLERGIC AGENTS

Sodium cromoglycate (Intal^{R}) and nedocromil sodium (Tilade^{R}) are anti-inflammatory agents used in the prophylaxis of asthma.

Pharmacology

Neither sodium cromoglycate (SCG) nor nedocromil sodium (NS) have direct bronchodilator or antihistamine properties, and neither is related to corticosteroids. When SCG is inhaled prior to challenge, it is capable of inhibiting both the early- and late-phase response to a variety of inhaled allergens, bronchoconstrictor agents such as sulphur dioxide, and exercise. It was originally thought that the mode of action of SCG was by inhibition of mediator release from activated mast cells, but its ability to block the bronchoconstriction caused by irritant stimuli and exercise suggests that this is not the sole mechanism. SCG obviously modifies the release of inflammatory mediators but the exact mode of action of remains to be determined.

Nedocromil sodium has been shown to inhibit the release of inflammatory mediators from a variety of inflammatory cells. Like SCG, when inhaled prior to challenge, it is capable of inhibiting the early- and late-phase response to inhaled allergens, bronchoconstrictor agents and exercise, and is thought to be more effective than SCG, especially in older patients.

Pharmacokinetics

Both drugs are taken by the inhaled route using either an aerosol or powder for SCG and in the form of an aerosol for NS. The plasma half-life is approximately 90 min for SCG and 2 h for NS. Since both drugs are topically active, there is no relationship between plasma levels and clinical effect. Neither drug undergoes any significant metabolism and both are excreted in urine and faeces.

Therapeutic use

Both drugs are used in the prophylaxis of asthma. Since neither drug has direct bronchodilator properties, they have no effect on the acute symptoms of asthma and it should be stressed that they are not to be used as 'rescue' therapy. When taken on a regular basis, both drugs will reduce the frequency of symptoms of asthma and may prevent asthma induced by a variety of stimuli including exercise, cold air and other inhaled irritants. SCG is taken in the dosage range 20–160 mg/day and NS 8–16 mg/day. Sodium cromoglycate seems to be more effective in younger patients, especially those that have a definite allergic element to their asthma. Nedocromil sodium is effective in adults and is thought to be equivalent to about 400 μg/day of beclomethasone dipropionate in the control of asthma, and is a possible alternative to inhaled corticosteroids in the initial management of mild asthma or can be used to reduce the requirements of inhaled corticosteroids.

Sodium cromoglycate is also available in a variety of preparations for the treatment of seasonal rhinitis and ocular symptoms due to hayfever.

Side-effects and overdosage

No serious side-effects from SCG or NS have been recorded. Some patients may complain of an odd taste following the inhalation of NS.

DOXAPRAM HYDROCHLORIDE

Doxapram hydrochloride (Dopram[R]) is a central nervous system stimulant (analeptic agent). It is used as a respiratory stimulant but has only a limited role in the management of respiratory failure. Formerly, nikethamide and ethamivan were used as respiratory stimulants but are no longer recommended because the effective doses were close to toxic levels.

Pharmacology

When given intravenously to normal subjects, it causes an increase in tidal volume and respiratory rate, thereby increasing minute volume with a concomitant fall in $Pa\text{CO}_2$ and rise in $Pa\text{O}_2$. This effect in animals is dependent upon an intact respiratory centre and is mediated by increased neuromuscular drive in a dose-dependent fashion. The main mode of action is thought to be due to specific stimulation of peripheral chemoreceptors, especially in the carotid body. Doxapram can antagonize the blunted ventilatory response to carbon dioxide caused by opiates and can also antagonize respiratory depression caused by ethanol.

Doxapram also has effects on the cardiovascular system including an increase in stroke volume and an increase in blood pressure. In higher dosages, there is non-specific stimulation of the central nervous system which may lead to convulsions.

Pharmacokinetics

Doxapram is given intravenously and has a half-life of about 3 h and has a mean volume of distribution of about 1.5 l/kg in adults. It is mainly metabolized by the liver and one of its main metabolites, keto-doxapram has slight pharmacological activity and accumulates during continuous intravenous infusion.

Therapeutic use

The use of doxapram in the management of acute hypercapnic respiratory failure is limited to those patients who are unsuitable for intubation and ventilation (i.e. patients with acute or chronic respiratory failure). When doxapram is used, it should be in conjunction with other supportive measures such as controlled oxygen therapy, nebulized bronchodilators, physiotherapy and more recently, nasal ventilatory support. Its short half-life requires that it is given as a continuous intravenous infusion and there is some evidence that there may be tachyphylaxis as the infusion rate may need to be increased with time to give an equivalent therapeutic effect, but this may just represent worsening of the underlying condition. The usual infusion rate is 1–4 mg/min according to clinical response and blood gas measurements. It should only be used where facilities for close patient monitoring are available. The use of doxapram is absolutely contraindicated in the treatment of respiratory failure secondary to acute severe asthma, pulmonary embolism, pulmonary oedema, pneumothorax and other causes of non-hypercapnic respiratory failure.

Doxapram is also used in the treatment of respiratory depression following general anaesthesia. It can antagonize the respiratory-depressant effects of opiate analgesics without inhibition of their analgesic properties. It is usually given as an intravenous injection of 1–1.5 mg/kg repeated after 1 h. If further injections are required, a continuous infusion may be necessary. The short duration of action after a single dose is due to redistribution of the drug rather than to metabolism.

Doxapram is also contraindicated in patients with epilepsy, severe hypertension, hyperthyroidism and ischaemic heart disease. It should not be used in respiratory depression due to intracranial pathology.

Side-effects and overdosage

General stimulation of the central nervous system may occur even within the therapeutic range. There may be muscle fasciculation or spasm and a risk of generalized seizures. There is often a slight rise in blood pressure and an increased incidence of dysrhythmias. Non-specific side-effects include headache, dizziness, agitation, confusion, nausea, vomiting and perineal warmth on intravenous injection. Side-effects may be more common if there is concomitant use of theophyllines, as is often the case. It should also be noted that doxapram cannot be given in the same infusion line as aminophylline as the two are incompatible. Because patients become more aroused with doxapram, they may become more aware of their dyspnoea and the increased respiratory drive may make bronchospasm more obvious and increase coughing. Toxic side-effects should be treated symptomatically.

FURTHER READING

Ali NJ, Capewell S, Ward MJ. Bone turnover during high dose inhaled corticosteroid treatment. *Thorax* 1991; **46:** 160–4.

Anderson JB, Jenson NH, Klausen NO. A pharmacologic respiratory stimulant, doxapram, used in acute deterioration in patients with chronic respiratory failure. *Ugeskr-Laeger* 1989; **151:** 1820–2.

Assoufi BK, Hodson ME. High dose salbutamol in chronic airflow obstruction: comparison of nebulizer with Rotacaps. *Respiratory Medicine* 1989; **83:** 415–20.

Barnes PJ, Pride NB. Dose response curves to inhaled β-adrenoceptor agonist in normal and asthmatic subjects. *British Journal of Clinical Pharmacology* 1983; **15:** 617–82.

Barros MJ, Rees PJ. Bronchodilator responses to salbutamol followed by ipratropium bromide in partially reversible airflow obstruction. *Respiratory Medicine* 1990; **84:** 371–5.

Bisgaard H, Nielson M, Andersson B, Andersson P, Foged N, Fuglsarg G, *et al.* Adrenal function in children with bronchial asthma treated with beclomethasone dipropionate or budesonide. *Journal of Allergy and Clinical Immunology* 1988; **81:** 1088–95.

Boe J, Rosenhall L, Alton M, Carlsson LG, Carlsson U, Hermansson BA, *et al.* Comparison of dose–response effects of inhaled beclomethasone dipropionate and budesonide in the management of asthma. *Allergy* 1989; **44:** 349–55.

Bone MF, Kubik MM, Keaney NP, Summers GD, Connolly CK, Sherwood Burge P, Dent RG, Allan GW. Nedocromil sodium in adults with asthma dependent on inhaled corticosteroids: a double blind, placebo controlled study. *Thorax* 1989; **44:** 654–9.

Brenner M, Berkowitz R, Marshall N, Strunk RC. Need for theophylline in severe steroid-requiring asthmatics. *Clinical Allergy* 1988; **18:** 143–50.

British Thoracic Society. Guidelines for the management of asthma in adults: I – Chronic persistent asthma. *British Medical Journal* 1990; **301:** 651–3.

British Thoracic Society. Guidelines for the management of asthma in adults: II – Acute severe asthma. *British Medical Journal* 1990; **301:** 797–800.

Brown PH, Blundell G, Greening AP, Crompton GK. Hypothalamo-pituitary-adrenal axis suppression in asthmatics inhaling high dose corticosteroids. *Respiratory Medicine* 1991; **85:** 501–10.

Capewell S, Reynolds S, Shuttleworth D, Edwards C, Finlay AY. Purpura and dermal thinning associated with high dose inhaled corticosteroids. *British Medical Journal* 1990; **300:** 1548–51.

Cheong B, Reynolds SR, Rajan G, Ward MJ. Intravenous β-agonist in severe acute asthma. *British Medical Journal* 1988; **297:** 448–50.

Clark TJH, Yernault JC eds. Proceedings of the first 'Serevent International Symposium'. *European Respiratory Journal* 1991; **1** (Review 4).

Corris PA, Neville E, Nariman S, Gibson GJ. Dose response study of inhaled salbutamol powder in chronic airflow obstruction. *Thorax* 1983; **38:** 292–6.

Ebden P, Jenkins A, Houston G, Davies BH. Comparison of two high-dose corticosteroid aerosol treatments, beclomethasone dipropionate (1500 mcg/day) and budesonide (1600 mcg/day), for chronic asthma. *Thorax* 1986; **41:** 869–74.

Fairfax AJ, Allbeson M. A double-blind group comparative trial of nedocromil sodium and placebo in the management of bronchial asthma. *Journal of International Medical Research* 1988; **16:** 216–24.

Franko BV, Ward JM. Nikethamide and doxapram effects on pentazocine and morphine induced respiratory depression. *Journal of Pharmacy and Pharmacology* 1971; **23:** 709–10.

Gordon ACH, McDonald CF, Thomson SA, Frame MH, Pottage A, Crompton GK. Dose of inhaled budesonide required to produce clinical suppression of plasma cortisol. *European Journal of Respiratory Disease* 1987; **71:** 10–14.

Grainger J, Woodman K, Pearce N, Crane J, Burgess C, Keane A, Beasley R. Prescribed fenoterol and death from asthma in New Zealand, 1981–7: a further case-control study. *Thorax* 1991; **46:** 105–11.

Grandordy BM, Thomas V, de Lauture D, Marsac J. Cumulative dose–response curves for assessing combined effects of salbutamol and ipratropium bromide in chronic asthma. *European Respiratory Journal* 1988; **1:** 531–5.

Grygiel JJ, Birkett DJ. Cigarette smoking and theophylline clearance and metabolism. *Clinical Pharmacology and Therapeutics* 1981; **30**: 491–6.

Hetzel MRH, Clark. Adult asthma. In: Clark TJH, Godfrey S eds. *Asthma*, 2nd edn. London: Chapman & Hall, 1983: 457–89.

Holgate ST. Reflections on the mechanism(s) of action of sodium cromoglycate (Intal) and the role of mast cells in asthma. *Respiratory Medicine* 1989; **83** (Suppl A): 25–31.

Jenne JW. Theophylline use in asthma: some current issues. *Clinics in Chest Medicine* 1984; **5**: 645–58.

Jonkman JHG, Upton RA. Pharmacokinetic drug interactions with theophylline. *Clinical Pharmacology* 1984; **9**: 309–34.

Kronig P, Hordvik NL, Kreutz C. The preventive effect and duration of action of nedocromil sodium and cromolyn sodium on exercise-induced asthma (EIA) in adults. *Journal of Allergy and Clinical Immunology* 1987; **79**: 64–8.

Kuzemko JA. Twenty years of sodium cromoglycate treatment: a short review. *Respiratory Medicine* 1989; **83** (Suppl A): 11–16.

Lawford P, Jones BJM, Milledge JS. Comparison of intravenous and nebulized salbutamol in the initial treatment of severe asthma. *British Medical Journal* 1978; **1**: 84.

Madsen BW, Tandon MK, Patterson JW. Cross-over study of the efficacy of four β_2-sympathomimetic bronchodilator aerosols. *British Journal of Clinical Pharmacology* 1979; **8**: 75–82.

Moser KM, Luchsinger PC, Adamson JS, McMahon SL, Schlueter DP, Spivack M, Weg JG. Respiratory stimulation with intravenous doxapram in respiratory failure. *New England Journal of Medicine* 1973; **288**: 427–31.

Nassif EG, Weinberger M, Thompson R, Huntly W. The value of maintenance theophylline in steroid-dependent asthma. *New England Journal of Medicine* 1981; **304**: 71–5.

Neville E, Gribbin H, Harrison BDW. Acute severe asthma. *Respiratory Medicine* 1991; **85**: 463–74.

Newman SP, Clarke SW. Therapeutic aerosols 1 – Physical and practical considerations. *Thorax* 1983; **38**: 881–6.

Newman SP, Miller AG, Leannard-Jones TR, Moren F, Clarke SW. Improvement of pressurised aerosol deposition with Nebuhaler spacer device. *Thorax* 1984; **39**: 935–41.

O'Driscoll BRC, Ruffles SP, Ayres JG, Cochrane GM. Long term treatment of severe asthma with subcutaneous terbutaline. *British Journal of Diseases of the Chest* 1988; **82**: 360–7.

Racineaux JI, Troussier J, Turcant A, Tuchais E, Allain P. Comparison of bronchodilation effects of salbutamol and theophylline. *Bulletin European de Physiopathologie Respiratoire* 1981; **17**: 799–806.

Reed CH. Aerosol glucocorticoid treatment of asthma. *American Review of Respiratory Disease* 1990; **141**: S82–S88.

Rossing TH, Fanta CH, Goldstein DH, Snapper JR, McFadden ER. Emergency therapy of asthma: comparison of the acute effects of parenteral and inhaled sympathomimetics and infused aminophylline. *American Review of Respiratory Disease* 1980; **122**: 365–71.

Smith MJ, Hodson ME. High-dose beclomethasone inhaler in the treatment of asthma. *Lancet* 1983; **i**: 265–9.

Stead RJ, Cooke NJ. Adverse effects of inhaled corticosteroids. *British Medical Journal* 1989; **298**: 403–4.

Tandon MK, Kailis SG. Bronchodilator treatment for partially reversible chronic obstructive airways disease. *Thorax* 1991; **46**: 248–51.

Tattersfield AE. Autonomic bronchodilators. In: Clark TJH, Godfrey S eds. *Asthma*, 2nd edn. London: Chapman & Hall, 1983: 301–35.

Thomson NC. Nedocromil Sodium: an overview. *Respiratory Medicine* 1989; **83**: 269–76.

Toogood JH. Complications of topical steroid therapy for asthma. *American Review of Respiratory Disease* 1990; **141**: S89–S96.

Ullah MI, Newman GB, Saunders KB. Influence of age on response to ipratropium and salbutamol in asthma. *Thorax* 1981; **36**: 523–9.

Ullman A, Svedmyr N. Salmeterol, a new long acting inhaled β_2-adrenoceptor agonist: comparison with salbutamol in adult asthmatic patients. *Thorax* 1988; **43**: 674–8.

Vozeh S, Kewitz G, Perruchoud A *et al.* Theophylline serum concentration and therapeutic effect in severe acute bronchial obstruction: the optimal use of intravenously administered aminophylline. *American Review of Respiratory Disease* 1982; **125**: 181–4.

Ward MJ, Fentem PH, Roderick Smith WH, Davies D. Ipratropium bromide in acute asthma. *British Medical Journal* 1981; **282**: 598–600.

Warner JO. The place of Intal in paediatric practice. *Respiratory Medicine* 1989; **83** (Suppl A): 33–7.

Weinberger M, Hendeles L. Slow-release theophylline: rationale and basis for product selection. *New England Journal of Medicine* 1983; **308**: 760–4.

Wolfe JD, Tashkin DP, Calvarese B, Simmons M. Bronchodilator effects of terbutaline and aminophylline alone and in combination in asthmatic patients. *New England Journal of Medicine* 1978; **298**: 363–7.

SECTION SIX

Drugs Acting on the Central Nervous System

20

Central Nervous System Pharmacology

PV Taberner

INTRODUCTION TO THE PHARMACOLOGY OF THE CENTRAL NERVOUS SYSTEM

Neuropharmacology can be defined as the study of drugs that act on the nervous system in general, but whereas the drugs that act on the peripheral nervous system are well understood in terms of their mode of action, those that act on the CNS (and they represent the majority of drugs in current use) are much less well understood. This lack of knowledge is reflected in the names given to the various groups of drugs. In the periphery, the autonomic drugs are classified in terms of their precise mechanism of action; so we talk of depolarizing neuromuscular blockers or adrenergic β-blockers. In the CNS the drugs are described in terms of their indications or uses: antidepressants, stimulants, sedative-hypnotics, neuroleptics, anxiolytics, and so on. These descriptions disguise the fact that, in most cases, the exact means by which the therapeutic benefit is brought about is still unclear.

It is only recently, with the development of microelectrodes, microdialysis, voltametry and non-invasive imaging techniques, that the brain has become accessible to experimental investigation to the extent that drug effects on specific neural pathways can be determined. The selectivity of action of CNS drugs is based on the fact that different groups of neurones employ different neurotransmitters. Consequently, the identification of the transmitters in specific pathways in the CNS is an important aspect of the development of potentially useful drugs.

CRITERIA FOR A NEUROTRANSMITTER ROLE

The traditional means of establishing the identity of a chemical neurotransmitter, that is, demonstrating release of the chemical from a nerve terminal following stimulation of the axon and stimulation of the postsynaptic neuron by application of the chemical, cannot be easily applied to the CNS. The complexity of the neuronal circuitry and the difficulty of applying a candidate transmitter sufficiently locally so as to excite a specific group of neurones make it almost impossible to conduct these crucial tests. To overcome this problem, a set of criteria has been developed for the identification of CNS transmitters.

1 Differential distribution of the transmitter, which should be localized in the terminals from which it is released. This can be demonstrated directly using histochemical and cytochemical techniques, or inferred from depletion of the transmitter due to neuronal degeneration following lesioning of the nerve cell bodies.
2 The presence of enzymes for the synthesis and degradation of the transmitter. This may apply to non-peptide transmitters, but peptides are synthesized in the nucleus of the cell body (which can be some distance from the terminal) and pass down the axon to the nerve terminal. Enzymes and peptides can be localized using immunocytochemical methods.
3 The existence of a storage system for the transmitter. This usually implies the presence of specific vesicles in the nerve terminal. Their existence is well established for acetylcholine and the monoamines

and has recently been shown in excitatory amino-acid releasing terminals.

4 A release mechanism that is Ca^{2+} dependent. This is important because chemical or electrical stimulation of nerves can lead to the calcium-independent release of a number of metabolites that are unrelated to the transmitter.

5 A mechanism for the rapid termination of the synaptic actions of the released transmitter. This may consist either of a highly active enzyme in the synaptic cleft (e.g. acetylcholinesterase), or a specific neuronal or glial uptake system (these have been demonstrated for the monoamine and amino acid transmitters).

6 Mimicry of the effects of the normal transmitter. This can be shown by micro-iontophoresis of the suspected transmitter through a multibarrelled pipette on to the appropriate cell, with simultaneous recording of the cell membrane potential. By including a selective antagonist in another barrel of the micropipette, confirmatory pharmacological evidence of specific receptor sites can be obtained. It should be noted, however, that a number of naturally occurring compounds, in particular the acidic amino acids, are capable of depolarizing the majority of CNS neurones. This evidence alone does not demonstrate a neurotransmitter role for these compounds.

An idealized nerve terminal illustrating all these features is shown in Fig. 20.1.

ORGANIZATION IN THE CENTRAL NERVOUS SYSTEM

In contrast to the peripheral nervous system where the principal function is to relay signals along afferent

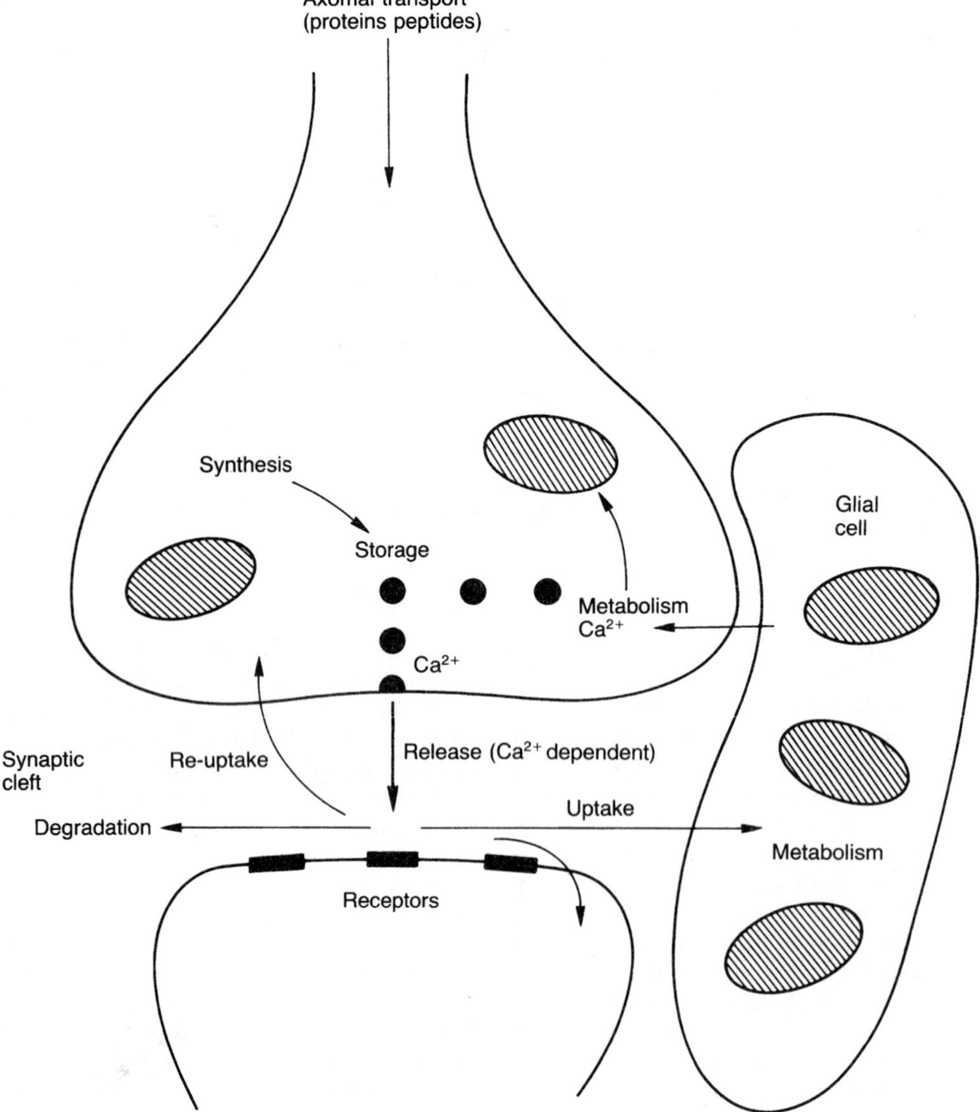

FIGURE 20.1 A generalized nerve terminal to show transmitter synthesis, storage, release, re-uptake, and metabolism.

(sensory) or efferent (effector) pathways, the CNS also has an integrative function in which a single neurone can have many branches (dendrites) and form synapses with very many other neurones. This branching is most clearly seen in the beautiful images obtained by Golgi staining of sections of the cerebellar cortex. The circuitry of the CNS can be conveniently divided into two general patterns: the hierarchical system, normally consisting of myelinated fibres that conduct signals along well-defined pathways, as in the sensory and motor pathways of the spinal cord and cerebellum; and diffuse pathways in which dendrites from specific groups of cell bodies innervate large areas of the brain. The noradrenergic cells originating in the locus coeruleus spread fine non-myelinated axons to extensive regions of the neocortex. The monoamines, dopamine, noradrenaline and 5-hydroxytryptamine (5-HT) seem to be the principal transmitters in these diffuse systems and are responsible for regulating the more global functions of the CNS such as sleeping, waking, mood and appetite.

EXCITATION AND INHIBITION IN THE CNS

Nerve cells are stimulated to fire an action potential by becoming depolarized. Briefly, the cell membrane is normally less permeable to sodium than potassium. Potassium levels are higher inside the cell than outside, whereas sodium levels are higher outside, due to the action of the membrane sodium pump which is actively transporting sodium ions out of the cell. The resting potential of the cell is normally about −70 mV with respect to the outside. What makes a nerve cell unique, however, is that if this resting potential is raised, either by depolarization using an intracellular electrode or by an increase in the membrane permeability to sodium so that the membrane potential rises to about −10 to −15 mV, there is a sudden influx of sodium and the potential overshoots to give a positive spike of up to 40 mV and which lasts for about 0.2–0.5 ms. This spike, or action potential, can be propagated along the axon. At the nerve terminal it causes a change in membrane permeability leading to the release of neurotransmitter from vesicles which fuse with the presynaptic cell membrane and discharge their contents into the synaptic cleft. The principal inhibitory mechanisms are illustrated diagrammatically in Fig. 20.2.

DISTRIBUTION AND FUNCTION OF THE PRINCIPAL CNS TRANSMITTERS

Acetylcholine (ACh)

Although ACh was the first neurotransmitter to be unequivocally identified in the peripheral autonomic nervous system, the visualization of central cholinergic pathways is a comparatively recent development, involving autoradiography using muscarinic receptor antagonists and immunohistochemical identification of choline acetyltranferase using specific antibodies to the enzyme. Choline acetyltransferase is present in all cholinergic nerve terminals and is responsible for the synthesis of the transmitter from acetyl CoA and choline, the latter being taken up by a high affinity sodium-dependent active transport system. ACh is stored in small, densely-staining vesicles in the nerve terminal and released in response to depolarization of the presynaptic cell membrane. The action of ACh on postsynaptic receptors is terminated by a specific acetylcholinesterase present in the synaptic cleft. An idealized cholinergic synapse is shown in Fig. 20.3.

If the concentration of choline acetyltransferase is taken as an indication of the density of cholinergic nerve endings, the greatest number of cholinergic endings are found in the interpeduncular nucleus, the caudate nucleus, and the ventral roots of the spinal cord. A number of ascending pathways from the brain stem and basal ganglia innervate the neocortex and ACh is also widely distributed within the hippocampus.

The role of ACh in the CNS can be inferred from observing the behavioural effects following the administration of drugs that alter cholinergic function and are capable of penetrating the blood–brain barrier. Thus, anticholinesterases, which will potentiate the actions of ACh, induce anxiety, aggression, affective changes, hallucinations and mental confusion. These effects can be blocked by the use of muscarinic antagonists, some of which have significant CNS effects following systemic administration (see p. 380). The large majority of ACh receptors in the CNS are of the muscarinic type and are unusual in that they act to reduce the membrane permeability to potassium.

Acetylcholine in disease states

Apart from the motoneurone disorder myasthenia gravis, the role of ACh in neurological disorders of the CNS is still open to question. Post-mortem studies in brains of patients suffering from Alzheimer's disease have shown significantly lower activity of choline acetyltransferase and high affinity choline uptake, particularly in the areas that possess a cholinergic input to the cortex. This is in addition to the other lesions that are evident in Alzheimer's disease and may of course only be a consequence rather than a cause of the disease. On the other hand, centrally acting muscarinic antagonists do have detrimental effects on cognitive functions and especially short-term memory, although the use of anticholinesterases or choline to treat the cognitive dysfunctions in Alzheimer's patients has not been particularly successful.

The central cholinergic system also plays a role in the control of voluntary movement and is intimately linked with the nigrostriatal dopaminergic pathways

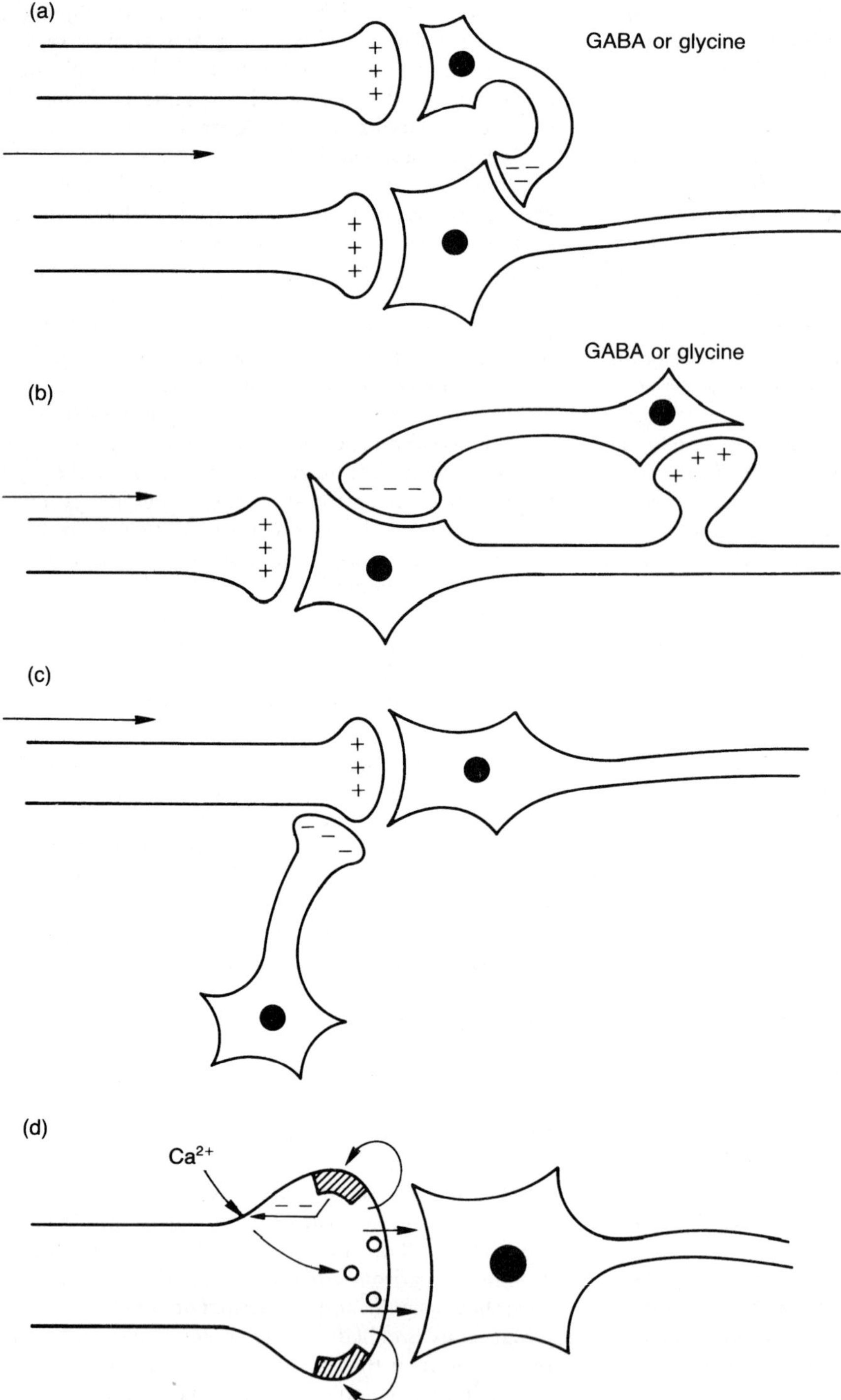

FIGURE 20.2 Types of inhibition in the CNS. (a) Feed forward postsynaptic. (b) Recurrent (feedback) postsynaptic. (c) Presynaptic. (d) Presynaptic autoreceptors (e.g. α_2-adrenoceptors, 5-HT_{1B}). Activation of these receptors inhibits neurotransmitter release by closing Ca^{++} channels. +, excitation; –, inhibition; GABA, γ-aminobutyric acid.

(see below). Since the muscarinic agonist tremorine was known to produce Parkinsonian symptoms in animals, and that anticholinesterases aggravated the condition of Parkinsonian patients, it seemed logical to use antimuscarinic drugs such as the belladonna alkaloids to treat Parkinsonism. The limitation of the use of drugs of this type (compared with the dopamine agonists) is their relative lack of specificity. Newer synthetic anticholinergic drugs such as *procyclidine* and *trihexylphenidyl HCl* have fewer side-effects, which may reflect their selectivity for different subtypes of the muscarinic receptor.

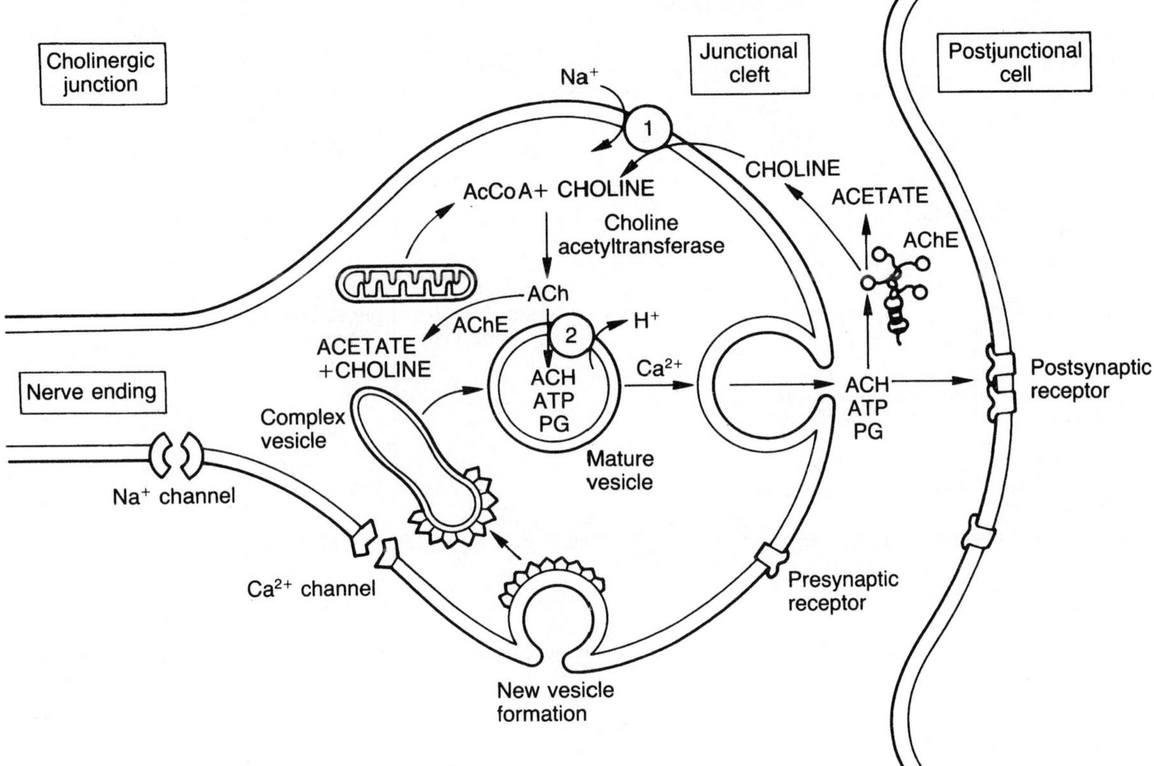

FIGURE 20.3 A cholinergic synapse, ACh, acetylcholine; PG, proteoglycan; AcCoA, acetylcoenzyme A; AChE, acetylcholinesterase.

Neurochemistry of the catecholamines

A number of neuroactive compounds are based on the parent catecholamine structure, including the neurotransmitters dopamine, noradrenaline and adrenaline. The common starting point is the essential amino acid tyrosine from which all the endogenous catecholamines are synthesized (Fig. 20.4). Adrenaline was first isolated from the adrenal glands, from which its name is derived: adrenaline in the UK, epinephrine in the USA. Noradrenaline (NA) is distributed throughout the soft tissues, with locally high concentrations in the brain. However, its immediate metabolic precursor, dopamine, shows a different pattern of distribution and this was the first clue to a separate transmitter role for dopamine. A large number of naturally occurring and synthetic sympathomimetic drugs are analogues of the endogenous catecholamines and compete with the endogenous catecholamines at the uptake, storage, and receptor sites.

Synthesis

Circulating tyrosine is taken up by catecholamine neurones and metabolized to dopamine and noradrenaline by enzymes present in the neurone (see Fig. 20.5). Tyrosine hydroxylase, which is unique to catecholamine-containing neurones, is the rate-limiting step in this synthetic pathway. A number of specific inhibitors have been developed; these will reduce transmitter synthesis and thereby diminish sympathetic neuronal activity. The only compounds to find clinical use in this respect are α-methyl-*p*-tyrosine (*metirosine*) and its esters. They have been used to treat patients with inoperable pheochromocytoma and also malignant hypertension.

Inhibitors of dihydroxyphenylalanine (DOPA) decarboxylase which do not cross the blood–brain barrier are employed as an adjunct to *levodopa* (L-DOPA) therapy in Parkinsonian patients. Since dopamine itself does not cross the blood–brain barrier it cannot be used to restore the depleted levels of dopamine in these patients. However, L-DOPA will enter the CNS and is taken up by dopaminergic neurones and converted to dopamine by DOPA decarboxylase. Unfortunately, this enzyme is widespread in the periphery and will destroy 95% of the administered L-DOPA before it has a chance to enter the CNS. The competitive inhibitor *carbidopa* prevents this peripheral destruction of L-DOPA and ensures that the precursor reaches the CNS in therapeutically effective concentrations (see p. 377).

The next enzyme in the pathway, dopamine-β-hydroxylase, is only found in noradrenergic neurones. Both DOPA decarboxylase and dopamine β-hydroxylase are relatively non-specific; they will convert phenylethylamines present in foodstuffs into catecholamine analogues that can subsequently be released as 'false' transmitters. Tyramine, for example, which is normally destroyed by monoamine oxidase

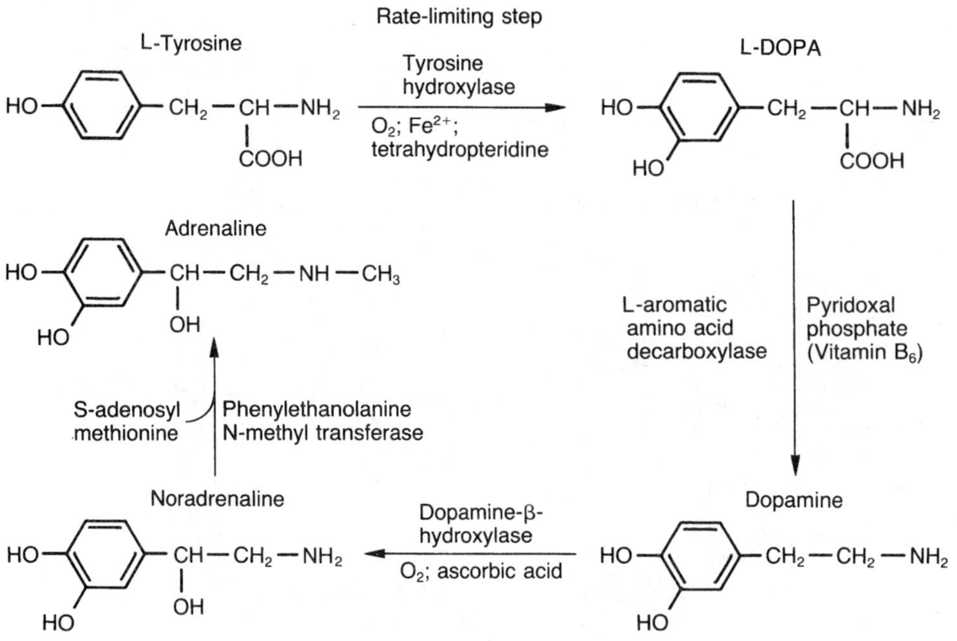

L-Tyrosine

HO–C₆H₄–CH_2–CH(COOH)–NH_2

Rate-limiting step

Tyrosine hydroxylase

O_2; Fe^{2+}; tetrahydropteridine

L-DOPA

(HO)₂C₆H₃–CH_2–CH(COOH)–NH_2

L-aromatic amino acid decarboxylase

Pyridoxal phosphate (Vitamin B_6)

Dopamine

(HO)₂C₆H₃–CH_2–CH_2–NH_2

Dopamine-β-hydroxylase

O_2; ascorbic acid

Noradrenaline

(HO)₂C₆H₃–CH(OH)–CH_2–NH_2

S-adenosyl methionine

Phenylethanolanine N-methyl transferase

Adrenaline

(HO)₂C₆H₃–CH(OH)–CH_2–NH–CH_3

FIGURE 20.4 Synthesis of the catecholamine transmitters. DA, dopamine; NA, noradrenaline; MAO, monoamine oxidase; COMT, catechol-O-methyl transferase.

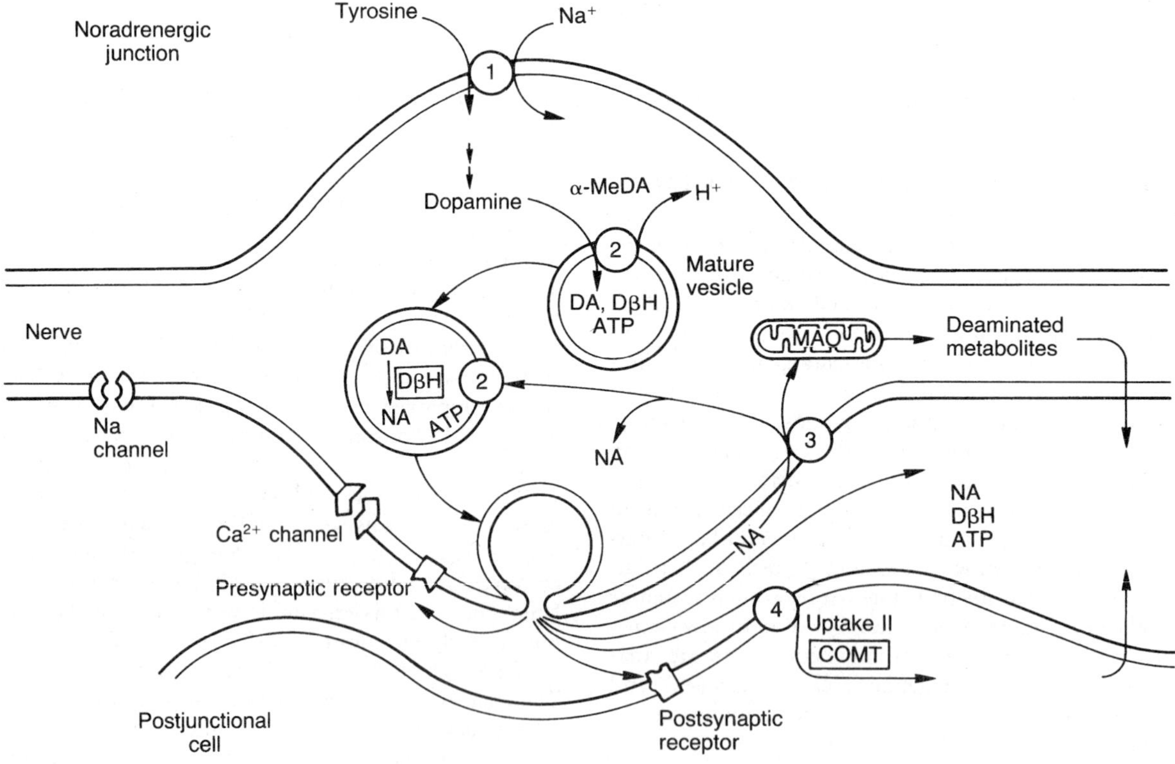

FIGURE 20.5 A noradrenergic nerve terminal varicosity and synapse. DβH, dopamine β-hydroxylase. Active transport (uptake) systems: (1) tyrosine; (2) dopamine (DA) into vesicles; (3) neuronal re-uptake of noradrenaline (NA) (uptake I); (4) uptake of NA (uptake II) into α-MeDA, α-methyldopamine.

(MAO) in the intestinal epithelium and the liver, is converted to octopamine. In the presence of monoamine oxidase inhibitors (MAOIs) significant amounts of octopamine will be produced and stored in place of NA in sympathetic nerve endings. Since octopamine is a less effective agonist at adrenoceptors, sympathetic tone will be decreased leading most obviously to a fall in blood pressure. This is believed to account for the hypotension often observed during chronic treatment with MAOIs. In contrast, if a large quantity of tyramine is ingested, for example in cheese or yeast extracts, sufficient tyramine enters the general circulation to produce an indirect pressor effect which can lead to a hypertensive crisis (see p. 350). The false transmitter principle is the basis for the action of the antihypertensive drug *methyldopa*. This is converted to methylnoradrenaline and released in place of the normal active transmitter.

Dopamine-β-hydroxylase is also inhibited by some MAOIs and the alcohol-aversive drug, *disulfiram*. Although the rationale for the use of disulfiram is based on its ability to inhibit aldehyde dehydrogenase, leading to a build up of acetaldehyde following the consumption of alcohol, it is possible that some of the effects of disulfiram are due to interference with catecholamine synthesis.

Storage and release

Since the catecholamines are released by exocytosis of storage granules in response to nerve stimulation, any disruption of this storage process that causes premature release intraneuronally will tend to reduce sympathetic activity. Most of the drugs that act in this way (bretylium, guanethidine) are highly polar quaternary bases that cannot cross the blood–brain barrier. Their actions are therefore confined to the periphery (see Chapter 13). Rauwolfia alkaloids, for example *reserpine*, prevent the packaging and storage of NA as well as dopamine and 5-HT, resulting in the depletion of all three monoamines. Not surprisingly these drugs have widespread central effects in addition to their hypotensive activity.

Metabolism

The catecholamines differ from ACh in that rapid enzymic breakdown is not responsible for terminating their synaptic actions. MAO is a non-specific enzyme, present within the nerve terminal, which will oxidatively deaminate a range of monoamines. Following the development of specific inhibitors it is now apparent that the MAO in dopaminergic terminals (MAO_B) differs from that found in NA and 5-HT neurones (MAO_A). The selective MAO_B inhibitor *selegiline* has therefore found use in the treatment of Parkinsonism (see Chapter 23). Although the non-specific inhibitors of MAO lead to increased tissue levels of the catecholamines and 5-HT, their effects on neuronal function are more subtle. The precise relationship between MAO inhibition and therapeutic response is still unclear.

Catechol-O-methyl transferase (COMT) is present in the synaptic cleft of catecholamine neurones. Although it is involved in the metabolism of the catecholamines, the inhibition of the enzyme does not significantly potentiate sympathetic activity. The pathways of the metabolism of dopamine and NA are shown in Fig. 20.6.

Uptake processes

Sympathetic nerves can take up NA against a concentration gradient by a high affinity sodium-dependent active transport process (uptake 1). A similar low affinity system is present in some non-neuronal tissues (uptake 2). Dopamine, tyramine and 5-HT are also substrates for the transport process. Uptake 1 is clearly important for terminating the synaptic actions of NA since drugs that block the process (*cocaine*, *amphetamine*) are potent sympathomimetics. The tricyclic antidepressants such as *desipramine* also block uptake 1, although their overall pharmacology is different from cocaine and amphetamine (see Chapter 22).

Dopamine

The central dopaminergic systems are fairly complex, although several well-defined long distance pathways can be recognized (see Fig. 20.7). The major pathways are the mesocortical projection which links the substantia nigra to the neostriatum (mainly the caudate and putamen) and accounts for about 75% of the dopamine in the brain, and the mesolimbic projection from the ventral tegmental region to the limbic structures (the septum, olfactory tubercle, nucleus accumbens, amygdala and piriform cortex). The former is involved in the initiation and control of voluntary movements; the latter is thought to be important in interactive and reactive behaviour. Shorter paths project from the arcuate and periventricular nuclei into the intermediate pituitary and the median eminence. These tuberohypophyseal dopamine neurones are important in the hypothalamic control of pituitary function, particularly prolactin and growth hormone secretion.

Dopamine receptors can be broadly divided into two classes:

- D_1 – coupled to adenylate cyclase, found in the CNS and periphery, possibly responsible for vasodilatation, require high concentration (10^{-6} M) of dopamine for activation.
- D_2 – not coupled to adenylate cyclase, mediate the pre- and postsynaptic action of dopamine in the CNS, activated by low concentrations (10^{-9} M) of dopamine, blocked by antipsychotic and neuroleptic drugs. The dopamine agonists apomorphine and bromocriptine have greater potency at D_2 receptors but are not completely selective. Similarly, the neuroleptic D_2 antagonists such as the phenothiazines and butyrophenones are non-selective. Sulpiride and spiperone, however, are D_2 selective.

It has been suggested that the presynaptic dopamine autoreceptor be classified as D_3, but this is still controversial.

Dopamine in disease states

The role of dopamine in the extrapyramidal motor disturbances associated with Parkinsonism and the

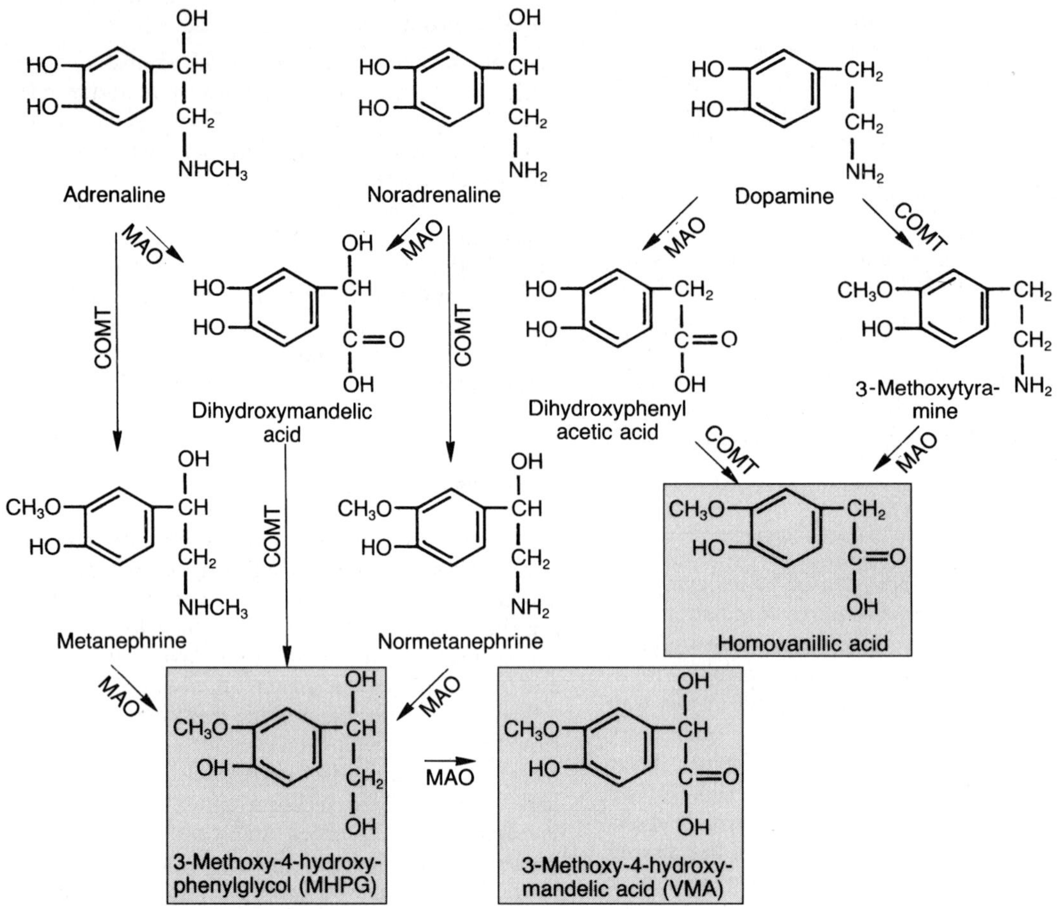

Adrenaline

Noradrenaline

Dopamine

MAO

COMT

Dihydroxymandelic acid

Dihydroxyphenyl acetic acid

3-Methoxytyramine

Metanephrine

Normetanephrine

Homovanillic acid

3-Methoxy-4-hydroxy-phenylglycol (MHPG)

3-Methoxy-4-hydroxy-mandelic acid (VMA)

FIGURE 20.6 Metabolism of dopamine and noradrenaline. Shaded areas, principal metabolites. MAO, monoamine oxidase; COMT, catechol-O-methyl transferase.

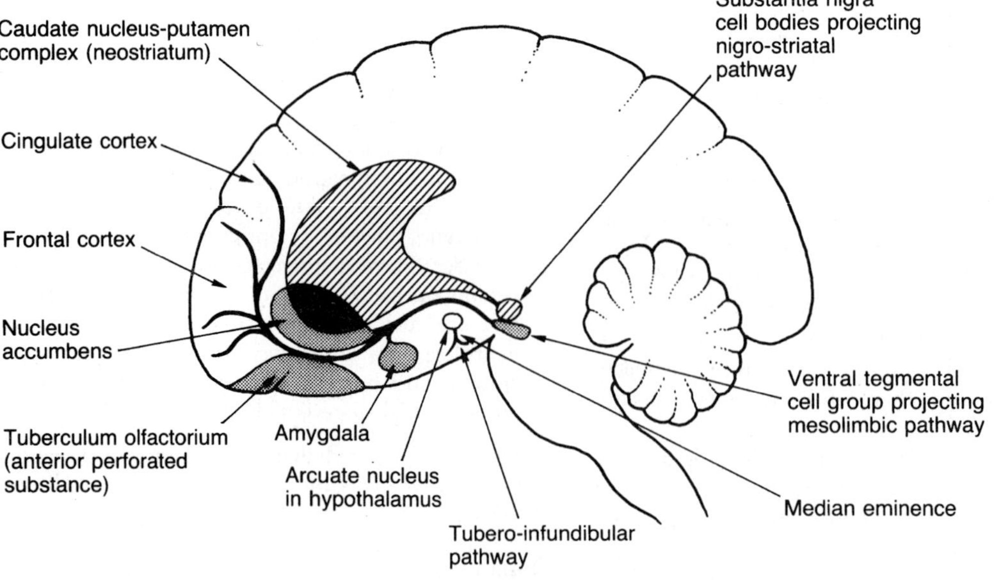

FIGURE 20.7 Dopaminergic pathways in the CNS. (From Kruk ZL, Pycock CJ. *Neurotransmitters and drugs*, 3rd edn. London: Chapman & Hall, 1991.)

tardive dyskinesias is considered in detail in Chapter 22. This involves the nigrostriatal and mesolimbic dopaminergic pathways. The role of dopamine as the prolactin release-inhibiting factor has clinical relevance in the treatment of prolactin-secreting pituitary tumours where the use of dopamine agonists such as bromocriptine can reduce circulating prolactin levels.

Noradrenaline (NA)

The noradrenergic pathways are more diffuse than those of dopamine and NA neurones project throughout the brain. However, the cell bodies from which they arise are restricted to the pons and medulla, the largest concentration being in the locus coeruleus (Fig. 20.8). The NA from these diffuse fibres usually produces inhibition of postsynaptic neurones by the activation of β-adrenoceptors. The function of these neurones has been more difficult to establish. Noradrenaline pathways in the medulla affect the responses to signals from the baroreceptors of the carotid sinus and thus have a regulatory influence on the central control of cardiac output and blood pressure. Noradrenergic neurones projecting to the limbic system are thought to be an important determinant of mood (see below). The activation of noradrenergic neurones in the locus coeruleus also produces behavioural arousal; there is a large sensory input into this area so that aversive or threatening stimuli induce firing of these neurones. The strong link that exists between state of mind (mood) and state of arousal is evidenced by the close association between behavioural depression and lethargy on one hand, and euphoria, arousal and even mania on the other. NA is one of several central neurotransmitters involved in the control of appetite and ingestive behaviour. Most sympathomimetic drugs are anorexic to some extent.

Noradrenaline in disease states

Endogenous noradrenaline is an important factor in the regulation of the normal sleep–wake cycle. Drugs such as reserpine, which deplete NA, tend to produce sedation and lethargy; sympathomimetics which stimulate release of NA or otherwise potentiate noradrenergic function (e.g. cocaine, amphetamine) produce excitation and insomnia. For this reason it is thought that imbalances in the noradrenergic system may be responsible for cases of idiopathic insomnia. The catecholamine theory of affective disorders (see Chapter 22) is similarly based on the association of depression with reduced noradrenergic activity and the mood-elevating properties of sympathomimetic drugs.

5-Hydroxytryptamine (serotonin)

5-HT is distributed in both peripheral tissues (enterochromaffin cells and platelets) and the CNS. The synthesis, storage and release of 5-HT is very similar to that of noradrenaline, except that the precursor in this case is the essential amino acid tryptophan. Like dopamine and noradrenaline, 5-HT is also oxidatively deaminated by MAO, the principal product being 5-hydroxy-indole-acetic acid (5-HIAA). An interesting point is that some of the minor metabolites of 5-HT have been shown to have hallucinogenic properties, leading to the theory that perturbations of 5-HT metabolism could be responsible for the delusional symptoms of schizophrenia. The metabolic pathways for 5-HT are shown in Fig. 20.9. As with the

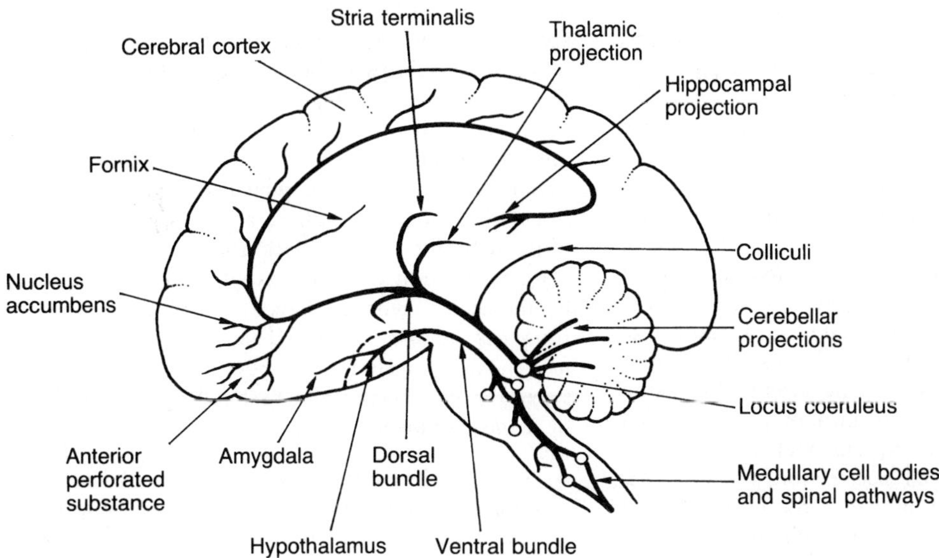

FIGURE 20.8 Noradrenergic pathways in the CNS. (From Kruk ZL, Pycock CJ. *Neurotransmitters and drugs*, 3rd edn. London: Chapman & Hall, 1991.)

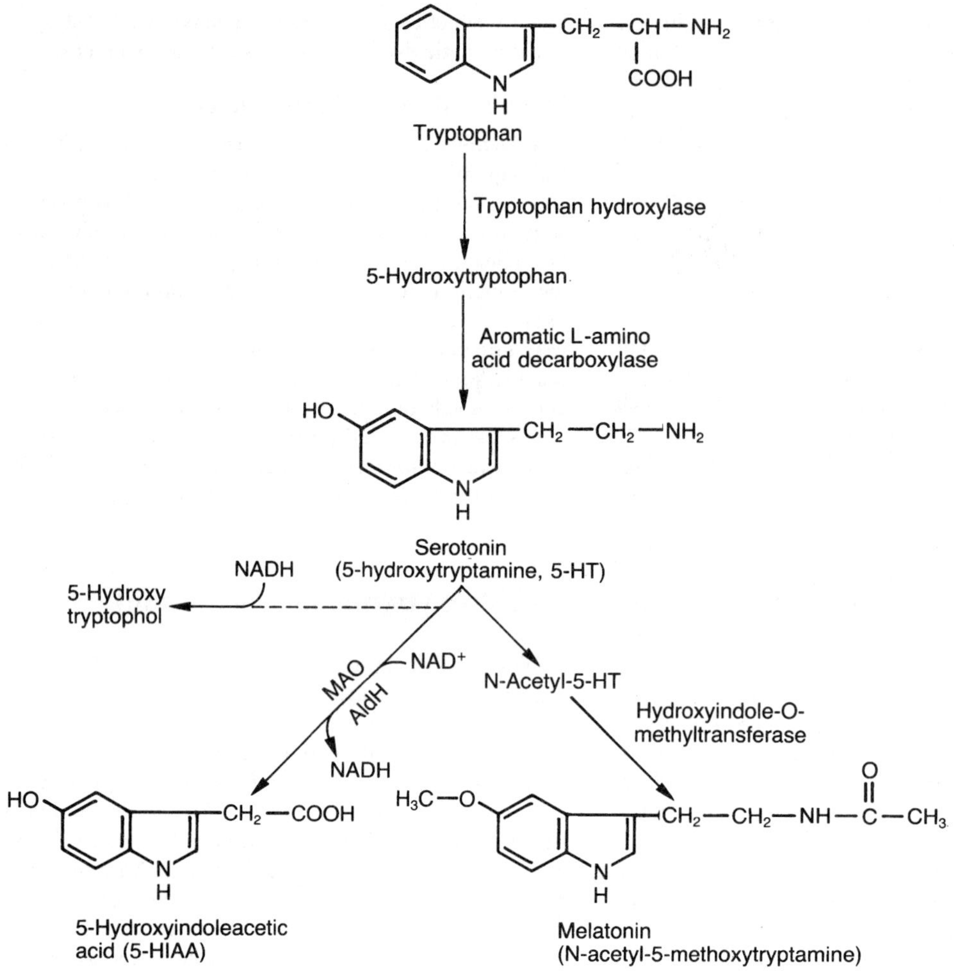

FIGURE 20.9 Synthesis and metabolism of 5-hydroxytryptamine (5-HT). AldH, aldehyde dehydrogenase; NADH, NAD^+, MAO, monoamine oxidase.

catecholamines, the re-uptake process is important for terminating the action of the transmitter. Some of the tricyclic antidepressants, particularly *clomipramine*, are very selective for the 5-HT uptake system.

5-HT containing cell bodies are clustered around the raphé regions of the pons and upper brain stem in a number of well-defined nuclei. Other groups of cells are present in the area postrema and interpeduncular nucleus. 5-HT produces both inhibition (hyperpolarization) and excitation (depolarization) of the neurones on to which serotonergic neurones project (Fig. 20.10). The role of 5-HT in the brain has not been fully elucidated, but it is implicated in a number of physiological and endocrine functions. The raphé nucleus is important in controlling sleep and wakefulness; depletion of 5-HT by chemical or surgical lesioning abolishes sleep in experimental animals and responses to sensory inputs (nociception) are enhanced. Descending 5-HT fibres influence the excitability of motoneurones; in the absence of 5-HT, monosynaptic reflexes become exaggerated. 5-HT has also been implicated in the control of emesis; some specific 5-HT antagonists have clear anti-emetic effects (see below).

The classification of 5-HT receptor subtypes is complicated by the regular discovery of ever more specific ligands which bind only to small proportions of the total number of binding sites. Historically, two peripheral receptor types were recognized: the D receptor, which could be blocked by dibenamine and the hallucinogen LSD (lysergic acid diethylamide), and the M type which acts by stimulating the release of acetylcholine, an effect that could be blocked by morphine. Apart from the pharmacological classification of 5-HT receptors, recent advances in molecular genetics have enabled a number of receptors to be cloned. The following simplified nomenclature includes the best established receptor types for which clinically useful drugs are available or in development:

- 5-HT_1. Presynaptic inhibitory effects on noradrenergic neurones to block NA release. Functional responses include behavioural changes, vasodilatation, selective vasoconstriction of the carotid vascular bed. (Subdivided into 5-HT_{1A}, 5-HT_{1B}, 5-HT_{1C} (which strictly belongs to the 5-HT_2 family),

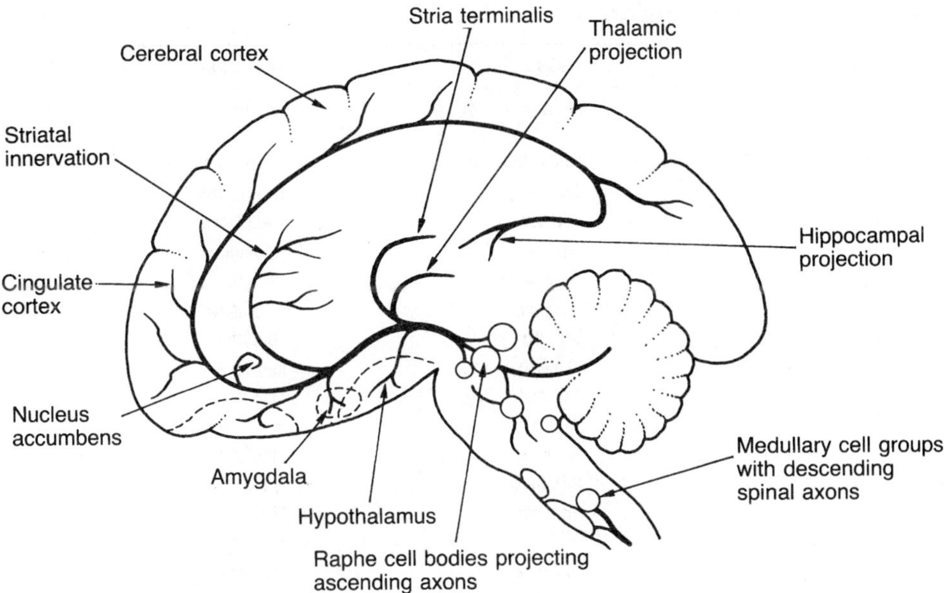

FIGURE 20.10 Serotonergic pathways in the CNS. (From Kruk ZL, Pycock CJ. *Neurotransmitters and drugs*, 3rd edn. London: Chapman & Hall, 1991.)

5-HT_{1D}, 5-HT_{1x}, etc. Some of these are only found in non-human species). Coupled through inhibitory G proteins and adenylyl cyclase. The 5-HT_{1A} agonist *buspirone* is used clinically as an anxiolytic; the 5-HT_{1D} agonist *sumatriptan* is used in migraine (see below).

- 5-HT_2 (D receptor). Postsynaptic excitation and inhibition. Functional responses include behavioural changes including mood, control of the level of arousal, sleep patterns and antinociception. Peripheral effects include bronchoconstriction, platelet aggregation, and vascular smooth muscle contraction. (Subdivided into 5-HT_{2A}, 5-HT_{2B}, 5-HT_{1C}). Coupled through G proteins and phospholipase C.
- 5-HT_3 (M receptor). Localized in the tractus solitarius and area postrema of the hind brain. Functional responses include behavioural changes, nausea and vomiting. Directly coupled to ion channels. The selective 5-HT_3 antagonists *ondansetron*, *granisetron* and *tropistron* are finding clinical use specifically for the treatment of the nausea associated with chemotherapy. Ondansetron is also used in the management of postoperative nausea and vomiting.
- 5-HT_4. Only recently characterized; present on CNS neurones, human atrial muscle and gastrointestinal smooth muscle. Selective agonists or antagonists for some of these receptor subtypes are summarized in Table 20.1.

Serotonin in disease states

Mention has already been made of one of the 5-HT theories of schizophrenia; namely, that the endogenously produced hallucinogen dimethyltryptamine is present in higher concentrations in schizophrenics. This has not been borne out by subsequent studies. Similarly, the view that a lack of 5-HT is responsible, based on the observation that the 5-HT antagonist LSD is hallucinatory, has been discredited. The antipsychotic activity of antischizophrenic drugs is not related to their ability to bind to 5-HT receptors. Raising brain 5-HT levels by administering 5-HT precursors such as tryptophan does not relieve the symptoms of schizophrenia nor has it proved effective in the treatment of insomnia or depression.

Migraine

There is now strong evidence to implicate 5-HT as an important trigger for migraine attacks. Although stress and specific dietary factors can provoke an attack, the precise stimulus responsible for releasing 5-HT in the first place is still not known. However, the pattern of events that follow 5-HT release is consistent with 5-HT receptor mediated effects. Secondary mediators include prostaglandins and NA. The prodromal visual disturbances result from the vasoconstriction of intracranial vessels. This is followed by severe headache, nausea and vomiting. The headache phase is associated with vasodilatation and inflammation of extracranial vessels. During an attack the level of 5-HT in blood platelets falls, and blood and urine levels of the 5-HT metabolite 5-HIAA are raised, suggesting an increased release of 5-HT.

The treatment of migraine is mainly symptomatic: analgesics such as aspirin or paracetamol to relieve the headache, vasoconstrictors such as *clonidine* and *ergotamine* (the latter being a partial agonist at 5-HT_2 receptors), and anti-emetics such as metoclopramide

TABLE 20.1 Agonists and antagonists acting at the principal receptor subtypes

TRANSMITTER	RECEPTOR	AGONIST	ANTAGONIST
Acetylcholine	Muscarinic M_1, M_2, M_3	Pilocarpine	Atropine
	Nicotinic	Suxamethonium	*d*-Tubocurarine
Adenosine	A_1	Adenosine	Theophylline
	A_2	Adenosine	Theophylline
Dopamine	D_1	Dopamine	Flupenthixol
	D_2	Dopamine	Sulpiride
GABA	$GABA_A$	*Muscimol*	*Bicuculline*
	$GABA_B$	Baclofen	*Phaclofen*
Glutamate	AMPA	Glutamate	Ketamine
	NMDA	Glutamate	MK801
	Kainate	Glutamate	—
Glycine		Glycine	*Strychnine*
Histamine	H_1	*Histamine*	Promethazine
	H_2	*Histamine*	Cimetidine
	H_3	*α-Methylhistamine*	*Thioperamide*
5-HT	$5\text{-}HT_{1A}$	Buspirone	*Spiperone*
	$5\text{-}HT_{1B}$	Methysergide	*Spiperone*
	$5\text{-}HT_{1D}$	Sumatriptan	*Methiothepin*
	$5\text{-}HT_2$	*Lysergic acid (LSD)*	Ketanserin
	$5\text{-}HT_3$	*Phenylbiguanide*	Ondansetron
Noradrenaline	α_1	Phenylephrine	Prazosin
	α_2	Clonidine	Yohimbine
	β_1	Dobutamine	Atenolol
	β_2	Salbutamol	Butoxamine
	β_3	BRL 35135	Propranolol
Opiates	μ	Fentanyl	Naloxone
	κ	Etorphine	Naloxone
	σ	Pentazocine	Naloxone

Compounds which have no current clinical usage are shown in italics. The drugs given as examples in the table have been selected on the basis of their relative potency at the receptor, but they are not necessarily completely selective.

(a non-specific dopamine and $5\text{-}HT_3$ antagonist) to relieve the nausea. Ergotamine canot be used prophylactically, but the more specific $5\text{-}HT_2$ antagonist *methysergide* can prevent the onset of a migraine attack. Unlike ergotamine, methysergide does not produce widespread vasoconstriction but acts more specifically as an agonist on $5\text{-}HT_1$ receptors on the carotid vascular bed. A relatively high incidence of toxicity is associated with the long-term use of methysergide. The antihistamine *cyproheptadine* also has $5\text{-}HT_2$ antagonist activity and is occasionally used in cases of migraine that have not responded to other treatments.

A number of increasingly specific 5-HT agonists and antagonists are currently being developed which may find use as therapeutic agents for migraine. Most notable among these is *sumatriptan* a $5\text{-}HT_{1D}$ agonist which appears to selectively contract the intracranial extracerebral blood vessels. It does not cross the blood–brain barrier and is therefore without centrally mediated side-effects. Early clinical studies found that 5-HT itself, administered intravenously, could abort an ongoing migraine attack, although it had no prophylactic value. It is likely that sumatriptan is acting in the same way.

Histamine

Although histamine appears to be a neurotransmitter in the CNS its functional role is still unclear. In contrast, in the periphery it has a well-established role as a mediator in the allergic response and as a stimulus for gastric acid secretion. Histamine is produced by the action of the enzyme histidine decarboxylase, which is localized in high concentrations in some nerve cells in the CNS. Breakdown of histamine in the first instance involves either oxidative deamination by a non-specific diamine oxidase or methylation catalysed by N-methyl-transferase (see Fig. 20.11).

The histamine receptor subtypes found in the CNS are the same as those found non-neuronally in the periphery. They have been characterized on the basis of the selectivity of histamine antagonists:

- *H_1 receptors*. These are blocked by all the early *antihistamines, chlorpheniramine, diphenhydramine, mepyramine* and *promethazine*. The receptors are coupled to phospholipase c by a G protein and operate via the second messengers diacylglycerol and inositol triphosphate.

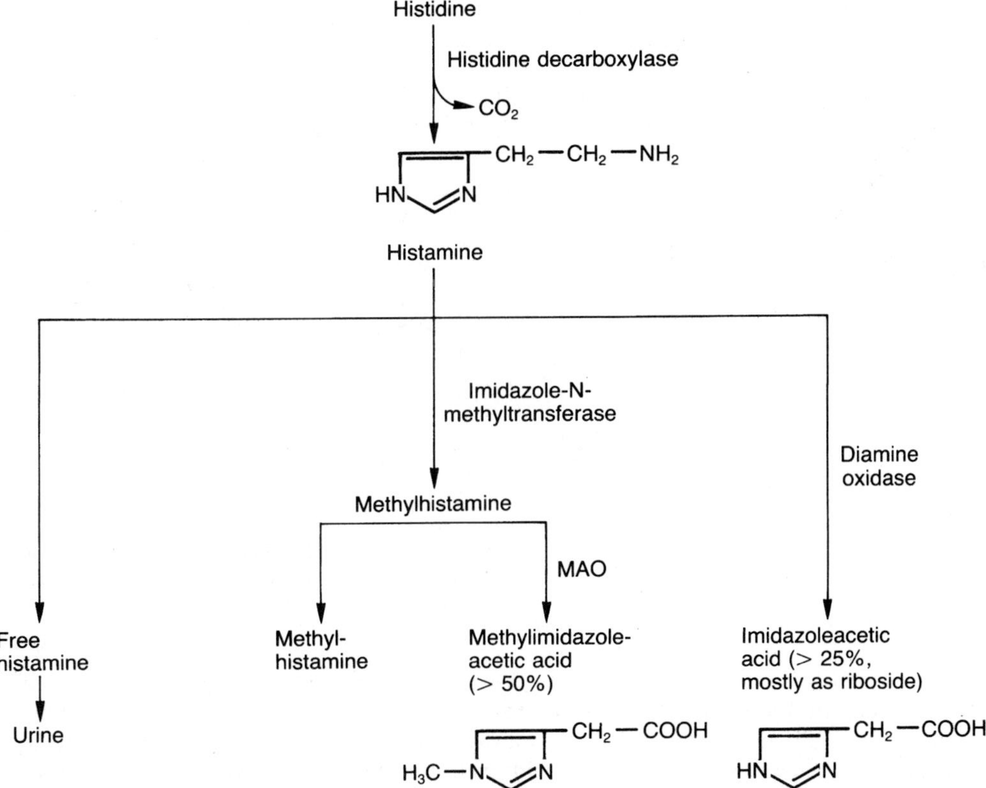

FIGURE 20.11 Synthesis and metabolism of histamine. (MAO: monoamine oxidase.)

- *H_2 receptors.* In the periphery they are responsible for stimulating gastric acid secretion, but their central function is unknown. They are blocked by *cimetidine* and *ranitidine.*
- *H_3 receptors.* These have been detected on histamine-containing nerve terminals where they appear to act as inhibitory autoreceptors. The experimental compound thioperamide is a competitive antagonist.

Central actions of H_1 antagonists

Several of the very large number of antihistamines on the market have marked sedative and anti-emetic properties. Several of these drugs are structurally similar to muscarinic, 5-HT and α-adrenoceptor antagonists, so it is not surprising that they also exhibit some antagonist activity at these sites in addition to their primary action. *Cyproheptadine*, for example, which is used mainly for the relief of allergic reactions, has also been used successfully as a treatment for migraine (see above). The sedative action of several antihistamines (notably promethazine and diphenhydramine) has led to the suggestion that endogenous histamine may be involved in controlling the level of arousal.

Amino acid neurotransmitters

Many amino acids have direct effects on the membrane potential of neurones, either to hyperpolarize or depolarize the cell and it is now recognized that the amino acids have specific transmiter functions in addition to their metabolic role in intermediary metabolism. In fact, they represent the major class of neurotransmitters in the CNS. From a neurochemical point of view it is very difficult to divorce their metabolic function from their transmitter role, but neurophysiologically they can be divided into the inhibitory amino acids γ-aminobutyric acid (GABA), glycine, and possibly taurine) and the excitatory amino acids (L-aspartate and L-glutamate). From their chemical structures (shown in Fig. 20.12), it can be seen that the excitatory amino acids have two carboxylic acid groups and the inhibitor amino acids only one.

Neurochemistry of the amino acids

Since all cells require glutamate and aspartate for metabolic purposes, and this represents a high proportion of the total cell content of these amino acids, their presence is ubiquitous and no obvious localization occurs. GABA and glycine on the other hand are

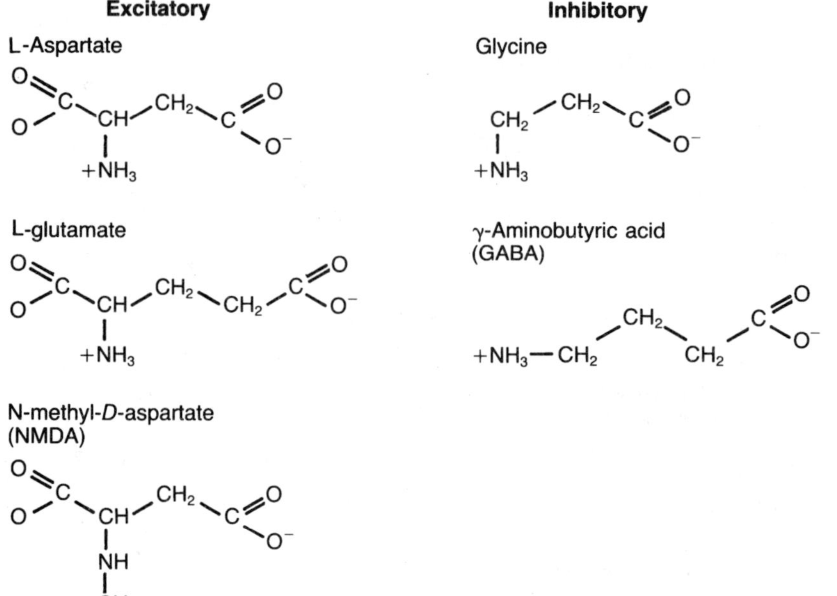

FIGURE 20.12 Structure of the inhibitory and excitatory transmitter amino acids.

unevenly distributed within the CNS. The highest concentrations of GABA are found in the hippocampus, the hypothalamus, the Purkinje cell layer of the cerebellum, the basal ganglia, and the grey matter of the dorsal horn of the spinal cord. Glycine is concentrated in the brainstem and the grey matter of the spinal cord.

Aspartate and glutamate can arise from a number of sources usually involving transaminase reactions in pathways that are linked closely to the tricarboxylic acid cycle (see Fig. 20.13). GABA is derived solely from glutamate by a specific decarboxylase (L-glutamic acid decarboxylase, GAD) which is found only in

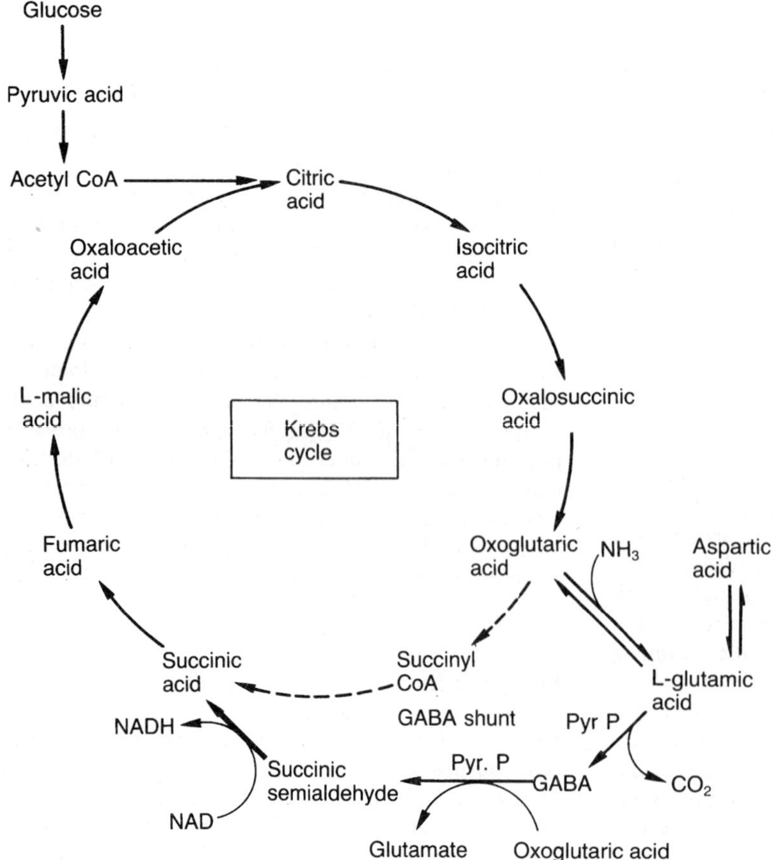

FIGURE 20.13 Synthesis and metabolism of the amino acids. Pyr. P, pyridoxal phosphate.

GABAergic nerve terminals. GABA is metabolized by a mitochondrial enzyme (GABA-aminotransferase, GABA-T) in a reaction coupled to α-ketoglutarate to yield glutamate and succinic semialdehyde. The latter is very readily oxidized by an NAD-coupled reaction to succinic acid which then re-enters the tricarboxylic acid cycle. This sequence of reactions is often referred to as the GABA shunt. Both GAD and GABA-T are pyridoxal phosphate (vitamin B_6) dependent reactions. GABA that has been released into the synaptic cleft can be taken up by active transport systems either back into the nerve terminal or into the surrounding glial cells.

Glycine can be derived from a number of sources (diet, protein breakdown, transamination of glyoxylic acid) so no discrete pathway appears to exist for its synthesis or breakdown. In fact, GABA is the only neurotransmitter amino acid that lends itself to neurochemical manipulation by enzyme inhibitors.

Compounds that inhibit GAD produce characteristic running fits and convulsions in experimental animals. These inhibitors have no clinical applications, but they have been useful in providing models for disease states involving GABA dysfunction (see below). Inhibitors of GABA-T, on the other hand, might be expected to potentiate the inhibitory actions of GABA by preventing its breakdown. A number of compounds have been specifically designed with this in mind; the irreversible GABA-T inhibitor γ-vinyl GABA has recently entered the clinic under the name of *vigabatrin* as a treatment for epilepsy. The earlier anti-epileptic sodium di-*n*-propyl acetate (*sodium valproate*) inhibits both GABA-T and succinic semialdehyde, but it is doubtful whether this is the basis for its anticonvulsant activity. The structures of some of these GABA-related drugs are shown in Fig. 20.14. Antagonists of vitamin B_6 will inhibit both GAD and GABA-T; the net result on GABA levels depending very much on the dose used. Disappointingly, the currently available inhibitors of GABA uptake have proved too toxic for clinical use.

γ-Aminobutyric acid (GABA)

GABA receptors can be divided into two subgroups on the basis of their sensitivity to the antagonist bicuculline, although a third subtype may also exist. Cloning studies have revealed a number of distinctive protein subunits that can be combined as hexamers in a bewildering array of potential receptor subtypes. Those of clinical relevance are:

- *$GABA_A$*. These are coupled to a chloride ion channel; their activation opens the chloride channel producing a hyperpolarization of the postsynaptic membrane. $GABA_A$ receptors on primary afferent neurone terminals are responsible for presynaptic inhibition (see Fig. 20.2). $GABA_A$ receptors are selectively stimulated by muscimol, THIP(4,5,6,7-tetrahydroxyisoxazolo [4,5-c]pyridin-3-ol) and 3-aminopropanesulphonic acid (homotaurine), and blocked by bicuculline.
- *$GABA_B$*. These are concentrated in the cerebellum and spinal cord and are not linked to a chloride channel. Stimulation of $GABA_B$ receptors produces hyperpolarization resulting from an increase in potassium conductance and a reduction in calcium conductance. They are insensitive to the $GABA_A$ agonists and to bicuculline, and are selectively stimulated by *baclofen* and blocked by phaclofen and saclofen.

$GABA_A$ receptors are part of a large complex formed from a number of protein subunits which include binding sites for benzodiazepines and barbiturates. These are discussed in detail in Chapter 21. Both GABA-receptor subtypes are involved in regulating neuronal excitability in the brain and spinal cord. The clinical effectiveness and selectivity of baclofen as an antispasticity agent (although it does have sedative and other properties) suggests that the $GABA_B$ receptors in the spinal cord have a role in controlling motoneurone outflow and hence, muscle tone. The actions of $GABA_A$ agonists are too non-specific for clinical use as sedative-hypnotics or anticonvulsants. However, the $GABA_A$ agonist *THIP* (4,5,6,7-tetrahydroxyisoxazolo [4,5,-c]pyridin-3-ol) has undergone clinical trials as a centrally acting analgesic. Rational drug design has yielded a number of GABA analogues, some of which have proved effective as anticonvulsants in epilepsy (see Fig. 20.14 and Upton, 1994).

GABA in disease states

Although it has long been speculated that a dysfunction in GABA transmission may be the underlying cause of epileptiform activity, this has not been convincingly demonstrated. Changes in GABA function have also been inferred from post-mortem studies of brains from schizophrenic, Parkinsonian or Alzheimer's patients, but it is difficult to distinguish the cause from the effect in this situation. The changes in GABA function may also reflect consequences of the long-term drug therapy used in the treatment of these conditions.

Specific loss of GABA neurones has clearly been associated with the symptoms observed in some of the rarer neurological disorders. In Huntington's chorea, the loss of GABA neurones removes the normal control exerted on nigrostriatal dopaminergic neurones resulting in choreiform movements and other dyskinesias. In stiff man syndrome, a progressive disorder in which the early symptoms are increased skeletal muscle tone, there is a more generalized loss of GABA neurones due to circulating autoantibodies.

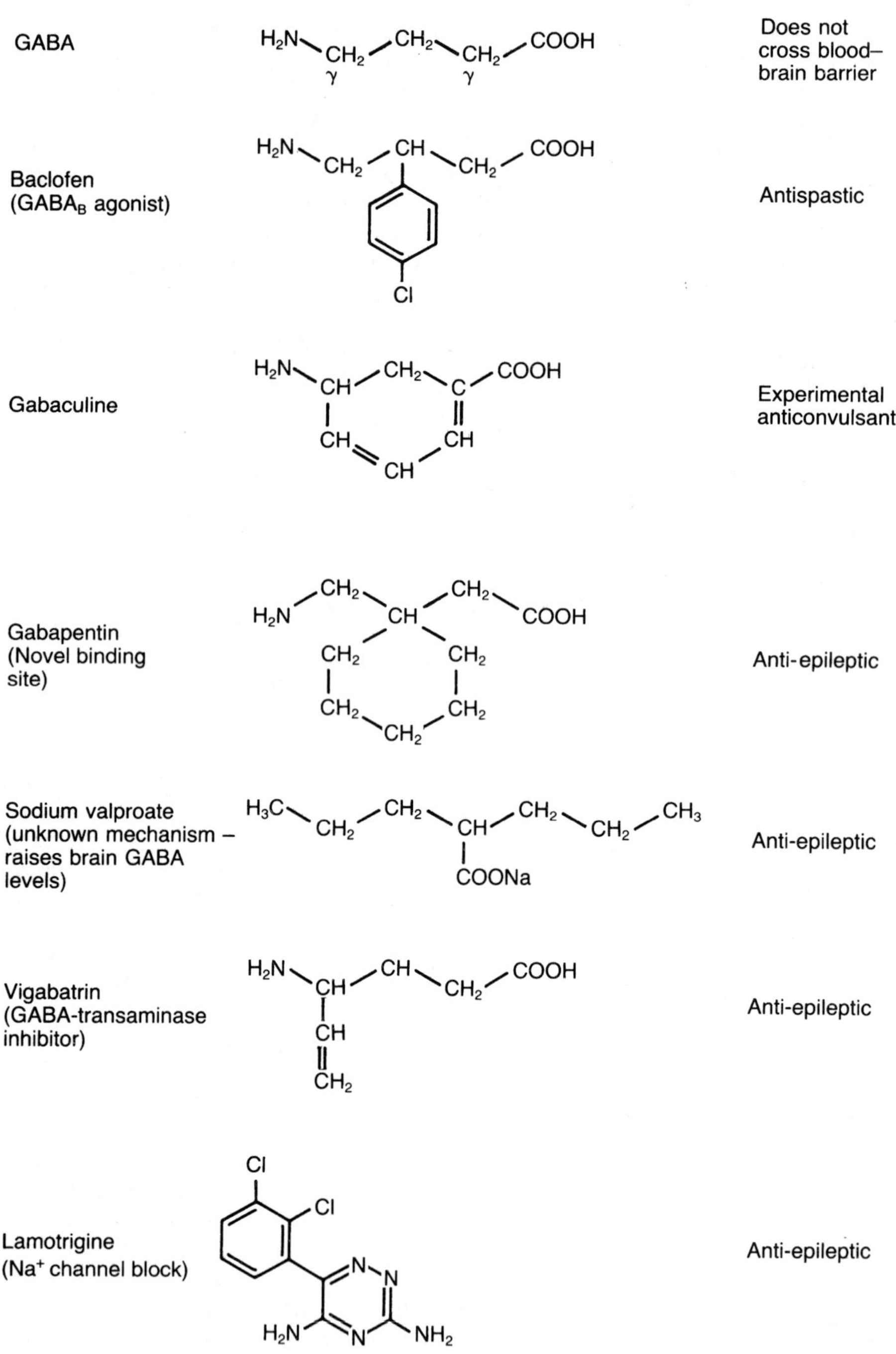

FIGURE 20.14 Structures of γ-aminobutyric acid (GABA)-related drugs. (Adapted from Upton N. *Trends in Pharmacological Sciences* 1994; 15: 456–63.)

Glycine

Glycine is an important postsynaptic inhibitor in the spinal cord; it is thought to be the transmitter released from the Renshaw cells onto the spinal motoneurone (see Fig. 20.2). It would seem that glycine, like GABA, has an important role in controlling muscle tone. In experimental animals it has been shown that spinal ischaemia resulting in spastic paraplegia is associated with a selective loss of glycine from the dorsal horn of the spinal cord. The release of glycine from inhibitory interneurones is blocked by tetanus toxin. The action of glycine is probably terminated by a specific high affinity uptake system. Glycine receptors can be blocked competitively by the convulsant *strychnine.* Not surprisingly, the convulsions resulting from strychnine poisoning resemble the symptoms of tetanus. Strychnine also produces stimulation of the vasomotor and vagal centres of the medulla and enhances sensory inputs to the cortex.

There are no agonist drugs available that act at glycine receptors and no compounds that can enhance glycine-mediated inhibition. At one time strychnine was regarded as a valuable constituent of medicinal tonics, but it, and the other convulsant analeptics, have now passed into virtual disuse as respiratory stimulants.

Excitatory amino acids

Although L-glutamate and L-aspartate excite most central neurones, the nature of the precise sites at which they act as transmitters is still being resolved. Specific agonists and antagonists have only been developed recently and it is likely that the designation of the various subtypes may yet change. Although the clinical potential of these receptors is still not fully understood, they are clearly important in explaining the action of the dissociative anaesthetics *phencyclidine* (PCP) and *ketamine*. At the present time there are believed to be four excitatory amino acid receptor subtypes, all of which respond to glutamate:

NMDA receptor

This is stimulated by aspartate and N-methyl D-aspartate (NMDA) and increases cell permeability to sodium, potassium and calcium ions in a voltage-dependent process mediated by magnesium. The action of the transmitter is potentiated by glycine, which binds to a closely related site on the receptor complex. Within the channel there is a phencyclidine-binding site to which opiates and ketamine can bind to block the ion channel. Agonist binding can be blocked by the competitive antagonist 2-amino-5-phosphonopentanoic acid (AP_5). The non-competitive ion channel blocker, MK801, was briefly used for the treatment of ischaemic neuronal damage under the name Dizocilpine. However, it proved to have serious side-effects that have precluded its continued clinical use.

AMPA (quisqualate) receptor

This is stimulated by α-amino-3-hydroxy-5-methylisoxazole (AMPA) and quisqualate but not aspartate, and blocked by the nitroquinoxaline derivatives BNQX and CNQX (FG9041). The associated ion channel permits the rapid flux of sodium and potassium ions resulting in depolarization. In its open configuration the ion channel can be blocked by barbiturates.

Kainate receptor

This is similar to the NMDA receptor except that it is not stimulated by aspartate. It is blocked by many of the same antagonists as the AMPA receptor. A further receptor subtype (metabotropic) linked to a G protein and triphosphoinositol, which is involved in the mobilization of intracellular calcium, has recently been discovered. The kainate and AMPA receptors are sometimes referred to jointly as non-NMDA receptors.

Neurotoxicity of excitatory amino acids

Direct application of glutamate or aspartate into the brain in the intact animal produces convulsions. At one time it was believed that monosodium glutamate, a widely used flavour-enhancer in food, was responsible for the so-called 'Chinese restaurant syndrome', but this now seems doubtful. Kainic acid is a selective and potent excitotoxin, destroying only those nerve cell bodies that possess excitatory amino-acid receptors. The rapid advance of research in this area, particularly with regard to the role of excitotoxicity in post-ischaemic cell death has implications for the future treatment of dementias and stroke. Antagonists at the NMDA receptor in particular may soon find clinical use as neuroprotective agents.

Adenosine

Adenosine is present in a large number of tissues in the body and has widespread physiological and metabolic actions. It affects the cardiovascular, renal and respiratory systems in addition to its actions in the CNS. Generally, it is released from metabolically active or stressed cells and acts in an inhibitory manner to restore normal function. This is achieved either through binding to adenosine (purinergic) receptors on the surrounding cell surfaces, or by the direct inhibition of intracellular adenylyl cyclase. Adenosine itself is used clinically, although the only current indication is in the diagnosis and treatment of supraventricular tachycardias (see Chapter 15, p. 219).

A number of adenosine receptor subtypes have now been recognized, currently designated A_1, A_{2A}, A_{2B} and A_3. The drug theophylline is a non-selective adenosine receptor antagonist and is used as a bronchodilator in the treatment of asthma (see Chapter 19). A number of other xanthine compounds, analogues of theophylline, have been synthesized in an attempt to produce more selective adenosine antagonists. The stimulation of adenosine A_1 receptors in the CNS results in an inhibition of neurotransmitter release. The behavioural manifestations of this action are sedation, reduced locomotor activity, and an anticonvulsant effect in animals. The insomnia associated with the use of theophylline in patients may be a reflection of the drug's antagonistic action at A_1 purinoceptors. Therapeutic applications for drugs acting on purinoceptors are limited at present, but the development of more selective agonists and antagonists should yield valuable novel drugs.

Neuropeptide transmitters

Neuropeptides represent the largest class of neurotransmitters and neuromodulators in the body, although their exploitation as drugs has hitherto been limited by their susceptibility to gastric acid hydrolysis and destruction by tissue proteases, and the expense involved in their manufacture. The neuropeptide transmitters are not essentially different from non-peptides in terms of the mechanism of neurotransmission. They are produced from inactive precursors (usually by the action of a selective protease cleaving a larger peptide chain), they are stored in nerve endings, released in response to an increase in intracellular Ca^{2+}, and act on specific receptors to produce excitatory or inhibitory responses. However, their actions tend to be neuromodulatory since peptide receptors are not linked directly to ion channels as are ACh, GABA, or glutamate, for example.

Opioid peptides

The discovery by Hughes and Kosterlitz in 1975 of two endogenous pentapeptides (which they christened enkephalins) possessing the ability to bind to morphine receptors heralded the beginning of the search for endogenous ligands for the various other drug-binding sites already known to be present in the CNS (barbiturates, benzodiazepines, cannabis). Cloning techniques have now made it far easier to identify the precursors of active peptides; in the case of the enkephalins the three parent peptides are prepro-opiomelanocortin (methionine enkephalin), prepro-enkephalin (also methionine enkephalin), and prepro-dynorphin (leucine enkephalin). The synthesis and function of the enkephalins is described in more detail in Chapter 24.

A number of non-opioid as well as opioid neuropeptides are locally concentrated in specific regions of the CNS. In many cases they are coreleased with one of the established neurotransmitters. The functional significance of this cotransmission is still unclear, but it is likely that the classical transmitter acts directly on the postsynaptic receptor while the other acts as a neuromodulator to influence the sensitivity of the receptor. The *enkephalins*, for example, are found in dopamine-, NA- and ACh-containing nerve endings. Other principal examples of cotransmission are summarized in Table 20.2.

Tachykinins

The first of these, substance P, was discovered over 60 years ago, but its structure was not elucidated until 1970. The name tachykinin derives from their ability to produce rapid contraction of smooth muscle, in contrast to bradykinin which produces a much slower response. Substance P is thought to be involved in afferent sensory transmission and pain sensation in particular. Other tachykinins include neurokinin A (NKA) and neurokinin B (NKB). Substance P and NKA are locally concentrated in particular regions of the CNS, implying a specific functional role. The tachykinins have excitatory effects on neurones and smooth muscle and also activate mast cells to release histamine. Tachykinin antagonists would therefore have potential as analgesic and anti-inflammatory drugs.

Cholecystokinin

Cholecystokinin (CCK) is a gastrin-like octapeptide which, in addition to its peripheral functions, appears to modulate dopamine neurotransmission in the

TABLE 20.2 Examples of co-transmission in the central and peripheral nervous system

LOCATION	CO-TRANSMITTER	FUNCTION
Sympathetic ganglia	Gonadotrophin releasing hormone (GnRH)	Co-transmitter with acetylcholine
Post-ganglionic sympathetic neurones (e.g. blood vessels)	ATP	Smooth muscle contraction
	Neuropeptide Y	Facilitates action of NA (vasoconstriction)
Pulmonary vessels	Nitric oxide (NO)	Vasodilatation
Corpus cavernosum	Nitric oxide	Facilitates penile erection
Post-ganglionic parasympathetic nerves to salivary glands	Vaso-active intestinal peptide (VIP)	Co-transmitter with acetylcholine
Non-myelinated sensory neurones	Calcitonin gene related peptide (CGRP)	Increased vascular permeability, neurogenic inflammation
(These co-transmitters are responsible for the well-established phenomenon of non-adrenergic, non-cholinergic (NANC) transmission observed in the autonomic nervous system.)		
Dopaminergic neurones in the substantia nigra and ventral tegmental areas of the CNS	Cholecystokinin (CCK)	Potentiation of DA-mediated behaviours including appetite and satiety

mesolimbic pathway and thereby influence ingestional and motivational behaviour. Strong evidence for the role of CCK in anxiety and panic attacks has arisen recently from both human and animal studies. Two CCK receptor subtypes have now been identified: CCK_A and CCK_B. The recent development of selective CCK antagonists makes this an exciting area of future research and the first results with CCK_B antagonists have indicated an anti-anxiety activity.

The lability of systemically administered peptides has stimulated the development of non-peptide antagonists. In the case of the opiates the drugs preceded the discovery of the relevant peptides; in the case of the neuropeptides mentioned above it is to be hoped that the drugs will follow on from the identification of the peptides.

FURTHER READING

General

Cooper JR, Bloom FE, Roth RH. *The biochemical basis of neuropharmacology*, 6th edn. Oxford: Oxford University Press, 1991.

Hokfelt T, Fuxe K, Pernow B (eds). Co-existence of neuronal messengers: new principle in chemical transmission. *Progress in Brain Research* 1987; **68**: 1.

Kruk ZL, Pycock CJ. *Neurotransmitters and drugs*, 3rd edn. London: Chapman & Hall, 1991.

Webster RA, Jordan CC eds. *Neurotransmitters, drugs and disease*. Oxford: Blackwell, 1989.

Catecholamines

Ungerstedt U. On the anatomy, pharmacology and function of the nigrostriatal dopamine system. *Acta Physiologica Scandinavica*. 1971 (Suppl 367).

Moore RY, Bloom FE. Central catecholamine neuron systems: anatomy and physiology. *Annual Review of Neuroscience* 1983; **2**: 113.

Excitatory amino acids

Iversen LL, Iversen SD, Snyder SH eds. *Psychopharmacology of the aging brain*. Handbook of Psychopharmacology **20**. New York: Plenum Press, 1988.

Lodge D ed. *Excitatory amino acids in health and disease*. Chichester: Wiley, 1988.

Meldrum BS ed. *Excitatory amino acid antagonists*. Oxford: Blackwell Scientific, 1991.

Monaghan DT, Bridges RJ, Cotman CW. The excitatory amino acid receptors: their classes, pharmacology, and distinct properties in the function of the nervous system. *Annual Review of Pharmacology and Toxicology* 1989; **29**: 365–402.

Watkins JC, Krogsgaard-Larsen P, Honore T. Structure–activity relationship in the development of excitatory amino acid receptor agonists and competitive antagonists. *Trends in Pharmacological Sciences* 1990; **11**: 25–33.

Yamamura T, Harada K, Kemmotsu O. Is the site of action of ketamine anaesthesia the *N*-methyl-D-aspartate receptor? *Anesthesiology* 1990; **72**: 704.

GABA

Olsen RW. Drug interactions at the GABA receptor–ionophore complex. *Annual Review of Pharmacology and Toxicology* 1982; **22**: 245.

Olsen RW. GABA–drug interactions. *Progress in Drug Research* 1987; **31**: 223.

Sieghart W. $GABA_A$ receptors: ligand-gated Cl-ion channels modulated by multiple drug-binding sites. *Trends in Pharmacological Sciences* 1992; **13**: 446–50.

Sivilotti L, Nistri A. GABA receptor mechanisms in the central nervous system. *Progress in Neurobiology* 1991; **36**: 92.

Upton N. Mechanism of action of new antileptic drugs: rational design and serendipitous findings. *Trends in Pharmacological Sciences* 1994; **15**: 456.

Verma A, Snyder SH. Peripheral type benzodiazepine receptors. *Annual Review of Pharmacology and Toxicology* 1989; **29**: 307–22.

5-Hydroxytryptamine

Julius D. Molecular biology of serotonin receptors. *Annual Review of Neuroscience* 1991; **14**: 335.

Parsons A. 5-HT receptors in human and animal cerebrovasculature. *Trends in Pharmacological Sciences* 1991; **12**: 310–15.

Peroutka SJ. 5-Hydroxytryptamine receptor subtypes. *Annual Review of Neuroscience* 1988; **7**: 45.

Histamine

Prell GD, Green JP. Histamine as a neuroregulator. *Annual Review of Neuroscience* 1986; **9**: 209–54.

Schwartz J-C, Arrang J-M, Garbarg M, Pollard H, Ruat M. Histaminergic transmission in the mammalian brain. *Physiological Reviews* 1991; **7**: 1–51.

Adenosine

Choi OH, Shamin MT, Padgett WL, Daly JW. Caffeine and theophylline analogues: correlation of behavioural effects with activity as adenosine receptor antagonists and as phosphodiesterase inhibitors. *Life Science* 1988; **43**: 387.

Collis MG, Hourani SMO. Adenosine receptor subtypes. *Trends in Pharmacological Sciences* 1993; **14**: 360.

Stone TW ed. *Purines: Pharmacology and physiological roles*. London: Macmillan, 1985.

Williams M. Purine receptors in mammalian tissues: pharmacology and functional significance. *Annual Review of Pharmacology and Toxicology* 1987; **27**: 315.

Peptides

Buck SH, Burcher E. The tachykinins: a family of peptides with a brood of receptors. *Trends in Pharmacological Sciences* 1986; 7: 65.

Eipper BA, Mains RE, Herbert E. Peptides in the nervous system. *Trends in Neurosciences* 1986; 9: 463.

Fredrickson RCA. Endogenous opioids and related derivatives. In: Kuhar MJ, Pasternak GW eds. *Analgesics: neurochemical, behavioral and clinical perspectives.* New York: Raven Press, 1984.

Harro J, Vasar E, Bradwejn J. CCK in animal and human research on anxiety. *Trends in Pharmacological Sciences* 1993; **14**: 244.

Woodruff GN, Hughes J. Cholecystokinin antagonists. *Annual Review of Pharmacology and Toxicology* 1991; **31**: 469.

21

Sedation

Part I Hypnotics and Sedatives

HJ Little

INTRODUCTION

The word 'hypnotic' means inducing sleep. The distinction between sleep and general anaesthesia is made on the basis of arousal, in that it is possible to wake someone from sleep but not from general anaesthesia. Sedation can be described as a decrease in all CNS activity, with a resultant calming effect. The main group of drugs in current use as sedative–hypnotic agents are the benzodiazepines, which have replaced the barbiturates in the treatment of anxiety and insomnia. This chapter concentrates on the mechanism of actions of the benzodiazepines, with some references to other types of agent. Other groups of drugs that also possess sedative properties are described in the last section of Part I.

BENZODIAZEPINES

The benzodiazepines have a spectrum of pharmacological actions including anxiolytic, sedative, anticonvulsant, amnesic and muscle relaxant properties. The first and the last of these actions contribute to their value as hypnotics, as much insomnia is due to anxiety and muscle tension. There is some selectivity in the anxiolytic actions of benzodiazepines, in that certain doses can produce this effect with only a small amount of sedation and ataxia; increasing doses produce increasing sedation, but the separation of these properties is far from complete (Fig. 21.1). Oral benzodiazepines on their own do not appear to cause the full state of general anaesthesia. They do not cause serious respiratory depression except at lethal doses, and they are not analgesic.

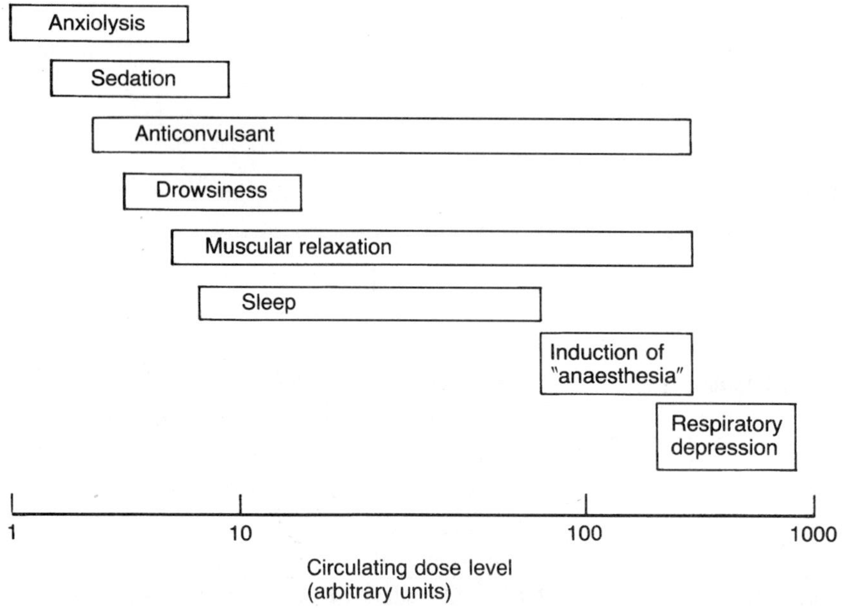

FIGURE 21.1 Relationship between dose and properties of benzodiazepines.

The anticonvulsant actions of benzodiazepines are utilized mainly in situations such as status epilepticus, where a rapid acute effectiveness is required. The development of tolerance to their anticonvulsant actions renders them unsuitable for routine anti-epileptic therapy. The amnesia actions of benzodiazepines can be useful, for example when they are used in premedication or for minor procedures. There is normally loss of memory for events that occurred during the time the drug remained in the CNS. The muscle relaxation properties of the benzodiazepine group of drugs are exerted centrally, as they are produced by actions on the spinal cord, not at the neuromuscular junction. The compounds cause ataxia at relatively low doses and this should be taken into account whenever they are prescribed.

In the past, barbiturates were used as hypnotic agents, but their low lethal doses and narrow safety margin make them quite unsuitable for this. The benzodiazepines have high therapeutic ratios, with the lethal doses being many 100-fold higher than the effective doses. In this respect they are far safer than the barbiturates. Although the benzodiazepines were initially thought to lack dependence liability, it is now obvious that this is not the case, and their addictive liability can be a serious problem.

BARBITURATES

These drugs were introduced early this century and were widely used as hypnotic sedatives until the advent of the benzodiazepines. Other compounds with non-barbiturate structures, such as the propanediol meprobamate, are also active at the same site as barbiturates (see below). Because of major hazards associated with the use and abuse of these drugs, they are rarely, if ever, used now. For example, mental confusion can be caused by therapeutic doses of barbiturates, particularly in the elderly, that could result in further doses being taken by mistake, with considerable danger to the patient. The only current indications for barbiturates are as anaesthetic induction agents (those in current use include methohexitone and thiopentone and are discussed in detail in Chapter 5) or as anticonvulsants.

MECHANISM OF ACTION OF BENZODIAZEPINES

The mechanism by which benzodiazepines produce most of their pharmacological effects are now well established. They potentiate the actions of the inhibitory neurotransmitter, γ-aminobutyric acid (GABA). GABA is the transmitter at a large proportion of inhibitory central synapses, and is released by interneurones in most areas of the brain. It acts at at least three types of receptors (see Chapter 20), but it is the $GABA_A$ type that is involved in the actions of benzodiazepines. The action of GABA at $GABA_A$ receptors is to increase the chloride conductance, thus increasing the flow of chloride ions (Fig. 21.2). In most locations this increase in conductance results in net entry of chloride, down the chemical gradient. This causes hyperpolarization and decreased excitability of the neurones. In some cells, however, the concentration gradient for chloride across the membrane is in the other direction, and there is a net outflow of chloride ions and depolarization.

When the effect of the benzodiazepines in potentiating the actions of GABA was first recognized, it was a

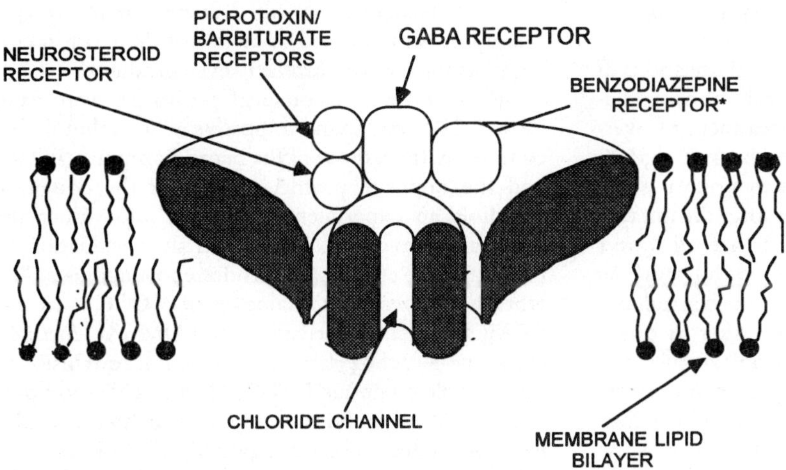

FIGURE 21.2 The GABA/benzodiazepine complex, showing the different binding sites for drugs acting on this complex.

novel concept, as they do not produce this effect by alteration of the uptake or metabolism of GABA, but by an allosteric action on the GABA-receptor protein. Since then, however, the receptor-mediated actions of several neurotransmitters are known to be altered by such allosteric actions of drugs. Benzodiazepines specifically increase the frequency of opening of chloride channels, although the mechanism by which this potentiation occurs is still not clear.

THE BENZODIAZEPINE-BINDING SITE

It was not until 1977 that high-affinity binding sites for benzodiazepines were demonstrated to exist in the CNS. The good correlation between the affinities of the benzodiazepine compounds for these sites and their pharmacological potencies provided evidence for a causal relationship. It is now known that these binding sites are on the same protein as the $GABA_A$ receptors and this protein is now known as the GABA–benzodiazepine receptor chloride ionophore complex (see Fig. 21.2). The distributions of benzodiazepine and $GABA_A$-binding sites in the CNS are very similar, but not identical, so it is possible that not all $GABA_A$ receptors are associated with benzodiazepine receptors.

Soon after the discovery of the high-affinity binding sites for benzodiazepines in the CNS it was suggested that these existed in multiple forms, called BZ_1 and BZ_2 subtypes. The BZ_1 subtype was found to predominate in certain regions, such as the cerebellum, while the hippocampus, for example, contained both BZ_1 and BZ_2 types. It was postulated that BZ_1 receptors mediated the anxiolytic and anticonvulsant actions and BZ_2 the sedative and ataxic properties. Newly developed compounds were reported to have selective affinities for one or other of these subtypes, and this explained apparent differences in their pharmacological properties. *Zolpidem* has an imidazopyridine structure and higher affinity for the BZ_1 receptor subtype than for the BZ_2 subtype. It has preferential hypnotic properties, with less potent ataxic and anticonvulsant actions. *Alpidem*, another imidazopyridine, that is selective for the BZ_2 receptor subtype, is said to be a selective anxiolytic, without sedative and ataxic actions.

Zopiclone, a cyclopyrrolone, that binds to an allosteric site on the benzodiazepine complex, is marketed as a sedative–hypnotic. It has a similar pharmacological profile to the benzodiazepines, with pronounced sedative, hypnotic, anticonvulsant and ataxic properties. The claim that it has less dependence liability than the benzodiazepines is still under scrutiny.

BENZODIAZEPINE ANTAGONISTS (FLUMAZENIL)

The next breakthrough came in 1981, when Haefely and coworkers reported that one of their compounds was a benzodiazepine antagonist. This drug, code number Ro 15-1788, now marketed as *flumazenil*, is an imidazobenzodiazepine. It antagonized virtually all the pharmacological effects of benzodiazepines except those produced at very high concentrations. It exhibited high-affinity binding and competition with the benzodiazepines for the receptor site. There was no antagonism of the effects of drugs such as the barbiturates that did not act directly at the benzodiazepine-binding site on the receptor complex, even though they bind to adjacent sites. At first, flumazenil was not thought to possess any pharmacological actions of its own, but it is now known to be a very weak partial agonist (see below).

Flumazenil is now available for clinical use and is of value for the rapid reversal of the effects of benzodiazepines. It has found a place in the treatment of overdose with benzodiazepines. One drawback is that its very short duration of action can lead to a return of the effects of the benzodiazepine agonists after the antagonist action disappears, as the agonists are all longer acting. Flumazenil will precipitate withdrawal in patients who are physically dependent on benzodiazepines, and there are reports of seizures after its use in patients who had overdosed on benzodiazepines and tricyclic antidepressants. Finally, it may cause severe anxiety in patients with panic disorder, which may indicate an abnormal benzodiazepine receptor sensitivity in this condition. However, when used to reverse the effects of short half-life agonists (e.g. midazolam), flumazenil has considerable value in speeding recovery from short procedures.

INVERSE AGONISTS AND THE 'TWO-WAY RECEPTOR'

When the benzodiazepine antagonists were first described, it appeared that the benzodiazepine receptor resembled a conventional receptor site, with the normal interactions between agonists and antagonists. In 1981, however, it became evident that the benzodiazepine receptor differed from all previously known receptor sites. The first indication of this came with the study of β-carboline-3-carboxylate ethyl ester (β-CCE). This compound was isolated from large quantities of human urine. It had a high affinity for the benzodiazepine receptor and was at first thought to be an endogenous ligand for the benzodiazepine receptor. This aspect was soon shown to be artefactual as the ethyl substituent had been added during purification and its removal resulted in loss of the receptor affinity. It soon proved to be one of the most interesting pharmacological artefacts ever produced.

When its pharmacological properties were examined, β-CCE was found to possess actions that differed completely from those of the benzodiazepines. In fact it had the opposite profile; it lowered the convulsion threshold in experimental animals, and rather than being anticonvulsant, it inhibited sleep induction and prevented the effects of benzodiazepine agonists. Later work has shown that analogues of β-CCE, such as β-CCM, the methyl derivative, and DMCM (methyl-β-carboline-3-carboxylate), can cause full convulsions. A more stable compound, FG7142, was given to human volunteers and found to produce a state that resembled extreme anxiety. These compounds all showed competition with benzodiazepine agonists in binding studies, suggesting that, despite their completely different properties, they might be acting through the same receptor sites.

When flumazenil, the benzodiazepine antagonist, was shown to prevent the proconvulsant and anxiogenic effects of β-CCE and its congeners, a new theory was required to explain these results. This was put forward in 1982, when it was suggested that ligands binding to the benzodiazepine receptor could either increase or decrease the actions of GABA, and that flumazenil could act as a competitive antagonist of either type (Fig. 21.2). The compounds that decrease the actions of GABA were named 'inverse agonists'.

PARTIAL AGONISTS

Some of the extensive range of compounds that interact with this fascinating receptor site are shown in Fig. 21.3 in the form of a spectrum of activity, from full agonist to full inverse agonist. Compounds with both types of action have also been found among the

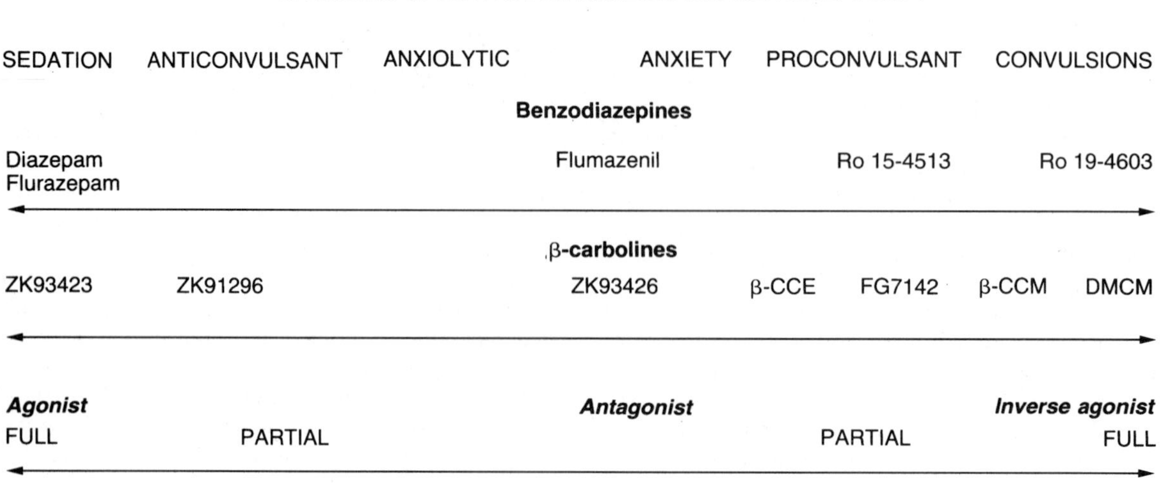

SPECTRUM OF ACTIVITY AT BENZODIAZEPINE RECEPTORS

SEDATION ANTICONVULSANT ANXIOLYTIC ANXIETY PROCONVULSANT CONVULSIONS

Benzodiazepines

Diazepam
Flurazepam
Flumazenil
Ro 15-4513
Ro 19-4603

β-carbolines

ZK93423 ZK91296 ZK93426 β-CCE FG7142 β-CCM DMCM

Agonist ***Antagonist*** ***Inverse agonist***

FULL PARTIAL PARTIAL FULL

FIGURE 21.3 Spectrum of activity of ligands acting at benzodiazepine receptors on the GABA/benzodiazepine complex.

pyrazoloquinolinones. It is now known that ligands with either type of action may be full or partial agonists, in exactly the same way as drugs acting at classical receptor sites. Partial inverse agonists decrease the effects of full inverse agonists and possess their pharmacological actions to a lesser extent. Partial agonists, similarly, have an antagonist effect when combined with an agonist of greater efficacy, and cause less effect than full agonists. The original benzodiazepines, such as diazepam and midazolam, are full agonists. Agonists and inverse agonists are, of course, mutually antagonistic. One theory postulates that agonists with low efficacy (partial agonists) have anxiolytic properties without the sedation and hypnotic actions of the full agonists. This was based on the suggestion that the anxiolytic effects were produced at lower receptor occupancy than the sedative and ataxic actions. Compounds with partial agonist properties are undergoing clinical trials as anxiolytic agents.

Antagonist properties were found among both the benzodiazepines (flumazenil) and the β-carbolines (ZK93426), but in all cases they appear to have extremely low efficacy, rather than being classical antagonists with no pharmacological effects in the absence of an agonist. At very high doses, flumazenil has agonist properties, while ZK93426 is a very weak inverse agonist.

MECHANISM OF ACTION OF BARBITURATES AND OTHER SEDATIVE DRUGS

The barbiturates bind to the GABA–receptor complex at a site distinct from that for benzodiazepines (Fig. 21.2). Barbiturate compounds have a dual action on the complex: they potentiate the effects of GABA on the chloride channel by prolonging channel opening and also, unlike benzodiazepines, have a direct effect in increasing the chloride conductance. Attempts have been made to correlate these actions with the anticonvulsant and anaesthetic actions of barbiturates, but the experimental results have been contradictory. It was originally thought that the convulsant *picrotoxin* and its congeners bound to the same site as the barbiturates, but these drugs are now thought to act at an adjacent site to decrease the chloride conductance. The two groups of compounds differ, however, in that the benzodiazepines have little action on any other sites at doses that produce the pharmacological effects, while barbiturates have other actions, such as blockade of calcium-dependent action potentials and antagonism of excitatory amino acids. This probably explains the greater selectivity of the benzodiazepines over the barbiturates, and the difference in the lethal doses. The non-barbiturate sedative drug, *etazolate*, competes with the barbiturates for binding.

Another group of compounds that potentiate GABA are the steroid anaesthetics, such as *alphaxalone*. This has been clearly demonstrated in electrophysiological studies, and they appear to bind to the GABA–benzodiazepine receptor ionophore complex (Fig. 21.2).

ETHANOL AND GABA

Ethanol has been found to have a potentiating effect on GABA transmission, in addition to its many other sites of action, but conflicting evidence has been found, and many electrophysiological studies did not demonstrate such an effect. This controversy may be explained by recent patch-clamp studies showing that ethanol increased the effects of GABA in some neurones bearing $GABA_A$ receptors, but not in others, and that some cells responding to benzodiazepines did not respond to ethanol. The involvement of the subunits of the complex (see below) will be of great interest, as the results so far suggest that ethanol may interact with only certain of the subunits. The benzodioizepine inverse agonist, Ro 15-4513 has been suggested to decrease the effects of ethanol.

ENDOGENOUS LIGANDS?

There has been much speculation about the possibility of an endogenous ligand for the benzodiazepine receptor, but whether such a ligand exists is still unclear. Early candidates included hypoxanthine, inosine, nicotinamide, thromboxane A and harmaline, but the affinities of these compounds for the receptor site were low compared with their synaptic concentrations, so it appeared unlikely that they would have much effect at the receptor sites in the physiological situation. Although the β-carboline derivative, β-CCE (see above), which has high receptor affinity, was originally isolated from human tissues, it does not exist in the body in this form, and so far no β-carboline has been found in the body that possesses such high-affinity binding for the benzodiazepine receptor site. Other synthetic benzodiazepine receptor ligands are described on p. 358.

There has been interest in the substance DBI ('diazepam-binding inhibitor'), a peptide isolated from CNS tissue that has some affinity for the receptor site, with a dissociation constant (Kd) value in the low micromolar range. This affinity is quite low, compared with the synthetic compounds, but the peptide appears to be present in sufficient concentrations in brain to have effects at the receptor site. Its concentrations in peripheral tissues are considerably lower. This substance has been reported to have anxiogenic-like activity in behavioural tests and to decrease the effects of GABA in electrophysiological studies. It may be present in some, but not all, neurones that use GABA as a neurotransmitter.

A compound with high-affinity binding at the benzodiazepine receptor was identified by a different approach from previous isolation studies, that of raising monoclonal antibodies to a benzodiazepine, then applying immunoaffinity chromatography purification that resulted in the isolation of a benzodiazepine-like molecule from brain tissue. This compound possessed a high affinity for the receptor site and agonist-like pharmacological properties, and had a molecular weight of around 1000. Further studies demonstrated that it was in fact N-desmethyldiazepam, a metabolite of certain benzodiazepines used in clinical practice. That the discovery of this compound in brain was not due to contamination with synthetic compounds was shown by its demonstration in human brain fixed years before benzodiazepines were first synthesized. The presence of similar compounds in food substances has led to the suggestion that the N-desmethyldiazepam could be of dietary origin.

NEW SELECTIVE COMPOUNDS?

Much recent research has been directed towards separation of the properties of the benzodiazepines, predominantly with the aim of producing drugs with selective anxiolytic effects, without the sedative and ataxic properties, although drugs with more selective sedative actions have been produced.

None of the compounds acting at the benzodiazepine receptor has proved as selective as anxiolytics as the buspirone series (see p. 356) or the new cholecystokinin antagonists. These do not possess sedative or hypnotic properties and do not potentiate the actions of other central depressants. Buspirone requires days or weeks to develop the full anxiolytic response and will not protect a patient from a benzodiazepine withdrawal syndrome (see p. 356).

GABA-receptor subunits

Explanations for the differential actions of the drugs described above may be found from studies of the subunit composition of the receptor protein. The GABA-receptor–ionophore complex is now known to be composed of at least five types of subunit, all of which are polypeptides of 48KDa–55KDa molecular weight. They have been divided into the α-subunits, of which six forms have been distinguished, β-subunits, of which four forms have been found so far, and two forms of the γ-subunit. There are also σ- and ϵ-subunits. The α-, β- and γ-subunits are needed for functional GABA–benzodiazepine interactions. The α-subunits carry the binding site for benzodiazepines, but the γ-subunits have been found to be required for stabilization of the binding at this site. The β-subunits carry the high-affinity GABA site. Combinations of these subunits are thought to compose up to twenty different forms of the GABA–benzodiazepine receptor complex, and there may be even more. Regional differences have been found in the distribution of the combinations of the subunits that may explain the existence of multiple receptor sites for benzodiazepine ligands.

PHARMACOKINETICS OF BENZODIAZEPINES

The individual benzodiazepine compounds differ mainly in their pharmacokinetic properties and hence their onset and duration of action, and these are the factors that principally determine their clinical indications (see Table 21.1). They can be considered to fall approximately into two groups: short-acting, such as midazolam, temazepam, lorazepam, triazolam and alprazolam with half-lives of 6–10 h, and long-acting, such as diazepam, and nitrazepam, which have half-lives of over 20 h (see Table 21.2). Some have equipotent metabolites that possess similar pharmacological properties, and these can prolong the duration of action (Fig. 21.4). The half-life of the main metabolite of flurazepam, for example, N-desalkyl-flurazepam, is about 50 h. While the short-acting compounds are considered to be more appropriate for night-time hypnosis, because they have fewer effects during the following day, morning rebound hyperexcitability can occur with these drugs. Alprazolam, a triazolobenzodiazepine, has been claimed to differ from the classical 1,4-benzodiazepines in having antidepressant as well as anxiolytic properties. Clobazam, with substituents in the 1 and 5 positions, may have fewer adverse psychomotor effects.

The rate of onset of action is important for both intravenously administered benzodiazepines and those taken orally as hypnotics. The relative lipid solubility is a significant factor here (see Table 21.3). Since diazepam is poorly soluble in aqueous media, the injectable form is prepared as an emulsion (diazemuls). This appears to produce fewer local complications than the formulation prepared in an organic solvent.

The hypnotic effects of drugs can be detected by measurements of sleep in experimental animals, but

TABLE 21.1 Properties and uses of the benzodiazepines

Pharmacological actions of benzodiazepines	
Anxiolytic	
Centrally acting muscle relaxants	
Sedative (tolerance)	
Anticonvulsant (tolerance)	
Amnesic	
Uses of benzodiazepines	
Premedication	Alcohol withdrawl
Anxiety	Spasticity
Insomnia	Night terrors
Status epilepticus	

TABLE 21.2 Pharmacokinetic properties of some commonly used sedative–anxiolytics

DRUG	BIOAVAILABILITY %	PLASMA-PROTEIN BINDING (%)	ELIMINATION HALF-LIFE (h)	ACTIVE METABOLITES
Benzodiazepines				
Midazolam	40	95	2–3.5	No
Oxazepam	95	100	4–12	No
Temazepam	>80	>95	5–11	No
Chlordiazepoxide	100	95	6–24*	Yes
Alprazolam	20	70	10–20	Yes
Lorazepam	90	90	10–20	No
Flunitrazepam	85	80	12–18	Yes
Clobazam	>90	90	17–50*	Yes
Nitrazepam	80	85	20–40*	Yes
Diazepam	100	>95	20–70*	Yes
Flurazepam	85	>95	>50*	Yes
Flumazenil (antagonist)	20	70	<1.0	No
Other sedative-anxiolytics				
Chlormethiazole	10	65	4–5	No
Chloral hydrate		75	4–9*	Yes
Meprobamate	80	<10	6–18	No

*Values include the half-lives of active metabolites.

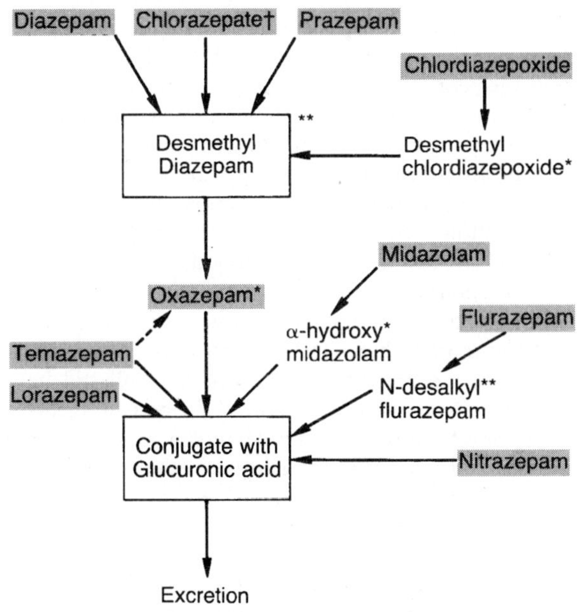

FIGURE 21.4 Metabolic pathway of the benzodiazepines. *Active metabolite (short half-life); **active metabolite (long half-life); †inactive precursor. Shaded text = clinically available drugs.

an important action used in screening for this effect is the ability to potentiate the sedative and general anaesthetic actions of other types of drug, such as alcohol and the barbiturates. The central depressant actions of benzodiazepines are additive with those of other drugs and they will all increase the depth of general anaesthesia.

TOLERANCE AND CROSS-TOLERANCE BETWEEN SEDATIVE–HYPNOTICS

Tolerance develops to most of the pharmacological actions of benzodiazepines, but tolerance to their different properties (see Table 21.1) develops at different rates. There is rapid loss of the sedative and anticonvulsant actions within a few days, but tolerance to the anxiolytic actions is less obvious and it was originally thought not to develop. It was difficult to investigate, owing to the possibility of changes in the underlying disorder, but it does appear that loss of anxiolytic action will take place after some months.

Cross-tolerance occurs between all the agonists that bind to the benzodiazepine receptor, so loss of effectiveness of one compound cannot be solved by its replacement with another. There is also cross-tolerance between benzodiazepines, barbiturates and ethanol. Alcoholics are likely to be less sensitive to benzodiazepines than other patients. On the other hand, the presence of high levels of alcohol in the circulation will potentiate the effects of any sedative–hypnotics administered. Importantly, cross-tolerance does not occur between benzodiazepines and buspirone.

Tolerance to benzodiazepines does not appear to be due to changes in metabolism, and they do not induce microsomal enzymes as do the barbiturates. Although decreases in receptor binding have been reported after chronic administration of benzodiazepines in experimental situations, the doses required to cause these changes were considerably higher than those needed to produce tolerance, so it is unlikely that this is the explanation for the loss of pharmacological activity. It

TABLE 21.3 Lipid solubilities and absorption of benzodiazepines

Relative lipid solubilities of benzodiazepines
Diazepam>oxazepam>lorazepam>temazepam>flunitrazepam>midazolam>alprazolam>clobazam
The rate of onset of action following intravenous administration is closely related to the lipid solubility of the drug
Relative absorption rates after oral administration
Diazepam>lorazepam>alprazolam>oxazepam>temazepam
The absorption rate will be a function not only of the lipid solubility of the drug but also the formulation of the preparation, the dietary state of the patient, and individual biological variation
Relative volumes of distribution
Diazepam>temazepam>midazolam>oxazepam>lorazepam>clobazam>alprazolam

appears that changes may occur in the coupling between the benzodiazepine receptor and the GABA receptor after repeated administration. Important alterations may also occur at the $GABA_A$ receptor site itself, as subsensitivity of this site has been reported that correlated with tolerance to benzodiazepine agonists.

DEPENDENCE LIABILITY OF BENZODIAZEPINES

Although original reports claimed that the benzodiazepines did not possess dependence liability, it is now known that this is not the case. When given over periods of months, they do cause physical dependence. The withdrawal signs include anxiety, dysphoria, hallucinations, characteristic disorders of perception, muscle pain and tremor and intestinal disorders. Epileptic fits and psychoses can occur. Many patients have found it extremely difficult to discontinue the use of these compounds.

The production of dependence is a function of the dose and duration of treatment, but has been reported after periods as short as 6 weeks. Experimentally, a withdrawal syndrome can be precipitated by the benzodiazepine antagonist, flumazenil, after prolonged benzodiazepine agonist administration. This interaction resembles that which occurs with opiate antagonists in patients dependent on opiates.

Recent studies, however, have suggested that flumazenil can have another effect during benzodiazepine dependence. In laboratory studies, it has been found that it can decrease the withdrawal syndrome if given during the intake of the benzodiazepine. This has been demonstrated experimentally with regard to the behavioural signs of withdrawal and the decrease in electrophysiological responses to GABA that occurs during the withdrawal phase. It appears to act by in some way 'resetting' the receptor complex. Trials in patients are under way to see if this effect can help those dependent on benzodiazepines.

OTHER GROUPS OF DRUGS WITH SEDATIVE PROPERTIES

Many other groups of compounds can produce sedation and these will have additive effects with general anaesthetics. As stated above, benzodiazepines are the most widely used hypnotics. Another compound in occasional use is *chlormethiazole*, a short-acting compound with barbiturate-like actions, that has been marketed for the treatment of alcohol withdrawal and the management of pre-eclamptic toxaemia. *Chloral hydrate* is little used today, owing to its propensity to cause irritation of the skin and gastrointestinal tract.

The sedative actions of opiates are well recognized, as is their production of respiratory depression. The antipsychotic (neuroleptic) agents, phenothiazines, typified by the original compound, chlorpromazine, have pronounced sedative actions. Other antipsychotic agents, such as the butyrophenones (e.g. haloperidol) and the thioxanthines (e.g. flupenthixol and thioridazine), are less potent as sedatives, but will still have additive effects with other central depressant agents.

Some of the tricyclic antidepressants have sedative actions and potentiate the effects of ethanol and other central depressants, including general anaesthetics. Monoamine oxidase inhibitors are less sedative, although they can be effective in correcting sleep disorders that are due to depression. Potentiation of the depressant actions of other central depressant drugs is due to interference by monoamine oxidase inhibitors with the metabolism of the compounds. Monoamine oxidase inhibitors can also cause severe reactions with pethidine.

Another group of compounds with pronounced sedative properties is the antihistamines, widely used in the treatment of allergies. With the older compounds (promethazine, diphenhydramine) this was a serious problem, but this has now been solved by the successful application of pharmacological principles to drug design. The new agents, such as terfenadine and astemizole, do not cause sedation because they do not penetrate the blood–brain barrier. Phenothiazine-based antihistamines such as trimeprazine, hydroxyzine and promethazine are used as hypnotics, especially for children. They may also be useful for premedication of children. These drugs have other side-effects (e.g. anticholinergic), and are not suitable for use as anxiolytics.

Among the antihypertensive agents in common use, clonidine is particularly liable to cause sedation, and guanfacine and methyldopa are also likely to do so. The vasodilators, such as hydralazine, minoxidil, sodium nitroprusside, and the organic nitrates and nifedipine, do not commonly have this effect.

FURTHER READING

Breimer DD. Pharmacokinetics and metabolism of various benzodiazepines used as hypnotics. *British Journal of Clinical Pharmacology* 1979; **8**, suppl 1: 7S–13S.

Brogden RN, Goa KL. Flumazenil. A preliminary review of its benzodiazepine antagonist properties. *Drugs* 1988; **35**: 448–467.

Ho IK, Harris RA. Mechanism of action of barbiturates. *Annual Review of Pharmacology and Toxicology* 1981; **21**: 83–111.

Lader M. Clinical pharmacology of benzodiazepines. *Annual Review of Medicine* 1987; **38**: 19–28.

Lader MH. Guidelines for the management of patients with generalised anxiety. *Psychiatric Bulletin* 1992; **16**: 560–5.

Owen RT, Tyrer P. Benzodiazepine dependence. A review of the evidence. *Drugs* 1993; **25**: 385–96.

Rodgers RJ, Cooper SJ (eds). *5-HT_{1a} agonists, 5-HT_3 antagonists and benzodiazepines: their comparative behavioural pharmacology*. Chichester: John Wiley, 1991.

Russell J, Lader MH. *Guidelines for the prevention and treatment of benzodiazepine dependence*. London: Mental Health Foundation, 1993.

Shapiro CM (ed). *ABC of sleep disorders*. London: British Medical Journal Publications.

Tallman JF, Gallager DW. The GABA-ergic system: a locus of benzodiazepine action. *Annual Review of Neuroscience* 1985; **8**: 21–44.

Taylor DP, Moon SL. Buspirone and related compounds as alternative anxiolytics. *Neuropeptides* 1991; **19** (suppl): 15–19.

PART II MANAGEMENT OF INSOMNIA

P Glue, SJ Wilson

CURRENT CONCEPTS IN ANXIETY DISORDERS

Anxiety is a mood state characterized by mental symptoms of fearful anticipation. As well as a discrete disorder, anxiety occurs as a component symptom in almost all psychiatric and in most physical illnesses. It is also a major component of drug withdrawal, especially from the opiates, benzodiazepines and ethanol.

The experience of anxiety is universal, in that it may be reported both as a normal emotion and also as part of a psychiatric disorder. Such diversity may be understood as a gradation of symptom severity, from normal to pathological anxiety; at the normal end of the spectrum, minor degrees of anxiety may lead to useful and performance-enhancing arousal, while at the pathological end of the spectrum, severe anxiety is maladaptive and disruptive. Another important concept is that of state and trait anxiety. State anxiety is a transient mood state and varies over short periods of time. When elevated, it is usually associated with transient stress, and settles once the stress disappears. In contrast, trait anxiety is an enduring feature. It appears to reflect aspects of personality and may have an inheritable component. Patients with anxiety disorders usually rate themselves highly on scales that assess both forms of anxiety, although for those with simple phobias, state anxiety may be quite low until confronted with their feared stimulus or situation.

Several different types of anxiety disorders have been distinguished in psychiatric practice on the basis of duration or nature of symptoms, or on the circumstances in which these occur. These are summarized in Table 21.4 (for more information, see Gelder *et al.*[1] and Nutt and Glue[2]). A significant recent change in diagnosing anxiety disorders is the distinction between generalized anxiety disorder and panic disorder, as in the USA-based DSM-III-R diagnostic scheme. This is based on pharmacological observations that both tricyclic and monoamine oxidase inhibitor (MAOI) antidepressant drugs will stop panic attacks, but have only

TABLE 21.4 Classification of anxiety disorders

Anticipatory anxiety:
Usually appropriate anxiety experienced while awaiting a stressful or unpleasant experience
Simple phobia:
Inappropriate anxiety in the presence of particular objects (e.g. spiders) or situations (e.g. heights). Avoidance behaviour (the tendency to avoid the unpleasant stimulus) is commonly present
Social phobia:
Inappropriate anxiety when contemplating or being in situations where there is a potential for being observed and criticized (e.g. in restaurants; while speaking in public). Avoidance behaviour is present
Agoraphobia:
Inappropriate anxiety (but not to the extent of panic attacks) displayed when away from home, in crowds, or in situations where escape is difficult (e.g. in queues). The subsequent refusal to leave home (avoidance behaviour) is termed agoraphobia.
Panic disorder:
The central symptom is the occurrence of panic attacks (sudden severe episodes of anxiety, with physical symptoms (e.g. shaking, shortness of breath), and expectations of imminent severe problems to explain the symptoms (e.g. death, heart attack)). These may occur spontaneously or be associated with certain situations. Avoidance behaviour (agoraphobia) often occurs if panic attacks happen in certain situations (e.g. supermarkets, when driving; see above)
Generalized anxiety disorder:
Persistent inappropriate anxiety symptoms out of context with life circumstances; associated with physical symptoms
Post-traumatic stress disorder:
Development of severe anxiety and other symptoms in response to a distressing event outside normal human experience (e.g. torture, kidnap, war)

limited effects on anxiety levels between attacks. The syndrome of anxiety that is accompanied by panic attacks has become known as panic disorder and patients with chronic high levels of anxiety who do not have panic attacks are referred to as having generalized anxiety disorder. The latter syndrome seems to respond best to sedatives such as benzodiazepines (see below). In view of the different treatments suitable for the range of anxiety disorders, it is important that a correct diagnosis is made prior to starting treatment. However, it is common for patients to report symptoms of more than one type of anxiety disorder and so a combination of therapeutic approaches may be needed.

As well as diagnostic subtypes within the range of anxiety disorders, patients may report different types of symptoms. Complaints can include lightheadedness or dizziness, which may not appear to be related to anxiety at all. A list of common symptoms is given in Table 21.5. It is difficult to categorize avoidance behaviour (avoidance of objects or situations associated with anxiety) as this involves both behavioural and cognitive components. It is possible that symptom differences may allow further subclassification of anxiety disorders, an example being the separation of panic and generalized anxiety disorders. Symptoms may also respond differently to drug treatments; for instance, benzodiazepines appear to be particularly good at treating anxiety-related insomnia whereas imipramine may be better for symptoms of tension.[3]

Theories on the aetiology of anxiety are wide ranging, and include genetic, biochemical, psychological and social factors.[1] A review of these is beyond the scope of this chapter. However, the mechanism of action of the above treatments may be understood better in light of recent research into the neurochemical bases of anxiety, especially with regard to noradrenergic and γ-aminobutyric acid (GABA)–benzodiazepine receptor abnormalities[4,5] (see Chapter 22).

TREATMENT GUIDELINES FOR ANXIETY DISORDERS

Current clinical practice recommends caution in the use of hypnotics or sedatives as initial treatment in anxious patients. Several techniques have been clearly shown to be of benefit in some anxiety disorders, and these are summarized in Table 21.6.

Benzodiazepines are indicated for the acute management of panic attacks, and may be of benefit early in the treatment of panic disorder with tricyclic antidepressants, as anxiety symptoms are often aggravated by this treatment. Recent research indicates that patients with panic disorder may have reduced sensitivity to benzodiazepines.[5] Clinically, this means that to consider using benzodiazepines in these patients means that relatively large doses of high potency drugs (e.g. clonazepam) must be used for any benefit to be noticed.

Benzodiazepines are also indicated for very short-term use in people with severe anticipatory anxiety, and in exacerbations of anxiety in other disorders (Table 21.6). It is possible that in generalized anxiety, when all other treatments have been exhausted, long-term use of benzodiazepines may be used as a last resort. Such an option should not be initiated lightly, with the risks of dependence and withdrawal to be considered. Barbiturates offer no useful advantage over benzodiazepines, either in terms of anti-anxiety effects, risk of tolerance, dependence or withdrawal, and have the major drawback of being lethal in over-

TABLE 21.5 Symptom subcomponents of anxiety

CATEGORY	SYMPTOM
Mood	Apprehension, worry, irritability
Cognitive	Thoughts of impending disaster or illness, social embarrassment
Physiological	Tachycardia, sweating, palpitations, flushing, nausea, diarrhoea, tremor, initial insomnia
Behavioural	Hand-wringing, pacing, scratching, hypervigilance, avoidance

TABLE 21.6 Established treatments for anxiety disorders

Anticipatory anxiety:	Reassurance; benzodiazepines; β-blockers
Simple phobia:	Behaviour therapy (desensitization/exposure)
Social phobia:	MAOIs; behaviour/cognitive therapy; ?benzodiazepines
Agoraphobia:	Behaviour therapy (exposure); antidepressants; benzodiazepines
Panic disorder:	Antidepressants; behaviour therapy; benzodiazepines
Generalized anxiety disorder:	Behaviour/cognitive/psychotherapy; benzodiazepines; antidepressants; buspirone
Post-traumatic stress disorder:	?Antidepressants; ?psychotherapy

dose. They should not be considered in the treatment of anxiety. Neuroleptics such as chlorpromazine or thioridazine may be useful in patients with anxiety associated with severe illnesses such as depression. Special care should be taken in treatment of elderly patients, as sensitivity to many drugs, including benzodiazepines, is increased.

As shown in Table 21.6, a range of other pharmacological or psychological therapies are preferable to hypnosedatives in the initial and long-term treatment of anxiety. Most research into treatment has been carried out in patients with simple phobias and with panic disorder. Behavioural treatment such as systematic desensitization or exposure has been demonstrated to be the treatment of choice for simple phobias. There is some controversy as to whether adjunctive treatment with benzodiazepines may help or hinder this type of treatment. The techniques available for treating panic disorder are more diverse. Treatment with tricyclic or monoamine oxidase inhibitor (MAOI) antidepressants is clearly effective in treating panic (episodic) anxiety, but much less effective in helping with generalized (persistent) anxiety in patients who have both disorders. There is a delay of at least several weeks before any antipanic effect is noted after starting antidepressant treatment, and tricyclic antidepressants frequently cause an exacerbation of anxiety symptoms early on. In these circumstances, a short course of benzodiazepines given concurrently with the antidepressants may be useful. There is also a large body of evidence showing that behavioural and cognitive psychotherapies are effective in reducing severity and frequency of panic attacks. Avoidance behaviour or agoraphobia is unaltered by antidepressant treatment, whether it occurs on its own or in combination with panic disorder, and must be dealt with by behavioural methods (exposure). Most research studies have emphasized that drug and behavioural treatment combined with patient education is more effective than one treatment in isolation.

There are several methods of treatment that have been reported to work in generalized anxiety disorder, but none is notably successful. A minority of patients may be helped by antidepressants or serotonin autoreceptor agonists such as buspirone (see Chapter 22, Part II). Similarly, a minority may be helped or supported with various types of psychotherapy. In cases where anxiety is prolonged and severe, long-term treatment with benzodiazepines in adequate doses may be the only way to produce symptomatic improvement (see above). β-Blockers may be useful for complaints of performance anxiety (tremor and tachycardia), but have little effect on anxious mood alone. There is little research into effective treatments for social phobia or post-traumatic stress disorder (PTSD). Social phobic symptoms appear to respond preferentially to MAOIs, although some success has been claimed for behavioural and cognitive techniques. While there is preliminary evidence that antidepressants may help in PTSD, benzodiazepines may disinhibit some of these patients.

The most common type of anxiety seen in anaesthetic practice will be anticipatory anxiety, in patients who are apprehensive about procedures or unfamiliar surroundings. Reassurance and explanation should be attempted before the use of drugs. If sedation is required, a long half-life benzodiazepine would be most suitable. If anxiety is extreme or sustained, or there is a history of anxiety disorder, drug or alcohol abuse or withdrawal, a more careful assessment will be required prior to consideration of treatment.

CURRENT CONCEPTS IN INSOMNIA

One-third of our lives is spent asleep, but the reasons that we sleep are not yet fully understood. Sleep is described as a state of inactivity accompanied by loss of awareness and a markedly reduced responsiveness to environmental stimuli. When a recording is made of the electrical activity of the brain (an electroencephalogram or EEG) and other physiological variables during sleep (a technique called polysomnography), a pattern of sleep consisting of five different stages emerges. This pattern varies from person to person, but usually consists of four or five cycles of quiet sleep alternating with paradoxical, or active sleep, with longer periods of paradoxical sleep in the latter half of the night (Fig. 21.5). The quiet sleep is divided further into four stages, each with a characteristic EEG appearance, with progressive relaxation of the muscles and slower, more regular breathing as the deeper stages are reached (Table 21.7). Most sleep in these deeper stages occurs in the first half of the night. During paradoxical sleep, the EEG appearance is similar to that of waking or drowsiness. There is irregular breathing, complete loss of tone of the skeletal muscles, and frequent phasic movements particularly of the eyes, consisting of conjugate movements which are mostly lateral but can also be vertical. This stage of sleep is called rapid eye movement (REM) sleep, and most dreaming takes place during this time (Table 21.7).

The time of day at which the usual long period of sleep takes place seems to be determined by an internal clock, influenced by the light cues of daylight and darkness. When these cues are missing humans tend to maintain an approximately 25-h clock, which helps to explain why it is less disruptive to lengthen our day on an east/west air trip than shorten it when travelling in the other direction. Many other factors including length of time since the last sleep period determine tendency to fall asleep. However, we are more likely to fall asleep at two particular times – at our usual nocturnal bedtime and in the post-lunch period.

The length of total sleep varies between 3 and 10 h in normal subjects with an average in the 20–45 age group of 7–8 h. Sleep time is decreased in older subjects, down to about 6 h in the over 70 age group, with

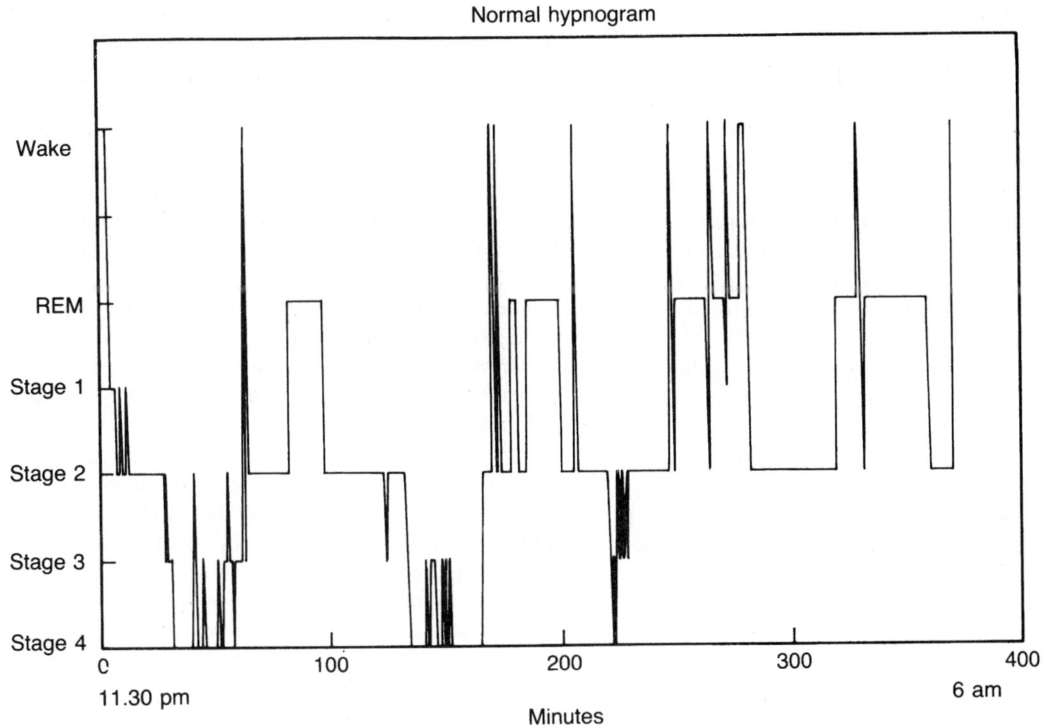

FIGURE 21.5 Hypnogram from a normal subject.

TABLE 21.7 Characteristics of sleep stages

SLEEP STAGE	EEG FEATURES	MUSCLE TONE	EYE MOVEMENTS
Awake	Low amplitude mixed frequency, α-rhythm	High tonic activity	Blinks, irregular
1	Low amplitude mixed frequency θ-activity	Slightly lower tonic activity	Slow rolling lateral
2	K complexes, sleep spindles, similar to stage 1	Tonic activity maintained	None
3	δ-Waves 20–50% of sleep record, with K complexes and sleep spindles	Tonic activity maintained	None
4	δ-Waves >50% of sleep record	Very low tonic activity	None
REM	Low amplitude, mixed frequency, similar to stage 1	No measurable tonic activity	Rapid phasic

increased daytime napping reducing the actual night time sleep block even more. The amount of time spent in each of the five stages will vary between subjects and particularly with age, with much less slow wave sleep in older people. Another sleep variable that increases with increasing age is the number of wakenings after the onset of sleep, which may be taken as a measure of sleep continuity.

After sleep deprivation experiments, where subjects were kept awake over one or more nights, subjects 'caught up' all of their deep quiet sleep (stages 3 and 4, or slow wave sleep) very quickly after sleep onset on the first night of recovery. Interestingly, the 'catching up' process recovered only about half of the REM sleep and very little of the lighter stages. In associated experiments, subjects who normally slept for 7–8 h had their sleep periods reduced gradually until they were regularly sleeping for about 6 h. This was satisfactory to the subjects but further reduction was difficult and proved unacceptable. The stages lost during these studies were REM and light sleep. These studies suggest that it is crucial to maintain a full quota of deep sleep and that the other sleep stages are less important.

Insomnia is the complaint of poor sleep, when a patient reports that the duration or subjective quality of their sleep is unsatisfactory. Insomnia may consist of difficulty in falling to sleep at night (initial insomnia) or difficulty in remaining asleep (maintenance insomnia), with either frequent awakenings or waking too early in the morning. Many patients complain of both. They may report that their sleep does not refresh them. Insomnia may or may not be accompanied by daytime fatigue.

Sleep parameters have been compared in insomniacs and subjects who are satisfied with their sleep ('good sleepers'). In one study, the overall distribution of sleep duration was found to be similar in both groups, although measures of trait anxiety were increased in the insomnia group. In another study using polysomnography, sleep in insomniacs was found to contain more interruptions and less stage 2 sleep than in good sleepers; however, there were a few patients with insomnia in whom a series of 7–8 h uninterrupted sleep periods were recorded. What causes patients to go to their doctors and complain of poor sleep remains unclear – either their sleep has changed in character or their ability to tolerate problems of sleep interruption or duration has decreased.

Insomnia may be further classified according to duration, as transient (lasting a few days), short term, or long term (lasting more than 3 weeks). Transient insomnia is usually situational, for example when subjects are sleeping in a novel environment (e.g. hospital), or when jet lag disrupts the day/night rhythm. Stress caused by factors such as examinations, impending surgical operations or situations requiring alertness can also cause this transient complaint. Short-term insomnia usually arises as a result of more substantial stress, such as that caused by major life events. Pain is one of the major causes of short-term insomnia; for instance postoperative pain is cited by patients as the main problem keeping them awake during their nights in hospital. Bereavement is another important cause of insomnia.

Pharmacological causes include use of drugs such as caffeine or alcohol. Although alcohol helps to reduce the time to onset of sleep, it often gives rise to disrupted sleep later in the night. Short-term insomnia is commonly seen after acute administration of certain antidepressants, especially serotonin reuptake inhibitors (e.g. fluoxetine, fluvoxamine), or monoamine uptake inhibitors. This is probably due to the increase in central serotonergic and/or noradrenergic activity (see Chapter 22). In such cases, it may be of some benefit to give the antidepressants during the day rather than at bedtime. Abrupt withdrawal of antidepressants may also lead to insomnia for several days. Withdrawal from hypnotic or anxiolytic drugs, particularly benzodiazepines, may cause 'rebound' insomnia which can last for 4–6 weeks; other causes must be sought if sleep has not improved after this time. Both transient and short-term insomnia are normally self-limiting, and once there is an improvement in the particular situation sleep is often perceived to improve spontaneously.

There are many factors associated with long-term insomnia. Physical factors that may lead to complaints of persistent poor sleep include discomfort due to pain, pregnancy, or constant coughing or wheezing. Sleep may be disturbed by the need to urinate. Nocturnal myoclonus (frequent jerks or twitches during the descent into deeper sleep), or the 'restless legs' syndrome where the subject has an unavoidable urge to keep moving the legs, may give rise to sleep problems in the patient but are more likely to cause them in the subject's sleeping partner.

Various cardiovascular and respiratory diseases with nocturnal symptoms may also disrupt sleep. A disorder that is becoming more widely recognized is obstructive sleep apnoea (sleep apnoeic syndrome), in which the patient's upper airway collapses during deeper sleep, causing loud snoring and eventually cessation of breathing. When the blood oxygen saturation decreases sufficiently, the patient wakes and starts breathing again, usually with a loud gasp. This can happen many times in a night, up to 200–300 times in some cases. Often the patient is only aware of excessive daytime sleepiness, and it is again the sleeping partner who suffers from insomnia. Obstructive sleep apnoea has been estimated to occur in 3/1000 middle-aged men.

Factors in the sleeping environment may also lead to long-term insomnia. If room temperature is too high or too low, sleep patterns may be substantially disrupted. Other common causes include excessive noise, or children waking. Subjects who have disturbed circadian rhythms, such as those involved in shift work, also frequently report insomnia.

Psychiatric disorders are commonly associated with long-term insomnia. Patients with depressive illnesses often have difficulty falling asleep at night and complain of restless, disturbed and unrefreshing sleep, and early morning waking. When their sleep is analysed by polysomnography, time to sleep onset is indeed prolonged, and there is a tendency for more REM sleep to occur in the first part of the night, with reduced deep quiet sleep in the first hour or so after sleep onset. Although the mechanism is unclear, weight loss occurring in severe depressive illness is associated with early morning waking. Anxiety disorders may cause patients to complain about their sleep, either because there is a reduction in sleep continuity or because normal periods of nocturnal waking are somehow less well tolerated. Early morning waking is commonly seen in patients with anorexia nervosa and is likely to be due to weight loss in this condition. Disrupted sleep records may be obtained from patients with schizophrenia or with various types of dementing illnesses, although insomnia is inconsistently reported. Although not a psychiatric disorder, bereavement, particularly involving a sleeping partner, often gives rise to long-term insomnia. This is not only because of grief but also because bedtime routines may be disrupted and a pattern of poor sleep satisfaction established.

Pharmacological factors are also important in long-term insomnia. Although alcohol may initially shorten the time taken to fall asleep, regular and excessive consumption disrupts sleep, particularly continuity. Indeed, insomnia is a key feature of alcohol withdrawal. Excessive intake of caffeine and theophylline, either in tea, coffee or cola drinks, also contributes to insomnia. As mentioned above, a minority of patients who are withdrawing from hypnotics and sedatives may report long-term insomnia. This is more likely to be due to the return of pretreatment anxiety or depressive symptoms rather than a persistent withdrawal effect. Other drugs which increase central noradrenergic and serotonergic activity also cause insomnia. These include stimulants such as amphetamine, cocaine and methylphenidate, and sympathomimetics such as the β-adrenergic agonist salbutamol and associated compounds.

TREATMENT GUIDELINES FOR INSOMNIA

Transient and short-term insomnia are self-limiting and should only require reassurance. For example, most surgical inpatients will report insomnia during their hospital stay, especially preoperatively. This is almost certainly in response to the novel environment of the hospital and due to anticipatory anxiety about procedures. The majority of these patients will not have had past problems with excessive trait anxiety or insomnia, and their symptoms can be regarded as minor and reversible responses to stress. Although reassurance and explanation may be all that is required for such insomnia, a brief course of short half-life benzodiazepines may be used symptomatically. These drugs should not be continued for more than 1 week to avoid any risk of dependency, and patients should be warned that brief rebound insomnia may be noted after stopping these drugs.

The steps for the treatment of long-term insomnia are summarized in Table 21.8. The first and most important step is explanation and reassurance. Patients should be informed that if there is an overwhelming physical need for sleep that this will occur whatever the circumstances, and that serious harm will not occur by them sleeping less than they think they should. This is particularly important where fear of insomnia is a factor. If the patient fears waking up unrefreshed because of poor sleep, this attitude alone may lead to a wakeful night.

Patients may worry about normal sleep-related phenomena such as hypnagogic hallucinations (either auditory or visual), or myoclonus in light sleep. They should be reassured that these are perfectly normal. Reassurance and education also plays a large part in dealing with complaints of insomnia in patients with anxiety disorders, so that informing patients that they will not suffer long-term damage from loss of sleep may leave them with one less problem to worry about. Elderly patients often benefit most from reassurance and education about the normal reduction in sleep time associated with advancing years. For instance, the average sleep time for 70-year-old subjects is about 6 h. Therefore, if an elderly subject is going to bed at 9 pm, he or she should expect to be awake at 3 am.

In insomniac subjects where no obvious factors can be identified, a programme of good sleep hygiene should be instituted. Most items in a sleep hygiene programme are common sense, but few patients who are dissatisfied with their sleep pay attention to all of them. Basically, sleep will be improved if there is regularity, comfort and satisfaction of physical needs, so the following checklist may be useful (see Table 21.8).

Patients should keep to regular bedtimes and rising times, paying attention to the realistically expected duration of sleep (about 6 h in the elderly). Rigorous adherence to these will usually result in an improvement. If more sleep is required at night, curtailing or missing daytime naps is advisable. Patients should be encouraged to exercise and to be exposed to daylight during the day. The use of stimulants, such as tea, coffee, or cola drinks during the hours before bedtime should be discouraged. The elderly seem to be more sensitive to the stimulant effects of tea than younger patients, and their consumption of it is fairly high; often the reaction to lack of sleep is to get up and make a cup of tea, which is not advisable. Alcohol should also not be consumed before bedtime. Although the mechanism is not clear, smokers tend to have poorer sleep than non-smokers, and abstinence should be encouraged.

A regular bedtime routine may also be helpful. An easily digested snack or milky drink before retiring

TABLE 21.8 Treatment of insomnia

TRANSIENT/SHORT-TERM	LONG-TERM
Reassurance	Reassurance and education
	Attention to sleep hygiene Regular bedtimes and rising times Reduce daytime napping Encourage daytime exercise and exposure to daylight Avoid stimulants, alcohol and cigarettes Establish bedtime routine; snack or milk drink may be helpful Avoid ruminating about problems in bed ? relaxation tape Bedroom temperature and noise levels should be controlled
	Treatment of physical and psychiatric contributing factors
Drug treatment – short-term benzodiazepines	Drug treatment – short-term benzodiazepines

may be included as part of this routine. Although it may be difficult, patients should be advised to try and avoid associating the bedroom with anxiety or other strong unpleasant emotions; for instance, worrying about bills or having arguments should not be done in bed. They should be encouraged to practise relaxation techniques, perhaps with a relaxation tape. If fear of insomnia has caused the bedroom to become associated with worries about sleep itself, then perhaps sleeping on the sofa or in the spare room for a while may help. It may be the presence of a clock beside the bed contributes to sleep anxiety, so that worrying about sleep is reinforced by continual referral to the time.

Attention should also be paid to the sleeping environment; this includes keeping the bedroom temperature comfortable, not being too hot or too cold, which may decrease sleep continuity. Noise in itself probably does not stop people sleeping; constant heavy traffic is ignored after a few nights. It is intermittent noise or noise causing anger which seems to cause problems. Earplugs may be a solution.

Children who do not sleep undoubtedly cause many of the complaints of poor sleep in adults, as do partners with loud snoring, sleep apnoea, restless legs or nocturnal myoclonus. When this problem becomes long term, the treatment of the subject's own insomnia may need to be preceded by treatment of the sleep disorder in the family member.

Pain is a major cause of sleep disruption, and analgesic treatment should improve sleep as a secondary effect. Symptomatic treatment of psychiatric disorders will also improve sleep. Antidepressant drugs cause major changes in the structure of sleep when given to normal subjects and depressed patients, some being relatively sedating and improving continuity of sleep, others causing more wakenings, as mentioned above. However, it is clear that when depressed patients improve in mood they report an improvement in their sleep, whether they are treated pharmacologically or with other methods. Treatment of anxiety improves sleep, and the hypnotic effects of anxiolytic drugs are described above. Complaints of poor sleep in dementia, however, are less open to treatment; once basic sleep hygiene has been attended to there is little scope for other measures apart from the use of hypnotic agents. Problems with these in the elderly patient, in particular increased sensitivity, are greater than in a younger population, and special care needs to be taken to ensure that iatrogenic toxicity is avoided.

Other disruptions caused by pharmacological intervention can be minimized by judicious timing of drugs. For instance, diuretics should not be administered in the evening, so that patients do not have to get up during the night to micturate. Sympathomimetic drugs used in asthma treatment sometimes cause increased arousal, but here a balance must be struck between adverse effects and constant waking due to asthmatic coughing or wheezing. Insomnia associated with other respiratory and cardiovascular disorders also improves when symptoms are treated, although sleep hygiene may have to be rigidly applied if poor sleep habits have become established during physical illness.

THE ROLE OF HYPNOSEDATIVES IN ANAESTHETIC PRACTICE

The main role for these drugs in anaesthesia is to reduce preoperative anxiety, to produce light sedation to allow minor procedures to be carried out, and as induction agents. The amnesia produced by benzodiazepines is a useful additional side-effect in these circumstances. The management of anxiety and insomnia in apprehensive patients is described above.

For premedication, benzodiazepines may be useful alternatives to opioids, especially for procedures requiring only light sedation. Indeed, for some procedures, benzodiazepines may be the only agents used (such as in endoscopy or dentistry), or they may be used in conjunction with local anaesthesia. Trimeprazine is an alternative in children, although there are no problems using benzodiazepines. If benzodiazepines are used for sedation during a procedure, these effects may be rapidly reversed with the antagonist flumazenil although whether this should be done routinely is not yet established (see above). Patients should be warned of the possibility that sedation may recur if a long half-life benzodiazepine is used.

Postoperatively, sedation or hypnosis may be required in patients who are being ventilated. Benzodiazepines are ideal for this purpose, because of their limited effects on respiratory function. Unfortunately, benzodiazepines are not analgesic, and additional analgesia is required. Night time sleep is often disrupted during the postoperative period when cues such as social interaction, light and other stimuli are similar throughout the 24h day. Surgery and anaesthesia interfere with normal sleep patterns, especially REM sleep on the first postoperative night and was associated with hypoxaemia.[6] However, once normal day/night patterns of activity are re-established, night time sleep will improve.

Interactions between commonly used anxiolytics and general anaesthetic or muscle-relaxant drugs are not a major problem. An interaction of note is between phenothiazines (such as thioridazine or chlorpromazine) and general anaesthetic agents, as the latter may potentiate these drugs' hypotensive effects. However, phenothiazines will be used rarely as sedatives or hypnotics in a general hospital setting. Patients who have been on barbiturates chronically, or are chronic heavy drinkers, will require increased amounts of anaesthetic induction agents. This may reflect reduced GABA sensitivity in response to chronic barbiturate or ethanol intake. Ethanol potentiates the actions of pethidine, causing profound respiratory depression and even coma, while the sympathomimetic effect causes extreme hypertension.

REFERENCES AND FURTHER READING

1 Gelder M, Gath D, Mayou R. *Oxford textbook of psychiatry*. Oxford: Oxford University Press, 1988.

2 Nutt DJ, Glue P. Clinical pharmacology of anxiolytics and antidepressants: a psychopharmacological perspective. *Pharmacology and Therapeutics* 1989; **44**: 309–34.

3 Kahn RJ McNair DM, Lipman RS, Covi L, Rickels K, Downing R, Fisher S, Frankenthaler LM. Imipramine and chlordiazepoxide in depressive and anxiety disorders. *Archives of General Psychiatry* 1986; **43**: 79–85.

4 Nutt DJ. The pharmacology of human anxiety. *Pharmacology and Therapeutics* 1990; **47**: 233–66.

5 Nutt DJ, Glue P, Lawson CW, Wilson SJ, Ball DM. Do benzodiazepine receptors have a causal role in panic disorder? In: British Association for Psychopharmacology Monograph *Psychopharmacology of Panic* Montgomery SA, ed. Oxford: Oxford University Press, Oxford, 1993.

6 Rosenberg J, Wildschiodt G, Pederson MH *et al.* Late postoperative nocturnal episodic hypoxaemia and associated sleep pattern. *British Journal of Anaesthesia* 1994; **72**: 145–50.

Carskadon M, Dement W, Mittler M, Guilleminault C, Zarcone VP, Spiegel R. Self-reports versus sleep laboratory findings in 122 drug-free subjects with the complaint of chronic insomnia. *American Journal of Psychiatry* 1976; **133**: 1382–8.

Gillin JC, Byerley WF. The diagnosis and managment of insomnia. *New England Journal of Medicine* 1990; **322**: 239–48.

Horne JA. *Why we sleep: the functions of sleep in humans and other mammals*. Oxford: Oxford University Press, 1988.

Williams RL, Karacan I, Moore CA. *Sleep disorders: diagnosis and treatment*, 2nd edn. New York: Wiley Interscience, 1988.

Zorumski, CF, Isenberg KE. Insights into the structure and function of GABA–benzodiazepine receptors: ion channels and psychiatry. *American Journal of Psychiatry* 1991; **148**: 162–73.

22

Psychiatry

PART I DRUGS AND THE TREATMENT OF PSYCHIATRIC DISORDERS

CJ Pycock

The monoamine neurotransmitters (noradrenaline, dopamine, 5-hydroxytryptamine (5-HT)) have been strongly implicated in the aetiology of many human psychiatric states, in particular schizophrenia[1] and depression.[2] Major support for their involvement derives from the fact that those drugs used to control the symptoms of these disorders exert powerful pharmacological actions on the brain monoamine systems. In addition, these agents often possess other well-documented pharmacological properties which explain the side-effects and drug interactions frequently encountered with use of these compounds. Drugs used to manage psychiatric disorders are not uncommonly encountered in anaesthetic practice.

THE PSYCHOSES

The psychoses are a collection of symptoms related to behavioural disturbances in which the patient loses insight into his illness. They can broadly be divided into two groups:

1 *Organic psychosis* occurs when the behaviour disorder is attributable to a physical illness, for example infection, electrolyte imbalance, drugs, cerebral lesions or hypoxia. Such states will present acutely either as delirium or chronically as dementia. Management should be directed towards the underlying cause, if possible; tranquillizers may be required to control agitation.
2 *Functional psychoses* are said to occur where there is no obvious systemic (or cerebral) pathology that is immediately identifiable. These states are divided broadly into the *affective disorders* where swings of mood such as depression and/or mania predominate, and *schizophrenia* characterized by disorders of thought, emotion and perception.[3]

Schizophrenia, depression, and the drugs used in their treatment, are the subject of this chapter.

CEREBRAL MONOAMINES AND SCHIZOPHRENIA

Most psychiatrists and neurochemists believe in the hypothesis that schizophrenia is related to the functional overactivity of certain cerebral dopamine systems.[4] Prior to the 1970s it had been suggested that psychotic and hallucinatory states may be due to the production in the brain of abnormal metabolites that possessed hallucinatory properties. These may have been compounds either found naturally within the body but being diverted through an adverse biochemical pathway, or those obtained from an exogenous source such as food substances. Indeed, it was well known that many methylated products of 5-HT and tryptamine had hallucinatory properties (e.g. lysergic acid diethylamide (LSD), psilocin and psilocybin). These methylated compounds could often be detected as a 'pink spot' on paper chromatograms when treated with Ehrlich reagent and ninhydrin, and so it was the vogue in the early 1960s to screen blood and urine from schizophrenics for the presence of N-methylated metabolites in order to refute or confirm the pink spot theory as the pathogenesis of mental illness.[5] Unfortunately for the advocates of the theory the findings were not substantiated and the pink spot idea was finally abandoned.

The close association between neurotransmitter dopamine and the aetiology of schizophrenia arose from two quite compelling sources. First, the administration of amphetamine to healthy human volunteers could provoke a psychotic state closely resembling paranoid schizophrenia.[6] Dexamphetamine is known to release dopamine (and other monoamines) from presynaptic nerve terminals, and this action, together with its ability to block neuronal re-uptake mechanisms (albeit weakly) causes the drug to stimulate indirectly postsynaptic dopamine receptors. In animal models it produces stereotyped behaviours and activation of the locomotor system which can be blocked by prior administration of neuroleptic (dopamine receptor blocking) drugs. Similarly dihydroxyphenylalanine (L-DOPA), an agent used to stimulate central dopamine systems in patients with Parkinson's disease (see Chapter 23), can precipitate psychotic states or aggravate pre-existing psychiatric symptoms.

The second major support for the dopamine hypothesis of schizophrenia comes from observation of those drugs used to control this disorder. There is a close association between the effectiveness of the antipsychotic drugs and the ability to block postsynaptic dopamine receptors both *in vitro* and *in vivo*. Using radioactively labelled compounds, experiments have been designed to study the potency with which neuroleptic drugs bind to dopamine receptors; this binding ability correlates remarkably well with their clinically reported antipsychotic efficacy.[7] One specific example comes from studies on the stereoisomers of the drug flupenthixol, the α (*cis*) isomer was noted as being some 1000 times more potent at blocking dopamine receptors compared with the β (*trans*) isomer. Clinical trials have established that *cis*-flupenthixol demonstrates marked antipsychotic activity: *trans*-flupenthixol had none.

Further support for the dopamine hypothesis of schizophrenia is provided from post-mortem findings which report raised concentrations of dopamine in striatal and limbic areas of brain in patients dying with schizophrenic illness. Receptor-binding studies have also shown an increased number of dopamine receptors in certain regions in the schizophrenic brain.[8]

Central dopamine systems: anatomy

The anatomy of the dopamine systems is comparatively well described in mammalian brain, and this is broadly linked with varying functional roles.[9] The system that is believed to be concerned with the control of emotion and behaviour is the limbic and reticular network. (The two other major dopaminergic systems are the ascending nigrostriatal pathway of the basal ganglia related to the initation and control of movement (described in Chapter 23), and the tubero-infundibular system of the hypothalamus with a neuroendocrine role.) The reticular-activating system is a network of nerve fibres and terminals, some of which contain noradrenaline, and these are found projecting from brain stem regions to the mesencephalon. The *mesolimbic forebrain dopamine system* arises from cell bodies in the ventral tegmentum of the mesencephalon, just medial to the substantia nigra. Axons project rostrally to terminate within the head of the caudate nucleus, the nucleus accumbens, the anterior perforated substance (tuberculum olfactorium of lower mammals), the frontal and cingulate cortex and the amygdaloid nuclei. It is changes in dopamine function within this system, with subsequent enhancement of neurotransmitter activity, that has been strongly implicated in the aetiology of schizophrenia.

Central dopamine systems: receptors

Over the last two decades, it has become apparent that more than one population of dopamine receptor exists.[10] Although the original classification subdivided the dopamine receptor into two main groups, the D_1 and D_2 receptors,[11] at the time of writing up to five types of dopamine receptor are now recognized (coded as D_1–D_5 subtypes).[12,13] From the original description,[11] the dopamine D_1 receptor is linked to an adenylate cyclase system on postsynaptic membranes such that stimulation of this receptor site with either dopamine or dopamine agonist drugs results in the generation of cyclic 3′,5′-adenosine monophosphate (cAMP) produced from adenosine triphosphate (ATP). cAMP is recognized as the secondary messenger that initates the train of postsynaptic events associated with receptor activation. Conversely, dopamine receptor antagonist drugs (the neuroleptic/antipsychotic drugs) will block this production of cAMP.[14]

The dopamine D_2 receptor is not linked to the adenylate cyclase system and this site is located either presynaptically or postsynaptically.

The subclassification of the dopamine receptor into further subtypes has been based largely on the specificity and selectivity by which various drugs and synthesized compounds bind to receptor subpopulations.[15] The five receptor subtypes have now been cloned and are facilitating the search for discovery of more selective dopaminergic drugs.[13] Dopamine itself is an agonist at all receptor subtypes but with varying affinity. The cloned D_5 receptor subtype has very similar characteristics to the D_1 receptor in native tissue, but the D_5 site is about ten times more sensitive to dopamine than the D_1 site. The D_2-like receptors, D_2, D_3 and D_4, have approximately similar sensitivity for dopamine. Likewise, various antipsychotic drugs show varying affinities for each of the receptor subtypes. The phenothiazines and thioxanthines tend to block all receptor subtypes (and thus cAMP formation), whereas the butyrophenones and the substituted benzamides appear as more selective antagonists at the D_2-like receptor group(s).

It would appear that all types of dopamine receptor are involved with the control of movement regulated by the basal ganglia, but that the D_2-like sites may be more exclusively associated with mood and behaviour control from mesolimbic regions.[16] Indeed, a recent report suggests that it is the D_4 site (a subgroup of the D_2 receptor) that is specifically elevated in the brains of schizophrenic patients.[17]

ANTIPSYCHOTIC DRUGS

The *antipsychotic drugs* (also known collectively as the neuroleptics or the major tranquillizers) have their major use in the management of schizophrenia and other psychotic states,[18] although they are also of clinical value (usually in smaller, more controlled doses) for treating mania and depression, as general sedatives for controlling acute psychotic or agitated states and in neuroleptanalgesia for terminal care. They can help reduce extrapyramidal dyskinetic movements associated with chorea or those which are drug-induced in the treatment of Parkinson's disease.

The antipsychotic drugs have the common pharmacological property of blocking cerebral dopamine receptors, but they are usually classified according to their chemical structure:

- *phenothiazines* (chlorpromazine, fluphenazine, thioridazine)
- *butyrophenones* (haloperidol, benperidol)
- *thioxanthines* (chlorprothixene, thiothixene, flupenthixol)
- *diphenylbutyl piperidines* (pimozide, fluspirilene)
- *substituted benzamides* (sulpiride)

The *Rauwolfia alkaloids* (e.g. reserpine) are often included as of historical interest only; they no longer have a clinical role and act pharmacologically by depleting CNS stores of monoamine transmitters.[19]

The phenothiazines

Structurally, the phenothiazines are divided into three chemical classes related to the chain substitution attached to the nitrogen grouping. These are molecules with:

- *aliphatic side chains* containing dimethylaminopropyl groups, e.g. chlorpromazine, promazine
- *piperidine side chains*, e.g. thioridazine
- *piperazine side chains*, e.g. trifluoperazine, prochlorperazine, fluphenazine, perphenazine

(In general it is this latter group that demonstrates the most potent antipsychotic properties.) The chemical structures of representative drugs are shown in Fig. 22.1.

Chlorpromazine is regarded as the prototype phenothiazine, discovered in the 1950s during the development of antihistaminic drugs. It was shown to have strong sedative properties and thus found use in calming the agitated, manic or aggressive patient. It was also noted as having definite antipsychotic effects. Pharmacologically, chlorpromazine has a broad spectrum of action, exhibiting antihistaminic (H_1-receptor blocking) actions, anticholinergic (antimuscarinic) activity, α-adrenergic blocking properties in addition to inhibiting dopamine receptors (D_1 and D_2 sites).

Pharmacokinetics of chlorpromazine

The most widely studied drug in terms of the pharmacokinetics of phenothiazines, and indeed of the major tranquillizers in general, is chlorpromazine. All of these drugs tend to be highly lipophilic but only about 30% appears to be absorbed following oral administration. Circulating chlorpromazine is 90–95% protein bound, with an active half-life in the range of 10–20 h. The primary site of metabolism occurs within the liver, although many other organs can metabolize the drug including the gut, lungs, kidneys and brain. Many metabolites of chlorpromazine and the other phenothiazines can be detected, each with varying degrees of bioactivity. The major metabolic routes include demethylation, oxidation, hydroxylation, or conjugation with glucuronic acid and these metabolites are excreted in the urine.

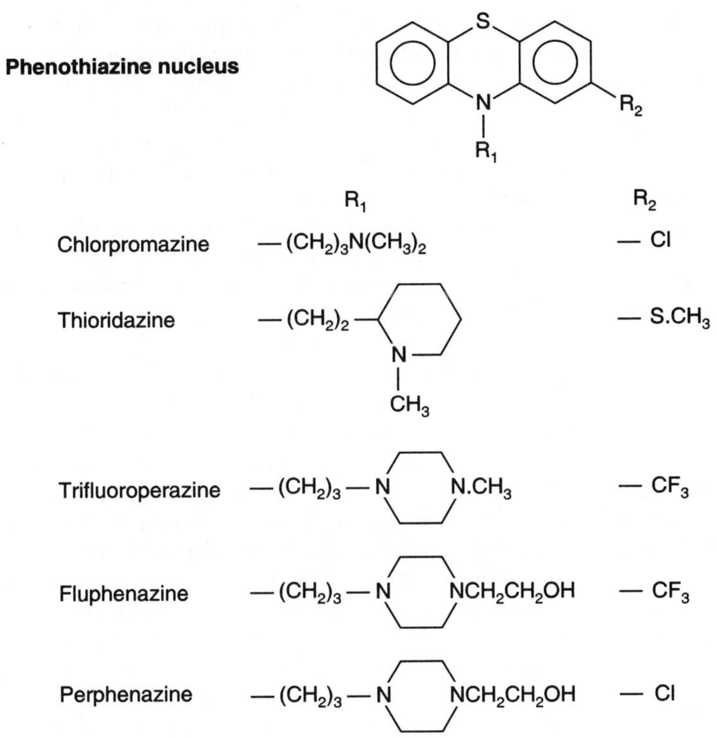

Phenothiazine nucleus

	R_1	R_2
Chlorpromazine	$—(CH_2)_3N(CH_3)_2$	— Cl
Thioridazine	$—(CH_2)_2$— (N-methyl-2-piperidyl; N–CH_3)	$— S.CH_3$
Trifluoroperazine	$—(CH_2)_3$— N (piperazine) $N.CH_3$	$— CF_3$
Fluphenazine	$—(CH_2)_3$— N (piperazine) NCH_2CH_2OH	$— CF_3$
Perphenazine	$—(CH_2)_3$— N (piperazine) NCH_2CH_2OH	— Cl

FIGURE 22.1. Structures of antipsychotic phenothiazine drugs (neuroleptics).

Clinical properties of the phenothiazines

Clinical properties of the phenothiazines include sedation; antipsychotic/antimanic/antidepressive effects; anti-emetic uses by blockade of dopamine receptors in the chemoreceptor trigger zone of the brainstem medulla; suppression of vestibular function in Menière's disease and other labyrinthine disorders; management of dyskinesias in chorea, Gilles de la Tourette's syndrome and in other extrapyramidal disorders by blockade of dopamine receptors within the basal ganglia; suppression of hiccoughs; control of alcohol-withdrawal hallucinations; control of sexually deviant behaviour (usually butyrophenones); and neurolept-analgesia in terminal care.

Those phenothiazines with the piperazine side-chain (e.g. *trifluoperazine*, *fluphenazine*, *perphenazine*) appear to be most potent as antipsychotic drugs having pharmacological activity more selectively directed towards blocking central dopamine receptors (both D_1 and D_2 sites) although there is an increased incidence of extrapyramidal side-effects (see below). With more potent antihistaminic and antimuscarinic activity, the phenothiazines with aliphatic side-chains tend to be more sedative, making drowsiness a problem.

However, both the phenothiazines *promethazine* and *trimeprazine* (Vallergan), which show potent antagonist activity at histamine H_1 and muscarinic sites making them strongly sedative drugs, have found use in anaesthetic premedication, and have also been thankfully blest by many weary mothers for providing nocturnal sedation to their apparently relentlessly sleepless child.

Side-effects of the phenothiazines

Many of the clinical side-effects of the phenothiazine drugs are directly related to the broad pharmacological properties of these compounds. Blockade of cerebral dopamine receptors (both D_1 and D_2 sites) especially within the basal ganglia can provoke extrapyramidal side-effects,[20] manifest in the form of abnormal involuntary movements including: bradykinesias, rigidity and drug-induced parkinsonism; tremor, motor restlessness (akathesia), catatonia; acute dystonias – often in the form of torticollis, facial grimacing, or oculogyric crises – which are occasionally seen at the onset of antipsychotic drug therapy and are thought to be possibly related to partial agonist action (and therefore stimulation of) at the dopamine receptors. Tardive dyskinesias are recognized complications of chronic drug therapy, thought to be related to 'disuse supersensitivity' whereby prolonged receptor inhibition leads to a general increase in the sensitivity of the receptor sites for neurotransmitter dopamine. Synaptic dopamine, released from presynaptic terminals whose synthesis and turnover has been enhanced by the continuous presence of the blocking agent, combines with the supersensitive postsynaptic receptor site resulting in an overstimulation of postsynaptic mechanisms; an action being manifest as abnormal movements or the tardive dyskinesias. Administration of higher doses of the dopamine-blocking drug in general inhibits these movements, but they are likely to then re-occur at the higher dosage of antipsychotic agent.[21]

Other side-effects of the phenothiazines (and antipsychotic drugs in general) that appear related to inhibition of dopaminergic activity associated with hypothalamic function include weight gain by action on the feeding/satiety centre, hyperprolactinaemia and subsequent amenorrhoea and galactorrhoea by blockade of prolactin inhibitory factor from the median eminence which itself is thought to be dopamine (see Chapter 20), and lack of temperature control by interference in function of the thermoregulatory centre.

On this latter point, chlorpromazine has a poikilothermic effect; it impairs the ability to thermoregulate and therefore the body may become hypothermic or hyperthermic depending upon the ambient temperature, an important consideration in the practice of anaesthesia. Chlorpromazine has therefore been usefully employed in the management of heat stroke whereby the overheated body is placed in a cool environment and the drug aids the reduction in body temperature.

The broader pharmacological properties of the neuroleptic drugs often explain the other documented side-effects:

- *anticholinergic actions* will cause the reported dry mouth, blurred vision, nasal stuffiness, constipation and urinary retention
- *anti-α-adrenergic* properties may evoke postural hypotension and cardiac arrhythmias
- *anti-histaminic* activity often results in undue sedation

Idiosyncratic drug reactions account for other side-effects such as:

- blood dyscrasias (uncommonly) – leucopenia, thrombocytopenia, agranulocytosis, haemolytic anaemia
- skin reactions – urticarial, maculopapular or petechial rashes, pigmentation, contact dermatitis, and light sensitivity reactions
- jaundice – due to intrahepatic cholestasis, occurs in 3% of patients taking chlorpromazine

The *neuroleptic malignant syndrome* is a rare complication of treatment with antipsychotic drugs characterized by catatonia, hyperpyrexia and autonomic instability. The disorder can be life-threatening, with cardiovascular collapse and extremely labile blood pressures which require aggressive and life-supportive management until the action of the neuroleptic drug has worn off.[22]

The butyrophenones

The butyrophenones – *haloperidol*, *droperidol* and *trifluperidol* – also possess potent antipsychotic properties. Benperidol is used in deviant and antisocial sexual behaviour but its value is not firmly established.

In general, they show better oral absorption (greater than 60%) than the phenothiazines. They are chiefly metabolized in the liver, metabolic pathways include oxidative dealkylation, and they are excreted in the bile and urine. The butyrophenones are extensively bound to plasma proteins; the half-life of haloperidol is long, in the order of 15–40 h. The half-life of droperidol is short (*c.* 2 h) and the drug must be given at more regular intervals. In addition to managing schizophrenia, these drugs can be used as anti-emetics, in neuroleptanalgesia, as premedicants, and in the control of agitation in active psychosis.

In general, they have less antimuscarinic and anti-α-adrenergic activity than the phenothiazines but their potent dopamine receptor blocking actions at both D_1 and D_2 sites can provoke more extrapyramidal reaction in the form of akathesia and dystonias. Initial biochemical and behavioural models, however, have suggested that the butyrophenones were more selective for the D_2 dopamine receptor, as much higher concentrations of these compounds were required to block the dopamine stimulated D_1 site mediated adenylate cyclase system than compared with the phenothiazines or thioxanthines.[14] The structures of haloperidol and droperidol are shown in Fig. 22.2.

The thioxanthines

Chemically, the thioxanthines are triple ring heterocyclic compounds and include *chlorprothixene*, *thiothixene*, *clopenthixol*, *flupenthixol* and *zuclopenthixol* (see Fig. 22.2). All exert potent antipsychotic properties but in general are less sedative and more antidepressant and anxiolytic than the phenothiazines. They exhibit good rapid absorption from the gastrointestinal tract. They are extensively metabolized in the liver, being excreted as numerous metabolites in the urine and faeces. Pharmacologically, they potently inhibit the dopamine-stimulated adenylate cyclase system indicating selectivity for D_1 sites.

Diphenylbutyl piperidines

This group of antipsychotic compounds includes *pimozide*, *fluspirilene* and *penfluridol*. Pharmacologically, they are claimed to be more selective at the D_2 (non-adenylate cyclase linked) dopamine receptor site and therefore are expected to exhibit less extrapyramidal side-effects, although this is not always the case in practice. Pimozide shows approximately 50% absorption from the gastrointestinal tract. There is significant first-pass metabolism, the major metabolic pathway of the liver being N-dealkylation. Metabolites and unchanged drug are excreted in the urine and faeces. The half-life of pimozide is long (in the order of 50 h) and so can be given by single daily dose.

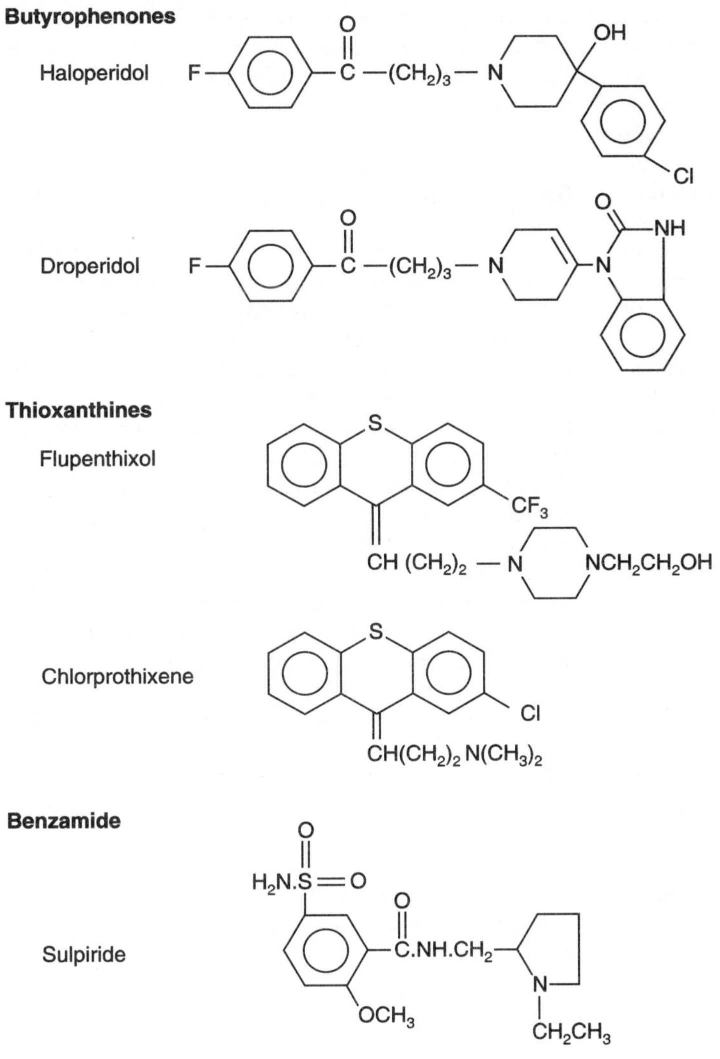

Butyrophenones

Haloperidol

Droperidol

Thioxanthines

Flupenthixol

Chlorprothixene

Benzamide

Sulpiride

FIGURE 22.2. Structures of non-phenothiazine neuroleptics.

Substituted benzamides (sulpiride)

Sulpiride (N-[1-ethyl-2-pyrrolidinylmethyl]-2-methoxy-5-sulphamoyl benzamide) is classed as a substituted benzamide compound and is thereby structurally distinct from the other antipsychotic drugs[23] (see Fig. 22.2). (It falls into the same chemical group as the anti-emetic *metoclopramide*.) It is quoted as controlling florid psychotic symptoms in high doses but in lower doses to alert the apathetic withdrawn schizophrenic. It is well absorbed from the gut and metabolized in the liver, metabolites being excreted in the urine and faeces. It has a half-life of 8–10 h, and therefore must be administered twice a day.

Sulpiride is claimed to be a selective blocker of the D_2 dopamine receptor (i.e. it has little action in blocking dopamine-stimulated adenylate cyclase), and thereby to have a reduced incidence of extrapyramidal side-effects in comparison to the more conventional antipsychotic agents (phenothiazines, thioxanthines), which act potently at both D_1 and D_2 receptor sites.

Dibenzodiazepines (clozapine)336

Clozapine[24] was originally introduced as a good potential antipsychotic agent but had to be withdrawn from general use owing to reports of bone marrow suppression and agranulocytosis. More recently it has been reintroduced but under strict control, and it is only indicated for treatment of schizophrenic patients unresponsive to, or intolerant of, conventional antipsychotic drugs. Regular blood tests must be taken, and the drug withdrawn if a leucopenia is observed.

Drug interactions with the antipsychotic drugs

As may be expected the neuroleptic drugs can interact with many other agents and such interactions can often be predicted knowing their pharmacological properties. They will interact with other anticholinergic compounds, potentiating the already documented antimuscarinic effects (e.g. with the tricyclic antidepressants, or anti-Parkinsonian medications). Delirium and confusional states may occur as a result of anticholinergic toxicity. This combination can be potentially hazardous in the elderly with narrow-angle glaucoma and prostatism. The antipsychotics can cause profound hypotension in combination with antihypertensives or diuretics by further blockade of α-adrenoceptors. Obviously, the antidopaminergic activity of the neuroleptic drugs will block the action of dopaminergic agents used in the treatment of Parkinson's disease.

Patients who take antihistamines may feel excessively drowsy if they are used in combination with antipsychotic drugs owing to the fact that these compounds often possess high intrinsic antihistaminergic activity.

The neuroleptics can potentiate the analgesic action of the opioid drugs, a property taken advantage of in the management of severe pain in neuroleptanalgesia. Alcohol, narcotic analgesics, anticonvulsants and respiratory depressants may all interact with the dopamine-receptor blocking antipsychotic drugs to potentiate their sedative properties and cause excessive drowsiness.

Lithium has occasionally been reported as interacting with antipsychotic drugs, particularly haloperidol, to cause neurotoxicity reactions and adverse extrapyramidal effects as well as very rarely precipitating the neuroleptic malignant syndrome. Phenytoin likewise may exacerbate neuroleptic-induced dyskinesias.

As the neuroleptics are, in general, substantially metabolized in the liver, they can often interfere with other drugs undergoing significant hepatic metabolism. Thus the phenothiazines can, for example, inhibit the metabolism of phenytoin resulting in increased serum anticonvulsant levels and subsequent signs of phenotoin toxicity.

Depot injections of antipsychotic drugs

More recently neuroleptics have been administered by deep intramuscular long-acting depot injections. Preparations available are *fluphenazine* (decanoate, enanthate), *flupenthixol* (decanoate), *fluspirilene*, *haloperidol* (decanoate) and *zuclopenthixol* (decanoate). In general, this route of administration offers better convenience and compliance for the schizophrenic patient. The fatty acid ester of the neuroleptic drug in an oily base allows a slow rate of absorption. For example, the half-life of oral fluphenazine is approximately 15 h; that of the depot decanoate is 3–9 days. However, these preparations usually give higher plasma drug levels than conventional oral administration as the initial first-pass hepatic metabolism is largely avoided. With these drugs, therefore, a higher incidence of extrapyramidal side-effects can occur. They should initially be given in a small test, for example 5–10% of normal concentrations, and the patient's response followed over 5–10 days, before the full higher dose is given at intervals of 2–4 weeks. Fluspirilene has a shorter duration of action than the other depot injections and therefore is given weekly.

A list of currently available antipsychotic drugs, their half-lives and usual daily oral dosages is given in Table 22.1.

TABLE 22.1 Clinically available antipsychotic drugs

CHEMICAL CLASS	DRUG	DAILY DOSAGE	HALF-LIFE
Phenothiazines			
Aliphatic side-chain	Chlorpromazine	75–300 mg	10–20 h
	Promazine	50 mg	
Piperidine side-chain	Thioridazine	150–600 mg	6–40 h
Piperazine side-chain	Trifluoperazine	5–10 mg	5 h
	Prochlorperazine	25–100 mg	7 h
	Fluphenazine	2.5–10 mg	15 h
	Perphenazine	4–12 mg	3–5 h
Butyrophenones	Haloperidol	5–20 mg	15–40 h
	Benzperidol	0.25–1.5 mg	
	Droperidol	5–20 mg	2 h
	Trifluperidol	0.5 mg	
Thioxanthines	Flupenthixol	5–15 mg	—
	Zuclopenthixol	20–50 mg	—
Diphenylbutylpiperidine	Pimozide	20 mg	50 h
	Fluspirilene	2–20 mg weekly	3 weeks
Substituted benzamides	Sulpiride	200–400 mg	8–10 h
Dibenzodiazepines	Clozapine	25–50 mg	12 h

CEREBRAL MONOAMINES AND MOOD

Depression describes a disorder characterised by a dominant feeling of sadness, unworthiness and despair. Like most syndromes in psychiatry, depression is an exaggerated response of a normal human emotion and can present as a wide spectrum of disorders ranging from mild despondency to abject despair.[3] Such feelings may be a primary symptom, or secondary to some other mental or physical illness. It is considered as being pathological when its severity or longevity interferes with normal lifestyle. Subjects become withdrawn, lose drive and energy, exhibit loss of appetite, motor slowness, diminished libido, disturbed menstrual function, flat affect, and disturbance of sleep pattern characterized by early-morning wakening.

Monoamine theories of depression

Early studies demonstrated that drugs producing a depletion of monoamine neurotransmitters from the brain (noradrenaline, NA; dopamine; 5-HT) often promoted the feeling of depression in man and assumed depression in animals.[2] For example, the use of reserpine to treat hypertension was often associated with depressive illness in a marked proportion of patients. This drug greatly lowers stores of monoamines within animal brains and hence the connection between depletion of cerebral monoamine neurotransmitters and assumed reduced function and clinical depression was made. The hypothesis gained further support from the fact that the stimulant drug amphetamine could elevate mood and pharmacologically it was known to stimulate potently the release of monoamines from nerve terminals and enhance neurotransmitter function. Additionally post-mortem studies from suicide victims who took their lives while known to be clinically depressed originally were reported as showing lower cerebral concentrations of 5-HT and decreased levels of its metabolite 5-HIAA (5-hydroxyindoleacetic acid) in cerebrospinal fluid (CSF) when compared with age-matched controls dying from other causes.

By the early 1960s the *biogenic amine theory of the affective disorders* was forwarded whereby the aetiology of depressive illness could be explained in terms of reduced functions of NA and 5-HT within the brain.[25] The precise anatomical location and possible defective biochemical pathways are still unknown despite 30 years of research, although areas of the limbic forebrain which are both believed to contribute to control of mood and behaviour and are rich in monoamine projections remain the prime sites under investigation.

Support for the biogenic amine theory of depression is provided from the fact that clinically effective antidepressant drugs – either the tricyclic antidepressants or monoamine oxidase inhibitors (MAOIs) – pharmacologically appear to act by enhancing brain monoamine systems (in particular NA and 5-HT) by blocking high-affinity transmitter uptake sites (e.g. tricyclics) or inhibiting enzyme degradation (MAOIs) (see Chapter 20).

More recently, however, research has directed itself towards changes in receptor action as an aetiology of depressive illness and a neurotransmitter receptor hypothesis is being considered to explain the mode of action of the tricyclic antidepressant drugs.[26] This evidence is being suggested from the more newly-introduced atypical antidepressant drugs (e.g. mianserin, trazodone, iprindole) which, although being clinically effective mood altering drugs, have little pharmacological action on presynaptic transmitter uptake. These drugs do, however, interact with pre- and postsynaptic adrenergic and serotonergic receptors. Another fact that has puzzled psychiatrists and neurochemists for many years is the question of why the tricyclics and MAOIs, which block monoamine mechanisms and enhance neurotransmission immediately, take at least 2–3 weeks or even longer to become clinically effective. This fact may lead to a problem of patient compliance with little motivation to persist with the medication (especially if side-effects predominate).

The *neurotransmitter receptor hypothesis of antidepressant drug action* proposes that the antidepressant drugs exert their clinical effect through central adrenergic (β_1 and α_2-adrenergic sites) and/or serotonergic receptors which are 'down-regulated' – that is, reduced in number and affinity for transmitter.[27] Thus the chronic treatment of animals with tricyclic drugs (or even electroconvulsive therapy) has been shown to reduce the number of both postsynaptic β_1-adrenergic and 5-HT_2 receptor sites. Therefore depression is now suggested as an illness related to an abnormality in the regulation of monoamine receptors, particularly noradrenergic[28] and serotonergic,[29] which can be corrected by the chronic administration of antidepressant drugs. Post-mortem studies have shown that depressed patients exhibit enhanced 5-HT_2 receptor binding.

Comparison of these two theories of depression reveals opposite proposals, the original *biogenic amine theory* hypothesizing underactivity of brain monoamines, the newer *receptor theory* suggesting that depression is associated with excessive 5-HT neurotransmission, and that antidepressant drugs act by reducing activity in this system. Further studies have identified high-affinity binding sites for radiolabelled tricyclic compounds in brain tissue and it is suggested that recognition sites exist in conjunction with the presynaptic uptake system. Whether this may serve to modulate re-uptake mechanisms is not fully known, but it has also been proposed that there may be an endogenous ligand in nervous tissue which acts naturally at these sites, and that such a compound could be involved in the aetiology of depressive illness.

The treatment of depression

Depressive illness is often loosely divided into *exogenous* (or *reactive*) *depression* whereby the change in mood occurs in response to an identifiable cause, for example social problems, loss of a relative, or systemic disease. Such depression is best managed by counselling and psychotherapy and, if possible, reversing the precipitating factors. In general, it does not respond well to drug therapy, although this may have to be considered if the depression induces a great degree of morbidity. *Endogenous depression* is recognized as occurring without identifiable cause or precipitating factors, and it is this type that responds best to drug treatment. When drug therapy fails or the depression is so severe that the patient's life is endangered, electroconvulsive therapy (ECT) under general anaesthesia is occasionally considered.

The drug treatment of depression is often said to be governed by the 'rule of thirds':

- one-third of patients will demonstrate a *full response*, responding well within 4–6 weeks and probably requiring continued treatment for up to 6 months to prevent relapse
- one-third of patients will have a *partial response* showing some improvement but probably requiring continued treatment for a year or more
- one-third of patients will have *resistant depression*, showing no significant response to drug therapy

The development of *antidepressant drugs* has, according to their major pharmacological actions, occurred in different phases with different 'generations' of agents now being available.

The *first-generation antidepressant drugs* were the originally described (and still highly used) *tricyclic antidepressants (TCAs)* (e.g. *imipramine*, *amitriptyline*, *desipramine*, *lofepramine*, etc.) and the (now lesser used) *MAOIs* (e.g. *isocarboxazid*, *phenelzine* and *tranylcypromine*). These drugs in the main interacted with cerebral monoamine systems, in particular enhancing brain noradrenaline and 5-HT mechanisms.

The *second-generation antidepressant drugs* were the *atypical non-tricyclic antidepressants* (including *trazodone*, *maprotiline*, *viloxazine* and *mianserin*), whose pharmacological actions appear to be related more to the regulation of monoamine neurotransmitter receptor sites, in particular those at presynaptic locations, than blockade of re-uptake systems as for the true TCAs.

The newest most recently introduced *third-generation antidepressant drugs* describe the *selective serotonin re-uptake inhibitors (SSRIs)* (e.g. *fluoxetine*, *paroxetine*, *sertraline* and *fluvoxamine*) which as their name implies are selective only at 5-HT presynaptic nerve terminals.

Not directly included in this classification are also *lithium* and the essential amino acid *tryptophan* which are still occasionally used in the treatment of this disorder.

Finally, an additional class of compound emerging for the drug treatment of depression is the *reversible inhibitor of MAO type A (RIMA)*, of which *moclobemide* is the currently available example. It is a specific MAOI selective at the type A isoenzyme with claimed antidepressant action but free of the prohibitive side-effects of the older, broader spectrum MAOI class.

The pharmacological actions and side-effects of these drugs, together with electroconvulsive therapy, are now considered.

TRICYCLIC ANTIDEPRESSANT DRUGS

Tricyclic and related antidepressants are considered as the drugs of choice for endogenous depression. They are generally safer and have less side-effects than the previously more extensively used MAOIs.[30] The *tricyclic antidepressants* are derivatives of dibenzazepine or dibenzocycloheptene, and as their name implies, originally referred to compounds with three cyclic carbon rings, for example amitriptyline, imipramine and lofepramine. Today, however, the term is used more broadly to include newer (second-generation)[31] agents with one, two and four ring structures, often classed as the *atypical antidepressants*, for example bicyclics – viloxazine; and tetracyclics – mianserin and maprotiline.

Mode of action of tricyclic antidepressant drugs

The first drug to be introduced in the tricyclic antidepressant class was *imipramine* which, being related to the phenothiazine chlorpromazine, was employed in mental institutions as an antipsychotic agent. However, although it did little for overt psychosis, it was noticed that this drug in general elevated patients' mood. Pharmacologically, at that time imipramine was known to possess antihistaminic activity, but later research concentrated on its interaction with cerebral monoamine systems, and it is this mechanism that is believed to be related to the drug's antidepressant activity. Currently used tricyclic compounds have been shown to enhance brain monoamine neurotransmission, particularly NA and 5-HT systems. The mechanism of action was originally principally believed to be by blockade of the high-affinity presynaptically-located re-uptake sites, and as this system is a potent mechanism for terminating the activity of released neurotransmitter, such inhibition allows more NA or 5-HT available in the synapse for prolonged interaction at the receptor.

More recent theories have advocated interaction of the tricyclic (and atypical) antidepressants at the level of the α-adrenergic and serotonergic receptors causing change in receptor numbers and sensitivities and thereby modifying neurotransmission.

Pharmacologically, the tricyclic drugs have been basically classified as to whether they have a preferential action on noradrenergic or serotonergic (5-HT) systems. All of the older tricyclics tend to inhibit NA reuptake, in particular desipramine, nortriptyline, viloxazine and maprotiline. Others are proposed as having greater effect on 5-HT uptake (amitriptyline, clomipramine, and the newer group of drugs, the SSRIs (see below) – fluvoxamine, fluoxetine and trazodone), although the major active metabolite of clomipramine – desmethylclomipramine – is a potent inhibitor of NA uptake. Protriptyline, imipramine and doxepin appear equipotent on both systems. A previously employed antidepressant agent, the drug nomifensin was noted for potently blocking the uptake of dopamine into presynaptic nerve terminals but having little action on NA or 5-HT systems. Mianserin appears to exert its pharmacological effect at the level of the transmitter receptor, blocking presynaptic α_2-adrenoceptors but having action on the uptake system.

A list of currently available tricyclic (and atypical) antidepressants is shown in Table 22.2. The structures of representative drugs from each class are shown in Figs. 22.3 and 22.4.

Pharmacokinetics of the tricyclic antidepressants

The tricyclic compounds are, in general, lipid soluble and show good oral absorption, peak plasma levels occurring 4–6 h after dosing. Serum protein binding is high (80–90%), and therefore there is liability of interaction and displacement of other protein-bound drugs. They are extensively metabolized in the liver, thereby being the subject of considerable (30–50%) first-pass metabolism. Metabolic pathways of the tricyclic antidepressants are mainly by demethylation, often into active products (see below) and by hydroxylation and N-oxidation. In this manner imipramine and lofepramine are both converted into desipramine (desmethylimipramine). Amitriptyline is converted into nortriptyline, which is, in turn, hydroxylated to the active metabolite 10-hydroxynortriptyline. Both trimipramine and clomipramine are demethylated into their

TABLE 22.2 Clinically available antidepressant drugs

CLASS	DRUG	DAILY DOSAGE	HALF-LIFE
Tricyclic antidepressant	Amitriptyline	50–100 mg	10–25 h
	Amoxapine	150–250 mg	
	Clomipramine	30–50 mg	18–28 h
	Desipramine	75–150 mg	30–40 h
	Imipramine	75–200 mg	4–18 h
	Lofepramine	70–140 mg	
	Nortriptyline	20–100 mg	
	Protriptyline	15–60 mg	18–90 h
	Trimipramine	75–150 mg	2–8 days
			24 h
Atypical antidepressants:			
Bicyclic compounds	Viloxazine	300 mg	2–8 h
Tetracyclic compounds	Maprotiline	50–150 mg	50 h
	Mianserin	30–90 mg	6–40 h
	Trazodone	150–300 mg	5–13 h
	Dothiepin	30–300 mg	20–30 h
	Doxepin	75–150 mg	8–24 h
Monoamine oxidase inhibitors	Isocarboxazid	10–20 mg	
	Phenelzine	15–30 mg	
	Tranylcypromine	10 mg	
Reversible inhibitor MAO type A (RIMA)	Moclobemide	150–600 mg	1–2 h
Selective serotonin re-uptake inhibitors (SSRIs)	Fluoxetine	20 mg	2–3 days
	Fluvoxamine	100–200 mg	15 h
	Paroxetine	20–30 mg	14–20 h
	Sertraline	50–100 mg	26 h
Lithium	Lithium carbonate	0.25–2 g	7–20 h
Tryptophan	Tryptophan	1–2 g	16 h
Thioxanthines	Flupenthixol	1–2 mg	

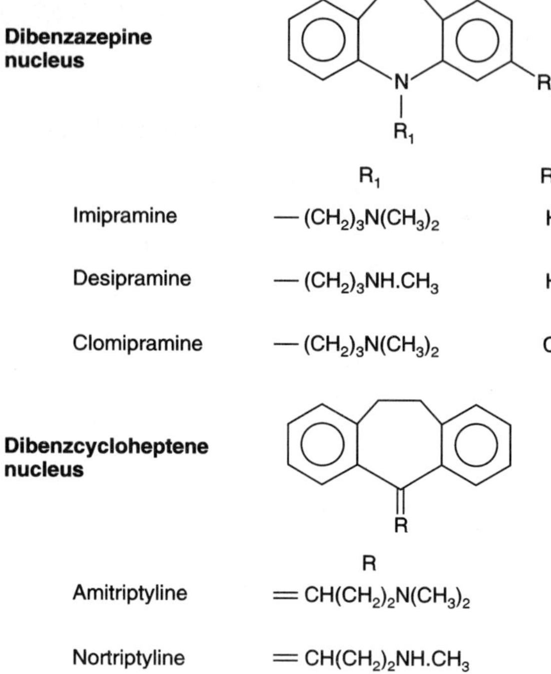

FIGURE 22.3. Structures of some tricyclic antidepressants.

Trazodone

Fluoxetine

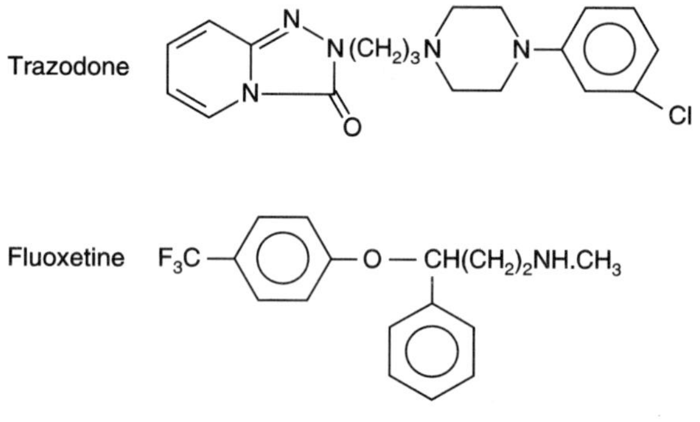

FIGURE 22.4. Structures of some atypical antidepressants.

active metabolites, desmethyltrimipramine and desmethylclomipramine respectively.

Patients with induced hepatic microsomal enzymes (e.g. from taking other drugs such as anticonvulsants or having a high regular alcohol intake) will have accelerated metabolic rates and lower effective drug concentrations.

The tricyclic antidepressants are excreted in the urine as their metabolites, either in free or conjugated form.

The half-lives of these drugs are variable, being short in the case of viloxazine (2–8 h) therefore requiring multiple dosing during the day, while others possess a slower metabolic rate and clearance – desipramine, amitriptyline (12–24 h), dothiepin (45–55 h); requiring single daily dosage only. Butriptyline and protriptyline have extremely long estimated half-lives of 2–6 days. Studies have shown, however, that there is a wide variation in plasma concentrations, and in general there is difficulty in achieving good correlation between plasma levels and effective clinical response with this group of compounds.

Uses of the tricyclic antidepressants

As expected, the tricyclic antidepressants are useful in the treatment of endogenous depression, characterized by symptoms of apathy, weight loss, early morning wakening and lowered daytime mood. Sometimes the tricyclic antidepressant drugs are classed as to whether they are sedative or non-sedative in action, or if they possess anxiolytic properties. These side-effects of the tricyclics can often be put to beneficial use. Amitriptyline, trimipramine, mianserin and trazodone have sedative properties and are thus useful in the management of the agitated patient to ensure a better sleeping pattern; imipramine, desipramine, clomipramine, viloxazine and protriptyline possess mild stimulant actions and help the withdrawn depressive. Doxepin and dothiepin have anxiolytic properties and are helpful in anxiety depressed states. Clomipramine can also be useful in phobic and obsessional states.

The tricyclic antidepressants are also employed in the management of nocturnal enuresis in children, amitriptyline, imipramine and nortriptyline being used in this respect. Occasionally amitriptyline is helpful in the control of migraine headaches, eating disorders, hiccough, chronic pain (e.g. postherpetic neuralgia, stroke pain, diabetic neuropathy) and in sleeping disorders including narcolepsy.

Side-effects of the tricyclic antidepressants

Although the mechanism of action of the tricyclic antidepressants is focused on the monoamine synapse, either by blocking re-uptake sites or presynaptic adrenergic receptors, the pharmacology of these compounds is in fact wide and varied. Knowledge of this aspect will lead to appreciation of the many side-effects and drug interactions that can occur with these compounds. Pharmacological properties of the tricyclic antidepressants include: (1) antihistaminic (H_1) actions; (2) anticholinergic (antimuscarinic) activity; (3) α_1-adrenergic blocking properties; and (4) monoamine uptake inhibition.

Most tricyclic drugs have significant antimuscarinic activity and therefore anticholinergic side-effects are not infrequently reported. These include actions on the gastrointestinal tract such as reduced gastric emptying and constipation due to slowed peristalsis, urinary retention – particularly if there were pre-existing symptoms of prostatism, dry mouth due to inhibition of salivary secretions, mydriasis and blurred vision by paralysis of accommodation precipitating narrow-angle glaucoma.

Actions through the sympathetic division of the autonomic nervous system by blockade of α-adrenoceptors can provoke postural hypotension, impotence, cardiac arrhythmias such as atrial fibrillation, ventricular tachycardia, atrioventricular block, flattening of T waves, ischaemic ST segment depression and prolongation of the QT interval. Because of these actions on the heart, the tricyclic antidepressants are best avoided in patients with known cardiac problems, especially ischaemic heart disease and susceptibility to arrhythmias. However, the more newly introduced tricyclic (and atypical) antidepressant drugs such as lofepramine, mianserin, trazodone and viloxazine are favoured as they are less antimuscarinic and less cardiotoxic than the earlier drugs and are therefore less prone to side-effects, especially in the elderly.

Reported central nervous system effects include tremor, sedation, convulsions (and so are best avoided in epileptics), confusion, precipitation of psychoses, depression of rapid eye movement (REM) sleep, ataxia, dysarthria and muscle twitching.

Allergic skin reactions are not infrequently noted; protriptyline, for example, can precipitate a photosensitive rash. Other side-effects reported with the tricyclic antidepressant drugs include cholestatic jaundice and PUO (pyrexia of unknown origin). Very rarely blood disorders occur, such as eosinophilia, thrombocytopenia, leucopenia, bone marrow depression and agranulocytosis.

Overdose of tricyclic antidepressants can provoke anticholinergic crisis, cardiac arrhythmias and conduction defects, convulsions, respiratory depression and coma. They are therefore potentially dangerous and lethal compounds if abused.

Amoxapine, classed as a tricyclic antidepressant, is a bibenzoxapin derivative related to the antipsychotic loxapine and possessing dopamine-receptor antagonist activity. As part of its noted side-effects it can cause drug-induced Parkinsonism and tardive dyskinesias on chronic dosing. Overdose can precipitate convulsions.

Dothiepin and doxepin

Dothiepin (3-(dibenzo-[b,e]thiepin-11-ylidene) propyldimethylamine) and *doxepin* (3-(dibenzo[b,e]oxepin-11-ylidene) propyldimethylamine) are useful tricyclic antidepressant drugs as they possess marked anxiolytic activity. They are readily absorbed from the gastrointestinal tract, and both are extensively metabolized in the liver to their primary desmethylated active metabolites – desmethyldothiepin and desmethyldoxepin. These metabolites and parent compounds are excreted free or in conjugated form in the urine. Their half-lives are in the range of 10–30 h.

ATYPICAL 'TRICYCLIC' ANTIDEPRESSANT DRUGS

Bicyclic compounds

Viloxazine

Viloxazine is an oxazine structure that is chemically distinct from the tricyclic and tetracyclic antidepressants. It is readily absorbed following oral administration, and extensively metabolized in the liver, the principal route of metabolism being hydroxylation and conjugation. It is not highly protein bound in plasma and is excreted in the urine as its metabolites, either in conjugated or in free form. It has a short half-life of 2–8 h, thereby warranting twice-daily dosing.

Pharmacologically, viloxazine has less intrinsic anticholinergic and adrenergic activity than the tricyclic drugs, and therefore causes less antimuscarinic and cardiovascular side-effects. It acts by inhibiting monoamine uptake into presynaptic nerve terminals, mainly noradrenaline.

Nomifensin

A previously used bicyclic antidepressant drug was *nomifensin.*[32] It was marketed as potently blocking the uptake of dopamine into presynaptic nerve terminals. Clinically, it possessed stimulant properties, but would exacerbate agitated depressives. However, this drug was associated with induced immunological reactions, presenting as fevers, malaise, myalgia and arthralgias. Nomifensin was also shown to cause blood dyscrasias and hepatic damage. On these grounds it has been withdrawn from clinical use in the UK.

Tetracyclic compounds

Mianserin

Mianserin[33] is indicated in depressive illness, particularly where a degree of sedation is required. It is rapidly absorbed from the gut, but by extensive first-pass metabolism its bioavailability is reduced to about 70%. It is metabolized by hydroxylation, N-oxidation and N-desmethylation; desmethylmianserin and 8-hydroxymianserin are pharmacologically active. It is extensively bound to plasma proteins, and has a calculated half-life of 6–40 h.

Mode of action of mianserin

Pharmacologically mianserin has been shown to block presynaptic α-adrenoceptors, which have a role in the regulation of NA synthesis. Its antidepressant action is believed to be related to the subsequent increase in cerebral NA turnover. Unlike the other tricyclic compounds, it does not block NA re-uptake sites, nor does it possess significant antimuscarinic properties.

Side-effects of mianserin

The major advantage of mianserin over the tricyclic antidepressants is the lack of serious cardiovascular toxicity and much less intrinsic anticholinergic activity. It does possess some mild antihistaminic effects to account for its sedating properties. It should be used with caution in the elderly as it can precipitate orthostatic hypotension, or cause convulsions, gynaecomastia, polyarthropathy or skin rashes.

Serious side-effects are the rare association of mianserin with bone marrow suppression, aplastic anaemia, agranulocytosis and granulocytopenia having been reported, especially in the elderly. Regular blood counts are therefore recommended, particularly in the first few weeks of initiating therapy.

Maprotiline

Maprotiline is slowly but completely absorbed from the gut. It is extensively deaminated to its principal active metabolite desmethylmaprotiline. The drug is highly protein bound in plasma, and is excreted unchanged or in the form of metabolites (free or conjugated) in the urine and faeces. It has a long half-life of 2 days.

Like mianserin, it is less antimuscarinic than the tricyclic compounds.

Trazodone

Trazodone[34] is a triazolopyridine antidepressant (see Fig. 22.4). It is rapidly absorbed from the gut, extensively metabolized in the liver by N-oxidation and hydroxylation. The major metabolite *m*-chloro-phenylpiperazine is biologically active. The drug and its metabolites are excreted in the urine. The half-life of trazodone is calculated at 5–13 h.

Pharmacologically, trazodone appears to be a selective inhibitor of 5-HT uptake; it does not inhibit NA uptake. It has also been noted as enhancing the turnover of brain dopamine. It has no significant antimuscarinic properties.

Side-effects of trazodone include drowsiness, headache, confusional states and nausea. Occasionally bradycardias and tachycardias are seen. It can cause disabling postural hypotension, especially in the elderly. Trazodone has been reported as provoking priapism and skin rashes.

Drug interactions with the tricyclic antidepressant drugs

Being active on the cerebral monoamine and autonomic systems, it is not surprising that a number of commonly used drugs show interaction with the tricyclic (and atypical) antidepressants. As the list is long, a few only are mentioned here:

1. Antihypertensives, including adrenergic neurone-blocking agents, methyldopa and clonidine, which all interact through the sympathetic nervous system (see Chapter 14).
2. MAOIs, discussed below.
3. Thyroxine – may induce a general stimulant effect and increase cardiotoxicity.
4. Sympathomimetic amines, for example adrenaline, phenylpropanolamine in 'cold cures' can precipitate hypertensive reactions. These are more fully discussed under the MAOIs below.
5. Alcohol – may exacerbate both cerebral and peripheral reactions.
6. Anticholinergics – will enhance the high intrinsic antimuscarinic activity of most tricyclic compounds, provoking effects by blockade of parasympathetic mechanisms.
7. Anticonvulsants – may alter metabolism of these drugs and lower the threshold for seizures.
8. Anti-Parkinsonian drugs, especially those with anticholinergic activity which will enhance antimuscarinic side-effects, and levodopa preparations can precipitate hyperpyrexia, agitation and convulsions.

SELECTIVE SEROTONIN RE-UPTAKE INHIBITORS (SSRIs)

The selective serotonin re-uptake inhibitors (SSRIs) are the newest 'third generation' antidepressant drugs which are claimed to selectively and potently affect 5-HT re-uptake into presynaptic nerve terminals.[35] The SSRIs have equivalent clinical efficacy to standard antidepressants such as the tricyclics, but their marketing point is an improved safety, a more acceptable side-effect profile and reduced risks with overdosage. SSRIs are also reportedly useful in the management of anxiety states, panic and obsessive-compulsive disorders, where serotonin appears to be involved although the precise mechanisms are unknown.

The currently important SSRIs are the aralkylketone derivative *fluvoxamine* (5-methoxy-4′-trifluoromethylvalerophenone); *fluoxetine*[36] (N-methyl-3-phenyl-3-(a,a,a-trifluoro-*p*-tolyloxy) propylamine) (see Fig. 22.4); the phenyl derivative *paroxetine*, and the naphthylamine derivative *sertraline*.[37]

All drugs show potent and selective inhibition of neuronal serotonin uptake (paroxetine the most potent) and some weak action at muscarinic cholinergic receptors. They have no detectable action at 5-HT receptors, and do not block NA uptake to any significant degree.

Pharmacokinetics of SSRIs

Fluoxetine, fluvoxamine and paroxetine are well and rapidly absorbed from the gastrointestinal tract following oral administration.[38] Sertraline is absorbed more slowly. Peak plasma concentrations of all drugs occur in 6–8 h following dosage. The SSRIs in general undergo desmethylation in the liver either into further biologically active or inactive compounds. The drugs are all extensively bound to plasma proteins and inactive products are excreted in the urine and faeces. All drugs have long half-lives (fluvoxamine, 15 h; paroxetine, 14–20 h; sertraline, 26 h; fluoxetine, 2–3 days – although its metabolite norfluoxetine is even longer at 7–9 days). The SSRIs therefore need to be given in once-daily dosage only.

Side-effects of SSRIs

Side-effects on the gastrointestinal tract are common and include nausea and vomiting, dry mouth (anticholinergic action), and diarrhoea. Other actions include drowsiness, dizziness, insomnia and agitation; headaches and skin rashes are also reported.

Cautions with use

At the time of their introduction, and in comparison with the older tricyclic drugs, the SSRIs are expensive to prescribe. They should be avoided in patients with hepatic or renal impairment, or with a history of epilepsy. They should also not be used in conjunction with the MAOIs for fear of precipitating the '*serotonin syndrome*' characterized by hyperthermia, rigidity, myoclonus and confusion, the outcome of which could be fatal.

MONOAMINE OXIDASE INHIBITORS (MAOIs)

In the early 1950s, analogues of isoniazid were used (and still are) for antituberculosis therapy. One such agent was iproniazid which was noted as exhibiting marked mood-elevating properties. Subsequent biochemical investigations demonstrated its potent inhibition of the enzyme complex monoamine oxidase (MAO). Since that time a number of drugs inhibiting MAO have been developed and used clinically in the treatment of depression. In modern practice, however, their use has declined, basically for two reasons: first the introduction of the more effective and safer tricyclic antidepressants, and secondly the MAOIs have a number of undesirable side-effects that restrict their use, especially regarding their interaction with sympathomimetic amines present in fermented food products and with other therapeutic drugs.

In modern day practice, the MAOIs are usually reserved for depressed patients not responding to the tricyclic antidepressants,[30] although they have also found use in the management of anxiety and phobic states, or mixed neurotic disorders. Like the tricyclic compounds, response to treatment is often delayed for up to 3 weeks or more. Four main MAOIs remain in clinical use today: *phenelzine*, *iproniazid*, *isocarboxazid* and *tranylcypromine* (see Fig. 22.5).

Mode of action of the MAOIs

These drugs strongly inhibit the enzyme MAO which normally degrades the active monoamine neurotransmitters NA, dopamine and 5-HT to inactive products within the synaptic cleft. MAO is a flavin-containing enzyme located on mitochondrial membranes. It is associated with nerve cell terminals, but also widely found in many other organs and tissues. It is important for regulating the activity of catecholamines and 5-HT in the body, and also other sympathomimetic substances taken in with foodstuffs which might otherwise cause problems in the portal and systemic circulations. Thus the MAO located in the gut wall is particularly important. Circulating amines so degraded include tyramine, phenylethylamine and metaraminol.

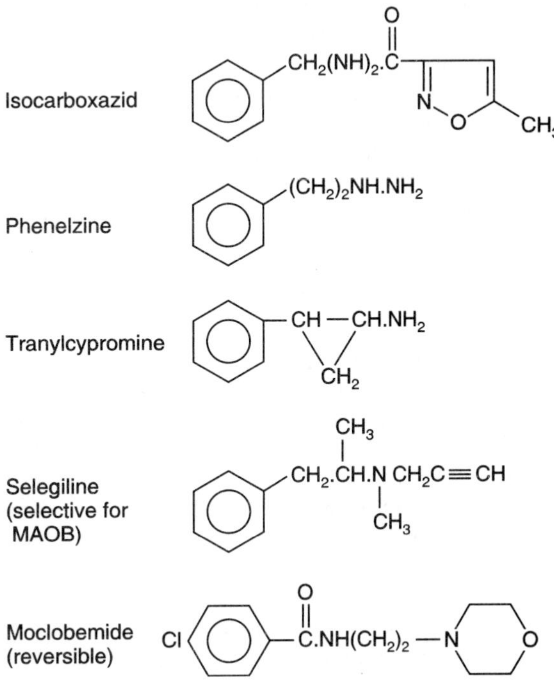

Isocarboxazid

Phenelzine

Tranylcypromine

Selegiline (selective for MAOB)

Moclobemide (reversible)

FIGURE 22.5. Structures of some monoamine oxidase (MAO) inhibitors.

MAO is a series of isoenzymes; the two most important being subgrouped A and B, depending on their preferences and affinities for various substrates and sensitivities to selective inhibitors. MAO_A combines more readily with NA and 5-HT as substrates and is potently inhibited by the experimental drug *clorgyline*. This isoenzyme is found mainly in the gut and human placenta.

MAO_B shows substrate preferences for phenylethylamine, tyramine and dopamine, and is selectively blocked by *selegiline* (*deprenyl*). This isoenzyme is the only MAO type detected in human platelets: both MAO_A and MAO_B are found in equal amounts in liver and brain.

The MAOIs are divided chemically into the hydrazine structures (*phenelzine*, *isoniazid*) that inhibit the enzyme non-competitively (irreversibly), and the non-hydrazine group (*tranylcypromine*) that cause competitive (reversible) inhibition. Although selective drugs do exist for the separate MAO isoenzymes, for example *clorgyline* and *moclobemide* inhibit MAO_A, while *selegiline* is claimed to be selective for MAO_B (see Chapter 23), the drugs discussed below and used in the treatment of depression show inhibitory action on both MAO subtypes. Following acute and chronic dosage with these MAOIs there is up to 90% inhibition of cerebral MAO, with subsequent elevation of brain NA and 5-HT (and dopamine) levels. These raised concentrations are believed to represent an enhanced functional neurotransmitter action which is taken to be the basis of their antidepressant effect. Although MAO shows highly significant inhibition after acute dosages, it is still not understood why a period of several weeks is generally needed to see an improvement in the depressive state. This fact would suggest that it is not just a direct effect on enzyme inhibition or of elevated NA or 5-HT levels, but more towards a change in neurotransmitter turnover, resetting a new balance, and of receptor sensitivity, as discussed in the neurotransmitter receptor theory of depression above.

Pharmacokinetics of the MAOIs

The MAOIs are in general lipid soluble, well absorbed following oral administration and penetrate the blood–brain barrier very readily. The hydrazine MAOIs are partially metabolized by hepatic acetylation, and therefore slow acetylators will be prone to drug toxicity. The MAOIs are excreted as their metabolites in the urine. The irreversible inhibitors of MAO (e.g. phenelzine) will exert signs of enzyme inhibition for up to 14 days after discontinuation of the drug until new enzyme is synthesized. Non-hydrazine, non-competitive inhibitors of MAO (e.g. tranylcypromine) demonstrate reversibility of enzyme action within 3–5 days of stopping the drug.

Side-effects of the MAOIs

Many of the side-effects of these drugs are exhibited either through the autonomic nervous system or represent toxic cerebral reactions. Most of the MAOIs show significant intrinsic anticholinergic (antimuscarinic) activity, and therefore autonomic effects can be manifest either through inhibition of the parasympathetic system or by stimulation of the sympathetic system by way of MAO-inhibiting properties. Anticholinergic effects cause dry mouth, blurred vision, urinary hesitancy and retention, and constipation and other gastrointestinal upsets. Hypertension or postural hypotension, flushing, sweating and cardiac arrhythmias are not uncommonly reported. Oedema, weight gain and skin rashes are occasionally noted.

Cerebral toxic effects include agitation, dizziness, anxiety, headache, tremor, convulsions, clonus and hyperreflexia, psychosis and acute confusional states. A peripheral neuropathy can occur with use of hydrazine derivatives; this is believed to be due to pyridoxine deficiency. Jaundice may be seen with these drugs, and in rare cases this is related to a hepatocellular necrosis.

Precautions on the use of MAOIs and potential drug interactions

Because of potentially dangerous side-effects and stimulation of the sympathetic nervous system, the MAOIs are best avoided in cerebrovascular and cardiovascular disease, hypertension, phaeochromocytoma, thyroid disease and hepatic disorders. Caution should also be exercised when considering administering these drugs to epileptic patients, or to the elderly or agitated persons. The use of MAOIs in patients with Parkinson's disease taking L-DOPA-containing compounds is to be avoided.

In view of potential hazardous reactions with sympathomimetic amines, patients should carry a card warning of possible interactions with food substances and various drugs (e.g. proprietary cough remedies and nasal decongestants). MAOIs can react with foods rich in sympathomimetic amines and, by blocking their natural metabolism (for example, by inhibition of gut MAO activity), a hypertensive crisis can be precipitated. Foods to be avoided in this manner include cheese, yeast protein extracts (Bovril, Oxo, Marmite) which contain tyramine; pickled herrings, nuts, bananas and broad beans which contain L-DOPA; and alcohol, especially Chianti, which has a very high tyramine content. A precipitous rise in blood pressure can also be provoked by inhibition of metabolism of ephedrine and phenylephrine in 'cold cures', or by interaction with the tricyclic antidepressants which will cause a further elevation of blood pressure. Such acute increases in blood pressure have led to subarachnoid haemorrhage or catastrophic intracerebral bleeds. The precipitation of a hypertensive crisis by interaction of a

MAOI and food substances has been become known as the '*cheese effect*'.

Although co-administration of the precursors of the biogenic amines, or of sympathomimetic amines available in foodstuffs, is associated with a greatly potentiated and prolonged response, it would appear that the direct administration of the catecholamines themselves has a less potentiated effect, since adrenaline and NA are mainly inactivated by re-uptake mechanisms and by interaction with catechol-O-methyl transferase (COMT).

Other drugs that may interact with the MAOIs by interfering with the detoxification mechanism either directly through enzyme inhibition or secondary to hepatic damage include general anaesthetic agents; antihistamines; alcohol; anticonvulsants, particularly *carbamazepine*; oral hypoglycaemics; antidepressant drugs; and some potent analgesics, especially *pethidine* which can precipitate both cerebral and cardiovascular instability.

To eliminate possibilities of hypertensive responses induced by interaction with either sympathomimetics or other agents, it is advised that the MAOI is withdrawn 2–3 weeks before anaesthesia if practical, but obviously a psychiatric opinion should be sought first, although tranylcypromine appears to be immune.

MOCLOBEMIDE: REVERSIBLE INHIBITOR OF MAO TYPE A (RIMA)

Moclobemide (*p*-chloro-N-(2-morpholinoethyl) benzamide) (see Fig. 22.5) is a reversible inhibitor of MAO preferentially of type A isoenzyme (RIMA).[39] It subsequently leads to increased concentrations of both NA and 5-HT in the brain. It is used for the treatment of major depressive illness, both of the endogenous and reactive type.

Pharmacokinetics of moclobemide

The drug is completely absorbed from the gastrointestinal tract, but undergoes considerable first-pass metabolism (20–40%). Approximately 50% is bound to plasma proteins (mainly albumin). Peak plasma drug levels are observed within 1 h of oral administration. Some 99% of the drug is metabolized, largely by oxidative reactions in the liver, before elimination from the body; less than 1% of dose is excreted renally in unchanged form. Drug dosage need not therefore be reduced in renal failure. Moclobemide has a calculated half-life of 1–2 h. Cimetidine prolongs the metabolism of moclobemide.

Side-effects of moclobemide

In general, moclobemide is well tolerated and has few reported side-effects, especially if compared with the classical tricyclics or irreversible MAOI antidepressants. Sleep disturbance, dizziness, nausea and headache may occur. Overdosing can produce drowsiness, hyporeflexia and disorientation but not cardiotoxicity.

As moclobemide is a reversible inhibitor of MAO type A it has less potentiation of tyramine and related compounds than the traditional irreversible MAOIs and does not necessitate special dietary restrictions.

OTHER DRUGS AND PROCEDURES

Tryptophan

Tryptophan[40] is an essential amino acid. It is readily absorbed from the gastrointestinal tract and extensively bound to serum albumin. Some is metabolized to 5-hydroxytryptophan and then subsequently to 5-HT within serotonergic nerves of the CNS. In this way it causes a functional increase in cerebral 5-HT, and this mechanism of action is claimed to be the cause of the drug's antidepressant effect. Its half-life is calculated at 16 h.

Side-effects include nausea, headache and drowsiness. Occasionally reversible dyskinesias and Parkinsonian-like rigidity is observed. There has been some association in animals between tryptophan and bladder tumours, and so it is best avoided in active bladder disease.

Lithium

Lithium (Li^+), administered in the form of either lithium carbonate or citrate, is a useful drug for the treatment of bipolar states where patients swing between manic and depressive phases, and also in mania alone.[41] The precise mechanism of action of lithium is unknown but it is suggested that it may substitute for the monovalent ions Na^+ and K^+, thereby disrupting the Na^+/K^+ membrane pump and carrier mechanisms. Lithium is readily and completely absorbed from the gastrointestinal tract with peak plasma concentrations occurring within 2 h. It is distributed throughout the body but is often particularly more concentrated in bone, thyroid and brain. The element is excreted at the kidney, but can also be detected in saliva and sweat. Lithium has quite a long half-life in the body (7–20 h) which is considerably increased in renal failure.

The serum therapeutic range for lithium is 0.8–1.2 mmol/l. The margin between therapeutic and toxic dosages is narrow and therefore it is important to monitor serum Li^+ levels reasonably regularly (especially if poor compliance is suspected), as the drug can induce many side-effects.

More recent biochemical studies have shown that Li^+ inhibits the hydrolysis of myoinositol-1-phosphate in the brain, thereby decreasing production of phosphatidyl inositols in the stimulated postsynaptic membrane associated with the 5-HT_2 receptor. Lithium consequently alters the 5-HT_2-receptor mediated response, and as this neurotransmitter system has been implicated in the aetiology of the affective disorders, this may be a potential mode of action of Li^+ in the control of manic depression.

Side-effects of lithium therapy

Lithium treatment has been associated with a number of recognized side-effects, but many of these are dose related. It can cause irritation of the gastrointestinal tract, provoking nausea and diarrhoea. Central nervous system signs include fine hand tremor, ataxia and incoordination, and hyperreflexia. Generalized muscle weakness is related to its action on the Na^+/K^+ muscle membrane pump. It is reported as producing peripheral oedema and subsequent weight gain. Lithium can occasionally provoke cardiac arrhythmias by a direct effect on the myocardium and interference with the K^+ channel, but this is more usually in association with toxic serum concentrations.

Other potentially more serious side-effects include:

- *Hypothyroidism*; lithium can interfere with thyroid function (being taken up and concentrated by the thyroid gland), causing a goitre, weakness, lethargy and low circulating thyroxine.
- *Nephrogenic diabetes insipidus*; lithium can disrupt ADH (antidiuretic hormone) action at the kidney tubule, resulting in polyuria and subsequent polydipsia. Other long-term effects on the kidney include interstitial fibrosis, glomerular sclerosis and tubular atrophy.
- *Hyperparathyroidism*; lithium can provoke a secondary hyperparathyroidism with elevated circulating levels of calcium and magnesium. More usually it is reported as inducing osteoporosis with loss of bone density and calcium.

Lithium clearance is reduced during treatment with diuretics. Serum lithium concentrations may also increase during treatment with tetracycline and NSAIDs. Rarely lithium can cause a lupus-like syndrome, with production of antinuclear antibodies.

In high toxic doses (greater than 4 mmol/l) confusion, spasticity, convulsions, coma and death can occur. Overdose is usually treated with intravenous fluids and cardiac monitoring: severe overdose may require haemodialysis.

ELECTROCONVULSIVE THERAPY (ECT)

Another and often very effective way of treating severe abject depression refractory to pharmacological therapies is ECT. The mechanism by which a course of ECT can reverse the most profound depressive symptoms is still obscure. However, animal experiments suggest that such procedures modify cerebral neurotransmitter biochemistry. Both 5-HT and dopamine function is generally enhanced, which appears to be a receptor-mediated change.[42] Conversely GABA turnover in brain limbic regions is reduced. Whether these noted changes are truly the mechanisms by which patients may get better is still widely debated.

REFERENCES

1 Spokes EGS. Biochemical abnormalities in schizophrenia: the dopamine hypothesis. In: Curzon G ed. *The biochemistry of psychiatric disturbances*. Chichester: John Wiley, 1980: 53–71.
2 Schildkraut JJ. The catecholamine hypothesis of affective disorders. A review of supporting evidence. *American Journal of Psychiatry* 1965; **122**: 509–22.
3 Gelder M, Gath D, Mayou R eds. *Oxford textbook of psychiatry*, 2nd edn. Oxford: Oxford Medical Publications, 1989: 217–323.
4 Snyder SH. The dopamine hypothesis of schizophrenia: focus on the dopamine receptor. *American Journal of Psychiatry* 1976; **133**: 197–202.
5 Friedhoff AJ, van Winkle E. Isolation and characterisation of a compound from the urine of schizophrenics. *Nature* 1962; **194**: 897–8.
6 Snyder SH. Amphetamine psychosis: a 'model' schizophrenia mediated by catecholamines. *American Journal of Psychiatry* 1973; **130**: 61–7.
7 Seeman P, Lee T, Chau Wong M, Wong K. Antipsychotic drug doses and neuroleptic/dopamine receptors. *Nature* 1976; **261**: 717–19.
8 Mackay AVP, Iversen LL, Rosser M, Spokes EGS, Bird ED, Arregui A, Creese I, Snyder SH. Increased brain dopamine and dopamine receptors in schizophrenia. *Archives of General Psychiatry* 1982; **39**: 991–7.
9 Moore RY, Bloom RE. Central catecholamine neuron systems: anatomy and physiology of the dopamine system. *Annual Review of Neuroscience* 1978; **1**: 129–69.
10 Seeman P. Brain dopamine receptors. *Pharmacology Review* 1980; **32**: 229–313.
11 Kebabian WJ, Calne DB. Multiple dopamine receptors. *Nature* 1979, **277**: 93–6.
12 Jarvie KR, Caron MG. Heterogeneity of dopamine receptors. *Advances in Neurology* 1993; **60**: 325–33.
13 Seeman P, Van Toh HH. Dopamine receptor pharmacology. *Current Opinions in Neurology and Neurosurgery* 1993; **6**: 602–8.
14 Miller RJ, Horn AS, Iversen LL. The action of neuroleptic drugs on dopamine-stimulated adenosine 3′,5′-monophosphate production in rat neostriatum and limbic forebrains. *Molecular Pharmacology* 1974; **10**: 759–66.
15 Creese I, Sibley DR, Hamblin MW, Leff SE. The classification of dopamine receptors: relationship to radioligand binding. *Annual Review of Neuroscience* 1983, **6**: 43–71.
16 Seeman P. Dopamine receptors and the dopamine hypothesis of schizophrenia. *Synapse* 1987; **1**: 133–52.
17 Seeman P, Guan HC, Van Toh HH. Dopamine D_4 receptors elevated in schizophrenia. *Nature* 1993; **365**: 441–5.
18 Davis JM, Garver DL. Neuroleptics: clinical use in psychiatry. In: Iversen LL, Iversen SD, Snyder SH eds. *Handbook of psychopharmacology*. New York: Plenum Press, 1978, Vol 10: 129–64.
19 Shore PA, Giachetti A. Reserpine: basic and clinical pharmacology. In: Iversen LL, Iversen SD, Snyder SH eds.

Handbook of psychopharmacology. New York: Plenum Press, 1978; Vol 10: 197–219.

20 Baldessarini RT, Tarsy D. Dopamine and the pathophysiology of dyskinesias induced by antipsychotic drugs. *Annual Review of Neuroscience* 1980; **3**: 23–41.

21 Tarsy D, Baldessarini RT. Clinical and pathophysiologic features of movement disorders induced by psychotherapeutic agents. In: Shah N, Donald A eds. *Movement disorders*. New York: Plenum Press, 1986: 365–89.

22 Levenson JL. Neuroleptic malignant syndrome. *American Journal of Psychiatry* 1985; **142**: 1137–45.

23 O'Connor SE, Brown RA. The pharmacology of sulpiride – a dopamine receptor antagonist. *General Pharmacology* 1982; **13**: 185–93.

24 Coward DM. General pharmacology of clozapine. *British Journal of Psychiatry* 1992; Suppl. pp. 5–11.

25 Coppin A. The biochemistry of the affective disorders. *British Journal of Psychiatry* 1967; **113**: 1237–64.

26 Stahl SM, Palazidou L. The pharmacology of depression: studies of neurotransmitter receptors lead the search for biochemical lesions and new drug therapies. *Trends in Pharmacological Science* 1986; 7: 349–54.

27 Heringer GR, Charney DS. Mechanisms of antidepressant treatment: Implications for the etiology and treatment of depressive disorders. In: Meltzer HY ed. *Psychopharmacology: The third generation of progress*. New York: Raven Press, 1987: 535–44.

28 Siever LJ. Role of noradrenergic mechanisms in the etiology of the affective disorders. In: Meltzer HY ed. *Psychopharmacology: The third generation of progress*. New York: Raven Press, 1987: 493–504.

29 Meltzer HY, Lowy MT. The serotonin hypothesis of depression. In: Meltzer HY ed. *Psychopharmacology: The third generation of progress*. New York: Raven Press, 1987: 513–33.

30 Maxwell RA, White HL. Tricyclics and monoamine oxidase inhibitor antidepressants: structure activity relationships. In: Iversen LL, Iversen SD, Snyder SH eds. *Handbook of psychopharmacology*. New York: Plenum Press, 1978, Vol 14: 83–155.

31 Enna SJ, Eison MS. Second generation antidepressants. In: Iversen LL, Iversen SD, Snyder SH eds. *Handbook of psychopharmacology*. New York: Plenum Press, 1987, Vol 19: 609–26.

32 Nicholson PA, Turner P eds. Symposium on nomifensin. *British Journal of Clinical Pharmacology* 1977; **4** (Suppl 2): 53S–248S.

33 Brogden RN, Heel RC, Speight TM, Avery GS. Mianserin: Review of pharmacology and therapeutic efficacy in depressive illness. *Drugs* 1978; **16**: 273–301.

34 Brogden RN, Heel RC, Speight TM, Avery GS. Trazodone: Review of pharmacological properties and therapeutic use in depression and anxiety. *Drugs* 1981; **21**: 401–29.

35 Hollister LE, Claghorn JL. New antidepressants. *Annual Review of Pharmacology* 1993; **33**: 165–77.

36 Stokes PE. Fluoxetine: A five-year review. *Clinical Therapeutics* 1993; **15**, 216–43.

37 Murdoch D, McTavish D. Sertraline. A review of its pharmacodynamic and pharmacokinetic properties, and therapeutic potential in depression and obsessive–compulsive disorder. *Drugs* 1992; **44**: 604–24.

38 van-Harten J. Clinical pharmacokinetics of selective serotonin re-uptake inhibitors. *Clinical Pharmacokinetics* 1993; **24**: 203–20.

39 Fitton A, Faulds D, Goa KL. Moclobemide. A review of its pharmacological properties and therapeutic use in depressive illness. *Drugs* 1992; **43**: 561–96.

40 Coppen A, Wood K. Tryptophan and depressive illness. *Psychological Medicine* 1978; **8**: 49–57.

41 Ramsey TA, Mendels J. Lithium as an antidepressant. In: Enna SH, Malick JB, Richardson E eds. *Antidepressants: Neurochemical, behavioral and clinical perspectives*. New York: Raven Press, 1981: 175–82.

42 Lerer B. Neurochemical and other neurobiological consequences of ECT: Implications for the pathogenesis and treatment of affective disorders. In: Meltzer HY ed. *Psychopharmacology: The third generation of progress*. New York: Raven Press, 1987: 577–88.

Part II Drug treatment for anxiety and panic attacks

SC Stanford

INTRODUCTION

The pharmacology of drugs used to treat anxiety is particularly pertinent in anaesthesia because acute anxiolysis is an important component of presurgical medication. Also, many patients will have been taking an anxiolytic agent, possibly on a chronic basis, before presenting for surgery.

Diagnostically,[1] anxiety is the major component of the following group of conditions:

- generalized anxiety disorder
- panic disorder (with and without agoraphobia)
- phobia
- obsessive–compulsive disorder
- post-traumatic stress disorder

Whereas generalized anxiety disorder involves continual anxious mood, panic disorder (with and without agoraphobia) is characterized by unpredictable surges of intense anxiety, culminating in extreme autonomic arousal with fear of dying or losing control. Anticipatory anxiety, often provoked by conditions associated with previous panic attacks, is a common feature of panic disorder.

Drug therapy is the predominant treatment for both generalized anxiety and panic; because traditional treatments for these two disorders have been quite distinct, their psychopharmacology is discussed separately. Psychotropic drugs are also an important adjunct to psychotherapy in treatment of phobias, obsessive–compulsive disorder (OCD) and post-traumatic stress disorder (PTSD). There are no specifically preferred treatments for these disorders and compounds reported to be effective are those commonly used to treat either anxiety or panic disorder.

Drugs noted for their anxiolytic effects all modify the actions of one or more neurotransmitters within the brain. This has drawn attention to the possibility that a disorder of chemical neurotransmission could underlie anxiety. Three neurotransmitters have been extensively researched in this respect and are discussed below: noradrenaline, 5-hydroxytryptamine (5-HT) and γ-aminobutyric acid (GABA). Recently, several new anxiolytic compounds have been investigated that interact with quite different (peptidergic) neurotransmitter systems. None of these latest compounds is yet available for clinical use, but they are important developments in preclinical research of anxiety and so are discussed briefly at the end of the chapter.

NORADRENALINE AND ANXIETY

Noradrenaline is the major neurotransmitter in the sympathetic division of the autonomic nervous system and is also found in the central nervous system (CNS), mainly within neurones arising from the nucleus locus coeruleus in the brainstem. These neurones project to many brain regions concerned with regulation of autonomic and cognitive function (hypothalamus, septum, hippocampus, amygdala and certain areas of the neocortex), collectively known as the 'limbic system'.

The symptoms of anxiety bear a striking resemblance to the response to stress or fear (Table 22.3). The locus coeruleus is thought to have an important role in this response, forming part of an 'alarm' or 'vigilance' system that alerts the individual to conspicuous stimuli.[2] A disorder of central noradrenergic transmission is a suspected cause of anxiety.[3] Reports that administration of anxiogenic drugs affects behaviour and the activity of central and peripheral noradrenergic neurones in ways that resemble the response to stress, are consistent with this view.[4]

Obviously, electrophysiological studies are not possible in man but the concentration of the noradrenaline metabolite, 3-methoxy-4-hydroxyphenylethyleneglycol (MHPG), circulating in the plasma can be used as an indirect measure of the activity of central noradrenergic neurones. Changes in plasma MHPG concentration are thought to parallel changes in the rate of release of noradrenaline from locus neurones. Also, levels of

TABLE 22.3 Major symptoms of anxiety

Motor tension:	Tremor, muscle tension, restlessness, rapid fatigue
Autonomic hyperactivity:	Shortness of breath, tachycardia, sweating, dry mouth, dizziness, abdominal distress, flushes or chills, frequent urination, difficulty with swallowing
Arousal:	Feeling on edge, exaggerated startle response, difficulty with concentration, insomnia, irritability

noradrenaline and adrenaline circulating in the plasma give an index of sympathetic arousal in anxiety. Drugs causing acute anxiety in non-human primates and man can increase the concentration of plasma noradrenaline and MHPG (among other factors), suggesting that this disorder is associated with increased central and peripheral noradrenergic neurotransmission.[3,5] Similar changes are induced by word association tests or mental arithmetic tasks which are used to model anxiety experimentally.

DRUGS THAT AFFECT ADRENOCEPTOR FUNCTION

α_2-Adrenoceptor agonists and antagonists: clonidine and yohimbine

Mode of action

The theory that increased release of noradrenaline has a pivotal role in anxiety and that anti-anxiety agents reduce release of this neurotransmitter is the basis of an explanation for the anxiolytic actions of the α_2-adrenoceptor agonist, clonidine. Clonidine has two actions that attenuate noradrenergic transmission. The first involves activation of presynaptic α_2-adrenoceptors on noradrenergic nerve terminals; these receptors operate a feedback mechanism that inhibits further release of transmitter. Under normal, physiological conditions, this feedback loop is activated by noradrenaline in the synapse. The second mechanism involves α_2-adrenoceptors on the cell bodies of noradrenergic neurones in the locus coeruleus; these are innervated by collaterals of axons projecting from the locus coeruleus and are sensitive to noradrenaline released from their terminals (Fig. 22.6). Activation of these feedback mechanisms by clonidine, both of which suppress release of noradrenaline in the brain, could explain the anxiolytic effects of this drug.

Clonidine also suppresses release of 5-HT by binding to α_2-adrenoceptors on serotonergic (5-HT releasing) cell bodies, in the raphe nuclei, and their nerve terminals (Fig. 22.6). This means that, in addition to the autoinhibition of noradrenaline release described above, α_2-adrenoceptors mediate synaptic interactions between different neurotransmitter systems. These effects of clonidine on serotonergic transmission could contribute to the anxiolytic effects of this drug since a disorder of serotonergic transmission may also underlie anxiety (see below).

Other pharmacological effects

Clonidine is not usually used to treat anxiety because it causes xerostomia, is highly sedative and has profound hypotensive effects. The hypotensive effect is mediated predominantly by postsynaptic α_2-adrenoceptors in the vasomotor centre of the medulla. There is also rebound hypertension on sudden withdrawal from chronic treatment. Nevertheless, in the context of anaesthesia, the anxiolytic and sedative effects of clonidine could be advantageous. Also, this drug reduces the dose requirements for anaesthesia, an interaction affecting volatile anaesthetics as well as thiopentone. Analgesic effects of anaesthetic agents are also potentiated by clonidine, which has some intrinsic analgesic activity, although this effect is strongly dose dependent. These analgesic effects are probably mediated by α_2-adrenoceptors in the spinal cord[6] lying on or near primary afferent nerve terminals and may involve intermediate secretion of the opioid peptide, dynorphin A.[7] The analgesic effects of clonidine and interactions with opioid analgesics are discussed in Chapters 5 and 25. In the light of all these actions, and since clonidine does not seem to prolong recovery from anaesthesia, this drug is gaining popularity as an adjunct to anaesthetic agents.[8]

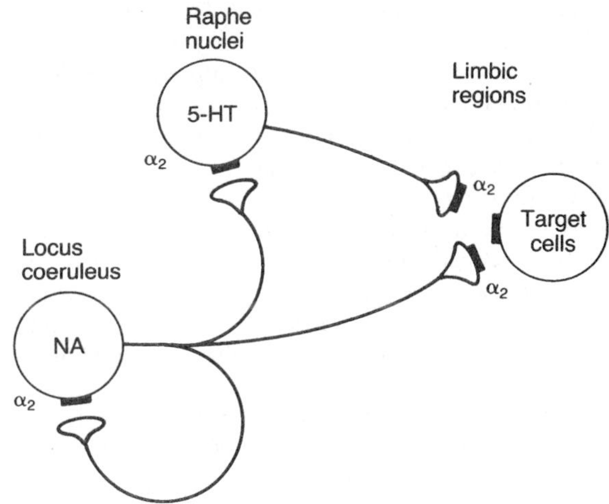

FIGURE 22.6 Modulation of noradrenergic (NA) and serotonergic (5-HT) release by terminal α_2-adrenoceptors. Axodendritic and axosomatic α_2-adrenoceptors also suppress neurotransmission by inhibiting cell firing.

Pharmacokinetics

Clonidine is well absorbed after oral administration and has a half-life of about 8.5 h. Approximately half the drug is excreted unchanged. Care is required when giving clonidine in combination with anaesthetic agents: time to peak plasma levels of clonidine can be as long as 60–90 min after oral administration and additive effects with anaesthetic agents will develop progressively over this period.

β-Adrenoceptor antagonists: propranolol

On the assumption that suppression of central noradrenergic transmission will reduce anxiety,

β-adrenoceptor antagonists, which block the postsynaptic actions of noradrenaline, have been used frequently as anxiolytic agents. Compounds such as propranolol have been especially recommended for relief of somatic symptoms of anxiety,[9] particularly those associated with situational anxiety (e.g. 'competition/performance nerves').[10] The efficacy of propranolol in treatment of generalized anxiety disorder is equivocal[11] and there are reports that this drug can even exacerbate depression and panic disorder. The main therapeutic advantage of β-blockers is that, unlike most other anxiolytics, they have minimal or no sedative actions.

Details of the pharmacology of β-blockers is discussed in Chapter 14 but, in the context of anaesthesia, it is important to note that all these drugs can cause bradycardia and hypotension and there is a risk of increasing airway resistance. For this reason, it has been suggested that cardioselective (β_1-adrenoceptor antagonist) agents such as metoprolol and atenolol may be more appropriate for blocking somatic components of anxiety, although they lose their selectivity at high doses. On the other hand, several points favour the use of non-selective agents. First, non-selective β-blockers (e.g. pindolol, timolol, nadolol and the prototypical propranolol) are more effective at reducing tremor than are cardioselective agents.[10] Secondly, non-selective β-blockers also suppress 5-HT transmission, probably by binding to 5-HT receptors, particularly of the 5-HT_{1A} subtype, and this could have a key role in the anxiolytic effects of these drugs (see below). Thirdly, there is a need for caution over adverse interactions between cardioselective β-blockers and anaesthetic agents; two situations give rise to such adverse interactions. The first is when stable cardiovascular function during anaesthesia depends on release of endogenous catecholamines, as is the case with cyclopropane, ether and possibly ketamine. Cyclopropane and ether are no longer in use in the UK. Obviously, essential effects of catecholamines on the cardiovascular system will be prevented by β-blockers. Secondly, the effects of agents with cardiosuppressant effects (enflurane, methoxyflurane, trichlorethylene) are all additive with those of propranolol.

5-HT AND ANXIETY

Neurones that release 5-HT in the brain arise in the brainstem raphe nuclei and project to many forebrain regions, particularly the limbic cortex and hippocampus. Despite the long-held belief that 5-HT has a key role in anxiety, evidence is not conclusive and pharmacological manipulation of serotonergic neurotransmission does not cause consistent changes in behaviour. Although benzodiazepines reduce the turnover of 5-HT in the CNS and, by implication, release of this neurotransmitter, it is not certain that this action is related to the anxiolytic effects of these drugs.[12]

The pharmacology of 5-HT has expanded rapidly in recent years with the identification of at least seven distinct receptor subtypes for this neurotransmitter (5-HT_{1A}, 5-HT_{1B}, 5-HT_{1D}, 5-HT_{2A}, 5-HT_{2B}, 5-HT_{2C}, 5-HT_3 and 5-HT_4 receptors.[13] Of these, 5-HT_{1A}, 5-HT_2, and 5-HT_3 are of particular interest in treatment of anxiety. Further genes have been cloned which encode further putative receptors: 5-ht_5, 5-ht_6 and 5-ht_7. As yet, these have no functional correlates.

5-HT_{1A} agonists: buspirone

Mode of action

Autoradiographic and electrophysiological studies have shown that 5-HT_{1A} receptors are located on the cell bodies of serotonergic neurones in the raphe nuclei. By analogy with α_2-adrenoceptors on noradrenergic neurones, they act as autoreceptors inhibiting neuronal firing and release of neurotransmitter. 5-HT_{1A} receptors are also found postsynaptically in limbic regions, particularly the cortex, hippocampus and septum, where they exert an inhibitory action.

The 5-HT_{1A} receptor partial agonist, buspirone (Fig. 22.7), has anti-anxiety effects in certain animal models and has recently been introduced for treatment of anxiety in man. Related compounds (azaspirodecanediones), gepirone and ipsapirone, have similar actions in animal models for anxiety, but their effects in man are less convincing and these drugs are not yet available clinically. The anxiolytic effects of these drugs have been attributed to suppression of serotonergic neurotransmission in the limbic system, although this is controversial. In contrast to other anxiolytic agents, the therapeutic actions of this drug are only apparent after chronic administration (approximately 2 weeks) and are most effective in patients who have not previously been exposed to benzodiazepine therapy.[14]

Buspirone is a potent dopamine receptor (D_2) antagonist, but this action is not thought to account for the anxiolytic effects of this drug. Involvement of α_2-adrenoceptors is also evident: the primary metabolite 1-2-(primidinyl)-piperazine (1-PP) is an effective α_2-adrenoceptor antagonist *in vivo*.[15] In preclinical studies (rodent), this compound has anxiolytic activity, albeit at high doses. Whether this affects the therapeutic actions of buspirone has yet to be resolved, particularly since relatively small amounts of 1-PP are produced in man (approximately 5% of dose) and

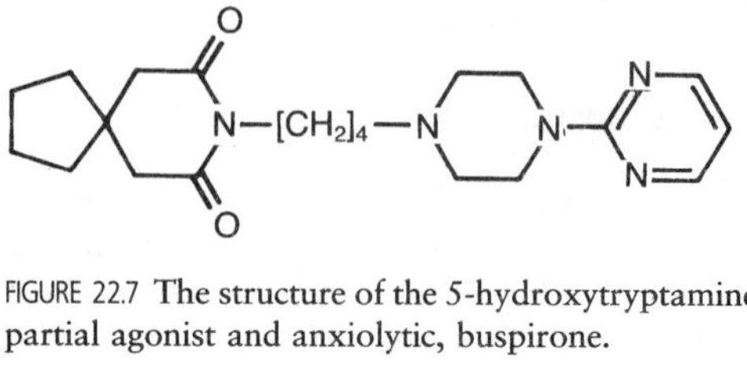

FIGURE 22.7 The structure of the 5-hydroxytryptamine (5-HT_{1A}) partial agonist and anxiolytic, buspirone.

because α_2-antagonists are normally anxiogenic (see below).

Other pharmacological effects

Buspirone has no appreciable, anticonvulsant, sedative or muscle-relaxant effects and its actions are not additive with those of hexobarbital or alcohol.[16] No CNS depressant interactions with anaesthetics would therefore be expected and none has yet been reported. The side-effects of buspirone include nausea, dizziness, light-headedness, diarrhoea and headaches.

Pharmacokinetics

Oral doses of buspirone are almost totally absorbed, but undergo extensive first-pass metabolism; bioavailability is approximately 4%. Metabolism is primarily by hydroxylation and N-dealkylation in the liver.[17] Excretion is via the kidneys, with some in the faeces; 50% of a single dose of drug is excreted as conjugated metabolites within 24 h.

5-HT_2 antagonists: ritanserin

5-HT_2 receptors are found postsynaptically in many brain regions, including the frontal cortex and mesolimbic areas. 5-HT_2 antagonists, such as ritanserin, are anxiolytic in certain animal models for this condition and possibly in man.[18] This compound also binds to 5-HT_{1C} receptors, however, and the extent to which these receptors are involved in the psychotropic actions of ritanserin is unknown. The effects of ritanserin are not additive with those of alcohol and it does not induce ataxia or affect total sleep time.[19] It does cause a large increase in slow wave sleep, with rebound insomnia on drug withdrawal. A reduced intake of alcohol in alcohol-dependent patients has also been reported with ritanserin. Confirmation of the anxiolytic and other potential therapeutic applications of this drug awaits the outcome of full clinical trials.

5-HT_3 receptor antagonists: ondansetron

5-HT_3 receptors have only recently been identified in the brain, and are particularly concentrated in the cortex, limbic regions and the dorsal vagal complex. Compounds acting selectively at these receptors have been developed (ondansetron, zacopride, granisetron, MDL 72222) and ondansetron is already used clinically as an anti-emetic in cancer chemotherapy. Also it is now available for the management of postoperative nausea and vomiting. The recommended dose is 4–8 mg given intravenously prior to induction of anaesthesia. The location of 5-HT_3 receptors (pre- or postsynaptic) is currently unknown but it is thought that there could be presynaptic 5-HT_3 receptors on dopaminergic nerve terminals. Activation of these receptors normally potentiates release of dopamine and ondansetron inhibits this potentiation; this effect of ondansetron could explain the anti-emetic actions of this drug.

In preclinical studies, ondansetron has been found to have anxiolytic activity in certain animal models and clinical trials are currently investigating this drug as a potential anxiolytic agent.[20] Ondansetron lacks anticonvulsant, ataxic and sedative activity and has no effects on pentobarbital sleeping time, so no additive interactions with anaesthetic agents would be expected.

GABA AND ANXIETY

GABA is found throughout the CNS, but neurones containing this neurotransmitter are generally intrinsic to each brain region (interneurones). There are few documented GABAergic pathways where activation of GABA-releasing neurones in one brain region directly influences the activity of nerve cells in another. Projections from cortical Purkinje cells and those of the striatonigral pathway are exceptions.

Two receptors for GABA have been characterized: $GABA_A$ and $GABA_B$. These are distinguished pharmacologically by the GABA agonist, muscimol, and the antagonist, bicuculline, which both act selectively at $GABA_A$ receptors. The muscle relaxant, baclofen, is a selective agonist of $GABA_B$ receptors. Evidence that GABA is involved in anxiety rests mainly on findings that benzodiazepines, barbiturates and even sodium valproate, all of which have potent anti-anxiety effects, potentiate $GABA_A$-receptor function. The $GABA_B$ receptor has not been linked with anxiety and is not affected by benzodiazepines.

The $GABA_A$ receptor: functional and structural subunits

The $GABA_A$ receptor comprises a multimolecular complex of functionally distinct subunits.[21,22] One of these subunits binds GABA itself and is coupled to a transmembrane Cl^- channel. When postsynaptic receptors at axosomatic or axodendritic synapses are activated by GABA, the Cl^- channel opens and Cl^- ions move down their electrochemical gradient from the extracellular fluid into postsynaptic cells. The resulting hyperpolarization inhibits cell firing. In addition, presynaptic $GABA_A$ receptors at axo-axonal synapses are thought to cause depolarization when activated by GABA; this reduces the amount of neurotransmitter released from the terminals when they are invaded by an incoming impulse. This is the basis of 'presynaptic inhibition'. Other functional components of the $GABA_A$ receptor bind benzodiazepines and barbiturates, both of which enhance GABAergic neurotransmission and are discussed in detail below.

Benzodiazepines

Benzodiazepines were introduced into clinical practice as anxiolytic agents in 1960 and rapidly replaced barbiturates and meprobamate which were more sedative at anxiolytic doses, less safe in overdose and well known for their ability to induce dependence with the associated potential for abuse. In contrast, benzodiazepines are generally regarded as extremely safe and with a large therapeutic index, although recent reports that these drugs can induce dependence have caused concern.[23]

All benzodiazepines have a broad therapeutic spectrum of CNS depression with actions ranging from anticonvulsant and anti-anxiety effects to muscle relaxation, sedation and hypnosis. Anterograde amnesia, which can be advantageous in the surgical context, is also induced by these drugs. The use of benzodiazepines in anaesthesia and as hypnotics or sedatives is discussed in detail in Chapter 21.

Mode of action

Specific binding sites for benzodiazepines have been identified and are prevalent in the cortex, cerebellum and limbic regions of the CNS. It is thought that the CNS depressant actions of these drugs are mediated exclusively by this receptor. Under optimal assay conditions, the affinity of different benzodiazepines for this binding site correlates strongly with their potency as CNS depressants *in vivo*, including their anxiolytic effects.[24]

Benzodiazepines do not influence the Cl^- channel of the $GABA_A$ receptor directly but induce changes in Cl^- conductance only in the presence of GABA. Benzodiazepine and GABA-binding sites are coupled in such a way that binding of agonists to the benzodiazepine receptor exerts an allosteric effect on the $GABA_A$ receptor complex and potentiates the effects of GABA on Cl^- channel opening. This potentiation is thought to involve an increase in the probability for opening of the channels, with no change in channel conductance or opening time. Studies showing that GABA potentiates binding of benzodiazepines to their receptor site provide further evidence for coupling of these two binding sites.

Several other agents cause similar potentiation of benzodiazepine binding. These include pyrazolopyridine anxiolytics, such as etazolate, hypnotic barbiturates and ethanol; all these compounds seem to exert their effects through the barbiturate binding site. Such potentiation could help explain why the CNS depression caused by benzodiazepines and barbiturates appears to be synergistic – that is, the effects of these drugs in combination are supra-additive. Examples include synergistic effects of midazolam when used in combination with either pentobarbitone or thiopentone in anaesthesia.[25,26] Interactions between midazolam or diazepam with halothane have also been reported.

Other ligands for the benzodiazepine receptor

Other families of compounds, in addition to benzodiazepines bind to the benzodiazepine receptor and have a similar spectrum of action. These include:

- Substituted benzodiazepines such as triazolobenzodiazepines and imidazobenzodiazepines: the 'new generation' benzodiazepines. The triazolobenzodiazepines, alprazolam and adinazolam are effective anxiolytics which cause relatively little sedation, amnesia or interaction with alcohol. They are unusual in that they are also effective in treatment of panic disorder and, possibly, mild depression (see below). Two imidazobenzodiazepines, bretazenil and flumazenil, are important clinically (see partial agonists and antagonists).
- Cyclopyrrolones (zopiclone and suriclone). These have actions that seem indistinguishable from benzodiazepines: zopiclone is already in clinical use as a hypnotic agent.
- Triazolopyridazines. None is available clinically.
- Quinolines. These bind to benzodiazepine receptors *in vitro* but do not have clear anxiolytic effects. This is almost certainly because of additional actions that mask the anxiolytic response.
- β-Carbolines. Many of these compounds have potent anxiolytic effects, but none is yet available clinically. β-Carboline-ethyl-carboxylate (β-CCE) and β-carboline-butyl-carboxylate (β-CCB) have been investigated as possible endogenous ligands for the benzodiazepine receptor; such a role for β-CCE, at least, has been ruled out. Although many β-carbolines have actions that resemble those of clinically useful benzodiazepines, β-CCE and β-CCB are interesting because they *induce* anxiety and seizures (see below, inverse agonists).
- Imidazopyridines. Two examples are being tested clinically: alpidem, which is predominantly anxiolytic, and zolpidem which is predominantly hypnotic.

Recent developments suggest that there are subtypes of benzodiazepine receptors that show different affinities for a range of ligands (type 1 and type 2); both are coupled to $GABA_A$ receptors. Although it is generally believed that similar mechanisms underlie the actions of all benzodiazepines, functional subdivision of benzodiazepine receptors is a possibility. An early suggestion was that type 1 receptors evoked the anticonvulsant and anxiolytic effects of benzodiazepines whereas type 2 receptors were responsible for the sedative and myorelaxant actions of these drugs; this possibility, which could lead to the development of non-sedative anxiolytics, has not been confirmed. Nevertheless, functional subdivision cannot be ruled out in the light of findings such as:

- In preclinical studies the non-benzodiazepine hypnotic, zolpidem, a selective type 1 receptor agonist, has sedative effects at much lower doses than those required to produce muscle relaxation, anticonvulsant effects or actions consistent with anxiolytic effects in man. A related compound, alpidem, is being promoted as an anxiolytic agent.
- 1,5 substituted benzodiazepines, clobazam and triflubazam, are effective anticonvulsant and anxiolytic agents, but are comparatively less potent amnesic, myorelaxant and sedative agents than the first generation, 1,4-substituted benzodiazepines.

Pharmacokinetics

The actions of benzodiazepines have always been considered to be qualitatively broadly similar; differences in their potency for CNS depression have been assumed to be related to their affinity for binding to benzodiazepine receptors. The suitability of individual compounds for their various therapeutic applications has been determined largely by their pharmacokinetics. Convention has dictated that drugs useful as hypnotics or premedicants should have actions that are fast in onset but short lasting (e.g. triazolam and temazepam) so as to minimize hangover effects. For long-term treatment of anxiety and prevention of seizures, a rapid onset of action is not critical. For such applications drugs should be either intermediate (e.g. lorazepam) or long-acting (e.g. clonazepam and diazepam) and these effects should be achieved with minimal sedation.

The rate of onset of action of benzodiazepines is dependent primarily on lipid solubility (Table 22.4) – compounds with the greatest solubility, typically diazepam, having the most rapid effects. Although high lipid solubility is an advantage for oral administration, it presents problems for intravenous administration since the inevitable low water solubility requires that the drug vehicle is usually an organic solvent (e.g. propylene glycol, polyethylene glycol); this can cause adverse tissue reactions at the site of injection and/or hypersensitivity reactions. Recently, vehicle comprised of emulsified soyabean oil and water has been introduced for intravenous injection of hydrophobic compounds such as diazepam. Midazolam and flurazepam are relatively water-soluble benzodiazepines.

Extensive binding to plasma proteins ensures that effective concentrations of these compounds are delivered to the CNS despite their low water solubility. High lipid solubility restricts renal excretion of these drugs and their duration of action is determined essentially by redistribution from the CNS and metabolism in the liver. Metabolism of benzodiazepines involves enzymic degradation by N-methylation, hydroxylation or nitroreduction to inactive metabolites followed by formation of soluble conjugates with glucuronic acid which can be excreted by the kidneys.

Some compounds, such as oxazepam, lorazepam and temazepam, are conjugated directly with no intermediate metabolites and have a relatively short duration of action. Others, such as diazepam and chlordiazepoxide, are converted into intermediate, active metabolites (commonly N-desmethyldiazepam) some of which have a half-life considerably longer than that of the parent compound. The half-life of desmethyldiazapam (65 h), for instance, is twice as long as that of diazepam itself (20–40 h).[27] As a consequence, liver function, age, sex and genetic factors can all affect the duration of action of benzodiazepines which are inactivated by enzymic degradation; conjugation is little affected by these factors. Although tolerance to the effects of benzodiazepines can develop, there is little evidence for increased metabolism through enzyme induction which is known to occur on repeated administration of barbiturates.

Benzodiazepine receptor partial agonists: bretazenil

The assumption that all benzodiazepines exert qualitatively the same effects on the $GABA_A$ receptor implies that all benzodiazepines act as full agonists at the benzodiazepine receptor. Under these conditions, the extent of drug-induced receptor activation would be dependent only on drug concentration and receptor

TABLE 22.4 Pharmacokinetic parameters of benzodiazepines commonly used with anaesthesia

DRUG	PLASMA $t_{\frac{1}{2}}$	% PROTEIN BOUND	OCTANOL : BUFFER PARTITION COEFFICIENT (LIPID SOLUBILITY)
Diazepam*	20–40	97–99	309
Lorazepam	9–22	85	73
Midazolam	1.3–3.1	94–97	475
Temazepam	8–24	96–98	62

*Active metabolites. Data derived from Refs 27–29.

affinity. This is now known not to be the case. In common with other receptor systems, compounds have been identified that bind with high affinity to the benzodiazepine receptor, but that do not evoke maximal potentiation of receptor function; these compounds have characteristics typical of partial agonists.

Specific therapeutic applications for benzodiazepine partial agonists have been suggested by investigations of the relation between the CNS depression and the proportion of benzodiazepine receptors that are occupied by drug. Relief of anxiety and prevention of seizures is thought to require relatively few receptors to be occupied by benzodiazepines (5–30%) and that a much greater receptor occupancy is required to achieve sedation or hypnosis. For full agonists, such as diazepam, it can be difficult to adjust the drug dose in order to achieve the correct balance between anxiolysis and sedation. With partial agonists, the therapeutic window is much broader: since these drugs have submaximal efficacy, it is possible that even when all benzodiazepine receptor sites are occupied by drug, the degree of $GABA_A$ receptor activation is insufficient to provoke sedation. Two such compounds, the imidazobenzodiazepine, bretazenil, and the pyrrolodiazepine, premazepam, are currently undergoing clinical trials as non-sedative, anxiolytic benzodiazepines. Bretazenil has an affinity for benzodiazepine-receptor binding which is approximately ten times that of diazepam and the anxiolytic dose is about one-tenth that of diazepam. Yet, this compound has no effects on motor co-ordination and no additive effects with ethanol.[30]

Bretazenil is also being investigated for prevention of panic attacks; to ensure a rapid onset of action, the drug is administered by the sublingual route at the onset of the attack. Such treatment could also be useful for rapid anxiolysis in day-case surgery, such as amnesic–sedative effects in dentistry, but interactions with other benzodiazepines must be taken into account if these are co-administered with bretazenil.

Benzodiazepine antagonists: flumazenil

Benzodiazepine receptor antagonists have little, or no, intrinsic effects but they block or reverse the actions of benzodiazepines. One such compound, the imidazobenzodiazepine flumazenil, is now used to reverse the sedation induced by benzodiazepines in anaesthesia or benzodiazepine overdose.[31] The lack of intrinsic activity at the $GABA_A$ receptor ensures that this drug has no anxiolytic activity and does not provoke a stress response.

Flumazenil does not affect the actions of drugs acting at other components of the $GABA_A$ receptor, notably barbiturates, but interactions with inhalational anaesthetics have not been ruled out. Flumazenil has an extremely short half-life (0.7–1.3 h) due to extensive first-pass metabolism and there is a significant risk of resedation unless repeated doses are given; longer-acting benzodiazepine antagonists are not yet available for clinical use.

Benzodiazepine inverse agonists

In addition to drugs that have the classical pharmacological profile of benzodiazepines (i.e. CNS depression), there are compounds which, although binding to the benzodiazepine receptor, have the opposite pharmacological effects. In animal models, these drugs reduce seizure threshold, are anxiogenic and attenuate the effects of GABA on Cl^- conductance. Such compounds are known as benzodiazepine inverse agonists. In the single study carried out in man, administration of an inverse agonist (FG 7142) caused profound anxiety which was relieved by iv injection of diazepam.[32] The severity of the anxiety was such that inverse agonists are regarded as inappropriate for induction of anxiety experimentally in man (see below).

Barbiturates

A testimony to the success of the benzodiazepines is the extent to which they have replaced the barbiturates and other anxiolytics such as meprobamate, chloral hydrate and paraldehyde. The pharmacokinetics and uses of barbiturates as sedative hypnotics and in anaesthesia are discussed in Chapters 5 and 21. Only a brief outline of their pharmacology is given here.

Mode of action

Barbiturates bind to the $GABA_A$ receptor complex but, unlike the benzodiazepine receptor, the binding site for barbiturates is thought to be a component of the Cl^- channel itself. Because they compete for binding with convulsant agents such as picrotoxin and pentylenetetrazol, this binding site is sometimes called the picrotoxin receptor.

Barbiturates modify $GABA_A$ receptor function in several ways: the duration of opening of the Cl^- channel is increased by barbiturates; they increase the number of binding sites available for GABA binding and potentiate the effects of GABA on Cl^- conductance. They may also have a direct effect on the Cl^- channel because, unlike benzodiazepines, high concentrations of barbiturates can increase Cl^- conductance in the absence of GABA. These direct actions are not blocked by the GABA antagonist, bicuculline.

Drugs that bind to the barbiturate receptor not only enhance the actions of GABA, but also, in the presence of GABA, potentiate binding of benzodiazepines to their receptor site; their potency for this effect correlates with their anaesthetic activity. These differences in the actions of benzodiazepines and barbiturates could explain why the latter group of compounds show greater CNS depressant effects and, unlike benzodiazepines, will induce anaesthesia in high doses.

Pharmacokinetics

Like the benzodiazepines, the clinical applications of barbiturates depend mainly on the pharmacokinetics of individual compounds. Compounds that are highly lipid soluble, and therefore have actions that are rapid in onset, are suitable for induction of anaesthesia; the prototypical agent with this action is thiopentone. Compounds with actions of longer duration, such as pentobarbitone and amylobarbitone, have anxiolytic and sedative actions which last several hours. These actions are terminated by metabolic transformation to inactive products which are then excreted by the kidney.

Over the first few days of administration, tolerance to the actions of barbiturates develops which is largely explained by a progressive increase in the rate of metabolism of these drugs. This is due to induction of the hepatic cytochrome P-450 and conjugating enzymes; this enzymic induction can affect the metabolism of other drugs which are treated in the same way, notably warfarin, contraceptive steroids, phenytoin and desmethylimipramine. Pharmacodynamic tolerance is also apparent, although the mechanisms underlying this process are not fully understood.

Meprobamate

This compound was the first to be developed specifically as an anxiolytic agent. Now rarely used, the mechanism of action of this compound has not been intensively researched. Although it has a pharmacological profile very similar to that of barbiturates and benzodiazepines, it does not interact with the $GABA_A$ receptor. It has been suggested that meprobamate inhibits uptake (inactivation) of adenosine, another inhibitory neurotransmitter within the CNS. This is an interesting possibility because adenosine antagonists can induce anxiety in man (see below, caffeine).

PANIC DISORDER

The view that panic disorder could be distinguished from generalized anxiety followed the discovery that tricyclic antidepressants, but not anxiolytic 1,4 benzodiazepines, effectively control panic attacks.[33] Benzodiazepines are used to prevent anticipatory anxiety associated with panic. Other antidepressants, the monoamine oxidase inhibitors (MAOIs) are also effective and phenelzine is widely used for this purpose. This clear distinction between treatment strategies for anxiety and panic has been brought into question by recent reports that the triazolobenzodiazepines, adinazolam and alprazolam, effectively control panic and widespread recognition that antidepressant drugs are also effective in treatment of generalized anxiety disorder.

Agents that induce panic attacks in man

Unlike generalized anxiety, the transient and unpredictable nature of panic disorder hinders research into this condition. For this reason, several procedures have been developed for inducing panic attacks in a controlled environment (Table 22.5); such procedures are used to investigate possible causes of this disorder. Ideally, these agents should induce panic only in panic patients, or have a much lower threshold for induction in panic patients than in control subjects. Validation of these procedures as models of panic disorder rests on finding that the symptoms induced by such procedures resemble those seen in spontaneous panic and that they are prevented by drug treatments with established clinical efficacy. Treatments that are used most commonly to induce panic are discussed below.

Adrenergic agents

The rationale for infusing catecholamines to induce a panic attack stems mainly from the theory that increased sympathetic tone, which causes increased heart rate, sweating and tremor, could serve as an internal (interoceptive) cue for triggering a panic attack. Adrenaline and noradrenaline have generally proved unconvincing in induction of panic, but the effects of the selective β-adrenoceptor agonist, isoprenaline, are more consistent both in terms of selectivity for panic patients and the nature of the symptoms experienced. Isoprenaline shows poor penetration of the blood–brain barrier, so it is possible that a major component of isoprenaline-induced panic is peripheral in origin.

The α_2-adrenoceptor antagonist, yohimbine, has been used widely and is fairly selective in inducing panic in patients, but not controls. A primary action of yohimbine is to block feedback inhibition of

TABLE 22.5 Agents which induce panic attacks in man

Frequently used:

- Adrenergic agents (particularly isoprenaline and yohimbine)
- Sodium lactate
- Caffeine

Others:

- Metachlorophenylpiperazine (mCPP; binds to 5-HT_1, 5-HT_2 and α-adrenoceptors)
- Benzodiazepine inverse agonists
- Carbon dioxide
- Dextrose

noradrenaline release, which is mediated by α_2-adrenoceptors on noradrenergic nerve terminals and on the cell bodies of neurones in the CNS. The anxiogenic actions of yohimbine support the view that overactivity of noradrenergic neurones has a key role in the cause of anxiety and panic.[3] This explanation may be an oversimplification because yohimbine, at least, also binds to 5-HT_{1D} and $GABA_A$ receptors and both these actions could contribute to the actions of this drug in panic.

Sodium lactate

Lactate, like isoprenaline, shows little penetration of the blood–brain barrier, yet commonly induces panic in panic patients; there is a much lower incidence in control subjects. The effects of lactate infusion are prevented by agents used clinically to treat panic disorder (alprazolam, imipramine and MAOIs), but are not affected by the β-adrenoceptor antagonist, propranolol. Mechanisms underlying the panicogenic effects of lactate are unknown.

Caffeine (1,3,7-trimethylxanthine)

Caffeine is well known for its anxiogenic effects and its ability to cause exaggerated responses to stress. Panic patients appear to have increased sensitivity to this drug; greater increases in plasma glucose, lactate and cortisol are seen in panic patients than in controls. All these changes are prevented by the antipanic agent, alprazolam.[34]

Several factors could underlie the actions of caffeine. Animal studies have shown that this compound activates noradrenergic neurones in the locus coeruleus. Inhibition of the enzyme phosphodiesterase, leading to enhanced postsynaptic β-adrenoceptor responses has been discounted. Caffeine is a potent inhibitor of adenosine receptors in the CNS at concentrations consistent with those causing a panic response. This could well underlie the anxiogenic effects of this drug since adenosine receptors are inhibitory in the CNS.

Drug treatments for panic disorder

Inhibitors of monoamine uptake

The tricyclic antidepressant, imipramine, was the first compound to be used successfully in treatment of panic disorder and remains the drug of choice. As in treatment of depression, there is a delay in improvement of the patients' symptoms and the drug has to be given on a chronic basis. Initially, in many patients, imipramine exacerbates the symptoms and the dropout rate for treatment is high in the first 2–3 weeks. Otherwise, imipramine is more effective than chlordiazepoxide and equieffective with alprazolam (see below) in relieving panic and anxiety. There is a high relapse rate if treatment is withdrawn prematurely. Imipramine also blocks panic attacks provoked by infusion of lactate or isoprenaline.

Clomipramine, a tricyclic antidepressant regarded as a relatively selective inhibitor of 5-HT uptake, is also used frequently and may be more effective than imipramine. There are reports that the 5-HT precursor, 1-5-hydroxytryptophan, (5-HTP) and the selective 5-HT uptake blockers, e.g. fluvoxamine and fluoxetine, have antipanic activity. Other uptake blockers (both selective and non-selective) that have been tested with moderate degrees of success include: zimeldine, trazodone, amitriptyline, nortriptyline, maprotiline, doxepine and desmethylimpramine.[35]

Monoamine Oxidase Inhibitors (MAOIs)

Phenelzine is the most widely used of this group of drugs and not only is this drug beneficial in treatment of panic but, unlike imipramine, is thought to be of benefit in preventing anticipatory anxiety. It is commonly used in combination with other agents. The major limitation in using MAOIs is the adverse side-effects of these compounds (postural hypotension, dizziness, dry mouth, disturbance of the gastrointestinal tract, blurred vision) and the risk of adverse drug interactions, particularly with indirectly acting sympathomimetic agents such as tyramine or ephedrine. Unlike the uptake inhibitors, these compounds do not seem to cause the initial aggravation of panic symptoms. Details of the pharmacology of MAOIs are given in Part I.

Benzodiazepines

The triazolobenzodiazepine, alprazolam, is thought to be as effective as imipramine or phenelzine if given in high enough doses and may act more quickly than the tricyclics or MAOIs. Although there are reports that propranolol can exacerbate panic attacks, alprazolam has also been tested in combination with propranolol and additive (possibly synergistic) effects shown. One advantage of alprazolam is that it has a much more rapid rate of onset than tricyclics and MAOIs. The high affinity of this drug for benzodiazepine receptors, coupled with relatively low sedative effects may explain its efficacy in panic. It has been suggested that other benzodiazepines, with a lower affinity, could have antipanic actions at high doses, but these are masked by sedation.

Theories to explain panic disorder

Several different theories have been proposed. Although each of these theories is based on changes in the function of one neurotransmitter system, only, it is equally likely that panic disorder involves disruption of neurotransmitter interactions within the brain.

Noradrenaline

Increased noradrenergic neurotransmission is one possible cause of panic; yohimbine is thought to induce panic by increasing release of noradrenaline, for instance (see above). In man, this is reflected by an increase in levels of plasma MHPG, the primary metabolite of noradrenaline, after a single yohimbine injection. Moreover, the levels of MHPG correlate with patient ratings of anxiety.[36] The increases in both plasma MHPG and panic ratings are prevented by alprazolam, but not by diazepam which has no effect in panic.[37] Nevertheless, increased release of noradrenaline does not seem to be essential for panic because a rise in plasma MHPG is not found in spontaneous panic or after isoprenaline- or lactate-induced panic.

Alternatively, the function of α_2-receptors may be exaggerated in panic. This could explain both why yohimbine can induce a panic attack in patients, but not controls and findings that panic patients have enhanced hypotensive responses to clonidine.[38] There are isolated reports of an increase in the number or affinity of α_2-adrenoceptors on platelets of panic patients, but these have not been confirmed. Disruption of receptor function beyond the transmitter binding site is also possible.

5-HT

There are several conflicting theories to explain the role of 5-HT in panic disorder. Since 5-HTP and drugs that block 5-HT reuptake are effective antipanic agents, it is possible that panic arises from a deficit in 5-HT function. Alternatively, it has been proposed that 5-HT receptors are hyperresponsive in panic disorder.[39] This would explain why the agonist metachlorophenylpiperazine (mCPP) induces panic and why panic patients report increased symptoms at the start of treatment with antidepressant drugs that increase levels of 5-HT in the synapse. Which subtype of receptor is involved remains conjectural. It is unlikely to be the (postsynaptic) 5-HT_2 receptor because the 5-HT_2 receptor antagonist, ritanserin, has no antipanic activity. 5-HT_{1A} receptors are a favoured candidate.

GABA

The efficacy of triazolobenzodiazepines in suppression of panic suggests that GABA_A receptor dysfunction may be a component of this disorder. Three lines of evidence have led to three different theories:

1 Benzodiazepine inverse agonists induce anxiety/panic in animal models (including primates) and man. Excess release of an endogenous ligand for the benzodiazepine receptor with characteristics of an inverse agonist could cause panic. There have been many candidates for such a ligand, but none is widely accepted.

2 Conversely, a deficit in an agonist ligand for the benzodiazepine receptor could cause anxiety. Again, many candidates for such a ligand have been proposed. The most interesting is desmethyldiazepam which has been found in post-mortem brain tissue of individuals for whom benzodiazepine intake can be excluded. It is thought that this compound, an active metabolite of diazepam, can be ingested in the diet. It is not widely believed to be an endogenous ligand.

3 GABA_A receptor function itself could be attenuated. A disruption in the coupling of the benzodiazepine- and GABA-binding sites has been proposed, such that actions of benzodiazepine agonists and antagonists are shifted towards those of inverse agonists. Evidence that flumazenil is anxiogenic in panic patients, but not control subjects, supports this theory.[40]

FUTURE TREATMENTS FOR ANXIETY AND PANIC DISORDER

The peptide, cholecystokinin (CCK), has recently been found in high concentrations in the brain. It is particularly prevalent in limbic regions and is thought to act as an excitatory neuromodulator. In some neurones, it may act as a cotransmitter with GABA. Administration of the tetrapeptide CCK-4 in man induces panic, even in subjects with no history of anxiety disorder. This action is thought to be mediated by central CCK receptors.[41]

Subtypes of the cholecystokinin receptor have been characterized (CCK-A and CCK-B) and a range of antagonists developed that are lipophilic and therefore cross the blood–brain barrier after oral administration.[42] These CCK-B antagonists have an anxiolytic profile in animal models without causing sedation.[43] The CCK-B receptor also promotes gastrin secretion, so CCK-B-receptor antagonists have prominent effects on gastric acid secretion.

Interestingly, benzodiazepine derivatives (devazepide and L-365, 260) are also ligands for the CCK-B receptor and panic caused by the agonist, CCK-4, is prevented by pre-administration of lorazepam but not meprobamate. Therefore, at least some of the anxiolytic actions of benzodiazepines could be attributed to interactions with the CCK-B receptor. It is possible that compounds acting in this way could be the next generation of non-sedative anxiolytics.

REFERENCES

1 American Psychiatric Association. *Diagnostic and statistical manual of mental disorders*, 4th edn. Washington, DC: American Psychiatric Association, 1994.

2 Clark CR, Geffen GM, Geffen LB. Catecholamines and attention II: pharmacological studies in normal humans. *Neuroscience and Biobehavioral Reviews* 1987, **11**: 353–64.

3 Charney DS, Heninger GR, Redmond DE. Yohimbine induced anxiety and increased noradrenergic function in humans: effects of diazepam and clonidine. *Life Sciences* 1983; **33**: 19–29.

4 Charney DS, Redmond DE. Neurobiological mechanisms in human anxiety. *Neuropharmacology* 1983; **22**: 1531–6.

5 Ninan PT, Insel TM, Cohen RM, Cook JM, Skolnick P, Paul SM. Benzodiazepine receptor-mediated experimental 'anxiety' in primates. *Science* 1982; **218**: 1332–4.

6 Yaksh TL. Pharmacology of spinal adrenergic systems which modulate spinal nociceptive processing. *Pharmacology, Biochemistry and Behavior* 1985; **22**: 845–58.

7 Fujimoto JM, Arts KS. Clonidine administered intracerebroventricularly in mice produces an anti-analgesic effect which may be mediated spinally by Dynorphin A (1–17). *Neuropharmacology* 1990; **29**: 351–8.

8 Mahoney A, Seeley H. Clonidine: old friend – new guises. *British Journal of Hospital Medicine* 1990; **44**: 358–61.

9 Tyrer P. Current status of β-blocking drugs in the treatment of anxiety disorders. *Drugs* 1988; **36**: 773–83.

10 Jefferson D, Jenner P, Marsden CD. Beta-adrenoceptor antagonists in essential tremor. *Journal of Neurology, Neurosurgery and Psychiatry* 1979; **42**: 904–9.

11 Hayes PE, Schulz SC. Beta-blockers in anxiety disorders. *Journal of Affective Disorders* 1987; **13**: 119–30.

12 Stephens DN, Kehr W, Duka T. Anxiolytic and anxiogenic β-carbolines: tools for the study of anxiety mechanisms. In: Biggio G, Costa E eds. *GABAergic transmission and anxiety*. New York: Raven Press, 1986: 91–106.

13 Fozard JR. 5-HT: the enigma variations. *Trends in Pharmacological Sciences* 1987; **8**: 501–6.

14 Schweizer E, Rickels K, Lucki I. Resistance to the anti-anxiety effect of buspirone in patients with a history of benzodiazepine use. *New England Journal of Medicine* 1986; **314**: 719–20.

15 Bianchi G, Garattini S. Blockade of α_2-adrenoceptors by 1-(2-primidinyl)-piperazine (PmP) *in vivo* and its relation to the activity of buspirone. *European Journal of Pharmacology* 1988; **143**: 343–50.

16 Riblet LA, Eison AS, Eison MS, Taylor DP, Temple DL, VanderMaelen CP. Neuropharmacology of buspirone. *Psychopathology* 1984; **17** (Suppl 3): 69–78.

17 Jajoo HK, Mayol RF, LaBudde JA, Blair IA. Metabolism of the antianxiety drug buspirone in human subjects. *Drug Metabolism and Disposition* 1989; **17**: 634–40.

18 Reyntjens A, Gelders YG, Hoppenbrouwers M-LJA, Bussche GV. Thymosynthetic effects of ritanserin (R 55667), a centrally acting serotonin-S2 receptor blocker. *Drug Development Research* 1986; **8**: 205–11.

19 Meert TF, Janssen PAJ. Psychopharmacology of ritanserin: comparison with chlordiazepoxide. *Drug Development Research* 1989; **18**: 119–44.

20 Jones BJ, Costall B, Domeney AM, Kelly ME, Naylor RJ, Oakley NR, Tyers MB. The potential anxiolytic activity of GR38032F, a 5-HT_3-receptor antagonist. *British Journal of Pharmacology* 1988; **93**: 985–93.

21 Olsen RW, Tobin AJ. Molecular biology of $GABA_A$ receptors. *FASEB Journal* 1990; **4**: 1469–80.

22 Schofield PR. The $GABA_A$ receptor: molecular biology reveals a complex picture. *Trends in Pharmacological Sciences* 1989; **10**: 476–8.

23 Petursson H, Lader MH. Withdrawal from long-term benzodiazepine treatment. *British Medical Journal* 1981; **283**: 643–5.

24 Braestrup C, Squires RF. Pharmacological characterisation of benzodiazepine receptors in the brain. *European Journal of Pharmacology* 1978; **18**: 263–70.

25 Short TG, Galletly DC, Plummer JL. Hypnotic and anaesthetic action of thiopentone and midazolam alone and in combination. *British Journal of Anaesthesia* 1991; **66**: 13–19.

26 Kissin I, Mason JO, Bradley EL. Pentobarbital and thiopental anesthesia interactions with midazolam. *Anesthesiology* 1987; **67**: 26–31.

27 Richens A. Clinical pharmacokinetics of benzodiazepines. In: Trimble MR ed. *Benzodiazepines divided*. Chichester: John Wiley, 1983; 187–207.

28 Pieri L, Schaffner R, Scherschlicht R, Polc P, Sepinwall J, Davidson A, Mohler H, Cumin R, Da Prada M, Burkard WP, Keller HH, Muller RKM, Gerold M, Pieri M, Cook L, Haefely W. Pharmacology of Midazolam. *Arzneimittelforschung/Drug Research* 1981; **31**: 2180–2201.

29 Greenblatt DJ, Divoll M, Abernethy DR, Ochs HR, Shader RI. Clinical pharmacokinetics of the newer benzodiazepines. *Clinical Pharmacokinetics* 1983; **8**: 233–52.

30 Martin JR, Pieri L, Bonetti EP, Schaffner R, Burkard WP, Cumin R, Haefely WE. Ro 16–6028: a novel anxiolytic acting as a partial agonist at the benzodiazepine receptor. *Pharmacopsychiatry* 1988; **21**, 360–2.

31 Geller E, Halpern P. Benzodiazepine antagonists and inverse agonists. *Current Opinion in Anaesthesiology* 1990; **3**: 568–72.

32 Dorow R, Horowski R, Paschelke G, Amin M, Braestrup C. Severe anxiety induced by FG7142, a β-carboline ligand for benzodiazepine receptors. *Lancet* 1983; **ii**: 98–9.

33 Klein DF, Fink M. Psychiatric reaction patterns to imipramine. *American Journal of Psychiatry* 1962; **119**: 432–8.

34 Uhde TW. Caffeine provocation of panic: a focus on biological mechanisms. In: Ballenger JC ed. *Frontiers of clinical science, Vol. 8. Neurobiology of panic disorder*. New York: Wiley-Liss, 1990: 219–42.

35 Nutt DJ, Glue P. Clinical pharmacology of anxiolytics and antidepressants: a psychopharmacological perspective. *Pharmacology and Therapeutics* 1989; **44**: 309–44.

36 Gurguis GNM, Uhde TW. Plasma 3-methoxy-4-hydroxyphenylethylene glycol (MHPG) and growth hormone responses to yohimbine in panic disorder patients and normal control. *Psychoneuroendocrinology* 1990; **15**: 217–24.

37 Charney DJ, Heninger GR. Noradrenergic function and the mechanism of action of antianxiety treatment: I. The effect of long-term alprazolam treatment. *Archives of General Psychiatry* 1985; **42**: 458–67.

38 Nutt DJ. Increased central α_2-adrenoceptor sensitivity in panic disorder. *Psychopharmacology* 1986; **90**: 268–9.

39 Kahn RS, Van Praag HM, Wetzler S, Asnis GM, Barr G. Serotonin and anxiety revisited. *Biological Psychiatry* 1988; **23**: 189–208.

40 Nutt DJ, Glue P. Evidence for altered benzodiazepine receptor in panic disorder. *Archives of General Psychiatry* 1990; **47**: 917–25.

41 De Montigny C. Cholecystokinin tetrapeptide induces panic-like attacks in healthy volunteers. *Archives of General Psychiatry* 1989; **46**, 511–17.

42 Singh L, Lewis AS, Field MJ, Hughes J, Woodruff GN. Evidence for an involvement of the brain cholecystokinin B receptor in anxiety. *Proceedings of the National Academy of Science, USA* 1991; **88**: 1130–1.

43 Horwell DC, Hughes J, Hunter JC, Pritchard MC, Richardson RS, Roberts E, Woodruff GN. Rationally designed 'dipeptoid' analogues of CCK. α-Methyltryptophan derivatives as highly selective and orally active gastrin and CCK-B antagonists with potent anxiolytic properties. *Journal of Medicinal Chemistry* 1991; **34**: 404–14.

23

Drugs and Neurological Disorders

CJ Pycock

INTRODUCTION

It is an unfortunate fact that a major portion of pathology within the central nervous system (CNS) is, by and large, irreversible. However, symptoms of neurological disease can often be greatly improved by pharmacological manipulation with drugs that act selectively in the brain. In general, damage to the peripheral nerves is less amenable to specific treatment although the function of the motor nerve synapse can be improved by, for example, anticholinesterase drugs for the management of myasthenia gravis (see Chapter 10).

This section deals with drugs employed in the treatment of neurological disorders, but in order to concentrate on specific pharmacological mechanisms, the chapter is mainly restricted to the discussion of agents used for the control of epilepsy and the extrapyramidal syndromes (Parkinson's disease, Huntington's chorea, dystonias). Other large areas of neurological disease whereby pathology is related to disturbance of vascular supply (e.g. stroke, migraine) or to inflammatory states (e.g. multiple sclerosis) have been omitted. Similarly, degenerative disorders such as Alzheimer's disease are not discussed.

THE EPILEPSIES

Epilepsy is a paroxysmal disorder of brain activity causing changes in motor, sensory, autonomic or mental function. It has a prevalence in the community of about 0.5%.

Classification of epilepsy

An epileptic attack begins as an abnormal electrical discharge from a group of neurones (called a focus). Such a discharge may be contained within a localized area producing either no effect or a *focal* or *partial seizure*, or it may spread to activate distal neurones and result in a *generalized* seizure. A clinical classification of the epilepsies, based on this scheme, is presented in Fig. 23.1. (Refer to Ref. 1. as a general text.)

Pathology of epilepsy

The causes of an epileptic fit are many. They may be related to neurological/neuroanatomical causes such as congenital defects or to structural abnormalities, head injury, vascular malformations, tumours or degenerative disease. Similarly, metabolic or toxic disturbances can be manifest as fits, including infections, heavy metal and drug poisoning (including alcohol), drug withdrawal, fever, and electrolyte and blood sugar imbalances. In many cases the cause of the convulsion is unknown, and is described as idiopathic epilepsy.

The neuropharmacology and neurochemistry of epilepsy is not well understood. Many cerebral neurotransmitter systems have been implicated in the aetiology, but to date the picture is far from clear. Certainly, it is well recognized that stimulation of brain excitatory transmitter systems or, conversely, inhibition of cerebral inhibitory transmitter systems will induce seizures in experimental animals. Thus it is well established that focal or general stimulation of cerebral acetylcholine (ACh) and the excitatory amino acids glutamate and aspartate mechanisms can provoke seizure activity. γ-Aminobutyric acid (GABA) and glycine are potent inhibitory amino acid neurotransmitters

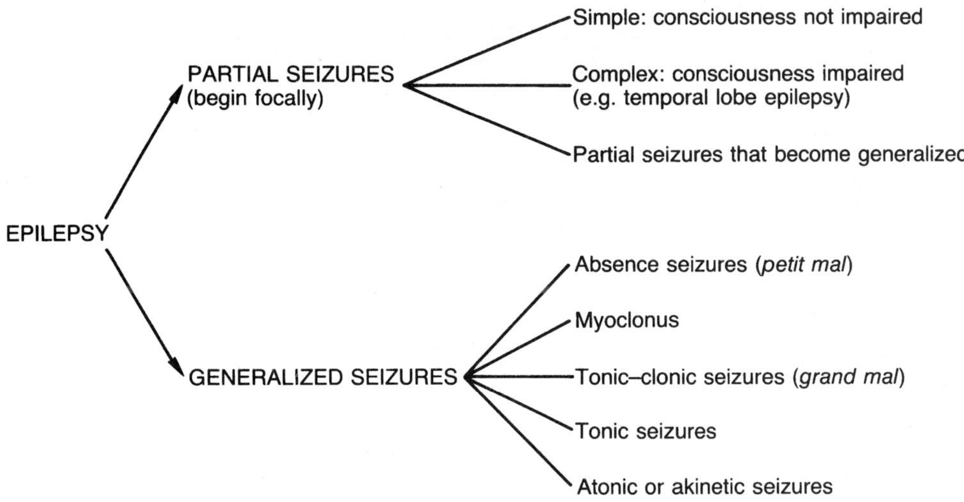

FIGURE 23.1 A clinical classification of the epilepsies.

within the brain and spinal cord, and blockade of their receptor systems with *picrotoxin* and *strychnine* respectively can cause generalized convulsions in laboratory animals. It has also been well demonstrated that enhancing cerebral GABA function either by stimulating postsynaptic receptors or by increasing synaptic GABA concentrations following blockade of its enzymatic degradation by GABA-transaminase, has a protective action against seizure activity. Similarly the benzodiazepine drugs, which partially interact at the GABA receptor site (see Chapter 21), possess anticonvulsant properties.

ANTICONVULSANT DRUGS

The first stage in the management of epilepsy is to confirm the diagnosis, and the second is to correct any treatable causes, for example infection, metabolic imbalance, alcohol withdrawal, cerebral lesions, etc. The action of the anticonvulsant drug is to increase the threshold of abnormal cerebral electrical discharges and thereby to reduce the frequency of epileptic attacks, and to prevent the spread of this electrical discharge through the brain substance. Some 10–12 anticonvulsant drugs are available in clinical practice to control both acute and chronic epilepsy. It is general consensus (and correctly so) that epileptics should preferentially be treated with one drug only when this single agent controls attacks and is largely free from side-effects. Unfortunately, in practice many patients with chronic epilepsy do not have their symptoms adequately controlled with a single medication and two or even more drugs are occasionally required to achieve reasonable control. Indeed, the newly introduced anti-epileptic drugs are being marketed as adjunctive therapy.

The precise mode of action of anticonvulsant drugs seems to have eluded pharmacologists for many years.[2] Broadly, such drugs can be divided into two basic groups: (1) those with non-specific general depressant actions on neuronal function; and (2) those that may act through a specific neurotransmitter system.

In general, the non-specific anticonvulsants are highly lipid soluble and will bind to the neuronal membrane, impairing transportation of calcium ions and decreasing membrane permeability to sodium ions, thereby raising the threshold to depolarization and preventing repetitive discharge. For some unexplained reason anti-epileptics do appear to retain some selectivity for an epileptic focus in the drug concentrations used, and are not generally depressant on normal impulse conduction.

Many anticonvulsant drugs have been explored in detail with respect to interactions with cerebral neurotransmitter systems implicated in epilepsy; in particular the inhibitory transmitters GABA, glycine and 5-hydroxytryptamine (5-HT). *Clonazepam* and *sodium valproate*, for example, have been shown to increase central 5-HT action, an effect that may be related to their anticonvulsant properties. The *benzodiazepines* are known to enhance GABA-receptor binding and this may be the mechanism of their anti-epileptic action (Chapter 21). Finally, a newly-introduced anticonvulsant *vigabatrin* is a potent GABA-transaminase (GABA-T) inhibitor which greatly increases brain GABA concentrations. It is proposed that its clinical effectiveness is manifest through this pathway (as indeed may be partly true for sodium valproate which also displays some weak antagonism of GABA-T).

Table 23.1 lists some of the more commonly used anticonvulsant drugs. It is recognized that different agents are more suitable for treating various types of epilepsy and this differentiation is indicated, together with the relative dosages, half-lives and proposed therapeutic serum concentrations. The chemical structures of representative drugs are shown in Fig. 23.2.

TABLE 23.1 Anticonvulsant drugs in clinical practice

DRUG	INDICATION	NORMAL DOSAGE	HALF-LIFE
Phenytoin	All seizure types *Grand mal* Partial focal Status (iv) (not *petit mal*)	200–400 mg single dose max 600 mg	20–100 h
Carbamazepine	All seizure types *Grand mal* Partial focal (not *petit mal*)	400–1200 mg given in 2–3 daily doses max 1600 mg	10 h
Phenobarbitone	*Grand mal* Temporal lobe Status (iv) (not *petit mal*)	60–180 mg single dose	100 h
Primidone	All seizure types *Grand mal* Partial focal (not *petit mal*)	125–250 mg single dose max 1.5 g	10 h
Sodium valproate	All seizure types including *petit mal* and myoclonic epilepsy Status (iv)	400–1000 mg given in 2–3 daily doses max 2.5 g	7–10 h
Clobazam	Adjunct to control of *grand mal*, partial focal and myoclonic epilepsy	20–30 mg single dose max 60 mg	30 h
Vigabatrin	All seizure types (those not well controlled with other medication)	1–2 g in single or two doses max 2.5 g	5–7 h
Lamotrigine	Adjunct therapy to control partial and generalized seizures	200–400 mg in two doses	29 h
Gabapentin	Adjunct therapy to control partial and generalized seizures	900–1200 mg in three doses	5–6 h

THERAPEUTIC SERUM LEVELS	MAJOR SIDE-EFFECTS	ADDITIONAL NOTES
40–80 µmol/l Useful to monitor	Cerebellar syndrome Hirsutism Gum hypertrophy Unsteadiness, rash Drowsiness Blood dyscrasias	Avoid in adolescent females and pregnancy Can be helpful in trigeminal neuralgia
20–50 µmol/l Related to last drug dose time	Sedation Unsteadiness Skin rash Blood dyscrasias Hyponatraemia	Probably drug of choice in pregnancy Helpful in trigeminal neuralgia and relief of chronic pain
60–180 µmol/l Useful to monitor to avoid drug toxicity	Excessive drowsiness Ataxia Behavioural change Nausea Blood dyscrasias Skin rashes	Best avoided nowadays unless epilepsy entirely refractory to other anticonvulsants
Monitor metabolites (phenobarbitone)	As for phenobarbitone	—
250–700 µmol/l related to last drug dose time	Sedation, hair loss Increased appetite + weight gain Behavioural change Blood dyscrasias Acute hepatitis Hyperammonaemia	Monitor liver function
Not applicable	Sedation Incoordination Hypotonia Paradoxical excitement	?Possibility of physiological and psychological dependence
Not helpful	Drowsiness Irritability Weight gain	—
Not routinely available	Diplopia Drowsiness Skin rashes	Halve dose in conjunction with sodium valproate
Not routinely available	Dizziness Nystagmus	—

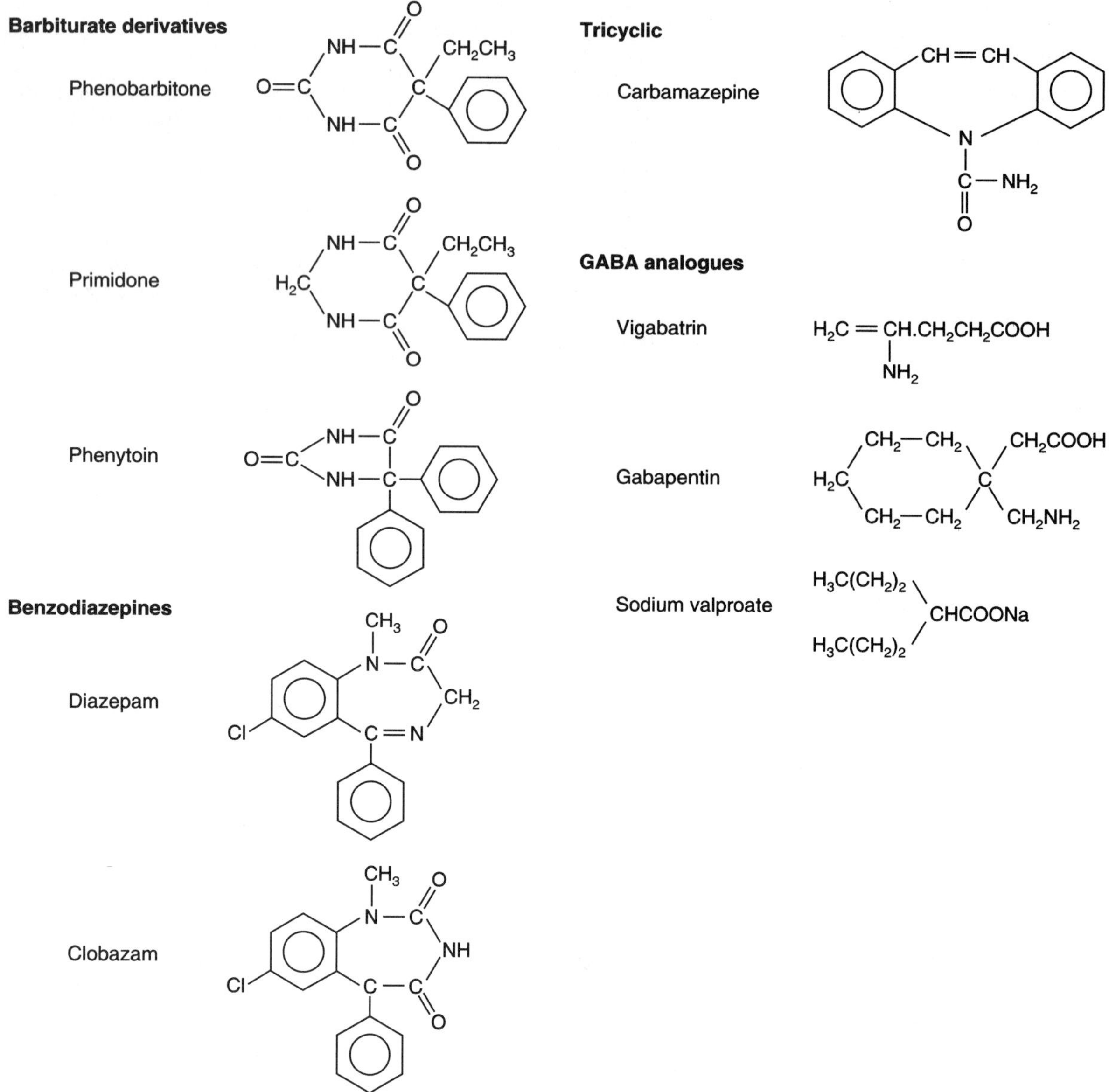

FIGURE 23.2 Structures of some anticonvulsant drugs

Serum monitoring of anticonvulsant levels

There are several reasons why the monitoring of serum levels of certain anticonvulsant drugs (most notably *phenytoin*, *carbamazepine* and *phenobarbitone*) is useful.[3] Phenytoin, for example, has a low therapeutic index, meaning that serum therapeutic and toxic levels lie close together. Drugs with long half-lives (e.g. phenytoin, phenobarbitone) usually give steady-state plasma concentrations which make for more reliable evaluation of therapeutic serum levels; other anticonvulsant drugs with shorter half-lives (e.g. carbamazepine, valproate) show greater variations in serum concentrations, more closely related to time of administration of the drug (if by oral route), and so monitoring of plasma drug levels and relation to therapeutic ranges is less reliable.

If seizures are not being adequately controlled, it is important to determine whether the drug serum levels are within the recognized therapeutic range. Toxic levels may also increase the frequency of fits or produce side-effects not obviously recognizable. Drug compliance is a problem not infrequently encountered among chronic epileptics and may often be confirmed if drug levels are very low or unrecordable. Another important point is that drug interactions with anticonvulsants occur not uncommonly, altering the rates of metabolism of these agents and thereby causing changes in circulating levels. Pregnancy can accelerate drug metabolism and therefore regular serum monitoring of anticonvulsant drugs is recommended if fits are to be avoided, and teratogenic risks reduced.

Anticonvulsant drugs in pregnancy

Because of the association of teratogenicity with the use of anticonvulsant drugs, the ideal situation is that anti-epileptics are best avoided in pregnancy and in women wishing to become pregnant. However, it is most often necessary that epileptic women continue anticonvulsant therapy throughout pregnancy. There is no single drug that is advised for this condition although *carbamazepine* is probably considered to be one of the safest, but of course not entirely without risk. The remote possibility of birth defects should be explained to women and their partners. The most hazardous time for teratogenicity is in the first trimester when major organs and tissues are being developed. Owing to enhanced metabolism and changes in plasma albumin levels, serum concentrations of anticonvulsant compounds are often lowered in pregnancy and so the routine monitoring may well suggest that dosages are regularly increased.

General side-effects of the anticonvulsant drugs

Unfortunately, all compounds that depress CNS function have the potential to induce unwanted side-effects, especially drowsiness and loss of concentration. Very broadly, the side-effects due to anticonvulsant drugs can be divided into three groups:

- *acute idiosyncratic reactions* – such as skin rashes, hirsutism, coarsening of facial features, drug-induced hepatitis, systemic lupus erythematosis (SLE)
- *reversible toxic effects* – (dose related) cerebellar syndrome with nystagmus, ataxia, dysarthria, tremor, drowsiness
- *chronic toxic effects* (not dose related) – e.g. bone marrow suppression, lymphadenopathy.

Many of the anticonvulsant drugs, administered for chronic therapy, can cause a mild folate deficiency that can occasionally (rarely) present as a macrocytic anaemia. Folate supplements are required. Vitamin D metabolism is also enhanced in patients taking anti-epileptic medication, by a mechanism of hepatic enzyme induction. Again vitamin D supplements may be required; symptoms of rickets and osteomalacia are very rare unless other deficiencies or malabsorption are precipitating their cause.

Phenytoin

Phenytoin is often considered as the drug of first choice for *grand mal* epilepsy and *partial* (*focal*) seizures. It does not, however, prevent simple absence attacks (*petit mal*).

Pharmacokinetics of phenytoin

The drug is highly lipid soluble and easily penetrates the blood–brain barrier.[4] It has fair oral absorption and a long half-life, although no single $t_{\frac{1}{2}}$ is stated because of zero-order kinetics but the range of 20–100 h is often quoted. It is therefore usually given as a single daily (nightly) dose. Phenytoin is highly protein bound in plasma (90% bound to albumin) and therefore serum levels are markedly lowered in hypoalbuminaemic states. The drug is extensively metabolized in the liver to the primary metabolite 5-(4-hydroxyphenyl)-5-phenyl-hydantoin, which is inactive. Phenytoin undergoes enterohepatic recirculation and is excreted in the urine, mainly as its hydroxylated product, in either free or conjugated form. It freely crosses the placental barrier and small amounts are excreted in breast milk, and so it should be used with caution in pregnancy. Absorption following intramuscular injection is much slower than by the oral route. Serum phenytoin levels can usefully be monitored.

Side-effects of phenytoin

In high (toxic) doses phenytoin can cause CNS-induced effects such as sedation and involuntary movements. It can also cause cerebellar dysfunction, manifest as cerebellar syndrome characterized by nystagmus, dysarthria, ataxia and an intention tremor. These symptoms are usually easily reversed by reducing drug dosage and thereby lowering serum levels into the therapeutic range.

Idiosyncratic reactions with phenytoin can occur not infrequently – skin rashes, pyrexias, acne and drug-induced hepatitis have been reported. Phenytoin can cause skin collagen changes resulting in exfoliative dermatitis, erythema multiforme, coarsening of facial features and gingival hypertrophy, and these factors, together with hirsutism, often make this drug undesirable for use initially in young females. Phenytoin can also induce an SLE-like syndrome.

Haematological problems reported with phenytoin include lymphadenopathy and folate-deficient megaloblastic anaemia, leucopenia, thrombocytopenia, agranulocytosis by a direct action on bone marrow, and very rarely aplastic anaemia. Endocrinologically the drug has been said to induce diabetes insipidus by inhibiting ADH (vasopressin) release, and to aggrevate pre-existing diabetes mellitus.

In keeping with other anticonvulsant drugs, phenytoin can be teratogenic, being associated with harelip and palate, congenital heart disease and microcephaly.

Drug interactions with phenytoin

Being a hepatic enzyme inducer, phenytoin enhances the metabolism (and thereby will reduce the clinical effectiveness) of a number of drugs including anti-infectives (chloramphenicol, griseofulvin), anticoagulants (dicoumarol, although action of warfarin is generally enhanced), anticonvulsants (primidone, phenobarbitone, carbamazepine, sodium valproate) and, very importantly, the oral contraceptive pill (especially the low-oestrogen formulations).

Conversely, it should be remembered that the metabolism of phenytoin itself is often changed by the co-administration of other drugs, in particular other anticonvulsants or hepatic enzyme inducers, and so therefore regular monitoring of serum drug levels is advised.

Carbamazepine

Although structurally related to the tricyclic antidepressants, carbamazepine is also considered as the drug of choice for *grand mal* and *temporal lobe* epilepsy.[5] It also finds clinical use for the control of neuralgic and phantom limb pain (believed to act on the pain control gating mechanisms at the level of the thalamus) and additionally in the control of diabetes insipidus.

Pharmacokinetics of carbamazepine

Carbamazepine is slowly but fairly completely absorbed from the gastrointestinal tract. The drug is 75% protein bound in plasma. It is extensively metabolized in the liver; one of its primary metabolites is carbamazepine-10,11-epoxide which possesses some anticonvulsant activity. As it is an inducer of hepatic microsomal enzymes, it will thereby induce acceleration of its own metabolism. Products are excreted in the urine. The half-life for carbamazepine is in the order of 10–20 h, being much shorter than those of phenytoin or the barbiturates, necessitating a twice-daily dosage regime although a modified release preparation is now available allowing once-daily dosing. Like other anticonvulsants, carbamazepine crosses the placental barrier and is excreted in breast milk.

Side-effects of carbamazepine

Side-effects with carbamazepine are common but not usually severe. Urticarial skin rashes (and occasionally erythema multiforme), sedation and gastrointestinal upsets are not infrequently reported. Ataxia, slurred speech, diplopia and nystagmus (i.e. cerebellar syndrome) are usually related to toxic drug effects. Rarely, a transient leucopenia and thrombocytopenia can occur, and the drug may cause water retention and hyponatraemia. Very rarely, carbamazepine-induced SLE is reported or the Stevens–Johnson syndrome may be provoked. Carbamazepine is believed to be the least likely anticonvulsant drug to cause teratogenic effects in man, and therefore is probably considered to be the safest agent for use in pregnancy if necessitated.

Drug interactions with carbamazepine

Carbamazepine tends to lower the serum concentrations of other drugs dealt with by hepatic metabolism, for example phenytoin, phenobarbitone, warfarin and oestrogens. Conversely, the metabolism of carbamazepine is inhibited by the antibiotics erythromycin and isoniazid, and by the analgesics dextropropoxyphene; carbamazepine levels may consequently rise to toxic values.

Phenobarbitone

The barbiturates were one of the first series of anticonvulsant drugs introduced into clinical practice. Despite newer superior compounds and many potential toxic effects, phenobarbitone is still quite widely used, and a number of elderly patients will have been taking the drug for decades. Its major use is in the control of *grand mal* epilepsy and in *status epilepticus* where first-line agents have failed. Barbiturates are highly lipid soluble, well absorbed from the gut, and approximately 50% bound to plasma proteins. They have long half-lives (up to 100 h) and therefore these drugs require to be given only once a day. Phenobarbitone is a potent hepatic enzyme inducer and its metabolism is mainly in the liver, where 50–75% of the drug is parahydroxylated, 10–40% is excreted unchanged at the kidney.

Side-effects of phenobarbitone

Phenobarbitone, in toxic doses, causes sedation, mental retardation and depression, and signs of cerebellar syndrome described above. The drug can evoke hyperkinesis in children, and rebound convulsions are documented on *rapid* withdrawal of barbiturates. Phenobarbitone can cause skin rashes, including exfoliative dermatitis, and haematological problems secondary to bone marrow suppression as has been observed with other anticonvulsant drugs.

Drug interactions with phenobarbitone

Phenobarbitone strongly induces hepatic enzymes and, as with phenytoin, will enhance the metabolism of a number of drugs including carbamazepine, phenytoin, warfarin, chloramphenicol and oestrogen in the contraceptive pill.

Primidone

Primidone is an anticonvulsant effective for *grand mal* and *partial* epilepsy. It is metabolized to phenobarbitone and phenylethylmalonamide – both of which possess anticonvulsant properties. Although the half-life of primidone is short (10 h), that of the active metabolites is long and so the drug can be given by once-daily dosage. The side-effects and drug interactions are as those documented for phenobarbitone.

Sodium valproate

Sodium dipropylacetate (valproate) was first licensed in the UK in 1974. It is recommended for many forms of epilepsy including *grand mal* and *petit mal*, myoclonic epilepsy and psychomotor epilepsy.[6]

Pharmacokinetics of sodium valproate

Sodium valproate shows a good oral absorption profile, and it is largely (90%) protein bound in the plasma. Its lipophilicity is in fact low, and together with a short half-life (7–10 h), means that comparatively large amounts of the drug have to be given daily in divided doses. Sodium valproate is extensively metabolized in the liver; it is excreted in the urine almost entirely in the form of its metabolites. A slow-release formulation is now available allowing once-daily dosing.

Side-effects of sodium valproate

Side-effects with sodium valproate can be common but not usually serious. Abdominal upsets such as pain, nausea, diarrhoea and vomiting can occur. Weight increase caused by an enhanced appetite and oedema may exacerbate pre-existing obesity. Temporary alopecia is occasionally reported, with the regrowth of characteristically curly hair on drug withdrawal. Rarely a hepatitis, pancreatitis and thrombocytopenia are seen, although it is suggested that liver function tests are initially monitored when a patient is commenced on valproate. There has been some concern regarding possible teratogenic effects of sodium valproate, the drug having been linked with spina bifida, but this connection is not entirely proven.

Clonazepam and clobazam

These benzodiazepines are often considered as second-line or adjunct therapy with wide ranging anticonvulsant activity against *grand mal* and *petit mal* seizures and *temporal lobe* epilepsy. Clonazepam is additionally recommended for myoclonic epilepsy. These benzodiazepines are well absorbed orally, the drugs being metabolized in the liver, clobazam to its active metabolite N-desmethylclobazam (see also Chapter 21).

Side-effects of clonazepam and clobazam

In keeping with the benzodiazepine group of drugs, clonazepam and clobazam frequently induce lethargy, somnolence and dizziness. Muscular incoordination and giddiness may be noticed and the drug prescriptions carry warnings about driving and working with machinery. The other side-effects, including possible psychological and physiological dependence, are considered in Chapter 21. Regarding this point of dependence, some neurologists are cautious in the use of regular benzodiazepines as anticonvulsant drugs. However, in part to avoid this problem, clobazam has found place for the control of intermittent seizure symptoms, such as in catamenial epilepsy in females, or in the management of cluster fits.

Ethosuximide

Ethosuximide has been described as the drug of choice for *petit mal* epilepsy. It has good oral absorption, with a long half-life (70 h) requiring once-daily dosage. It is mainly degraded in the liver to inactive metabolites; these metabolites and some unchanged ethosuximide (20%) are excreted in the urine. The drug will cross the placental barrier and is excreted in breast milk.

Side-effects of ethosuximide

These are few, but include skin rashes, gastrointestinal disturbances and dizziness. Rarely haematological complications and lupus-like reactions are encountered.

Acetazolamide

This drug is a carbonic anhydrase inhibitor which by way of its biochemical action raises the cerebral P_{CO_2} and lowers brain pH. This, together with the associated local rise in chloride ions, is believed to have a membrane-stabilizing effect. Acetazolamide is reported as being useful in catamenial epilepsy.

Acetazolamide is fairly rapidly absorbed from the gastrointestinal tract, reaching peak plasma concentrations at 2 h after oral administration. It binds tightly to carbonic anhydrase, particularly in erythrocytes and in renal cortex. In serum it is bound to plasma proteins, and is excreted unchanged in the urine. Its half-life is estimated at 3–6 h.

Side-effects of acetazolamide

In high doses acetazolamide can cause drowsiness and anorexia, and by its action on carbonic anhydrase in the renal tubules it reduces salt and water retention and causes an alkaline diuresis (with loss of Na^+, K^+ and HCO_3^- in the urine) which may provoke a metabolic acidosis. Hypersensitivity reactions can occur, and blood dyscrasias are rarely reported to include aplastic anaemia, agranulocytosis, leucopenia, thrombocytopenia and thrombocytopenic purpura.

Vigabatrin

This is one of the newer anticonvulsant drugs introduced in the UK in 1989. Its chemical structure is γ-vinyl-γ-aminobutyric acid (γ-vinyl GABA) (see Fig. 23.2), a stable analogue of GABA which specifically and non-competitively inhibits GABA transaminase, the enzyme that metabolizes cerebral GABA. It is thereby assumed that this drug's anticonvulsant activity is directly related to this enzyme inhibition with subsequent enhancement of brain GABA concentrations. Indeed, animal studies readily demonstrate that γ-vinyl GABA greatly increases brain GABA levels.[7,8]

In man, vigabatrin is well absorbed following oral administration, with a bioavailability of 60–80%, and peak plasma concentrations being achieved in 1–2 h. It is not protein bound in serum: it has a half-life in serum of 5–7 h, although its enzyme inhibiting activity is considerably longer. Most of the drug (80%) is excreted unchanged by the kidney. As it is an irreversible enzyme inhibitor, monitoring of serum drug levels is unhelpful. Vigabatrin is recommended for the control of all types of epilepsy, and is especially employed in patients not previously satisfactorily controlled by other anticonvulsant medications.[9]

Side-effects of vigabatrin

The side-effects of vigabatrin are in line with those of other anticonvulsant drugs – drowsiness, fatigue and dizziness. Weight gain is occasionally reported; as also irritability, headache, confusion and mood changes in early trials. Possible interactions with other drugs have not yet been fully evaluated.

Lamotrigine

Lamotrigine is now newly licensed as adjunctive therapy for the management of *partial* seizures and *generalized tonic–clonic* convulsions not satisfactorily controlled with other anti-epileptic drugs. Pharmacologically, lamotrigine acts by blocking the excessive release of excitatory amino acids from presynaptic nerve terminals in the brain, especially glutamate, and this is how it is believed to exert its anticonvulsant effect.[10]

Pharmacokinetics of lamotrigine

After oral administration lamotrigine is completely and rapidly absorbed with negligible first-pass effect. Time to peak plasma concentrations is 2–3 h; the half-life of elimination from the bloodstream in otherwise healthy individuals is approximately 29 h. However, the presence of other anticonvulsant drugs (with which it is always used) will accelerate lamotrigine metabolism (excepting valproate which slows it), which necessitates the drug to be taken twice daily. Metabolism by glucuronidation in the liver is slow but extensive; only a few per cent is excreted unchanged in the urine. Approximately 55% of lamotrigine is protein bound in plasma.

Side-effects of lamotrigine

Reported side-effects of lamotrigine include skin rashes, diplopia, blurred vision, drowsiness, headache, ataxia, gastrointestinal upset and irritability. However, remember that it is most often administered in combination with other anti-epileptic agents.

Gabapentin

Gabapentin is an analogue of the potent central inhibitory neurotransmitter GABA. Like lamotrigine, it is used as an add-on anticonvulsant for patients with poorly controlled epilepsy, particularly *partial* seizures alone and partial seizures with secondary generalization.[11]

Although structurally related to GABA, the precise pharmacological mechanism of action of gabapentin is unclear. It does not appear to alter brain GABA concentrations, affect GABA-transaminase activity, block neuronal or glial re-uptake mechanisms or bind to GABA receptors.

Pharmacokinetics of gabapentin

The drug is rapidly absorbed following oral administration, peak plasma levels occurring within 1–3 h. Gabapentin is not bound to plasma proteins and is eliminated solely by renal excretion. Its half-life is calculated at 5–6 h and therefore is required to be taken three times a day. There is no interaction between phenytoin, carbamazepine, sodium valproate or phenobarbitone.

Side-effects of gabapentin

The side-effects of gabapentin are those reported for other general anticonvulsant drugs (including somnolence, dizziness, ataxia, fatigue, nystagmus, diplopia and gastrointestinal upsets), but remember that, like lamotrigine, it is most often administered in combination with other anti-epileptic medications.

Management of status epilepticus

Status epilepticus – that is, continuous tonic–clonic seizures that follow each other without remission, is a life-threatening situation that should be brought under control in the shortest time possible to avoid irreversible cerebral damage, usually by use of systemically administered agents. Often *diazepam* (Valium, Diazemuls) is used to good effect to control status epilepticus – given intravenously in dosages of 5–10 mg over 2–5 min, repeated if necessary, or rectally in enema form (5–10 mg), especially in children. Benzodiazepines can also be given by intravenous infusion if a single bolus is insufficient to abort the episode and maintain a controlled state (e.g. infusions of diazepam or clonazepam).

Another successful treatment of status epilepticus is infusion of *phenytoin* (dosage 750–1500 mg; i.e. 10–15 mg/kg) over 20–30 min (rate 15 mg/min, not exceeding 50 mg/min). As cardiac arrhythmias can very occasionally be a problem, loading should ideally be done with continuous cardiac monitoring.

Other drugs used in the control of this medical emergency include paraldehyde, thiopentone and chlormethiazole, but due to high degrees of respiratory depression by the first two drugs, infusions should be conducted only when ICU facilities are available.

Sodium valproate has more recently been introduced in intravenous formulation in this country and its efficacy in controlling status epilepticus is being established. *Phenobarbitone*, given by the intravenous route, can be a very effective drug for stopping seizure activity where, for example, phenytoin has failed.

Anaesthetic agents and convulsant activity

Although it is generally accepted that anaesthetic agents will of course induce depression of cerebral neuronal activity, some drugs can in fact precipitate convulsions and should be used with extreme caution in the epileptic patient.

The inhaled agent *enflurane* normally, in keeping with its anaesthetic properties, produces depression of electroencephalic (EEG) activity, although higher doses can induce paroxysmal spike wave formation. Therefore it is best avoided in the epileptic patient. Its isomer *isoflurane*, however, is basically free of this action.

With *methohexitone*, epileptiform activity has been demonstrated on EEGs of epileptic patients. Similarly, *propofol*, while generally provoking CNS depression, has through several reports to the CSM (Committee on Safety of Medicines) been cited as inducing convulsions in epileptics and thereby it is recommended that extreme caution be exercised when this drug is used in this group of patients.

EXTRAPYRAMIDAL MOVEMENT DISORDERS

The basal ganglia are a collection of subcortical cell nuclei and interconnections which control motor activity. Changes in function are characteristically associated with disturbances of posture and movement.[12] Over the last three decades this area of the brain has been the subject of much intensive research, resulting in a better understanding of its neurophysiology, neurochemistry and neuropharmacology.[13,14] The central focus of the basal ganglia appears to be the corpus striatum (caudate nucleus and putamen), receiving inputs from the cerebral cortex and pars compacta of the substantia nigra, via the important dopaminergic nigrostriatal pathway. In turn the corpus striatum projects neurones to the globus pallidus and to pars reticulata of the substantia nigra, both sites seemingly to be major outlets of the basal ganglia. Human movement disorders are often associated with degeneration of neuronal pathways within the basal ganglia – an observation made from both post-mortem studies and animal models. In the early 1960s it was recognized that in Parkinson's disease there is a deficiency of striatal dopamine[15] and further work established that this disorder is associated with degeneration of the nigrostriatal pathway with subsequent loss of the pigmented (melanin-containing) cell bodies within substantia nigra, pars compacta.[16] Support for this hypothesis was soon found when the neurotoxin *6-hydroxydopamine*, which can selectively destroy dopaminergic fibres, when injected directly into the substantia nigra produced biochemical and behavioural models resembling Parkinson's disease in laboratory animals.[17] More recently in 1983 it was recognized that a drug of abuse, MPTP (1-methyl-4-phenyl-1,2,3,6-tetra-hydropyridine) could act as a probable human neurotoxin that would destroy dopamine cells of the substantia nigra in unfortunate drug addicts, and in so doing would produce neuropathological and neurochemical changes in the basal ganglia very similar to those seen in Parkinson's disease, and clinically a Parkinsonian-like syndrome.[18] Certainly animal models of Parkinson's disease can be developed by the administration of MPTP.[19] It is believed that the true neurotoxin is the oxidative metabolite of MPTP, MPP^+(1-methyl-4-phenyl-pyridinum) which is produced at the mitochondria containing monoamine oxidase subtype B (MAO_B). It is thereby further suggested that the selective monoamine oxidase inhibitor (MAOI) *selegiline* (see below) may have a protective effect by blocking the oxidation of MPTP. Current theories propose that idiopathic Parkinson's disease may be due to an environmental or endogenous toxin similar to MPTP, or to a deficiency in mitochondrial handling, possibly genetically determined, which increases the vulnerability of some patients to develop this neurological disorder.[20]

Almost the clinical reverse of Parkinson's disease is Huntington's chorea, an inherited disorder characterized by wild choreic movements and pathologically in which there is atrophy of the basal ganglia with loss of corpus striatum substance. In particular there is degeneration of GABA-containing interneurones from the caudate nucleus, putamen and globus pallidus.[21]

PARKINSON'S DISEASE

The triad of symptoms commonly characteristic of the akinetic-rigid syndrome are limb tremor – usually more prominent at rest and disappearing when the limb is put to use or during sleep; limb rigidity – said to be cogwheeling in nature; and a bradykinesia – producing difficulty for the initiation and control of movement.[22] Normally no apparent aetiology is recognized – that is, *idiopathic Parkinson's disease*, although a postencephalitic cohort is well documented following the epidemic of encephalitis lethargica in the 1920s. As detailed above, idiopathic Parkinson's disease is associated with degeneration of neurones of the nigrostriatal tract and subsequent depletion of neurotransmitter dopamine from the corpus striatum. Drugs that either deplete the brain of dopamine (e.g. reserpine) or block cerebral dopamine receptors (e.g. antipsychotic drugs, the phenothiazines or butyrophenones – see Chapter 22) can cause symptoms of Parkinson's disease (drug-induced Parkinsonism).

Principles and management of Parkinson's disease

Prior to the discovery of the close association between brain dopamine concentrations and neurological symptoms, anticholinergic drugs were the mainstay for the management of this difficult condition. Indeed, and perhaps rather too simplistically, a reciprocal balance between dopamine and ACh is described, whereby reduction in dopamine function (from degenerating nigrostriatal neurones) results in a secondary overactivity of ACh systems and vice versa.[23] Hence quelling this now enhanced cholinergic function with anticholinergic drugs will effectively restore the pharmacological balance and reverse the symptoms of this extrapyramidal disease.

However, it is the connection between loss of basal gangliar dopamine and the symptoms of Parkinson's disease that has revolutionized the treatment of this disorder. For the last 25 years attention has thereby been focused on methods to 'replete' lost dopamine stores and in so doing to functionally restore dopaminergic mechanisms within the nigrostriatal system.[24,25] To achieve this either the synthetic precursor of dopamine, *levodopa* (L-DOPA; 3,4-dihydroxyphenylalanine), is administered, or directly-acting *dopamine receptor agonists* such as *bromocriptine*, or more recently *lysuride*, *pergolide* or *apomorphine* can be given.[26] Dopamine itself is not very lipid soluble and therefore will not cross the blood–brain barrier; it is also very rapidly metabolized by the enzyme MAO in the gut and liver.

More specifically in the brain, dopamine either found naturally or that newly synthesized from exogenous L-DOPA, is broken down by the isoenzyme of MAO, subtype B (MAO_B). A drug that selectively inhibits MAO_B is *selegiline*, which also has some benefit in the therapy of Parkinson's disease.[27] *Amantadine*[28] is another agent that can be helpful for a few patients with this condition.

The last few years have seen another milestone in the management of Parkinson's disease. Current work is in hand to establish the possible benefits of implantation of adrenal gland grafts or human fetal nigral cells into the head of the caudate nucleus in patients with Parkinson's disease, or indeed of other neurosurgical procedures.[29] Initial claims of great success do not unfortunately appear to have been substantiated in larger patient groups; it is still too early to reliably comment on trials of fetal cell implantation but the issue remains very controversial.

Levodopa (L-DOPA)

L-DOPA was first introduced into the management of Parkinson's disease in the early 1960s with initially very encouraging effects, backed by claims that previously chair- or bed-bound patients could now walk. L-DOPA is the direct precursor of dopamine, the conversion aided by a rather non-specific enzyme L-aromatic amino acid decarboxylase (L-DOPA decarboxylase) which is present in virtually all tissues in the body, but importantly in brain glial cells. The pathway is depicted in Figure 23.3.

Unfortunately the early use of levodopa was thwarted by several problems. To have a good therapeutic effect, the drug had to be administered in high concentrations, several grams a day. At these doses there were often disabling side-effects such as involuntary movements and severe nausea which often limited its use.

Mechanism of action

Levodopa can cross the blood–brain barrier, enter the brain and be decarboxylated into dopamine by DOPA decarboxylase.[30] The newly synthesized dopamine

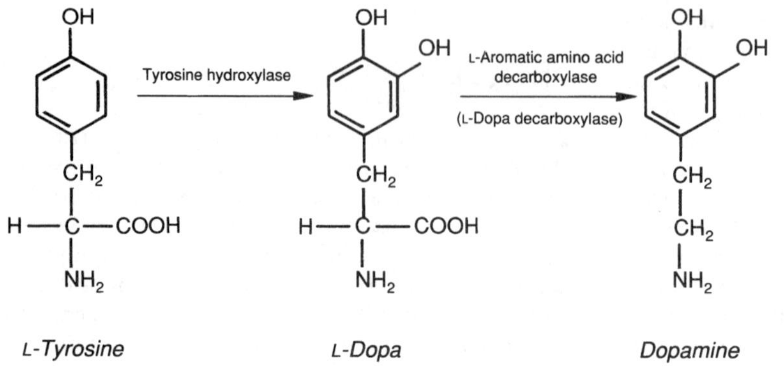

OH
Tyrosine hydroxylase
OH
OH
L-Aromatic amino acid decarboxylase
(L-Dopa decarboxylase)
OH
OH
CH2
H—C—COOH
NH2
CH2
H—C—COOH
NH2
CH2
CH2
NH2
L-Tyrosine
L-Dopa
Dopamine

FIGURE 23.3 The synthesis of dopamine.

helps to functionally restore brain concentrations of this neurotransmitter lost by degeneration of the nigrostriatal pathway in Parkinson's disease. It is believed that much of the conversion of L-DOPA into dopamine occurs within glial cells, and other non-neuronal tissues (e.g. endothelium of blood vessels), as many of the dopaminergic terminals would be non-functional in this condition. While some newly formed dopamine can be stored within remaining functional neuronal terminals, that which is synthesized within glial cells cannot as no form of storage mechanism exists at such sites. This dopamine will presumably diffuse out on to the synapse and have an action at the postsynaptic dopamine receptor (both D_1 and D_2 sites – see Chapter 22), hopefully thereby reversing some of the symptoms of Parkinson's disease.

Peripheral decarboxylase inhibitors

When given by mouth, only a small fraction of the oral dosage of L-DOPA will reach the brain. DOPA decarboxylase is found in many tissues (e.g. liver, kidneys, gut, lungs), and this means that much of the drug (90%) will be converted in the periphery before reaching the cerebral circulation, hence the initial high doses of L-DOPA required before a therapeutic effect is seen. In order to reduce peripheral decarboxylation, L-DOPA is today combined with a second drug – an inhibitor of peripheral decarboxylase. In the late 1960s two peripheral decarboxylase inhibitors were developed – *carbidopa* (1-α-methyldopa hydrazine) and *benserazide* (1-DL-seryl-2-(2,3,4-dihydroxybenzyl)-hydrazine). Neither drug crosses the blood–brain barrier and therefore is not active centrally.

These drug combinations are the current drug treatment of choice for patients with Parkinson's disease, particularly where bradykinesia is the prominent symptom. Carbidopa is combined with L-DOPA as the preparation *Co-careldopa* (Sinemet tablets) in a ratio of L-DOPA to decarboxylase inhibitor of either 4 to 1 or 10 to 1. Benserazide is formulated with L-DOPA in a ratio of 1 to 4 in *Co-beneldopa* (Madopar preparations). These combinations have allowed a marked lowering of the total dosage of L-DOPA, and therefore have effectively reduced the incidence of side-effects. An added advantage of Sinemet and Madopar is that in general the time to therapeutic effect after oral dosage is sooner (particularly with the soluble Madopar formulation) and that a clinically smoother response is usually obtained. A further recent development in this field is the introduction of 'controlled release' preparations in order to try and achieve more steady plasma levels of L-DOPA.

Side-effects of L-DOPA therapy

Nausea and vomiting

A problem not uncommonly encountered, particularly in the early stages of development of L-DOPA, is that of nausea and vomiting, principally caused by direct action of the dopamine agonist (L-DOPA) on the chemoreceptor trigger zone in the medullary area postrema which remains outside the blood–brain barrier. The incidence of this side-effect has been lessened since the introduction of the L-DOPA/decarboxylase inhibitor combinations. If particularly troublesome, the symptoms can often be controlled with the simultaneous administration of *domperidone*, a peripheral dopaminergic D_2 receptor blocker which itself does not interfere with the anti-Parkinsonian action of L-DOPA.

On–off phenomenon

The variability and unpredictability in response to L-DOPA preparations can be a major problem for some patients. It is suggested that 5 years after starting this drug, 50% of patients will experience fluctuations in response. Most report rapid swings from adequate mobility (with or without dyskinetic movements) to immobility or freezing – the so-called on–off phenomenon. This does not appear related to plasma L-DOPA levels but may represent changes in receptor sensitivity. The development of the controlled, sustained release formulation is an attempt to produce a less variable plasma drug concentration with the hope that it may stabilize receptor sensitivity and smooth out the variance in response.

L-DOPA dyskinesias

Abnormal involuntary movements not infrequently occur with usage of L-DOPA preparations. Most appear at peak action of the drug: others are not dose related. Dyskinesias observed include limb and trunk choreic or dystonic movements, orofacial dyskinesias, and myoclonus. They are usually, but not always, associated with overstimulation of cerebral dopamine receptors, and usually (but not always) subside when the effects of the L-DOPA wear off.

Psychiatric disturbances

Excessive stimulation by L-DOPA can, especially if there is a previous history of mental disorder, provoke psychiatric disturbances and confusion. This is more commonly seen in the elderly. Hallucinations and delusions are reported, occasionally frank psychosis. Mania and heightened sexual drive have also been described, even drug-induced depression.

Cardiovascular reactions

Postural hypotension can be a common complaint, again particularly in the elderly. The mechanism is believed to be mediated through noradrenergic function at the brain stem vasomotor systems. Cardiac arrhythmias have, uncommonly, been reported.

Autonomic dysfunction

L-DOPA therapy can result in excessive sweating and pupillary dilatation, again presumably mediated through noradrenergic mechanisms and the sympathetic nervous system.

Specific drug interactions with L-DOPA

Pyridoxine

Pyridoxine, a vitamin B_6 derivative, acts as a cofactor for DOPA decarboxylase. This agent will enhance the enzymatic destruction of L-DOPA and thereby greatly reduce effective circulating L-DOPA concentrations.

Antipsychotic drugs

These agents are dopamine receptor antagonists, acting at both D_1 and D_2 sites, and will therefore block the action of administered L-DOPA. Indeed the phenothiazines and butyrophenones are the most common cause of drug-induced Parkinsonism.

MAOIs

The antidepressant MAOIs (see Chapter 22) may produce a hypertensive reaction if given concurrently with L-DOPA due to stimulation of noradrenaline mechanisms in the sympathetic system.

Dopamine Receptor Agonists

Dopamine receptors occur in high density within the putamen and caudate nucleus – that is, the terminal projection of the nigrostriatal pathway. They also occur in mesolimbic forebrain regions (discussed in Chapter 22) as well as in the median eminence of the hypothalamus where dopamine is believed to function as the prolactin inhibitory factor controlling prolactin release (see Chapter 30). The direct activation of D_1 and D_2 receptors within the basal ganglia would be expected to have a similar net action as stimulation of the nigrostriatal system, thereby relieving the symptoms of Parkinson's disease related to degeneration of this neuronal tract. Several synthetic compounds are known to act as directly acting dopamine agonists and some of these have found use in the management of Parkinson's disease. These drugs include *bromocriptine*, *lysuride*, *pergolide* and *apomorphine* (see Fig. 23.4).[31]

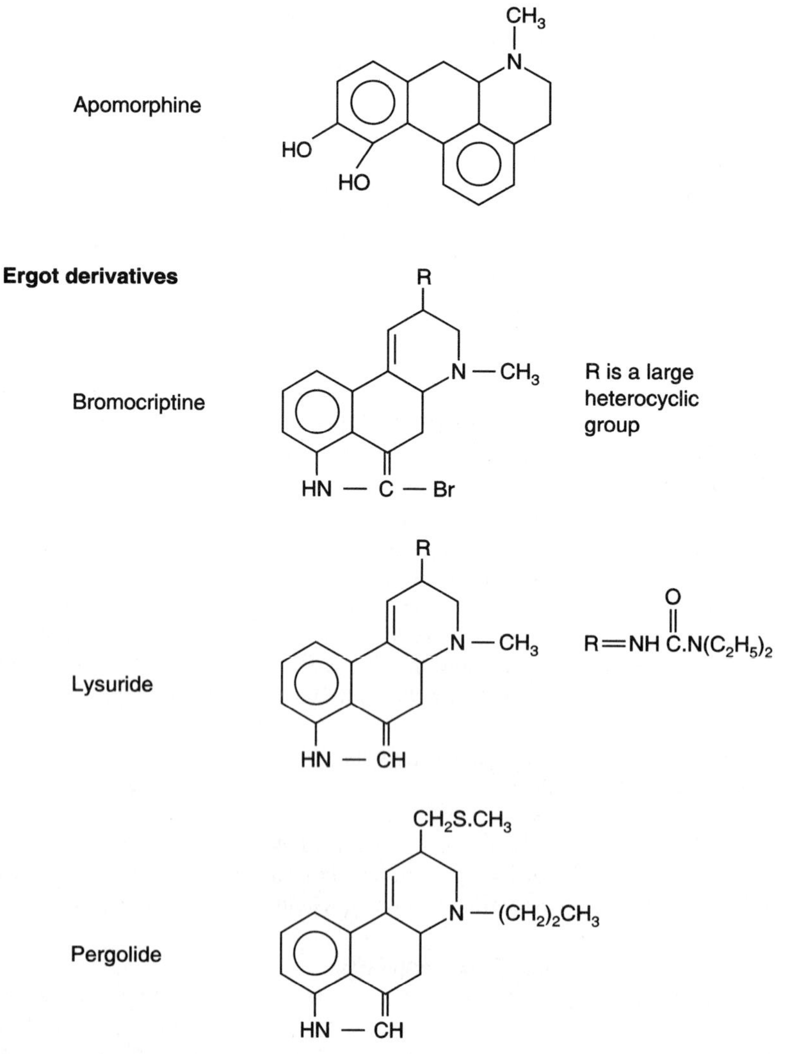

Apomorphine

CH_3 N HO HO

Ergot derivatives

Bromocriptine

R N — CH_3 HN — C — Br

R is a large heterocyclic group

Lysuride

R N — CH_3 HN — CH

R=NH C(=O).N$(C_2H_5)_2$

Pergolide

$CH_2S.CH_3$ N — $(CH_2)_2CH_3$ HN — CH

FIGURE 23.4 Structures of some dopamine agonists.

Bromocriptine

Bromocriptine is a semisynthetic ergot derivative with good absorption from oral dosing. It is extensively metabolized in the liver, showing a very high degree of first-pass metabolism so that only a small proportion of the administered drug is available for cerebral activity. It is mainly excreted in the bile, with some enterohepatic recirculation. It has a half-life in the range of 6–8 h and therefore needs at least twice or three times daily dosages.

Mechanism of action

Bromocriptine shows a preference for D_2 (non-adenylate cyclase linked) dopamine receptors found in the corpus striatum, located in healthy tissue both pre- and postsynaptically. Bromocriptine also binds to D_2 receptors located at other brain sites such as mesolimbic areas, the hypothalamus and pituitary, but it is at sites within the basal ganglia that the drug presumably exerts its anti-Parkinsonian effects. Actions at the pituitary and hypothalamic level are related to its neuroendocrine properties (see Chapter 30). The drug is occasionally of benefit to Parkinsonian patients refractory to L-DOPA treatment.[32]

Side-effects of bromocriptine

This drug can cause gastrointestinal upsets such as dry mouth, metallic taste, nausea and vomiting, and constipation. As with L-DOPA, postural hypotension can be pronounced. In keeping with its central dopamine receptor agonist action, bromocriptine can provoke dyskinesias and psychiatric disorders including visual and auditory hallucinations and confusion. On the cardiovascular side cardiac arrhythmias and peripheral vasospasm have been reported. Cutaneous livedo reticularis may occur.

Lysuride and pergolide

The synthetic ergot derivatives, lysuride[33] and pergolide[34] which stimulate central dopamine receptors, predominantly D_2 sites, have recently been introduced in the management of Parkinson's disease. It is hoped that such drugs will reduce the degree of on–off fluctuations associated with L-DOPA therapy. It is suggested that in this neurological disorder the simultaneous stimulation of both D_1 and D_2 receptor sites is required. Thus treatment with preferentially D_2 agonists such as lysuride, pergolide and bromocriptine may also need a small priming dose of L-DOPA, but that the presence of the D_2 agonist would allow for a reduction in L-DOPA dosage.

Apomorphine

Although apomorphine was initially widely used in animal models of Parkinson's disease, it was formerly avoided in man due to its short duration of action and its potent emetic properties by direct effect on the chemoreceptor trigger zone (vomiting centre) in the brainstem medulla. Pharmacologically, apomorphine stimulates both D_1 and D_2 receptor subtypes, and the compound is currently being re-evaluated for use in the management of Parkinson's disease.[35] Owing to its poor oral absorption, it must be given systemically, usually by subcutaneous injection either in repeated boluses or by continuous infusion from a motor-driven syringe pump. Patients usually need, at least initially, concurrent administration of domperidone to reduce the incidence of nausea. Other side-effects associated with apomorphine use include orthostatic hypotension and bradycardia, pallor, sweating, weakness, lacrimation and salivation. The full value of apomorphine in this disorder has still to be fully established.

Monoamine oxidase B inhibitor: selegiline

Selegiline is an amphetamine derivative (see Fig. 22.5) that blocks the enzyme MAO.[27] It is absorbed from the gastrointestinal tract, metabolized in the body to methylamphetamine and *l*-amphetamine (which also possess weak MAO blocking actions) and these are then excreted in the urine.

Mode of action

Selegiline is an irreversible inhibitor of MAO_B, whose endogenous substrate is mainly dopamine. Animal and post-mortem studies confirm approximately 80–90% inhibition of cerebral MAO_B, following drug administration. Selegiline also, to some degree, blocks the re-uptake of dopamine into presynaptic nerve terminals. Both of these pharmacological actions result in an increase in concentration of dopamine in the synaptic cleft, and thereby presumably enhances transmitter–receptor interaction.

Therapeutic value of MAO_B inhibitors

Selegiline was introduced as an adjunct to L-DOPA therapy, with the hope that it would smooth out the unpredictable fluctuations in L-DOPA response, thereby to minimize the on–off effect by reducing the 'off' time and improving the end-of-dose deterioration. It was also suggested that it could allow for a small reduction in dosage of L-DOPA (or the combination medications).

From the results of some experimental work it is claimed that selegiline may slow the natural progression of Parkinson's disease.[36] In animal studies, pretreatment with selegiline inhibits the neurotoxic action of MPTP, by blocking its conversion to its toxic metabolite MPP^+ (l-methyl-4-phenyl pyridine) by MAO_B. If human Parkinsonism results from the action of either an exogenous or endogenous neurotoxin, it is conceivable that this drug could slow the pathogenesis of idiopathic Parkinson's disease. It has thereby been claimed that selegiline should be used early in the management of Parkinson's disease when it may delay the need for L-DOPA preparations.

Another advantage of selegiline is that, being an MAOI, it is reported to improve the endogenous depression that can often be associated with Parkinson's disease.

Side-effects of selegiline

Side-effects with selegiline are, in general, uncommon, but nausea, dizziness, dry mouth and non-specific abdominal discomfort have all been reported. Centrally stimulant side-effects include insomnia, vivid dreams and hallucinations, and confusion and agitation, particularly in the elderly. The incidence of L-DOPA related dyskinesias is often enhanced initially, but these often improve with reduction of L-DOPA dosage. Unlike other MAOIs, especially of the type A specificity (see Chapters 13 and 22), selegiline does not cause hypertension and is not subject to rigorous dietary restrictions.

Amantadine

Amantadine was originally used as an antiviral agent. By serendipity it was employed in Parkinsonian patients for protection against influenza, and improvement in their extrapyramidal symptoms was noted. It is now considered that the drug causes mild improvement in tremor, rigidity and akinesia of some patients.[28] The mode of action of amantadine in this respect is uncertain, but it has been shown to enhance presynaptic dopamine synthesis and release and therefore presumably requires intact and functional nerve terminals to be effective.

Pharmacokinetics of amantadine

Amantadine is readily absorbed from the gut, reaching peak plasma levels 4 h after oral dosage. The drug is not metabolized, the majority of amantadine is excreted unchanged in the urine. Its half-life has been estimated at between 10–30 h.

Side-effects of amantadine

The drug is reported as causing restlessness, insomnia, dizziness and an inability to concentrate. However, the most common side-effects appears to be livedo reticularis, particularly in women. It can induce ankle oedema and thereby may precipitate pre-existing heart failure. Rarely convulsions can be provoked.

Anticholinergic drugs

Anticholinergic agents were one of the first groups of drugs recognized to be of some benefit for the control of symptoms of Parkinson's disease. In particular the limb rigidity and occasionally tremor was reduced by these compounds; bradykinesis is the symptom that is benefited least. They can be helpful in relieving symptoms in drug-induced Parkinsonism and in patients with postencephalitic Parkinsonism. Anticholinergic drugs used in Parkinson's disease include *benzhexol*, *benztropine*, *orphenadrine*, *methixene*, *biperiden* and *procyclidine*.

Mechanism of action

Obviously the major pharmacological mechanism of action of these agents is by way of their anticholinergic (antimuscarinic) properties. Their usefulness in Parkinsonism was, however, established before it was recognized that there is a functional inverse balance between dopaminergic and cholinergic activity within the basal ganglia.[23] Loss of nigrostriatal dopamine projections results in functional hyperactivity of cholinergic neurones within the corpus striatum. Blockade of this now overactive neurotransmitter system helps to restore the balance and so theoretically reverse symptoms of the Parkinson's disease (as it also does by enhancing dopaminergic neurotransmission).

In addition, some of the antimuscarinic drugs employed in the treatment of this disorder possess the ability to block the presynaptic re-uptake sites for dopamine, thereby increasing synaptic concentrations of dopamine and hopefully prolonging postsynaptic receptor interaction. *Benztropine* and *benzhexol* in particular possess significant dopamine uptake blocking activity.

Side-effects of anticholinergics

Unfortunately it is not possible to design antimuscarinic drugs that act solely on central cholinergic receptors without blockade at peripheral sites: side-effects are therefore common and inevitable. Problems with the gastrointestinal system include dry mouth (which is sometimes advantageous as it controls distressing sialagosis and dribbling often encountered in Parkinsonian patients), delaying of gastric emptying and constipation (often a pre-existing problem in Parkinsonism). In the eye, blurred vision can result due to pupillary dilatation, and these drugs are contraindicated in narrow-angle glaucoma where they can cause blindness. They may provoke urinary retention, especially in males with pre-existing symptoms of prostatism. In the cardiovascular system, antimuscarinic drugs may precipitate tachycardia and other arrhythmias. Central nervous system effects of anticholinergics include dizziness, memory impairment and confusional states – particularly in the elderly where their usage should always be monitored with caution. Uncommonly dyskinesias can occur, in the form of involuntary limb movements or orofacial dyskinesias.

Drug interactions of the anticholinergics

The pharmacological actions of these agents will obviously be enhanced by interaction with any other drugs possessing anticholinergic activity. Accordingly, the antimuscarinic drugs used in Parkinson's disease may provoke excessive anticholinergic activity, in particular the antipsychotic phenothiazines and thioxanthenes and the tricyclic antidepressants.

HUNTINGTON'S DISEASE

Huntington's disease is an autosomal dominant inherited disorder which does not usually manifest its symptoms of progressive dementia and wild bizarre involuntary choreiform movements often until middle adult life.[37] Early suspicion may be aroused by the strong family history. Neuronal degeneration is widespread throughout the brain, as evidenced by its small size and enlarged ventricular system, but particularly there is marked cell loss from the basal ganglia. Neurochemically, this is associated with a generalized loss of all neurotransmitter systems, but most obvious is depletion of the inhibitory amino acid neurotransmitter GABA.[21] Disruption of such a controlling inhibitory system results in a generalized overactivity of remaining basal gangliar networks, being thought to be manifest as the uncontrolled choreic movements which are the hallmark of this extrapyramidal disorder.

Principles of management of Huntington's disease

Unfortunately there is no known treatment in the primary sense for Huntington's chorea,[38] and the neurologist is therefore left to attempt to control the dyskinetic movements. Working on the hypothesis that this disorder is due to an overactive basal ganglia (resultant from loss of inhibitory GABA mechanisms), control is best achieved by blocking the now excessively active dopamine systems. Huntington's disease is therefore often considered to be the clinical and neurochemical reverse of Parkinson's disease. Drugs used in Huntington's chorea either deplete presynaptic monoamine stores (*tetrabenazine*) or block postsynaptic dopamine receptors (*pimozide, haloperidol*). The benzodiazepines may be useful to control restlessness, insomnia, hypertonicity and agitation.[38]

Tetrabenazine

Tetrabenazine is one of the few drugs helpful in controlling the dyskinetic movements of Huntington's chorea. Tetrabenazine disrupts the storage vesicles of noradrenergic and dopaminergic nerve terminals, greatly depleting brain concentrations of both these catecholamines. A consequence of such depletion can result in drug-induced Parkinsonism, depression and drowsiness.

Pimozide

Pimozide potently blocks postsynaptic dopamine receptors (see Chapter 22). In this manner it helps to control the motor restlessness of Huntington's chorea, but can of course result in the development of tardive dyskinesias instead.

THE DYSTONIAS

The dystonias are a collection of involuntary movements caused by uncoordinated but sustained muscle contractions resulting in twisting or repetitive gestures or abnormal postures.[39] These movements can affect any part of the body including face (e.g. blepharospasm), neck (spasmodic torticollis), limbs and trunk (axial dystonia). In many cases (often 60%) the pathological cause is never identified, in others pathology within the CNS is present, for example ischaemic damage, degeneration or tumour, or hereditary, metabolic or drug-induced (e.g. neuroleptics, L-DOPA) problems are identified.

Treatment is very difficult, often impossible.[40] Virtually every drug has been tried in this distressing condition. However, agents occasionally providing some beneficial effects are the anti-Parkinsonian drugs, particularly L-DOPA in combination with a peripheral decarboxylase inhibitor (e.g. *carbidopa*) or anticholinergic compounds (e.g. *benzhexol*). The benzodiazepines (e.g. *diazepam*) may provide general muscle relaxation as will *baclofen* (a $GABA_B$-receptor antagonist) and *carbamazepine* (anticonvulsant). Drugs also blocking cerebral dopamine mechanisms such as the receptor antagonists (e.g. *phenothiazines, haloperidol, pimozide* – see Chapter 22) or *tetrabenazine* which depletes synaptic dopamine stores, may provide some symptomatic relief.

A more recent advance to the treatment of refractory persistent dystonias, particularly blepharospasm and spasmotic torticollis, is the injection of *botulinum toxin* locally into the muscle in spasm. This drug binds tightly to presynaptic cholinergic nerve terminals and thereby blocks the release of ACh. Its use in other dystonias such as writer's cramp is to be established. The effect of the botulinum toxin often only lasts a few months after which the injections have to be repeated as the muscle may well return to its previous state of spasm. As a last resort surgery to divide the neuronal input or even cut the muscle itself may be required.

REFERENCES

1 Laidlaw J, Richens A, Oxley J eds. *A textbook of epilepsy*, 3rd edn. Edinburgh: Churchill Livingstone, 1983.

2 Macdonald RL. Mechanism of anticonvulsant drug action. In: Pedley TA, Meldrum BS eds. *Recent advances in epilepsy*. Edinburgh: Churchill Livingstone, 1985: 1–23.

3 Hvidberg EF. Monitoring anticonvulsant drug levels. In: Frey H-H, Janz D eds. *Antiepileptic drugs. Hdbk exp pharmacology*. Berlin: Springer-Verlag, 1985; **74**: 725–65.

4 Yaari Y, Selzer ME, Pincus JH. Phenytoin – mechanism of its anticonvulsant action. *Annals of Neurology* 1986; **20**: 171–84.

5 Schmitz M. Carbamazepine. In: Frey H-H, Janz D eds. *Antiepileptic Drugs. Handbook of experimental pharmacology*. Berlin: Springer-Verlag, 1985; 74: 479–506.

6 Dreifuss FE. Sodium valproate: a re-appraisal. In: Pedley TA, Meldrum BS eds. *Recent advances in epilepsy*. Edinburgh: Churchill Livingstone, 1983; 35–46.

7 Palfreyman MG, Schechter PJ, Buckett WR, Tell GP, Kochweser J. The pharmacology of GABA-transaminase inhibitors. *Biochemical Pharmacology* 1981; **30**: 817–24.

8 Meldrum BS. Pharmacological considerations in the search for new anticonvulsant drugs. In: Pedley TA, Meldrum BS eds. *Recent advances in epilepsy*. Churchill Livingstone: Edinburgh, 1983; 75–92.

9 Reynolds EH. Vigabatrin. *British Medical Journal* 1990; **300**: 277–8.

10 Leach MJ, Marsden CM, Miller AA. Pharmacological studies on lamotrigine, a novel antiepileptic drug. II. Neurochemical studies on the mechanism of action. *Epilepsia* 1986; **27**: 490–7.

11 Goa KL, Sorkin EM. Gabapentin. A review of its pharmacological properties and clinical potential in epilepsy. *Drugs* 1993; **46**: 409–27.

12 Hallet M. Physiology of basal ganglia disorders: an overview. *Canadian Journal of Neurological Science* 1993; **20**, 177–83.

13 Young AB, Penney JB Jr. Biochemical and functional organisation of the basal ganglia. In: Jankovic J, Tolosa E eds. *Parkinson's disease and movement disorders*. Baltimore: Urban & Schwarzenberg, 1988; 1–11.

14 Phillips JG, Bradshaw JL, Jansek R, Chiu E. Motor functions of the basal ganglia. *Psychological Research* 1993; **55**: 175–81.

15 Hornykiewicz O 1975. Parkinson's disease and its chemotherapy. *Biochemical Pharmacology* 1975; **24**: 1061–5.

16 Agid Y, Javoy-Agid F, Ruberg M. Biochemistry of neurotransmitters in Parkinson's Disease. In: Marsden CD, Fahn S eds. *Movement disorders 2*. London: Butterworths, 1987: 167–230.

17 Kopin IJ. The pharmacology of Parkinson's disease therapy: an update. *Annual Reviews of Pharmacology* 1993; **33**, 467–95.

18 Langston JW, Irwin I. MPTP: Current concepts and controversies. *Clinical Neuropharmacology* 1986; **9**: 485–507.

19 Jenner PG, Marsden CD. MPTP-induced parkinsonism as an experimental model of Parkinson's disease. In: Jankovic J, Tolosa E eds. *Parkinson's disease and movement disorders*. Baltimore: Urban & Schwarzenberg, 1988: 37–48.

20 Kopin IJ, Markey SP. MPTP toxicity: Implications for research in Parkinson's disease. *Annual Reviews of Neuroscience* 1988; **11**: 81–96.

21 Spokes EG. Neurochemical alterations in Huntington's chorea. A study of post-mortem brain tissue. *Brain* 1980; **103**: 179–210.

22 Marsden CD. Parkinson's disease. *Lancet* 1990; **i**: 948–52.

23 Duvoisin RC. Cholinergic-anticholinergic antagonism in parkinsonism. *Archives of Neurology* 1967; **17**: 124–36.

24 Calne DB. Treatment of Parkinson's disease. *New England Journal of Medicine* 1993; **329**: 1021–7.

25 Yahr MD. Parkinson's disease: new approaches to diagnosis and treatment. *Acta neurologica scandinavica* 1993; (Suppl) **146**: 22–5.

26 Riederer P, Lange KW, Youdim MB. Recent advances in pharmacological therapy of Parkinson's disease. *Advances in Neurology* 1993; **60**: 626–35.

27 Wessel K, Szelenyi I. Selegiline – an overview of its role in the treatment of Parkinson's disease. *Clinical Investigations* 1992; **70**: 459–62.

28 Schwab RS, Poskanzer DC, England AC, Young RR. Amantadine in Parkinson's disease: Review of more than two years' experience. *Journal of the American Medical Association* 1972; **222**: 792–5.

29 Widner H, Rehncrona S. Transplantation and surgical treatment of parkinsonian syndromes. *Current Opinions in Neurology and Neurosurgery* 1993; **6**: 344–9.

30 Wooten GF. Pharmacokinetics of levodopa. In: Marsden CD, Fahn S eds. *Movement disorders 2*. London: Butterworths, 1987: 231–48.

31 Montastruc JL, Rascol O, Senard JM. Current status of dopamine agonists in Parkinson's disease management. *Drugs* 1993; **46**, 384–93.

32 Laihinen A, Rinne UK, Suchy I. Comparison of lisuride and bromocriptine in the treatment of advanced Parkinson's disease. *Acta neurologica scandinavica* 1992; **86**: 593–5.

33 Rinne UK. Lisuride, a dopamine agonist in the treatment of early Parkinson's disease. *Neurology* 1989; **39**: 336–9.

34 Fuller RW, Clemens JA. Pergolide: a dopamine agonist at both D_1 and D_2 receptors. *Life Sciences* 1991; **49**: 925–30.

35 Lees AJ. Dopamine agonists in Parkinson's disease: a look at apomorphine. *Fundamentals of Clinical Pharmacology* 1993; **7**: 121–8.

36 Vezina P, Mohr E, Grimes D. Deprenyl in Parkinson's disease: mechanisms, neuroprotective effect, indication and adverse effects. *Canadian Journal of Neurological Science* 1992; **19** (Suppl): 142–6.

37 Harper PS ed. *Huntington's disease. Major problems in neurology*. London: WB Saunders, 1991; Vol 22.

38 Morris MR, Tyler A. Management and therapy. In: Harper PS ed. *Huntington's disease. Major problems in neurology*. London: WB Saunders, 1991; Vol 22, 205–49.

39 Marsden CD, Quinn NP. The dystonias. *British Medical Journal* 1990; **300**: 139–44.

40 Fahn S, Marsden CD. The treatment of dystonia. In: Marsden CD, Fahn S eds. *Movement disorders 2* London: Butterworths, 1987: 359–82.

SECTION SEVEN

Drugs Used in the Management of Pain and Inflammation

24

Endogenous Mediators of Pain and Inflammation

M Ehrenstein, DA Isenberg, M Seed

...inflammation is an action produced for the restoration of the most simple injury in sound parts...Inflammation is to be considered only as a disturbed state of parts which require a new but saluting mode of action to restore them to that state wherein a natural mode of action is necessary,...but when it cannot accomplish that salutary purpose as in cancer, scrofula, venereal disease etc., it does mischief.

John Hunter (1794)

INTRODUCTION

In 1794 John Hunter[1] reported in his treatise on the blood, inflammation and gunshot wounds many of the fundamental principles of inflammation. One of these was to restore the affected parts 'to that state wherein a natural mode of action is necessary...', that is, the restoration of normal function. However, this healing process could malfunction and do harm, 'but when it cannot accomplish that salutary purpose...it does mischief'. Inflammation can thus be regarded as an individual's cellular and humoral reaction used in defence against a wide variety of substances that may be introduced into living tissues. These may include bacteria, viruses, fungi, parasites and other particles and soluble substances. The immune system invokes an elegant system of innate and adaptive responses to recognize and eliminate foreign substances, and then to repair those tissues that have been damaged by them. The innate response deals primarily with the clearance of microbes and biological debris while the adaptive response develops recognition and memory that allows the amplification of the response, and improves its specificity. Both of these systems interact to produce acute and chronic inflammation, which are dependent on the persistence of the initiating factor. The elimination of the factor results in the termination of acute inflammation, while failure of the innate system is followed by the chronic response. A foreign body reaction can follow, resulting in granuloma formation. Activation of the adaptive response follows the recognition of a foreign antigen and the development of an epithelioid granuloma. Once the foreign agent has been eliminated, or isolated, tissue repair processes are activated.

It should be noted that these processes are continuous. Clinically relevant inflammation occurs when there is an excess or persistence of antigen, or where there is a cross-reaction between the initiating antigen and an endogenous epitope, which may be present in a particular location, such as the joint in rheumatoid arthritis, or the central nervous system as in multiple sclerosis. In other disease processes, widespread immunoregulatory abnormalities occur as in systemic lupus erythematosis or acquired immunodeficiency syndrome.

The treatment of acute inflammation relies generally on the modulation of the synthesis and action of the various soluble mediators released by the inflammatory cells and surrounding tissues, using agents such as the non-steroidal anti-inflammatory drugs (NSAIDs) and antihistamines. That of the adaptive response and chronic inflammation relies on attempts to modify cellular behaviour using drugs such as the anti-inflammatory steroids and slow-acting antirheumatic drugs.

The common mediators and their cellular sources are listed in Table 24.1.

TABLE 24.1 The cellular sources of inflammatory mediators and their relationship to acute and chronic inflammation

TYPE OF IMMUNE RESPONSE	CELLS	SOLUBLE FACTORS/MEDIATORS
INNATE	PLASMA	Bradykinin Complement (alternative) Acute phase proteins
	Neutrophils	T and P kallikrein Kininogens Lysosomal enzymes Neutral proteases Reactive oxygen species LtB_4, PGE_2, PAF
	Mast/basophils	Histamine LtB_4, SRSA, PAF (basophils) Kininogenase Heparin
	Macrophages	PGE_2 (major source) PAF Interleukin-1 Tumour necrosis factor Complement Plasminogen activator Proteases Nitric oxide (NO) Reactive oxygen species
	Platelets	TxA_2, PAF 5-Hydroxytryptamine
	Endothelial cells	NO, PAF, PGI_2
	PLASMA	Complement (classical) Antigen/antibody complexes
ADAPTIVE	T lymphocytes	Interleukin-2
	B lymphocytes	Antibody
	Macrophages	PGE_2 PAF Interleukin-1 Tumour necrosis factor Complement Plasminogen activator Proteases NO Reactive oxygen species

Acute inflammation

Acute inflammation can still be described by the four classical signs of Celsus – heat, pain, swelling and redness – which are the result of vasodilatation, sensitization of nociceptors, oedema formation and cellular recruitment. The fifth sign, defined by Vilnius as loss of function, is a result primarily of oedema and pain though tissue destruction as seen in rheumatoid arthritis is also a major factor.

The primary tissue insult results in an immediate and transient vasoconstriction followed by vasodilatation mediated by histamine from mast cells, and kinins from the circulation. The increased capillary pressure results in tissue fluid accumulation which in turn increases blood viscosity. Concurrent with this, the margination, jamming and adhesion of leucocytes to the capillary vascular endothelium is enhanced by the increased viscosity and also by the expression of cell adhesion molecules. Fibrin deposition in association with platelet activation may occur, and kinin formation is raised further. Increased vascular permeability leads to more extravasation of plasma leading to a raised osmotic pressure within the tissue, further accelerating the movement of fluid into the tissue.

The release of histamine, kinins, prostaglandins and potassium from damaged cells results in the sensitization and stimulation of sensory nerve endings and hyperalgesia. The swelling resulting from oedema also induces pain. Polymorphonuclear leucocyte neutrophils (PMNs) push between the endothelial cells, followed by monocytes, and migrate along a concentration gradient of chemotactic mediators, such as prostaglandins and leukotrienes, to the inflammatory stimulus. These cells then phagocytose cellular debris and infective agents, releasing further mediators, lysozymes, proteases and reactive oxygen species into the extracellular compartment.

Chronic inflammation

Chronic inflammation is characterized by granuloma formation with the recruitment of monocytes, followed by differentiation and division into macrophages, and then activation of a variety of macrophage functions. If the foreign particles are antigenic, such as found with micro-organisms or autoantigens, the adaptive response can be superimposed leading to a delayed-type hypersensitivity reaction and the formation of an epithelioid granuloma.

This involves antigen processing and presentation by antigen-presenting cells such as macrophages, dendrocytes, endothelial cells and B lymphocytes, to T helper lymphocytes. The macrophages secrete interleukin-1 in response to antigen or T lymphocyte products which, in conjunction with antigen, induce the T helper cells to release interleukin-2. Under the influence of interleukin-2 T lymphocytes proliferate and differentiate into helper, suppressor and cytotoxic T lymphocytes (Fig. 24.1). The release of various cytokines then leads to a further recruitment of macrophages and lymphocytes. Macrophages are instrumental in the repair process, and the ingress of histiocytes and fibroblasts completes healing.

Other types of delayed-type hypersensitivity include contact hypersensitivity, the tuberculin reaction and Jones Mote reactions and are outside the scope of this chapter; however more detailed texts on inflammation are recommended.[2,3]

HISTAMINE

The pioneering work of Dale, Lewis, Willoughby, Feldberg and Black has illustrated the pharmacology of histamine, identified its relevance to inflammation and discovered the receptor subtypes leading to the therapy of minor allergic reactions to shock and gastric ulceration. When injected intradermally, histamine induces three of the five cardinal signs of inflammation, namely swelling, redness and pain in

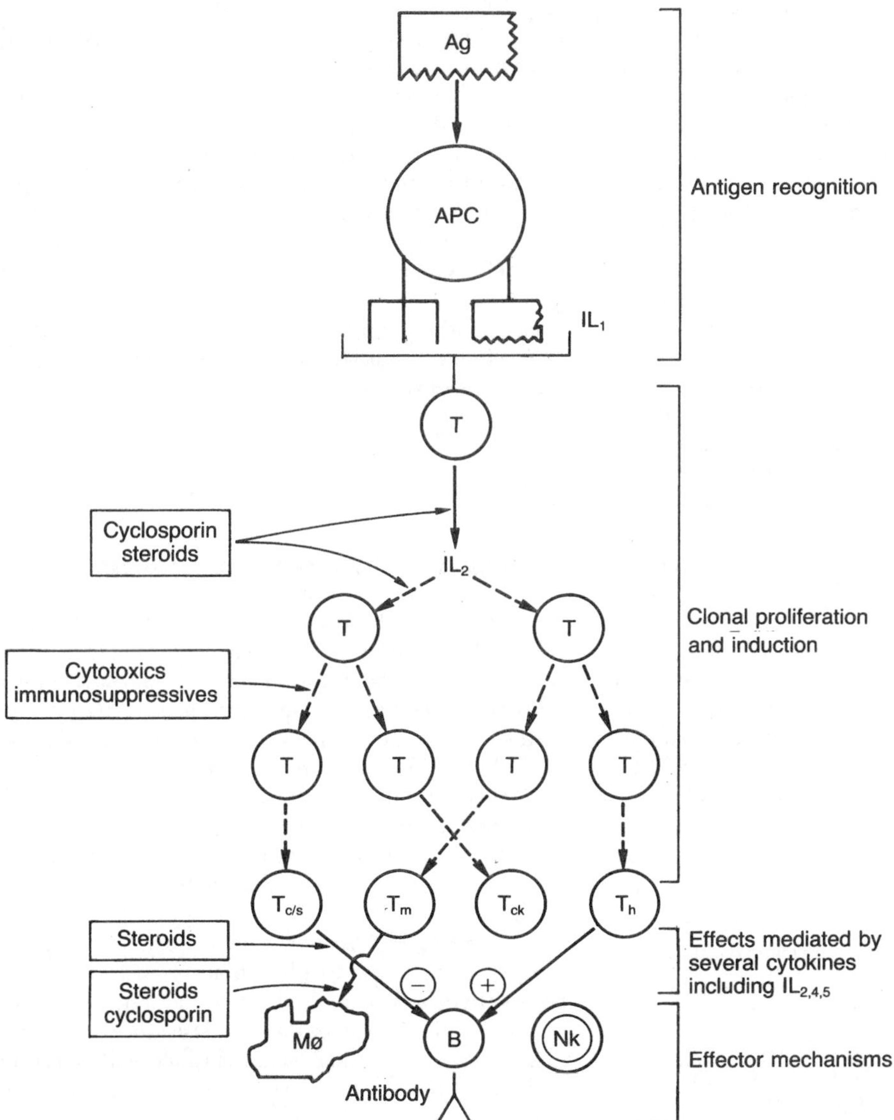

FIGURE 24.1 The induction of the adaptive immune response. The antigen (Ag) is processed by antigen-presenting cells (APC), commonly macrophages, endothelial cells or fibroblasts, and presented in conjunction with the multiple histocompatibility complex to T lymphocytes (T) bearing T lymphocyte receptors. Interleukin-2 (IL-2) released by these cells induces clonal proliferation of T lymphocytes and development into $T_{cytotoxic/suppressor}$ ($T_{c/s}$), T_{memory} (T_m), $T_{lymphokine\ secreting}$ (T_{lk}), and T_{helper} (T_h) lymphocytes. The T_h lymphocytes induce antibody production from B lymphocytes, and $T_{c/s}$ lymphocytes suppress them. Nk, natural killer cell; MO macrophage (see text).

the characteristic wheal and flare reaction. It therefore has a similar role in many respects to the kinins, inducing vasodilatation and extravasation. However, there are substantial differences in its modulation of the immune response and its significance in allergenic reactions.

Synthesis, release and metabolism

2(4-Imidazolyl) ethyl amine (5β-amino ethylimidazole, histamine) is synthesized from histidine by the action of histidine decarboxylase and is stored in conjunction with the proteoglycan matrix of cytoplasic granules of mast cells and basophils. The turnover is very low and once degranulation has occurred, some weeks are required before levels are fully restored. Epidermal cells, gastric mucosa and CNS neurones synthesize histamine *de novo*, while the main sites where mast cells are found are skin, lung and the gastrointestinal tract. Gastric histaminocytes are the main cellular source of histamine in the gastric mucosa and are found within the acid secreting glands (see Chapter 29).

Histamine is released from mast cells and basophils by many of the factors which are released at the site of inflammation as well as many other chemicals (Table 24.2). In conditions such as urticaria pigmentosa, systemic mastocytosis and myelogenous leukaemia, allergens and histamine-releasing agents will elicit systemic effects at considerably lower doses than in unaffected individuals. Complement factors C3a and C5 act via specific receptors, and allergens react by cross-linking cell surface immunoglobulin E (IgE) bound to Fc receptors on presensitized cells, in an allergic (immediate)-type hypersensitivity reaction. These induce a gross influx of calcium ions as a result of phospholipase C activation, adenosine triphosphate formation, diacylglycerol release and protein kinase C activation. This results in the release of not only histamine but also the other granular contents such as heparin, eosinophil and neutrophil chemotactic factors, acid hydrolases, neutral proteases and superoxide dismutase. The stimulation of protein kinase C also results in the synthesis of the lipid mediators of inflammation such as platelet-activating factor (PAF), eicosanoids and leukotrienes (see later this chapter).

TABLE 24.2 Agents known to induce the systemic release of histamine

LIGAND	ALLERGEN
Organic bases	Amides, amidines, quaternary ammonium compounds, pyridinium compounds, piperidines, alkaloids, basic antibiotics
Drugs	Tubocurarine, succinylcholine, morphine, radiocontrast media, dextran, carbohydrate plasma expanders, 40/70
Polypeptide bases	Bradykinin, substance-P, polymixin B, luteinizing hormone RH

The granular contents are released from mast cells by two differing mechanisms. Human skin mast cells release whole granules by exocytosis following activation of actin by calcium, while lung and nasal mucosal mast cells solubilize the granules and release the solubilized fraction through channels formed by fused granular membranes that ultimately combine with the cell membrane. The release of histamine from exocytosed granules is as a result of cation exchange with sodium and calcium since histamine, being a base, is combined with the acidic groups of the heparin proteoglycans.

There are two pathways of metabolism in man, one via histamine -N methyl transference to produce N-methyl (histamine) which is then converted to N-methyl imidazole acetic acid by monoamine oxidase (MAO). The other pathway involves oxidative deamination by diamine oxidase to give imidazole acetic acid. Metabolites are secreted in the urine.

Histamine release from mast cells can be inhibited by agents that raise intracellular cyclic AMP (cAMP) such as catecholamine and β-adrenergic receptor agonists. Histamine acts in a negative feedback loop to act on H_2 receptors (see later) to inhibit or reduce further release. Other agents that raise intracellular cAMP, such as phosphodiesterase inhibitors and eicosanoids, may reduce histamine release.

Actions

Inflammation and the cardiovascular system

Pioneering work by Black has resulted in the pharmacological identification of the two histamine receptor subtypes termed H_1 and H_2 receptors.[4] Subsequently a third class, H_3, has been identified as presynaptic regulatory receptors on histaminergic neurones in the CNS. While H_2 receptors were originally thought to be concerned with the induction of gastric acid secretion, they are now recognized to have a profound role in the regulation of the various cells involved in the immune response and cardiovascular system (see Table 24.3).

In general, H_1 receptors are linked, probably via specific G proteins, to phospholipase C and induce events characteristic of this pathway and the H_2 receptors are linked to adenylate cyclase and, therefore, raise intracellular AMP levels. Intradermal injection induces a typical triple response (dermographism), where a small central vasodilatation occurs at the site of injection, due to the direct action of histamine on the arterioles, within 15 s, followed by a slow flare as a result of antidromic axon reflex induced vasodilatation and 1–2 min later by the wheal, which is oedema formation occurring due to the increased capillary permeability. Various nerve endings are also stimulated by

TABLE 24.3 Tissue histamine receptors and effects of activation

TISSUE	RECEPTOR	EFFECT
Vascular smooth muscle		
Large veins	H_1	Contraction
Large arteries	H_1	Contraction
Arterioles and venules	H_2	Slow onset and sustained dilatation
Arterioles and venules	H_1	Rapid onset, short duration, EDRF dependent
Small calibre/arterioles	H_2	Increased permeability venules/capillaries
Endothelium	H_1	Retraction
		Increased permeability
Cardiovascular system	H_1/H_2	Profound hypotension
		Allergic shock
Extravascular smooth muscle		
Bronchial	H_1	Severe contraction
	H_2	Mild relaxation
Gut	H_1	Contraction
Uterus	H_1	Contraction
	H_2	Relaxation
Exocrine glands		
Adrenal	H_1	Corticosteroid release
Gastric mucosa	H_2	Gastric acid release
Myocardium	H_2	Increased contractility and heart rate (SA node)
		Responses overcome by reflex responses and decreased venous return
	H_1	Decreased A-V conduction

EDRF, endothelium-derived relaxing factor.

histamine, such that the intradermal injection or release of histamine induces itch alone. The effects of iv-administered histamine is dependent on species; however, in man this as well as endogenous release stimulated by allergen in allergic anaphylaxis produces a profound hypotension, characterized by a reduction in the total peripheral resistance, blush response and increased capillary permeability.

The action on the resistance vessels in man is complex and the degree of vasodilatation is dependent on the vascular bed concerned and the type of histamine receptor. H_2 receptors are generally restricted to the microvascular smooth muscle and induce vasodilatation via the intracellular release of AMP. This effect is slow in onset and of a long duration. However, H_1 receptors are restricted to endothelial cells and induce a rapid-onset vasodilatation by the release of endothelium-derived relaxing factor (EDRF, nitric oxide) and eicosanoids, which is short lived. Since H_1 receptors have a higher Ka for histamine than the H_2 receptor, H_1 receptor antagonists will antagonize low levels of histamine, but will only have moderate actions on the profound H_2-mediated vasodilatation to higher concentrations of histamine. This is one reason why H_1 antagonists are not used in the treatment of acute anaphylactic shock (see later).

Capillary permeability is increased at the same time, via H_1 receptor mediated endothelial cell retraction. This, coupled with the dilatation of the microcirculation, results in the passage of plasma fluid, and even platelets between the endothelial cells and accumulation in the extravascular space.

The direct cardiac effects of histamine (H_2-induced positive chronotropic and inotropic actions, H_1 receptor mediate negative inotropic) are overshadowed by the reflex increases in heart rate compensating for the hypotension. However, with large doses, such as found in a severe anaphylactic reaction, cardiac output is reduced since peripheral blood pooling, and increased capillary permeability, reduce venous return (see Chapter 38).

Extravascular smooth muscle

Extravascular smooth muscle also responds to histamine, the most relevant in man being H_1-dependent bronchoconstriction (see Chapter 19), since very low doses of histamine will induce intense bronchoconstriction in patients suffering from asthma. H_2 receptors mediate bronchodilatation, such that H_2-receptor antagonists may marginally potentiate histamine induced bronchoconstriction. H_1 antagonists are of minor importance in the treatment of asthma.

Immune regulation

Histamine has a variety of effects on cells that make up the immune system, mostly being inhibitory at the low concentrations normally found at the site of inflammation (10^{-4}–10^{-7} M), and mediated by H_2 receptors. However, higher doses (10^{-2}–10^{-3} M) exhibit immune stimulatory actions via H_1 receptors. It appears that the responsiveness of cells to histamine increases after immunization, and this therefore increases the negative feedback. The immunosuppressant activity of histamine is mostly induced by the release of T-cell derived histamine releasing factors (HSF) in the presence of monocytes or interleukin-1 (see Fig. 24.2). HSF has a wide range of activities leading to a suppression of the immune response and induces prostaglandin E_2 (PGE_2) release by monocytes which may further inhibit T cell proliferation. HSF has relevance to the clinic since it has been found that atopic subjects synthesize reduced quantities of this factor, while interleukin-1 levels and T suppressor and helper cell ratios appear normal.[5] The lymphocytes appear to be less responsive to HSF-induced PGE_2 release.

Cimetidine, an H_2-receptor antagonist, increases delayed-type hypersensitivity reactions to antigen in duodenal ulcer patients, increases antibody production in hypogammaglobulinaemia, increases T-suppressor cell function, reverses immunosuppression in cholecystectomy patients, ovarian carcinoma, melanoma, colorectal cancer and also enhances natural killer cell activity. It is clear that histamine has a significant role to play in the adaptive, as well as the innate, immune response.

Antihistamines

Histamine-dependent effects can be modulated therapeutically by four main mechanisms: (1) prevention of synthesis; (2) prevention of release; (3) functional antagonism; and (4) H_1-receptor antagonism. Common antihistamines are listed in Table 24.4.

Tritoqualine and fluoromethylhistidine, inhibitors of histidine decarboxylase, inhibit the formation of histamine. While tritoqualine can be used as an anti-

TABLE 24.4 Histamine antagonists

Arylalkylamines	Acrivastine Brompheniramine Chlorpheniramine Clemastine Pheniramine Triprolidine
Ethanolamines	Bromphenhydramine Dimenhydrinate Diphenhydramine Trimethobenzamide
Ethylenediamines	Chlorpyrilene Histapyrrodine Mepyramine Thonzylamine Tripelenamine
Phenindenes	Dimethindene Mebhydrolin Phenindamine
Phenothiazines	Isothipendyl Mequitazine Promethazine Trimeprazine
Piperazines	Cetirizine Chlorcyclizine Cyclizine Hydroxyzine Oxatomide
Piperidines	Astemizole Bamipine Diphenylpyraline Terfenadine Thenalidine

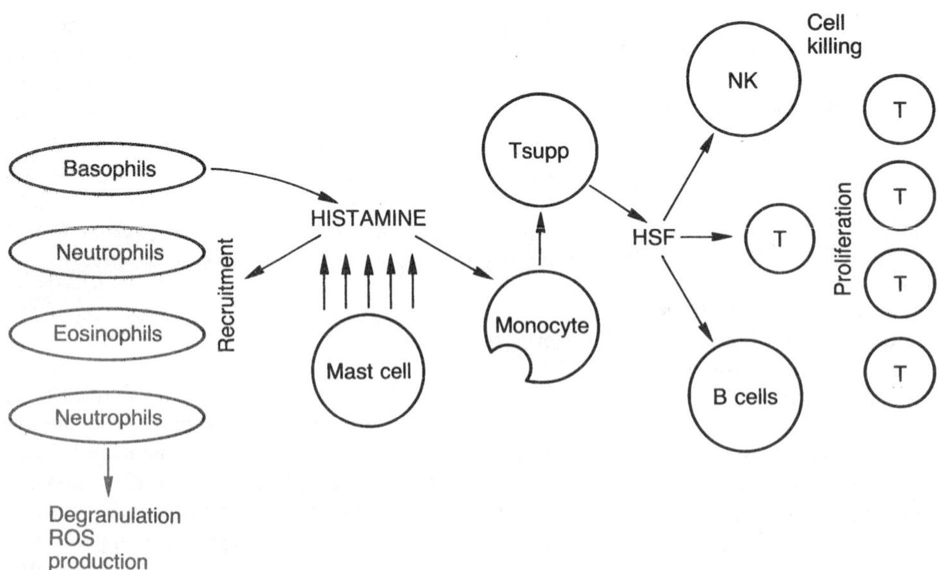

FIGURE 24.2 The effects of histamine on the inflammatory cells in the inflammatory lesion. Mast cell degranulation results in the release of histamine which influences inflammatory cell recruitment and activation as well as the induction of histamine suppressor factor which inhibits natural killer (NK) cell killing, T lymphocyte proliferation, and B lymphocyte function (see text).

histamine,[6] fluoromethylhistidine appears to be ineffective in allergic rhinitis[7] but effective in ice-induced urticaria[8] in clinical trials. The prevention of histamine release can be elicited by sodium cromoglycate which may stabilize the mast cell membrane. Because of their mode of action, these agents are given prophylactically. Functional antagonism is used in the emergency treatment of acute anaphylaxis (see Chapter 38) and angioedema in the form of adrenaline (see later).

H_1-receptor antagonists (commonly known as antihistamines) are used therapeutically in the symptomatic treatment of various inflammatory states.[9] H_2-receptor antagonists are used primarily for the treatment of gastric disorders (see Chapter 29) but therapeutic uses for H_3 antagonists have yet to be defined. Many H_1 antagonists also have profound local anaesthetic and antimuscarinic activity (see Table 24.5). Because of the latter activity, those that cross the blood–brain barrier are used for sedation and the suppression of motion sickness. A substantial potentiation of these effects by alcohol is a common problem. H_1 antagonists have their main therapeutic value in the treatment of histamine-dependent allergic reactions. They can be administered topically or parenterally, and iv in severe anaphylaxis as an adjunct to adrenaline. H_1 antagonists are often more useful as a prophylactic treatment of anticipated reactions.

It should be noted that there are several other classes of drugs that have potent H_1-antagonist activity which are not taken advantage of therapeutically such as tricyclic antidepressants, phenothiazines, 5-hydroxytryptamine (5-HT) antagonists, and anticholinergic agents.

Allergy

Exudative allergies are the most amenable to H_1-antagonist therapy such as allergic rhinitis, hay fever, acute and chronic urticarias, conjunctivitis and other acute mild allergic reactions. The acute urticarias respond well, especially the pruritis which is reduced by the local anaesthetic activity, the oedema and erythema being less well controlled. Although effective in many instances with chronic urticarias, this type responds less well when compared with the acute form. Contact and atopic dermatitis are often responsive to H_1 antagonists, but corticosteroids are more effective (see later). It should be remembered that H_1-antagonist therapy should be discontinued prior to skin allergy testing! Iatrogenic allergies are responsive to H_1 antagonists as well as serum sickness, where the signs of itch, urticaria and oedema are involved. Systemic anaphylaxis accompanied by angioedema, however, always indicates the use of adrenaline which reverses the bronchoconstriction and hypotension while reducing capillary calibre and permeability, as well as inhibiting histamine release. Secondary therapy with H_1 antagonists may be required.

Hay fever responds very well to H_1 antagonists unless nasal congestion has developed as a result of chronic exposure to allergen, when their effectiveness is reduced. Asthma rarely responds to this approach, though the antimuscarinic activity may account for the therapeutic effects reported (see Chapter 19).

The use of H_2-receptor antagonists in allergic disease is purely experimental. Late phase allergic reactions to timothy grass and ragweed challenge have been tested in various combinations of H_1 and H_2 antagonists.[10] The H_1 antagonist clemastine inhibits the early phase only, while the H_2 antagonist cimetidine alone has no effect. Both drugs together increase the immediate response but inhibit the late response.

Disorders of the central nervous system

Histamine antagonists of certain classes are very effective in the treatment of motion sickness as well as antiemetics, especially the ethanolamines, phenothiazines and piperazine derivatives (Table 24.5). Those modern antagonists such as terfenadine,[11] astemizole[12] and loratidine have no CNS activity due to their designed inability to cross the blood–brain barrier. Diphenhydramine and promethazine are useful in labyrinthine disorders, such as Ménière's syndrome, relieving vertigo and nausea. Those H_1 antagonists with potent antimuscarinic activity, such as diphenhydramine, have been found to be effective in the early stages of Parkinson's disease. Diphenhydramine can also reverse phenothiazine-induced extrapyramidal side-effects. H_1 antagonists are also used for their sedative effects.

Side-effects

The single most problematic side-effect of the H_1 antagonist is sedation. The few exceptions are terfenidine, astemizole and loratidine which do not enter the CNS. The interaction with alcohol and other CNS depressants can be quite dramatic, and impairs motor skills substantially. Children, however, are prone to CNS stimulation prior to sedation. The phenindines are unusual in that there may be CNS stimulation as opposed to sedation, and some arylalkylamines have lower sedative activity and even some paradoxical CNS stimulatory actions which can lead to insomnia. With many of the agents there are the classical antimuscarinic effects such as dry mouth, blurred vision and urinary retention. Digestive tract effects, such as nausea, vomiting, diarrhoea and epigastric pain, are very common. The ethanolamines as a class appear to have fewer problems in this respect, and terfenadine and astemizole do not appear to have these effects, having few antimuscarinic actions.

Contact dermatitis to H_1 antagonists is common, especially on topical administration, but occasionally orally. Cross-sensitization occurs within chemical

TABLE 24.5 A profile of the additional and significant actions of the common classes of H_1 antagonists

	ANTIMUSCARINIC ACTIVITY	ANTI-EMETIC ACTIVITY	SEDATIVE ACTIVITY	LOCAL ANAESTHETIC ACTIVITY	OTHER
Arylalkylamines	Pronounced activity	Pheniramine antiemetic	Whole class some activity, more suitable for daytime use than other classes Still some sedation Some prone to paradoxical CNS stimulation, e.g. chlorphenyramine	None	Potent H_1 antagonists
Ethanolamines	Pronounced activity	Diphenhydramine, bromdiphenhydramine, trimethobenzamide mild activity	Pronounced sedative activity	Diphenhydramine marked activity	Whole class low gastrointestinal effects. Diphenhydramine anti-Parkinson activity Trimethobenzamide weak H_1 antagonist activity
Ethylenediamines	Some activity	Mepyramine some activity	Less severe sedative activity	Tripelenamine marked activity, histapyrodine some, and mepyramine less	Gastrointestinal side-effects and skin sensitization common
Phenindenes	Phenindamine some activity	None	Less pronounced sedative activity. Dimethindine some activity, phenindamine CNS stimulant activity	Dimethindine some activity	—
Phenothiazines	Pronounced activity	Mostly used as anti-emetics	Pronounced sedative activity, e.g. schizophrenia Mequitazine no or minor sedation	Promethazine marked activity	Photosensitivity reactions Adverse effects in hepatic disease Cause extrapyramidal syndromes
Piperazines	Meclozine marked activity Cyclizine some activity	Often used as anti-emetics and for motion sickness	Cetirizine no or minor sedation	Cyclizine some activity Chlorcyclizine, cinnarizine mild activity	—
Piperidines	Little activity	None, except diphenylpyraline moderate activity	Bamipine marked activity, diphenylpyraline less Astemizole, loratadine and terfenidine no sedation	Thenalidine and diphenylpyraline only	Astemizole, loratidine and terfenadine have poor penetration into the CNS
Other agents	None	No sedation	Sodium chromoglycate, ketotifen and triprolidine no sedation	None	Sodium chromoglycate and ketotifen inhibit histamine release Triprolidine inhibits histamine synthesis

classes. Photosensitization can be a severe problem, especially with the phenothiazines.

LIPID-DERIVED AUTACOIDS

Prostaglandins, leukotrienes, lipoxins and platelet-activating factor make up the prevalent family of lipid-derived autacoids which have profound activities in inflammation, the immune response, smooth muscle function and haemostasis. The recognition by Vane,[13] and Smith and Willis[14] that prostaglandin production was inhibited by anti-inflammatory agents that have been in use since the last century, namely the aspirin-like drugs, provided an insight into their primary mechanism of action, and allowed the investigation of the role of cyclo-oxygenase products in the physiology and pathology of disease. The pharmacology has since expanded to provide a wide variety of choice of agents available for the therapy of inflammatory disease, such as the selective inhibitors of prostaglandins synthesis, the NSAIDs: agonists and antagonists.

Synthetic and metabolic pathway

Prostaglandins and leukotrienes are acidic lipids derived from eicosatetraenoic acid (eicosa=twenty, enoic=double bonds, or more commonly termed arachidonic acid) which is released from the 2-position of membrane phospholipids, such as phosphatidylcholine, serine or inositol, by phospholipase-A_2. The ubiquitous nature of both the substrate and enzyme ensures that there is the widest possible availability of arachidonic acid. The range of products derived from this common precursor is determined by the presence of cyclo-oxygenase and/or lipoxygenase, their state of activation, and the presence of further specific synthetic enzymes[15] (Fig. 24.3).

Cyclo-oxygenase has now been recognised to have two forms, termed cyclo-oxygenase-1 and -2. The first is considered at present to be mainly a constitutively expressed enzyme, whilst the second is inducible by cytokines and mediators. Cyclo-oxygenase-1 is considered to be the isoform found in the stomach, its products being cytoprotective, and the renal system, modulating tubule function.

Cyclo-oxygenase has dual activities, namely endoperoxide synthetase to produce the cyclic endoperoxide prostaglandin-G_2 (PGG_2), and peroxidase activity to reduce the 15 hydroperoxide of PGG_2 to the 15 hydroxyl group which defines PGH_2. Further differentiation of the prostaglandins endoperoxides is determined by the presence of either thromboxane (TxA_2) synthetase, prostacyclin (PGI_2) synthetase, PGE_2 isomerase or PGD_2 isomerase. The formation of $PGF_{2\alpha}$, the 9-keto reduced form of PGE_2, may be via a reductase.

5-Lipoxygenase, as its name implies, oxidizes arachidonic acid at the 5 position to form 5-hydroperoxy eicosatetraenoic acid (5-HPETE). Leukotriene-A_4 synthetase acts on 5-HPETE to produce LtA_1, the precursor of LtB_4 (via LtA hydrolase), and the leukotrienes LtC_4, LtD_4 and LtE_4 which are the cysteinyl-peptido leukotrienes derived from the action of glutathione-*S*-transferase and a series of peptidases. The 12-hydroperoxy derivative of arachidonic acid is formed by the action of 12-lipoxygenase. As with the prostaglandin synthetases, the presence or absence of the enzymes within the cells determines the profile of leukotrienes released.

The action of phospholipase-A_2 also deacylates 1-O-alkyl-2-acyl-sn-glycero-3-phosphorylcholine. The lysophospholipid product is acetylated by a specific acetyltransferase to form 1-O-alkyl-2-acetyl-glycero-3-phosphorylcholine, namely, platelet-activating factor (PAF, named after its first discovery). PAF is metabolized by acetyl hydrolysis which results in the unusual formation of the inactive precursor which can subsequently be reacylated to PAF or the original phospholipid precursor.

Prostaglandins are rapidly metabolized or hydrolysed to inactive derivatives. Initially PGE_2, $PGF_{2\alpha}$ and PGD_2 are metabolized by a specific 15-hydroxy prostaglandin dehydrogenase (PGDH) found in vessel walls, kidney and lung to give the corresponding 15-keto prostaglandins which are then reduced by prostaglandin 13-reductase. The resulting fatty acids are then degraded by β and ∞ oxidation. PGI_2 is hydrolysed in aqueous solution or blood to 6-keto-$PGF_{1\alpha}$ and then follows the normal pattern followed by the other prostaglandins. TxA_2 spontaneously degrades to the inactive hydrolysis product TxB_2, 2,3-dinor TxB_2 being the final urinary metabolite. LtB_4 is degraded by ∞ oxidation and intracellular LtC_4 is inactivated by peptidase conversion to LtD_4 and LtE_4, depending on the cell type. Extracellular cysteinyl-leukotrienes can be oxidized into their respective sulphoxides by myeloperoxidase-dependent oxidation, in the extracellular inflammatory locus in the presence of neutrophils and eosinophils.

Eicosanoid interactions

Transcellular metabolism of arachidonic acid metabolites can occur, enabling cells that are deficient in certain enzyme pathways to release products from precursors unavailable from their own synthetic processes. For example, platelets and neutrophils contain 12-lipoxygenase and 5-lipoxygenase respectively. On incubation under controlled conditions, platelet-derived 12-HETE can be converted to 5,12-diHETE (namely LtB_4) by neutrophils, and the same product derived from platelets supplied with 5-HETE from neutrophils.[16] Platelets and erythrocytes also contain glutathione-*S*-transferase, and are therefore able to transform LtA_4 into the cysteinyl-leukotrienes, without being able to produce LtA_4 endogenously. Neutrophils will also utilize platelet arachidonic acid, and mast cells may convert neutrophil derived LtA_4 to LtC_4. This phenomenon is not only isolated to the leukotrienes. Platelet-derived arachidonic acid is utilized by endothelial cells to enhance PGI_2 formation, and thus inhibit platelet aggregation,[17] and is utilized by neutrophils to synthesize LtB_4.

Control of release

The lipid-derived autacoids are all released *de novo*. Prostaglandins may be released from tissues disturbed by injury, membrane perturbation or receptor activation. Leukotrienes and PAF release, on the other hand, are associated with receptor activation. Phospholipase-A_2 (PLA_2) and 5-lipoxygenase are both calcium-dependent enzymes, and because of this prostaglandin and leukotriene release is calcium dependent.

The signal transduction pathway (Fig. 24.4) after receptor activation is the activation of a series of phosphatidylinositol-

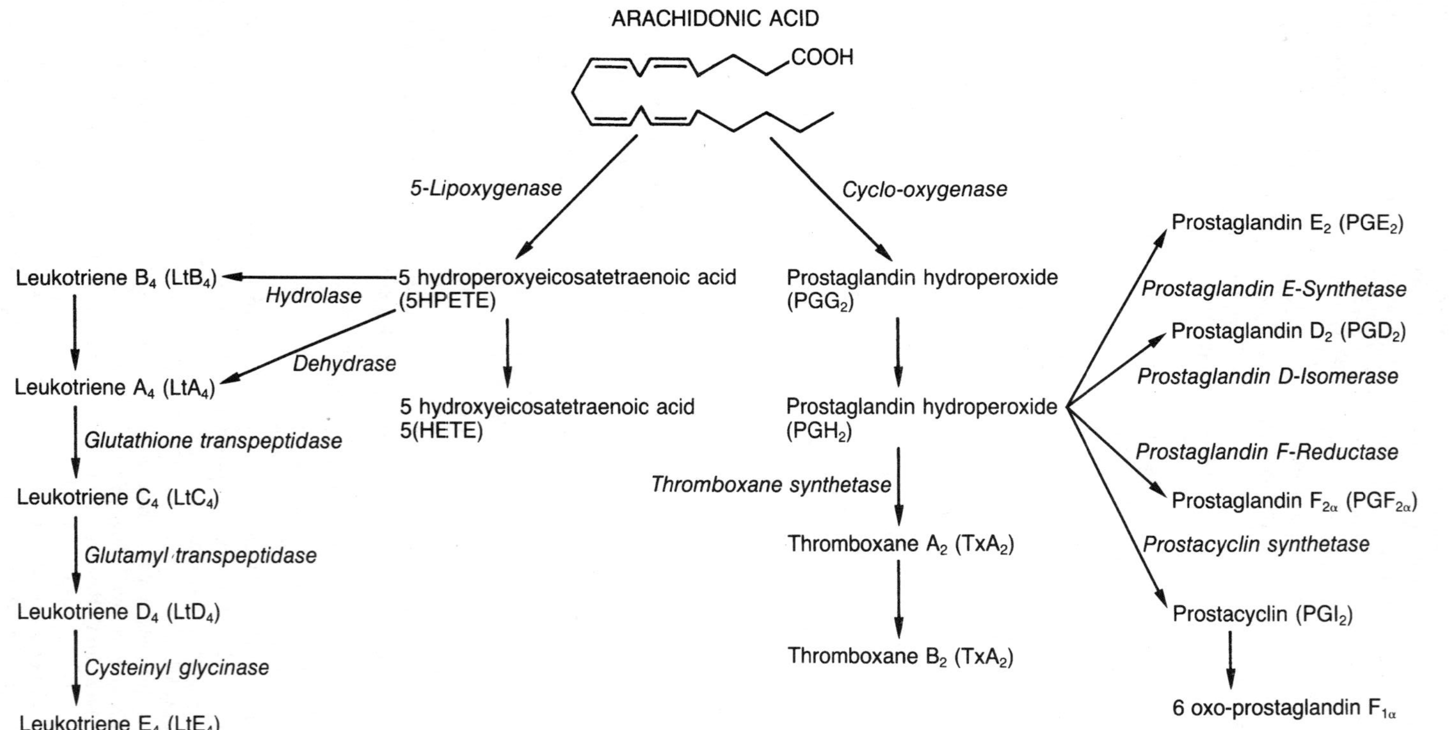

FIGURE 24.3 The synthetic pathway of eicosanoids derived from arachidonic acid divided into the lipoxygenase and cyclo-oxygenase pathways.

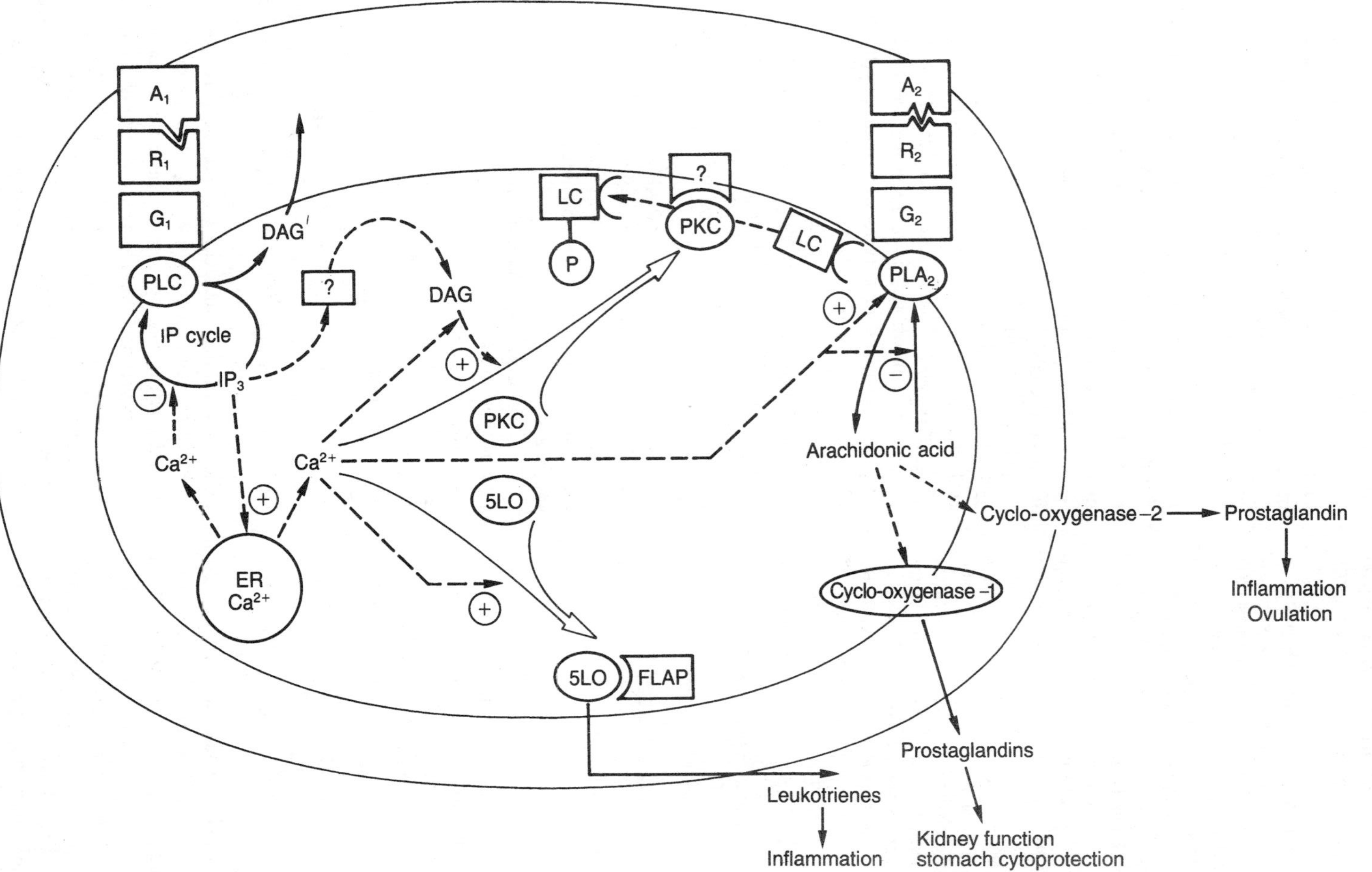

FIGURE 24.4 The release of arachidonic acid is mediated by various intercellular mechanisms which are stimulated by the occupation by various agonists (A_1 & A_2) of receptors (R_1 & R_2) linked to phospholipase C (PLC) or phospholipase A_2 (PLA_2) via G proteins (G_1 & G_2). PLC activation results in the production of inositoltriphosphate (IP_3) which induces the release of calcium (Ca^{2+}) from endoplasmic reticulum (ER) and the intracellular release of diacylglycerol (DAG) from an unknown source. The combination of DAG and Ca^{2+} results in the activation and translocation of protein kinase C (PKC) to the plasma membrane, to bind to a putative docking protein, and it is postulated that PLA_2 is then disinhibited by the resulting phosphorylation of lipocortin (LC). Raised intracellular calcium levels also induce the translocation of 5-lipoxygenase to a docking protein in the plasma membrane, 5-lipoxygenase activating protein (FLAP), and it is activated to convert arachidonic acid to 5-hydroperoxy-eicosatetraenoic acid leading to the synthesis of leukotrienes. PLA_2 is also a calcium-dependent enzyme which cleaves arachidonic acid from membrane phospholipids which is then diverted to the cyclo-oxygenase pathway to form the prostaglandins. Both IP_3 and arachidonic acid are rapidly reincorporated into the membrane phospholipids, and this process is inhibited by raised intracellular calcium, further increasing their intracellular availability.

specific phospholipase C_s (PLC_s) which release inositol triphosphate (IP_3) from the phospholipid, with diacylglycerol (DAG) which remains membrane bound. The subsequent formation of IP_3 induces intracellular calcium mobilization which, along with DAG from an extra membrane source, results in protein-kinase C (PKC) translocation to the plasma membrane, and activation. It is believed that phospholipase-A_2 may be disinhibited by the PKC or tyrosine kinase dependent phosphorylation and inactivation of the membrane-bound PLA_2 inhibitor lipocortin.[18] This will therefore result in a greatly enhanced release of arachidonic acid and PAF. Phospholipase A_2 is also receptor linked and can be activated independently of PLC.

The liberation of arachidonic acid is not the only prerequisite for eicosanoid release. The presence of cyclo-oxygenase is vital, and can be induced in the form of cyclo-oxygenase-2 in order to maximize prostaglandin release, as is found in the pregnant uterus prior to labour. 5-Lipoxygenase also requires activation prior to the formation of LtA_4. 5-Lipoxygenase is a calcium-dependent cytosolic enzyme and as such has no access to membrane phospholipids. Raised intracellular calcium levels, induced by PLC activation, result in the translocation of the enzyme to the plasma membrane and are associated with a docking protein termed 5-lipoxygenase activating protein (FLAP).[19] The discovery of this novel pathway was a result of the finding that an inhibitor of 5-lipoxygenase, MK0886, being only active in whole cell preparations, bound to a specific 5-lipoxygenase binding protein thus preventing the formation of LtA_4. Future work will determine if the molecules such as FLAP may co-operate with other enzymes, such as phospholipase-A_2, and thus regulate eicosanoid production. PLC and PKC are both enzymes that translocate and may associate with similar ‘docking’ proteins. It must be noted that arachidonic acid levels may also be regulated by the degree of reacylation into the phospholipids of the plasma membrane, a process that is also inhibited by calcium.

The role of lipid-derived autacoids in inflammation

Eicosanoids

The cyclo-oxygenase products are a further series of mediators that contribute to the cardinal signs of inflammation,[20] and the systemic manifestation of inflammation, namely hyperpyrexia. They are detected in all inflammatory lesions tested, including rheumatoid arthritis, sunburn, eczema, psoriasis, ulcerative colitis and gout. The major product formed is PGE_2, though the products of PGI_2, TxA_2, and $PGF_{2\alpha}$ are found in lower quantities. The widespread detection of prostaglandins in inflammatory exudates indicates an important role for them in the inflammatory process and the development of NSAIDs has confirmed this thesis. There is a good correlation between PGE_2 synthesis *in vivo* and oedema formation in inflammatory lesions. PGE_2 and PGI_2 are both potent vasodilators but do not appear to increase vascular permeability directly. They have an additive effect with histamine and bradykinin, and a permissive effect on C5a and neutrophil-dependent vascular permeability. These prostaglandins markedly enhance neutrophil infiltration due to the vasodilatation, not directly. Neutrophils are a significant source of LtB_4, a powerful chemoattractant that further potentiates neutrophil-dependent vascular permeability and PGE_2 synthesis. However, it is unlikely that leukotrienes contribute to the changes in vascular tone seen in inflammation. TxA_2 released from platelet aggregates may also increase vascular injury by inducing neutrophil adhesion to endothelial cells.

The inducible nature of cyclo-oxygenase-2 means that the site at which it is induced will have a profound influence on the actions of its products. Macrophages are the major inflammatory cells expressing cyclo-oxygenase-2, as well as fibroblasts, in chronic inflammation.[21] In acute inflammation, neutrophils have been found to express cyclo-oxygenase-2 transiently during the early stages. It is therefore the predominant isoform in inflammation, and its selective inhibition may provide a safer form of NSAID therapy than those currently available, cyclo-oxygenase-1 being found in the gastric mucosa and renal tubules.

PGE_2, however, as well as the pro-inflammatory actions mediated by its vasodilator action, has varied and significant negative immunomodulatory effects. PGE_2 suppresses interleukin-1 production by macrophages and fibroblasts in a negative feedback loop since it is released in conjunction with interleukin-1. PGE_2 inhibits neutrophil LtB_4 release and the oxidative burst, and inhibits T-lymphocyte proliferation.[22] Mast-cell dependent allergy in the hamster cheek pouch is inhibited by PGE_2, as mediator release is inhibited by raised intracellular cAMP. Cyclo-oxygenase inhibition potentiates the inflammation in this model.[23] One of the explanations for the enhancement of cartilage degradation by NSAID therapy in animal models of inflammatory joint disease has been that the inhibition of PGE_2 release may relieve the immune response of one of the major negative homeostatic mechanisms.

The detection of leukotrienes in inflammatory lesions has been less forthcoming. However, LtB_4 and LtC_4 are present in synovial fluids from rheumatoid arthritic patients and can be isolated from psoriatic lesions while LtB_4 is found in gout effusions. Their actions and extreme potency indicate a significant role in inflammatory cell functions. The cysteinyl-leukotrienes LtC_4, LtD_4 and LtE_4, are potent bronchoconstrictor agents (see Chapter 19) being constituents of slow-reacting substance of anaphylaxis (SRSA). LtC_4 and LtD_4, unlike prostaglandins, directly increase vascular permeability, and the leukotrienes are the only arachidonic acid metabolites to be directly chemotactic. LtB_4 is the most potent in this respect. LtB_4 also induces neutrophil aggregation, degranulation, and adhesion to endothelium and induces neutrophil-dependent increases in vascular permeability.

Pain is modulated by arachidonic acid metabolites; PGE_2 can induce deep, long-lasting pain when injected intradermally in sufficient doses. It is most widely recognized that in the inflammatory locus prostaglandins do not induce pain, but induce hyperalgesia in combination with histamine, bradykinin and may induce hypersensitivity to nociceptive stimuli such as that found in sunburn. LtB_4 induces hyperalgesia, which is neutrophil dependent; however, LtB_4, LtC_4 and LtD_4 inhibit bradykinin-induced algesia. The role of leukotrienes in hyperalgesia therefore remains unclear.

Platelet-activating factor (PAF)

The phospholipid product of PLA_2 action, PAF, also has potent actions consistent with a mediator of inflammation.[24] PAF, again, induces the characteristic wheal and flare response with pain, indicating vasodilatation and increased vascular permeability. However, it appears these actions are mediated by histamine. In the presence of H_1 antagonists and cyclo-oxygenase inhibitors, PAF directly induces vasodilatation and endothelial cell retraction in postcapillary venules. These effects, unlike those of prostaglandins, are independent of the presence of neutrophils, although neutrophil, monocyte and platelet accumulation occurs at the site of PAF injection. PAF induces neutrophil aggregation, degranulation, accumulation, the oxidative burst, PLA_2 activation and eicosanoid release, including LtB_4. PAF directly increases immunoglobulin production by B lymphocytes.

In vivo, the systemic administration of PAF induces bronchoconstriction and hypotension similar to that found with IgE anaphylaxis. This is accompanied by, and is dependent on, platelet aggregation and accumulation in the lungs, and neutropenia induced by increased margination and lung accumulation. The inhalation of PAF induces eosinophilia and bronchoconstriction independent of platelet aggregation and occurs in the presence of systemic PAF desensitization, indicating a direct effect on bronchiolar smooth muscle. It is considered that PAF plays a major role in allergy.

Haemodynamics

PGI_2 is not only a potent vasodilator, but also inhibits platelet aggregation and disaggregates platelets. In these senses, being synthesized in large quantities by endothelial cells, it acts as the endogenous antagonist to TxA_2 derived from circulating and aggregating platelets. The association of platelets with vascular endothelium can induce PGI_2 release not only by contact, but also by the donation of platelet-derived arachidonic acid to endothelial PGI_2 synthetase. This results in a reduced platelet adhesion and aggregation. Platelets mixed with aspirin-treated endothelial cells will not aggregate to thrombin, illustrating this point.

Endothelial cells *in vivo* overcome cyclo-oxygenase inhibition by aspirin by the *de novo* synthesis of cyclo-oxygenase, unlike platelets, which do not have this capacity being anucleate. Low-dose aspirin therapy takes advantage of this phenomenon resulting in the selective and irreversible inhibition of platelet thromboxane synthesis while the endothelium retains the capacity to synthesize PGI_2, prolonging bleeding time.

Mechanism of action

The action of eicosanoids is mediated by specific receptors.[25,26] There are eight subtypes of prostanoid receptor that have been characterized so far. These have been defined by the use of synthetic and natural agonists, and named after the principal natural ligand. The secondary messengers for the PGD receptor (DP), IP, EP_2 receptors, and possibly the EP_3 receptor is cAMP, and those for EP_1, FP and TxA_2, (TP_α and TP_τ) is the phospholipase-C dependent inositol-triphosphate cycle. There is evidence that the TP receptor may have up to three subtypes which may differentiate vascular and aggregatory actions. These generally relate to the pharmacological actions of the prostaglandins, raised cAMP levels being associated with the relaxation of smooth muscle and the inhibition of platelet aggregation, while the phospholipase-C system is associated with platelet aggregation and smooth muscle contraction. There is, however, little evidence that EP receptors are present on platelets. PGE_1 and PGE_2 are anti-aggregatory, PGE_2 being much less potent than PGE_1, and probably act via the IP receptor. However PGE_2 can enhance the actions of pro-aggregatory agents by an unknown mechanism. The receptors for lipoxygenase products are of three types for LtB_4, LtC_4 and LtD_4/LtE_4 which activate PLC. PAF has a specific receptor which is also linked to PLC. Receptors for the lipoxins, HETEs and hepoxilins remain uncharacterized at present.

Synthetic prostaglandin agonists, such as misoprostol, rioprostil, epoprostanol and iloprost, have been synthesized and are used in the clinic. The use of PGD_2 or PGI_2 agonists as antiplatelet agents is limited by the vasodilator actions, and thus a selective agonist for the platelet IP receptor would be a significant advance. The pharmacological dissociation of the vasodilator and immune regulatory actions of PGE_2 would also be very beneficial and are being pursued. TxA_2 antagonists[27,28] are being developed for use as antithrombotic agents, prolonging bleeding time, but have otherwise been disappointing. Perhaps this is due to the very high local concentrations of TxA_2 at the site of release displacing the antagonists, which are competitive. The actions of TxA_2 synthetase inhibitors also may be overcome by the excess of PGH_2 which acts on the same receptor. Combination therapy is promising, and dual TxA_2 antagonists/synthetase inhibitors are being developed and are nearing clinical use. Orally active leukotriene antagonists reduce antigen-induced bronchoconstriction. Clinical trials of specific PAF antagonists are at present being carried out. It acts via a specific receptor; however, those antagonists that have been developed up to the present have not shown dramatic therapeutic promise, despite significant actions such as antagonizing bronchoconstriction and improving survival in animal models of anaphylaxis and allergy.

The use of these antagonists will provide powerful tools for finally determining the role and significance of these mediators in inflammation and disease.

KININS

The kinins are a group of structurally and pharmacologically related peptides, of which bradykinin and kallidin are two. They are products of the enzymes tissue kallikrein and plasma kallikrein, and are released from plasma and tissue respectively. They are found at sites of inflammation and in inflammatory exudates. They contribute to the acute phase of inflammation by inducing oedema, vasodilatation and pain, while there is some evidence that they may play a role in chronic inflammation (for review see Proud and Kaplan[29]).

Synthesis and metabolism

The kinins are released as a result of activation of plasma and tissue enzyme cascades which, as is usual in such systems, undergo considerable amplification (Fig. 24.5). Simply, the cascade centres on the conversion of kininogens to kinins by the action of kallikreins which have been converted from their inactive precursor prekallikreins. The plasma cascade is initiated by the contact of pre-Hageman factor with anomalous negatively charged surfaces such as collagen, proteoglycans, glass, bacterial cell walls and urate crystals. This cleaves a portion from the plasma prekallikrein (which is complexed to a high molecular weight kininogen, MW 88–114 kDa) leading to activation and cleavage of the complexed kininogen and then plasma kininogen of the same form to release bradykinin. Plasma kallikrein (MW 90–100 kDa) has the ability to profoundly activate pre-Hageman factor and thus acts as a potent positive feedback mechanism. Complement factor C1NA and α_2-macroglobulin are potent inhibitors of plasma kallikrein, and α_1-macroglobulin is less so, acting to reduce the formation of plasma kinins.

Tissue kallikrein (MW 25–45 kDa) on the other hand, is released by various glands and tissues such as the kidney, salivary glands, bronchi and pancreas (kinin is derived from the Greek kallikreas, meaning pancreas). However, the identity of the activating protease is unknown. Tissue kallikrein and prekallikrein may be synthesized or released under hormonal or neuronal influence dependent upon the tissue. Once released, tissue kallikrein releases kallidin from a low molecular weight kininogen (MW 50–68 kDa). Other sources of kallikreins and kininogens include neutrophils which are recruited to the site of inflammation.

The kinins are rapidly metabolized ($t_{1/2}$ 15 s) via the kininases, by cleavage of the C-terminal Arg,Phe dipeptide or C-terminal Arg, respectively (see Table 24.6). An aminopeptidase has been identified which may convert kallidin to bradykinin; however, this

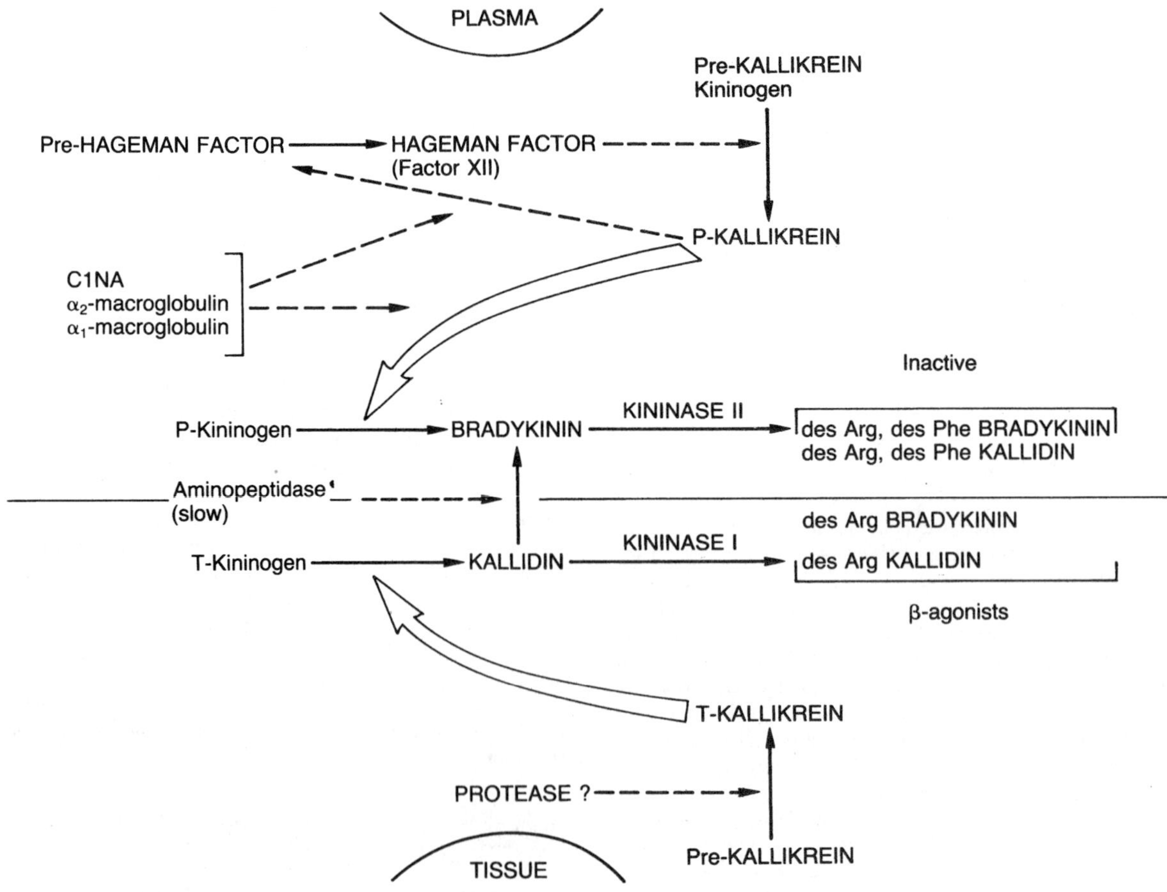

FIGURE 24.5 The enzymic pathways leading to the release and metabolism of bradykinin and kallidin.

TABLE 24.6 The metabolic products of kallidin and bradykinin, and their activity on bradykinin receptor subtypes (B_1 and B_2), in comparison with synthetic analogues

SUBSTRATE	ENZYME	PRODUCT	PRODUCT STRUCTURE	B_1	B_2
Plasma kininogen	Plasma kallikrein	Bradykinin	Arg-Pro-Pro-Gly-Phe-Ser-Pro-Phe-Arg	+	+++
Tissue kininogen	Tissue kallikrein	Kallidin	Lys-Arg-Pro-Pro-Gly-Phe-Ser-Pro-Phe-Arg	+	+++
Bradykinin	Kininase I	Des-arg bradykinin	Arg-Pro-Pro-Gly-Phe-Ser-Pro-Phe	+++	0
Kallidin	Kininase I	Des-arg kallidin	Lys-Arg-Pro-Pro-Gly-Phe-Ser-Pro-Phe	+++	0
Bradykinin	Kininase II	Des-arg-des-phe bradykinin	Arg-Pro-Pro-Gly-Phe-Ser-Pro	0	0
Kallidin	Kininase II	Des-arg-des-phe kallidin	Lys-Arg-Pro-Pro-Gly-Phe-Ser-Pro	0	0
	Synthetic	D-arg[hyp^{2,3}thi^{5,8}D-phe^{7}]bradykinin	D-Arg-Hyp-Hyp-Gly-Thi-Ser-D-Phe-Thi-Arg	0	− − −

0 = Inactive; − = antagonist; + = agonist; − − − = Potent antagonist; + + + = potent agonist.

activity is markedly slower than that of the kininases. Circulating kinins are deactivated mainly by kininase II (angiotensin-converting enzyme) found in vascular beds and lung. The action of kininase I, however, does not result in the complete loss of biological activity, and may even induced an altered profile of kinin activity (see below).

Actions

The physiology of the kinins is poorly understood in comparison to our knowledge of their synthesis and metabolism. Bradykinin and kallidin act on receptors which have been distinguished by their selectivity for various vascular preparations[30] and compared with the respective kininase I metabolites (Table 24.6), in the presence and absence of various antagonist peptides. Briefly, the vascular contractile effects of kinins on the rabbit aorta and mesenteric vein are mediated by B_1 receptors and the vascular relaxation of preparations such as the dog carotid artery and the contraction of the rabbit jugular vein are mediated by the B_2 receptor. The kinins bradykinin and kallidin have selectivity for the B_2 receptor while the kininase I derivatives have selectivity for the B_1 receptor.

From this it can be seen that the kinins may play an important role in vascular tone or blood pressure regulation. Bradykinin induces a profound fall in systemic blood pressure on iv administration via an action on systemic arteriolar endothelial B_2 receptors which induce the release of EDRF and vasodilator prostaglandins.[31] Most large arteries and veins are contracted. The blush response is induced, and blood vessels in muscle, viscera and kidney are dilated. This, coupled with the systemic arteriolar dilatation and venoconstriction increases venous return and induces a reflex increase in cardiac output and heart rate. The arteriolar vasodilatation may be, in part, mediated by the induction of histamine release.

The tissue kinin pathway is involved in the regulation of blood pressure since stimulation of sensory nerve endings in rabbit ear, dog's splenic and carotid arteries significantly alters systemic blood pressure. On the other hand, the use of antagonists has not provided corroborative evidence, but has revealed that the kinin system may act to reduce the actions of pressor agents.[32] Aldosterone increases renal tissue kallikrein activity, and bradykinin receptors found on the collecting duct, coupled with increased chloride transport, suggest a local role for kinins in renal function.

By far the most important actions of the kinins, however, are those regarding pain and inflammation. Plasma kallikrein itself has potent effects on neutrophil function, namely potent chemotactic activity, it primes the release of reactive oxygen species, induces elastase release and activates collagenase from procollagenase. Neutrophils are also capable of releasing kallikreins and kinins. Injected intradermally, the kinins produce the wheal and flare reaction, and pain. The action of bradykinin already described on arterioles and venules leads to oedema formation and this can be compounded by the induction of endothelial cell retraction, as with histamine. Plasma kinin synthesis is accelerated at the inflammatory locus, as in urate crystal or carageenin-induced inflammation for example,[33] and kininogen formation by the liver in various animal models of inflammation is significantly raised. Bradykinin is also a potent inducer of histamine release from mast cells and basophils, as well as prostaglandins from fibroblasts and endothelial cells.

It is interesting to note that B_1 receptor expression occurs in animal models of inflammation, such that the inactive kininase I metabolite of bradykinin, des-Arg-bradykinin, has vasodilator activity in lipopolysaccharide(LPS)-treated rabbits.[34] Triton X-100 chemical inflammation in the rat bladder also induces B_1-receptor expression. It is also feasible that kininase-II inhibition by angiotensin-converting enzyme inhibitors may lead to kininase-I derived kinin products that retain B_1 agonist activity and produce related side-effects. This remains to be proven.

The effect of kinins released at the inflammatory site on nociception is well documented. B_2 receptors are localized at those sites involved in nociception. Bradykinin produces pain when applied to a blister base, and when injected intradermally, giving a burning sensation.

A role for the kinin pathway in the chronicity of disease is being recognized. There are indications that T-lymphocyte proliferation and tumour necrosis factor release from monocytes can be stimulated by kinins along with interleukin-1. It has also been noted that whilst the half-life of kinins in exudate is very short, the slower inhibition of kallikrein could allow the sustained formation of kinins. Also at the inflammatory site, the acid conditions would reduce kininase activity and thus prolong the duration of kinin action.

Kinins in disease states

The lack of effective modulators of kinin production or action in the clinic has limited the exploration of the role of kinins in human disease. Our present knowledge is reviewed elsewhere.[29,32] Their presence and increased synthetic capacity have remained as the only indicators. Bradykinin has been assayed during rhinitis in allergic individuals challenged with ragweed pollen. Certain protozoal infections are coupled with the activation of the kinin pathway which also occurs following burns. Bradykinin is formed, and kininogen depletion occurs, during episodes of laryngeal oedema in hereditary angioedema resulting from C1NA defects since C1NA inhibits plasma kallikrein (see Fig. 24.5). Kinin participation in disseminated vascular coagulation and endotoxic shock has also been proposed. Bradykinin is found in the synovial fluid of patients suffering from rheumatoid arthritis, and levels of kinins are raised during acute phases of gout.[35]

The use of the B_1- and B_2-receptor antagonist *d*-Arg[4-hydroxyPro-^{3}dPhe]bradykinin (HOE 140)[29,36] has been assessed in initial clinical studies and shows promise in the relief of rhinovirus-induced cold symptoms, pain from burns and certain clinical measurements in allergic asthma.

SUBSTANCE-P

Peptidergic neurones contain a variety of neuropeptides such as substance-P, calcitonin-derived growth factor and the neurokinins, which are involved in the mediation of pain and inflammation. These can be released under the influence of mechanical or chemical stimuli, including the consequences of inflammation. It is becoming increasingly apparent that these peptides, especially substance-P, play a significant role in the mediation of pain and inflammation.[37]

Substance-P is an undecapeptide that is localized in preformed granules within primary sensory neurones. It is a vasodilator *in vitro* and induces extravasation. Work with analogues has illustrated that there are at least two receptors for substance-P, though they are poorly characterized. Its action is terminated by an enkephalinase that is membrane bound to the presynaptic neurone and which generates the inactive nonapeptide of amino acids 1–10. Specific inhibition of this enzyme may potentiate the action of substance-P.

When injected intradermally, substance-P induces the wheal and flare response in skin, as well as itch and hyperalgesia. This is consistent with its localization within the nociceptive neurones, and its involvement in the axon reflex stimulating peripheral fibres that terminate near blood vessels, connective tissue and smooth muscle. However, substance-P also provokes histamine release from mast cells.[38] The H_1 antagonists diphenhydramine and chlorcyclizine,[39] as well as mast cell depletion, inhibit the reaction. Treatment of human skin with capsaicin, which depletes unmyelinated sensory fibres of substance-P, inhibits the vasodilatation of the flare but not the oedema of the wheal induced by histamine.[40] There are therefore complex interactions that interfere with the interpretation of such findings. However, *in vitro* studies with inflammatory cells illustrate that substance-P released during inflammation may have profound actions on the inflammatory response, stimulating immunoglobulin release from B lymphocytes, reactive oxygen species from macrophages, neutrophil activation as well as fibroblast and T-lymphocyte proliferation.[33]

The involvement of substance-P in inflammatory joint disease is an example where its role is being seriously considered. Rheumatoid synoviocytes release collagenase and PGE_2 in response to substance-P. Studies with hemiplegic patients suffering from rheumatoid arthritis show that the hemiplegic limb remains unaffected. Animal studies, concentrating on adjuvant-induced arthritis, have shown that severe disease is associated with increased levels of substance-P within the joint, and that mild disease can be exacerbated by substance-P administration. Administration of capsaicin reduces the disease severity. These data are taken to suggest the importance of neurogenic inflammation in the maintenance of inflammatory disease.[41]

NON-STEROIDAL ANTI-INFLAMMATORY DRUGS (NSAIDs)

Aspirin, the predecessor of all the NSAIDs, has been recognized as an analgesic (in the form of extracts of willow bark) since ancient times. However, it was not until 1876 that salacin, the principal active ingredient in willow bark, was shown to have anti-inflammatory effects.[42,43] In the 1940s aspirin was employed in sufficient dosages to achieve maximum anti-inflammatory and analgesic properties. With these doses came the full spectrum of side-effects and the search to find a safer NSAID. The first step forward was the observation that the pure salicylate forms of salicylic acid – that is, those without acetylation – were significantly less gastrotoxic. The search has progressed: the 1990 edition of the *Extra Pharmacopoeia* lists approximately 150 currently available NSAIDs. Figure 24.6 classifies them according to their chemical structure.

In 1989, 23 million prescriptions were written for NSAIDs. These agents may now be self-prescribed in the form of ibuprofen (Nurofen^R). The fact that NSAIDs are consumed in enormous quantities, and that they are used only for the relief of symptoms in the majority of the conditions for which they are prescribed, focuses our attention on the side-effects of these agents. These range from the trivial (e.g. skin irritation) to the severe, even life-threatening (e.g. gastric ulceration and renal toxicity). What has therefore come to shape the usage of these drugs is not their superiority in terms of efficacy (although there are differences between them) but their comparative toxicity,

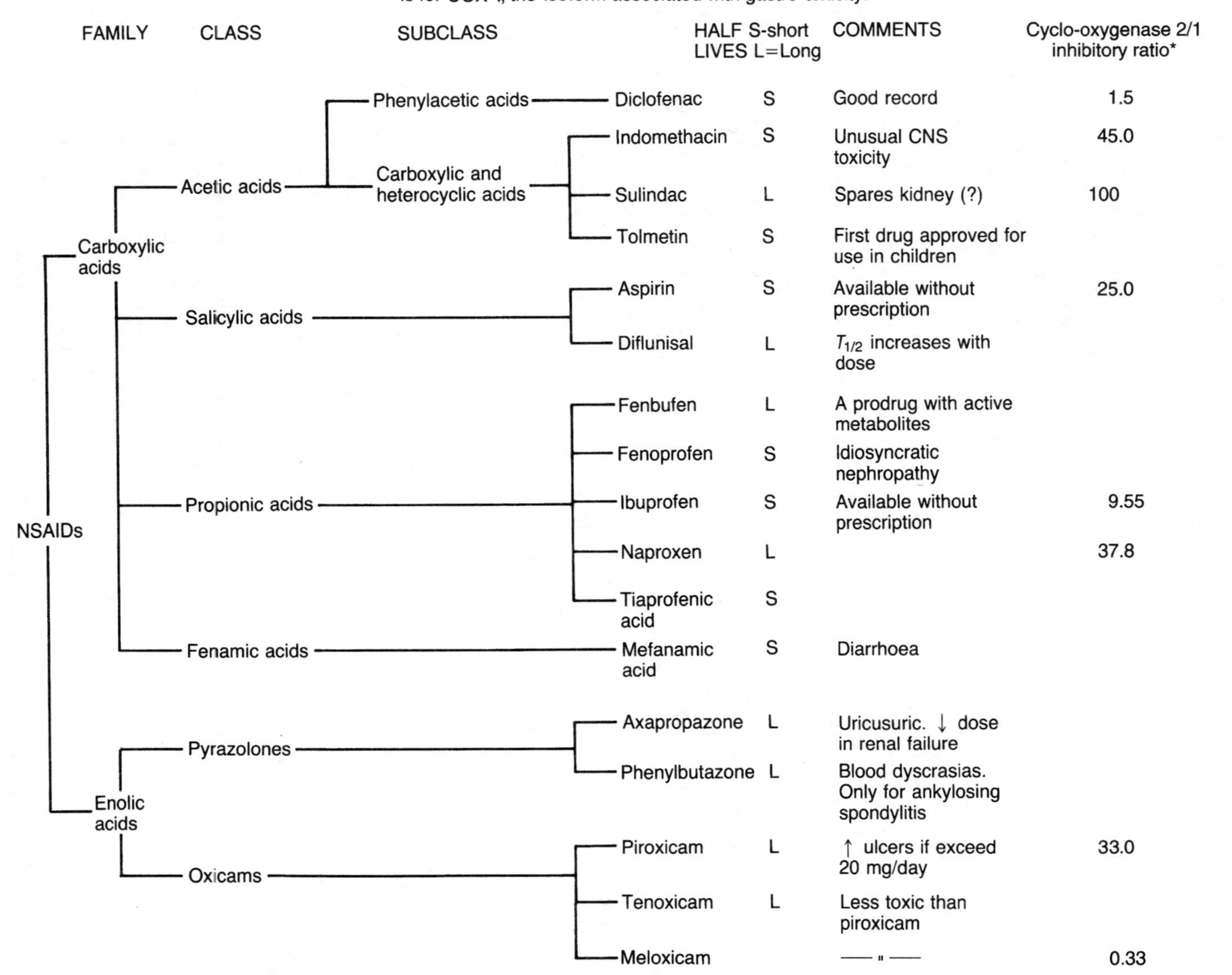

FIGURE 24.6 The non-steroid anti-inflammatory drugs (NSAIDs).

in particular, which NSAID causes the least gastrointestinal irritation.

The NSAIDs are used alone, or in combination with other drugs, to provide consistent analgesia and suppression of inflammatory events. They are effective in a wide range of conditions (Table 24.7) and thus are prescribed by a wide range of physicians.[44] (The use of NSAIDs in the management of chronic pain is described in Chapter 26.) These drugs are also available in a wide range of formulations including slow release and intradermal, thus increasing the likelihood of patient compliance. The emergence of other agents (which will be described later) that modify the destructive rheumatic processes has not replaced the NSAIDs, but they are invariably complementary to them. While there is no doubt of their effectiveness, it has been more difficult to determine their mechanism of action.

Mechanism of action

Although the usefulness of aspirin has been recognized throughout this century, the biological basis for its action eluded understanding until 1971. It was found that indomethacin, aspirin, and sodium salicylate inhibited prostaglandin (PG) synthesis *in vitro* (Fig. 24.4). Aspirin irreversibly acetylates cyclo-oxygenase whereas the other NSAIDs do so in a reversible manner. These effects apply to both forms of cyclo-oxygenase, though different NSAIDs have varying affinities for cyclo-oxygenase-1 (COX-1) and cyclo-oxygenase-2 (COX-2) (see Fig. 24.6). This inhibition accounts for both the anti-inflammatory effect as well as many of the important side-effects (see below). The analgesic effect of NSAIDs is most apparent where pain is secondary to inflammation or injury. Prostaglandins can induce pain directly but this occurs only in high concentrations not expected *in vivo*. However, PGs can enhance the sensitivity of nociceptors to bradykinin and histamine when they are present in minute concentrations.

Aspirin and NSAIDs are also effective antipyretic agents in situations where the fever is secondary to an inflammatory condition; the elevation in temperature is due to an increase in the synthesis of PGE_2 in the hypothalamus that is inhibited by NSAIDs.[45]

Gastrointestinal mucosal lesions with a notable propensity for bleeding, and also impact on clotting mechanism and platelets are known to be due to the inhibition of cyclo-oxygenase-1 and the blockade of PG synthesis.[46] Thus the fact that the non-acetylated form of sulphasalicylic acid inhibits PG synthesis far less than the acetylated form explains why it is less gastrotoxic. However, acetyl sulphasalicylic and sulphasalicylic acid are equipotent in efficacy. Furthermore, the discrepancy between the dose of aspirin needed to inhibit PG formation *in vitro* and *in vivo* and the higher dose required to induce an anti-inflammatory effect *in vivo* provides additional evidence against PG suppression as the sole mechanism of action of NSAIDs. The differential inhibition of COX-1 and COX-2 by various NSAID might explain further the varying effects of these drugs.

Inhibition of neutrophil activation has been proposed as an alternative for NSAID activity.[47] During the inflammatory process neutrophils migrate to inflamed sites such as joints. They then release a variety of inflammatory mediators. This process has been shown to be inhibited by a wide variation of NSAIDs such as ibuprofen and indomethacin *in vitro* and this inhibition is not PG dependent. Other possible mechanisms that have been proposed include the effects on lymphokine production, inactivation of lysosomal enzymes and scavenging free oxygen radicals. Salicylates and other NSAIDs have been found to inhibit the lipoxygenase pathway. Benoxaprofen was a powerful inhibitor of lipoxygenase formation but had to be withdrawn because of toxicity.[48] Agents that inhibit only the lipoxygenase pathway have been developed and are known to be effective anti-inflammatory drugs. However, problems with toxicity have prevented them from being used in the clinical setting at present.

TABLE 24.7 Diagnosis for which NSAIDs have a role

Osteoarthritis
Rheumatoid arthritis
Gout
Bursitis
Sprains/strains/fractures
Surgical aftercare
Dysmenorrhea
Back pain
Headache and non-specific pains, e.g. cramp

Pharmacokinetics

The pharmacokinetics of different NSAIDs vary to some degree among the subgroups. Absorption of NSAIDs is achieved by rapid passive diffusion through the upper gastrointestinal tract mucosa. Appreciable concentrations are found in the plasma in 30 min and levels peak at 2 h with most NSAIDs. These figures vary according to which type of preparation is used: liquid preparations are absorbed most rapidly; time-released and enteric-coated preparations are absorbed more slowly. Other factors influencing the rate of absorption, include gastric emptying time, the contents of the stomach, rate of tablet disintegration, solubility and concurrent drug therapy. Drugs are not absorbed as well in the elderly with diminished gastrointestinal blood flow and motility, delayed gastric emptying and reduced acid production.[49]

The half-life differs between the NSAIDs; most NSAIDs can be grouped according to whether they have a short or long half-life (see Fig. 24.6). NSAIDs are avidly bound by serum albumin. At normal concentrations, between 1 and 20% are available for tissue distribution depending on the particular NSAID. Some NSAIDs, such as diclofenac and phenylbutazone, accumulate in the synovial fluid but this has not been shown to improve their effectiveness. The hypoalbuminaemia seen in chronic rheumatic disease and in the elderly results in a higher unbound concentration. In the case of salicylates, as drug concentration increases proportionately less is bound to albumin unlike other drugs where the fraction of protein-bound drug remains constant (it is assumed, though not proven, that this is the case for other NSAIDs). Therefore at higher concentrations more drug is available for distribution into the tissues – an important consideration when evaluating acute intoxication. A patient may be clinically ill despite relatively low serum salicylate levels due to the amount of salicylate present in the tissues. The acidosis seen in salicylate poisoning increases further the volume of distribution.

In the case of salicylates biotransformation proceeds via hepatic microsomal enzymatic pathways. Five metabolites are formed and then excreted by the kidney. The enzymes that are involved are divided into those that follow zero-order kinetics and those that follow first-order kinetics.[50] The result is that at moderate and high doses of salicylate the concentration rises rapidly. Some NSAIDs undergo substantial first-pass metabolism: only 50% of diclofenac is available systemically.

Urinary excretion of salicylic acid and its metabolites occurs through a combination of glomerular filtration and proximal tubular secretion. The excretion is increased by an alkaline urine and by a high urine flow rate. It is affected by other drugs that compete for proximal tubular transport and of course by the overall renal function. As is mentioned below, salicylates will, via their effect on renal blood flow, decrease their own excretion, although this is only of significance where renal function is already compromised. A significant proportion of some NSAIDs is excreted in the faeces, for example 25% in the case of sulindac.

Side-effects

The side-effects of NSAIDs have been recognized for many years. They account for 25% of all the reports of adverse reactions received by the Committee on Safety of Medicines (CSM). Many of these reports were of gastrointestinal haemorrhage. In England it has been estimated that NSAIDs cause 4000 deaths per year.[51] As with many drugs, the elderly are more susceptible to the development of adverse effects of these drugs. As alluded to earlier, the pharmacokinetics are altered so that drug elimination time is prolonged. Both the elderly and NSAIDs are a heterogeneous group and treatment has to be individualized. Brater suggests, for instance, that the dose of ibuprofen should not be changed in the elderly but that the dose of naproxen should be halved.[52]

By far the most important of these side-effects are those related to the gut. About 60% of these reports received by the CSM report dyspepsia. It has been confirmed in several trials that there is a close correlation between NSAID ingestion and ulceration; this is especially true in the elderly who are more likely to be hospitalized or die as a result. There is no correlation between symptoms and signs.[51]

The manner in which NSAIDs cause gastric mucosal injury has been studied extensively.[53] Initial damage is thought to occur via an acid-mediated topical effect. This initiates the breakdown of mucosal defence which is accelerated by the back diffusion of hydrogen ions entering the epithelial and subepithelial cell layers. These cells are normally surrounded by a neutral pH environment and are rapidly destroyed by acid. PGs synthesised from arachidonic acid by cyclo-oxygenase-1 are thought to play an even more important role, particularly PGE_2. They are considered central to maintaining blood flow; they enhance the secretion of mucus and bicarbonate and may increase hydrophobic lipids. The inhibition of cyclo-oxygenase-1 by non-selective NSAIDs is therefore a major cause of gastric toxicity. In addition to the inhibition of PG synthesis, NSAIDs inhibit platelet thromboxane synthesis increasing the risk of bleeding still further. Not surprisingly, therefore, the risk factors for gastrointestinal bleeding include old age, cirrhosis, coagulation abnormalities and platelet disorders.

Several therapeutic approaches have been used to try and overcome the gastrointestinal mucosal damage caused by NSAIDs. Simple manoeuvres such as using enteric-coated tablets significantly reduce the incidence of gastric ulcers. H_2 antagonists only protect the gastric mucosa to a limited extent but the most promising agent is misoprostol, a synthetic PG analogue. This has been shown to protect against gastric ulcers in patients taking NSAIDs and aids healing of both gastric and duodenal ulcers. Interestingly, misoprostol does not interfere with the therapeutic action of NSAIDs.

NSAIDs impair platelet aggregation, thereby prolonging the bleeding time via its inhibition of endoperoxides and thromboxane A_2. This inhibition is reversible in the case of NSAIDs, but not with aspirin. This effect should be carefully considered in patients undergoing surgery and those already affected by bleeding disorders. Preoperatively, these drugs should be stopped for a long enough time to allow for the drug to be excreted – that is, about four or five times the half-life of the drug. Drugs such as ibuprofen can be discontinued 18–24 h preoperatively, whereas drugs with a longer half-life, such as piroxicam, require 8 days for complete elimination.

Patients with normal renal function are not usually affected by NSAIDs, but when the glomerular filtration rate falls these agents can have serious effects. This is particularly true in the elderly being treated with diuretics but other groups can also be affected, such as patients with heart failure or with cirrhosis of the liver. Inhibition of the synthesis of PGs removes the control exerted on the vasoconstrictive effects of angiotensin II and catecholamines, which leads to a reduction in renal blood flow. Moreover, these drugs promote sodium and water retention and can have a profound effect on diuresis, natriuresis and potassium homeostasis. In addition to impairing renal function severe hypertension can be precipitated, particularly in those patients already taking antihypertensive medication. Other mechanisms of NSAID toxicity have been implicated and include direct tubular toxicity, immunological mechanisms and precipitation of uric acid crystals.[54] These untoward actions may induce the development of renal papillary necrosis, acute tubular necrosis, functional renal insufficiency, chronic interstitial nephritis, obstructive nephropathy or glomerulonephritis. The so-called analgesic nephropathy, which is characterized by the progression of renal papillary necrosis to end-stage renal failure, can be induced by numerous NSAIDs though it is rare. Sulindac, a prodrug converted to its active form in the liver, is the one NSAID thought to have limited effects on blood pressure and renal function. Indomethacin, on the other hand, has a worse reputation for exacerbating renal impairment and hypertension.

Some form of hepatic dysfunction can occur with all the NSAIDs.[55] Most cause mild, reversible damage revealed by elevation of transaminases. Rarely more severe hepatic lesions may ensue, capable of causing fatal liver failure. Diclofenac, sulindac and phenylbutazone have a higher potential toxicity than other NSAIDs. In contrast, mefanamic acid and ibuprofen are particularly safe. Benoxaprofen had to be withdrawn because of hepatotoxicity; it resulted in over sixty deaths from cholestatic jaundice and consequent renal failure. Reye's syndrome, characterized by acute encephalopathy and fatty degeneration of the liver, has a strong epidemiological association with aspirin ingestion in children. This uncommon but frequently fatal disease has declined in incidence as most western countries have curtailed its use in children, especially as an antipyretic.

Intolerance reactions to NSAIDs are secondary only to gastrointestinal side-effects in incidence and importance. These effects involve mainly the respiratory tract and skin, for example asthma, laryngeal oedema, urticaria and Stevens–Johnson syndrome. Occasionally, complete respiratory and vasomotor collapse can occur requiring intravenous adrenaline. These reactions are not generally thought to involve allergic mechanisms. An individual who reacts to one NSAID may show intolerance to other NSAIDs of diverse chemical classes. It is more likely that inhibition of PG synthesis plays a role, for example by diverting arachidonic acid through the lipoxygenase pathway.

Central nervous system side-effects are particularly frequent with indomethacin and this is attributed to the unique serotonin-like ring structure of indomethacin. These side-effects include headaches, giddiness and confusion. Other NSAIDs have also caused CNS side-effects in elderly patients which range from cognitive function to paranoid ideation.

Other side-effects that may occur include bone marrow depression. Although phenylbutazone is the principal offender (a death rate of 47 patients per 1 million patients has been reported), indomethacin and dipyrone have also been implicated.[56] NSAIDs (particularly pyrazolone derivatives and indomethacin) have been shown to have an adverse effect on the fetal circulation, delay the progression of labour, and via the mothers' milk, to cause cyanotic crises and haemolytic anaemia in breast-fed infants. A wide range of cutaneous side-effects has also occurred including benign morbilliform reactions, vesiculobullous eruptions and erythema multiforme.

In recent years it has been suggested that the use of NSAIDs in osteoarthritis might favour the progression of the disease by inhibiting repair mechanisms. A recent trial comparing indomethacin, a strong prostaglandin inhibitor, with azapropazone, a weak prostaglandin inhibitor, showed that indomethacin hastened the development in osteoarthritis faster than azapropazone.[57] However the trial has been criticized in many respects. These include the trial design (it was not double blinded) and the type of prostaglandin measured in the synovial fluid, and it has been pointed out that NSAIDs can affect bone remodelling by mechanisms other than prostaglandin synthesis inhibition such as their effect on osteocyte activity.

The recent discovery of cyclo-oxygenase-2 has led to an explosion of research[58] into the differential effects of NSAIDs on the two isoforms. Compounds in preclinical research that are selective for cyclo-oxygenase-2 (in excess of 1000 times) exhibit gastro toxicity, which is very low or even absent in rats. Meloxican, a new NSAID, which has three-fold activity against cyclo-oxygenase-2 (Fig. 24.6) as opposed to cyclo-oxygenase-1 appears to have promise, and may be superseded by more selective drugs within a matter of years.

Drug interactions

NSAIDs have the potential to interact with a variety of other drugs (Table 24.8).[59] Even in young subjects clinically important interactions occur. These usually take the form of kinetic interactions but pharmacodynamic interactions can occur as well. NSAIDs can reduce the glomerular filtration rate, particularly in the already compromised kidneys. This can lead to a reduction in the excretion of drugs that are eliminated

TABLE 24.8 NSAID interactions

DRUG AFFECTED	EFFECT
Anticoagulants, warfarin	Inhibition of metabolism
Antidiabetics, sulphonylureas	Enhanced effect
Antiepileptics, phenytoin	Enhanced effect due to increased plasma displacement
Antihypertensives	Antagonism of effect; risk of hyperkalaemia; increased risk of renal failure on administration of captopril
Cardiac glycosides filtration	Exacerbation of heart failure, reduced glomerular rate, and increased digoxin concentration
Diuretics effect	Increased risk of nephrotoxicity and reduction in diuretic
Methotrexate	Excretion delayed

by glomerular filtration. This is a potential mechanism whereby NSAIDs can interact with methotrexate leading to increased plasma concentrations. Competition for binding sites on albumin rarely leads to any significant interactions. One example that has recently been documented involves the interaction with phenytoin. In this case the displacement of phenytoin from albumin leads to an increased clearance rate resulting in the depletion of folate. This in turn leads to a reduction in the clearance of phenytoin and an increased concentration.

The majority of NSAIDs are metabolized by the liver and thus have the potential to interact with other drugs that are metabolized by the same hepatic enzymes. Two important examples are the ability of some NSAIDs (e.g. phenylbutazone, azapropazone) to interact with tolbutamide and warfarin due to the inhibition of their metabolism. The hypoglycaemic effect and the anticoagulant effect are potentiated respectively. Interestingly, while the tolbutamide concentration rises when coprescribed with a NSAID, the warfarin concentration does not. This is because only the metabolism of the potent S-isomer is inhibited, while the metabolism of the less effective R-isomer is induced. A dynamic interaction is also possible via the direct effect NSAIDs have on clotting mechanisms through the platelet.

The effect of certain diuretics is decreased by NSAIDs. For instance, the ability of bumetanide to induce water and sodium excretion is reduced by 20% by indomethacin. This is achieved via two different mechanisms: first by PG-mediated inhibition of renal blood flow and second by limiting chloride delivery to the distal tubule. This latter property is made use of therapeutically in Bartter's syndrome where a defect of chloride absorption occurs.

GOUT

Gout is unique among the common inflammatory rheumatic conditions in that it is potentially curable. It is caused by the precipitation of urate crystals in joints, which is related to the level of urate in the blood. The inflammatory response involves local infiltration of granulocytes which phagocytose the urate crystals. This leads to the release of a chemotactic protein, the initiation of the kallikrein system, the activation of complement, and the disruption of intracellular lysosomes with the release of pro-inflammatory mediators. How the crystals form in the joint is not completely understood.

Drugs used in the therapy of gout can be divided into those that are employed in prophylaxis (i.e. to reduce the serum level of urate) and those for acute gout. This division is important since the main drug used for prophylaxis, allopurinol, can precipitate an attack of gout or make an attack of acute gout worse.

Acute gout

The standard therapy for acute gout includes NSAIDs (e.g. indomethicin) and colchicine. High doses of NSAIDs are frequently employed for this exquisitely painful condition. If this approach is unsuccessful, or causes side-effects (much more likely), then colchicine is the drug of choice. The drug was recognized for the treatment of gout by the ancient Greeks, but its use has always been limited by its side-effects.

Colchicine works by interfering with neutrophil function, particularly migration. This is achieved by its effects on microtubular systems within the cell leading to its disaggregation. It is thought that colchicine binds to tubulin and prevents its polymerization. An additional effect of importance is its inhibition of chemotactic factors such as leukotriene B_4. The observation that the earlier the colchicine is started in the attack, the more effective it is, may be the clinical correlate of the finding that colchicine interferes with the initial mechanisms of inflammation. Colchicine works in about 12 h compared with NSAIDs which can take up to 24–48 h.

The dose of colchicine has been limited by its side-effects.[60] About 60–80% of patients on a full therapeutic dose develop diarrhoea, abdominal pain and vomiting. In chronic usage bone marrow depression, peripheral neuritis, hair loss, amenorrhoea and azoospermia have been reported. Even more important is the cumulative toxicity that can result unwittingly if colchicine is given to patients with diminished renal or hepatic function. This is particularly true when intravenous colchicine is given (not now licensed for routine use in Britain) as well as oral colchicine. This toxicity includes cytopenias, hepatocellular failure, renal shut down and seizures.

The pharmacokinetics explain why cumulative toxicity occurs. After rapid absorption from the gastrointestinal tract, colchicine swiftly leaves the plasma and passes into cells. Interestingly, cells previously exposed to the drug are more sensitive to its effects. After a single dose, only 10% of the drug is excreted during the first 24 h. In healthy patients colchicine can be detected in the cells 10 days after a single dose, implying a half-life of 30 h. Colchicine is excreted in the bile, faeces and urine. Although classically associated with the treatment of gout, it has also been used successfully in familial Mediterranean fever, and its use is being evaluated in Behçet's disease, amyloidosis, cutaneous necrotizing vasculitis, and the skin manifestations of scleroderma. Colchicine has no clinically significant drug interactions.

Prophylaxis of gout[61]

Allopurinol has now been in use for over 20 years and has done much to reduce the incidence of uncontrolled hyperuricaemia and gout. Initially tested unsuccessfully as an anticancer drug, it was shown to protect the development of hyperuricaemia when cytotoxic agents were used. As an analogue of hypoxanthine, it reduces urate production, first by its action in blocking xanthine oxidase, which increases the concentration of urate precursors xanthine and hypoxanthine, and second by blocking the production of new purines (Fig. 24.7).

Allopurinol is completely absorbed in the gastrointestinal tract. It is detectable in plasma for only a few hours. Most of the allopurinol is converted to oxipurinol (also a potent inhibitor of xanthine oxidase) which has a longer half-life ranging from 14 to 28 h. Both allopurinol and oxipurinol inhibit the metabolism of allopurinol to alloxanthine and therefore the half-life of allopurinol increases with the inhibition of xanthine oxidase. Both allopurinol and oxipurinol are excreted in the kidney with a renal clearance of around 20 ml/min. The renal excretion of oxipurinol is increased by uricosuric compounds.

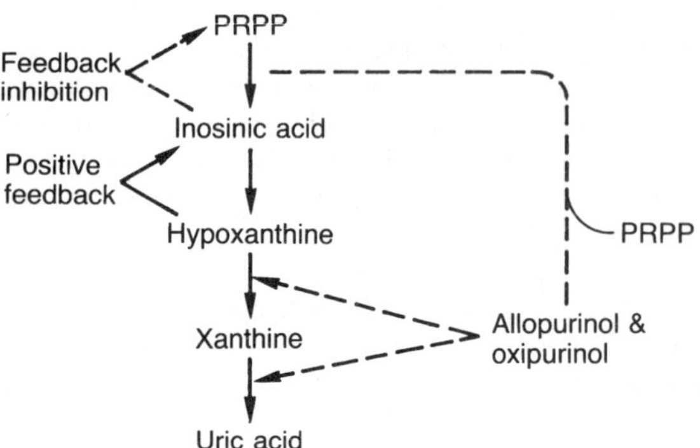

FIGURE 24.7 Effects of allopurinol treatment on uric acid synthesis. Dashed lines represent inhibition. PRPP, phosphoribosylpyrophosphate.

The purine analogue chemotherapeutic (and anti-inflammatory) agents, such as 6-mercaptopurine and azathioprine, are inactivated by xanthine oxidase. When these drugs are given with allopurinol, their blood level may rise, leading to toxicity. Allopurinol inhibits hepatic microsomal enzymes and enhances the effects of anticoagulants such as warfarin and nicoumalone. The half-life of probenecid is prolonged by 50% through the same mechanism.

The most frequent side-effect of allopurinol is a maculopapular rash occurring in about 5% of patients. Interestingly, this skin rash is more frequently seen in those patients also taking ampicillin. Hypersensitivity reactions are usually manifested by rashes but also include fever, eosinophilia, leukocytosis, deteriorating renal function, and hepatocellular injury. Death occurs in about 20% of these patients reported with hypersensitivity reactions. Bone marrow suppression may also occur. Untoward consequences of normal therapeutic effects deserve special mention, particularly precipitation of an acute attack. Formation of xanthine stones is also included in this category. Side-effects are more frequently seen in renal insufficiency and with the concomitant administration of thiazide diuretics.

Uricosuric drugs are also used in the prophylaxis of gout; however, their use is declining because of the acceptability and efficiency of allopurinol. Although there is a wide variety of drugs that can act in this way, the two most commonly used in this country are probenecid and sulphinpyrazone. Both these agents work by inhibiting the tubular reabsorption of filtered urate.

Probenecid

The increase in renal clearance of urate can be substantial but does not exceed 50% even with high concentrations of probenecid. The uricosuria is effectively blocked by salicylates in low dosages and in chronic renal failure. Probenecid is rapidly absorbed by the gastrointestinal tract. The half-life is about 6–12 h and is increased by allopurinol. It is highly protein bound and is rapidly metabolized by the liver. Probenecid interacts with a variety of other drugs by altering their metabolism. For instance, it reduces the excretion of a number of drugs such as indomethacin and penicillin. This latter effect is used to advantage in the therapy of infections. Side-effects are few and include hypersensitivity reactions and gastrointestinal complaints. Untoward consequences of normal therapeutic effects include acute gout and nephrolithiasis. In the latter case, where uric acid stones may be formed, it is advisable to alkanilize the urine in high-risk patients (those with normal renal function who are overproducers of uric acid).

Sulphinpyrazone

This drug is a derivative of phenylbutazone though it has no anti-inflammatory properties. It is about three to six times more potent than probenecid. It is rapidly absorbed from the gastrointestinal tract and has a half-life of 3 h. In addition to its uricosuric effects, it also has a beneficial effect on platelet function resulting in reduction of thrombotic events. This effect is thought to be mediated through the inhibition of PG synthesis. The uricosuric effects are blocked by salicylates and by a reduction in renal function. It has a similar side-effects profile to probenecid although being a derivative of phenylbutazone it rarely affects the bone marrow. Sulphinpyrazone has a number of drug interactions. The effects of warfarin and sulphonylureas are enhanced, the plasma concentration of phenytoin is increased and the plasma theophylline concentration is decreased.

CORTICOSTEROIDS

Corticosteroids have a long-standing role in the treatment of rheumatic diseases. Their introduction in 1949 for use in the treatment of rheumatoid arthritis transformed a disease that had no other effective treatment at the time. It was realized soon afterwards that their side-effects were substantial and dosage regimes have had to be modified. However, they still retain an important role in the treatment of this and many other rheumatic diseases. Alternate day therapy, which reduces the incidence of side-effects, is known to be effective in certain situations but in diseases such as systemic lupus erythematosis and dermatomyositis high daily doses are often required. In addition, the intravenous route may be used to administer high doses rapidly.

Mechanism of action

Corticosteroids have a wide range of actions on the immune system.[62] It has not been possible to identify which are clinically relevant, nor has it been possible to deduce a single mechanism of action by which these numerous effects occur. It is known that corticosteroids enter the cell and bind to a receptor by displacing a heat shock protein, HSP 90. The receptor/steroid complex passes to the nucleus and activates genes that affect the rate of synthesis of different proteins. There is no correlation between the number of receptors, their density or the binding constants and the efficacy of corticosteroids. HSP 90 is a highly conserved protein whose basal rate of synthesis is dramatically increased in conditions of heat and other forms of stress.

Probably the most important net effect of corticosteroids is the reduction of the number of effector cells at the inflammatory site. This occurs first by altering cellular traffic. Though there are more neutrophils in the circulation fewer egress into sites of inflammation. This is achieved in a number of ways. Corticosteroids inhibit the release of chemotactic factors from macrophages and neutrophils, including leukotriene B_4 and macrophage migration inhibition factor, and they reduce the synthesis of factors that increase vascular permeability such as PAF. There are fewer circulating lymphocytes, particularly T helper cells, due to redistribution to other lymphoid compartments. This is thought to be of benefit in autoimmune diseases by restoring the balance between helper and suppressor T cells.

The cells that are sequestered into the inflammatory site are made less effective by corticosteroids. Corticosteroids interfere with the immune network as outlined in Fig. 24.8. The balance of interleukins secreted by T cells is completely changed by corticosteroids; IL-2 production is suppressed while the release of IL-4 is enhanced. IL-4 inhibits many of the functions of macrophages. There is some evidence that T cells become resistant to all these effects through changing the type of T-cell receptor expressed on the cell surface. Monocytes are generally more sensitive to corticosteroids, depressing bactericidal activity and inhibiting release of mediators such as interleukin 1. As mentioned previously (see Fig. 24.4) corticosteroids

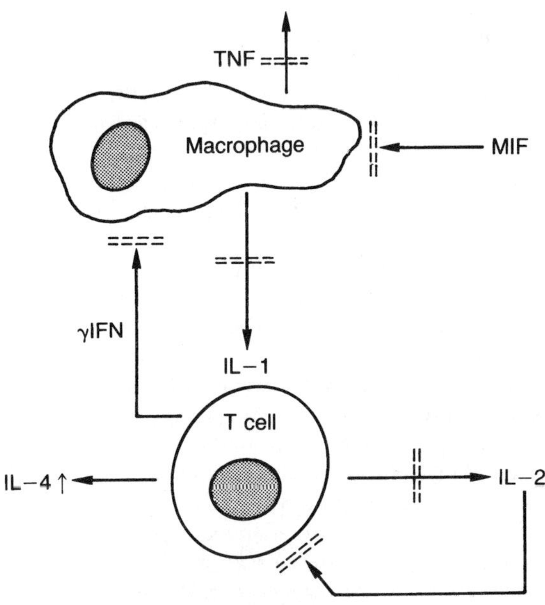

FIGURE 24.8 Effects of corticosteroids on the immune response. ⟶, inhibition of synthesis; ⟶, inhibition of effect; MIF, macrophage migration inhibition factor; TNF, tumour necrosis factor; γIFN, γ-interferon; IL, interleukin.

inhibit both prostaglandin and leukotriene production by inhibiting arachidonic acid release from phospholipids via the synthesis of lipocortin (as distinct from NSAIDs which inhibit prostaglandin production alone via its effect on cyclo-oxygenase).

Corticosteroids have also been shown to inhibit the synthesis of several complement components including C_3, and factors D and H.

Side-effects

The side-effects of corticosteroids are mentioned in detail elsewhere in the book. However, certain side-effects are worth emphasizing in the context of rheumatic diseases. Some of them can be caused by, or are more likely to occur in, the underlying disease while others mimic the disease process itself. In addition, many of the patients with rheumatic disease may be on long-term treatment, increasing the cumulative risk.

Perhaps the most important long-term side-effect is osteoporosis. This appears to relate to total cumulative dose and is more prominent in children and postmenopausal women. This is typically seen when more than 10 mg of steroid is used per day; whether osteoporosis occurs at lower dosages is disputed.[63,64] This is compounded by the fact that certain rheumatic diseases, particularly rheumatoid arthritis, can themselves lead to osteoporosis. The debilitating nature of rheumatoid arthritis with often profound functional impairment results in less exercise and often a poor diet, both of which can cause osteoporosis. Moreover, rheumatoid arthritis is relatively common in postmenopausal women who are also more prone to osteoporosis. Steroids induce osteoporosis both by reducing bone formation and by increasing bone resorption. In addition, they reduce the calcium absorption from the gut. The spine and ribs are affected at an early stage. The former explains the tendency to sustain vertebral compression fractures. A variety of agents have claimed to retard bone loss, the most recently introduced of these drugs, the biphosphonates, have been shown to be moderately effective.

Avascular necrosis is less common than osteoporosis and is thought to occur because of changes in bone microvasculature. As with osteoporosis, some of the rheumatic diseases, in particular systemic lupus erythematosus, may precipitate the condition.[65]

Steroid myopathy is frequently seen in patients who are maintained on high doses of steroids for long periods of time. Patients with inflammatory myositis often require large doses of steroids for a prolonged period of time. Ironically, it may be difficult to distinguish between the proximal muscle weakness of the disease and that caused by the corticosteroids. A muscle biopsy may be needed to distinguish them. The mechanism of action of steroid myopathy is unknown.

A natural extension of the mechanism of action of steroids is the reduced resistance it confers to infection. This very important consequence can increase both morbidity and even mortality in patients with rheumatic disease whose susceptibility to infection is increased by the underlying disease. Moreover, the usual signs of infection may be masked by the steroids. The consequences of this side-effect are particularly noticeable in systemic lupus erythematosis. As deaths from renal disease have fallen, those due to infection have risen and are closely related to the dose of steroids and other immunosuppressives prescribed.

Finally, corticosteroids can induce psychiatric effects in patients.[66] The commonest of these are mild elevation of mood and sleep disturbance. However, more profound changes can occur such as hypomania, depression and schizophrenia which are seen when high doses are used. This can lead to diagnostic confusion in patients with systemic lupus erythematosus who may suffer similar psychiatric problems due to the disease itself. In practice, however, steroids are rarely the cause of frank psychosis in these patients.

SLOW-ACTING ANTIRHEUMATIC DRUGS IN RHEUMATOID ARTHRITIS

A variety of slow-acting antirheumatic drugs (SAARD) have been developed for the treatment of rheumatoid arthritis. Because the cause of the disease is unknown, therapy has largely been directed at suppressing the inflammatory response, with the aim of diminishing symptoms and preventing joint damage. None of these compounds was developed specifically to treat rheumatoid arthritis but chance observations showed them to be effective. The mechanism of action that achieves this effect has not been delineated and therefore the principles guiding the use of these drugs are based on accumulated clinical experience. There is a wide variation in the way these drugs are employed. Table 24.9 summarizes the information about these drugs. Some of them are discussed in the text.

A characteristic feature of these drugs is a delayed onset of clinical effect. This applies both to the desired therapeutic effect and the side-effects both of which may not be apparent until months after the initiation of therapy and may persist for weeks or months after the therapy has been discontinued. This contrasts with the action of NSAIDs which are prompt and last only as long as the drug is continued.

Many, but not all, patients will respond to therapy with SAARD. No serological or clinical indicator will predict which patient will respond to any particular agent. Moreover, it is not possible to predict which patient will develop toxicity to these agents though it is thought (there have been no studies on this point) that those patients who are antinuclear antibody positive are more likely to develop side-effects when treated with gold or penicillamine. The decision as to which agent to use first is up to the clinician and is far from

TABLE 24.9 The slow-acting antirheumatic agents

DRUG	CHEMISTRY	PHARMACOKINETICS	MECHANISM OF ACTION	SIDE-EFFECTS	INTERACTIONS
Sulphasalazine	5-aminosalicylic acid linked to ⟶ sulphapyridine ⟶	5% absorbed 90% absorbed: metabolized in the liver ⟶	Unknown (Active moiety)	Gastrointestinal disturbance Rashes Neutropenia	Can interact with highly protein bound drugs
Gold	Sodium aurothiomalate: intramuscular	$t_{1/2}$ ↑ with duration of therapy Accumulates in body: 60% retained after 1g cumulative dose Excreted in renal and biliary tract	?Interferes with macrophage and T cell activation	Membranous nephropathy Rash (potential exfoliative dermatitis) Stomatitis Neutropenia	None relevant
	Auranofin: oral	Less retained in tissues than im preparation Almost all excreted in faeces	Unknown	As above but less common Diarrhoea in 30%	
Penicillamine	Analogue of cysteine plus extra methyl groups	Rapidly absorbed, half the dose rapidly excreted via the kidney Persists in body 3 months after stopping the drug	? Predominant effect on T helper cells	Membranous nephropathy Thrombocytopenia Rash Myasthenia	Antacids and iron decrease absorption
Antimalarials	Quinoline derivatives: hydroxychloroquine, chloroquine	Rapidly absorbed Persists in tissues up to 5 years after cessation of therapy Localizes to the eye	Unknown ? ↓ synthesis of arachidonic acid Interferes with antigen presentation	Retinal damage. More commonly seen with chloroquine though rare even with this drug	Antagonism of neostigmine. Antacids reduce absorption

being universally agreed but there a number of pharmacological considerations that are central to this issue. The most important of these is the efficacy/side-effects ratio of these drugs.

A number of successes have been reported with the use of combination therapy, particularly in severe disease.

Sulphasalazine

Sulphasalazine is frequently the first agent that is tried for control of rheumatoid arthritis when NSAIDs alone do not control the symptoms. Sulphasalazine is a conjugate of 5-aminosalicylic acid and sulphapyridine, which are linked by an azo band. Unlike ulcerative colitis and Crohn's disease, where the 5-aminosalicylic acid is known to be the effective moiety, the sulphapyridine moiety is thought to be the active compound though the activity of the parent molecule has not been discounted.[67] The mechanism of action is, however, unknown. The immunological effects of sulphasalazine are negligible but sulphasalazine has been shown to inhibit the lipoxygenase and cyclo-oxygenase pathway in neutrophils.[68] It also inhibits endothelial cell proliferation in synovium.

About one-third of the sulphasalazine is absorbed in the small intestine. The remainder is split in the distal small intestine and passes into the colon. Only a small proportion (<5%) of the 5-aminosalicylic acid is absorbed, whereas more than 90% of the sulphapyridine enters the circulation. Sulphapyridine undergoes N-acetylation, ring hydroxylation, and conjugation with glucuronic acid in the liver.[69] The rate of the acetylation is genetically determined and the slow acetylators have a higher incidence of adverse effects but no apparent difference in antirheumatic efficacy.

Side-effects are frequently seen with sulphasalazine though these are more annoying than serious. Nevertheless, they lead to the withdrawal of the drug in up to 30% of patients.[70] Almost all of these side-effects are seen in the first 3 months of therapy. The most common side-effects relate to the gastrointestinal tract (i.e. nausea, heartburn and epigastric discomfort). By using enteric-coated tablets and by slowly increasing the dose these can be avoided. A variety of skin rashes including maculopapular eruptions, urticaria and rarely toxic epidermal necrolysis can occur. Haematological effects are the most frequent serious reactions. Neutropenia, agranulocytosis, and megaloblastic anaemia have all been observed. Megaloblastic anaemia is most frequently seen during the first 3 months of treatment due to the antifolate activity of sulphasalazine.

Drug interactions with the 5-aminosalicylate moiety do not occur since the blood levels achieved are negligible. Sulphapyrazone, however, does achieve appreciable serum levels. Because it is highly protein bound it has the potential to interact with other protein-bound drugs such as warfarin and the sulphonylureas. Sulphasalazine can reduce the bioavailability of digoxin; the mechanism is unknown.

Gold

Forestier pioneered the use of gold for rheumatoid arthritis in 1924 in the belief that it had a common aetiology with tuberculosis for which gold therapy was then in vogue (it was later found to be of no value). He reported that 70–80% of 550 patients with chronic rheumatoid arthritis responded favourably to gold therapy.[71] There was no control group in his trials but, subsequently, appropriately controlled trials have confirmed this experience. Today it is used in both an intramuscular and oral form, the former being the only SAARD that has been shown to retard bone changes.

The chemistry of gold compounds is reviewed elsewhere.[72] The intramuscular form most commonly used is sodium aurothiomalate and this is rapidly absorbed into the circulation. The half-life of a 50 mg dose of sodium aurothiomalate is 7 days but with cumulative dosages the half-life lengthens into weeks and months reflecting the binding with tissues. After a cumulative dose of 1 g, 60% is retained in the body. Most of the gold is stored in the bone marrow, liver, skin and bone. Its excretion occurs via the renal and biliary routes, the former being the most important.

Auranofin is the oral preparation used but only 25% of the administered dose is absorbed slowly from the stomach. Much less is found in the synovium compared with injectable gold and a smaller proportion is retained in the body in other sites.

All significant preparations of intramuscular gold contain a gold sulphur bond and through this moiety gold is thought to exert its action by interfering with sulphydryl systems. At the cellular level the most likely explanation of its mechanism of action is that it interferes with the maturation and activation of macrophages.[73] Both antigen- and mitogen-induced responsiveness is suppressed due to the inhibitory action of gold on antigen presenting cells (such as macrophages) and lymphocytes. Moreover, gold accumulates in macrophages in synovial tissue. However, numerous studies have shown that gold has a wide variety of other effects on the immune system which may be directly due to the gold or may be epiphenomena.

Auranofin exerts its effects through its triethylphosphine group. It also has effects on macrophages, while other cell types are less affected.[74] The speed of action of these effects is swifter than observed with intramuscular gold due to the lypophilicity conveyed by the triethylphosphine group.

The side-effects of gold occur in about one-third of patients taking the drug and are the major limitation to therapy. Most reactions are trivial and consist of dermatitis, transient haematuria and proteinuria. More serious reactions include effects on the haemopoietic system, such as neutropenia, and on the liver and kidney. The incidence of serious reactions decreases as therapy is prolonged. Although auranofin is less often associated with these serious side-effects, about 40% of patients cannot tolerate it because of diarrhoea. All forms of gold should be avoided in renal impairment (glomerular filtration rate <50 ml/min), pregnancy and while breast feeding.

Penicillamine and antimalarials are used less often compared with gold and sulphasalazine (Table 24.9). The antimalarials have found a place in the arthropathy seen in systemic lupus erythematosus.

CYTOTOXIC AGENTS

Cytotoxic agents have been employed in the use of rheumatic diseases since the 1960s. These drugs are used in autoimmune rheumatic diseases such as in systemic lupus erythematosus, rheumatoid arthritis and myositis, especially when they are complicated by vasculitis. The use of these drugs is quite different from their use in neoplastic diseases (see Chapter 35). It is not the intention to destroy all abnormal cells with the often life-threatening consequences that ensue but to suppress the inflammatory response. In other words, whereas life-threatening side-effects are almost inevitable in the treatment of cancer they are not in the treatment of rheumatic diseases. However, the therapeutic window is narrow with all these drugs and side-effects are more likely to occur whenever these drugs are used. Moreover, although they are used in lower dosages, cytotoxic drugs may be used for much longer periods than in neoplastic diseases. Table 24.10 summarizes the pharmacology of the major cytotoxic agents. Methotrexate and cyclophosphamide are discussed in more detail below.

Methotrexate

Methotrexate, an antifolate compound, is now commonly used for the treatment of rheumatoid arthritis. Furthermore, it is being used much earlier in the course of the disease. It was initially found that the folic acid antagonist, aminopterin, was useful in rheumatoid and psoriatic arthritis in the 1950s.[75] In the next two decades several trials showed that methotrexate was effective in rheumatoid arthritis. Early in its development it was noted that weekly regimes were beneficial and that the toxicity profile with the weekly regime was markedly different from that seen with the high doses used in cancer chemotherapy. There is continuing debate as to when to employ the drug in rheumatoid arthritis – that is, whether to use the drug earlier than other slow-acting drugs or to keep it in reserve when other drugs fail to achieve a therapeutic response. Advocates point to its comparatively rapid onset of action (about 4 weeks), its excellent success in controlling the most aggressive disease and the relatively few side-effects. Opponents, however, point out the lack of knowledge regarding long-term side-effects and the absence of evidence regarding its ability to retard bone changes (unlike intramuscular gold).

Pharmacokinetics

Absorption of oral methotrexate in the low doses used was previously thought to be complete but is now known to be variable and erratic. A mean bioavailability of 0.67 with a range of 0.4–1.0 has been reported.[76] It can be affected by food as well as a number of drugs, such as non-absorbable antibiotics. After undergoing limited metabolism methotrexate and its metabolites are excreted renally, both by glomerular filtration and active tubular secretion. In addition, it is metabolized in the cell to polyglutamated derivatives which are more potent and increase the duration of action. Lymphocyte precursors tend to accumulate more of these polyglutamated derivatives than the myeloid precursors or gastrointestinal cells. If oral methotrexate is not tolerated it can be given intramuscularly, which has the advantage of ensuring compliance.

Mechanism of action[77]

Methotrexate is classified as an antimetabolite. It interferes with the biosynthesis of thymidilic acid, inosinic acid and other purine metabolites by binding to dihydrofolate reductase. This interferes with nucleic acid synthesis and protein synthesis. In the doses used in cancer chemotherapy, it is the interference with nucleic acid synthesis that is the key to its action; however, in the lower doses used in the rheumatic diseases it is the protein synthesis that is significantly altered. Thus it is thought by some that methotrexate is more anti-inflammatory than immunosuppressive. Although much needs to be learnt about the way in which methotrexate exerts its effects, some observations have been made. It inhibits the release of interleukin-1 and -6, other inflammatory cytokines and collagenolytic proteases. It also reduces macrophage chemotaxis by reducing their sensitivity to leukotriene B_4 and by reducing the synthesis of leukotriene B_4 itself which occurs 24 h after the dose is administered. Of interest is the phenomenon of resistance that occurs in cancer patients when treated with methotrexate. This is rarely found in rheumatoid patients treated with low dose regimes.

Side-effects

The side-effects seen in patients treated with low dose regimes for long periods differ from those (oncology) patients prescribed higher doses for shorter periods. Despite the high frequency of adverse experiences

TABLE 24.10 Cytotoxic agents used in rheumatic diseases

DRUG	CHEMISTRY	PHARMACOKINETICS	MECHANISM OF ACTION	SIDE-EFFECTS	INTERACTIONS
Methotrexate	Folic acid analogue	Absorption erratic $t_{1/2} < 10$ h Renal excretion Weekly dose	Folic acid antagonist Antimetabolite Inhibits protein synthesis > nucleic acid synthesis at low doses	Oral and gastrointestinal ulceration Neutropenia Hepatic fibrosis Pneumonitis	Coadministration of cotrimoxazole → additive antifolate effect
Azathioprine	Purine analogue	Rapid absorption $t_{1/2}$ 90 min Liver metabolism: converted to the active drug 6-mercaptopurine Renal excretion	Inhibition of nucleic acid synthesis. Predominant effect on lymphocytes. Also anti-inflammatory	Neutropenia Abnormal liver function ?Oncogenicity	Allopurinol: enhancement of effect: ↑ toxicity
Cyclophosphamide	Alkylating agent	Well absorbed $t_{1/2}$ 6–7 h Renal excretion and liver metabolism	Cross-link DNA. Profound immunosuppressive action.	Neutropenia Gonadal dysfunction Haemorrhagic cystitis Alopecia Oncogenicity	Enhances effect of suxamethonium. Allopurinol: enhancement of effect: ↑ toxicity

with long-term methotrexate therapy they have been generally mild.

Hepatic fibrosis has been the main concern with long-term use. It was first identified with patients with psoriasis and studies performed with these psoriatics have shown that hepatic fibrosis occurs in 10% of patients who have received more than 1.5 g. However, evidence from trials using rheumatoid patients has shown a much lower incidence. In one trial involving 82 patients who had received more than 3 g of methotrexate only one patient was shown to have developed fibrosis.[78] In one prospective 5-year trial, one out of 123 patients with rheumatoid arthritis developed cirrhosis.[79] Risk factors for hepatic toxicity in patients receiving methotrexate therapy include diabetes, obesity, cumulative dose of drug, and alcohol consumption.

Pneumonitis is also seen in patients treated with methotrexate, though unlike hepatic fibrosis it is more commonly seen in patients with rheumatoid arthritis than psoriasis. Other side-effects include oral and gastrointestinal ulceration, which is common but often minor, and neutropenia. Some of the side-effects, particularly the nausea and stomatitis, can be alleviated with folinic acid which is the fully reduced metabolically active folate coenzyme and thus does not need the dihydrofolate reductase for activation. This drug should also be used in cases of overdose and in acute haematological side-effects. Alternatively the use of weekly folic acid supplements has been shown to reduce side effects.

Drug interactions

It has been suggested that NSAIDs reduce the renal clearance of methotrexate but evidence for clinically important interactions is still awaited. The co-administration of cotrimoxazole (trimethoprim/sulphamethoxazole) and methotrexate leads to additive antifolate effects and therefore an increased risk of neutropenia and thrombocytopenia.

Cyclophosphamide

Cyclophosphamide is well absorbed orally but is also used intravenously. Its use is mainly in the more serious manifestations of autoimmune rheumatic diseases. It is the most powerful of the immunosuppressive agents in common use for the rheumatic diseases and has the most significant side-effects.

The drug is inert and is activated by metabolism in the liver. The metabolites are excreted in the kidney.

Cyclophosphamide acts primarily on rapidly dividing cells (i.e. those in the S phase of the cycle) though it does affect other phases as well. It inhibits almost all components of the humoral and cellular immune system. It profoundly inhibits antibody production while T-cell function is affected to a lesser extent. The effects of cyclophosphamide on T cells seem to be selective rather than global which may be an advantage in terms of preserving host defences.[80]

Cyclophosphamide given in boluses of 1 g has been found to be very effective in controlling disease flares in systemic lupus erythematosus, particularly with renal involvement. Several trials have shown that when intravenous cyclophosphamide and intravenous steroids are combined for treating systemic lupus erythematosus they have an additive therapeutic effect. Recovery of lymphocytes to their normal function can take up to 4 months with this treatment.

The most important side-effects pertain to the bone marrow where any or all of the blood-forming elements of the blood can be suppressed. Neutropenia is the most frequent toxic effect of cyclophosphamide. Gonadal suppression is almost invariable with chronic administration of cyclophosphamide. In both sexes this may be irreversible. Haemorrhagic cystitis occurs in about 15% of patients due to the action of acrolein, a metabolite of cyclophosphamide, and may eventually lead to bladder cancer. This occurs less commonly with intravenous regimes especially if large volumes of fluid are administered concurrently. Mesna (sodium-2-mercapto-ethane sulphonate) specifically prevents toxic effects to the bladder by reacting with the acrolein in the urinary tract and converting it into a harmless compound. With long-term use all types of malignancies have been reported and must be taken into account when prescribing this agent for non-malignant disease.

REFERENCES

1 Hunter J. Fundamental principles of inflammation. In: Hunter J ed. *A treatise on the blood, inflammation and gunshot wounds*. London: George Nicol bookseller to His Majesty, 1794: 221–6.

2 Lewis GP. *Mediators of inflammation*. Bristol: Wright, 1986.

3 Gallin JI, Goldstein IM, Snyderman R. *Inflammation. Basic principles and clinical correlates*. New York: Raven Press, 1988 and 1992.

4 Black JW, Duncan WAM, Durant CJ, Ganelli CR, Parsons EM. Definition and antagonism of histamine H_2-receptors. *Nature* 1972; 236: 385–90.

5 Matloff SM, Kiselis IK, Rochlin RE. Reduced production of histamine-induced supressor factor (HSF) by atopic mononuclear cells and decreased prostaglandin E_2 output by HSF-stimulated atopic monocytes. *Journal of Allergy and Clinical Immunology* 1983; 72: 359–64.

6 Sonneville A. Hypostamine (tritoqualine), a synthetic reference anti-histaminic. *Allergie et Immunologie Paris* 1988; 20: 365–8.

7 Pipkorn U, Granerus G, Proud D, Kagey-Sobotka A, Norman PS, Lichtenstein LM, Naclerio RM. The effect of a histamine synthesis inhibitor on the immediate nasal allergic reaction. *Allergy* 1987; 42: 496–501.

8 Niettaanmaki H, Fraki JE, Harvima RJ, Forstrom L. Alphafluoromethyl-histidine in the treatment of idiopathic cold urticaria. *Archives of Dermatological Research* 1989; 281: 99–104.

9 Rocha e Silva M. Histamine II and Antihistaminics. Chemistry, metabolism and physiological and pharmacological actions. *Handbuch der Experimentellen Pharmakologie*. Berlin: Springer-Verlag, 1978; **18** (2).

10 Smith JA, Mansfield LE, deShazo RD, Nelson HS. An evaluation of the pharmacologic inhibition of the immediate and late cutaneous reaction to allergen. *Journal of Allergy and Clinical Immunology* 1980; **65**: 118–21.

11 Sorkin EM, Heel RC. Terfenadine: a review of its pharmacodynamic properties and therapeutic efficacy. *Drugs* 1985; **29**: 34–56.

12 Krstenasky PM, Cluxton RJ. Astemizole: a long-acting, non-sedating antihistamine. *Drug Intelligence and Clinical Pharmacy* 1987; **21**: 947–53.

13 Vane JR. Inhibition of prostaglandin synthesis as a possible mechanism of action of aspirin-like drugs. *Nature* 1971; **231**: 232–5.

14 Smith JB, Willis AL. Aspirin selectively inhibits prostaglandin production in human platelets. *Nature* 1971; **231**: 235–7.

15 Needleman P, Turk J, Jakschik BA, Morrison AR, Leftowith JB. Arachidonic acid metabolism. *Annual Review of Biochemistry* 1986; **55**: 69–102.

16 Marcus AJ, Broekman MJ, Safier LB, Uuman HL, Islam N, Serhan CN, Rutherford LE, Korchak HM, Weissman G. Formation of leukotrienes and other hydroxyacids during platelet-neutrophil interactions in vitro. *Biochemical and Biophysical Research Communication* 1982; **109**: 130–7.

17 Marcus AJ, Weksler BB, Jaffe EA, Broekman T. Synthesis of prostacyclin from platelet-derived endoperoxides by cultured human endothelial cells. *Journal of Clinical Investigation* 1980; **66**: 979–86.

18 Billah M. Regulation of phospholipase A_2. *Annual Reports in Medicinal Chemistry* 1987; **22**: 223–33.

19 Ford-Hutchinson AW. FLAP: a novel target for inhibiting the synthesis of leukotrienes. *Trends in Pharmacological Sciences* 1991; **12**: 68–72.

20 Williams KI, Higgs GA. Eicosanoids and inflammation. *Journal of Pathology* 1988; **156**: 101–10.

21 Appleton I, Tomlinson A, Mitchell JA, Willoughby DA. Distribution of cyclooxygenase isoforms in murine chronic granulomatous inflammation. Implications for future anti-inflammatory activity. *Journal of Pathology* 1995; **176**: 413–20.

22 Goldyne ME, Stobo JD. Immunoregulatory role for prostaglandins and related lipids. *Critical Reviews in Immunology*. 1981; **2**: 189–223.

23 Hedquist P, Raud J, Dahlen S-E. Microvascular actions of eicosanoids in the hamster cheek pouch. *Thromboxane and Leukotriene Research* 1990; **20**: 153–60.

24 Braquet P, Touqui L, Shen TY, Vargaftig BB. Perspectives in platelet activating factor research. *Pharmacological Reviews* 1987; **39**: 97–145.

25 Kennedy I, Coleman RA, Humphrey PPA, Levy GP, Lumley P. Studies on the characterisation of prostanoid receptors: a proposed classification. *Prostaglandins* 1982; **24**: 667–89.

26 Halushka PV, Mais DE, Mayeux PR, Morinelli TA. Thromboxane, prostaglandin and leukotriene receptors. *Annual Review of Pharmacology and Toxicology*. 1989; **29**: 213–19.

27 Gresele P, Deckmyn H, Nenci GG, Vermylen J. Thromboxane synthetase inhibitors, thromboxane receptor antagonists and dual blockers in thrombotic disorders. *Trends in Pharmacological Sciences* 1991; **12**: 158–63.

28 Lane IF, Lumley P, Michael MF, Peters AM, McCollum CN. An initial study with intravenous GR32191, a thromboxane receptor blocking agent, in healthy volunteers. *Thrombosis Haemostasis* 1990; **64**: 369–73.

29 Proud D, Kaplan AP. Kinin formation: mechanisms and role in inflammatory disorders. *Annual Review of Immunology* 1988; **6**: 49–83.

30 Regoli D. Kinins. *British Medical Bulletin* 1987; **43**: 270–84.

31 Furchgott RF, Vanhoutte PM. Endothelium-derived relaxing and contracting factors. *FASEB Journal* 1989; **3**: 2007–18.

32 Burch RM, Farmer SG, Steranka LR. Bradykinin receptor antagonists. *Medical Research Reviews* 1990; **10**, 143–75.

33 Lewis GP. Kinins in inflammation and tissue injury. *Handbook of Experimental Pharmacology* 1970; **25**: 516–30.

34 Marceau F, Lussier A, Regoli D, Giroud JP. Pharmacology of kinins: their relevance to tissue injury and inflammation. *General Pharmacology* 1983; **14**: 209–29.

35 Melmon KL, Webster ME, Goldfinger SE, Seegmiller JE. The presence of a kinin in inflammatory synovial effusions from arthritides of varying etiologies. *Arthritis and Rheumatism* 1967; **10**: 13–20.

36 Steranka LR, Farmer SG, Burch RM. Antagonists of B_2 bradykinin receptors. *FASEB Journal* 1989; **3**: 2019–25.

37 Kidd BL, Gibson SJ, Mapp PI, Zhao PI, Polak JM, Blake DR. Neuropeptides as mediators of inflammation and chronic pain. *European Journal of Rheumatology and Inflammation* 1991; **11**: 46–65.

38 Shanahan F, Denburg JA, Fox J, Bienenstock J, Befus D. Mast cell heterogeneity: effects of neuroenteric peptides on histamine release. *Journal of Immunology* 1985; **135**: 1331–7.

39 Jorrizo JL, Coutts AA, Eady RAJ, Greaves MW. Vascular response of human skin to injection of substance P and mechanisms of action. *European Journal of Pharmacology* 1983; **87**: 67–76.

40 Lundblad L, Lundberg JM, Angaard A, Zetterstrom O. Capsaicin pretreatment inhibits the flare component of the cutaneous allergic reaction in man. *European Journal of Pharmacology* 1985; **113**: 461–2.

41 Levine DJ, Clark R, Devor M, Helms C, Basbaum AI. Intraneuronal substance P contributes to the severity of experimental arthritis. *Science* 1984; **226**: 547–9.

42 MacLagan T. The treatment of acute rheumatism by salacin. *Lancet* 1876; i: 342–83.

43 Rodman GP. The early history of anti-rheumatic drugs. *Arthritis Rheumatism* 1976; **13**: 145–65.

44 Baum C, Kennedy D, Forbes M. Utilization of NSAID. *Arthritis Rheumatism* 1985; **28** (6): 686–9.

45 Dascombe MJ. The pharmacology of fever. *Progress in Neurobiology* 1985; **25**: 327–73.

46 Vane J. Evolution of NSAID and their mechanism of action. *Drugs* 1987; **33**: 18–27.

47 Altman RD. Neutrophil activation: An alternative to prostaglandin inhibition as the mechanism of action for NSAIDs. *Seminars in Arthritis and Rheumatism* 1990; **19**(4) (Suppl 2): 1–6.

48 Dawson W, Boot JR, Harvey J, Walker JR. The pharmacology of benoxaprofen with particular reference to effects on lipoxygenase product formation. *European Journal of Rheumatology and Inflammation* 1982; **5**: 61–5.

49 Roth SH. Pharmacological approaches to musculoskeletal disorders. *Clinical Geriatric Medicine* 1988; **4** (2): 441–61.

50 Levy G, Tsuchiya T. Salicylate accumulation kinetics in man. *New England Journal of Medicine* 1972; **287**: 430–2.

51 Hazleman BL. Incidence of gastropathy in destructive arthropathies. *Scandinavian Journal of Rheumatology* 1989; (Suppl 78): 1–4.

52 Brater DC. Drug–drug and drug–disease interactions with NSAID. *American Journal of Medicine* 1986; **80** (Suppl 1A): 62–77.

53 Shorrock CJ, Rees WDW. Mechanisms of gastric damage by NSAID. *Scandinavian Journal of Rheumatology* 1989; (Suppl 78): 5–11.

54 Vrhovac B. Anti-inflammatory analgesics and drugs used in gout. In: Dukes MNG ed. *Meyler's side effects of drugs*, 8th edn. Amsterdam: Elsevier, 1988: 170–204.

55 Prescott LF. Effects of non-narcotic analgesics on the liver. *Drugs* 1986; **32** (Suppl 4): 129–47.

56 International Agranulocytosis and Aplastic Anemia Study. Risks of agranulocytosis and aplastic anemia: a first report of their relation to drug use with special reference to analgesics. *Journal of the American Medical Association* 1986; **256**: 1749–57.

57 Rashad S, Revell P, Hemingway A, Rainsford K, Walker F. Effect of NSAID on the course of osteoarthritis. *Lancet* 1989; ii(8662): 519–22.

58 Battistini B, Botting R. Bahkle YS. Cox-1 and Cox-2: Toward the development of more selective NSAIDs. *Drug News and Perspectives* 1994; **7**: 501–12.

59 Furst DE. Clinically important interactions of NSAID with other medications. *Journal of Rheumatology* 1988; **15** (Suppl 17): 58–62.

60 Roberts WN, Liang MH, Stern SH. Colchicine in acute gout. *Journal of the American Medical Association* 1987; **257**: 1920–7.

61 Rodnan GP. Treatment of the gout and other forms of crystal-induced arthritis. *Bulletin of Rheumatic Diseases* 1982; **32**: 43–53.

62 Bowen DL, Fauci AS. Adrenal corticosteroids. In: Gallin JI, Goldstein IM, Snyderman R eds. *Inflammation: Basic principles and clinical correlates*. New York: Raven Press, 1988: 877–95.

63 Joffe I, Epstein S. Osteoporosis associated with rheumatoid arthritis: Pathogenesis and management. *Seminars in Arthritis and Rheumatism* 1991; **20** (4): 256–72.

64 Butler RC, Davie MWJ, Worsfold M, Sharp CA. Bone mineral content in patients with rheumatoid arthritis: relationship to low dose steroid therapy. *British Journal of Rheumatology* 1991; **30**: 86–90.

65 Zizic TM, Marcoux C, Hungerford DS, Dancereau JV, Stevens MB. Corticosteroid therapy associated with ischemic necrosis of bone in systemic lupus erythematosus. *American Journal of Medicine* 1985; **79**: 596–604.

66 Lewis DA, Smith RE. Steroid induced psychiatric syndromes. *Journal of Affective Disorders* 1983; **5**: 319–32.

67 Pullar T, Hunter JA, Capell HA. Which is the active component of sulphasalazine in rheumatoid arthritis? *British Medical Journal* 1985; **290**: 1535–80.

68 Peppercorn MA. Sulphasalazine. Pharmacology, clinical use, toxicity, and related new drug development. *Annals of Internal Medicine* 1984; **101**: 377–86.

69 Azad Khan AK, Truelove SC. The disposition and metabolism of sulphasalazine in man. *British Journal of Clinical Pharmacology* 1982; **13**: 523–8.

70 Jones EJ, Jones JV, Woodbury JFL. Response to sulphasalazine in rheumatoid arthritis: Life table analysis of a 5-year follow-up. *Journal of Rheumatology* 1991; **18**: 195–8.

71 Forestier J. Rheumatoid arthritis and its treatment by gold salts. The results of six years experience. *Journal of Laboratory and Clinical Medicine* 1924; **20**: 827–40.

72 Sadler PJ. The comparative evaluation of the physical and chemical properties of gold compounds. *Journal of Rheumatology* 1982; **9** (Suppl 8): 71–8.

73 Ugai K, Ziff M, Lipsky PE. Gold induced changes in the morphology and functional capacity of human monocytes. *Arthritis and Rheumatism* 1979; **22**: 1352–60.

74 Salmeron G, Lipsky PE. Modulation of human immune responsiveness *in vitro* by auranofin. *Journal of Rheumatology* 1982; **9** (Suppl 8): 25–32.

75 Gubner R, August S, Ginsberg V. Therapeutic suppression of tissue reactivity. II. Effect of aminopterin in rheumatoid arthritis and psoriasis. *American Journal of Medicine and Science* 1951; **22**: 176–82.

76 Furst DE. Clinical pharmacology of very low dose methotrexate for use in rheumatoid arthritis. *Journal of Rheumatology* 1985; (Suppl 12): 11–14.

77 Segal R, Yaron M, Tartovsky B. Methotrexate: mechanism of action in rheumatoid arthritis. *Seminars in Arthritis and Rheumatism* 1991; **20**(3): 190–9.

78 Mackenzie AH. Hepatotoxicity of prolonged methotrexate therapy for rheumatoid arthritis. *Cleveland Clinics Quarterly* 1985; **52**: 129–35.

79 Weinblatt ME, Kaplan H, Germain BF, Block S, Solomon SD, Merriman RC, Wolfe F, Wall B, Anderson L, Gall E, Torretti D, Weissman B. Methotrexate in rheumatoid arthritis. A five year prospective multicenter study. *Arthritis and Rheumatism* 1994; **37** 1492–8.

80 McCune WJ, Fox D. Intravenous cyclophosphamide therapy of severe SLE. *Rheumatic Disease Clinics of North America* 1989; **15**(3): 455–77.

25

Opioid Analgesics and Antagonists

Part I Opioid analgesics and antagonists (non-clinical)

A Livingston

INTRODUCTION

The history of opioids is almost as long as the history of pain itself.[1] Opium is derived from the milky, viscous fluid (latex) which is obtained from the unripe seed capsule of the poppy, *Papaver somniferum*, the word 'opium' being the Greek name for fluid or juice. Its use for the relief of pain was recorded on Sumerian stone tablets of around 4000 BC, but it first achieved popularity during Roman and Greek times. The first 'written' reference to poppy juice was by Theophrastus in the third century BC.

During the middle ages use of the drug spread from the East, but its popularity diminished due to its inherent toxicity. However, it was repopularized in Europe by Paracelsus (1493–1541) and in the 17th century Thomas Sydenham introduced 'laudanum' or 'tincture of opium'. This was a highly efficacious (and toxic) mixture of opiate alkaloids, so much so that in 1680 Sydenham was able to report that 'among the remedies which it has pleased Almighty God to give to man to relieve his sufferings, none is so universal and so efficacious as opium' (see Jaffe and Martin[2]). The alkaloid content of 'opium' is shown in Table 25.1.

The main active ingredient, morphine, was not isolated and extracted from opium until 1803 by Serturner. He named the compound after Morpheus,

TABLE 25.1 The alkaloid content of opium

Morphine	9–17%
Noscapine (narcotine)	2–9%
Codeine	0.3–4%
Thebaine	0.1–0.8%
Papaverine	0.5–1%

NB. Noscapine (contained in papaveretum and Nepenthe R and some proprietary cough suppressants) has recently been implicated as being genotoxic, as it induces polyploidy in mammalian cell lines maintained *in vitro*. In the UK, the current preparation of papaveretum does not contain noscapine

Ovid's god of dreams, the son of sleep. Its widespread use in the American Civil War led to a major spread of addiction. The development of the syringe by Pravaz in 1853 and the hollow needle by Wood in 1855 allowed it to be employed parenterally. By the turn of the century morphine was being used both for premedication and anaesthesia although limitations of efficacy on the one hand (many patients were not adequately anaesthetized) and toxicity (due to respiratory depression) hampered its widespread use (see Moldenhauer[3]).

Despite its ability to relieve pain and suffering, two problems had already emerged which limited the use of morphine – addiction and respiratory depression. In the absence of techniques for controlled ventilation, the latter was frequently accompanied by the demise of the patient. In the belief that allyl compounds were respiratory stimulants, Pohl[4] in 1915 studied *n*-allylnorcodeine and found that it both antagonized morphine and produced respiratory stimulation. This allowed larger doses of morphine to be administered with lessened danger of respiratory depression. Pohl's work indirectly led to the development in the 1940s and thereafter of other *n*-allyl versions of parent opioids, for example *n*-allylnormorphine (nalorphine) and *n*-allyloxymorphone (naloxone). The discovery of nalorphine's analgesic properties led to the development of the agonist/antagonist and partial agonist opioids in an attempt to improve the profile of the parent compound, morphine, both in reduction of addiction potential and lessened risk of toxicity.

Despite the eventual elucidation of its structure in 1923 and synthesis in the 1950s, morphine is still produced from the naturally occurring compound derived from *Papaver somniferum* (see Casy and Parfitt[5]).

There are, thus, two distinct groups of compounds: 'opiates' which are natural derivatives of opium and 'opioids' which can refer both to the 'opiates' *and* synthetic compounds whose structural similarity to morphine is tenuous, although still possessing most of its characteristics. Since the term 'opioid' can properly refer to both groups of drugs it will be used as the basic term for all opiates and opioids in this chapter. The word 'narcotic', although still appearing in some standard texts to refer to opioids, usually only refers to illicit use of opioids and also to various governmental agencies around the world which are designated to combat it.

It is over 30 years since the demonstration of specific opioid-receptor binding in nervous tissue and more than 25 years since the description of the endogenous peptide opioid transmitter agents and at that time it was felt that these discoveries would open the door to a whole new spectrum of specific, side-effect free, non-toxic, opioid-based analgesics. Today the most widely used and clinically most popular opioid analgesic is . . . morphine! So what has happened in the intervening years? Where are all the new compounds? We now know a lot more about how the endogenous opioids are formed, how the opioids interact with their receptors, where these receptors are, and how the receptors stimulate cellular responses, but there are still some areas where the picture is unclear.

OPIOID RECEPTORS

Early studies on the relative potencies and side-effects of various opioid analgesics had suggested that they might act at more than one type of receptor, but it was not until the studies of Martin and his coworkers[6] that a real classification was made, and Martin's classification forms the basis of that used today. This study used a series of substitution tests in opioid-dependent spinalized dogs to group the known opioid drugs into three divisions which, they suggested, represented three opioid receptor subtypes. These opioid receptors were designated the morphine-like or μ-receptor, the ketocyclazoline-like or κ-receptor and the SKF10,047 (*n*-allylnormetazocine)-like or σ-receptor, and they were characterized by mainly analgesic, sedative and psychotomimetic effects respectively.

This classification broadly still characterizes the majority of opioid drugs in use today (Table 25.2) but two major developments have modified its modern use. The first major modification concerns the σ-receptor, which is now no longer considered an opioid receptor due to its insensitivity to naloxone reversal and the second major modification involves the inclusion of the δ-receptor as an opioid receptor following the discovery of the endogenous peptides.

TABLE 25.2 Action of opioids at receptors

	μ-RECEPTOR	κ-RECEPTOR
Morphine	+++	+
Fentanyl	+++	0
Pethidine	++	++
Meptazinol	++	0
Codeine	+	0
Dextropropoxyphene	+	0
Diamorphine	+++	+
Methadone	++	+
Pentazone	–	++
Nalbuphine	––	++
Phenazocine	+++ (partial)	+
Naloxone	–––	––

+, agonist; – antagonist.

The availability of numerous ligands has led to the proposition of further opioid receptor types and subtypes. There has been a proposal for an ϵ-receptor to account for the activity of the endogenous peptide β-endorphin at the receptors in the rat vas deferens and there have been proposals for the subdivision of the μ-receptor into μ_1 and μ_2 subgroups with the μ_1 site being associated with analgesia and the μ_2 site with some of the side-effects, based on the activity of meptazinol. There have also been suggestions of the division of the κ-site into κ_1, κ_2 and κ_3 sites on the basis of binding activity and differences in actions of various κ-agonists.

The clinical significance of the discovery and proposal of various receptor subtypes is not immediately clear; however, the investigations of the activity of the various ligands has the object of increasing the desirable effects of these compounds while hopefully reducing the unwanted side-effects and so we can hope eventually for additional clinically useful drugs to come from these studies.

As with all drugs, these compounds can act as agonists or antagonists at the various receptors. One of the problems with some of the clinically used opioids like pentazocine is that they can act as an agonist at one receptor and as an antagonist at another, or as an agonist at both, like pethidine, producing a mixture of effects that can be dependent on dose if the affinities at the two receptors are different. Furthermore, several clinically used opioids such as buprenorphine are partial agonists – that is, they are not capable of producing a maximal effect whatever the dose.

The opioid group of drugs do have antagonists among them that are clinically relevant, perhaps the best known of these is naloxone which, dependent on dose, is capable of reversing μ-, δ- and κ-agonists in that order of sensitivity and, as indicated earlier, is used experimentally as the type of drug for defining opioid activity. Although naloxone has been defined as the typical opioid antagonist there are experimental reports that it can, at low doses, actually induce analgesia itself, so the picture is clearly complicated.

The range of side-effects and multiplicity of actions of the opioids is not really surprising when we remember that these drugs are acting on a variety of receptors, to a variety of endogenous transmitters which interact to modify the effects of a range of other transmitters in the brain and periphery. We must not forget that suppression of the processing of pain information is only one of the many neuronal pathways in which these transmitters are involved and while it would be most useful if we could obtain drugs that only acted on pain pathways it is unlikely that such compounds will ever be found (Table 25.3).

TABLE 25.3 Actions of opioid receptor stimulation

μ-RECEPTOR	κ-RECEPTOR
Spinal and supraspinal analgesic	Spinal analgesia
Euphoria	Sedation/hallucination
Strong respiratory depression	Weak respiratory depression
Strong tolerance and addiction	Weak tolerance and addiction
Miosis	Weak tolerance and addiction
Naloxone reversible	Naloxone reversible
Emesis	No emesis
Cardiovascular depression	Some cardiovascular stimulation
Constipation	Diuresis

ENDOGENOUS OPIOIDS

The demonstration of specific opioid-binding sites in the brain led to an intensive search for the endogenous ligands for these receptors and in 1975 two pentapeptides were described that fulfilled the criteria. These peptides were named met- and leu-enkephalin, depending on whether there was a methionine or leucine residue in the fifth amino acid position. Shortly after this, a much larger peptide of thirty-one amino acids in length was described. This larger peptide consisted of part of the sequence of an already described polypeptide known as β-lipotropin from the anterior pituitary, and was named β-endorphin. This peptide was also found to fulfil the criteria for an endogenous ligand for the opioid-receptor sites. Endorphin is derived from 'endogenous morphine'.

Met-enkephalin and β-endorphin give similar responses to morphine and can be classed as acting on the μ-receptor, the responses to leu-enkephalin are different, and act on another receptor, the δ-receptor. The investigations into the occurrence of endogenous opioid substances continued and further peptides were isolated. These included α-neo-endorphin which showed activity at μ- and δ-receptors and most importantly the discovery of dynorphin which, although it contained the amino-acid sequence for leu-enkephalin, showed activity at the κ-site and seemed to be the endogenous κ-ligand. The total number of peptides isolated from various body tissues with opioid activity now stands at about twenty, but the major breakthrough in these studies came with the isolation and sequencing of the precursor molecules for these peptides, which together with some other hormones, are produced from just three large precursor molecules. These are known as pro-opiomelanocortin (POMC), first characterized from pituitary tissue, pro-enkephalin first characterized from adrenal medulla and pro-dynorphin first characterized from the hypothalamus. These precursors are all about 270 amino acids long and the possible cleavage sites have been identified, allowing the identification of other potentially active peptide sequences (Fig. 25.1) Pro-opiomelanocortin is not only the precursor of β-endorphin but also β-lipotropin, adrenocorticotrophic hormone (ACTH) and melanocyte-stimulating hormone (MSH). The precursor is processed differently in different tissues to produce different proportions of the various peptides. Pro-enkephalin contains the sequences for both met- and leu-enkephalin in the ratio of six to one, as well as other peptides, and several studies have found met- and leu-enkephalin present in the CNS in this ratio. Pro-dynorphin contains the sequence for the neo-endorphin and leu-enkephalin as well as dynorphin. These findings suggest that post-translational proteolytic processing may be an important factor for regulating the endogenous opioid activity in different tissues and regions of the nervous system, since the regional brain content of the various peptides varies considerably (Table 25.4).

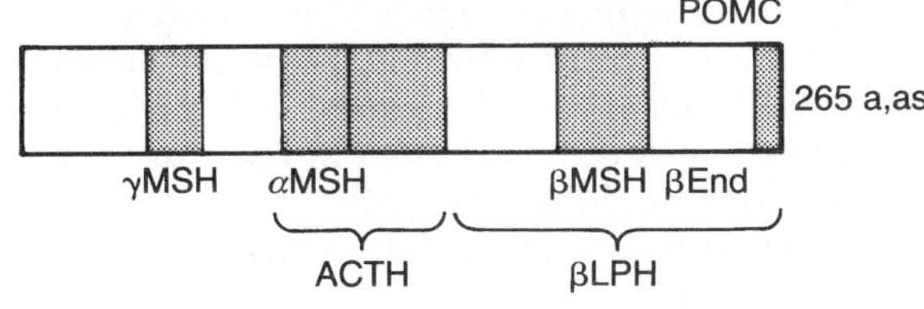

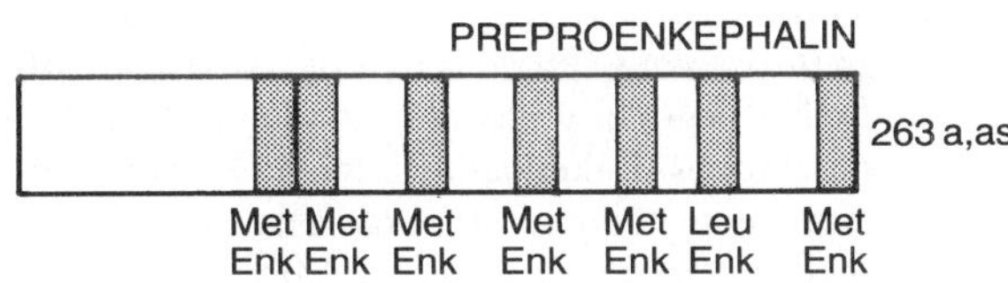

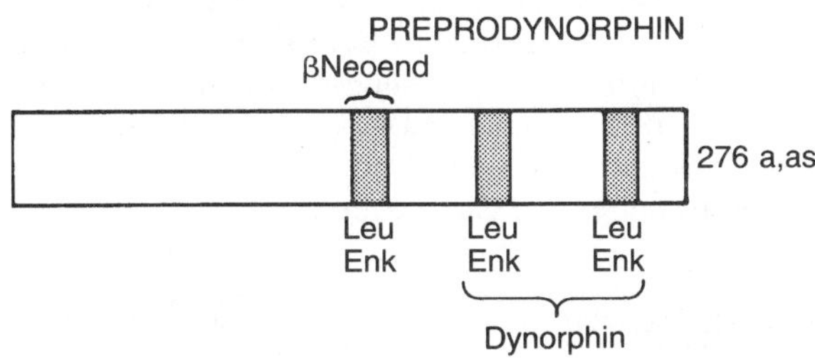

FIGURE 25.1 Structure of precursor molecules of endogenous opioids.

TABLE 25.4 Endogenous opioids and sites of location in the central nervous system

	POMC	PRO-ENKEPHALIN	PRO-DYNORPHIN
Cortex	0	++	+
Amygdala	+++	+++	+
Hippocampus	0	++	+++
Caudate	0	+++	++
Hypothalamus	++++	+++	++
Thalamus	0	+++	0
Substantia nigra	0	+	+++
Pons/medulla	++	+++	++
Dorsal horn of spinal cord	++	++++	+++

POMC, pro-opiomelanocortin.

MECHANISMS OF ACTION

At the simplest level, starting with studies on the guinea-pig ileum, it has been shown that opioids can act by inhibiting transmitter release from neurones. A wide variety of neurotransmitters can be affected in this way, including acetylcholine, noradrenaline and dopamine.

Furthermore, it has been suggested that these actions are longer lasting than those seen with inhibitory neurotransmitters such as γ-aminobutyric acid (GABA) and glycine and so it has been proposed that the endogenous opioids should be referred to as 'neuromodulators' rather than neurotransmitters. These inhibitory effects of opioids are normally associated with a hyperpolarization of the cell membrane which appears to be mediated either by an increased potassium ion conductance in the case of μ- and δ-receptor activation or by decreased calcium ion conductance in the case of κ-receptor activation, which result in an inhibition of the excitatory transmitter release. However, the picture may not be as simple as this, and some authors have described excitatory effects of opioid ligands on neurones.

The most significant change in recent years in the use of opioids to control perioperative pain has come, not from the development of more powerful analgesics, but from the modified use of them. This has happened because of a better understanding of the physiology of clinical pain. The concept of giving the analgesic before the infliction of tissue damage in elective surgery, in order to reduce the postoperative pain sensitization, has been called 'pre-emptive analgesia'. This has led to the consideration of 'balanced analgesia', where different classes of analgesics are used at what would seem to be the most appropriate stage of the pre-, peri- and postoperative situations. (See review by Woolf and Chong, 1993.)

TOLERANCE

The chronic use of opioids has always been associated with the problem of addiction in so far as the two things have become linked in the minds of the public. Addiction, however, is a complex phenomenon involving psychology, physiology and pharmacology and is beyond the scope of this chapter, but certain aspects such as tolerance and withdrawal are worthy of comment.

Tolerance is the situation whereby the body's responses to a given dose of drug become reduced on subsequent redosing. Studies in laboratory animals suggest that these effects can be seen within a few hours of initial opioid administration and on repeated dosing can give rise to the situation whereby doses of opioid that would be lethal in the naive patient produce little or no effect in the tolerant individual. Thus we have the situation where both the euphoric effects and the respiratory depressant effects show tolerance. In the case of the opioids the position is complicated by the existence of homologous tolerance – that is, to the particular receptor type – and heterologous tolerance where changes can take place which respond to both opioid and non-opioid drugs. The position can be complicated still further by the multiple-drug abuser, an individual who is sadly becoming encountered more frequently. The treatment of opioid tolerance is made more difficult by the occurrence of the phenomenon of withdrawal. Withdrawal symptoms appear when the body has adjusted to the constant presence of a drug and if that drug is rapidly removed then the body broadly displays a range of symptoms that represent the opposite of the normally produced effects of that drug. In the case of the opioids these could include hyperalgesia, intestinal hyperactivity and dysphoria, all of which are highly distressing and would reinforce the desire to continue abusing the drugs.

In the case of opioid tolerance it has been possible to study the effects in laboratory animals and cultured cells. Studies in laboratory animals have shown that, following opioid administration over a prolonged period, changes take place in the numbers of opioid receptors in the various neuronal tissues, normally in terms of a reduction in the numbers; this is referred to as 'down-regulation' of receptors. However, this change is probably too slow to account for some of the effects of tolerance although it may contribute to the whole-animal picture in the long term and may be involved in the withdrawal symptoms. Studies in cultured cells have shown much more rapid changes and these are probably associated with the effects that can be seen in a few hours. These changes seem to be associated with effects such as the functional uncoupling of the agonist-occupied receptors and their associated guanine-nucleotide binding proteins.

DEVELOPMENT OF TOLERANCE, DEPENDENCE AND ADDICTION

The phenomenon of tolerance, whereby increasing dosage is required to maintain clinical effectiveness, is a feature of most of the opioids studied to date. There is increasing evidence that tolerance can develop *acutely* and this could interfere with quality of analgesia in the postoperative period, particularly following high efficacy, short-acting, opioids administered intraoperatively. Tolerance to morphine in the rat develops within 20 min of a single dose.[7] Subjective effects of the drug such as euphoria and sedation are believed to correlate closely with their abuse potential. Thus, following *prolonged* administration, the patient becomes dependent on continuing opioid administration which, if stopped, leads to symptoms of withdrawal and drug seeking behaviour. The latter, where the patient may seek drugs illicitly to ameliorate effects of withdrawal, is a particular feature of full μ-agonist opioids and is one of the major limitations of their clinical use.

The role of the adrenergic system

α_2-Agonists, such as clonidine, and opioids potentiate each other for analgesia both systemically and intrathecally.[8] Cells made tolerant to the action of μ-agonists are still sensitive to α_2-agonists. Antinociception, such as is produced by clonidine, is independent of opioid-receptor mechanisms, as it is not reversible by naloxone.[9] This property may be useful in the clinical situation of chronic pain patients who have become tolerant to morphine[10] and demonstrates a role of the adrenergic system in the development of tolerance.[11] A number of α_2-agonists, such as xylazine and medetomidine, are established in veterinary practice as analgesics. Their potential chemical use in patients as adjuncts in general anaesthesia is currently being evaluated.

One other recent development that has influenced our views on the mode of action of endogenous opioid peptides in the nervous system is that of co-existence of these and other peptides with conventional neurotransmitters in neurones. Enkephalins have been shown to occur in dopamine-containing, noradrenaline-containing, adrenaline-containing and acetylcholine-containing cells in various regions of the body. The functional significance of this co-existence is not completely clear but experiments have shown that opioid peptides can modify the responses produced by conventional neurotransmitters in these tissues and may well act to alter the time course of the action of the neurotransmitter (see Chapter 20).

DRUGS USED PERIOPERATIVELY

Morphine

Introduction

Morphine has long been regarded as the 'type' of drug of opioid analgesics (Fig. 25.2). This means that all the other opioid drugs are compared with morphine in terms of effectiveness and toxicity as well as clinical convenience. It is interesting, as pointed out earlier, that although morphine is the oldest drug in this group it is still probably the most popular clinical choice for medium to severe pain control. Morphine shows a wide range of side-effects. However, this is not

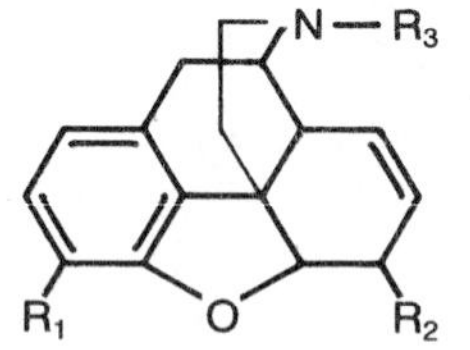

	R_1	R_2	R_3	Other
Morphine	OH	OH	CH_3	
Diamorphine	CH_3COO	CH_3COO	CH_3	
Codeine	CH_3O	OH	CH_3	
Naloxone	OH	O	CH_2CHCH_2	
Nalbuphene	OH	OH	CH_2–◇	No O in ring

FIGURE 25.2 Morphine-like opioids.

unexpected when it is remembered that, as a μ-opioid agonist, morphine will be acting to mimic the endogenous enkephalins that act as neuromodulators at many other sites, besides the pain pathways, in the control and peripheral nervous systems. One other interesting aspect of the actions of morphine is that it appears that a considerable proportion of its activity is mediated via its active metabolite, morphine-6-sulphate, which, like morphine, is a potent agonist at the μ-receptor. Thus, following hepatometabolism, there is still an appreciable analgesic effect seen that accounts for the relatively long duration of action of the drug, which can be between 4 and 5 h.

Analgesic actions

Morphine acts by mimicking the inhibitory actions of enkephalins on the various neuronal pathways in the central nervous system associated with the passage of pain information to the higher centres. This central mode of action means that morphine and similar opioids are particularly relevant in the treatment of medium to severe pain, particularly in relation to visceral pain. This is in contrast to the non-steroid anti-inflammatory drug (NSAID) analgesics (Chapter 24) whose effectiveness is best demonstrated in skeletomuscular and superficially originating pain. The nature of the pain to be treated will obviously affect the dose and schedule of the administration of morphine since a clear difference will exist, for instance, in perioperative use and the use in chronic intractable or terminal pain.

Side-effects

Morphine, in common with the opioids, has a wide range of effects in addition to analgesia and these can be of both central and peripheral origin reflecting the wide distribution of receptors for the endogenous transmitters.

The behavioural side-effects, such as feelings of euphoria and wellbeing are normally shown, but occasionally individuals will experience dysphoria often in association with higher dose levels. These feelings of euphoria form the basis of the abuse of morphine and related drugs which, combined with the problems of tolerance and dependence (see later), give rise to the social problem of morphine addiction. The high risk of opioid abuse and addiction has led to legislative control of these drugs, which results in the added complication in clinical use of storage and recording of usage. There is also the occasional problem of the need for clinical use in addicted patients and the consequent problems associated with establishment of realistic dose regimes in these cases. The other centrally mediated side-effects of morphine include respiratory depression, vomiting (Chapter 29 Part II) and bradycardia and papillary constriction (which will all be relevant in the perioperative use of morphine), cough suppression (Chapter 19 Part II) and drowsiness. The peripheral side-effects of morphine include urinary retention, which again could be relevant following perioperative use in visceral surgery, but is also significant in the chronic use for control of intractable pain as is the well-known effect of morphine on the bowel (Chapter 29 Part II) resulting in severe constipation. It also causes spasm of the Sphincter of Oddi and is contraindicated in the presence of biliary stones.

The induction of tolerance and dependence to morphine is unlikely to be a major problem in the perioperative acute use of morphine although the potential for this must always be considered; however, in the chronic use of morphine the problem becomes much more significant. If the pain condition is severe and terminal then the ethical considerations of pain control can well overcome the problems associated with the induction of tolerance and dependence and under these situations the level of dosage can be assessed in terms of need, rather than according to proposed regimes. One factor that is relevant here, however, is that it appears that although tolerance to the analgesic doses of morphine can develop, these are not reflected in tolerance to some of the side-effects, such as constipation. There are various conditions in which use of morphine requires care. These include patients taking monoamine oxidase inhibitors (MAOIs) (Chapter 22, p. 350) since morphine interacts with many monoamines in the nervous system, and in hypotension, asthma, respiratory problems and hypothyroidism. Clearly any hepatic or renal impairment will affect metabolism and excretion and pregnancy or nursing could give rise to tolerance and dependence in the newborn. Care must also be taken when used in conjunction with head injury since impairment of the pupillary response could make diagnosis and prognosis, using this criterion, difficult.

Preparations

One of the advantages of morphine as an analgesic is the wide variety of formulations available. It is available as an injection for intramuscular or subcutaneous administration, as suppositories, and as oral solutions, compound elixirs, tablets or slow-release preparations. This wide range of formulations allows a wide range of dose schedules and treatments for a wide range of analgesic indications, although for perioperative use the injectable form is obviously the route of choice.

Papaveretum

Papaveretum is not a single drug but a mixture of the hydrochloride salts of morphine, codeine and papaverine, which are alkaloids of opium (in the proportions 253:20:23). Noscapine has been removed from the mixture because it may be genotoxic. The actual content of the various opioid alkaloids may vary slightly. The majority of effects seen are similar to those seen with morphine, although a greater degree of sedation is normally seen. The preference of papaveretum to morphine is usually based on the particular clinical requirement of the anaesthetist.

Alfentanil and fentanyl

These two drugs are phenylpiperidine derivatives (Fig. 25.3) like pethidine (see later) and are potent (50 × morphine as an analgesia) and short acting (about 30–45 min), which has made them very popular for perioperative use. Like morphine, they are μ-agonists and hence share the actions and side-effects of morphine. They are extremely lipid soluble and rapidly enter the central nervous system, thus the effects seen on this system are profound. Apart from their potent analgesic effects, they cause a severe respiratory depression, hypotension, bradycardia and vomiting. However, the duration of these effects is normally short, like the analgesia. Thus, because of the pharmacology and clinical indications the more chronic side-effects are not normally noted; however, the contra-indications associated with the use of morphine are applicable to these drugs.

The short duration of action has made these drugs very popular for perioperative use and thus they are frequently given intravenously, although the intramuscular route is also used. One unusual effect that has been reported for these drugs is that high doses have been seen to cause muscular rigidity, possibly from an interaction with central dopamine mechanisms.

Pethidine

Pethidine was one of the earliest synthetic analgesics and has several interesting characteristics. Its analgesic actions are similar to morphine and its range of activities have led to suggestions that it may interact as an agonist at both μ- and κ-receptors. It also has certain actions which are atropine-like, which is what it was originally intended to be by the chemists who synthesized it (Fig. 25.3). Clinical observations suggest that for equianalgesic doses pethidine has less constipating and urinary retention effects and appears to cause less respiratory depression in the newborn when used at parturition. The duration of analgesia seen with pethidine is similar to that of morphine, namely 2–4 h, although the time to peak effect varies with the route of administration. The most common unwanted side-effects tend to appear when pethidine is administered to ambulatory patients. This can take the form of nausea and dizziness, associated with effects on the middle ear or syncope associated with hypotension. However, both of these effects can be alleviated by lying down. Pethidine can be administered orally or by injection,

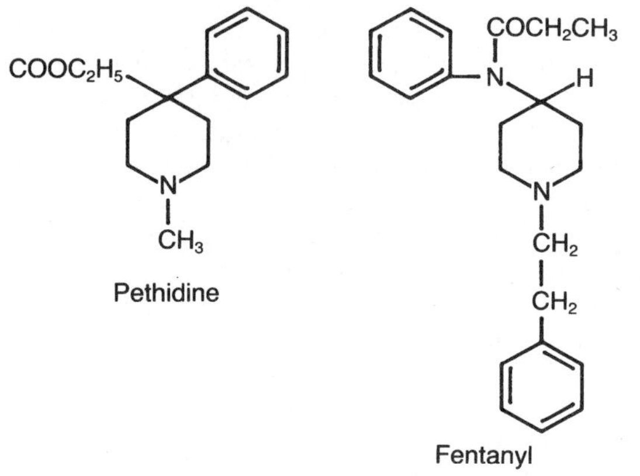

$COOC_2H_5$
N
CH_3
Pethidine

$COCH_2CH_3$
N
H
N
CH_2
CH_2
Fentanyl

FIGURE 25.3 Pethidine-like opioids.

either intramuscularly or intravenously. Pethidine is a popular perioperative analgesic and sedative and is often used as an adjunct to anaesthesia. It is also popular in obstetrics due to the reduced respiratory depression in the neonate compared with other opioids. It is often the drug of choice in biliary and renal colic. In overdose with pethidine, patients may show excitatory symptoms, with muscle twitching, dilated pupils, tremors and convulsions. These effects are more like those seen with atropine, than morphine and other opioids, and can be difficult to interpret. Confusion and hallucinations may be as a result of one of the breakdown products, norpethidine. Pethidine should not be prescribed in patients who are on MAOIs.

Phenoperidine

Phenoperidine is a drug with morphine-like actions, related to pethidine. In fact, it is partially metabolised to pethidine. It is a potent analgesic frequently used to promote analgesia during surgery, and combined with major tranquilizers, it can produce neurolepsis. Since it produces respiratory depression at higher doses, it is often used with assisted ventilation. It is given by intravenous injection and lasts for about one hour.

Meptazinol

Meptazinol, like morphine, is an opioid that acts mainly on μ-receptors although it has been claimed that equianalgesic doses cause less respiratory depression and constipation. The duration of effect is similar to morphine and pethidine and the drug has been used for perioperative pain, obstetric pain and renal colic. As well as respiratory depression and constipation, the other side-effects seen with morphine are said to be less apparent although dizziness, nausea, vomiting and sweating are still commonly seen. The drug is available in oral or injectable form and the latter may be given by the intramuscular or intravenous routes.

DRUGS USED FOR PAIN CONTROL

Of the drugs discussed in the first section, morphine, papaveretum, meptazinol and pethidine are all used for chronic or on-going pain control, more usually by the oral route, but on occasions by injection. In all cases, these drugs are hepatometabolized and renally excreted and if repeated dosing is to be utilized then the integrity of the elimination systems must be taken into account when establishing a dose schedule. Other opioid drugs that can be used for pain control are listed below.

Codeine/dihydrocodeine

Codeine, like morphine (Fig. 25.2), is a natural alkaloid and is far less active than morphine as an analgesic, with its use being mainly confined to mild and medium pain levels. Codeine is, interestingly, relatively more effective by the oral route than morphine and the other opioids which are far more potent when given by injection, whereas codeine is nearly equipotent by the two routes. A proportion of codeine is metabolized to morphine and it was suggested that this was the mode of action of the drug; however, the good antitussive actions of the drug suggest that either this is not true, or that a separate form of receptor exists for the antitussive effects. Apart from the antitussive effects, the other opioid side-effects such as respiratory depression, nausea, constipation and sedation are seen in proportion to the analgesic effects, namely that under normal dose regimes they are, like the analgesia, much milder. The drug is available in oral and injectable forms and can be given intravenously or intramuscularly. It has been suggested that dihydrocodeine can be used in more severe pain states than codeine is normally recommended for.

Dipipanone

Dipipanone is an analgesic related chemically to methadone, used for moderate to severe pain. It is normally used orally and has a duration of action of 5–6 h. Intravenous use of this drug has been reported to produce a precipitous fall in blood pressure. Prolonged use of dipipanone has been associated with the development of dependence. Dipipanone has been widely used for the control of mild postoperative pain.

Dextropropoxyphene

Dextropropoxyphene is another morphine-like drug that has relatively low analgesic activity compared with morphine. It is normally given orally and has a similar range of effects and activities to codeine and dihydrocodeine although rather less potent. There have been reports of CNS excitation and hepatotoxicity following high doses. The drug is specifically contraindicated in cases of porphyria. The compound is structurally related to methadone (see later).

Diamorphine (diacetylmorphine, heroin)

Diamorphine (Fig. 25.2) exerts extremely potent analgesic effects. It is thought that this relates to the high lipid solubility of diamorphine resulting in rapid accumulation in the CNS followed by rapid hydrolysis to morphine, by which it exerts its analgesic effects. This rapid CNS accumulation gives increased euphoria and hence the great potential of this drug for creating addiction. This high CNS activity also tends to give less constipation than morphine and the rapid distribution may also relate to the lower incidence of nausea and hypotension. Since it is believed that the majority of the analgesic effects of diamorphine are produced by morphine then the range of effects will be similar but the pharmacokinetics will differ due to the high lipid affinity. Diamorphine is used much less now for pain control in the form of compound elixirs with cocaine and chlorpromazine and is either given orally as tablets or by injection. One interesting point is that the drug can be used intravenously to treat myocardial infarction or acute pulmonary oedema.

Methadone

Methadone is a synthetic morphine-like analgesic acting mainly as an agonist at the μ-receptors (Fig. 25.4). Thus many of the actions of morphine are seen with methadone. Perhaps the greatest difference from morphine lies in the degree of protein binding exhibited by methadone, which causes a gradual build-up in certain tissues, including brain, following repeated injections. This means that on cessation of treatment a slow release occurs from tissues into the plasma. This in itself means that the drug can produce mild and protracted withdrawal symptoms; however, it does mean that the drug is well-suited as replacement therapy for withdrawal treatment of morphine and diamorphine

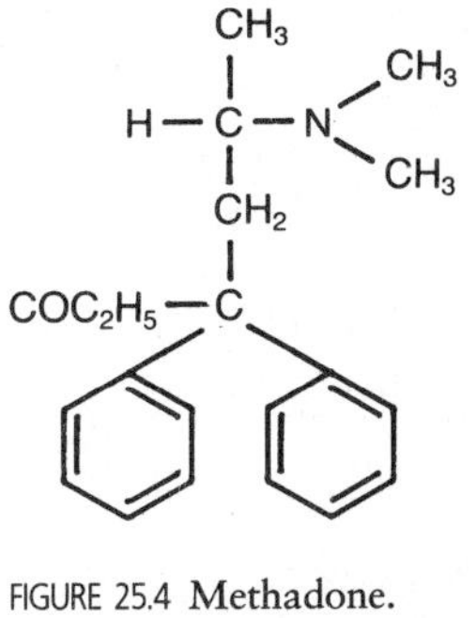

FIGURE 25.4 Methadone.

addicts. It is active against severe pain states and is available in oral or injectable forms and can be given subcutaneously and intramuscularly. Its duration of action as an analgesic is similar to morphine.

Pentazocine

Pentazocine differs from most of the previously mentioned opioids in that it has mixed effects on opioid receptors (Fig. 25.5). It is generally accepted to act as a weak antagonist at the μ-receptor and a strong agonist at the κ-receptor. While in clinical use it resembles the other opioids by having analgesic, sedative and respiratory depressant actions, experimental studies indicate that the nature of the analgesia produced is different and is probably mediated through κ-receptor effects. Other differences are that although respiratory depression can occur at therapeutic doses, it does not seem to increase proportionally with dose thereafter. There are also different effects on the cardiovascular system with large doses producing hypertension and tachycardia and thus the drug is contraindicated in patients with hypertension and heart failure, or after myocardial infarction. This drug is also capable of causing hallucinations. The drug is hepatometabolized like all opioids, has an effective duration of action of 2–4 h and is available as oral and injectable forms as well as suppositories. Injections can be given subcutaneously, intramuscularly or intravenously.

Nalbuphine

Nalbuphine (Fig. 25.2), like pentazocine, is an antagonist at μ-receptors and an agonist at κ-receptors; however, the μ-antagonist effects are much more apparent. Thus the analgesic effects seen with nalbuphine are κ-mediated and, like pentazocine, although it produces respiratory depression the effect does not increase beyond a certain level with increasing doses. Many other side-effects are similar to pentazocine with the exception of the effects on the cardiovascular system, which seem to be very low, and consequently the drug is used in cases of myocardial infarction and has little effect on cardiac index or blood pressure. At high doses dysphoria and other central disturbances have been reported. The duration of action of the drug is 3–6 h.

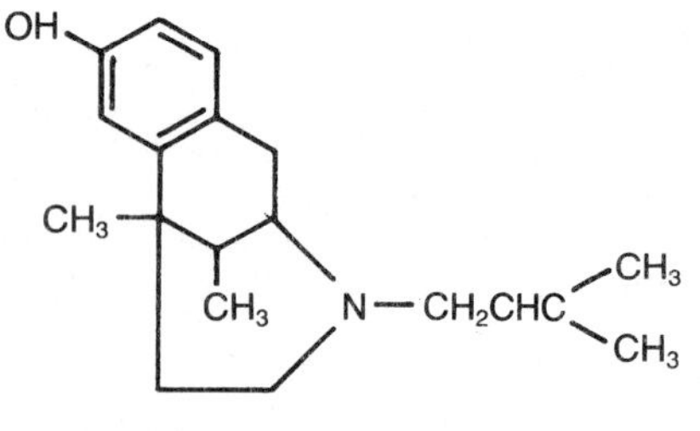

OH
CH_3
CH_3
$N-CH_2CHC(CH_3)_2$

FIGURE 25.5 Pentazocine.

Phenazocine

Phenazocine is another μ-antagonist κ-agonist drug with weaker μ-antagonist activity than nalbuphine. Its activity as an analgesic is quite good and it can be used in cases of biliary colic and other viscerally mediated pain conditions. High doses can cause dysphoria and behavioural changes. Its duration of activity is 4–6 h.

Buprenorphine

Buprenorphine reacts differently from other opioid drugs with regard to the opioid receptors, in as much as it seems to act as a partial agonist at the μ-receptors (see Table 25.7) and may have some agonist activity at other receptor types. It also appears that this drug associates and dissociates very slowly from the μ-receptors which means that its onset time may be delayed and that reversal with antagonists is not as rapid or complete as with other opioids. The drug produces good analgesia with less respiratory depression than morphine and other side-effects are also reduced. The commonest side-effects reported include sedation, dizziness and nausea. The drug is well absorbed and can be used sublingually as well as injection by the intramuscular or intravenous routes. The duration of action of this drug is greater than 6 h and this may be associated with the unusually high plasma binding exhibited compared with other opioids.

Tramadol

Tramadol is a synthetic analgesic not related to the other opioids, but is reported to exert at least some of its analgesic actions via μ-receptors. It is also reported to interact with noradrenaline and serotonin re-uptake, which may also produce analgesic effects. There is also a biologically active metabolite which is proposed to interact with the μ-receptors. Reported side-effects and contra-indications include cardiovascular disturbances, anaphylaxis and convulsions. This drug is not recommended during lactation or pregnancy, nor in cases of epilepsy. Some commonly reported side-effects include dizziness, nausea, constipation, headache and somnolence. The drug can be given orally or by intramuscular or intravenous injection. The duration of action is 4–6 h.

This drug is not recommended for analgesia during light anaesthesia since there have been reports of increased operative recall.

DRUGS THAT ACT AS OPIOID ANTAGONISTS

Naloxone

Naloxone (Fig. 25.2) is a competitive opioid antagonist acting at all opioid receptor types, but is most effective at the μ-site. It is the drug of choice for reversing the effects of opioids and is mainly used for antagonizing respiratory depression. The effect following intravenous use is seen rapidly and, apart from buprenorphine and similar partial agonist drugs, will completely reverse all the effects of the opioids, including the analgesic effects. Normally the drug shows little in the way of effects on its own, but it has been reported high doses may cause hypertension and hyperalgesia. These effects may be associated with antagonism of endogenous opioid transmitters. The drug is presented as an injectable form which can be given by subcutaneous, intramuscular or intravenous routes, although for emergency use the intravenous route is favoured. The drug is capable of producing profound withdrawal symptoms in addicted or dependent patients. There has been some controversy as to the period of activity and some reports suggest that it may be as short as 1 h following intravenous administration, thus care may be needed when used to antagonize longer acting opioids. Normally the drug is given incrementally to effect reversal of opioids in cases of emergency.

FURTHER READING

Basbaum AI, Bessan JM. *Towards a new pharmacology of pain.* New York: John Wiley, 1991.

Gilman AG, Rall TW, Nies AS, Taylor P, eds. *The pharmacological basis of therapeutics*, 8th edn. New York: Pergamon Press 1990.

Johnson SM, Fleming WW. Mechanism of cellular adoptive sensitivity changes application to opioid tolerance and dependence. *Pharmacological Reviews* 1989; **41**: 435–88.

Woolf CJ, Chong MS, Pre-emptive analgesia-treating post-operative pain by preventing the establishment of central sensitization. *Anesthesia Analgesia*, 1993; 77: 352–79.

REFERENCES

1 Bonica JJ. History of pain concepts and pain therapy. *Seminars in Anesthesia* 1985; **4**: 189–208.

2 Jaffe JH, Martin WR. Opioid analgesics and antagonists. In: Gilman AG, Rall TW, Nies AS, Taylor P eds. *The Pharmacological basis of therapeutics.* New York, Pergamon Inc. 1990; 485–521.

3 Moldenhauer CC. New narcotics. In: Kaplan JA ed. *Cardiac anesthesia*, Vol 2. *Cardiovascular pharmacology.* New York: Grune & Stratton, 1985: 31–78.

4 Pohl J. Uber das n-allylnorecodeine, einen antagonisten upon morphine. *Experimental Pathology and Therapeutics* 1915; **17**: 370–82.

5 Casy AF, Parfitt RT. *Opioid analgesics. Chemistry and receptors.* New York, Plenum Press, 1986.

6 Martin WR, Eades CG, Thompson JA, Huppler RE, Gilbert PE. The effects of morphine- and nalorphine-like drugs in the non-dependent and morphine dependent chronic spinal dog. *Journal of Pharmacology and Experimental Therapeutics*, 1976; **197**: 517–32.

7 Kim DH, Fields HL, Barbaro NM. Morphine analgesia and acute physical dependence: Rapid onset of two opposing, dose-related processes. *Brain Research* 1990; **516**: 37–40.

8 Kitahata LM. Spinal analgesia with morphine and clonidine. *Anesthesia and Analgesia* 1989; **68**: 191–3.

9 Ossipov MH, Suarez LJ, Spaulding TC. Antinociceptive interactions between α_2-adrenergic and opiate agonists at the spinal level in rodents. *Anesthesia and Analgesia* 1989; **68**: 194–200.

10 Eisenach JC, Lysak SZ, Viscomi CM. Epidural clonidine analgesia following surgery: Phase 1. *Anesthesiology* 1989; **71**: 640–6.

11 Kihara T, Kaneto H. Important role of adrenergic function in the development of analgesic tolerance to morphine in mice. *Japanese Journal of Pharmacology* 1986; **42**: 419–23.

PART II PHARMACOLOGY OF THE CLINICAL USE OF OPIOID AGONISTS AND ANTAGONISTS

DW Green

OPIOID PHARMACOLOGY

Expoxymorphinans derivatives

Morphine and related opioids are described as 4,5 expoxymorphinans, characterized by an epoxy bridge between carbon 4 and 5 (see Fig. 25.6). The basic phenanthrene ring structure is typical of many opioids. Morphine has an —OH group on both C_3 and C_6 carbon atoms. Masking of the 3—OH of morphine by the methyl ether group CH_3O results in codeine, a naturally occurring compound of lower potency and addiction potential than morphine and with greater oral bioavailability.

Modification of the morphine nucleus and the development of totally new congeners has been carried out in an attempt to increase analgesic potency while at the same time reducing side-effects such as respiratory depression and addiction potential. Acetylation of both —OH groups represented the first attempts at modification to produce a compound with more desirable properties.[1] Diacetylmorphine (diamorphine, heroin) is inactive and must first be hydrolysed by an esterase to 6-monoacetylmorphine (four times more potent than morphine) and thence to morphine. Unfortunately, its early promise was not fulfilled and its *increased* addiction potential (owing to its more rapid onset and greater euphoric action) has led to its use being illegal in the majority of countries, the UK being a notable exception.

Substitution for CH_3 on the nitrogen has led to the development of opioid antagonists and is discussed on p. 441.

Thebaine derivatives

The thebaine nucleus has two —CH_3O substitutions on C_3 and C_6. Clinically useful compounds in this series are distinguished by reversion to an —OH group on C_3, lipophilic

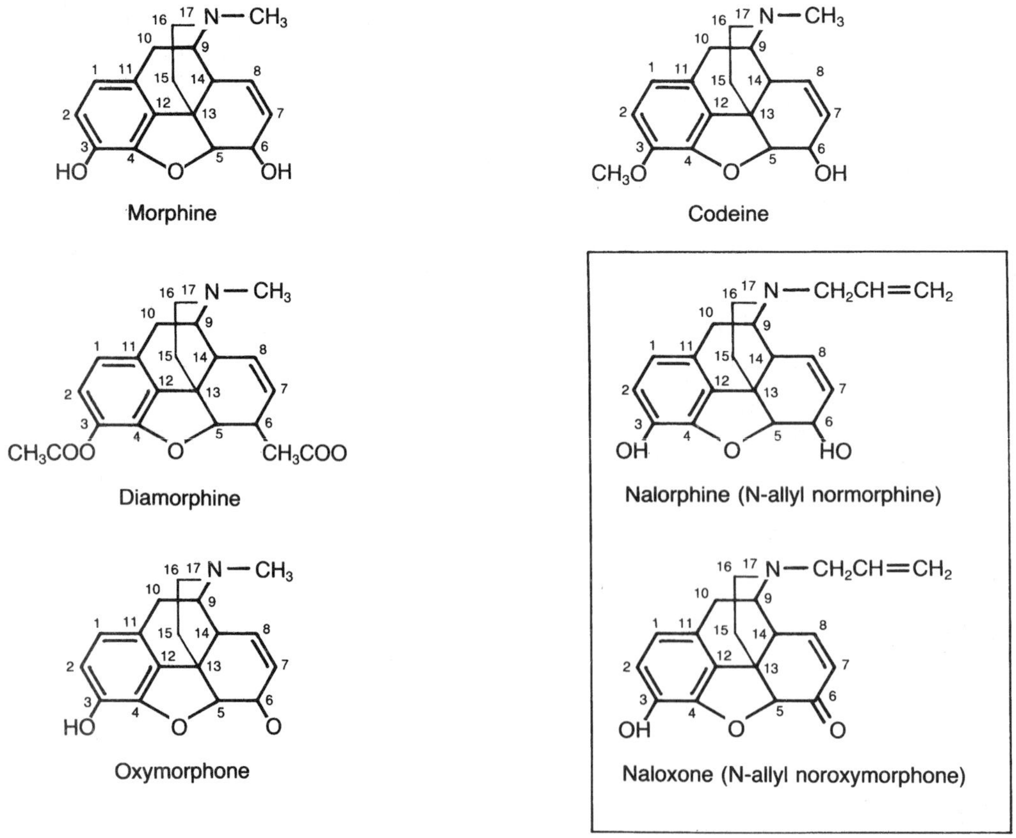

Morphine

Codeine

Diamorphine

Nalorphine (N-allyl normorphine)

Oxymorphone

Naloxone (N-allyl noroxymorphone)

FIGURE 25.6 The 4,5 epoxymorphinans and associated antagonists, nalorphine and naloxone.

substitution on C_7 and changes to the N—CH_3 grouping at C_{17} (Fig. 25.7). Etorphine and buprenorphine are identical save for the differing substitution on the nitrogen. Etorphine retains the traditional N—CH_3 grouping and is an exceptionally potent μ-agonist being up to 10 000 times more potent than morphine. It is used in veterinary medicine to immobilize large animals (Immobilon^R). The N-cyclopropylmethyl (N-CPM) group of buprenorphine results in a compound of lessened potency and partial agonism at the μ-receptor. Of great interest in this series is how the small change in the substitution on C_7 of buprenorphine (see Fig. 25.7) results in the extremely powerful antagonist of etorphine, diprenorphine (Revivon^R).

Benzomorphan derivatives

Following the development of nalorphine, it was clear that compounds could be synthesized that had greater separation of analgesia from addiction potential than morphine. The benzomorphans were developed by simplification of the morphine structure with eventual exclusion of the morphine D ring. Here, substitution at the N atom was crucial to the profile of the compound. Phenazocine (Narphen^R) was one of the first compounds to be developed, showing traditional morphine-like activity but being five times as potent with increased oral bioavailability. Change from an N-phenol to a N-dimethylallyl or a N-CPM grouping led to the development of two compounds, pentazocine (Fortral^R) and cyclazocine. Both these compounds demonstrate increased antagonistic properties at the μ-receptor with agonist effects at the κ-receptor (receptor dualism). Pentazocine was the first clinically acceptable agonist/antagonist analgesic with low addiction potential. Synthesis of *keto*cyclazocine resulted in a compound with little antagonist activity and predominant agonist action at the κ-receptor. This was Martin's prototype κ-agonist. N-allyl substitution (as is found with epoxymorphinan antagonists such as naloxone) resulted in the antagonist *n*-allyl normetazocine, Martin's prototype sigma agonist.[2]

4-Phenylpiperidine and 4-anilinopiperidine derivatives

Pethidine, an ethyl methyl phenylpiperidine, was developed by chance. The 4-phenylpiperidine compounds were being examined as spasmolytics on the basis of their clinical similarity to atropine. Pethidine showed activity in antinociceptive tests and was introduced clinically in the 1940s. It was the first non-opium derived opioid (see Casy and Parfitt[3]). Although initially thought to be non-addictive, this hope was not fulfilled in clinical practice. The Janssen company in Beerse, Belgium have been responsible for developing a remarkable series of compounds based on the 4-piperidone nucleus (the anilino-piperidines) which have included the butyrophenone tranquillizers (e.g. droperidol) as well as the fentanyl, alfentanil, sufentanil series of analgesics (Fig. 25.3).

CLINICAL ASPECTS OF OPIOID USE

Opioid pharmacokinetics

Lack of knowledge of the pharmacokinetics of conventional opioids means that they may be used inappropriately.[4] This is one of the main reasons that 75% of patients sampled from five Chicago hospitals stated that they had moderate to severe pain postoperatively, despite opioids.[5]

A knowledge of pharmacokinetics involves understanding how the body handles the drug (see Chapter 2). For example, when an opioid is given orally we have to consider not only how well it is absorbed from the gut, but also how much of it undergoes 'first-pass metabolism' in the gut and liver. Absorption and first-pass metabolism determine the bioavailability of the drug. The fraction that is bioavailable is calculated by measuring the 'area under

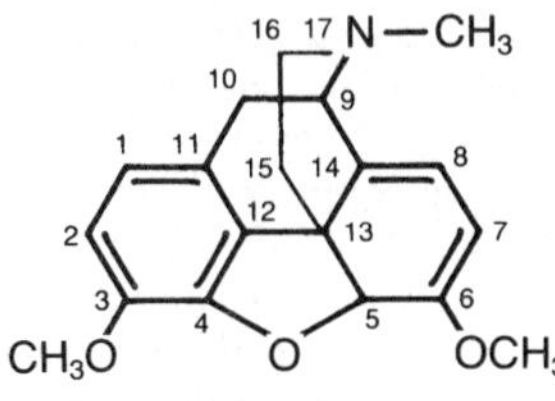

Thebaine

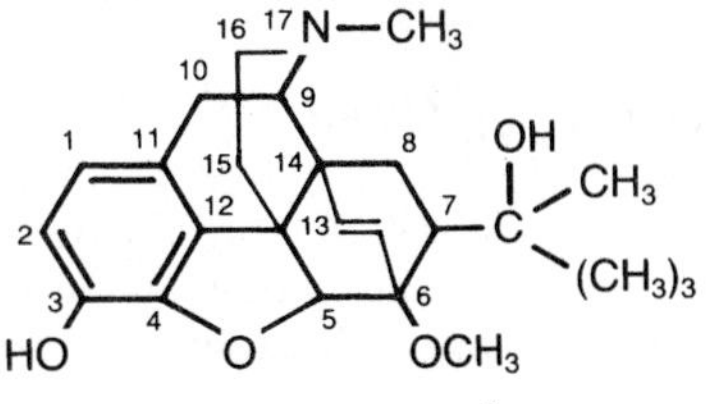

Etorphine (Immobilon^R)

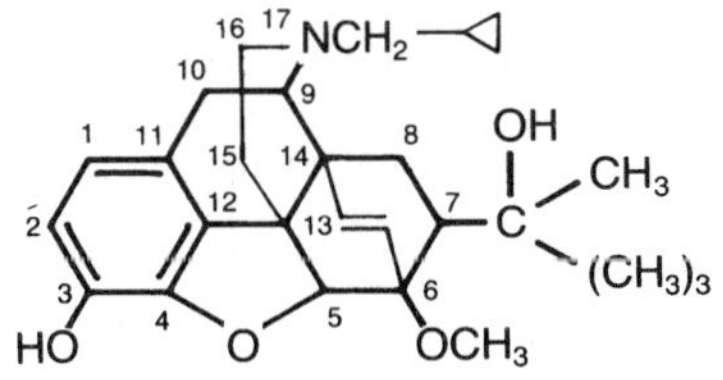

Buprenorphine (Note cyclopropyl methyl substitution on NCH_2 and the lipophilic moiety on C7

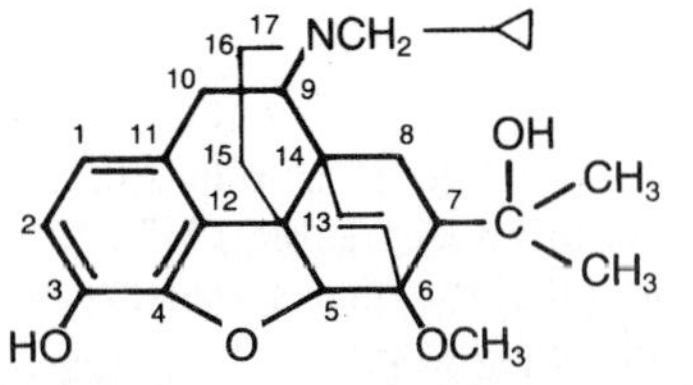

Diprenorphine (Revivon^R). NB how the change from $(CH_3)_3$ to CH_3 on C7 converts the analgesic buprenorphine to this potent antagonist of etorphine.

FIGURE 25.7 The 4,5 epoxymorphinans thebaine derivatives etorphine, buprenorphine and the antagonist, diprenorphine.

the curve' of the drug concentration/time curve following oral administration and dividing that by the area obtained with the same dose of the drug given intravenously at a later date (by definition the iv route has a bioavailability of 1 or 100%).

Most opioids are well absorbed from the gut, but undergo significant first-pass metabolism, leaving a bioavailability in the range of 0.2 (morphine) to 0.5 or greater (pethidine, pentazocine phenazocine, codeine and levorphanol). This means that only one-fifth to one-half of the oral dose reaches the systemic circulation so the oral dose must be large in relation to an equivalent parenteral dose.

When the drug is given parenterally, especially intravenously, we can ignore these effects and concern ourselves with administering sufficient drug to achieve and maintain an effective concentration in the plasma (C_{eff}). There is considerable variation in the C_{eff} between the opioids (see pethidine below).

Volume of distribution (V_d) (see Chapter 2)

For opioids, the initial V_d (I_{vd}) is usually about 20–50 l and represents the distribution volume associated with those organs that have high blood flow, for example brain, heart and splanchnic organs. Further distribution then occurs to areas of the body less well perfused, such as muscle and skin. Finally, large quantities of opioid may be taken up into fat, especially if administration of the drug continues for long periods (e.g. opioid infusions in ICU). This slow distribution occurs over many hours and results in a further fall in drug concentration independent of metabolism. This will result in a higher volume of distribution which is known as the volume of distribution of steady state (here simply referred to as V_d). It is about 150–250 l (in a 60-kg patient).

Total body clearance (Cl) (see Chapter 2)

Clearance (Cl) is approximately equal to hepatic blood flow in the majority of opioids and is thus about 1 l/min in a 60-kg patient (exceptions being methadone and alfentanil).

Half-life (see Chapter 2)

The redistribution half-life ($t_{\frac{1}{2}\alpha}$) is measured in minutes for the majority of opioids, while the elimination half-life ($t_{\frac{1}{2}\beta}$) is usually about 3–5 h (see Table 25.5).

It is important to note that the three factors, $t_{\frac{1}{2}\beta}$, V_d and Cl are related by the equation:

$$t_{\frac{1}{2}\beta} = \frac{V_d}{Cl} \times 0.693$$

Thus an increase in half-life of a drug may be due to an increase in the volume of distribution or a fall in clearance or a combination of the two. It is noteworthy that the short $t_{\frac{1}{2}\beta}$ of alfentanil is due to a low V_d not high Cl which is actually less than the majority of opioids (see Table 25.5).

Calculating the loading dose of an opioid

The loading dose is determined by multiplying the volume of distribution of the drug by the required effective concentration (C_{eff}). An initial bolus (for I_{vd}) is followed by a loading infusion (for the total V_d).

Thus, if for pethidine, the I_{vd} is 50 l and the C_{eff} is 0.6 mg/l, the initial bolus is about 30 mg (50 × 0.6). If the total V_d is 250 l, then this should be followed by a loading infusion over about an hour of 200 × 0.6 = 120 mg (200 is 250 − 50).

In this way, the requisite C_{eff} will be achieved. In fact the actual C_{eff} varies considerably amongst different subjects (0.2–0.8 mg/l), but is fairly reproducible in the same subject.[4]

Calculating the maintenance dose

Having achieved the C_{eff}, it must be maintained to sustain effective analgesia. Since opioids are metabolized according to first-order kinetics, then:

Metabolism is proportional to concentration of drug (C_{eff})
or, Metabolism = clearance (l/h) × C_{eff}

Thus, to maintain C_{eff}, maintenance dose must equal the amount metabolized, that is:

= Clearance × C_{eff} (see later)

The clearance of pethidine is about 700 ml/min (40 l/h), so the hourly maintenance dose will be 40 × 0.6 = 25 mg.

Effect of the half-life

If a maintenance infusion, maintenance im injections at 3–4 h intervals, or patient-controlled analgesic apparatus is started *without* a loading dose, $t_{\frac{1}{2}\beta}$ tells us how long it will take to achieve steady-state levels (i.e. C_{eff}). In the case of pethidine, with a $t_{\frac{1}{2}\beta}$ of 5 h, a maintenance regime will only begin to achieve half effectiveness at 5 h, 3/4 at 10 h, 7/8 at 15 h, and so on. Final steady state is usually achieved at $t_{\frac{1}{2}\beta}$ × 5 (e.g. 25 h in the case of pethidine). No wonder patients complain of inadequate pain relief with a conventional postoperative regime that has neglected to use a loading dose!

Similarly, a concentration of 20 ng/ml is considered sufficient to keep the patient unaware during high-dose fentanyl regimes for cardiac surgery. However, postoperatively, a level of about 1 ng/ml is needed to allow the patient to breathe spontaneously. On discontinuation of the infusion, 5 half-lives (15 h) will be needed before the level drops to this value (see Moldenhauer[6]).

Effect of changes in liver blood flow on rate of elimination, extraction ratio and clearance of opioids

The examples quoted above take no account of the effects of changes in liver blood flow on metabolism of opioids and thus on the amount required to maintain steady-state

TABLE 25.5 Pharmacokinetic data for commonly used opioids (doses refer to 60-kg adult)

DRUG	EQUIVALENT iv DOSE (mg) AND DURATION OF ACTION (h)	pKa	% UNIONIZED AT pH 7.4 (%)	% UNBOUND	PARTITION COEFFICIENT AT pH 7.4	TYPICAL C_{eff} (ng/ml)	Cl (l/ min/60 kg)	VOLUME OF DISTRIBUTION IN LITRES (TOTAL)	$t_{\frac{1}{2}\beta}$(h)
Morphine	10/3	7.9	24	65	1	10–65	0.8–1.2	100–300	1–4
Pethidine	100/2	8.7	7	35	24	200–800	0.4–0.8	170–300	2–5
Methadone	10/12	9.3	1	11	116	100	0.1–0.2	200–400	25–45
Alfentanil	0.5/0.2	6.5	89	8	130	100–300	0.2–0.6	50	1–3
Fentanyl	0.1/0.4	8.4	9	16	960	1–3	0.8–1.3	240–400	2–7
Sufentanil	0.02/1	8.1	20	7	1730	?	0.5–1.0	100	2–4
Buprenorphine	0.3/6	8.4	9	4	2320	1–2	1.1–1.5	120–250	2–5

concentrations appropriate for adequate analgesia without serious toxicity. Although changes in liver blood flow do not affect the loading dose required, changes occurring as a result of myocardial depression, anaesthetic agents (particularly halothane and β-blockers), during abdominal surgery and hypovolaemia can have profound effects on the rate of opioid metabolism. Failure to appreciate these changes and to make suitable adjustments in the dosing schedule can lead to serious problems in the spontaneously breathing patient, particularly in the perioperative period when the greatest changes are likely to take place.

Alternative routes of opioid administration

Opioids can be administered by routes other than iv, im or orally. Avoiding the possibility of complications with high peak levels obtained with the iv route, avoiding the pain of im injections and the poor bioavailability of the oral route are obviously to be welcomed.

Sublingual (sl)

The high first-pass effect can be avoided by using the sublingual route. Absorption is best in those opioids that have high lipophilicity and potency, and is favoured by an alkaline medium in the mouth which increases the proportion of the unionized (lipophilic) fraction. Compared with morphine (18% absorption), buprenorphine (55%), fentanyl (51%) and methadone (34%) are absorbed to a significantly greater extent.[7] In practice, buprenorphine is the only opioid that is routinely given thus. In another study using 0.4 mg, 0.8 mg and placebo, levels peaked at 200 min and absorption was complete at 5 h with overall bioavailability of 55%.[8]

Buccal and transmucosal route

Several groups have looked at the possibility of using morphine by the buccal route in an effort to avoid both parenteral injection and high first-pass effect of the oral route. As would be predicted by the low potency and lipophilicity of morphine, absorption has been erratic and unpredictable with bioavailability similar or inferior to the oral route.[9–11]

Fentanyl is well absorbed by the oral (transmucosal) route and has been utilized in the form of a 'lollipop' for premedication in volunteers.[12] However, since the 'lollipop' contains a potent opioid, this description is best avoided and the term 'lozenge' is more appropriate in the clinical context.[13]

Transnasal

The kinetics and systemic bioavailability of intranasally administered buprenorphine have been investigated in nine healthy volunteers in an intranasal/intravenous cross-over study. Each subject received a nominal 0.3 mg dose of buprenorphine intranasally followed 1 week later by a matched dose intravenously. For the intranasal administration mean t_{max} and mean C_{max} were 30.6 min and 1.77 ng/ml, respectively. Mean intranasal bioavailability was 48.2 ± 8.35% (mean ± SEM) of the intravenous value. Intranasal administration may represent a valuable new delivery route for buprenorphine.[14]

Transdermal

Fentanyl is effectively absorbed from a patch by the transdermal route, with a long duration of onset and offset suitable for providing stable blood levels over a period of days. The fentanyl patch was removed after 24 h. Plasma fentanyl concentrations increased to a plateau 14 h after application of the patch and thereafter relatively stable concentrations were maintained. After removal of the patch, fentanyl concentrations declined with an average terminal half-life of 17 + 2.3 h (mean + SD). This increased duration is presumed to result from continued absorption of fentanyl from the depot in the skin. The fentanyl patches were designed to deliver 100 μg/h fentanyl; the calculated delivery rate being 92 + 26 μg/h. The bioavailability of fentanyl was 92%. The results indicate that transdermal fentanyl may be a useful technique for management of patients with pain after surgery. However, the wide variability in the delivery of fentanyl may be a problem and further studies are needed, including ones where the patch remains for longer periods.[15]

Nebulized

Although this is an unsuitable route of administration for systemic effects,[16] topical opioids may have a role in the management of airway disease. Mucus secretion is reduced by morphine, possibly by inhibiting substance-P release in response to irritation.[17] In addition, opioids are efficacious in reducing airway excitation by a mechanism involving not only the cholinergic, but also another undefined system.[18] However, opioid inhalation can also be associated with occupational asthma.[19]

For the spinal route, see p. 437.

Factors affecting opioid pharmacokinetics

Anaesthesia

Decrease in splanchnic blood flow during general anaesthesia, particularly for abdominal surgery, could be expected to decrease metabolism of opioids with high hepatic clearance. The situation is exacerbated by hypovolaemia and concomitant use of halothane and β-blockers. In general, however, the effect of general anaesthesia on morphine metabolism is minimal, but metabolite accumulation is presumably due to reduced renal excretion.[20] However, Hudson *et al.*[21] determined the pharmacokinetics of sufentanil, 12.5 μg/kg iv in ten patients undergoing abdominal aortic surgery. They found that the volume of distribution was greater and the elimination half-life longer than values reported in previous studies on the pharmacokinetics of sufentanil.

Renal failure

Deterioration of renal function leads to build-up of hydrophilic metabolites of morphine. A reduced volume of distribution is also noted.[22] In the case of active metabolites, such as morphine-6-glucuronide, accumulation could lead to toxic effects such as respiratory depression.[23]

With buprenorphine, no difference in pharmacokinetics was noted between healthy and renally impaired patients. No metabolites were detected (buprenorphine-3-glucuronide and norbuprenorphine) with a single iv dose. Infusion in ITU patients (161 μg/h average) showed similar clearance to normals (1 l/min) but increased levels of norbuprenorphine (four times) and buprenorphine-3-glucuronide (fifteen times).[24]

Sufentanil pharmacokinetics are not affected by renal failure.[25]

Liver disease

Metabolism of most opioids is flow limited (methadone is the exception). A decreased *Cl*, prolongation of $t_{\frac{1}{2}\beta}$ and increased duration of action has been shown for morphine,[26] although not for sufentanil.[27] In mild to moderate liver disease, a reduction in oral dosage is needed as there is an increase (up to three-fold) in oral opioid bioavailability, not only due to decreased extraction by the liver but also to portosystemic shunting. This applies particularly to pethidine and pentazocine. Drugs given by the sublingual route (such as buprenorphine) or parenterally require little adjustment of dosage in mild to moderate disease. However, in moderate to severe liver disease, hepatic blood flow and plasma *Cl* fall still further leading to a marked prolongation of $t_{\frac{1}{2}\beta}$. Increase in the dosage interval together with careful titration is then required.

Neonates, infants and children

The pharmacokinetics of fentanyl have been studied in a number of centres and in general the clearance is increased. A greater decrease in plasma concentration has been noted in infants versus adults,[28] but the effects of abdominal surgery must be taken into account as these can have a deleterious effect on fentanyl clearance.[29,30]

Buprenorphine (3 μg/kg) was given intravenously as premedication to small children (age 4–7 years) undergoing minor surgery. Because of the rapid decline of the plasma buprenorphine concentrations, the terminal elimination half-life could not be estimated reliably. Given this constraint, values of clearance appeared to be higher than those in adults but values of V_d were similar.[31]

Old age

Limited pharmacokinetic data are available for opioid use in the elderly patient. The main effect in the elderly is a fall in opioid clearance due to a reduction in liver blood flow, which may be up to 50%. Thus $t_{\frac{1}{2}\beta}$ is prolonged up to three-fold.[32,33] A reduction in the volume of distribution has been shown for morphine[34] which, taken together with the prolongation of $t_{\frac{1}{2}\beta}$, suggests that both loading and maintenance doses should be reduced.

Enzyme inhibition

High clearance drugs are less affected by changes in enzyme activity than liver blood flow. The clearance of alfentanil is lower than other commonly used opioids (with the exception of methadone) and in a controlled, cross-over study in six volunteers it was demonstrated that a 7-day course of erythromycin significantly inhibits the metabolism of alfentanil.[35] It would be expected that other inhibitors such as cimetidine and metronidazole would have similar effects.

Influence of opioid physical characteristics

In order to be effective, opioids have to cross the blood–brain barrier. However, it is important to appreciate that although only the unionized fraction (free base) is lipophilic, individual opioids vary considerably in the lipid solubility of the unionized fraction (see Table 25.5). Increasing lipophilicity of the free base of the drug (octanol/water (O/W) partition for free base), tends to increase protein binding. Thus, buprenorphine has an O/W of 2320 with 96% bound to protein whereas morphine has an O/W of 1, with only 35% bound.

Only the unbound, free base of the drug (diffusible %) is able to penetrate the biophase to exert its effect at the receptor, for example morphine is 24% unionized free base at body pH with 65% unbound to protein. Therefore, 16% of the total is available for diffusion across the blood–brain barrier.

In the case of buprenorphine, the diffusible percentage is 0.35%. The actual lipid-diffusing potential (LDP) of the drug overall is the product of this diffusible per cent multiplied by the octanol/water partition coefficient. The lipid-diffusing index (LDI) is the ratio of the LDP of the drug to the LDP of morphine (see Table 25.6). Thus, the ability of fentanyl to diffuse through lipid (LDI) is eighty-four times that of morphine, which accounts for its more rapid onset of action. Despite its high LDI, buprenorphine has a delayed onset of action due to slow receptor *association* (see p. 432).

Types of opioid receptors and the development of agonist/antagonists

Following the development of *n*-allyl norcodeine and then nalorphine (*n*-allyl normorphine) (1940) as a morphine antagonist, the subsequent discovery of nalorphine's analgesic properties[36] made it clear that it was not essential for an effective 'opioid-like' analgesic to be strongly addictive or exhibit dose-dependent respiratory depression. The limitations on the use of nalorphine as an analgesic relate to its propensity to cause dysphoric effects (see p. 443).

TABLE 25.6 Diffusibility of morphine, buprenorphine and fentanyl

DRUG	DIFFUSIBLE % (FB% × UB%)	PARTITION COEFFICIENT at pH 7.4	LDP	LDI
Morphine	16	1	16	1
Fentanyl	1.4	960	1344	84
Buprenorphine	0.35	2320	812	51

FB, freebase; UB, unbound.
LDP, lipid-diffusing potential; LDI, lipid-diffusing index.

The benzomorphan group of drugs exhibited similar properties to nalorphine and led to the development of phenazocine (μ-agonist), ketocyclazocine (κ-agonist) and pentazocine (μ-antagonist, κ-agonist). The latter represented the first clinically acceptable strong analgesic which was (at the time) uncontrolled, although still exhibiting dysphoria. Drugs such as pentazocine and nalbuphine have an analgesic potential which is more divorced from dangerous side-effects (respiratory depression and addiction) than the conventional opioids. However, if respiratory depression does occur with pentazocine, it is not reversed by nalorphine. Although this could be explained on the assumption that both these drugs were simply partial μ-agonists, other facts made this untenable. Pentazocine is unable to substitute for morphine in morphine addiction making it unlikely to be a partial μ-agonist. In addition, although naloxone *is* capable of reversing respiratory depression of both morphine and pentazocine, it is markedly less effective in the latter.

The opioid buprenorphine is a partial agonist, but closely resembles the full agonist end of the spectrum. In most situations it is indistinguishable from a full agonist, showing little tendency for its efficacy to tail off at high dosage (e.g. drug A in Fig. 25.8). However, since the peak (ceiling) effect is less than with the agonist (e.g. drug B in Fig. 25.8), it can act like an antagonist following prior administration of the agonist at high dose levels. Thus, a patient with respiratory depression following a large dose of the opioid fentanyl, may have this reversed (but not the analgesia) by administration of buprenorphine.[37a] On the other hand, if a small dose of agonist has been given first, buprenorphine will act in tandem and increase analgesia and vice versa.[37b]

For this reason, buprenorphine is often classified incorrectly as an agonist/antagonist analgesic, but it is more correctly referred to as a high efficacy partial agonist. The true agonist/antagonist drugs, such as nalbuphine and pentazocine, exert their agonist (analgesic) effects on the κ-receptor and their antagonist effects on the μ-receptor (receptor dualism, see pp. 424 and 443). They have a completely different profile from buprenorphine, although often receiving a similar classification (see Table 25.7).

The ability of the μ-antagonist–κ-agonist drugs to also produce dysphoria (nalorphine > pentazocine > nalbuphine) is due to their action on σ-receptors. These are also thought responsible for the same effects seen with the induction agents phencyclidine (PCP) and ketamine. Whether these receptors are one and the same is still disputed by some. The term 'sigma' derives from the SKF benzomorphan compound, *n*-allyl normetazocine, which causes σ-effects *par excellence* (see Table 25.7).

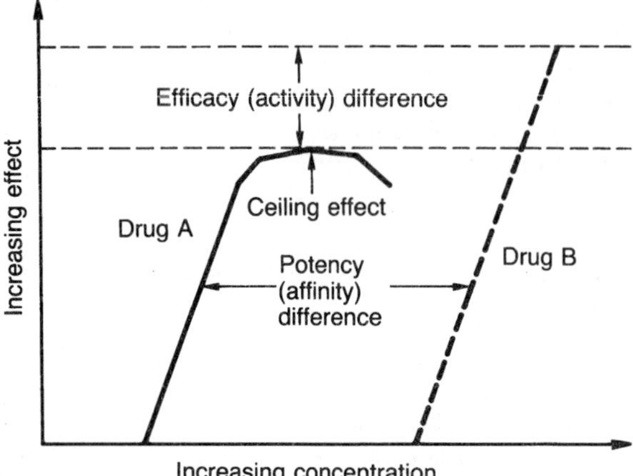

FIGURE 25.8 Opioid efficacy and potency differences. Drug A is more potent than drug B (e.g. buprenorphine). Drug B is more efficacious than drug A (e.g. morphine).

Age-related pharmacodynamic changes

Neonates

Although pharmacokinetic data suggest that neonates and infants handle opioids in the same way as older children and adults, they seem significantly more sensitive to the pharmacodynamic effects, especially respiratory depression. This makes pain relief involving the use of opioids problematical. A retrospective review of 131 neonates admitted to a surgical ICU showed that there is a high risk of sudden apnoea and respiratory obstruction when opioids are used in the spontaneously breathing patient.[38] Other methods of pain relief besides opioids are recommended unless the patient can be nursed in a high dependency environment with facilities for rapid resuscitation should respiratory arrest occur.[39]

Infants older than 3 months are no more sensitive than older patients to the ventilatory depressant effects of fentanyl when assessed by cutaneous $Pa{CO_2}$ and ventilatory pattern recording using impedance pneumography. Elevation of $Pa{CO_2}$ correlated with increasing plasma fentanyl concentrations but did not differ between groups.[29]

Older children show no differences in response to equipotent doses of opioids.

Effect of old age

Provided that alteration in pharmacokinetics of opioids is taken into account in this age group, there is no evidence to support the premise that the elderly are more 'sensitive' pharmacodynamically to opioids.

TABLE 25.7 Opioid agonist and agonist/antagonist drugs

	μ-RECEPTOR	κ-RECEPTOR	σ-RECEPTOR
Receptor effects	Supraspinal analgesia Euphoria Respiratory depression *** Tolerance and addiction *** Drug seeking behaviour *** Miosis *** Reversible with naloxone ***	Spinal analgesia Sedation Respiratory depression * Tolerance and addiction * Drug seeking behaviour * Miosis * Reversible with naloxone *	Not analgesic Dysphoria Respiratory stimulation – – Mydriasis Reversible with naloxone *
Drug effects			
Morphine	+++	+	0
Fentanyl	+++	0	0
Buprenorphine	(+++)	–	0
Nalorphine	– –	(++)	++
Pentazocine	–	(++)	+
Nalbuphine	(+)	(++)	0 – +
Cyclazocine	– –	++	++
Ketocyclazocine	0	+++	0
Naloxone	– – –	– –	– –
N-allyl normetazocine	?	?	+++

KEY
+++ Strong agonist.
++ Moderate agonist.
+ Weak agonist.
– – – Strong antagonist.
– – Moderate antagonist.
– Weak antagonist.

(+++) Strong partial agonist.
(++) Medium partial agonist.
0 No effect.
? Effect disputed.

*** Strong effect.
** Medium effect.
* Weak effect.

For fuller explanation, see text.

Other drug interactions and concomitant drug therapy

The effect of alcohol, smoking and caffeine

There is evidence to suggest that chronic consumption of alcohol, smoking and caffeine significantly increase patient requirement for fentanyl.[40] The effect of alcohol intake on the pharmacodynamics of alfentanil was studied in six females with an average daily consumption of 20–40 g alcohol and eight females who were abstainers. The plasma concentrations of alfentanil needed to suppress responses to surgical stimulation were twice as high in the alcohol consumers as in the abstainers. A similar difference was found for the plasma concentration associated with adequate spontaneous ventilation at the end of surgery.[41]

The effect of anticonvulsants

An increased requirement for fentanyl by infusion has been noted in a carefully controlled trial in patients on anticonvulsants undergoing craniotomy. Although this was presumed due to a pharmacodynamic interaction, it is possible that enzyme induction could have been responsible for this effect.[42]

PHYSIOLOGICAL EFFECTS OF OPIOIDS

Central nervous system (CNS)

Apart from those effects already mentioned, such as analgesia, euphoria and sedation, opioids exert other effects on the CNS which have important clinical implications. In addition, they may adversely affect the CNS indirectly, for example opioid-induced carbon dioxide retention causing increased intracranial pressure in head-injured patients.

Respiration

Respiratory depression is the most important adverse CNS effect and is seen in intimate association with the use of all opioid drugs.[43,44] High-dose opioids used intraoperatively may result in a large proportion of patients requiring naloxone at the end of the procedure.[45] In the postoperative period the danger of hypoxaemia in association with respiratory depression is evident whichever route of administration is used, but is especially common if used intrathecally (see p. 439). In a direct comparison with iv (patient controlled analgesia, PCA) and im, respiratory depression and epochs of hypoxaemia were found to be quantitatively more severe with the extradural route.[46]

Pain is a significant antagonist to the respiratory depressant effects of opioids. Sudden alleviation of the pain by addition of local anaesthetic blockade may precipitate hypoxaemia and apnoea. Sleep can have similar effects.[47]

Long-acting barbiturates such as thiopentone may be associated with a higher risk of respiratory depression from the use of some opioids in the perioperative period. This effect is not seen with etomidate, a shorter-acting induction agent.[48] Several workers have noted an increased tendency for sedation and respiratory depression with the associated use of benzodiazepines (as premedicants or induction supplements) and buprenorphine [48–52] although the effects have not been quantified. This 'additive' or 'synergistic' effect has been associated with a number of fatalities when opioids such as pentazocine are combined with benzodiazepines for sedation during endoscopy.

Nausea and vomiting

Nausea and vomiting are a feature of the use of all opioids. It is caused by a dopamine-like agonist action of the drug at the chemoreceptor trigger zone (CTZ) in the area postrema. This, in turn, causes activation of the emetic centre (EC) in the floor of the IV ventricle. Although dopamine antagonist anti-emetics, such as metoclopramide and droperidol, are theoretically the most appropriate choice for prevention and treatment, there is also a significant labyrinthine component. This is manifest by a much higher incidence of nausea and vomiting in ambulant patients. It is rare for opioid premedication to produce nausea and vomiting in the recumbent patient preoperatively. Thus, drugs that reduce motion sickness, such as cyclizine and hyoscine, are useful in these cases. There is no evidence that there is any separation of analgesic efficacy from propensity of a particular opioid to cause nausea and vomiting.[51,53–55] It is much commoner if opioids are given spinally (see p. 439).

Opioid-induced anaesthesia

A resurgence in interest in opioid *anaesthesia* stemmed from the work of Lowenstein and colleagues in the late 1960s.[56] Morphine (0.5–3.0 mg/kg) was combined with oxygen to produce anaesthesia which was remarkably free of cardiovascular depression, thus especially useful for cardiac surgery.[57,58] The concomitant use of neuromuscular blockade and intermittent positive pressure ventilation in the intubated patient ensured that this technique had a considerably higher success rate than when it was used in the late 19th century!

Nevertheless, problems emerged when the technique came into more widespread use. Use of morphine was associated with vasodilatation, which required massive concomitant fluid therapy to avoid hypotension, and prolonged recovery. Fentanyl (75–150 μg/kg) and subsequently alfentanil and sufentanil have been employed instead, but there is still doubt as to whether this technique reliably produces *anaesthesia* as cases of awareness have been reported.[59] Studies have not demonstrated a dose-related increase in anaesthetic effect which therefore makes it impossible to guarantee unconsciousness.[60,61] As a result, other agents such as nitrous oxide[62] and diazepam[63] are frequently added, reducing awareness *and* opioid dose requirement, but at the expense of mild to moderate cardiac depression (see Moldenhauer[6]).

It is pertinent to note that high-dose *spinal* morphine may, paradoxically, produce hyperaesthesia (increased sensitivity to pain and/or non-noxious stimuli perceived as being 'painful') in the experimental animal. This may be due to accumulation of the antagonist metabolite morphine-3-glucuronide.[64,65]

Stress-free anaesthesia

The metabolic responses to anaesthesia and surgery include increased output of catecholamines, growth hormone, renin–angiotensin–aldosterone, antidiuretic hormone, adrenocorticotrophic hormone (ACTH) and cortisol and a resultant varying degree of insulin resistance. These result in the common accompaniments of surgery such as hypertension, tachycardia, sodium and water retention and immune depression. Hyperglycaemia results from increased mobilization of hepatic glucose stores and decreased peripheral utilization, the insulin response being abnormal and ineffective. Although these 'responses' are neurally mediated and can be blocked by regional anaesthetic techniques, blockade is usually only partial suggesting an additional local response from the injured tissue. This local 'wound factor' is thought to be the cytokine interleukin-1 (see Hall[66]).

It is not clear that these 'stress responses' to surgery are unequivocally bad,[67] indeed *specific* abolition of steroid production by the 11-β-OHase blocking action of etomidate has been associated with *increased* mortality in ICU patients. Nevertheless, stress-free anaesthesia seemed a goal worth striving for. The introduction of high-dose morphine (1 mg/kg) and morphine anaesthesia (as above) produce a partial blockade of these responses.[68] Fentanyl provided a more rational opioid to use for this purpose and has been extensively studied in pelvic[66] and cardiac surgery (see Moldenhauer[6]). Although high-dose opioids are able to abolish the stress response to sternotomy, effects during bypass are less predictable. To have a consistent effect, fentanyl should be administered in high dosage (50–100 μg/kg) prior to surgery. Prolonged respiratory depression and sedation are major problems (except in cardiac anaesthesia) and could be overcome by the use of buprenorphine to reverse these effects at the end of surgery, but allowing continuation of analgesia well into the postoperative period. This aspect remains to be evaluated.

Cardiovascular system

Haemodynamic effects

Evidence is accumulating that endogenous opioid peptides may have a significant role in haemodynamic regulation.[69] Exogenous opioids, such as morphine, produce peripheral vasodilatation and a fall in sensitivity of baroreceptor reflexes. In the absence of hypovolaemia and severe cardiac dysfunction little effect on cardiovascular haemodynamics is seen in the supine patient. However, hypotension can occur on assuming the upright position. A fall in peripheral resistance is used to good effect in patients with acute left ventricular failure where a fall in impedance to ventricular ejection results in improved cardiac output and a fall in pressure in the pulmonary circuit. Although vasodilatation may, in part, be due to histamine release with morphine and other opioids, it is rarely completely reversible with histamine antagonists. These sometime profound effects are specifically reversible with naloxone.[70] Agonist/antagonist drugs such as pentazocine[71] and partial agonists such as buprenorphine do not extensively release histamine and the effects are therefore less marked.[72]

Bradycardia

Bradycardia, due to a central opioid vagotonic action, is a common accompaniment of potent opioids such as fentanyl and sufentanil.[57] Severe bradycardia may still occur in patients given these drugs despite prophylactic glycopyrrolate when the baseline resting heart rate is low.[73] Not surprisingly, both propranolol and diltiazem are found to enhance the bradycardia induced by sufentanil and vecuronium.[73,74]

Antidysrhythmic effects

The dysrhythmias accompanying dental extraction may be circumvented by the judicious use of small doses of intravenous fentanyl. In addition, μ-agonists such as fentanyl and buprenorphine raise the myocardial fibrillatory threshold to both ischaemia and hypovolaemia in the animal model.[75] The former may be related to an anticholinergic effect as it is reversed by atropine.[76,77]

Effects on the pulmonary circulation

Although pentazocine was initially popular with general practitioners as a potent analgesic with little addiction potential, its use to relieve the pain of myocardial infarction was associated with an increase in pulmonary artery pressure.[78] This detrimental effect, probably σ-related, is a distinctive feature of the drug and is not found with conventional μ-opioids such as morphine,[79] pethidine[80] or the agonist/antagonist, nalbuphine.[81] Pentazocine is no longer advocated for use in this situation.

Gastrointestinal system

Opioids significantly delay gastric emptying, an effect that is reversed by naloxone and iv metoclopramide.[82] This may increase the risk of gastric aspiration, especially during induction of anaesthesia for emergency surgery (see Duthie and Nimmo[83]). In addition, there is an overall delay in gut transit time and this effect is demonstrable by both μ- and κ-agonists.[84] This effect on gut motility manifests itself as an adynamic ileus in the ICU patient receiving opioid sedation and as troublesome constipation in the chronic pain patient maintained on oral morphine.

Sphincter of Oddi

Injection of morphine results in constriction of the sphincter of Oddi with 10–15-fold increases in pressure in the common bile duct. This can precipitate or worsen symptoms of biliary colic in some patients (see Staritz[85]). Other opioids, particularly the piperidine analogues pethidine and fentanyl, are much less likely to cause this problem. Buprenorphine has been found to have no undesirable effects on the biliary tract.[86]

NATURALLY OCCURRING OPIOID ANTAGONISTS

Clinical use of opioid analgesics preceded the discovery of endogenous opioid *agonists*. Recent work has demonstrated the presence of endogenous opioid *antagonists*, which are likely to have increasing clinical relevance. Cholecystokinin octapeptide (CCK), closely related to the gastrin family of peptides, is an important neuropeptide in the CNS and is involved in nociception.[87] Although in large doses it is capable of producing analgesia, at physiological levels it antagonizes opioid analgesia mediated by μ- and κ- but not δ-receptors in the spinal cord of the rat.[88] Indeed, opioids and endogenous opioid peptides may release CCK from nerve terminals in the spinal cord, thus diminishing analgesia.

On the other hand, the use of CCK *antagonists* such as proglumide[89,90] and L-365, 260[91] can enhance opioid analgesia and prevent tolerance. The clinical significance of CCK and related compounds remains to be elucidated.

The role of opioid metabolites

During chronic therapy with morphine, there is accumulation of the major metabolite of morphine, morphine-3-glucuronide. This has been implicated as an antagonist/inverse agonist in that it may produce hyperaesthesia in the experimental animal.[65]

INTRAOPERATIVE OPIOIDS

The concept of 'balanced anaesthesia' was introduced by Lundy in 1926 to describe a technique whereby the different components of premedication, general and regional anaesthesia were combined so that analgesia and unconsciousness were provided by a 'balance' of different techniques.[92] Following the introduction of curare, pethidine was added to nitrous oxide to produce the forerunner of the 'balanced' anaesthetic technique still in widespread use today.[93] This technique was subsequently extended to children.[94]

Opioids are now widely used intraoperatively as part of a balanced anaesthetic technique. Although different opioids have been used for this purpose, very few controlled studies outside cardiac surgery have looked at the comparative effects of one opioid versus another in the quality of anaesthesia obtained. In a rigorously controlled, double-blind, study Flacke and others[45] studied four commonly used opioids, morphine, pethidine, fentanyl and sufentanil in major surgery (e.g. hip, spine and abdominal). Using moderate doses of opioid (e.g. fentanyl 7.5 μg/kg), they looked at quality of induction (additional thiopentone was used), cardiovascular stability, catecholamine production, recovery and resumption of spontaneous respiration and requirement for naloxone (1.5 μg/kg iv increments if respiratory rate was less than 12/min or $Paco_2 > 50$ mmHg). Morphine (0.6 mg/kg) was least satisfactory both in controlling haemodynamics (additional inhalation agents were used as necessary) and for slowness of recovery. Pethidine (5.0 mg/kg) was least satisfactory at induction due to histamine release, hypotension and tachycardia. Sufentanil (1.5 μg/kg) was most satisfactory overall, no patients requiring inhalational supplementation, although 40% of patients required a single dose of naloxone postoperatively.

In a double-blind study using more modest doses of opioid (morphine 0.15 mg/kg or buprenorphine 5 μg/kg) no differences were detected in intraoperative cardiovascular stability or quality of anaesthesia for major gynaecological surgery.[95] No patients required naloxone.

Since anaesthetists should be concerned with the quality of postoperative analgesia it is pertinent to consider the carry-over effect of the intraoperative analgesic and the time to administration of first postoperative analgesic. Buprenorphine has been compared in this regard with fentanyl given intraoperatively.[96] Although intraoperative conditions were equally satisfactory, there was a longer period of postoperative analgesia with buprenorphine (12 h to first postoperative analgesic versus 2.8 h with fentanyl). If the latter drug *is* used, recovery room staff *must* be in a position to rapidly regain analgesia, preferably by the use of iv opioids. Casual use of im opioids on an ordinary ward is unlikely to be sufficient.

OPIOIDS FOR POSTOPERATIVE PAIN

There is evidence that prescribing habits are resulting in patients receiving less analgesia than they need. But, patients are usually uncomplaining, so just because they do not make a fuss does not mean that they are not in pain.[97] Various methods of drug delivery are available in the postoperative period.

Nurse administered

Although a prn (pro re nata) prescription of an opioid may seem simple to the prescriber, in practice it may be fraught with difficulties. Unfortunately, to give a controlled drug on a general ward may take up to 30 min involving:

- complicated protocols and extra staff due to controlled drug regulations
- the use of syringes and needles (adding to expense, time and patient discomfort)
- if the drug is short acting (e.g. 2 h for pethidine) then up to 25% of the nurse's time may be engaged in administering postoperative pain-relieving drugs.
- the onset time of an im drug (30–60 min) may be too slow to catch up with the rapidly declining analgesia of a short-acting intraoperative opioid (see p. 428)

The result is that the patient ends up in pain. In addition, doctors underprescribe analgesics and nurses reduce these doses still further.

Pharmacokinetic and pharmacodynamic principles dictate that there is no way that 3–4 hrly prn im regimes of parenteral opioids (except buprenorphine and methadone) can be expected to produce good postoperative analgesia. A better solution is to use either a long-acting (due to pharmacodynamics) analgesic such as buprenorphine which consistently gives equivalent (or better) analgesia to controlled drugs with less administrative effort[53,95,98,99] or to titrate iv a long-acting (due to pharmacokinetics) analgesic such as methadone.[100]

Regular pre-emptive opioids

A number of studies have assessed the analgesia obtainable by *regular* (pre-emptive) use of opioids in the postoperative period. This has included a variety of techniques and agents, such as by im injection, sl or by nurse-controlled iv infusion.[48,101–106] The results have generally been good, with both sl buprenorphine and im morphine proving equally satisfactory to PCA techniques (see next section). However, these techniques, particularly the iv infusions, have the inherent danger of respiratory depression and must only be carried out in a high-dependency environment with nurse/patient ratios much higher than is to be found on a normal ward.

Patient-controlled analgesia (PCA)

Patient-controlled analgesic techniques were first introduced in 1970,[107] the implication being that an improvement in analgesic efficacy is obtained by allowing the patient (rather than the nurse) to manage analgesic requirements. Following introduction of the concept, it became a useful medium for comparing efficacy of different opioids for postoperative pain relief.[108] Although the availability of custom-made apparatus, with in-built safety features, increased the popularity and applicability of the technique,[109] the cost of the apparatus remained prohibitive.[110] The normal route of administration is iv, but the im[111] and epidural routes (see p. 438) have also been employed. The patient must be given clear instructions on how to use the apparatus for maximal benefit. To avoid inadvertent toxicity, the following parameters must be preset by the operator:

- Correct dose and concentration of opioid setup in the machine.
- Demand dose administered (e.g. 15 mg for iv pethidine)
- Lockout interval. The time interval from an administered dose until the next dose will be given by the machine despite patient requests (e.g. 9 min for pethidine). This prevents repeated doses at short intervals and thus limits toxicity but also the amount of drug the patient can receive.
- Maximum hourly dose (e.g. 75 mg/h for pethidine)

Much effort has been expended on coming up with suitable doses of analgesics and the time intervals of administration.[112] For maximum efficacy a loading dose of the appropriate analgesic must be administered before allowing the machine to take over as these regimes only cater for maintenance requirements.

Once the apparatus is satisfactorily set up, the great advantage claimed for PCA over techniques of postoperative analgesia such as opioids by infusion, regular administration and by spinal techniques is absence of need to monitor the patient in a high-dependency environment.

Although the technique has proved acceptable,[50,113,114] the results have not always been convincingly in favour of PCA when compared with *regular* sl buprenorphine[103] or *regular* im morphine.[104] Poor results for PCA may be explained by:

- Failure to adequately explain the apparatus to the patient.
- Failure to give a loading dose.
- The patient choosing pain rather than adverse effects of opioids, for example nausea and excessive sedation.
- Excessive pain following a period of sleep during which there has been no administration of analgesic. During the 'catching up' period, the patient will be in pain.

The latter problem is partially addressed by utilizing apparatus that has the ability to provide a background infusion of opioid, but this is not entirely effective and leads to increased opioid consumption.[112]

Thus, although finding favour with some,[107] PCA techniques did not come into widespread use for two reasons:

- the expense and complexity of the apparatus
- the introduction, at about the same time, of spinal opioid techniques that were 'automatically' assumed to be more efficacious

It is only in the last few years that direct comparison has been made between PCA and epidural opioids, the former being slightly less efficacious but equally if not more acceptable to the patient (see p. 440). It was not long before the patient was also able to control the administration of opioids by the epidural route.[115]

Is PCA the ideal way to administer opioids for postoperative pain relief?[107] The very narrow dividing line between serious respiratory depression, good analgesia and no pain relief at all, suggests that it might be. However, it must be said that regular sublingual buprenorphine or im morphine give equivalent analgesia to iv pethidine or fentanyl via PCA. There is no convincing evidence that PCA is better than other forms of postoperative analgesia in the trial situation.

Spinal opioids

The discovery of endogenous opioid receptors and ligands in the brain and spinal cord led to the feasibility of their use spinally. Intrathecally applied narcotics produced a long-lasting elevation in the nociceptive threshold.[116,117] Clinical use of this technique in man followed with first reports by Behar *et al.*[118] (epidural) and Wang *et al.*[119] (intrathecal) in 1979. At the outset, it is most important to establish the rationale for the spinal administration of opioids. There must be firm evidence that this route is preferable, in terms of analgesic effectiveness, without an increase in side-effects such as respiratory depression, when compared with the simpler and less invasive oral or parenteral administration. If questioned, patients may not wish to accept increased risks for the possible benefit of improved analgesia.[120] It should also be remembered that none of the opioids is licensed for use by the epidural or intrathecal route in acute pain.

Crucial to the subsequent popularity of spinal opioids was the observation that the effects were primarily limited to pain perception, *selective spinal analgesia*, with little effect on motor, sensory (e.g. pin prick) and autonomic function.[121] Adverse effects of spinal opioids, however, are extremely important and are noted later.

When given epidurally, opioids can reach the cord and brain:

- by penetrating the dura
- by gaining access via arachnoid granulations
- via the posterior radicular artery direct to the cord
- via systemic spread

Pharmacokinetics of intrathecal opioids

A study of the pharmacokinetics of intrathecal morphine was carried out by Nordberg *et al.*[122] Using two groups of patients (twelve in all) receiving either 0.25 or 0.5 mg of morphine, they measured cerebrospinal fluid (CSF) levels of morphine at 1, 3, 5 and 18 h postinjection. The CSF levels at 1 h postinjection averaged 4200 and 10 400 ng/ml respectively. Finding that the terminal elimination half-life ($t_{\frac{1}{2}\beta}$) of 180 min and relative clearance of morphine from CSF were similar to that from plasma, they concluded that the long duration of action of morphine by the intrathecal route must therefore result from the high concentrations of morphine found in the CSF. Plasma levels were very low (<1 ng/ml).

Sjostrom *et al.*[123] compared the plasma and CSF kinetics for 6 h in two groups of patients who received either morphine (0.3 mg) or pethidine (10 mg) intrathecally. The CSF levels achieved were very variable (C_{max} of 6400 ± 1290 ng/ml for morphine) with a $t_{\frac{1}{2}\beta}$ of 90 min for morphine and 68 min for pethidine. The more rapid elimination of pethidine was thought due to its increased lipid solubility and could thus explain its lessened tendency to produce late respiratory depression.

Pharmacokinetics of epidural opioids

Sjostrom *et al.*[124] reported on the pharmacokinetics of epidural morphine and pethidine. There were 5 groups of 6 patients each, with measurements being made of the appearance of the opioids in the plasma and CSF. With morphine, the influence of volume of injectate (3 mg in 1 ml or 10 ml) was also studied. t_{max} was 5–10 min for the appearance of morphine in the plasma (C_{max} 39.5 +/– 2.9 ng/ml), with a $t_{\frac{1}{2}\beta}$ of 90 min. For CSF, the t_{max} was 60 – 90 min (C_{max} 1290 +/– 182 ng/ml) with a $t_{\frac{1}{2}}$ (absorption) of 22 min. Overall dural transfer rate was 3.6% and elimination showed a biphasic pattern with a $t_{\frac{1}{2}}$ of 1 h and 6 h.

They concluded that there were large interindividual differences with respect to both plasma and CSF kinetics and pain relief in all groups. The volumes of the bolus (1 or 10 ml) with morphine was not of major importance. It seems that the increased area of absorption with the larger volume is balanced by the reduced concentration gradient. Despite similar kinetics, the duration of morphine was longer than with pethidine, but, notably, the CSF concentration of opioid at which analgesia was requested was extremely variable.

Sjostrom *et al.* calculated that the minimum effective analgesic concentration of morphine in the CSF was about 50 ng/ml. Obviously the peak concentrations obtained with both epidural and intrathecal morphine greatly exceed this. It is interesting that morphine is not detectable in the CSF even when given chronically by the oral route in high doses up to 24 h prior to sampling.[125]

Choice of intrathecal opioid

Although large individual series of intrathecal opioids have been reported, there has been little work comparing their use with more conventional techniques in randomized, double-blind, prospective studies. Diamorphine and low-dose intrathecal morphine (0.1–0.3 mg) are effective and may be less prone to respiratory depression than larger dose techniques.[126–128]

Choice of epidural opioid

Morphine

Morphine has moderate *in vitro* dural permeability but low lipophilicity. Its overall dural transfer rate is 3.6%.[124] It has a slow onset of action, with a modest contribution from systemic uptake. The long duration of action is due to low systemic concentration and metabolism and high receptor affinity, with a low epidural/systemic dose requirement ratio. It is a reasonable choice, but more likely to migrate rostrally with the possibility of delayed respiratory depression.

Diamorphine

Diamorphine also has moderate *in vitro* dual permeability but is more lipophilic than morphine. It has thus a faster onset of action, with a large (early) contribution from systemic uptake. Duration of action is less than with morphine (although its conversion to morphine makes it longer than would be expected from the physical properties), with a 1 : 1 epidural/systemic dose requirement ratio. Little advantage would seem to accrue from epidural use, except for a moderate increase in duration of action over the systemic route. Addition of adrenaline may be advantageous (qv). CSF data are difficult to obtain and interpret due to its rapid conversion to morphine.

Fentanyl

Fentanyl has excellent *in vitro* dural permeability and high lipophilicity. It has thus a very rapid onset of action, but due to its high dural permeability there is no need to maintain a high concentration gradient in the epidural space. This tends to negate the otherwise high systemic absorption of the drug. Duration of action is short (owing to rapid receptor dissociation) requiring continuous infusion. Recent studies comparing iv and epidural fentanyl have cast doubt on improved efficacy for the epidural (thoracic or lumbar) versus simpler iv administration. Most studies have shown no (or only slight) advantages, sometimes with increased side-effects with the epidural route, sometimes with the iv route.[130–135] Only one trial has discerned advantages in terms of a lower dose and reduced side-effects in patients after thoracotomy.[136] The role of epidural fentanyl must now be seriously questioned.

Buprenorphine

Buprenorphine has poor *in vitro* dural permeability with very high lipophilicity, high receptor affinity but limited activity (partial agonist). It is as effective epidurally as morphine but the manufacturers do not recommend its use in this fashion. It is possibly too lipophilic, which together with poor dural penetration, results in significant systemic uptake.

Conclusions

Sjostrom *et al.*[124] concluded that the ideal epidural opioid should be lipophilic with a strong affinity for the opioid receptor. This would ensure a rapid onset, long duration of action and low risk of rostral transport.

Toxicity

The most feared complication of spinal opioids is severe respiratory depression and there is evidence that this is more likely when opioids are given by this route.[46] The subject has been comprehensively reviewed.[137]

Respiratory depression

Intrathecal route

Many reports followed the initial clinical use of intrathecal opioids in 1979 (e.g. Davies[129]) with an incidence of approximately 0.36%.[138] Respiratory depression may occur even up to 24 h postinjection. Aggravating factors include adjuvant use of depressant drugs, for example benzodiazepines, concomitant use of other opioids, nursing in the supine position postoperatively and rapid injection. It is pertinent to observe that almost all cases have followed intrathecal morphine when used for postoperative analgesia. Rostral spread of opioid in the CSF to the respiratory centre is thus favoured for a hydrophilic drug (such as morphine) that does not have high cord penetrability. Thus, more of the drug may be available for spread, and this increases if the patient is nursed in a supine position.

Epidural route

Results of the nationwide Swedish survey[138] suggest a 0.09% incidence of clinically obvious respiratory depression, but this is probably an underestimate, and certainly less than their report of 1982.[139]

Early onset of respiratory depression usually occurs within an hour and probably represents a bolus effect from epidural vein systemic absorption. It may also follow inadvertent direct venous injection or spinal tap. (Remember that the dose of opioid used is often large, e.g. pethidine 100 mg.)

Late onset of respiratory depression occurs for similar reasons to intrathecal opioids (see above). Respiration depression is usually evident if ventilatory response to carbon dioxide is measured.[140] It is not quite clear whether severe respiratory depression occurs to the same extent with all opioids.

Effect of chronic use

Chronic administration of epidural opioid seems to protect the patient against respiratory depression, although it has been described following accidental intrathecal injection of morphine during chronic epidural use.[141]

Treatment of respiratory depression

See also sections on monitoring and opioid antagonists.

Use of antagonists

Patients receiving spinal opioids must be closely monitored (see p. 440). Naloxone is the antagonist of choice for spinal opioid-induced respiratory depression. Other antagonists have been used and are effective, such as naltrexone which can be given orally.[142] Nalbuphine, a κ-agonist analgesic with partial agonist (or antagonist) effects on the μ-receptor, is also effective in humans[143–145] (see p. 424).

Adverse effects of antagonists

Naloxone and naltrexone, although effective in treating respiratory depression, have been shown in carefully controlled studies to produce a dose-related reversal of analgesia.[142,146,147] It is also important to remember that sudden reversal of intense opioid action (e.g. with naloxone) can lead to serious side-effects such as pulmonary oedema[180] and cardiac arrest.[148] Analgesics, such as buprenorphine, nalbuphine and possibly butorphanol, which have partial agonist activity at the μ-receptor, may act like full antagonists in the presence of excess opioid. It should be noted here that, when substituting epidural for oral opioids in chronic pain conditions where the latter has become ineffective, withdrawal symptoms can occur unless the oral component is reduced very slowly.

Nausea and vomiting

The incidence following intrathecal opioids is very high,[149] but appears to be lower epidurally, the incidence decreasing with chronic use. However, the incidence following epidural opioid for postoperative pain control is often higher than following the same opioid systemically.[150,151] It is not clear whether naloxone consistently ameliorates nausea and vomiting.[151] In parturients, the incidence of nausea and vomiting can be reduced by transdermal scopolamine.[152]

Pruritus

This is noted very commonly after epidural and intrathecal administration of opioids, notably of morphine, diamorphine, pethidine and fentanyl. An overall incidence of 8.5% after epidural opioid (15 272 cases) and 46% after intrathecal opioid (264 cases) using these drugs has been reported.[153] The symptom probably reflects the role of endogenous opioids in enhancing as well as suppressing protective reflexes, itch being a manifestation of the enhanced scratch reflex. It is less common after buprenorphine,[154] if bupivacaine is mixed with the opioid, and is not reported with the use of β-endorphin.[155] Spinal opioid-induced itch can sometimes be abated by nalbuphine[143,144,156] and systemic opioid antagonists such as naloxone.[151,157]

Retention of urine

This is a more common complication when spinal opioids are used in volunteers rather than in patients with opioid-sensitive pain. The incidence varies widely.[158] Opioids and specific opioid receptors are known to play a role in mediation of bladder activity and bladder reflexes both at spinal and supraspinal levels. This may be utilized to good effect by reducing detrusor activity and improving postoperative analgesia in patients following prostatic surgery.[128]

Spinal haematoma

The increasing use of prophylactic (rather than therapeutic) heparinization prior to major surgery and the increasing use of low-dose aspirin has placed enormous constraints on the use of epidural and spinal techniques.[159] Many anaesthetists feel very wary about the safety of spinal blockade in these circumstances. The subject has been reviewed by Owens *et al.*[160] It is important for anaesthetists to weigh up the risk benefit ratio for any patient who is on anticoagulants and for whom spinal opioids are contemplated. The problem is discussed in detail by Horlocker *et al.*[161]

Clinical experience of spinal opioids

Introduction

A casual perusal of the literature reveals the explosion of clinical work, anecdotal to carefully controlled, that has been performed in the last 10 years. The majority has centred around postoperative and chronic pain control.

Monitoring

At the outset, it cannot be overemphasized that the ever-present spectre of respiratory depression, particularly with intrathecal morphine, necessitates that these patients are closely monitored (e.g. blood pressure, respiratory rate and pulse oximetry) for at least 12 h in a high dependency or intensive care unit (HDU, ICU). Apparatus and skilled personnel for oxygenating and ventilating the apnoeic patient and dealing with cardiovascular collapse must be immediately available. It is important to remember other risk factors that might be present, particularly additional systemic opioids. This requirement greatly restricts their routine use postoperatively.

In addition, perception of the effectiveness and safety of this technique may be overestimated by the anaesthetist. In a prospective trial, follow-up of patients with epidural opioids for postoperative analgesia was carried out by a pain team. The study revealed four out of fifteen patients with severe respiratory depression, despite all having been managed in ICU for the first 24 h postoperatively. The anaesthesiologist responsible for the regime was unaware of the trial or the complications that ensued. The trial was terminated and closer follow-up instituted.[162]

However, it has to be recognized that some centres which have employed epidural opioids for many years, have abandoned the requirement for all patients to stay for prolonged periods in HDU postoperatively. Instead, they have emphasized the requirement for strict protocols to be observed by nursing, surgical and anaesthetic staff for the management of these patients.

Use in obstetrics for labour and delivery

Intrathecal morphine produces adequate analgesia in the majority of parturients (varying from 50% pain relief to complete). The duration of analgesia is quoted as being from 2 to 10 h with an average of 6 h. Doses used have varied from 0.5 mg[163] to 2 mg.[164] Unfortunately, a high incidence of side-effects is described including pruritus, nausea and vomiting in about 50% of patients. Only pruritus is reliably reduced by naloxone.[165] Although maternal progress and fetal well-being do not seem to be compromised,[164] this technique would not seem to confer any advantage over more conventional epidural techniques using local anaesthetics.

Epidural fentanyl has been used extensively by the St Thomas' group in London. It is undoubtedly effective, with little contribution claimed from systemic absorption. However, it is considered less effective than local anaesthetics and its use is reserved principally for perineal pain which is unrelieved by bupivacaine 0.25%.[166]

As epidural opioids on their own are relatively ineffective in labour, combined opioid and local anaesthetic techniques are being used increasingly. Their use is supported by experimental evidence suggesting that local anaesthetics potentiate spinal morphine antinociception.[167] Continuous infusion of 0.125% bupivacaine plus alfentanil 5 μg/ml was compared with 0.25% bupivacaine, both at 10 ml/h in twenty patients. Both regimes were equally satisfactory, but there was less motor block with the alfentanil regime (30% versus 80%) due to lower bupivacaine usage.[168]

Comparisons with PCA suggest little difference in either analgesia achieved or patient satisfaction.[169,170]

Conclusion

Despite the profound enthusiasm for spinal opioids alone in postoperative pain relief in some quarters, there is conflicting evidence as to whether they are definitely superior to optimally administered parenteral opioids, especially PCA.

Some advantages would appear to be:

- longer duration of action
- the necessity for smaller doses (particularly with morphine)
- less incidence of hypotension compared with epidural local anaesthetics

Balanced against this are the following disadvantages:

- technical difficulty and time to insert catheter
- risk of spinal haematoma with sc heparin therapy
- higher incidence of side-effects, nausea, vomiting, urinary retention and pruritus
- risk of respiratory depression (particularly intrathecal) necessitating at least 12 h high-dependency observation
- there is no compelling evidence that spinally administered opioids are more efficacious than optimally administered parenteral opioids.

It is not clear whether the advantages outweigh the disadvantages, except perhaps in the instances where an epidural catheter is already in place, for example following caesarean section.

Use of spinal opioids in chronic pain conditions

Introduction

The use of spinal opioids in chronic pain conditions has highlighted that natural reluctance to inject agents of any sort epidurally, particularly intrathecally, for long periods. The spectre of toxicity has loomed large ever since the famous Wooley and Roe case of paraplegia following contamination with phenol of intrathecal local anaesthetic.[171] Coombs and Fratkin[172] have briefly reviewed the evidence for toxicity of agents placed both intrathecally, such as methotrexate, metrizamide, steroids, and also epidurally, such as 2-chloroprocaine. Obviously, potential toxicity will be exacerbated by long-term therapy as is necessary with chronic pain conditions. Happily, toxicity has not been a problem with the spinal opioids in common use, as have been described so far.

The place of spinal opioids

The treatment schedule of the patient with chronic pain is complex and requires a multidisciplinary approach. As far as 'analgesics' are concerned (in contradistinction to other modes of therapy such as antidepressants), therapy is begun with simple nonsteroidal analgesics and progresses upwards to high-dose opioids, usually by the oral or sublingual route. It is only when tolerance develops and these simpler methods fail that the decision is made to switch to spinal opioids, although these may not always prove effective.[173]

Clinical experience with epidural morphine in chronic cancer pain patients is now extensive with many patients receiving the drug through tunnelled catheters for prolonged periods. [174] The main complication seems to be pain on injection and catheter obstruction due to epidural space fibrosis, particularly in longer term use (greater than a month). This is less of a complication with subarachnoid catheters which is preferred for patients expected to live for longer than a month.[175] In another larger series, infection was reported in 8% of patients in long term use.[176]

Conclusion

There seems little doubt that epidural opioids provide significant pain relief when the conventional route has become ineffective.

Concluding remarks on the use of spinal opioids

Any method of providing analgesia must meet three basic criteria: effectiveness, safety and feasibility. Although the first criterion is met, the incidence of complications alluded to above means that patients receiving spinal opioids must be kept under close surveillance (and, by implication, closer than after conventional routes of administration) for at least 12 h. It therefore follows that these methods are not feasible for the vast majority of patients suffering pain in the postoperative period.[177] Do they have a place at all? Certainly in those small numbers of chronic pain patients who have become tolerant to opioids administered by conventional routes, the answer is yes. A dispassionate review of well-controlled trials in which spinal opioids have been used suggests caution in their burgeoning use. After the initial enthusiasm, deficiencies in analgesia obtained with spinal opioids on their own have become evident. It is unfortunate that this 'spinal opioid band wagon' effect may have diverted attention away from other less invasive means of obtaining good analgesia (see Green[178]).

OPIOID ANTAGONISTS

Clinical pharmacology

Pharmacokinetics and duration of action

The short duration of action of naloxone ($t_{\frac{1}{2}\beta}$ 1–1.5 h[179]) means that there is a danger of recurrence of respiratory depression despite initially adequate reversal.[37,180,181] Thus doses may have to be repeated or an infusion set up. Naltrexone, the N-CPM variant of oxymorphone, has a much longer duration of action with a $t_{\frac{1}{2}\beta}$ of 8 h (see Pinkert[182]). It is also orally active and is thus useful for maintenance therapy in addicts undergoing treatment. Nalmefene is another long-acting antagonist, which is not yet commercially available in the UK (Table 25.8).[181,183]

Effects in the absence of exogenous opioids

Considering that there exists an *endogenous* opioid peptide system, it is perhaps surprising that opioid antagonists have so little an effect in normal man. Experimental pain thresholds induced by electric current and heat were measured in twenty-four volunteers under controlled experimental conditions. Drug treatments, administered double blind, were 5 and 20 mg of naloxone and placebo. The authors did not demonstrate any anti-analgesic effect by naloxone and concluded that in the absence of pain a tonically active endogenous opioid system does not exist in healthy humans.[184] However, in patients with congenital insensitivity to pain, naloxone does restore normal sensitivity. Naloxone reverses analgesia consequent on placebo medication and following acupuncture; that produced by hypnosis is not affected (see Jaffe and Martin[185]).

Many conditions are thought to result from, or be exacerbated by, excess release of *endogenous* opioid, such as stroke and spinal cord trauma.[186,187] Of

TABLE 25.8 **Agonist/antagonist pairs**

μ-AGONIST	ANTAGONIST AND N-SUBSTITUTION	EFFECT OF ANTAGONIST AT μ-RECEPTOR	EFFECT OF ANTAGONIST AT κ-RECEPTOR	EFFECT OF ANTAGONIST AT σ-RECEPTOR
Codeine	N-allyl norcodeine	–	0	0
Morphine	N-allyl normorphine (nalorphine)	– –	(++)	++
Levorphanol	N-allyl levorphanol (levallorphan)	– –	?	?
Oxymorphone	N-allyl oxymorphone (naloxone)	– – –	– –	– –
Oxymorphone	N-cyclopropyl-methyl oxymorphone (naltrexone)	– – –	– –	– –

KEY
+++ Strong agonist. – – – Strong antagonist.
++ Moderate agonist. – – Moderate antagonist.
+ Weak agonist. – Weak antagonist.
(+++) Strong partial agonist. 0 No effect.
(++) Medium partial agonist. ? Effect disputed.

Note that n-allyl substitution of agonists of increasing potency (oxymorphone > levorphanol > morphine > codeine) results in antagonists with a decreasing agonist profile and an increased antagonist profile.

greater relevance to the anaesthetist are the effects of antagonists in shock, especially due to sepsis.

Effects in shock

Naloxone has been shown to antagonize the cardiovascular-depressant effects of increased output of endogenous opioids, such as β-endorphin, seen after haemorrhage,[188] severe stress, pancreatitis or septic shock.[189] In animals with experimental endotoxaemia, the use of naloxone was associated with improved blood pressure and skeletal muscle perfusion at lower lactate levels, versus controls.[190] Although sepsis-induced hypotension in humans is reversed by naloxone in some instances, very high doses may be necessary. Despite haemodynamic improvement and increased survival in some animal models following naloxone or naltrexone,[191] overall survival in humans is not improved (see Hinds[192]). It should be noted that, since the preservatives in 'Narcan' are pharmacologically active, in high-dose therapy it may be these that are producing beneficial effects in septic shock.[193]

Effects in the presence of excess exogenous opioid agonist

Narcotic antagonists are primarily used to reverse the acute effects of opioid overdose either relative or absolute. Small doses of naloxone (0.05 mg increments up to 0.4 mg iv in a 60-kg patient) consistently reverse the effects of μ-opioid agonist drugs. This applies to sedation, respiratory depression and analgesia. Respiratory rate and blood pressure return promptly to normal (or above, see adverse effects). Respiratory depression or σ-dysphoric effects due to κ-agonist analgesics such as pentazocine require larger doses of naloxone for reversal (see Brogden *et al.*[71]).

A large proportion of patients receiving high-dose opioid analgesia during surgery will require judicious use of naloxone in the early postoperative period to reverse respiratory depression.[37a,45] Following chronic use of opioids or in the addicted subject, administration of an opioid antagonist may precipitate withdrawal.

Effect with buprenorphine

The effect of naloxone in the presence of the avidly associating partial μ-agonist buprenorphine suggests that difficulties may be encountered in reversing respiratory depression, should it occur.[194] In a placebo-controlled study the ability of three doses of naloxone (1.0, 5.0 and 10 mg) to antagonize the respiratory depression produced by buprenorphine, 0.3 mg/70 kg, was investigated. While 1 mg naloxone had little effect on respiratory depression, both 5 and 10 mg produced reversal, being more complete after the larger dose. It did not occur immediately, reaching a maximum effect 3 h after administration.[195] Doxapram would seem a viable alternative in these circumstances although quantitative assessment and duration of effect has not been studied. In addition, naloxone is unable to reverse the inhibitory effects of buprenorphine on C-fibre evoked responses in the rat spinal cord, in sharp contrast to etorphine and fentanyl.[196]

Treatment of opioid abuse

The mainstay of treatment of opioid addiction is first to replace the illicitly obtained drug with methadone or buprenorphine and then gradually reduce the replacement opioid over a period of months or even years.[197–199] Despite fractional declines in dosage (e.g. by 10% per week), most addicts experience withdrawal symptoms as the dose is reduced. Clonidine, as

α_2-adrenergic agonist is useful to suppress some of the symptoms (see Jaffe[200]).

Narcotic antagonists are primarily used for maintenance therapy following successful opioid withdrawal. This is based on the premise that occupation of the opioid receptor by antagonist prevents the 'pleasurable' effects of exogenous opioids which led to the addicted state in the first place. As an orally active compound, naltrexone is the drug of choice in this regard (see Pinkert[182]).

Adverse effects of opioid antagonists

Many of the adverse effects of opioid antagonists may represent an acute withdrawal phenomenon resulting in overshoot of pain perception, blood pressure and respiratory rate.[201] In subjects who are known to be chronically physically dependent on opioids, small doses of naloxone may precipitate the withdrawal syndrome. These effects have constrained the routine use of antagonists such as naloxone to reverse the effects of opioid-supplemented anaesthesia.

Effect on pain perception

Pure antagonists

There is clear evidence that reversal of *systemic* opioid-induced respiratory depression with a pure antagonist such as naloxone is associated with an increase in pain which sometimes is severe.[37,147] Although antagonists such as naltrexone significantly decrease side-effects such as pruritus and nausea without affecting analgesia if given before *spinal* morphine,[157] initial work seemed to suggest that one could also reverse respiratory depression *without* reversing analgesia. Recent studies have not substantiated this.[142,157] Following epidural opioid, Gowan and others[147] demonstrated an unacceptable incidence of inadequate analgesia in the naloxone groups and no difference in the side-effects.

Agonist/antagonists and partial agonists

In an effort to avoid the precipitate effects of sudden reversal of excess agonist by pure antagonists such as naloxone and naltrexone, several investigators have studied the effects of nalbuphine and buprenorphine.

Nalbuphine, as a μ-antagonist and κ-agonist, would be expected to reverse respiratory depression but still maintain analgesia.[202] Although this has been demonstrated in clinical practice and in volunteers following systemic opioids,[203,204] a recent report has cast doubts on the safety of the use of nalbuphine for this purpose. Nalbuphine was used to reverse the respiratory depressant effects of high-dose fentanyl (50–75 μg/kg) for abdominal aortic surgery in four patients. Hypertension, increased heart rate and significant increase in analogue pain scores accompanied reversal of respiratory depression in all cases. Agitation, nausea, vomiting and cardiac dysrhythmias were also observed frequently. The authors do not recommend the use of nalbuphine in this way.[205] In a randomized trial following cardiac surgery, nalbuphine caused similar side-effects unless the dose was very carefully titrated. Residual analgesia from nalbuphine was insufficient in eight of the eighteen patients studied.[206] This and the previous study suggest that nalbuphine reversal of respiratory depression following high-dose opioids is a technique possessing few material advantages.

Nevertheless, several studies have also shown reversal of respiratory depression and other side-effects such as pruritus following *epidural* opioids *without* reversal of analgesia.[143–145,156,207] This has been substantiated by carefully controlled animal work.[202]

Following earlier work with pentazocine, buprenorphine has been used to *reverse* the respiratory depressant effects of intraoperative high-dose fentanyl and sufentanil while at the same time allowing prolongation of analgesia.[208] In a more recent study, following high-dose fentanyl sufficient to cause respiratory depression and sedation, buprenorphine was found to be indistinguishable from naloxone in its ability to reverse these effects. However, the latter led to increased pain in the first 15 min following administration when compared with buprenorphine.[37]

Further work is needed in this area, particularly documenting the haemodynamic effects of agonist/antagonist and partial agonists when used in this way.

Cardiovascular effects

Apart from the problem of analgesia, the cardiovascular effects of sudden reversal of high-dose opioids by antagonists such as naloxone and nalbuphine should not be underestimated. This may lead to hypertension,[205,206,209] acute left ventricular failure and pulmonary oedema[180] cardiac dysrhythmias[205,206] or even death due to cardiac failure.[148]

CONCLUSION

The discovery that patients suffered postoperative pain despite opioids revealed that they were being improperly prescribed due to lack of understanding of opioid pharmacology. This prompted intensive research into opioid pharmacokinetics and pharmacodynamics in an attempt to improve drug efficacy. Although this has probably led to an increase in the quality of opioid analgesia, it is now emerging that, provided opioids are given to the maximum of their effectiveness in a particular patient (whether by regular administration, PCA apparatus or spinal routes), no *route* of administration is definitely superior to another. Opioids are not the panacea for the treatment of severe pain and, to limit toxicity, must be combined with other drugs if pain relief is to be maximized.

REFERENCES

1 Sawynok J. The therapeutic use of heroin: a review of the pharmacological literature. *Canadian Journal of Physiology and Pharmacology* 1986; **64**: 1–6.

2 Martin WR. Pharmacology of opioids. *Pharmacological Review* 1983; **35**: 283–323.

3 Casy AF, Parfitt RT. *Opioid analgesics. Chemistry and receptors.* New York: Plenum Press, 1986.

4 Mather LE. Pharmacokinetic and pharmacodynamic factors influencing the choice, dose and route of administration of opiates for acute pain. In: Bullingham RES ed. *Clinics in anaesthesiology*, Vol. 1, No. 1. London: WB Saunders, 1983: 17–40.

5 Marks RM, Sachar EJ. Undertreatment of medical inpatients with narcotic analgesics. *Annals of Internal Medicine* 1973; **78**: 173–81.

6 Moldenhauer CC. New narcotics. In: Kaplan JA ed. *Cardiac anesthesia*, Vol 2. *Cardiovascular pharmacology*. New York: Grune & Stratton, 1985: 31–78.

7 Weinberg DS, Inturrisi CE, Reidenberg B, Moulin DE, Nip TJ, Wallenstein S, Houde RW, Foley KM. Sublingual absorption of selected opioid analgesics. *Clinical Pharmacology and Therapeutics* 1988; **44**: 335–42.

8 Bullingham RES, McQuay HJ, Porter EJB, Allen MC, Moore RA. Sublingual buprenorphine used postoperatively: ten hour plasma drug concentration analysis. *British Journal of Clinical Pharmacology* 1982; **13**: 665–73.

9 Manara AR, Shelly MP, Quinn KG, Park GR. Pharmacokinetics of morphine following administration by the buccal route. *British Journal of Anaesthesia* 1989; **62**: 498–502.

10 Hoskin PJ, Hanks GW, Aherne GW, Chapman D, Littleton P, Filshie J. The bioavailability and pharmacokinetics of morphine after intravenous, oral and buccal administration in healthy volunteers. *British Journal of Clinical Pharmacology* 1989; **27**: 499–505.

11 Simpson KH, Tring IC, Ellis FR. An investigation of premedication with morphine given by the buccal or intramuscular route. *British Journal of Clinical Pharmacology* 1989; **27**: 377–80.

12 Stanley TH, Hague B, Mock DL, Streisand JB, Bubbers S, Dzelzkalns RR, Bailey PL, Pace NL, East KA, Ashburn MA. Oral transmucosal fentanyl citrate (lollipop) premedication in human volunteers. *Anesthesia and Analgesia* 1989; **69**: 21–7.

13 Diaz JH. Opioid premedicants are not candy, lollipops, or funny stickers. *Anesthesiology* 1990; **72**: 208.

14 Eriksen J, Jensen NH, Kamp-Jensen M, Bjarno H, Friis P, Brewster D. The systemic availability of buprenorphine administered by nasal spray. *Journal of Pharmaceutical Pharmacology* 1989; **41**: 803–5.

15 Varvel JR, Shafer SL, Hwang SS, Coen PA, Stanski DR. Absorption characteristics of transdermally administered fentanyl. *Anesthesiology* 1989; **70**: 928–34.

16 Chrubasik J, Wust H, Friedrich G, Geller E: Absorption and bioavailability of nebulized morphine. *British Journal of Anaesthesia* 1988; **61**: 228–30.

17 Rogers DF, Barnes PJ. Opioid inhibition of neurally mediated mucus secretion in human bronchi. *Lancet* 1988; **8644**: 930–1.

18 Johansson IGM, Grundstrom N, Andersson RGG. Both the cholinergic and non-cholinergic components of airway excitation are inhibited by morphine in the guinea-pig. *Acta Physiologia Scandinavica* 1989, **135**: 411–15.

19 Agius R. Opiate inhalation and occupational asthma. *British Medical Journal* 1989; **298**: 323.

20 Sear JW, Hand CW, Moore RA, McQuay HJ. Studies on morphine disposition: influence of general anaesthesia on plasma concentrations of morphine and its metabolites. *British Journal of Anaesthesia* 1989; **62**: 22–7.

21 Hudson RJ, Bergstrom RG, Thomson IR, Sabourin MA, Rosenbloom M, Strunin L. Pharmacokinetics of sufentanil in patients undergoing abdominal aortic surgery. *Anesthesiology* 1989; **70**: 426–31.

22 Sear JW, Hand CW, Moore RA, McQuay HJ. Studies on morphine disposition: influence of renal failure on the kinetics of morphine and its metabolites. *British Journal of Anaesthesia* 1989; **62**: 28–32.

23 Hasselstrom J, Berg U, Lofgren A, Sawe J. Long lasting respiratory depression induced by morphine-6-glucuronide? *British Journal of Clinical Pharmacology* 1989; **27**: 515–18.

24 Hand CW, Sear JW, Uppington J, Ball MJ, McQuay HJ, Moore RA. Buprenorphine disposition in patients with renal impairment: single and continuous dosing, with special reference to metabolites. *British Journal of Anaesthesia* 1990; **64**: 276–82.

25 Fyman PN, Reynolds JR, Moser F, Avitable M, Casthely PA, Butt K. Pharmacokinetics of sufentanil in patients undergoing renal transplantation. *Canadian Journal of Anaesthesia* 1988; **35**: 312–15.

26 Crotty B, Watson KJR, Desmond PV, Mashford ML, Wood LJ, Colman J, Dudley FJ. Hepatic extraction of morphine is impaired in cirrhosis. *European Journal of Clinical Pharmacology* 1989; **36**: 501–6.

27 Chauvin M, Ferrier C, Haberer JP, Spielvogel C, Lebrault C, Levron JC, Duvaldestin P. Sufentanil pharmacokinetics in patients with cirrhosis. *Anesthesia and Analgesia* 1989; **68**: 1–4.

28 Singleton MA, Rosen JI, Fisher DM. Plasma concentrations of fentanyl in infants. *Canadian Journal of Anaesthesia* 1987; **34**: 152–5.

29 Hertzka RE, Gauntlett IS, Fisher DM, Spellman MJ. Fentanyl-induced ventilatory depression: Effects of age. *Anesthesiology* 1989; **70**: 213–18.

30 Koehntop DE, Rodman JH, Brundage DM, Hegland MG, Buckley JJ. Pharmacokinetics of fentanyl in the neonate. *Anesthesia and Analgesia* 1986; **65**: 227–32.

31 Olkkola K, Maunuksela EL, Korpela R. Pharmacokinetics of intravenous buprenorphine in children. *British Journal of Clinical Pharmacology* 1989; **28**: 202–4.

32 Bentley JB, Borel JD, Nenad RE. Age and fentanyl pharmacokinetics. *Anesthesia and Analgesia* 1982; **61**: 968–71.

33 Kent AP, Dodson ME, Bower S. The pharmacokinetics and clinical effects of a low dose of alfentanil in elderly patients. *Acta Anaesthesiologica Belgica* 1988; **39**: 25–33.

34 Owen JA, Sitar DS, Berger L, Brownell L, Duke PC, Mitenko PA. Age related morphine kinetics. *Clinical Pharmacology and Therapeutics* 1983; **34**: 364–8.

35 Bartkowski RR, Goldber ME, Larijani GE, Boemer T. Inhibition of alfentanil metabolism by erythromycin. *Clinical Pharmacology and Therapeutics* 1989; **46**: 99–102.

36 Lasagna L, Beecher HK. The analgesic effectiveness of nalorphine and nalorphine–morphine combinations in

man. *Journal of Pharmacology and Experimental Therapeutics* 1954; **122**: 356–63.

37 (a) Boysen K, Hertel S, Chraemmer-Jorgensen B, Risbo A, Poulsen NJ. Buprenorphine antagonism of respiratory depression following fentanyl anaesthesia. *Acta Anaesthesiologica Scandinavica* 1988; **32**: 490–7.
(b) Green DW, O'Connor L, Hanna M. Efficacy of post-operative pain treatment regimens employing both buprenorphine and papaveretum in sequential use after abdominal hysterectomy. *British Journal of Anaesthesia* 1993; **70**: 626–30.

38 Purcell-Jones G, Dormon F, Sumner E. The use of opioids in neonates. A retrospective study of 933 cases. *Anaesthesia* 1987; **42**: 1316–20.

39 Lloyd-Thomas AR. Pain management in paediatric patients. *British Journal of Anaesthesia* 1990; **64**: 85–104.

40 Stanley TH, de Lange S. The influence of patient habits on dosage requirements during high dose fentanyl anaesthesia. *Canadian Journal of Anaesthesia* 1984; **31**: 368–76.

41 Lemmens HJM, Bovill JG, Hennis PJ, Gladines MPRR, Burm AGL. Alcohol consumption alters the pharmacodynamics of alfentanil. *Anesthesiology* 1989; **71**: 669–74.

42 Tempelhoff R, Modica PA, Spitznagel EL. Anticonvulsant therapy increases fentanyl requirements during anaesthesia for craniotomy. *Canadian Journal of Anaesthesia* 1990; **37**: 327–32.

43 Jordan C. Assessment of the effects of drugs on respiration. *British Journal of Anaesthesia* 1982; **54**: 763–82.

44 Shook JE, Watkins WD, Camporesi EM. Differential roles of opioid receptors in respiration, respiratory disease, and opiate-induced respiratory depression. *American Review of Respiratory Disease* 1990, **142**: 895–909.

45 Flacke JW, Bloor BC, Kripke BJ, Flacke WE, Warneck CM, Van Etten AP, Wong DHW, Katz RL. Comparison of morphine, meperidine, fentanyl and sufentanil in balanced anesthesia. A double-blind study. *Anesthesia and Analgesia* 1985; **64**: 897–910.

46 Wheatley RG, Somerville ID, Sapsford DJ, Jones JG. Postoperative hypoxaemia: comparison of extradural, i.m. and patient-controlled opioid analgesia. *British Journal of Anaesthesia* 1990; **64**: 267–75.

47 Catley DM, Thornton C, Jordan C, Lehane JR, Jones JG. Pronounced episodic desaturation in the postoperative period: its association with ventilatory pattern and analgesic regimen. *Anesthesiology* 1985; **63**: 20–8.

48 Fry ENS. Postoperative analgesia: a technique using continuous infusion of buprenorphine. *Anaesthesia* 1984; **39**: 1134–5.

49 Papworth DP. High dose buprenorphine for postoperative analgesia. *Anaesthesia* 1983; **38**: 163.

50 Gibbs JM, Johnson HD, Davis FM. Patient administration of i.v. buprenorphine for postoperative pain relief using the 'Cardiff' demand analgesia apparatus. *British Journal of Anaesthesia* 1982; **54**: 279–84.

51 Cook PJ, James IM, Hobbs KEF, Browne DRG. Controlled comparison of i.m. morphine and buprenorphine for analgesia after abdominal surgery. *British Journal of Anaesthesia* 1982; **54**: 285–90.

52 Korttila K, Hovorka J. Buprenorphine as premedication and as analgesic during and after light anaesthesia. A comparison with oxycodone plus fentanyl. *Acta Anaesthesiologica Scandinavica* 1987; **31**: 673–9.

53 Cuschieri RJ, Morran CG, McArdle CS. Comparison of morphine and sublingual buprenorphine following abdominal surgery. *British Journal of Anaesthesia* 1984; **56**: 855–9.

54 Downing JW, Leary WP, White ES. Buprenorphine: a new potent long-acting synthetic analgesic. Comparison with morphine. *British Journal of Anaesthesia* 1977; **49**: 251–4.

55 Edge WG, Cooper GM, Morgan M. Analgesic effects of sublingual buprenorphine. *Anaesthesia* 1979; **34**: 463–7.

56 Lowenstein E. Morphine 'anesthesia' – a perspective. *Anesthesiology* 1971; **35**: 563–5.

57 Bovill JG, Sebel PS, Stanley TH. Opioid analgesics in anesthesia: With special reference to their use in cardiovascular anesthesia. *Anesthesiology* 1984; **61**: 731–55.

58 Janssen P. The past, present, and future of opioid anesthetics. *Journal of Cardiothoracic Anaesthesia* 1990; **4**: 259–66.

59 Mummaneni N, Rao TLK, Montoya A. Awareness and recall with high dose fentanyl–oxygen anesthesia. *Anesthesia and Analgesia* 1980; **59**: 948–9.

60 Philbin DM, Roscow CE, Schneider RC, Koski G, D'Ambra MN. Fentanyl and sufentanil anesthesia revisited: How much is enough? *Anesthesiology* 1990; **73**: 5–11.

61 Hug CC Jr. Does opioid 'Anesthesia' exist? *Anesthesiology* 1990; **73**: 1–4.

62 Lunn JK, Webster LR, Stanley TH, Woodward A. High dose fentanyl anesthesia for coronary artery surgery: Plasma fentanyl concentration and influence of nitrous oxide on cardiovascular responses. *Anesthesia and Analgesia* 1979; **58**: 390–5.

63 Stanley TH, Webster LR. Anesthetic requirements and cardiovascular effects of fentanyl–oxygen and fentanyl–diazepam–oxygen anesthesia in man. *Anesthesia and Analgesia* 1978; **57**: 411–16.

64 Woolf CJ. Intrathecal high dose morphine produces hyperalgesia in the rat. *Brain Research* 1981; **209**: 491–5.

65 Yaksh TL, Harty GJ, Onofrio BM. High doses of spinal morphine produce a nonopiate receptor mediated hyperesthesia: Clinical and theoretical implications. *Anesthesiology* 1986; **64**: 590–7.

66 Hall GM. The anaesthetic modification of the endocrine and metabolic response to surgery. *Annals of the Royal College of Surgeons of England* 1985; **67**: 25–9.

67 Editorial. Analgesia and the metabolic response to surgery. *Lancet* 1985; **i: 1018–19.**

68 George JM, Reier E, Lanese RR, Rower JM. Morphine anaesthesia blocks cortisol and growth hormone response to stress in humans. *Journal of Clinical Endocrinology and Metabolism* 1974; **38**: 736–9.

69 Sander GE, Lowe RF, Given MB, Giles TD. Interactions between circulating peptides and the central nervous system in hemodynamic regulation. *American Journal of Cardiology* 1989, **64**: 44C–50C.

70 Green DW. Severe cardiovascular collapse following phenoperidine. *Anaesthesia* 1981; **36**: 617–19.

71 Brogden RN, Speight TM, Avery GS. Pentazocine: a review of its pharmacological properties, therapeutic efficacy and dependence liability. *Drugs* 1973; **5**: 6–91.

72 Hayes MJ, Fraser AR, Hampton JR. Randomised trial comparing buprenorphine and diamorphine for chest

pain in suspected myocardial infarction. *British Medical Journal* 1979; **2**: 300–2.

73 Dobson JAR, Davies JM, Hodgeson GH. Bradycardia after sufentanil and vecuronium. *Canadian Journal of Anaesthesia* 1988; **35**: S121.

74 Schmeling WT, Kampine JP, Warltier DC. Negative chronotropic actions of sufentanil and vecuronium in chronically instrumented dogs pretreated with propranolol and/or diltiazem. *Anesthesia and Analgesia* 1989; **69**: 4–14.

75 Freye E. Effects of high dose fentanyl on myocardial infarction and cardiogenic shock in the dog. *Anesthesiology* 1974; **3**: 105–13.

76 Saini V, Carr DB, Verrier RL. Comparative effects of the opioids fentanyl and buprenorphine on ventricular vulnerability during acute coronary artery occlusion. *Cardiovascular Research* 1989; **23**: 1001–6.

77 Boachie-Ansah G; Sitsapesan R; Kane KA; Parratt JR. The antiarrhythmic and cardiac electrophysiological effects of buprenorphine. *British Journal of Pharmacology* 1989; **97**: 801–8.

78 Jewitt DE, Maurer BJ, Sonnenblick EJ, Hubner PJ. Increased pulmonary arterial pressures after pentazocine in myocardial infarction. *British Medical Journal* 1970; **1**: 795.

79 Alderman EL, Barry WH, Graham AF, Harrison DC. Hemodynamic effects of morphine and pentazocine differ in cardiac patients. *New England Journal of Medicine* 1972; **27**: 623–7.

80 Lee G, De Maria AN, Amsterdam EA, Realyvasquez F, Angel J, Morrison S, Mason DT. Comparative effects of morphine, meperidine and pentazocine on cardiocirculatory dynamics in patients with acute myocardial infarction. *American Journal of Medicine* 1976; **60**: 949.

81 Trouton TG, Adgey AJ. High dose nalbuphine in early acute myocardial infarction. *International Journal of Cardiology* 1989; **23**: 53–7.

82 McNeill MJ, Ho ET, Kenny GNC. Effect of i.v. Metoclopramide on gastric emptying after opioid premedication. *British Journal of Anaesthesia* 1990, **64**: 450–2.

83 Duthie DJR, Nimmo WS. Adverse effects of opioid analgesic drugs. *British Journal of Anaesthesia* 1987; **59**: 61–77.

84 Culpepper-Morgan J, Kreek MJ, Holt PR. Orally administered κ- as well as μ-opiate agonists delay gastrointestinal transit time in the guinea pig. *Life Sciences* 1988; **42**: 2073–6.

85 Staritz M. Pharmacology of the sphincter of Oddi. *Endoscopy* 1988; **20** (Suppl 1): 171–4.

86 Cuer JC, Dapoigny M, Ajmi S. Effects of buprenorphine on motor activity of the sphincter of Oddi in man. *European Journal of Clinical Pharmacology* 1989, **36**: 203–4.

87 Baber NS, Dourish CT, Hill DR. The role of CCK, caerulein and CCK antagonists in nociception. *Pain* 1989, **39**: 307–28.

88 Wang XJ, Wang XH, Han JS. Cholecystokinin octapeptide antagonized opioid analgesia mediated by μ- and κ- but not δ-receptors in the spinal cord of the rat. *Brain Research* 1990, **523**: 5–10.

89 Bodnar RJ, Paul D, Pasternak GW. Proglumide selectively potentiates supraspinal μ_1-opioid analgesia in mice. *Neuropharmacology* 1990, **29**: 507–10.

90 Suh HH, Tseng LF. Differential effects of sulfated cholecystokinin octapeptide and proglumide injected intrathecally on antinociception induced by β-endorphin and morphine administered intracerebroventricularly in mice. *European Journal of Pharmacology* 1990; **179**: 329–38.

91 Dourish CT, O'Neill MF, Coughlan OJ, Kitchener SJ, Hawley D, Iversen SD. The selective CCK-B receptor antagonist L-365, 260 enhances morphine analgesia and prevents morphine tolerance in the rat. *European Journal of Pharmacology* 1990, **176**: 35–44.

92 Lundy JS. Balanced anesthesia. *Minnesota Medical Journal* 1926; **9**: 299.

93 Neff W, Mayer EC, Oerales M. Nitrous oxide and oxygen anesthesia with curare relaxation. *California Medicine* 1947; **66**: 67–9.

94 Auld W. Pethidine, curare, nitrous oxide–oxygen anaesthesia in children. *Anaesthesia* 1952; **7**: 161–5.

95 Green DW, Sinclair JR, Mikhael MS. Buprenorphine versus morphine. A comparison of intraoperative and postoperative analgesia. *Anaesthesia* 1985; **40**: 371–5.

96 Kay B. A double blind comparison between fentanyl and buprenorphine supplemented anaesthesia. *British Journal of Anaesthesia* 1980; **52**: 453–7.

97 Donovan BD. Patient attitudes to postoperative pain relief. *Anaesthesia and Intensive Care* 1985; **11**: 125–9.

98 Kamel MM, Geddes IC. A comparison of buprenorphine and pethidine for immediate postoperative pain relief by the iv route. *British Journal of Anaesthesia* 1978; **50**: 599–602.

99 Fry ENS. Relief of pain after surgery. A comparison of sublingual buprenorphine and intramuscular papaveretum. *Anaesthesia* 1979; **34**: 549–51.

100 Gourlay GK, Willis RJ, Wilson PR. Postoperative pain control with methadone: influence of supplementary doses and blood concentration response relationships. *Anesthesiology* 1984; **61**: 119–26.

101 Fry ENS, Deshpande S. Postoperative analgesia by titration of papaveretum. *British Medical Journal* 1977; **2**: 870.

102 Church JJ. Continuous narcotic infusions for relief of postoperative pain. *Britiish Medical Journal* 1979; **1**: 977–9.

103 Ellis R, Haines D, Shah R, Cotton BR, Smith G. Pain relief after abdominal surgery – a comparison of i.m. morphine, sublingual buprenorphine and self-administered i.v. pethidine. *British Journal of Anaesthesia* 1982; **54**: 421–8.

104 Welchew EA. On-demand analgesia: a double-blind comparison of on-demand intravenous fentanyl with regular intramuscular morphine. *Anaesthesia* 1983; **38**: 19–25.

105 Bullingham RES, O'Sullivan G, McQuay HJ, Poppleton P, Rolfe M, Weir L, Moore RA. Mandatory sublingual buprenorphine for postoperative pain. *Anaesthesia* 1984; **39**: 329–34.

106 Chraemmer Jorgensen, Schmidt JF, Risbo A, Pedersen J, Kolby P. Regular interval preventive pain relief compared with on demand treatment after hysterectomy. *Pain* 1985; **21**: 137–42.

107 White PF. Patient controlled analgesia: A new approach to the management of postoperative pain. *Seminars in Anesthesia* 1985; **4**: 255–66.

108 Ved S, Dubois M, Carron H, Lea D. Sufentanil and alfentanil pattern of consumption during patient-controlled analgesia: a comparison with morphine. *Clinical Journal of Pain* 1989; **5 (Suppl 1): S63–S70.**

109 Evans JM, Rosen M, MacCarthy J, Hogg MIJ. Apparatus for patient controlled administration of intravenous narcotics during labour. *Lancet* 1976; i: 17.

110 Owen H, Glavin RJ, Reekie RM, Trew AS. Patient-controlled analgesia: Experience of two new machines. *Anaesthesia* 1986; **41**: 1230–5.

111 Harmer M, Slattery PJ, Rosen M, Vickers MD. Intramuscular on demand analgesia: double blind controlled trial of pethidine, buprenorphine, morphine and meptazinol. *British Medical Journal* 1983; **286**: 680–2.

112 Owen H, Szekely SM, Plummer JL, Cushnie JM, Mather LE. Variables of patient-controlled analgesia 2. Concurrent infusion. *Anaesthesia* 1989; **44**: 11–13.

113 Tamsen A, Hartvig P, Dahlstrom B, Lundstom B, Holmdahl MH. Patient controlled analgesic therapy in the early postoperative period. *Acta Anaesthesiologica Scandinavica* 1979; **23**: 462.

114 Harmer M, Slattery PJ, Rosen M, Vickers MD. Comparison between buprenorphine and pentazocine given iv on demand in the control of postoperative pain. *British Journal of Anaesthesia* 1983; **55**: 21–4.

115 Marlowe S, Engstrom R, White PF. Epidural patient-controlled analgesia (PCA): an alternative to continuous epidural infusions. *Pain* 1989, **37**: 97–101.

116 Yaksh TL, Rudy TA. Chronic catheterisation of the spinal subarachnoid space. *Science* 1976; 1357–8.

117 Yaksh TL. Spinal opiate analgesia: Characteristics and principles of action. *Pain* 1981; **11**: 293–346.

118 Behar M, Magora F, Olshwang D, Davidson JT. Epidural morphine in treatment of pain. *Lancet* 1979; i: 527–9.

119 Wang JK, Nauss LA, Thomas JE. Pain relief by intrathecally applied morphine in man. *Anesthesiology* 1979; **50**: 149–51.

120 Tigerstedt I. Postoperative pain. *Current Opinion in Anaesthesiology* 1990; **3**: 771–6.

121 Cousins MJ, Mather LE, Glynn CJ, Wilson PR, Graham JR. Selective spinal analgesia. *Lancet* 1979; **i**: 1141–2.

122 Nordberg G, Hedner T, Mellstrand T, Dahlstrom B. Pharmacokinetic aspects of intrathecal morphine analgesia. *Anesthesiology* 1984; **60**: 448–54.

123 Sjostrom S, Tamsen A, Perrson MP, Hartvig P. Pharmacokinetics of intrathecal morphine and meperidine in humans. *Anesthesiology* 1987; **67**: 889–95.

124 Sjostrom S, Hartvig P, Persson P, Tamsen A. Pharmacokinetics of epidural morphine and meperidine in humans. *Anesthesiology* 1987; **67**: 877–88.

125 Hanna MH, Peat SJ, Woodham M, Knibb A, Fung C. Analgesic efficacy and CSF pharmacokinetics of intrathecal morphine-6-glucuronide: comparison with morphine. *British Journal of Anaesthesia* 1990; **64**: 547–50.

126 Kaufman L. Intraspinal diamorphine: epidural and intrathecal. In: Scott DB ed. *Diamorphine: its chemistry, pharmacology and clinical use.* New York: Woodhead-Faulkner, 1987: 82–96.

127 Yamaguchi H, Watanabe S, Motokawa K, Ishizawa Y. Intrathecal morphine dose–response data for pain relief after cholecystectomy. *Anesthesia and Analgesia* 1989; **70**: 168–71.

128 Kirson LE, Goldman JM, Slover RB. Low-dose intrathecal morphine for postoperative pain control in patients undergoing transurethral resection of the prostate. *Anesthesiology* 1989; **71**: 192–5.

129 Davies GK, Tolhurst-Cleaver CL, James TL. Respiratory depression after intrathecal narcotics. *Anaesthesia* 1980; **35**: 1080–3.

130 van Lersberghe C, Camu F, de Keersmaecker E, Sacre S. Continuous administration of fentanyl for postoperative pain: a comparison of the epidural, intravenous, and transdermal routes. *Journal of Clinical Anesthesia* 1994; **6**: 308–14.

131 Sandler AN, Stringer D, Panos L, Badner N, Friedlander M, Koren G, Katz J, Klein J. A randomized, double-blind comparison of lumbar epidural and intravenous fentanyl infusions for postthoracotomy pain relief. Analgesic, pharmacokinetic, and respiratory effects. *Anesthesiology* 1992; **77**: 626–34.

132 Glass PS, Estok P, Ginsberg B, Goldberg JS, Sladen RN. Use of patient-controlled analgesia to compare the efficacy of epidural to intravenous fentanyl administration. *Anesthesia and Analgesia* 1992; **74**: 345–51.

133 Guinard JP, Mavrocordatos P, Chiolero R, Carpenter RL. A randomized comparison of intravenous versus lumbar and thoracic epidural fentanyl for analgesia after thoracotomy. *Anesthesiology* 1992; **77**: 1108–51.

134 Baxter AD, Laganiere S, Samson B, Stewart J, Hull K, Goernert L. A comparison of lumbar epidural and intravenous fentanyl infusions for post-thoracotomy analgesia. *Canadian Journal of Anaesthesia* 1994; **41**: 184–91.

135 Welchew EA, Breen DP. Patient-controlled on-demand epidural fentanyl. A comparison of patient-controlled on-demand fentanyl delivered epidurally or intravenously. *Anaesthesia* 1991; **46**: 438–41.

136 Salomaki TE, Laitinen JO, Nuutinen LS. A randomized double-blind comparison of epidural versus intravenous fentanyl infusion for analgesia after thoracotomy. *Anesthesiology* 1991; **75**: 790–5.

137 Etches RC, Sandler AN, Daley MD. Respiratory depression and spinal opioids. *Canadian Journal of Anaesthesia* 1989; **36**: 165–85.

138 Rawal N, Arner S, Gustafsson LL, Allvin R. Present state of extradural and intrathecal opioid analgesia in Sweden. A nationwide follow-up survey. *British Journal of Anaesthesia* 1987; **59**: 791–9.

139 Gustafson LL, Schildt B, Jacobsen K. Adverse effects of extradural and intrathecal opiates: Report of a nationwide survey in Sweden. *British Journal of Anaesthesia* 1982; **54**: 479–86.

140 Rawal N, Watwill M. Respiratory depression after epidural morphine – an experimental and clinical study. *Anesthesia and Analgesia* 1982; **63**: 8–14.

141 Krantz T, Christensen CB. Respiratory depression after intrathecal opioids. Report of a patient receiving long-term epidural opioid therapy. *Anaesthesia* 1987; **42**: 168–70.

142 Norris MC, Leighton BL, DeSimone CA. Naltrexone and subarachnoid morphine following cesarean section. *Anesthesiology* 1989; **71**: A873.

143 Henderson SK, Cohen H. Nalbuphine augmentation of analgesia and reversal of side effects following epidural hydromorphone. *Anesthesiology* 1986; **65**: 216–18.

144 Penning JP, Samson B, Baxter A. Reversal of epidural morphine induced respiratory depression and pruritus with nalbuphine. *Canadian Journal of Anaesthesia* 1988; **35**: 599–604.

145 Cheng EY, May J. Nalbuphine reversal of respiratory depression after epidural sufentanil. *Critical Care Medicine* 1989, **17**: 378–9.

146 Rawal N, Schott U, Dahlstrom B, Inturrisi CE, Tandon B *et al.* Influence of naloxone infusion on analgesia and

respiratory depression following epidural morphine. *Anesthesiology* 1986; **64**: 194–201.

147 Gowan JD, Fraser RA, Kitts J. Naloxone infusion after prophylactic epidural morphine: effects on incidence of post-operative side effects and quality of analgesia. *Canadian Journal of Anaesthesia* 1988, **35**: 143–8.

148 Andree RA. Sudden death following naloxone administration. *Anesthesia and Analgesia* 1980; **59**: 782–4.

149 Jacobson L, Chabal C, Brody MC, Ward RJ, Wasse L. Intrathecal methadone: a dose–response study and comparison with intrathecal morphine 0.5 mg. *Pain* 1990; **43**: 141–8.

150 Bromage PR, Camporesi E, Chestnut D. Epidural narcotics for postoperative analgesia. *Anesthesia and Analgesia* 1980; **59**: 473–80.

151 Thind GS, Wells JC, Wilkes RG. The effects of continuous intravenous naloxone on epidural morphine analgesia. *Anaesthesia* 1986; **41**: 582–5.

152 Loper KA, Ready LB, Dorman BH. Prophylactic transdermal scopolamine patches reduce nausea in postoperative patients receiving epidural-morphine. *Anesthesia and Analgesia* 1989; **68**: 144–6.

153 Ballantyne JC, Loach AB, Carr DB. Itching after epidural and spinal opiates. *Pain* 1988; **33**: 149–60.

154 Zenz M, Piepenbrock S, Glocke M. A double-blind comparison of epidural buprenorphine and morphine in postoperative pain. Buprenorphine and anesthesiology. *Royal Society of Medicine* 1984; **65**: 115–24.

155 Oyama T, Jin T, Yamaya R, Ling N, Guillemin R. Profound analgesic effects of beta endorphin in man. *Lancet* 1980; **i**: 122–4.

156 Davies GG, From R. A blinded study using nalbuphine for prevention of pruritus induced by epidural fentanyl. *Anesthesiology* 1988; **69**: 763–5.

157 Abboud TK, Afrasiabi A, Davidson J, Zhu J, Reyes A, Khoo N, Steffens Z. Prophylactic oral naltrexone with epidural morphine: effect on adverse reactions and ventilatory responses to carbon dioxide. *Anesthesiology* 1990; **72**: 233–7.

158 Cousins MJ, Mather LE. Intrathecal and epidural administration of opioids. *Anesthesiology* 1984; **61**: 276–310.

159 Macdonald R. Aspirin and extradural blocks. *British Journal of Anaesthesia* 1991; **66**: 1–3.

160 Owens EL, Kasten GW, Hessel EA. Spinal subarachnoid hematoma after lumbar puncture and heparinisation: a case report, review of the literature and discussion of anaesthetic complications. *Anesthesia and Analgesia* 1986; **65**: 1201–7.

161 Horlocker TT, Wedel DJ, Schlichting JL. Postoperative epidural analgesia and oral anticoagulant therpay. *Anesthesia and Analgesia* 1994; **79**: 89–93.

162 Kabat K, Preble L, Sinatra R, Silverman D. Anesthesiologist followup of intraoperative epidural narcotics: seeing is believing. *Anesthesiology* 1989; **71**: A963.

163 Abboud TK, Shnider SM, Dailey PA, Raya JA, Sarkis F, Grobler NM, Sadri S, Khoo SS, DeSousa B, Baysinger CL. Intrathecal administration of hyperbaric morphine for the relief of pain in labour. *British Journal of Anaesthesia* 1984; **56**: 1351–60

164 Baraka A, Noueihid R, Hajj S. Intrathecal injection of morphine for obstetric analgesia. *Anesthesiology* 1981; **54**: 136–40.

165 Dailey PA, Brookshire GL, Shnider SM, Abboud TK, Kotelko DM, Noueihid R, Thigpen JW, Khoo SS, Raya JA, Foutz SE. The effects of naloxone associated with the intrathecal use of morphine in labor. *Anesthesia and Analgesia* 1985; **64**: 658–66.

166 Vella LM, Willatts DG, Knott C, Lintin DJ, Justins DM, Reynolds F. Epidural fentanyl in labour. An evaluation of the systemic contribution to analgesia. *Anaesthesia* 1985; **40**: 741–7.

167 Akerman B, Arwestrom E, Post C. Local anesthetics potentiate spinal morphine antinociception. *Anesthesia and Analgesia* 1988; **67**: 943–8.

168 Huckaby T, Gerard K. Scheidlinger J, Johnson MD, Datta S. Continuous epidural infusion of alfentanil-bupivacaine vs bupivacaine for labor and delivery. *Anesthesiology* 1989; **71**: A847.

169 Eisenach JC, Grice SC, Dewan DM. Patient-controlled analgesia following caesarean section: a comparison with epidural and intramuscular narcotics. *Anesthesiology* 1988; **68**: 444–8.

170 Harrison DM, Sinatra R, Morgese L, Chung JH. Epidural narcotic and patient-controlled analgesia for post-caesarean section pain relief. *Anesthesiology* 1988; **68**: 454–7.

171 Cope RW. The Wooley and Roe case, Wooley and Roe versus Minstry of Health and others. *Anaesthesia* 1954; **9**: 249–70.

172 Coombs DW, Fratkin JD. Neurotoxicology of spinal agents. *Anesthesiology* 1987; **66**: 724–6.

173 Tanelian DL, Cousins MJ. Failure of epidural opioid to control cancer pain in a patient previously treated with massive doses of intravenous opioid. *Pain* 1989; **36**: 359–62.

174 Erdine S, Aldemir T. Long-term results of peridural mophine in 225 patients. *Pain* 1991; **45**: 155–9.

175 Crul BJ, Delhaas EM. Technical complications during long-term subarachnoid or epidural administration of morphine in terminally ill cancer patients: a review of 140 cases. *Regional Anesthesia* 1991; **16**: 209–13.

176 Plummer JL, Cherry DA, Cousins MJ, Gourlay GK, Onley MM, Evans KH. Long-term spinal administration of morphine in cancer and non-cancer pain: a retrospective study. *Pain* 1991; **44**: 215–20.

177 Morgan M. Editorial. *Anaesthesia* 1982; **37**: 527–9.

178 Green DW. The clinical use of spinal opioids. In: Kaufman L ed. *Anaesthesia Review* 9. Edinburgh: Churchill Livingstone. 1992; 80–111.

179 Ngai SH, Berkowitz BA, Yang JC *et al.* Pharmacokinetics of naloxone in rats and in man: Basis for its potency and short duration of action. *Anesthesiology* 1976; **44**: 398–401.

180 Flacke JW, Flacke WE, Williams GD. Acute pulmonary edema following naloxone reversal of high-dose morphine analgesia. *Anesthesiology* 1977; **47**: 376–8.

181 Barsan WG, Seger D, Danzl DF, Ling LJ, Bartlett R, Buncher R, Bryan C. Duration of antagonistic effects of nalmefene and naloxone in opiate-induced sedation for emergency department procedures. *American Journal of Emergency Medicine* 1989, **2**: 155–61.

182 Pinkert TM, Ginzburg HM. Naltrexone. In: Bullingham RES ed. *Clinics in anaesthesiology*,Vol. 1, No. 1. London: WB Saunders, 1983; 168–72.

183 Konieczko KN, Jones JG, Barrowcliffe MP, Jordan C, Altman DG. Antagonism of morphine induced respiratory depression with nalmefene. *British Journal of Anaesthesia* 1988; **61**: 318–23.

184 Stacher G, Abatzi TA, Schulte F, Schneider C, Janotta GS, Gaupmann G, Mittelbach G, Steinringer H.

Naloxone does not alter the perception of pain induced by electrical and thermal stimulation of the skin in healthy humans. *Pain* 1988; **34**: 271–6.

185 Jaffe JH, Martin WR. Opioid analgesics and antagonists. In: Gilman AG, Rall TW, Nies AS, Taylor P eds. *The Pharmacological basis of therapeutics*. New York, Pergamon Inc. 1990; Ch. 21, 485–521.

186 Caudle RM, Isaac L. Intrathecal dynorphin (1–13) results in an irreversible loss of the tail flick reflex in rats. *Brain Research* 1987; **435**: 1–6.

187 Bakshi R, Faden AI. Competitive and non-competitive NMDA antagonists limit dynorphin A induced rat hind-limb paralysis. *Brain Research* 1990; **507**: 1–5.

188 Reynolds DG, Gurll NJ, Holaday JW, Lechner RB. The therapeutic efficacy of opiate antagonists in hemorrhagic shock. *Resuscitation* 1989; **18**: 243–51.

189 Satake K, Hiura A, Nishiwaki H, Ha SS, Chang YS, Umeyama K. Plasma β-endorphin and the effect of naloxone on hemodynamic changes during experimental acute pancreatitis in dogs. *Surgery, Gynaecology and Obstetrics* 1989; **165**: 402–6.

190 Law WR, Ferguson NL. Naloxone alters organ perfusion during endotoxin shock in conscious rats. *American Journal of Physiology* 1988, **255**: 5(2): H1106–H1113.

191 Murray MJ, Offord KP, Yaksh TL. Physiologic and plasma hormone correlates of survival in endotoxic dogs: effects of opiate antagonists. *Critical Care Medicine* 1989; **17**: 39–47.

192 Hinds CJ. Opiate antagonists in shock. *British Journal of Hospital Medicine* 1985; **34**: 233–4.

193 Soulioti A. Naloxone for septic shock. *Lancet* 1988; **ii**: 1113–34.

194 Knape JTA. Early respiratory depression resistant to naloxone following epidural buprenorphine. *Anesthesiology* 1986; **64**: 382–4.

195 Gal TJ. Naloxone reversal of buprenorphine-induced respiratory depression. *Clincial Pharmacology and Therapeutics* 1989; **45**: 66–71.

196 Dickenson AH, Sullivan AF, McQuay HJ. Intrathecal etorphine, fentanyl and buprenorphine on spinal nociceptive neurones in the rat. *Pain* 1990; **42**: 227–34.

197 Jasinski DR, Fudala PJ, Johnson RE. Sublingual versus subcutaneous buprenorphine in opiate abusers. *Clinical Pharmacology and Therapeutics* 1989; **45**: 513–19.

198 Johnson RE, Cone EJ, Henningfield JE, Fudala PJ. Use of buprenorphine in the treatment of opiate addiction. I. Physiologic and behavioral effects during a rapid dose induction. *Clinical Pharmacology and Therapeutics* 1989; **46**: 335–43.

199 Fudala PJ, Johnson RE, Bunker E. Abrupt withdrawal of buprenorphine following chronic administration. *Clinical Pharmacology and Therapeutics* 1989; **45**: 186.

200 Jaffe JH. Drug addiction and drug abuse. In: Gilman AG, Rall TW, Nies AS, Taylor P eds. *The pharmacological basis of therapeutics*. New York: Pergamon, 1990: 522–73.

201 Heishman RJ, Stitzer ML, Bigelow, GE, Liebson IA. Acute opioid physical dependence in postaddict humans: naloxone dose effects after brief morphine exposure. *Journal of Pharmacology and Experimental Therapeutics* 1989; **248**: 127–34.

202 Kumar V, Ness TJ, Gebhart GF. Does systemic nalbuphine antagonise visceral or cutaneous antinociceptive effect of intrathecal morphine in rats. *Anesthesiology* 1989; **71**: A1148.

203 Moldenhauer CC, Roach GW, Finlayson DC, Hug CC, Kopel ME, Tobia V, Kelly S. Nalbuphine antagonisation of ventilatory depression following high dose fentanyl anesthesia. *Anesthesiology* 1985; **62**: 647–50.

204 Latasch MD, Teichmuller T, Dudziak R, Probst S. Antagonisation of fentanyl-induced respiratory depression by nalbuphine. *Acta Anaesthesiologica Belgica* 1989; **40**: 35–40.

205 Blaise GA, Nugent M, McMichan JC, Durant PA. Side effects of nalbuphine while reversing opioid-induced respiratory depression: Report of four cases. *Canadian Journal of Anaesthesia* 1990; **37**: 794–7.

206 Jaffe RS, Moldenhauer CC, Hug CC Jr, Finlayson DC, Tobia V, Kopel ME. Nalbuphine antagonism of fentanyl induced ventilatory depression. *Anesthesiology* 1988; **68**: 254–60.

207 Baxter AD, Samson B, Penning J, Doran R, Dube LM. Prevention of epidural morphine-induced respiratory depression with intravenous nalbuphine infusion in post-thoracotomy patients. *Canadian Journal of Anaesthesia* 1989; **36**: 503–9.

208 De Castro J, Parmentier P. Buprenorphine in analgesic anaesthesia. VI World Congress of Anaesthesiology, Mexico City 1976; Section 5: 3.

209 Patel K, Gelman S. Pressor responses to naloxone and physostigmine. *Anesthesia and Analgesia* 1980; **59**: 517.

26

Drug Management of Acute, Severe and Chronic Pain

I Power

INTRODUCTION

Pain is a complex sensation involving physical, neuronal, emotional and psychological factors. The physiology of pain involves nociceptors, afferent nerves and sympathetic nerves, all interacting and being impinged upon by descending influences from the central nervous system. Pain can result from disorder in any of these components. There is also good evidence that peripheral and central sensitization of pain pathways leads to hyperalgesia so that, after the initial insult, even mild stimuli can be painful.[1] The pharmacology of pain relief encompasses not only the obvious opioids and non-steroidal anti-inflammatory drugs (NSAIDs) but also antidepressants and anticonvulsants which can be very effective in certain circumstances. The full panoply of analgesic drugs can be presented by a discussion of the management of three pathological states; acute pain, chronic neurogenic pain, and chronic cancer-related pain. The drug treatment of other pain states can then be deduced from a knowledge of these three different clinical problems. The relief of acute and cancer-related pain in children is also addressed in this chapter.

The treatment of acute pain, including that after surgery, is dominated by the use of opioids, NSAIDs and local anaesthetic techniques. Chronic neurogenic pain results from some disorder of the central, peripheral or sympathetic nervous components of the pain pathway and antidepressants and anticonvulsants can be of great value. The pain resulting from cancer can be of many aetiologies and the use of various different therapeutic agents may be of benefit, but the basis of management remains the use of appropriate doses of oral opioids, usually morphine.

DRUG TREATMENT OF ACUTE PAIN

Acute pain most often results from tissue damage, either as a result of trauma or surgical incision, and may alternatively be described as nociceptive pain. It is now known that tissue damage initiates inflammatory processes that produce pain and sensitize the neuronal components of the system to further stimuli.[2] Substances released at the site of tissue damage include histamine, bradykinin, prostaglandins and thromboxanes. Acute pain usually lasts a matter of hours or days; the causation is clear, the outcome relatively obvious, associated problems are uncommon, and the long-term psychological effects are minimal.

The main drugs used to relieve acute pain are the opioids and the non-steroidal anti-inflammatory analgesics. Various adjuncts, including the α_2-adrenoceptor antagonists, may be of benefit in certain circumstances. As nerve conduction, both in the somatic and sympathetic systems, is important in the sensation of acute pain, it should be obvious that local anaesthetics have an integral role in analgesia, especially after surgery. Local anaesthetic drugs are not discussed in detail in this chapter, but the evidence for their place in balanced analgesia is presented.

Opioids

The opioids currently available in clinical practice are listed in Table 26.1, and the activity of some at opioid receptors is described in Table 26.2.[3,4] Analgesia is thought to involve μ-receptors at supraspinal sites and κ-receptors within the spinal cord. Most opioids used to treat acute pain are μ-receptor agonists. The agonist/antagonist drugs are active at κ-receptors and antagonists at μ-receptors. The partial agonist, buprenorphine, has high affinity for μ-receptors, but is a weaker agonist than true agonists like morphine. The mode of action of meptazinol is not well understood, although it is thought to be a selective agonist at μ_1-receptors and has a central cholinergic effect. The hope was that the discovery of different opioid receptors and agonists would lead to the development of potent analgesics with less side-effects than morphine but, disappointingly, this has not been the case.

The choice of an opioid for the relief of acute pain depends on many factors including efficacy, side-effects and the preparations available. The detailed pharmacology of opioids has been dealt with in Chapter 25, and the aim of this section is to present their clinical use. Accordingly, the formulations and doses of the main opioids used are shown in Table 26.3 and their relative merits discussed below.

TABLE 26.1 Classification of the opioids

Agonists

Morphine and derivatives
- Morphine
- Papaveretum
- Diamorphine
- Codeine
- Dihydrocodeine
- Levorphanol

Phenylpiperidines
- Pethidine
- Phenoperidine
- Fentanyl
- Alfentanil
- Sufentanil
- Remifentanil

Methadone and congeners
- Methadone
- Dextromoramide
- Dipipanone
- Dextropropoxyphene

Benzomorphan derivatives
- Phenazocine

Mixed agonists/antagonists and partial agonists

Pentazocine
Butorphanol
Nalbuphine
Meptazinol

Buprenorphine

TABLE 26.2 Summary of the actions of agonists, agonist/antagonists, partial agonists, and antagonists at the μ- and κ-opioid receptors

	μ	κ
Morphine	++	+
Fentanyl	+++	+
Pentazocine	−	++
Butorphanol	−	++
Nalbuphine	−	++
Buprenorphine	P	−
Naloxone	−	−

+ agonist; − antagonist; P, partial agonist.

Efficacy

The agonist/antagonist and partial agonists tend to be less potent analgesics than the pure agonists. The weaker analgesia and dysphoria, nausea and vomiting associated with higher doses of pentazocine, butorphanol, nalbuphine, meptazinol and buprenorphine limit their application for the relief of acute pain.

Onset and duration of action

Highly lipophilic drugs like fentanyl have a more rapid onset than hydrophilic drugs like morphine. Alfentanil has a low ionization constant, is present in plasma mainly as the non-ionized diffusible form (90%) and has a rapid onset of action. Remifentanil has the shortest duration of the opioids as it is metabolized by plasma cholinesterases and will have to be used by infusion. Methadone has the longest elimination half-life of these drugs (17–24 h) but is normally still prescribed on a 6–8 hourly basis indicating a separation between the clinical effects and the pharmacokinetic parameters.

Absorption and routes of administration

Morphine is absorbed well from the gastrointestinal tract but significant first-pass hepatic metabolism means that the bioavailability of oral morphine is only 30% after a single dose. Oral doses of morphine have therefore to be significantly higher than the parenteral for a given effect (Table 26.3). Although oral formulations of opioids are not often used for acute pain relief, sublingual buprenorphine has been introduced to avoid first-pass hepatic metabolism. Codeine, dihydrocodeine and dextropropoxyphene are all effective when given orally.

TABLE 26.3 Summary of the available preparations, dose and frequency of administration of the opioids

	ROUTE	DOSE (mg)	FREQUENCY (h)	COMMENTS
Morphine	im, iv, sc	10	3–4	
	Oral	30	3–4	
Papaveretum*	im, iv, sc	10–20	4	Noscapine removed
Diamorphine	im, iv, sc	5	4–5	More soluble
Codeine	im	30–60	4–6	Histamine release on iv administration
	Oral	30–60	4	
Dihydrocodeine	im, sc	50	4–6	
	Oral	30	4–6	
Levorphanol	im, sc	2	4–5	
	Oral	4	4–5	
Pethidine	im, iv, sc	100	4	Less constipating than morphine. Toxic metabolite
	Oral	200	4	
Phenoperidine	iv	1–2	1	
Fentanyl	iv	0.1	–	
Methadone	im, iv, sc	10	6–8	
	Oral	20	6–8	
Dextromoramide	Oral	5–20	2–3	Less sedating than morphine; shorter action
	pr	10		
Dipipanone	Oral	10	6	Usually in combination with cyclizine
Dextropropoxyphene	Oral	65	6–8	Used in combination with paracetamol
Phenazocine	Oral, sl	5	4–6	
Pentazocine	im, iv, sc	30–60	4–6	Dysphoria
	Oral	50	4–6	
Butorphanol	im	2	4–6	
Nalbuphine	im, iv, sc	10–20	3–6	Ceiling analgesic effect
Meptazinol	im, iv	50–100	2–4	
	Oral	200	3–6	
Buprenorphine	im	0.3	6–8	Only partially reversed by naloxone
	sl	0.4	6–8	

*Noscapine is no longer present in papaveretum, which consists only of morphine, papaverine and codeine. There is one strength of papaveretum, 15.4 mg/ml, and the drug is now prescribed by volume.

Central nervous system effects

Morphine produces analgesia, sedation, euphoria, respiratory depression and miosis. High doses of opioids can produce muscular rigidity probably due to dopaminergic effects in the central nervous system, and this can occur when high doses of fentanyl are used for general anaesthesia. Pethidine produces less sedation than morphine, and may have an atropine-like effect on the pupillary sphincter. Pentazocine produces dreams and hallucinations in about 20% of patients, possibly as a consequence of activity at σ-receptors.

Metabolic products and their effects

Morphine is metabolized to morphine-6-glucuronide and to morphine-3-glucuronide. Morphine-6-glucuronide is more active than morphine itself and has a longer elimination half-life. There is some evidence that morphine-3-glucuronide, previously thought to be inactive, may be involved in the development of morphine tolerance. This metabolite may be important in the normal action of morphine and may accumulate in patients with renal impairment leading to side-effects.[5] Diamorphine has no affinity for opioid receptors and has to be metabolized to monoacetylmorphine and morphine before it has any effect. Approximately 10% of administered codeine is converted to morphine, which may be responsible for the clinical effect. A metabolite of pethidine, norpethidine, has a long elimination half-life of 15–20 h and can accumulate in patients with renal failure or after prolonged administration, producing tremors, muscle twitches, dilated pupils, hyper-reflexia and convulsions.

Cardiovascular effects

Administration of morphine is associated with a slight fall in blood pressure and heart rate. The release of histamine by morphine may explain the fall in blood pressure after morphine, and the bradycardia may be a direct vagal effect. Like morphine, pethidine also produces histamine release and a fall in blood pressure, but instead may result in a tachycardia due to its atropine-like effect. The other phenylpiperidines, including fentanyl, do not release histamine even when given in high doses, but can produce bradycardia.

Smooth muscle effects

Morphine reduces propulsive activity in the gut, and produces spasm of the sphincter of Oddi in the biliary tract and the ureter. Pethidine, fentanyl and some of the agonist/antagonist agents may produce smaller increases in biliary pressure.

Drug interactions

Dangerous interactions may occur between monoamine oxidase inhibitors and pethidine, probably due to the accumulation of norpethidine. Sequelae include mental confusion, cerebral excitation, hyperpyrexia and hypertension or circulatory collapse. Clinically important drug interactions are much less common with other opioids.

Dependence

Opioids are common drugs of abuse, but dependence as a result of medical treatment is uncommon and should not be used as an excuse for failure to alleviate pain effectively.

Opioids used for acute pain relief

The pure agonists are most often used for the relief of acute severe pain, because of the disadvantages of the agonist/antagonists and the partial agonists. Alfentanil, fentanyl and sufentanil are used as components of general anaesthesia, but are rarely employed specifically for acute or postoperative pain apart from by the epidural route. The parenteral drugs of choice for relief of acute severe pain remain morphine, pethidine, papaveretum (now formulated without noscapine) and, in some countries, diamorphine. When it is appropriate to treat acute pain with oral opioids then the weaker drugs codeine, dihydrocodeine and dextropropoxyphene can be employed usefully, either alone or in combination preparations with paracetamol.

Intravenous, intramuscular and patient-controlled analgesia

The intravenous route is most commonly used for the initial control of acute pain and then intramuscular administration is used for continuing control of severe pain. Unfortunately, intramuscular doses are often given inappropriately with large doses being given infrequently. Whatever the route of administration, it is necessary to adjust the dose of an opioid to the individual patient's needs. This can be done with impressive success by making regular formal pain scores and constructing clear and sensible protocols for the administration of small doses of opioids on a frequent basis.[6] Patient-controlled analgesia (PCA) allows the prescription of effective and safe analgesia primarily under the control of the patient, usually by the intravenous route. There is good evidence that PCA provides better analgesia and is associated with less respiratory side-effects than other routes of opioid administration.[7] Typically, morphine is used for intravenous PCA in a dose of 1 mg, with a lockout time between doses of 5 min and no background infusion. Pethidine, papaveretum and diamorphine can all be used in this way.

Spinal opioids and patient-controlled epidural analgesia

Opioids given by the spinal route are thought to act, at least to a degree, on receptors in the substantia gelatinosa. Different drugs and doses tend to be used intrathecally and epidurally. Morphine, pethidine, diamorphine and buprenorphine have been used intrathecally in doses of one-tenth of the intramuscular dose and it is probable that the site of action is the level of the spinal cord. One milligram or less of morphine or diamorphine or 30–45 μg of buprenorphine given intrathecally can give long-lasting analgesia. When opioids are given epidurally the effect may be partly spinal and systemic. The epidural dose of hydrophilic opioids is similar to those given parenterally (e.g. fentanyl 50–100 μg), but hydrophilic drugs are given in lower doses epidurally (e.g. morphine 1–2 mg).

Epidural opioids are now being combined with low concentrations of local anaesthetics in epidural infusions. Most recently, combinations of lipophilic opioids (fentanyl 2 μg/ml or sufentanil 0.8 μg/ml) with low concentrations of local anaesthetics (bupivacaine 0.1%) have been used to impressive effect as patient-controlled epidural analgesia (PCEA).[8]

The side-effects of spinal opioid administration include respiratory depression, nausea and vomiting, pruritus, and urinary retention. These effects, together with the analgesia, can be reversed by naloxone, but the hope that spinal opioid administration would provide analgesia with no side-effects has not been confirmed. Risk factors for respiratory depression, which may have been of late onset, include the use of hydrophilic drugs, large doses and simultaneous systemic opioid administration. It is thought that hydrophilic opioids may produce late respiratory depression because they slowly ascend rostrally in the cerebrospinal fluid without being taken up at spinal level.

Tramadol

Tramadol has been in use for a number of years in Germany and is now being introduced into various other countries. Reports indicate that it is a useful analgesic with minimal sedative effects or abuse potential, but it is weaker than morphine. The mechanism of action of tramadol is not understood fully, but it is an agonist at opioid receptors and has also a spinal action on noradrenergic pathways.[9] Tramadol is available in oral and parenteral forms, and it may be that it will be useful for mild to moderate pain.

Non-steroidal anti-inflammatory drugs (NSAIDs)

NSAIDs have the same analgesic, antipyretic and anti-inflammatory effects as aspirin and are being used for the treatment of acute, severe pain. NSAIDs do not have the side-effects normally associated with opioids of respiratory depression, sedation, addiction, inhibition of gastrointestinal motility, or nausea and vomiting. Unfortunately, NSAIDs can have serious side-effects as they inhibit the tissue enzyme prostaglandin endoperoxide synthase. These side-effects are similar to those encountered with aspirin, and include inhibition of platelet function, peptic ulceration, impairment of renal function, and precipitation of bronchospasm in some asthmatics. There are many NSAIDs now available, with a spectrum of anti-inflammatory, antipyretic and analgesic properties. A chemical classification of these antipyretic analgesics is given in Table 26.4, together with paracetamol which is devoid of any anti-inflammatory effect, and the recommended doses and preparations available are presented in Table 26.5.

NSAIDs used for acute pain relief

Diclofenac is available as a preparation for injection, as well as tablets and suppositories. There have been a

TABLE 26.4 The antipyretic analgesics

Carboxylic acids
Salicylates – acetylsalicylic acid, diflusinal, salsalate
Propionic acids – ibuprofen, naproxen, fenbufen, fenoprofen, ketoprofen, flurbiprofen
Acetic acids:
Indolacetic acids – indomethacin, sulindac, etodolac
Pyrroloacetic acids – ketorolac, tolmetin
Phenylacetic acids – diclofenac
Anthranilic acids – mefenamic acid, floctafenine
Pyrazolones
Phenylbutazone, azapropazone
Oxicams
Piroxicam, tenoxicam
Naphthylalkalones
Nabumetone
Para-aminophenols
Paracetamol

TABLE 26.5 Summary of the available preparations and doses of the NSAIDs and paracetamol

DRUG	PREPARATIONS AVAILABLE	DAILY DOSE (mg)	DOSING INTERVAL (h)
Salicylates			
Aspirin	Oral	1800–3600	4
Propionic acids			
Ibuprofen	Oral	1200–2400	6–8
Ketoprofen	Oral, pr, im	100–200	6–8
Naproxen	Oral, pr	500–1000	12
Acetic acids			
Diclofenac	Oral, iv, pr	150	12
Indomethacin	Oral, pr	50–200	6–12
Ketorolac	Oral, iv, im	120	6
Anthranilic acids			
Mefenamic acid	Oral	1500	8
Pyrazolones			
Phenylbutazone	Oral	300–400	6–8
Oxicams			
Piroxicam	Oral, pr, im	20	24
Tenoxicam	Oral, iv, im	20	24
Naphthylalkalones			
Nabumetone	Oral	1000	24
Para-aminophenols			
Paracetamol	Oral, pr	2000–4000	6

considerable number of studies reporting the successful use of diclofenac after surgery.[10] Diclofenac has also been shown to be very effective at relieving pain associated with smooth muscle spasm, including renal and biliary colic, conditions for which it may be the analgesic of choice. Unfortunately the parenteral form of diclofenac is irritant to tissues and should be given by deep intramuscular injection. Ketorolac is available as tablets and as a parenteral preparation. As is the case for all NSAIDs, ketorolac alone is unsuitable for the treatment of severe pain present immediately after major surgery, but is adequate for the relief of mild to moderate pain.[11] Recently, the use of ketorolac has been associated with reports of adverse effects, and, in the UK, the initial parenteral dose has been reduced to 10 mg and any anticoagulant therapy, including subcutaneous heparin, is now a contraindication. It is probable that such restrictions will reduce significantly the use of ketorolac. Indomethacin has marked anti-inflammatory activity, and is normally used for the treatment of medical conditions such as gout. A number of studies have successfully assessed indomethacin as a postoperative analgesic, but the lack of an intramuscular preparation has been a restriction on the use of this drug for acute pain. Piroxicam has a long half-life, allowing once-daily administration and prophylactic use before surgery is effective.[12] Early reports suggest that tenoxicam, another oxicam with an even longer elimination half-life, may also be useful. Ibuprofen and ketoprofen have also been used for pain relief after operation.

Side-effects of NSAIDs

Unfortunately, the NSAIDs do have undesirable effects as a consequence of their mechanism of action, inhibition of tissue prostaglandin and thromboxane production, and they are a major cause of serious adverse reactions reported to the regulatory authorities. Prostaglandins act as local hormones, regulating tissue function, and interference with them can produce problems. Essentially these effects are well recognized in association with long-term aspirin or NSAID therapy. In surgical patients the main concerns are the possibility of peptic ulceration, interference with platelet function, renal impairment and bronchospasm in some asthmatics. A significant proportion of patients are susceptible to such effects and should not be given NSAIDs.

The use of NSAIDs for acute pain

NSAIDs have an important role in the management of acute pain, and they may be superior to opioids for the relief of biliary and renal colic. In general, NSAIDs are not sufficient in themselves for the relief of severe pain and have to be combined with opioids or local anaesthetic techniques.

α_2-Receptor antagonists

The adrenergic α_2-agonist, clonidine, has sedative and analgesic properties in addition to its antihypertensive and sympatholytic effects. Central α_2-adrenoreceptors seem to be responsible for the sedative effect, while analgesia is due to spinal α_2-activation by clonidine. Clonidine can be shown to have analgesic effect when given systemically or epidurally, but its clinical use is limited by the principal side-effects of hypotension and bradycardia. Dexmedetomidine is a more highly selective α_2-agonist than clonidine and may be of more use as an analgesic.[13]

Inhalational agents

Inhalational agents such as 50% nitrous oxide in oxygen (entonox) are used in obstetrics and also for changing painful dressings.

Balanced analgesia

The pharmacological relief of acute severe pain is now based on the concept of using combinations of opioids, NSAIDs and local anaesthetics to produce balanced analgesia. Using this technique it is possible to control pain effectively after surgery with the minimum of side-effects.[14] Moreover, in clinical anaesthetic practice attempts are now being made to prevent the known sensitization of pain pathways by using prophylactic or pre-emptive analgesia before any surgical incision is made.[1,15]

The treatment of acute pain in children

The management of acute postoperative pain in children comprises combinations of the same drugs and techniques used for adults.[16] Paracetamol may be sufficient for the relief of mild pain, but NSAIDs are now being used in children, either alone or in combination with opioids or local anaesthesia. In the UK, diclofenac is available as a 12.5 mg paediatric suppository and this has proved very useful. There has been a tendency to underutilize opioids in children, perhaps due to fear of side-effects, but they are necessary for severe pain. The sensitivity of the newborn to morphine is due to their slow metabolism of opioids, but this matures by about 3 months of age. Continuous morphine infusions are often used in younger children at rates of around 25 μg/kg/h, which is reduced to 10 μg/kg/h in infants younger than 6 months. PCA can be used safely and effectively by children as young as 6 years of age. Alternatively, opioids may be administered via an indwelling subcutaneous catheter to avoid the discomfort of repeated intramuscular administration. For the relief of pain after major surgery, opioids are now given to children by the epidural route, usually in combination with local anaesthetics.

DRUG TREATMENT OF CHRONIC NEUROGENIC PAIN

Neurogenic pain is due to a disorder of the nervous system in the absence of nerve terminal stimulation by trauma or disease. For the purposes of this discussion, the drug treatments of trigeminal neuralgia, postherpetic neuralgia, painful diabetic neuropathy, phantom limb pain, reflex sympathetic dystrophy and causalgia, and central poststroke pain are presented here. Chronic neurogenic pain can be extremely severe; it may last for months and years, the prognosis is unpredictable, and depression and anxiety may be associated problems. The differential diagnosis is important and organic disease should be excluded before drug therapy is instituted. A characteristic of this pain state is that it is often insensitive to opioid therapy, but instead can be treated successfully with antidepressants and anticonvulsants.

Trigeminal neuralgia

This normally appears suddenly in elderly patients as a facial stabbing, shooting or lancinating pain in the distribution of the second or third division of the nerve. The initial attack may be only brief, but the frequency and severity increase rapidly. Carbamazepine is specific for the relief of trigeminal neuralgia. At first, 100 mg a day should be given and the dose increased slowly over 2 weeks; most patients need 200 mg three or four times daily, but some require up to 1600 mg a day. Plasma concentrations should be monitored when high doses are given. Dizziness and drowsiness are common side-effects, gastrointestinal disturbances can occur, and the drug should be stopped if an erythematous rash develops. Some benefit should be seen after 2 weeks' treatment; patients should not expect an immediate analgesic effect after one or two doses. Unfortunately, most cases of trigeminal neuralgia eventually become refractory to carbamazepine, and, although there may be some response to phenytoin, valproate or baclofen at this point, percutaneous radiofrequency coagulation may be required.

Postherpetic neuralgia

As postherpetic neuralgia occurs after 10% of cases of herpes zoster, every effort should be made to prevent the problem by giving acyclovir 800 mg five times daily for 7 days as soon as the rash appears and the diagnosis is made. Once the burning pain of this neuralgia is established, amitriptyline or imipramine are used, not as antidepressants, but for their recognized benefits in reducing the peripheral nervous component of neurogenic pain.[17] In younger patients, the initial dose of amitriptyline should be 25 mg and can be gradually increased to 75 mg a day. In the elderly the starting dose of amitriptyline is 10 mg, and then 50 mg a day in divided doses. The analgesic effect may take a week to appear. Side-effects of tricyclic antidepressants include drowsiness, dry mouth, blurred vision, constipation, urinary retention, sweating and arrhythmias and heart block. If there is also a 'shooting pain' component to the neuralgia, then anticonvulsant therapy can be added in the form of sodium valproate up to 800 mg a day. Dihydrocodeine may also be useful as an additional analgesic.

Painful diabetic neuropathy

Treatment for this disorder is similar to that for postherpetic neuralgia. In refractory cases, oral mexilitene may be used under initial careful monitoring (400 mg, then 200 mg 6-hourly) after a trial of intravenous lignocaine.

Phantom limb pain

Drug therapy consists of the use of low dose amitriptyline with simultaneous anticonvulsant therapy if shooting pains are present.

Reflex sympathetic dystrophy and causalgia

Intravenous regional sympathetic blocks using guanethidine may give temporary relief of these conditions. The normal dose given to the affected limb is 15–20 mg of guanethidine in 40 ml of saline using an arterial tourniquet which is kept inflated for 10 min. Systemic administration of phenoxybenzamine, propranolol, calcium-channel antagonists and corticosteroids have also been reported to improve this condition.

Central poststroke pain

This severe pain may affect up to 2% of patients after a stroke. Again drug treatment is based on the use of low-dose amitriptyline, and anticonvulsants are added if the pains have a shooting quality.

Summary of neurogenic pain

There is considerable controversy over the medical treatment of neurogenic pain, indicating that the available drugs are not completely successful, but, as described here, antidepressants and anticonvulsants are used in preference to conventional analgesics.[18]

DRUG TREATMENT OF THE CHRONIC PAIN OF MALIGNANCY

Pain associated with malignancy may be mild, moderate or severe and is of unpredictable duration. The prognosis is of increasing discomfort and deterioration in health; there are many associated problems including fear and depression, and drug treatment is the basis of the management. With all the drugs used, it is again important to tailor therapy to the needs of the individual patient.[19] Opioid analgesics are used most often in advanced cancer pain, but the much higher doses and routes of administration are quite different from those given for acute pain.

The aetiology of the pain of malignancy and specific therapy

Patients with cancer may have pain for many reasons, and some respond to specific therapy. For example, nerve invasion may require the antidepressants and anticonvulsants used for neurogenic pain; bone pain responds well to NSAIDs; anticholinergics may be indicated for gastrointestinal spasm; and laxatives may be needed for constipation. In adults with cancer, pain is most often due to direct tumour involvement including metastatic bone disease and nerve invasion. A significant number of patients also have pain related to cancer surgery, chemotherapy or radiation therapy and these may require the use of the drugs described in the sections of this chapter dealing with acute and neurogenic pains. Indeed, in children with malignancy, treatment for the cancer is the most common source of discomfort. It should be remembered that the most effective analgesia for some patients may be specific antitumour chemotherapy or radiotherapy to reduce the size of the lesion. The aetiology, severity and quality of pain can change quickly, as in the sudden appearance of a painful pathological fracture, and therapy should be flexible enough to take account of this.

The analgesic ladder

A protocol has been recommended by the World Health Organization (WHO) for the relief of cancer pain, consisting of a three-step ladder. The first step is for mild to moderate pain and consists of non-opioid drugs; NSAIDs and paracetamol (Tables 26.4 and 26.5). The second step is for moderate to severe pain and requires the addition of codeine or an analogue (Table 26.3); usually the non-opioid is given regularly and the opioid is titrated until pain relief is satisfactory. The third step of the ladder is for severe pain and a strong opioid, usually morphine, replaces the weaker codeine. Adjuvant drugs, described below, may be used at all the steps on the analgesic ladder.

The use of opioids in cancer pain

In general, the pure agonist opioids are used for cancer pain (Table 26.1) as the mixed agonist/antagonists are not as potent and have few advantages. Morphine is used for severe pain and in most cases the oral administration is effective. The dose range is very wide, but the majority of patients find relief with less than 200 mg a day, although much higher doses may be required in some cases. Morphine elixirs give peak plasma concentrations within 1 h; tablets take a little longer, but both preparations produce an effect that lasts 4 h. Using such 'immediate release' formulations severe pain can be controlled quickly by prescribing oral morphine 10 mg 4-hourly, and increasing the dose by 2.5 mg each 4 h until the desired effect is achieved or undesirable side-effects are produced. Once the daily dose of morphine required to control pain has been identified, the frequency of administration can be reduced to twice daily by substituting equivalent amounts of controlled release preparations (e.g. MST Continus). Provision must then be made for 'breakthrough' or pain related to movement, and a suitable oral dose of immediate-release morphine can be given. Nausea and vomiting occur in up to two-thirds of adult patients taking oral morphine, but may either settle with time, or usually can be controlled with standard anti-emetics. Constipation is a common problem and laxatives may be prescribed. Respiratory depression is unusual in such patients with severe pain, but sedation is common at the start of therapy although it usually resolves within days.

If troublesome side-effects occur with morphine then alternative strong opioids can be substituted, including methadone and phenazocine, but pethidine is avoided because of the risk of norpethidine toxicity with chronic use (Table 26.3). Once opioid requirements have been identified, transdermal fentanyl patches may also be useful in selected cancer patients who experience side-effects, or cannot take oral preparations.

Patients may be unable to take oral opioids, and rectal administration or morphine or dextromoramide may then be of use. Alternatively, intravenous or subcutaneous opioid infusions can be instituted and maintained for considerable periods, and diamorphine may be useful because it can be prepared in smaller volumes due to its high solubility. Spinal opioids may be indicated for intractable pain, and the development of new catheter materials and implantable epidural or intrathecal systems allows administration for weeks or months.

Adjuvants

The tricyclic antidepressants, anticonvulsants and steroids can be used at all stages of the WHO analgesic ladder. The tricyclic antidepressants and anticonvulsants are used for similar indications and in the doses recommended in this chapter for neurogenic pain, but an additional benefit of the former drugs is that some patients with cancer pain may well be depressed. Steroids may lower pain perception, reduce opioid requirements, and improve appetite and mood in cancer patients, and prednisolone may have these effects even at low doses of 5–10 mg. Steroids are also of use in reducing pain of metastatic bone disease and spinal cord compression by tumours. NSAIDs should be avoided if steroids are prescribed as the combination increases the risk of gastrointestinal complications.

Children

The three-step analgesic ladder is also appropriate for children with pain from cancer, and morphine may be required when weaker drugs are no longer sufficient. The main opioid side-effects seen in children with malignancy are sedation and constipation. Respiratory depression is uncommon in children older than 3 months of age given opioids for malignancy, and nausea is less of a problem than in adults. Sedation is common, but often improves after a couple of days of therapy. Constipation can be a prolonged problem, and regular laxatives should be prescribed. Morphine can be given orally in 4-hourly doses of 0.3 mg/kg, or, preferably, twice daily as a slow release preparation.

SUMMARY OF THE DRUG MANAGEMENT OF ACUTE, SEVERE AND CHRONIC PAIN

The management of acute, chronic neurogenic and cancer-related pain has been presented to describe the clinical use of the variety of analgesics available. Acute pain, as present after surgery, is best managed by combination therapy of opioids, NSAIDs and local anaesthetic techniques, perhaps given in a pre-emptive fashion. Completely different drugs are indicated for chronic neurogenic pain which responds best to agents originally developed as antidepressants and anticonvulsants. Pain associated with cancer should be treated in a stepwise fashion using mild to powerful analgesics according to the severity of pain and progression of the disease.

REFERENCES

1 Woolf CJ. Recent advances in the pathophysiology of acute pain. *British Journal of Anaesthesia* 1989; **63**: 139–46.

2 Dray A, Bevan S. Inflammation and hyperalgesia: highlighting the team effort. *Trends in Pharmacological Sciences* 1993; **14**: 287–90.

3 Lutz RA, Pfister HP. Opioid receptors and their pharmacological profiles. *Journal of Receptor Research* 1992; **12**: 267–86.

4 Pleuvry BJ. Opioid receptors and their relevance to anaesthesia. *British Journal of Anaesthesia* 1993; **71**: 119–26.

5 Portenoy RK, Thaler HT, Inturrisi CE, FriedlanderKlar H, Foley KM. The metabolite morphine-6-glucuronide contributes to the analgesia produced by morphine infusion in patients with pain and normal renal function. *Clinical Pharmacology and Therapeutics* 1992; **51**: 422–31.

6 Gould TH, Crosby DL, Harmer M, Lloyd SM, Lunn JN, Rees GAD, Roberts DE, Webster JA. Policy for controlling pain after surgery: effect of sequential changes in management. *British Medical Journal* 1992; **305**: 1187–93.

7 Wheatley RG, Somerville ID, Sapsford DJ, Jones JG. Postoperative hypoxaemia: comparison of extradural, i.m. and patient-controlled opioid analgesia. *British Journal of Anaesthesia* 1990; **64**: 267–75.

8 Cohen S, Amar D, Pantuck CB, Pantuck EJ, Goodman EJ, Widroff JS, Kanas RJ, Brady JA. Postcesarean delivery epidural patient-controlled analgesia: Fentanyl or sufentanil? *Anesthesiology* 1993; **78**: 486–91.

9 Driessen B, Reimann W, Giertz H. Effects of the central analgesic tramadol on the uptake and release of noradrenaline and dopamine *in vitro*. *British Journal of Pharmacology* 1993; **108**: 806–11.

10 Todd PA, Sorkin EM. Diclofenac sodium. A reappraisal of its pharmacodynamic properties, and therapeutic efficacy. *Drugs* 1988; **35**: 244–85.

11 Power I, Noble DW, Douglas E, Spence AA. Comparison of i.m. ketorolac trometamol and morphine sulphate for pain relief after cholecystectomy. *British Journal of Anaesthesia* 1990; **65**: 448–55.

12 Serpell MG, Thomson MF. Comparison of piroxicam with placebo in the management of pain after total hip replacement. *British Journal of Anaesthesia* 1989; **63**: 354–6.

13 Proctor LT, Schmeling WT, Warltier DC. Premedication with oral dexmedetomidine alters hemodynamic actions of intravenous anesthetic agents in chronically instrumented dogs. *Anesthesiology* 1992; **77**: 554–62.

14 Dahl JB, Rosenberg J, Dirkes WE, Mogensen T, Kehlet H. Prevention of postoperative pain by balanced analgesia. *British Journal of Anaesthesia* 1990; **64**: 518–20.

15 McQuay HJ. Pre-emptive analgesia. *British Journal of Anaesthesia* 1992; **69**: 1–3.

16 Burrows FA, Berde CB. Optimal pain relief in infants and children. *British Medical Journal* 1993; **307**: 815–16.

17 McQuay HJ, Carroll D, Glynn CJ. Low dose amitriptyline in the treatment of chronic pain. *Anaesthesia* 1992; **47**: 646–52.

18 Davies HTO, Crombie IK, Macrae WA. Polarised views on treating neurogenic pain. *Pain* 1993; **54**: 341–6.

19 Ashburn MA, Lipman AG. Management of pain in the cancer patient. *Anesthesia and Analgesia* 1993; **76**: 402–16.

SECTION EIGHT

Drugs Affecting Peripheral Organ Systems

27

Blood

Part I Pharmacology of Blood and Blood-forming Organs

PL Cervi, AH Goldstone

THE FUNDAMENTALS OF COAGULATION

Disruption of vascular integrity initiates a well-co-ordinated series of physical and biochemical events that plug the initial vessel breach, produce a clump of platelets held together by a mesh of fibrin, strengthen and contract the clot, and provide a base for endothelial repair. Normally these events occur with astounding efficiency and, more importantly, are restricted to the site of injury by a complex system of regulatory mechanisms that prevents the uncontrolled extension of thrombus. The following is a brief overview of the cellular and soluble participants in this process.

Role of the platelets

Platelets are produced in the bone marrow by the cleavage of specialized membrane components of megakaryocytes and are released into the circulation under the control of the growth factor, thrombopoietin. Platelets have an average lifespan of 9 days and their production can increase by six- to eight-fold in situations of chronic platelet loss. At rest, one-third of the platelet population resides in the spleen and these platelets exchange freely with the remaining two-thirds in the circulation. In certain situations, such as hypersplenism and immune thrombocytopenia, 90% of platelets are sequestered in the spleen.

The structure of the platelet is shown schematically in Fig. 27.1. A peripheral zone composed of glycocalyx, a complex system of at least five glycoproteins (GP) which have important receptor and signal transduction functions, lies superficial to the plasma membrane. The plasma membrane of these disc-shaped cells is extensively invaginated to form a canalicular system of tubules and, just beneath this membrane, lies a system of microfilaments that is important in maintaining resting platelet shape. A circumferential band of microtubules lies in the equatorial plane and following platelet activation, their contraction results in the characteristic platelet shape change: discoid to spheroid. Within the cells lies a system of 'dense tubules,' so-called because they appear electron dense on electron microscopy, and probably act as the principal cellular store of calcium. Platelets also contain two specialized organelles, α-granules and dense bodies, and these act as storage sites for metabolites important in platelet aggregation.

When platelets are exposed to subendothelial collagen, as occurs at the time of vessel wall injury, surface receptors are activated and this reduces the repellent negative surface

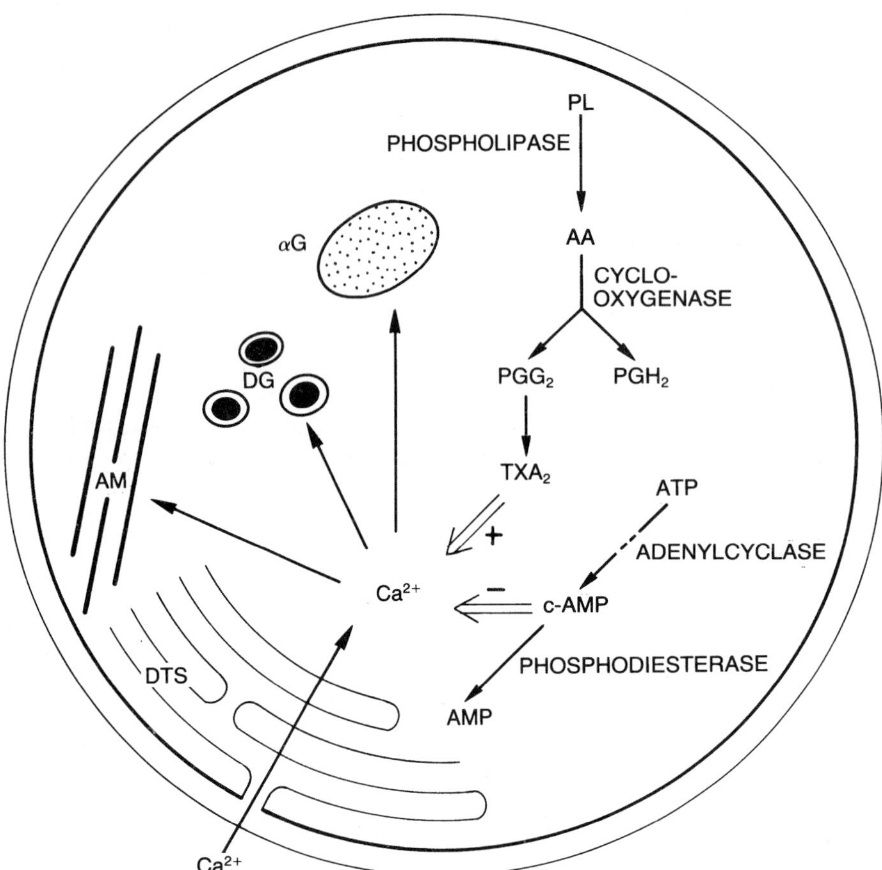

FIGURE 27.1 Schematic representation of platelet structure and metabolism. PL, membrane phospholipid; AA, arachidonic acid; PGG_2, PGH_2 prostaglandins G2 and H2; TXA_2, thromboxane A_2; ATP, adenosine triphosphate; (c)AMP, (cyclic) adenosine monophosphate; DTS, dense tubular system; AM, actin myosin; DG, dense granules; αG, α-granules.

charge and the platelets adhere to the injured surface. Von Willebrand's Factor (VIII–VWF), produced by endothelial cells, is necessary to allow the adhesion of platelets to the endothelial surface. This is followed by the shape change, which encourages further interaction with other cells. Finally, flattening and discharge of cytoplasmic granule contents, with the release of ATP, ADP, Ca^{2+}, platelet factor IV (which has a heparin-neutralizing effect) and fibrinogen results in further amplification by activating nearby platelets. Released fibrinogen enables a firm platelet plug to be produced. Platelet membrane phospholipids (PL) are exposed during activation and they provide a catalytic surface for the interaction between the coagulation cascade and platelet activation. These PL interact with the clotting cofactors V and VIII-C in the enzymatic conversion of the vitamin-K dependent factors, mainly X and II (prothrombin) to their active forms. Contraction of platelet microfilaments, in conjunction with factor XIII, leads to clot retraction.

Platelet metabolism is complex and not completely understood. A large amount of energy, provided by the hydrolysis of ATP, is required to induce the shape changes and the discharge of granule contents. Intracytoplasmic free Ca^{2+} levels are closely regulated by an ATP-dependent calcium pump. It is thought that the release of free Ca^{2+} ions from the dense tubular system is the trigger for the contractile events. In addition, free Ca^{2+} trigger the activation of the α-granules and dense bodies which further stimulates platelet receptors and recruits more platelets into the platelet plug. Ca^{2+} ions activate phospholipase which in turn induces the release of arachidonic acid from the cell membrane. The enzyme cyclo-oxygenase converts arachidonic acid to prostaglandins PGG_2 and PGH_2, which in the platelets are largely converted into the pro-aggregant TXA_2 by thromboxane synthetase; and in the vascular endothelium are largely converted to prostacyclin or PGI_2, a potent inhibitor of platelet aggregation. Thus the same process of cyclo-oxygenase activation elegantly results in a counterbalancing effect such that local amplification of platelet aggregation is achieved near the site of endothelial damage, but extension of thrombus is tightly restricted by the normal adjacent endothelium.

Role of the soluble clotting factors

The coagulation cascade is composed of twelve primary factors, has two pathways of activation and results in the conversion of soluble fibrinogen to fibrin and ultimately to a stable fibrin clot. (The clotting factors are enumerated I–XIII and are followed by the suffix -a when activated.) Figure 27.2 shows how either the intrinsic pathway, activated by contact with negatively charged surfaces, or the extrinsic

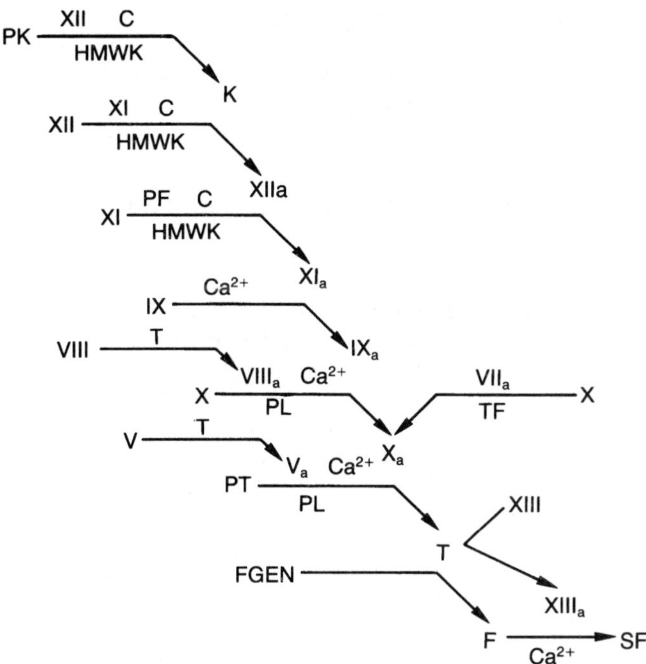

FIGURE 27.2 The coagulation cascade. PK, prekallikrein; K, kallikrein; HMWK, high molecular weight kininogen; C, contact factor; PF, platelet factor; PT, prothrombin; T, thrombin; PL, phospholipid; FGEN, fibrinogen; F, fibrin monomer; SF, stable fibrin; TF, tissue factor.

pathway, activated by the release of thromboplastin from damaged cells, will result in the conversion of factor X to Xa, which is the first step in the final common (shared) pathway to fibrin formation. The prothrombin time (PT) and the activated partial thromboplastin time (APTT) are used to assay the function of the extrinsic and the intrinsic pathways respectively.

The intrinsic pathway sequence usually begins when factor XII is activated by exposure to a negatively charged surface, such as collagen or vascular basement membrane. In addition to factor XII, high molecular weight kininogen (HMWK) and kallikrein constitute the 'contact factors' which are involved in a reciprocating mechanism of activation following contact with a negatively charged surface. Factor XI is then activated by XIIa (or directly by platelet metabolites, which may explain why deficiencies in the contact factors do not always result in a bleeding diathesis). Factor XIa then cleaves a single polypeptide bond of factor IX to form factor IXa. Activated factor IX then complexes with factor VIII-C to bring about the activation of factor X. Factor VIII-C is activated in turn to factor VIII-Ca, a cofactor 500 times more active, by the action of thrombin, which is produced later in the sequence. The activation of factor X also requires Ca^{2+} and PL which are provided from the platelet surface as platelet factor III.

In the extrinsic pathway, factor X is activated directly by a complex of tissue thromboplastin, Ca^{2+} and factor VIIa. In the final common pathway, factor Xa complexes with factor V, Ca^{2+} and PL to bring about the conversion of prothrombin to thrombin. Thrombin catalyses the hydrolysis of four specific arginyl–glycine bonds of fibrinogen to bring about the liberation of fibrinopeptides A and B. The remaining fibrin monomers polymerize spontaneously to form a loose fibrin gel. This in turn is stabilized by activated factor XIII which catalyses the formation of peptide bonds between adjacent fibrin monomers which ultimately results in visible clot retraction.

The cascade system has evolved so that a fibrin clot will be generated with sufficient speed and specificity to prevent significant haemorrhage from an injured vessel. However, such a powerful system must be restricted by an equally effective set of regulatory or inhibitory factors, otherwise uncontrolled activation would result: prostaglandin I_2 (prostacyclin or PGI_2) is synthesized by the endothelium in response to injury and activation of clotting and, as discussed, it is a powerful inhibitor of clot extension. Thrombomodulin, which is also produced by the endothelial cells, binds and modulates the action of thrombin. This interaction results in the production of protein C (Prot C) and its cofactor protein S (Prot S). These vitamin K-dependent cofactors result in the inactivation of factors Va and VIIIa. Antithrombin III (ATIII) is a cofactor of heparin that inhibits factor Xa and thrombin. The antithrombotic activity of heparin is largely dependent on the presence of adequate ATIII.

Role of the fibrinolytic system

The fibrinolytic system has evolved to dissolve thrombus after repair of the vascular breach. It is now apparent that it is also intimately involved in the prevention of inappropriate accumulations and extensions of fibrin. It is also important in the repair and remodelling process following injury and may activate the complement cascade. As in the coagulation system, the major proteolytic enzymes within the fibrinolytic system circulate as inert pro-enzymes and their activity is enhanced by conformational or spatial alterations following interaction with the target molecule. The major fibrinolytic enzyme is plasmin, which is responsible for the digestion of fibrin. Plasmin circulates as its inactive precursor, plasminogen. Conversion of plasminogen to plasmin is effected by the plasminogen activators (PA) of which there are two basic types: tissue type (tPA), which is produced in most cells and vascular endothelium and its action on plasminogen is restricted to fibrin, and urokinase-like (uPA), found in urine and other secretions, which can activate plasminogen in the absence of fibrin. The vascular endothelium also produces an inhibitor of tPA, plasminogen-activator inhibitor (PAI). Kallikrein, released as a result of contact activation, is also capable of converting plasminogen to its active form. Plasmin digests fibrin into soluble fibrin degradation products (FDPs) which are cleared by the reticuloendothelial system. Any free plasmin in the circulation is quickly mopped up by α_2-antiplasmin and similar molecules. The fibrinolytic system is the subject of intense research as its function is central to the pathophysiology of important disease processes such as coronary artery disease, thrombophilia and mechanisms for tumour extension.

DISORDERS OF COAGULATION

Coagulation defects can be divided into congenital and acquired and further subdivided according to whether the defect results in inadequate haemostasis and hence bleeding, or excessive haemostasis resulting in unwanted thrombosis or thrombophilia. The pharmacological approach to these disorders is directed at identifying the underlying abnormality using the facilities of a modern haematology laboratory, the correction of deficiencies with the most appropriate products or the reversal of excess thrombosis using anticoagulants or fibrinolytic agents. All of these agents require close monitoring and good liaison between the primary team and the haematologist.

Congenital disorders of coagulation factors

Congenital deficiencies of all of the factors in the coagulation cascade have been described. Table 27.1 summarizes the most important ones describing their principal manifestations, inheritance and incidence. The most important are haemophilia A and B, which are both inherited as X-linked recessive disorders and result in deficiencies of factors VIII-C and IX respectively. Both disorders have similar clinical presentations depending on whether the degree of the deficiency is mild (factor levels 5–25% of normal); moderate (1–5% of normal); or severe (<1% of normal). Patients with mild disease or female carriers lead relatively normal lives requiring factor replacement only at times of high risk of bleeding such as trauma, surgery, dental work or childbirth. Patients with severe deficiencies may be subject to recurrent spontaneous haemorrhage into joints, muscles and renal tract. The ready availability of the appropriate moderately purified intravenous factors, derived from large pools of plasma donations, led to the practice of home self-administration of treatment. Like most other concentrates, factor VIII is supplied as a freeze-dried powder which is reconstituted with a small volume of sterile water before intravenous injection. This revolutionized the lifestyle of many of these patients. It both prevents and stops bleeding and prevents crippling arthropathy. Unfortunately, following the infusion of these products, many haemophiliacs have become infected with hepatitis non-A non-B virus and human immunodeficiency virus (HIV). The introduction of heat treatment in 1985 has virtually eliminated this risk.

TABLE 27.1 The congenital coagulation disorders

DEFICIENT FACTOR	PRINCIPAL MANIFESTATIONS	INHERITANCE (COMMONEST)	INCIDENCE (APPROX.)
I	Serious neonatal bleeding	AR	$<1:2\times10^6$
II	Serious neonatal bleeding	AR	$<1:2\times10^6$
V	Mild excessive bleeding in early life	AR	$1:1\times10^6$
VII	Mild to moderate bleeding	AR	$1:4\times10^5$
VIII-C	Mild to serious bleeding in males from age 6 months: deforming haemarthroses, haematomata and intra-abdominal bleeding	SLR	1 : 25 000
VIII-VWF	Epistaxis, menorrhagia, postoperative bleeding	AD	$1:1\times10^4$
IX	As for VIII-C	SLR	$1:1\times10^5$
X	Mild to moderate bleeding	AR	$1:4\times10^5$
XI	Excessive delayed bleeding following trauma. More common in Jews	AR	$1:1\times10^6$
XII	Seldom causes bleeding	AR	$1:1\times10^6$
XIII	Neonatal bleeding	AR	$1:2\times10^6$

AR, autosomal recessive; AD, autosomal dominant; SLR, sex-linked recessive.

Although haemophilia A is a rare disease, demand for factor VIII-C is the main force behind the world's plasma fractionation industry, and the economics of supply of all other plasma products are critically dependent on this demand. Recombinant (synthetic) factor VIII-C has recently been introduced in clinical trials. Although it may take several years for it to become generally available, it has the potential for causing serious imbalances in the fractionation industry with possible adverse affects on the supply and cost of other plasma products.

The principles behind the administration of specific plasma-derived products in order to control or prevent bleeding in these disorders are similar. The desired increment of the factor concerned is judged clinically and is based on the extent and site of trauma and the likely duration of bleeding; the correct dose can be calculated from the knowledge of the concentration of specific factor in the product to be administered, the level required to achieve full haemostasis and its recovery in the plasma after infusion; and the frequency of administration is determined by the half-life of the factor in the circulation (Table 27.2). For instance, in the case of a severe haemophilia A sufferer about to undergo abdominal surgery, one would need to sustain factor VIII-C levels above 60–100%, beginning preoperatively and continuing for 10–14 days. As factor VIII-C has a high recovery and each unit of factor VIII per kilogram administered results in a rise of factor VIII-C level of 2 iu/dl (normal plasma concentration of VIII-C is 40–200 iu/dl), the dose required to achieve a desired increment can be easily calculated. Factor VIII is administered twice daily as its half-life is 12 h in the circulation.

Additional guidance as to the adequacy of therapy is obtained by the clinical state of the patient and frequent monitoring of pre- and postinfusion levels of factor VIII-C. If the level actually achieved is less than that predicted, then increased consumption (shortened half-life) should be suspected. In the case of factor VIII-C, this may be due to the development of antifactor VIII-C antibodies (inhibitors), which can inactivate the transfused product almost immediately. Alternative products may have to be used in these circumstances: porcine factor VIII; products that bypass VIII-C in the coagulation cascade such as factor IX (which also contains factor Xa); or similar commercial products such as FEIBA (factor eight inhibitor bypass activity) or Autoplex. Specialist assistance is mandatory in such cases.

The most common congenital disorder of coagulation is von Willebrand's disease (VWD), which is usually milder than haemophilia and is caused by a deficiency of factor VIII – von Willebrand's factor (VIII-VWF). The inheritance is autosomal dominant in the mild type I VWD (the commonest form). Several distinct types have been described depending on the precise molecular abnormality. VIII-VWF plays an important role in the initiation of haemostasis, being responsible for the adherence of platelets to the exposed subendothelial collagen following vessel wall damage. It also acts as a carrier protein for VIII-C, protects it from degradation, and delivers it to the site of injury. Patients with VWD present with bleeding from mucosal surfaces, similar to patients with thrombocytopenia. VIII-VWF is found in cryoprecipitate and intermediate purity factor VIII concentrates and administration of these products will be needed to treat or prevent excessive bleeding. High purity VIII-VWF concentrates are now available.

In mild VWD (and mild haemophilia A), minor surgery can be 'covered' by using DDAVP (1-deamino-8D-arginine vasopressin). This vasopressin analogue has the property of releasing stored, functionally active VIII-VWF and VIII-C. A single intravenous infusion of 0.4 μg/kg over 20 min is well tolerated and provides reasonable cover for 6–10 h. It is also commonly given as a nasal snuff (in conjunction with inhibitors of fibrinolysis such as tranexamic acid) to control menorrhagia in female patients with VWD. DDAVP is contraindicated in type IIB VWD because the abnormal VIII-VWF released in this variant of the disease may precipitate intravascular platelet aggregation. It is not suitable in cases of prolonged bleeding as its effectiveness diminishes markedly after 3–4 days.

It is now apparent that a significant proportion of cases of recurrent thrombosis are due to inherited deficiencies of inhibitors of coagulation such as AT-III, Prot C or Prot S. In addition, the inheritance of a mutant factor V, called V-Leiden, which results in a factor V molecule, which is resistant to degradation by activated Prot C, is now believed to be responsible for a large proportion of otherwise unexplained cases of familial thrombophilia. The identification of such cases is important as there may be indications for life-long anticoagulation and there may be implications for other family members. The investigation of these disorders is best carried out in reference laboratories. Specialized products that may be used in the

TABLE 27.2 *In vivo* properties of important clotting factors

FACTOR	% NORMAL CONCENTRATION REQUIRED FOR HAEMOSTASIS	HALF-LIFE	RECOVERY (% TRANSFUSED DOSE)
I	10–25	4–6 days	50
V	10–15	12 h	80
VII	5–10	4–6 h	75
VIII-C	10–40	12 h	65
IX	10–40	18–24 h	25–50

replacement of the specific deficient factor/inhibitor are under investigation.

Acquired disorders of coagulation factors

Cases of acquired non-mechanical bleeding are commonly encountered by the anaesthetist managing patients on the intensive care unit. The cause is usually deficient production, dilution or excessive consumption of clotting factors or platelets.

Vitamin K

Vitamin K is a fat-soluble vitamin which is found in two forms: vitamin K_1 (phytomenadione), derived from dietary green vegetables and vitamin K_2 produced by bacteria present in the gastrointestinal tract. The daily adult requirement is 1 μg/kg body weight. It is an essential cofactor in the post-translational modification (by γ-carboxylation of certain glutamic acid residues) of factors VII, IX, X and prothrombin and the inhibitory proteins S and C. The carboxylation of these factors enables them to bind Ca^{2+} and lipid surfaces. Vitamin K deficiency is caused by decreased dietary intake, malabsorption, or antibiotic therapy, which can alter the normal gastrointestinal flora – a secondary source of vitamin K in the infant. In the absence of the vitamin, non-functioning molecules are produced. This may result in a bleeding tendency that may be characterized in the laboratory as a prolonged PT. Ten milligrams of vitamin K_1, administered parenterally, once or twice weekly will prevent this problem. The PT normalizes within 6 h of administration as the functionless proteins are replaced by their active counterparts (assuming normal hepatic synthetic function). Intravenous administration of vitamin K_1 should not exceed a rate of 1 mg/min.

The hepatocyte is the site of synthesis of all the clotting factors with the exception of VIII-C and VIII-VWF. The liver is also largely responsible for the clearance of fibrin degradation products, which can act in themselves as anticoagulants. Hepatic synthetic failure is associated with a prolonged PT, APTT and thrombin clotting time (TT) and this will contribute to a bleeding tendency. This abnormality cannot be corrected by the administration of vitamin K, a fact that helps distinguish it from biliary obstruction, which if prolonged will result in vitamin K deficiency through malabsorption. Treatment of factor deficiencies secondary to liver disease consists of factor replacement with fresh frozen plasma, cryoprecipitate, or factor IX or VII concentrates.

In patients undergoing massive transfusion (greater than one blood volume in 4 h), where fresh blood is being replaced by red cell concentrates and colloid or albumin, it is possible that additional bleeding will result simply because of the dilution of clotting factors and platelets. Some authors recommend that one to two units of fresh frozen plasma be transfused with each four to six units of blood, but there is no general agreement on this subject. Regular monitoring of coagulation and platelet count is mandatory in this situation so that rational replacement therapy can be planned. The often attendant problems of hypothermia, acidosis and poor tissue perfusion contribute to the coagulopathy.

Increased consumption of clotting factors and platelets, often accompanied by increased fibrinolytic activity occurs in disseminated intravascular coagulopathy (DIC). This can be triggered by a variety of stimuli including infections such as Gram-negative septicaemia, obstetric emergencies such as abruptio placentae or amniotic fluid embolism, malignancies such as acute promyelocytic leukemia, shock, intravascular haemolysis and major tissue damage. The patient may bleed spontaneously from venepuncture sites and there will be a prolongation of the PT, APTT and TT, a falling platelet count and fibrinogen level, and a rise in FDPs. Treatment of DIC involves the removal of the precipitating cause, and replacement with fresh frozen plasma and platelets. In some cases, the judicious use of heparin can inhibit excessive procoagulant activity.

Platelet disorders

As with the coagulopathies, platelet disorders can be either congenital or acquired or they may result from underproduction or increased consumption. The common causes of underproduction include marrow infiltrations such as by acute leukemia, drug effects such as cytotoxic therapy, and radiotherapy. In general, where thrombocytopenia results from underproduction, then platelet transfusions will correct the bleeding tendency. The causes of increased platelet consumption include hypersplenism, severe infection, active bleeding and diseases such as immune thrombocytopenic purpura (ITP), which may be idiopathic or due to drugs, and thrombotic thrombocytopenic purpura (TTP). Treatment in these cases is best directed at the underlying cause.

DRUGS USED TO MODIFY BLOOD COAGULATION AND THEIR PHARMACOLOGY

The most widely used oral anticoagulant is warfarin, a coumarin derivative, which acts by interfering with vitamin K metabolism. Anticoagulants such as phenindione, of the inanedione family, are usually selected when warfarin-specific side-effects have occurred. These drugs are well absorbed and are 95% bound to albumin in the circulation. Only the unbound fraction is metabolically active. Warfarin is a racemic mixture of two isomers, R^+ and S^-. The S^- form is the more active isomer but is metabolized more quickly by the hepatic microsomes. Peak warfarin concentrations are achieved 2–4 h following ingestion with a half-life of 35 h in the circulation. The inactive metabolites are excreted in the urine and faeces.

It is thought that the oral anticoagulants interfere with the cyclic interconversion of the reduced and oxidized forms of vitamin K by inhibiting the activity of the enzyme vitamin K epoxide-reductase. The peak inhibitory effect of the oral anticoagulants is not achieved until the previously formed active clotting factors have been depleted according to their decay half-lives and replaced by their inactive counterparts. This usually takes 2–3 days and injectable anticoagulants will be needed initially if immediate anticoagulation is required.

The principal indication for oral anticoagulation is in the secondary prophylaxis of venous thromboembolism following deep vein thrombosis or pulmonary embolism. Warfarin is also widely used in the prevention of thromboembolism in patients with valvular heart disease, prosthetic heart valves, atrial fibrillation and recurrent stroke.[1,2] Therapeutic levels are maintained for 6 weeks to 6 months depending on the site and extent of the thrombosis and the individual risk factors for recurrence. These risks are increased in patients with malignant disease; the obese; the elderly; pregnancy; those on steroid therapy or oestrogen-containing oral contraceptives; smokers; or at the time of surgery, trauma or prolonged stasis. Oral anticoagulation is used in some centres as primary prophylaxis of deep venous thrombosis (DVT) and pulmonary embolism (PE) before high-risk surgery such as hip replacement in the elderly.[3] Occasionally, patients such as those with prosthetic heart valves or recurrent pulmonary embolism are advised to take life-long anticoagulation. Long-term oral anticoagulation is recommended for some patients with cardiac dysrhythmias or cardiomyopathy where there is a large left atrium, low cardiac output and paroxysmal or established atrial fibrillation.[4] In addition, symptomatic patients identified as having a congenital predisposition to thromboembolism, such as ATIII, Prot C or Prot S deficiency, and some patients with the antiphospholipid antibody syndrome are advised to be anticoagulated for life. Although the oral anticoagulants appear to be most effective in the management of venous thrombosis, there is increasing evidence that they may be useful in preventing arterial thrombosis and they are sometimes prescribed following myocardial infarction, acute arterial occlusion, thromboembolic stroke and arterial bypass grafting.[5,6]

Because of the risks of haemorrhage, oral anticoagulation is absolutely contraindicated in patients who have undergone recent neurosurgery, eye surgery, nonembolic stroke, or liver or kidney biopsy. Relative contraindications include chronic disorders likely to be complicated by bleeding such as active gastrointestinal ulceration, acute pancreatitis, subacute bacterial endocarditis, renal failure and thrombocytopenia. Reduced dosage is required in liver disease as hepatic synthetic function may already be impaired. In addition, because of the potentially serious risks of bleeding and the need for close control with laboratory monitoring, these drugs should be avoided in unreliable patients or those unable to comply.

There is considerable variation between individuals in the maintenance doses of warfarin required to establish therapeutic anticoagulation. This is because of the highly variable interindividual rates of protein binding and metabolism and the effects of drug interactions. As there is a narrow therapeutic : toxic ratio, regular monitoring of the PT is required for the duration of therapy. It is accepted that VII levels (to which the PT is most sensitive) are the best measure of oral anticoagulation. Because PT results vary according to the laboratory techniques used, and in particular to the type of thromboplastin used in the test, it has become normal practice to convert PT ratios to international normalized ratios (INR) when compared with an international standard reference preparation. The recommended therapeutic range of INR for different situations is shown in Table 27.3. All patients should be advised to report any excessive bruising, nosebleeds, melaena or haematuria to their doctors without delay.

Because of the delay of 48–72 h before full anticoagulation is achieved after the initiation of warfarin, an overlap period of 4–5 days is recommended when converting patients from heparin to warfarin therapy. Most clinicians administer a loading dose of 10–15 mg warfarin daily on the first 1–2 days and then continue with a maintenance daily dose of about 6 mg (range 3–20 mg). Several algorithms exist which help to predict the maintenance dose, but these are little used in practice. If a patient is over-anticoagulated and there is a danger of serious bleeding, then temporary reversal of oral anticoagulation can be achieved immediately by the administration of factor IX and VII concentrates (or fresh frozen plasma if the above concentrates are not available). If the risk of bleeding is less, then the slow iv injection of vitamin K (0.5–2 mg) will result in correction of the INR within about 6 h. Care should be taken not to administer too much vitamin K because there may be considerable resistance to re-anticoagulation. When the course of oral anticoagulation is complete, it is preferable to tail off the drug

TABLE 27.3 Recommended therapeutic ranges of international normalized ratios (INR). (Based upon *Guidelines on oral anticoagulants*, British Society for Haematology, 1984)

CLINICAL INDICATION	RECOMMENDED RANGE
Prophylaxis of DVT	2.0–2.5
Prophylaxis of DVT for hip surgery	2.0–3.0
Treatment of DVT and PE	3.0–4.5
Prophylaxis of prosthetic heart valves	3.0–4.5
Prophylaxis of arterial grafts	3.0–4.5
Prophylaxis of recurrent VT	3.0–4.5

DVT, deep venous thrombosis; PE, pulmonary embolism; VT, venous thromboembolism.

gradually rather than to stop it abruptly to prevent a rebound rise in VII levels which can occur and may render the patient susceptible to a recurrence of thrombosis.

The oral anticoagulants are uniquely susceptible to drug interactions such that even minor changes in medication can result in a loss of therapeutic control. Any changes in medication should be accompanied by increased frequency of monitoring of the INR. Drugs such as cholestyramine, which interfere with the absorption of fat-soluble vitamins such as vitamin K, will potentiate the effects of warfarin. Other drugs that share albumin-binding sites with the oral anticoagulants may cause alterations in the free, active form of the drug especially at the time of initiation and discontinuation of therapy. Barbiturates and rifampicin induce the activity of the hepatic microsomal enzymes which will result in increased hepatic metabolism of the anticoagulants. Other drugs, such as the tricyclics and major tranquillizers, inhibit the liver microsomal enzymes and reduced dosage will be required. Commonly used drugs, such as cimetidine, cotrimoxazole and metronidazole, tend to potentiate the effect of warfarin by inhibiting the metabolism of the more active S isomer of the drug. Self-medication is important and patients should be advised to avoid proprietary preparations such as aspirin which may induce gastric erosions, inhibit platelet function and displace warfarin from protein-binding sites and they should also avoid excessive alcohol intake.

Warfarin is rarely associated with idiosyncratic reactions but rashes and acute skin necrosis may occur rarely. The latter is thought to be due to an allergic vasculitis which usually begins 2–3 days after the start of treatment and may eventually lead to scarring if not recognized early. The inanediones are much more frequently implicated in causing rashes and in some patients will cause red discoloration of the urine, which can be confused with haematuria.

Particular problems arise during and after pregnancy because warfarin crosses the placenta freely and can enter breast milk in small amounts. Warfarin is teratogenic and can cause chondrodysplasia punctata, a condition that causes stippling of the vertebral bones, skeletal deformities such as nasal hypoplasia and, occasionally, microcephaly. The risk is greatest in the first trimester but occasional cases have occurred following the use of warfarin in the second and third trimesters. For this reason, warfarin is contraindicated in early pregnancy. The use of warfarin is not desirable in late pregnancy because of the increased risk of intracranial haemorrhage in the fetus.

The alternative therapy, namely long-term parenteral heparin, carries other risks to the mother such as thrombocytopenia and osteoporosis and in some situations where the indication of continuation of anticoagulation is absolute (such as maternal prosthetic heart valve) the risks to the fetus from warfarin may be outweighed by the risks to the mother from the underlying disease and the heparin.

Heparin

Unfractionated heparin

Unfractionated or standard heparin has powerful anticoagulant properties and consists of a mixture of negatively charged sulphated mucopolysaccharide polymers whose molecular weight ranges from 2000 to 40 000; it is available either as the sodium or calcium salt. Heparin is derived from beef lung or porcine intestinal mucosa. When given subcutaneously, heparin is absorbed into the circulation reaching peak concentrations at 4 h and disappearing by about 8 h. Once in the circulation, about 40% is sequestered, probably by endothelial cells. The remainder is protein bound, some of it by ATIII, Xa and other coagulation components. The mean heparin plasma half-life is 30–120 min. It is metabolized by desulphation probably in the reticuloendothelial system prior to excretion in the urine. Heparin binds ATIII, altering its configuration and thus potentiating its activity. The effectiveness of heparin as an anticoagulant is therefore dependent on the presence in the circulation of adequate amounts of ATIII.

The main clinical uses of heparin are to prevent venous thromboembolism in high-risk situations when it is usually given in low dosage subcutaneously (5000 units 8–12 hourly). This 'low dose' heparin regimen is commonly used preoperatively in patients undergoing major abdominal, gynaecological or orthopaedic surgery. Many clinical trials have shown significant reductions in postoperative venous thrombosis and probably also fatal pulmonary embolism and the postphlebitic syndrome. Low-dose heparin is also used to prevent DVT in patients immobilized for long periods and post myocardial infarction.[2] Monitoring of anticoagulation is not mandatory with low-dose heparin.

The other main use of heparin is to prevent the extension of established thrombosis and during endarterectomy when it is best administered by continuous intravenous infusion (20 000–40 000 units per 24 h) following an intravenous loading dose (5000–10 000 units). Four-hourly intravenous boluses will also achieve anticoagulation but this is more difficult to monitor and the risk of unwanted bleeding is greater. Intramuscular injections while on heparin therapy are contraindicated because of the risk of haematoma formation.

Monitoring of heparin anticoagulation is mandatory except when used for prophylaxis. The most commonly used coagulation assay to monitor heparin's effect is the APTT, which should be prolonged to 1.5–2 times the patient's control value. Other tests such as the TT are in use. The TT should be prolonged to greater than 60 s and should be correctable to within 3 s of the control value by prior addition of 1% protamine sulphate to the assay. In certain circumstances, such as cardiac bypass surgery when there are rapid disturbances in haemostasis, there is inadequate time to utilize these laboratory tests as they all depend on the prior separation of cells from plasma before performing the assay. In these cases, the crude whole blood clotting time can be used and newer techniques, such as thromboelastography, may find a place in the future.

Therapeutic heparin is usually maintained for 4–7 days with an overlap period of 4–5 days when both heparin and warfarin are used together. Once warfarin is started, the PT is used to monitor anticoagulation, and the dose of heparin should be maintained at the established therapeutic dose for that patient.

Heparin is contraindicated in situations where there is a high risk of bleeding such as malignant hypertension, active bleeding due to surgery or trauma, or recent neurological or eye surgery. Pregnant women must not be considered for epidural anaesthesia if heparin was used within the previous 24 h. For normal vaginal delivery, heparin should be stopped 6 h beforehand.

Bleeding that arises while on heparin often responds to withdrawal of the drug because of the short plasma half-life. In extreme cases, protamine sulphate can be administered according to the principle that 1 mg of protamine will neutralize 100 units of heparin. Caution should be exercised if this drug is used as hypotensive reactions may occur if it is administered too quickly and if given in overdose, it has an endogenous anticoagulant effect.

Thrombocytopenia is now recognized as a common complication of sustained heparin therapy. The rarer but more severe 'late onset type' presents with a rapidly declining platelet count after 7–10 days of exposure. It is associated with an increase of platelet-bound IgG and is reversed after heparin is withdrawn. Arterial thrombosis caused by a tendency for increased platelet aggregation may also be a feature of this syndrome. Hypersensitivity reactions to heparin are rare and include skin reactions and alopecia. Long-term heparin (15 000 units daily for 6 months or more) carries the risk of osteoporosis especially when used during pregnancy and this is thought to be due to the inhibition of the conversion of vitamin D to its active 1,25 dihydroxy derivative. Heparin resistance is said to occur if high doses of heparin fail to produce the expected prolongation of the APTT. This may be due to congenital or acquired ATIII deficiency, which should be identified as ATIII concentrates are available and may be of use in conjunction with heparin.

Low-molecular-weight heparins (LMWHs)

In order to reduce the variation in molecular weight of unfractionated or standard heparin, and to increase the number of molecules with affinity for ATIII, attempts have been made to depolymerize the long chains of heparin using enzymatic or chemical cleavage. The resulting product, now called low-molecular-weight heparin (LMWH), remains polydisperse with molecular weights ranging from 2000 to 12 000 Da (mean 5000 Da). LMWH binding to ATIII results in greater inhibition of Xa than of thrombin compared with the effects of the parent compound. This is said to result in a more specific anticoagulant effect with reduced haemorrhagic risk resulting in a wider therapeutic : toxic ratio and therefore reduced need to monitor therapy. Other advantages include reduced effect on platelet function (most patients who experience thrombocytopenia while on standard heparin, can continue to be anticoagulated with LMWH); and a significantly longer half-life in the circulation following subcutaneous injection (3–4 h). This has permitted the development of convenient once-daily dose schedules, which is of particular value where long-term or home treatment is contemplated. The major disadvantages of LMWH compared with standard heparin include the need for special factor Xa assays (the standard APTT is more sensitive to thrombin levels than Xa levels) which are not always available, and the increased cost of the drug which results from increased production costs. It is uncertain whether LMWH carries a reduced risk of osteoporosis compared with standard heparin. Numerous clinical trials have been published which show that LMWH was at least equal, if not superior to, standard heparin when administered subcutaneously for the prophylaxis of deep venous thrombosis in general surgery. In orthopaedic hip surgery, LMWH used at about twice the dose used in general surgery prophylaxis, is more effective than adjusted dose standard heparin prophylaxis (which required regular measurement of the APTT). At the time of writing, there are insufficient data to recommend the use of MLWH in other clinical situations such as for treatment of venous or arterial thrombosis, in high-risk medical patients or during pregnancy. Other compounds, related to heparin and belonging to the family of glycosaminoglycans, such as heparan sulphate and dermatan sulphate, have similar anticoagulant properties and are the subject of further investigation.

Antiplatelet agents

Antiplatelet agents are commonly used in the secondary prevention of myocardial infarction, unstable angina and transient ischaemic attacks. An understanding of the major metabolic pathways leading to platelet activation is needed to classify these agents.

Drugs interfering with prostaglandin metabolism

The production of TXA_2 from arachidonic acid can be inhibited by a number of agents. Arachidonic acid is derived from meat products in the western diet. Eskimo diets, on the other hand, are rich in fish oils such as eicosapentaenoic acid which replace arachidonic acid as an alternative substrate for prostaglandin metabolism. This results in the production of TXA_3 which lacks the platelet aggregating properties of TXA_2. In the vessel wall, PGI_3 is formed instead of PGI_2, also a potent anti-aggregant. The net result of the ingestion of a diet rich in fish oil is a platelet anti-aggregant effect which may explain why Eskimos have a low rate of coronary artery disease. This approach, although promising, has not been widely utilized in the West because of the vast quantities of unpalatable fish oil necessary to have a measurable effect on platelet function, the fishy smell secreted from the skin and the cost.

β-Blockers are capable of inhibiting the enzyme, phospholipase, which is responsible for the release of arachidonic acid from the inner platelet membrane. Their activity in this regard is low and similar drugs in this category are under investigation.

Aspirin is the best known and most widely used antiplatelet agent and interferes with prostaglandin metabolism by irreversibly acetylating cyclo-oxygenase, the enzyme that converts arachidonic acid into cyclic endoperoxides. It is well absorbed orally within 20 min unless an enteric-coated form is used. The plasma half-life is 20 min. As platelets have no means of replacing the inactivated enzyme, the antiplatelet effect will persist for the full lifespan of the platelet (9 days). Indeed, *in vitro* platelet aggregation in response to ADP and adrenaline may remain impaired for up to 2 weeks after a single dose of aspirin. It is believed that the use of low-dose aspirin (75–150 mg/day) inhibits platelet cyclo-oxygenase preferentially and that higher doses may in fact be counterproductive as they may inhibit endothelial cyclo-oxygenase, resulting in reduced PGI_2 production. Much of the published work on the use of aspirin related to doses in the range 300–1300 mg/day, and there is doubt cast as to the relevance of this work today as doses of 75 mg per day are currently recommended. Nevertheless, even at these higher doses, several randomized controlled studies have shown aspirin to be effective in the primary and secondary prevention of myocardial infarction, unstable angina, peripheral vascular disease and the secondary prevention of transient ischaemic attack and stroke.[7–10] Aspirin is in widespread use because of the low cost of the drug, the lack of any need for monitoring, and the safety profile when compared with the oral anticoagulants. The side-effects of aspirin are well known and include gastrointestinal haemorrhage, rash, nausea and vomiting. Toxic levels can cause tinnitus and severe metabolic disturbances including metabolic acidosis, which can lead to hyperventilation and dehydration. Other non-steroidal anti-inflammatory drugs, such as indomethacin and ibuprofen, also interfere with platelet function by reversibly inhibiting platelet cyclo-oxygenase.

Sulphinpyrazone is a uricosuric agent derived from phenylbutazone but lacks the anti-inflammatory activity and the bone marrow toxicity associated with this drug. It is believed to irreversibly inhibit cyclo-oxygenase but its use has largely been superseded by aspirin.

Prostacyclin itself is now available for therapeutic use and is known as epoprostenol. It has to be infused intravenously and has a short half-life of 2–3 min in the circulation as it is rapidly metabolized and its effects disappear within 30 min of stopping the infusion. It is used as a vessel wall protectant and platelet anti-aggregant during extracorporeal blood circulation such as during charcoal haemoperfusion, renal dialysis and cardiopulmonary bypass. The major side-effects are reversible hypotension, flushing, headache and gastrointestinal symptoms.

Drugs affecting platelet membranes

Drugs that interfere with the ability of platelets to interact, or that block surface receptors thus inhibiting signal transduction, are the subject of intense research.

Dextran is the best known drug that has significant platelet surface effects. Dextran is used primarily as a plasma expander (see below) and is composed of a mixture of branched chain polysaccharides of varying molecular weights. In the circulation, dextran molecules interfere with fibrin polymerization, platelet–fibrinogen interaction and hence platelet cross-linking. Dextrans also affect platelet–VIII-VWF interactions as well as reducing plasma viscosity which in turn reduces the opportunity for platelet–platelet interactions.

Ticlopidine is a thienopyridine derivative with broad antiplatelet activity which results in a dose-dependent prolongation of the bleeding time, reaching peak levels after 3 days and persisting for up to 10 days after withdrawal of the drug. The exact mechanism of action of this promising drug is unclear but one theory is that it blocks ADP-induced exposure of the fibrinogen-binding site of the glycoprotein IIb–IIIa complex. Two large North American studies have shown that ticlopidine 250 mg twice daily results in a 20–30% risk reduction of recurrent stroke, an effect greater than aspirin alone.[11,12] Other studies suggest it may find a place in the secondary prevention of myocardial infarction and the treatment of angina. The commonest side-effects are gastrointestinal disturbance and rash. Severe neutropenia arises in about 1% of patients within 3 months of starting ticlopidine, but this appears to resolve spontaneously on stopping the drug. Regular monitoring of the blood count and liver function is necessary at the start of treatment.

Newer agents, including monoclonal antibodies with high affinity for certain platelet receptors, are under investigation as several of these compounds modulate platelet function and may be of value in combination with thrombolytic therapy following myocardial infarction.

Drugs that reduce Ca^{2+} availability

The level of free Ca^{2+} ions within the platelet cytoplasm [free Ca^{2+}] is critical as high levels result in platelet activation by stimulating actin–myosin induced shape changes, TXA_2 synthesis and the release of activators from storage granules. Cyclic AMP (cAMP) is the second messenger that reduces [free Ca^{2+}], dampening the proactivating tendency of this system. Thus, drugs that inhibit the enzyme, phosphodiesterase, which normally catabolizes cAMP have an antiplatelet effect by reducing [free Ca^{2+}]. Dipyrimadole is a clinically used orally active phosphodiesterase inhibitor. Its effects are thought to be synergistic with those of aspirin. However, it should be noted that the overall evidence supporting dipyrimidole as an effective antiplatelet agent has been questioned.

Drugs that alter fibrinolytic activity

Antifibrinolytic agents

The amino acids, aminocaproic acid (EACA) and tranexamic acid, have the ability to bind plasminogen by its lysine binding site, preventing its association with fibrin and therefore its activation to plasmin. Tranexamic acid is more potent but less well absorbed orally than EACA. Both drugs are distributed widely and are excreted unchanged in the urine; dosage reduction is indicated in renal impairment. Both agents are useful in conditions where there is an unwanted external bleeding tendency, such as normal women and patients with VWD suffering from menorrhagia. They are commonly used following prostatic or uterine surgery, gastrointestinal bleeding and as adjunctive therapy in patients with haemophilia and VWD. Primary systemic fibrinolysis is rare but can be treated with antifibrinolytics if DIC is excluded. Side-effects are more frequently seen with EACA and include gastrointestinal symptoms and dizziness. Prolonged use of EACA rarely causes acute necrotizing polymyositis with myoglobinuria. Antifibrinolytics should not be used in patients with renal haematuria because of the risk of clots forming in the ureters and subsequent hydronephrosis. In general, they should also be avoided when bleeding is into an enclosed compartment because clot reabsorption after the cessation of bleeding may be delayed. Antifibrinolytics should be avoided during DIC or in conditions such as hepatic impairment where DIC is a common complication.

Aprotinin is a serine protease inhibitor with specificity for plasmin and kallikrein. As well as its antifibrinolytic effects, it also has poorly defined antiplatelet activity. It is indicated in the treatment of life-threatening haemorrhage associated with hyperplasminaemia. There is increasing evidence that its use is beneficial in controlling the bleeding tendency created during cardiac bypass and liver transplant surgery resulting in drier operating fields and markedly reduced blood product requirements.

Thrombolytic (fibrinolytic) therapy

Thrombolytic therapy has the important advantage over conventional anticoagulation in that it is capable of dissolving thrombi rather than simply preventing further propagation of formed thrombus. It has therefore earned a valuable place in the management of common conditions such as myocardial infarction and severe pulmonary embolism. The agents currently available act primarily by activating plasminogen to plasmin. Much recent research has been directed at finding thrombolytic agents that are specific for fibrin-bound plasminogen rather than plasma plasminogen and therefore less likely to cause a generalized bleeding tendency. This occurs when excessive free plasmin is formed in the circulation, overcoming the natural defences of the circulating antiplasmins. The proteolytic activity of plasmin is not restricted to fibrin, and degradation of fibrinogen, clotting factors V and VIII and other plasma proteins may occur. It has yet to be demonstrated conclusively in clinical trials that the so-called fibrin-specific agents result in improved patient survival.

Streptokinase is still the most widely used drug in this category. It is a single chain protein with a molecular weight of 48 000. It is derived from the filtrate obtained from cultures of β-haemolytic streptococci and invokes an intense fibrinolytic response when injected intravenously. Most normal individuals will have preformed antistreptococcal antibodies, the quantity of which will depend on previous exposure to the drug or recent streptococcal infection. It is customary to administer a loading dose of about 250 000 units over 30 min to swamp the preformed antistreptokinase antibodies. (In circumstances where the antistreptococcal antibodies are likely to be very high, such as previous exposure within 6 months, alternative agents should be considered as very high doses of streptokinase may be needed and adverse reactions are more likely.) Once the antibodies have been neutralized, the remaining drug is metabolized and has a half-life of 80–100 min in the circulation. The infusion can be maintained at about 100 000–150 000 units per hour for about 4–10 days if necessary, before further anamnestic rises in antibodies neutralize its effect. Streptokinase can also be applied directly to the thrombus where facilities for angiography exist. Streptokinase forms a 1 : 1 stoichiometric complex with plasminogen, which causes a conformational change that can activate other plasminogen molecules to the activated form, plasmin. Allergic reactions such as fever and rash (which may respond to steroids) and, rarely, anaphylactic reactions occur. Other agents should be used in patients with a history of streptokinase allergy.

Urokinase is a single chain β-globulin molecule of molecular weight 54 000. It is extracted from human urine or produced by the culture of fetal kidney cells. It is non-antigenic and does not cause allergic reactions and is said to have a higher affinity for fibrin-bound rather than soluble-phase plasminogen compared with streptokinase. It must be administered intravenously, starting with a loading dose followed by a continuous infusion; its half-life is 10–16 min; and it is excreted via the liver and kidneys. Its use on a wide scale is limited by its high cost.

More recently developed fibrinolytic agents include tissue plasminogen activator (rt-PA (alteplase)) and acylated plasminogen streptokinase activated complex (APSAC (anistreplase)). t-PA is a normal human product and can be produced in large quantity using recombinant gene technology by the cloning of the t-PA gene followed by mammalian tissue culture. rt-PA has a low affinity for circulating plasminogen except in large doses when it may cause a mild reversible hypocoagulable state. The half-life of rt-PA is 5–8 min. This product has been used successfully following intravenous administration to patients suffering myocardial infarction. APSAC is also produced using recombinant gene technology; it is a preformed inactive acylated complex of plasminogen and streptokinase with affinity for fibrin-bound clots. Once bound, the plasminogen becomes activated by hydrolysis and the fibrin is lysed. It has the advantage of a longer half-life (90 min) and can be administered by bolus injection. Other agents such as stanozolol, a derivative from anabolic steroids, are known to increase plasminogen-activator levels by lowering PAI. Such agents have not yet found a place in routine management of thromboembolism because of the high incidence of masculinizing and hepatic side-effects and uncertainties over efficacy.

Indications for thrombolytic therapy

Although thrombolytic therapy can be more effective than conventional anticoagulant therapy, it should only be administered after serious consideration of the potential risks and benefits for the individual patient. Many uncertainties still remain about the optimal dose schedules and precise indications for use.[8,13,14] In general, treatment should be started as soon as possible after thrombus formation: up to 24 h for arterial occlusion and up to 72 h for venous occlusion. In the case of serious deep venous thrombosis, the principal advantage of thrombolysis over conventional anticoagulation is thought to be a reduction in the incidence of postphlebitic limb syndrome rather than a reduction in the risk of pulmonary embolism. Lytic therapy is indicated in the management of pulmonary embolism of sufficient magnitude to cause shock. In both DVT and PE, thrombolytic therapy should be followed by conventional anticoagulation. Other indications for thrombolytic therapy include peripheral arterial occlusion, retinal vein thrombosis, arteriovenous cannula occlusion and priapism.

The recent widespread availability of coronary angiography has highlighted the importance of thrombosis in the pathogenesis of acute myocardial infarction and this has rekindled interest in the use of thrombolytic therapy in the management of this common disease. Furthermore the technique has allowed the direct visualization of the site of thrombosis, the local administration of the thrombolytic agent and the assessment of the efficacy of treatment. Because of the impracticability of providing angiography on the scale necessary for routine management of myocardial infarction, attention has shifted to the administration of thrombolytic therapy via peripheral veins and this has been the subject of several large randomized controlled studies.[8,14] These studies have shown that the prompt use of thrombolytic therapy, ideally within 6 h of thrombosis, will result in reperfusion of the occluded vessel in up to 80% of cases. This results in improved cardiac function and prolonged survival in patients suffering a myocardial infarction, especially when followed up promptly by a definitive procedure such as coronary angioplasty or bypass surgery. Re-occlusion is a problem after the infusion has stopped, and this has led to further studies such as GISSI-2 and ISIS-3 which are examining the usefulness of heparinization following thrombolytic therapy. Thrombolytic therapy has become routine in the initial therapy of myocardial infarction and studies are in progress to evaluate its effectiveness when administered by general practitioners or ambulance crews in the acute situation. Because of the risks of bleeding and in particular intracerebral haemorrhage, the following contraindications apply to the use of thrombolytic therapy: surgical procedure within the previous 10 days including invasive biopsy, thoracentesis and paracentesis; active gastrointestinal bleeding or any condition with a high potential for bleeding; defective haemostasis; stroke within the previous 2 months; diseases with a high potential for cerebral embolism such as mitral valve disease; recent trauma or external cardiac massage; intracranial neoplasia; severe hypertension; hepatic or renal disease and pregnancy.

For all patients receiving these drugs, close clinical monitoring for bleeding is mandatory. Whatever the results of laboratory monitoring, treatment should be stopped if excessive bleeding occurs. If thrombolytic therapy is to be sustained for longer than 2–4 h, then laboratory monitoring and the advice of a haematologist should be sought. Up to 50% of patients treated over 12 h suffer haemorrhage, which occurs most commonly at venepuncture sites or from the gastrointestinal or genitourinary tracts. The thrombin time should be prolonged to two to five times the control value to achieve a therapeutic effect. A value of more than five times the control value, suggests the need to stop therapy which can be reintroduced at a lower dose when the TT is in the therapeutic range. During treatment, all invasive procedures should be avoided: fine needles should be used in preference to large ones; and arterial stabs should be restricted to the radial or brachial arteries. If haemorrhage occurs the infusion is stopped, resulting in a rapid fall in the level of the agent. If the haemorrhage is life-threatening, the fibrinolytic activity can be reversed by using intravenous EACA or tranexamic acid, and fibrinogen replaced by infusion of cryoprecipitate or fresh frozen plasma. When the infusion is completed, a heparin infusion is started after the TT falls to less than twice the control value which usually takes 2–4 h. Heparin is continued for 5–7 days while warfarinization is achieved.

Although thrombolytic therapy can be more effective than conventional anticoagulation, it should only be administered after thorough consideration of the potential risks and benefits for the individual patient.

PRODUCTS USED FOR REPLACEMENT OF BLOOD AND ITS COMPONENTS

The transfusion of products derived from human donation differs from conventional pharmacological preparations because of the difficulties of standardization and the potential for immunological, allergic and infectious hazards. Adverse reactions to such products may have implications for the donor as well as the recipient. Each alternative product must be considered in terms of the clinical need and the potential risks.

Replacement of red blood cells

There is as yet no suitable synthetic substitute for red blood cells in their ability to transport oxygen and carbon dioxide between the tissues and the lungs. The red cell membrane and protoplasm provides a unique environment that facilitates the function and survival of haemoglobin, an iron-containing protein that elegantly and effectively acts as the carrier molecule in both directions. Although artificial haemoglobin solutions are currently under development and are discussed in more detail below, the replacement of red blood cells is almost wholly effected by the use of homologous donated blood. This has resulted in the development of a blood transfusion industry whose main aim is the provision of safe and effective blood products.

The immunological reactions to red cell transfusion include reactions to the red cell antigens of which the ABO and Rhesus systems are the most important. Because of the presence of naturally occurring isohaemagglutinins, ABO compatibility is essential. The administration of an ABO incompatible blood is a rare event (about 1:10 000 units) but can lead to acute hypotension, renal failure, DIC and even death within minutes of beginning the transfusion. The signs of such reactions are often missed if the patient is already anaesthetized. It is the responsibility of the transfusion service and the blood bank to provide matched blood, and of the nurse or doctor or anaesthetist to make the appropriate checks before administering blood products. The majority of such erroneous transfusions are due to clerical errors, the majority of which arise at the time of administration of blood.[15] Because of the antigenicity of the Rhesus D antigen (80% of Rhesus D negative individuals will make anti-D antibodies after the transfusion of a Rhesus D positive unit of blood), red cells are routinely matched for the Rhesus D antigen also but this is really only essential in female recipients of child-bearing capacity. The pretransfusion checks include antibody screen or cross-matching at 37°C to detect the presence of antibodies in the recipient to atypical red cell antigens. These occur in about 3% of recipients and unless antigen-negative blood is given, a delayed haemolytic transfusion reaction, a normally mild illness in which the transfused red cells are haemolysed 4–11 days after the transfusion of the offending blood, may occur. Other immunological reactions due to leucocytes or plasma proteins may arise following red cell transfusions. Rarely, allergic reactions arise in recipients due to the presence of allergenic substances such as drugs in the transfused blood.

Donor selection procedures and pretransfusion microbiological screening tests are designed to minimize the risks of infectious complications of blood transfusion. Viral infections remain the most important cause. So far, inactivation methods are only available for certain products made from pooled plasma. Inactivation of HIV (and probably non-A, non-B hepatitis virus) is achieved by heat treatment (or chemical inactivation) of plasma products but this technique cannot be applied to red cells or platelets. In the UK, there is mandatory screening for hepatitis B surface antigen, and antibodies to hepatitis C virus and HIV. It must be remembered that infections caused by these agents will still rarely arise because the tests are not 100% sensitive, especially in early infection of the donor. Vaccination against hepatitis B virus will protect the previously unexposed recipients of pooled plasma products (such as newly diagnosed haemophiliacs) or of regular blood transfusions (such as those with thalassaemia). Screening for other viruses, such as human T-cell leukaemia virus I and HIV II, is performed in some countries with a high prevalence. Screening of donors for the absence of exposure to cytomegalovirus is only necessary when transfusing immunocompromised recipients such as some bone marrow transplantation recipients and very low birthweight preterm infants. Other viruses that can cause blood-borne transmission, such as parvovirus, are not routinely screened out as they are not usually pathogenic.

Rarely, bacterial and parasitic infections of donors can be transmitted to recipients. These agents include syphilis, brucellosis, *Plasmodium* species, *Trypanosoma cruzi*, *Toxoplasma gondii* and *Babesia microti*. Of these, only antibody to *Treponema pallidum* is mandatorily searched for because of the high association with other more serious sexually transmitted diseases and the medicolegal and sociological implications. Rarely, individual donations may become contaminated at the time of donation or during the processing of blood. Such cases can be rapidly fatal if not discovered before transfusion. For this reason, all packs should be inspected to ensure they are intact, have been stored at the right temperature and for the absence of haemolysis or clot formation.

Despite the myriad of possible complications of blood transfusion, patients are at much greater risk if they do not have transfusions when they really need them. The risks of serious adverse reaction are minute as long as proper precautions are observed.

The following is a discussion of red cell products or substitutes currently available.

Whole blood

Over recent years whole blood transfusions have become less popular. This is because of the rising demand for plasma-derived products (which are still largely derived from whole blood donations) and because in many clinical situations it is becoming clear that the replacement of the deficient component is often more effective and less hazardous than the 'blunderbuss' use of whole blood. When available, whole blood is the preferred product in acute massive blood loss (greater than one blood volume in 4 h) but care should be taken to monitor for dilutional coagulopathy as under normal storage conditions at 4°C there is a rapid loss of the 'labile' clotting factors V and VIII-C, and of platelets. Fresh whole blood (less than 24 h old) is now rarely available because of the time required for pretransfusion screening and testing.

Red cell concentrates

Red cell concentrates comprise a single donor unit of blood from which some or most of the plasma has been harvested by centrifugation or sedimentation. They are the most commonly used red cell products and are indicated in patients with chronic blood loss or anaemia. In those cases where nearly all the plasma has been removed, the cells are resuspended in an optimal additive solution to maintain the cellular viability and improve storge life (up to 5 weeks at 4°C). In the UK, the commonest additive is SAG-M which contains sodium chloride 140 mmol/l, adenine 1.5 mmol/l, glucose 50 mmol/l and mannitol 30 mmol/l. The resulting suspension has a packed cell volume of 50–70% and because of the lack of plasma, has a low viscosity and can be transfused rapidly. Red cells in optimal additive solution should not be used in neonates or for exchange transfusion. Specialized red cell products are available for specific purposes: leucocyte depleted red cell components are given to prevent human leucocyte antigen (HLA) alloimmunization, an important cause of platelet refractoriness and bone marrow graft failure in patients with aplastic anaemia; washed red cells (where virtually all the plasma proteins and leucocytes are removed) are indicated in patients with paroxysmal nocturnal haemoglobinuria and patients with IgA deficiency; frozen, thawed and washed red cells are extremely expensive to produce and their use is largely restricted to patients with rare blood groups or with antibodies against public antigens.

Autologous blood transfusion

The term 'autologous' is applied where the transfusion recipient is also the transfusion donor. This practice is becoming more widespread and has obvious advantages for the donor–recipient over homologous transfusion. These include the prevention of transfusion reactions and of alloimmunization to HLA antigens. Autologous transfusion is practised prior to elective surgery when up to four units of blood can be harvested during the preoperative month. The techniques of preoperative haemodilution, intraoperative and postoperative blood salvage are other forms of autologous transfusion. So-called 'speculative' predeposit where there is no defined medical need and where blood is harvested and frozen for autologous use at some time in the future, is being increasingly practised in North America despite its high cost and the inaccessibility of frozen blood in an emergency. Autologous transfusion is time consuming, requires close co-ordination between surgeon and transfusion centre and meticulous attention to recipient identification and labelling.

Recombinant erythropoietin

Erythropoietin (EPO) is a glycoprotein hormone (composed of 166 amino acids) of primarily renal origin that promotes the proliferation and differentiation of erythroid precursors. It can be produced in quantity using recombinant DNA technology. *In situ* hybridization studies have shown that EPO production in the hypoxic kidney occurs primarily in the peritubular cells, most likely endothelial cells. EPO has found a place in the management of anaemia associated with chronic renal failure and patients on long-term renal dialysis programmes. It is administered thrice weekly intravenously or subcutaneously and normally results in a reticulocytosis within 10 days and a significant dose-dependent increase in the blood haemoglobin by the fourth week of therapy. The correction of anaemia by EPO has consistently been associated with reduced transfusion requirement, and an improved sense of wellbeing in dialysis patients, including improvements in appetite, energy, sleeping patterns and exercise. A proportion of patients receiving EPO develop hypertension which limits its use. Further studies are in progress in the evaluation of EPO in the management of other chronic anaemic states such as patients with malignancy, rheumatoid arthritis and HIV infection.

Artificial haemoglobin solutions

Homologous red cell transfusions remain the mainstay of transfusion practice. Some of the many disadvantages associated with homologous blood could be overcome by the development of an effective red cell substitute. Ideally, such a substitute should not provoke immunological reactions, or transmit infection; it should be isotonic with blood, have a long shelf-life, and a long half-life when infused; it should be safe and effective at delivery of oxygen to the tissues with the patient breathing room air; it should be readily excreted and it should be acceptable to certain religious groups who find human blood products an unacceptable form of therapy. Such a red cell substitute does not exist at this time but many groups are actively involved in this research.

One approach is the development of modified haemoglobin solutions. The haemoglobin is extracted from donated red blood cells and the contaminating stroma removed. The haemoglobin is polymerized to prolong its intravascular persistence and reduce the osmotic effect and is conjugated to pyridoxine-5-phosphate which corrects its oxygen affinity. An alternative to polymerization is to encapsulate the haemoglobin molecules in a synthetic lipid membrane. These solutions have been used in animal experiments and have been shown capable of sustaining life even when over 90% of the red cells have been removed. Their circulation half-life is about 20 h.

An alternative approach is the development of synthetic compounds with oxygen carrying capacity. Perfluorochemicals are produced in the form of emulsions and have the capacity of binding oxygen molecules at high oxygen tensions and releasing them again at low oxygen tensions. Owing to the simple straight-line relationship between oxygen content and partial pressure with perfluorochemicals, a high oxygen content is only achieved at an inspired oxygen fraction of 0.7–1.0. Other disadvantages include a short intravascular persistence, the need to store at −20°C and the high cost relative to homologous blood. With regard to *in vivo* storage and complete elimination from the body, the recently developed compounds are definitely better than the earlier fluorocarbons. However, the elimination by excretion through the lungs of the material stored is protracted and the long-term sequelae have not been identified. Nevertheless, because of their low viscosity, they may improve microcirculatory oxygen flow and they have already found a place in the distal perfusion of obstructed coronary arteries during angioplasty and may become of value in limb salvage procedures or in patients with myocardial infarction.

Replacement of platelets and granulocytes

Platelet and granulocyte transfusions may be derived either by differential centrifugation of whole blood packs or a blood cell processor may be used to collect the cell of interest.

Platelet transfusions are indicated in patients with thrombocytopenia due to bone marrow failure or dilutional thrombocytopenia and in patients with platelet dysfunction. Platelet transfusions have little place in the management of thrombocytopenia due to peripheral destruction of platelets. Platelets are usually chosen to observe ABO and Rhesus compatibility because of the red cell and plasma contents of these components. Platelet transfusions are normally administered as batches of five or six single donor packs, which is equivalent to a single donor apheresis pack. The recovery of platelets 1 hour after transfusion is 50–80% and the half-life in the circulation is about 4 days. The principal unwanted effect of repeated platelet transfusion is alloimmunization to HLA antigens which can affect up to two-thirds of recipients and may result in platelet refractoriness. Refractoriness may be defined as the failure of two consecutive transfusions to give a corrected platelet increment of greater than 7.5×10^9/l 1 h after transfusion in the absence of fever, infection, severe haemorrhage, splenomegaly or DIC. A search should be made for HLA or platelet-specific antibodies in the recipient's serum and, if positive, appropriately matched platelets should be given. Prevention of platelet refractoriness can be achieved by consistently transfusing less than 10^7 leucocytes in all platelet and red cell transfusions but this requires the regular use of leucocyte filters and this practice has not been proven as yet to be cost-effective.

Indications of granulocyte transfusions are very few because of the difficulties in obtaining enough neutrophils to have a meaningful effect, the short life-span of the neutrophil, the high rate of adverse reaction, and the cost of production. They are indicated in patients where the neutrophil count is persistently less than 0.2×10^9/l (but expected to recover) and there is clear evidence of bacterial or fungal infection and there is failure to respond to the appropriate antibiotic therapy after 48–72 h. They may also be used in patients with proven neutrophil dysfunction and persistent infection. Granulocyte transfusions must be ABO compatible and cross-matching with the recipient's serum is undertaken. Because of the high antigenic load, HLA alloimmunization is common and severe febrile reactions occur regularly. These can be treated by slowing or stopping the transfusion and in mild cases, hydrocortisone and chlorpheniramine intravenously may help. Other adverse reactions to granulocytes include pulmonary infiltrations and graft versus host disease in susceptible individuals as well as the hazards of red cell and plasma transfusion.

Myeloid growth factors

Myeloid growth factors are glycoprotein hormones that regulate the differentiation and proliferation of myeloid progenitor cells and the function of mature blood cells. Several of these factors have been molecularly characterized and produced in quantity via recombinant DNA technology. In particular, granulocyte-macrophage colony stimulating factor (GM-CSF), granulocyte colony stimulating factor (G-CSF), macrophage colony stimulating factor (M-CSF) and interleukin-3 (IL-3) have been developed as potential therapeutic agents and their effects on myelopoiesis and mature blood cell function are currently being investigated in clinical trials. Their main function *in vivo* may be to recruit and activate mature cells of the myeloid lineage and the main stimulus for their production is exposure to bacterial lipopolysaccharide and other endotoxins, or following damage to the producing cells by chemical or physical agents.

Intravenous GM-CSF results in a significant rise in circulating neutrophils, eosinophils and monocytes. G-CSF results in a dramatic dose-dependent rise (12–15-fold normal values) of neutrophils (and a smaller rise in monocytes). Both of these agents have been shown to be of value in reducing the severity and duration of chemotherapy induced neutropenia and in some studies this resulted in reduced febrile episodes, lower antibiotic use and shorter hospital stay. These drugs should make chemotherapy more tolerable; improve the likelihood of maintaining dose schedule and possibly permit increased dose intensity thereby improving long-term survival outcomes. In addition myeloid growth factors may be used to hasten recovery from neutropenia in patients with severe fungal infections, or patients with bone marrow graft failure following bone marrow transplantation. They have been shown to improve marrow cellularity and neutrophil count in patients with HIV infection, congenital neutropenias and myelodysplastic syndromes. Possible inadvertent biological effects include recruitment and exhaustion of stem cells, lineage competition and tumour transformation. In general, these agents appear to be well tolerated with only occasional patients withdrawn from therapy because of adverse effects. Clinical experience with M-CSF and IL-3 is not as extensive as that with GM-CSF and G-CSF. Thrombopoeitin has been identified and cloned recently and will soon be available for clinical trial. It is hoped that thrombopoeitin will become an invaluable platelet growth factor.

Replacement of plasma and its components

All products made from large pools of donor plasma are derived from individually screened donors and made by processes that inactivate or remove any contaminating viruses. Table 27.4 lists the products currently available and the indications for their use. Factor VIII concentrates are discussed on p. 464. Human albumin solutions are discussed in the next section. This discussion will be restricted to the other more important products.

Fresh frozen plasma (FFP) is obtained by separation of plasma from whole blood or by plasmapheresis. It must be frozen as soon as possible and used immediately after thawing to maximize its effect as factors V and VIII decay rapidly at room temperature. It is not heat treated and therefore carries a risk of viral contamination. Despite its widespread use in patients who have multiple coagulation defects (such as severe liver disease, DIC and following massive transfusion) its effects are poorly defined and justification for its continued use must be based on clinical improvement in the patient and a correction of the coagulopathy *in vitro*. Factor IX and VII concentrates are now the preferred treatment of warfarin toxicity as they have lower infective risk compared with FFP. FFP is indicated in the treatment of overdose of thrombolytic therapy, TTP, and certain congenital clotting factor deficiencies where there is no specific concentrate available. There is no justification for its use as a volume expander.

Cryoprecipitate is prepared from FFP by slow thawing at 4–6°C; the resulting precipitate (cryo) is then separated from the supernatant and refrozen for storage. Cryoprecipitate contains factor VIII-C, fibrinogen, VIII-VWF, XIII and fibronectin in higher concentrations than those found in plasma. In the past, cryoprecipitate was considered to be safer than factor concentrates in the treatment of coagulopathy since it is derived from a much smaller pool of donors. With the advent of heat treatment, this is no longer the case, and the risk is greater with cryoprecipitate. This product is used in a variety of conditions but it is uncertain which of the various components is functionally active. When used in VWD, the high proportion of high molecular weight VWF multimers may be of key importance. Its use is indicated also in the coagulopathy associated with renal failure, severe liver disease and some congenital platelet disorders.

Factor IX concentrate (prothrombin complex concentrate) of intermediate purity, is heat treated and contains substantial amounts of X and II. In addition

TABLE 27.4 Plasma products and indications for their use

PLASMA PRODUCT	MAIN INDICATIONS
Factor VIII (human)	Haemophilia A, von Willebrand's disease
Factor VIII (porcine)	Factor VIII inhibitors
Factor IX	Haemophilia B, reversal of oral anticoagulation, factor II & X deficiency, factor VIII inhibitors, liver disease
Factor VII	Factor VII deficiency, reversal of oral anticoagulant overdose, liver disease
Antithrombin III	Antithrombin III deficiency
Factor XI	Factor XI deficiency
Factor XIII	Factor XIII deficiency
Activated prothrombin complex concentrate	Factor VIII inhibitors
Protein C	Protein C deficiency
C1 esterase inhibitor	Hereditary angioedema
α_1-Antitrypsin	α_1-Antitrypsin deficiency
Immunoglobulins	Passive prophylaxis, hypogammaglobulinaemia, immune thrombocytopenia, viral infections, Kawasaki syndrome

to treating deficiencies of these factors, it is also of value in oral anticoagulant overdose, liver disease and in patients with haemophilia A with inhibitors. Used in high doses, factor IX concentrate may result in thrombotic episodes.

Immunoglobulins can be extracted from plasma by cold ethanol fractionation and heat treated to reduce the risk of viral infection. When pooled from unselected donors, these preparations contain all the antibodies to infectious micro-organisms prevalent in the community and they have a place in the management of hypogammaglobulinaemia and the passive prophylaxis of hepatitis A. Their use has broadened recently with the discovery that they have a beneficial effect on certain autoimmune disorders such as ITP and Kawasaki syndrome. Their mode of action is not certain, but probably includes the blockade of receptors for the non-antigen binding part of the immunoglobulin molecules (Fc receptors) on mononuclear phagocytes. Specific immunoglobulins can be obtained from donors whose plasma contains selected high titre IgG antibodies as a result of previous infection or active immunization. Preparations are available for the passive prophylaxis of varicella-zoster, tetanus, hepatitis B, cytomegalovirus and others. Anti-Rhesus D is prepared in this way for the prevention of haemolytic disease of the newborn.

Replacement with intravenous fluids

The development of the technology to transfuse safely a wide number of intravenous fluids including crystalloids, colloids, nutritional compounds, blood products and blood substitutes has been fundamental to the advancement of the support care of modern therapeutics.

Isotonic crystalloid solutions are the mainstay of treatment of patients requiring intravenous rehydration or correction of electrolyte abnormalities. They are used commonly in the initial management of acute blood loss and shock. Once infused, they are widely distributed throughout the body as they lack any water retaining properties, and fluid overload and oedema are the main risks. This is usually rapidly reversed if renal function is normal. For this reason, synthetic colloid solutions that can exert an oncotic effect are often used in combination with crystalloids. Having said this, there is little evidence from randomized controlled trials that colloid solutions are superior to crystalloids in the management of traumatic or septic shock and also in patients undergoing major vascular surgery who require large volumes of fluid replacement during the operation.[16] However, many of these studies were carried out on fit young adults and may not be relevant to a more elderly debilitated population where the risks from pulmonary oedema are greater.

Dextrans are high molecular weight polysaccharides consisting of glucose molecules connected by 1–6 glucosidic linkages. Dextran 70 (6% solution) and dextran 40 (10% solution) are the most important dextran preparations and as their names suggest have mean molecular weights of 70 000 and 40 000 respectively. Dextran 70 exerts an oncotic effect of 20–25 ml per gram of polymer and has an intravascular persistence of 6 h. It is therefore particularly suitable for primary volume replacement and maintenance of intravascular volume over several hours. Dextran 40 (10% solution) is hyperoncotic compared with plasma and for this reason the initial volume effect is about twice the volume infused. The transcapillary shift in fluid from the interstitial space to the intravascular space is said to improve microcirculatory flow and dextran 40 is therefore indicated in patients with protracted shock and microcirculatory disorders. Because of its lower mean molecular weight, its intravascular persistence is short (2–3 h). Both dextrans possess antithrombotic properties (see section on antiplatelet agents) and this limits its use as a plasma expander to 20 ml/kg of body weight per day. In common with all colloid solutions, there is a small risk (less than 0.1%) of anaphylaxis. This risk can be greatly minimized in the case of dextran by prior injection of 20 ml of dextran 1 (monovalent hapten–dextran) which acts as a hapten and neutralizes any preformed antidextran antibodies.

Modified fluid gelatin or urea-linked gelatin solutions have an advantage over dextrans in that they have no antithrombotic effect and can be used in larger quantities. They have a lower mean molecular weight and the resulting short intravascular persistence (2–3 h) limits their usefulness.

Hydroxyethylstarch (HES) is manufactured from amylopectin and consists of hydroxylated glucose molecules linked by α–1–4 bindings; it may be stored in the cells of the reticuloendothelial system before it is degraded by serum α-amylase in the circulation. There are reports that it may interfere with the clotting mechanism by decreasing factor VIII activity and recent reports suggest that large and repeated doses should be used with caution to avoid bleeding complications.

Human albumin solutions were developed in the USA during the Second World War to provide an alternative to blood or dried plasma for resuscitating military casualties. The method of cold ethanol fractionation is still used in its production from pooled plasma. The final product is filtered and heat treated to inactivate any contaminating viruses. Albumin has a molecular weight of 68 000 and the 4.5% solution has the best pharmacokinetic characteristics of the colloid solutions commonly available in that it is retained in the circulation for 2–4 days (this may not apply to patients with pulmonary oedema); it is a natural compound so it does not stimulate any allergic reaction.

However, its use is not without problems. It can rarely cause anaphylactic reactions due to other contaminating plasma proteins such as prekallikrein activators; it is relatively expensive to produce (five to ten times the cost of dextran). For these reasons, human albumin solutions should not be used for routine plasma volume replacement: they should be reserved for those hypovolaemic patients with significant hypoproteinaemia. Hyperoncotic solutions (such as 20% albumin) must be used carefully as they may result in volume overload. This may precipitate acute pulmonary oedema, especially if the pulmonary capillary bed is already damaged. The use of 20% albumin should be largely restricted to patients with hypovolaemia and hypoproteinaemia caused by increased loss of plasma proteins through the kidneys or gut which leads to oedema resistant to usual diuretic therapy. Albumin should not be used routinely as a volume expander or as a source of parenteral nutrition as there are cheaper, more effective alternatives available.

FUTURE PROSPECTS

There is no doubt that advances in biotechnology will continue to supply us with new and varied products of human derivation in high purity. Recombinant VIII-C, VIIa and albumin solutions have already been produced and will eventually replace the pooled plasma concentrates. Recombinant haematopoietic growth factors are finding their place in the management of disorders such as anaemia associated with haemodialysis and renal failure, and haematological malignancies and will become an invaluable adjunct to chemotherapy. Red cell substitutes such as the perfluorochemicals have already found a place in assisting distal coronary artery perfusion during angioplasty. Platelet substitutes are actively being researched. Human monoclonal antibodies offer numerous therapeutic possibilities. Clearly, we are entering an exciting and challenging era in the pharmacology of blood and bone marrow.

REFERENCES

1 Gallus AS. Anticoagulants in the prevention of thromboembolism. In: Hirsh J ed. *Clinical haematology: Antithrombotic therapy*. London: Ballière Tindall, 1990: 651–84.

2 Verstraete M, Vermylen J. Guidelines for the use of heparin and oral anticoagulants. In: Verstraete M, Vermylen J eds. *Thrombosis*. Oxford: Pergamon Press, 1984: 113–28.

3 Paiement GD, Bell D, Wessinger SJ, Harris WH. New advances in the prevention, diagnosis and cost effectiveness of venous thromboembolic disease in patients with total hip replacement. In: Brand RA ed. *The hip*. St Louis: CV Mosby, 1987: 94–119.

4 John RM, Swanton RH. Anticoagulants in cardiovascular diseases. *British Journal of Hospital Diseases* 1990; **43**: 207–14.

5 Chalmers TC, Matta RJ, Smith H Jr, Kunzler AM. Evidence favoring the use of anticoagulants in the hospital phase of acute myocardial infarction. *New England Journal of Medicine* 1977; **297**: 1091–5.

6 Gohlke H, Gohlke-Barwolf C, Sturzenhofecker P, Gornandt L, Ritter B, Reichelt M, Buchwalsky R, Schmuziger M, Roskamm H. Improved graft patency with oral anticoagulant therapy after aortocoronary bypass surgery: a prospective randomized study. *Circulation* 1981; **64** (Suppl II): 22–7.

7 Cliveden PE, Salzmann EW. Platelet metabolism and the effects of drugs. In: Walter Bowie EJ, Sharp AA eds. *Haemostasis and thrombosis*. London: Butterworths, 1985: 1–35.

8 ISIS-2 (Second International Study of Infarct Survival). Randomized trial of intravenous streptokinase, oral aspirin, both or neither among 17187 cases of suspected acute myocardial infarction. *Lancet* 1988; **ii**: 349–60.

9 Lewis HD, Davis JW, Archibald DG, Steinke WE, Smitherman TC, Doherty JE 3rd, Schnaper HW, LeWinter MM, Linares E, Pouget JM, Sabharwal SC, Chesler E, DeMors H. Protective effects of aspirin against acute myocardial infarction and death in men with unstable angina: Results of a Veterans Administration Cooperative Study. *New England Journal of Medicine* 1983; **309**: 396–403.

10 Canadian Co-operative Study Group. A randomized trial of aspirin and sulphinpyrazone in threatened stroke. *New England Journal of Medicine* 1978; **299**: 53–9.

11 Gent M, Blakely JA, Easton JD and the CATS Group. The Canadian–American Ticlopidine Study (CATS) in thromboembolic stroke. *Lancet* 1989; **i**: 1215–20.

12 Hass WK, Easton JD, Adams HP Jr, Pryse-Phillips W, Molony BA, Anderson S, Kamm B. for the Ticlopidine Aspirin Study Group. A randomized trial comparing ticlopidine hydrochloride with aspirin for the prevention of stroke in high risk patients. *New England Journal of Medicine* 1989; **321**: 501–7.

13 Samama M, Szwarcer E, Conrad J, Harellou J. Thrombolysis. In: Pullar L ed. *Recent advances in blood coagulation*. Edinburgh: Churchill Livingstone, 1985: 267–300.

14 GISSI. Long-term effects of intravenous thrombolysis in acute myocardial infarction. Final report of the GISSI study. *Lancet* 1988; **ii**: 349–60.

15 Sazama K. Reports of 355 transfusion-associated deaths: 1975 through 1985. *Transfusion* 1990; **30**: 583–90.

16 Lowe RJ, Moss GS, Jilek J, Levine HD. Crystalloid vs. colloid in the etiology of pulmonary failure after trauma, a randomized trial in man. *Surgery* 1977; **81**: 676–83.

PART II BLOOD TRANSFUSION, COLLOIDS, CRYSTALLOIDS AND PARENTERAL NUTRITION

W Aveling, C Bullen, AR Webb

BLOOD TRANSFUSION

Indications

Haemorrhage is the main indication for blood transfusion in surgery. The loss of volume can be made up with colloid or crystalloid solutions but blood is necessary to restore the lost oxygen carrying capacity. Loss of more than 30% of the circulating blood volume requires the use of blood. Other indications are severe anaemia, blood clotting disturbances and exchange transfusion, for example in sickle cell disease or Rhesus autoimmunization.

Blood and blood products

It is unusual to give patients whole blood because much better use of scarce donated blood can be made by fractionating it into the various components listed in Table 27.5.

The standard anticoagulant in the UK is citrate–phosphate dextrose adenine (CPD-A1). Plasma and platelets are removed from this anticoagulated blood and saline–adenine–glucose–mannitol (SAGM) is added to the concentrated red cells. At this time the haematocrit of the product will be about 65%. The addition of the SAGM will have added nutrients and reduced the viscosity of the product making it transfusable. The shelf-life of banked blood at a storage temperature of 4–6°C is 35 days. During this time less than 1% of the red cells will have haemolysed. Levels of 2,3-diphosphoglycerate (2-3 DPG) in the red cells will fall during storage, increasing the cells' affinity for oxygen, making less oxygen available to the tissues. Acid–citrate–dextrose (ACD) when used as an anticoagulant in blood results in the loss of 90% of the 2-3 DPG during 2 weeks of storage. In contrast, using CPD-A1 anticoagulated blood, only 20% of the 2-3 DPG leaves the cells. This will have less effect on the oxygen dissociation curve but will reduce the P_{50} from normal (3.6 kPa) to about 2.4 kPa during rapid transfusion. Following transfusion there is a delay of some 24 h before intracellular levels of 2–3 DPG return to normal in the transfused red cells.

Failure of the sodium pump in stored blood is inevitable resulting in high plasma concentrations of potassium. However, the sodium pump recovers on rewarming the blood, extracorporeally or following transfusion, and the complications of hyperkalaemia are rarely encountered. Citrate acts as the anticoagulant in all stored blood by chelating the ionized calcium but there is excess citrate to requirements and following transfusion serum ionized calcium levels may fall.

Lactic acidosis from anaerobic glycolysis in combination with the citric acid from the anticoagulant results in an acid product. Following transfusion this is quickly buffered, but in the compromised patient with poor cardiac output or severe peripheral vasoconstriction it may exacerbate a metabolic acidosis. In the patient with normal hepatic function the citrate is metabolized to bicarbonate which can result in a metabolic alkalosis. However, in practice this is rarely seen.

TABLE 27.5 Blood components

Plasma reduced blood	Packed cells
Washed red cells	If high risk of transfusion reaction
Plasma protein fraction	No useful clotting factors
Fresh frozen plasma (FFP)	FFP contains dilute clotting factors
Cryoprecipitate	Rich in factor VIII
Factor VII concentrate	Even richer in VIII
Factor II VII IX X concentrate	
Factor XI concentrate	
Fibrogen	
Platelet concentrate	

Hazards of transfusion

Table 27.6 lists the hazards associated with any transfusion even of only one unit. All blood donated in the UK is screened for HIV, hepatitis and syphilis and

TABLE 27.6 Hazards of any transfusion

Transmission of disease, e.g. AIDS, malaria, syphilis, hepatitis
Bacterial contamination
Pyrogenic reactions (antibodies to white cells)
Haemolysis due to incompatibility reactions (clerical error the commonest cause)

recent travel to areas where malaria is endemic precludes donation. Cytomegalovirus (CMV) is transmissible by transfused blood. It may persist in a latent state in the lymphoid cells and may become a source of infection in immunocompromised patients. Filtration of blood may reduce the incidence of post-transfusion CMV seroconversion and infection.

Minor pyrogenic reactions are quite common but serious incompatibility reactions leading to haemolysis and acute renal failure are rare and are usually due to human error. The importance of very careful cross-checking and matching of patient and blood cannot be overemphasized.

Transfusion of small amounts of banked blood does not cause metabolic disturbances but when large volumes are transfused rapidly a number of problems arise. Massive transfusion is defined as giving half the circulating volume in half an hour or 500 ml in 5 min. The problems associated with it are listed in Table 27.7

Microaggregates are formed rapidly in stored blood from platelets, white cells and fibrin precipitate. They may cause pulmonary dysfunction and have been implicated in the development of adult respiratory distress syndrome. Filtering the blood through a 40-μm filter reduces the likelihood of this. Removal of the microaggregates also helps minimize the falls in platelet and fibronectin levels that have been measured following transfusion of 5–9 units of stored blood. Fibronectin is a plasma glycoprotein that has major opsonin properties preparing invading bacteria and debris for phagocytosis by macrophages. A decrease in this compound may result in a reduced capacity for host defence.

The hazards, expense and difficulty of ensuring regular supplies of blood products has led to an increase in various blood and plasma substitutes collectively known as the colloids.

COLLOIDS

Colloids and electrolyte solutions may be used in certain circumstances instead of blood for transfusion but have many more indications for expansion and replenishment of the various body fluid compartments. A brief discussion of the physiology of the fluid compartments and the barriers between them is therefore appropriate at this point.

TABLE 27.7 Hazards of massive transfusion

Hypothermia
Hyperkalaemia
Citrate toxicity
Acidosis
Air embolism
Microaggregate embolism, 'shock lung'
Accidental overload
Dilution and consumption of clotting factors

Fluid compartments

An adult male is 60% water, a female having more fat is 55% water, newborn infants are 75% water. The most important compartments are the intracellular fluid (ICF) – 55% of body water – and the extracellular fluid (ECF) – 45%. ECF is further subdivided into the plasma (part of the intravascular space), the interstitial fluid, the transcellular water (e.g. fluid in the gastrointestinal tract, the CSF and aqueous humour) and water associated with the bone and dense connective tissue which is much less readily exchangeable and of much less importance. The partitioning of the total body water (TBW) with average values for a 70-kg male, who would contain 43 l of water, is shown in Fig. 27.3.

The capillary membrane

The barrier between the plasma and the interstitium is the capillary endothelium, which allows the free passage of water and electrolytes but restricts the passage of larger molecules such as proteins (the natural colloids). Although no one has demonstrated holes in the membrane, capillaries behave as if they had pores of 4–5 nm in most tissues. The osmotic pressure generated by the presence of colloids on one side of a membrane that is impermeable to them is known as the colloid osmotic pressure (COP). Albumin (MW 69 000 Da) crosses the membrane relatively slowly and is mainly responsible for the difference in COP between the plasma and interstitium (normally about 25 mmHg).

The balance of hydrostatic and osmotic pressures across the capillary membrane was first described by Starling. Staverman introduced the concept that different molecules will be 'reflected' to a different extent by the membrane. This term, the reflection coefficient, varies between zero (all molecules passing through the membrane) and +1 (all molecules reflected). In disease states when the capillary membrane becomes leaky the reflection coefficient will fall. Flow across the membrane is represented in the equation:

$$J_v = K_f S[(P_c - P_{if}) - \sigma(\pi_p - \pi_{if})]$$

where J_v is the rate of movement of water, K_f the capillary filtration coefficient, S the surface area, P_c and P_{if} the capillary and interstitial pressures, π_p and π_{if} the plasma and interstitial colloid osmotic pressures, and σ the reflection coefficient.

The cell membrane

The barrier between the ECF and ICF is the cell membrane. This is freely permeable to water but not to sodium ions, which are actively pumped out of the

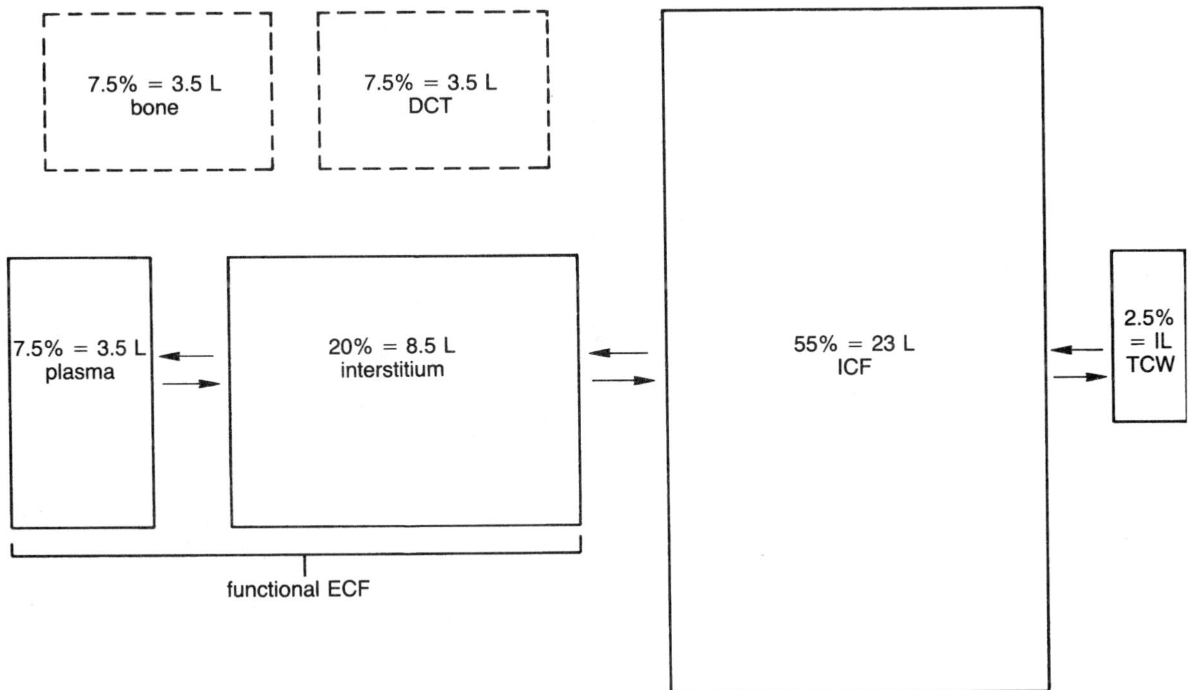

FIGURE 27.3 Distribution of total body water in a 70-kg man. ECF, extracellular fluid; ICF, intracellular fluid; DCT, dense connective tissue; TCW, transcellular water.

cells. Sodium is the chief extracellular cation and potassium the principal intracellular one. Water will move across the cell membrane in either direction if there is a difference in osmolality between the two sides. Osmolality expresses the potential of a solution to develop an osmotic pressure across a semipermeable membrane. It depends on the number of particles in solution rather than their size. Normal osmolality of ECF is 280–295 mOsmol/kg.

Properties of colloid solutions

These are summarized in Table 27.8. *Human albumin solution* is prepared by separating red cells from donated blood. A bottle contains plasma from several donors and has been pasteurized to prevent the transmission of disease (e.g. hepatitis or HIV). It contains 4.5% albumin, has no clotting factors and is stable at room temperature. All the molecules are the same size (MW 69 000 Da) and, provided the capillary membrane is healthy and not leaking, the infused solution will stay within the intravascular compartment. The problem is that in many conditions where expansion of the plasma compartment is required (e.g. septic shock) the capillaries leak (the reflection coefficient falls).

All the synthetic colloids are heterodisperse solutions – that is, there is a great range of molecular weights. The smaller molecules will pass easily into the interstitium, the larger ones will remain in the plasma compartment. The number average (or simple average) molecular weight gives some idea as to how likely the solution is to stay in the plasma. Note that manufacturers generally quote the weight average molecular weight, which is larger for all heterodisperse colloids and looks more favourable. The ideal synthetic colloid would be large enough to stay within even leaky capillaries and have a narrow range of molecular weight. Such a solution is not commercially available at the present time.

Another approach to this problem is to compare the COP of colloids across an artificial membrane that retains molecules larger than 10 000 Da (COP_{10}) and one of 50 000 Da – that is, which allows molecules smaller than 50 000 Da to leak through (COP_{50}). The ratio of COP_{50} to COP_{10} is then analogous to the reflection coefficient of Staverman for the more porous membrane and is a relative index of the ability of each solution to stay in the plasma (see Table 27.9).

The *dextrans* are glucose polymers available in preparations of different molecular weights. Dextran 70 is so called because it has a weight average MW of 70 000 Da but the number average MW, which is more relevant, is 38 000 Da. Dextran 40 has smaller molecules and can be nephrotoxic. Dextran 110 has higher average MWs. Neither of these will be considered further. Dextran 70 is quite a good plasma substitute but has declined in popularity because of its adverse effects on coagulation and the relatively high incidence of allergic reactions.

TABLE 27.8 Characteristics of colloid solutions

NAME	BRAND NAME	NUMBER AVERAGE MW	MW RANGE	Na^+ (mmol/l)	K^+ (mmol/l)	Ca^{2+} (mmol/l)	$t_{\frac{1}{2}}$ IN PLASMA	ADVERSE REACTIONS MILD (%)	ADVERSE REACTIONS SEVERE (%)	EFFECT ON COAGULATION	UK COST 1991
Human albumin solution		69 000	69 000	150	5	2	20 days	0.02	0.004	Dilution effect	£40
Dextran 70 in saline 0.9% or glucose 5%	Macrodex Lomodex Gentran	38 000	<10 000–>250 000	150	—	—	12 h	0.7	0.02	Inhibit platelet aggregation Interfere with cross-match	£3.60–£4.10
Polygeline (urea-linked gelatin)	Haemaccel	24 500	<5 000–>50 000	145	5	6.25	2.5 h	0.12	0.04	Dilution effect	£3.80
Succinylated gelatin	Gelofusin	22 600	<10 000–>140 000	154	0.4	0.4	4h	0.12	0.04	Dilution effect	£3.20
Hydroxyethyl starch 6% in saline	Hespan	70 000	<10 000–>10^6	154	—	—	25 h	0.09	0.006	Reduced W factor Fibrinolytic effect	£15.40

TABLE 27.9 Colloid osmotic pressure of colloid solutions

COLLOID	COP_{10} (mmHg)	COP_{50}/COP_{10} RATIO
Human albumin solution	17.6	0.36
Dextran 70	56.2	0.25
Gelofusin	42.3	0.37
Haemaccel	26.5	0.18
Hespan	30.5	0.58

Dextrans are not metabolized intravascularly; that which is not filtered by the kidney passes to tissues and is completely hydrolysed by the enzyme dextran-1, 6-glucosidase.

Gelatin solutions are prepared by the hydrolysis of bovine collagen. They have the advantage over the dextrans of not affecting coagulation and having a low incidence of allergic reactions. Being of smaller average particle size they stay in the plasma a shorter time. Haemaccel contains potassium and calcium ions, which can cause coagulation if mixed with citrated blood in a giving set. Haemaccel has the lowest COP_{50}/COP_{10} ratio of any of the colloids and it has been shown that 30% of the molecules of an infused solution have dispersed to the interstitial tissues in 30 min. Gelofusin is probably preferable from that point of view.

Little is known about the metabolism of gelatins since direct assay is not possible. The smaller molecules are rapidly eliminated through the kidneys.

Hydroxyethyl starch solutions (Table 27.10) have the highest MWs and the highest COP_{50}/COP_{10} of all the solutions; they therefore stay in the circulation longest. The smaller molecules are rapidly eliminated by glomerular filtration so that 40% of the starch is excreted within 24 h. The larger polymers are slowly hydrolysed by plasma α-amylase and cleared once their size has fallen below the renal threshold. Hydrolysis by α-amylase depends on the proportion of glucose units in the polymer which are substituted by hydroxyethyl groups (degree of substitution – ds); the higher the ds the greater the protection against α-amylase. About 30% of the dose infused leaves the vascular compartment and is taken up by the reticuloendothelial system without apparently affecting its function.

Hetastarch reduces the release of von Willebrand's factor, decreases factor VIII, and has a fibrinolytic effect. Doses up to 1.5 g/kg/day have not been shown to produce clinically significant haemostatic defects.

TABLE 27.10 Hydroxyethyl starch solutions

TRADE NAME	CONCENTRATION (%)	MW_n	MW_w	ds
Hespan	6	70 000	450 000	0.7
Pentaspan	10	60 000	264 000	0.45
Elohes	6	60 000	200 000	0.62

Indications and choice of colloid

Loss of circulating volume has a critical effect on cardiac output and organ perfusion. This may be due to blood loss in acute haemorrhage or plasma loss in acute burns or the many circumstances where plasma leaks into the interstitial tissues, for example septic shock. Different situations require different solutions. Where blood is not available for transfusion, crystalloid may be used but because it rapidly disperses throughout the ECF which is four times larger than the plasma compartment 4 l of crystalloid is needed to expand the blood volume by 1 l. Usually blood will be available within a few hours, in which case succinylated gelatin is a good substitute because it will be leaving the circulation at the time that blood is given and it is of low cost.

In continuing hypovolaemia, hetastarch gives a more prolonged expansion and its larger molecules are better retained when the capillaries are leaky.

Hazards

Anaphylactoid reactions can occur with any of the colloids and their true incidence is difficult to determine. Severe reactions are probably commonest with dextrans and least common with hetastarch and human albumin solution (frequencies are quoted in Table 27.8). The effects on coagulation have been mentioned above.

CRYSTALLOIDS

Crystalloid solutions are available for intravenous use both for the maintenance of normal water and electrolyte balance and for the restoration of various deficits. A large number of solutions are made in 1 l and 0.5 l bags and the contents of the principal ones are listed in Table 27.11.

Correct use of the crystalloids depends on an understanding of their distribution between the various body fluid compartments when infused (see Fig. 27.3) as well as a knowledge of which compartments have been depleted in different kinds of dehydration.

Consider what happens when a patient takes in water, either by drinking or as intravenous 5% glucose whose glucose is soon metabolized. It will rapidly distribute through the ECF with a resultant fall in ECF osmolality. Since osmolality must be the same inside and outside the cells, water will move from ECF to ICF until the osmolalities are the same. Thus 1 l of 5% glucose will distribute itself throughout the body water. By a converse argument one can see that a man marooned on a life-raft with no water will lose water from all compartments.

Normal saline (0.9%) contains Na^+ 150 mmol/l and Cl^- 150 mmol/l with an osmolality of 300 mOsmol/l. If

TABLE 27.11 Content of crystalloid solutions

NAME	KNOWN AS	Na^+	Cl^-	K^+	HCO^{3^-}	Ca^{2+}	CALCULATED mOsmol/l
Sodium chloride 0.9%	Normal saline	150	150	—	—	—	300
Sodium chloride 0.9%, potassium chloride 0.3%	Normal saline + KCl	150	190	40	—	—	380
Sodium chloride 0.9%, potassium chloride 0.15%	Normal saline + KCl	150	170	20	–	—	340
Ringer's lactate	Hartmann's	131	111	5	29 as lactate	2	280
Glucose 5%	5% dextrose	—	—	—	—	—	280
Glucose 5%, potassium chloride 0.3%	5% dextrose + KCl	—	40	40	—	—	360
Glucose 5%, potassium chloride 0.15%	5% dextrose + KCl	—	20	20	—	—	320
Glucose 4%, sodium chloride 0.18%	Dextrose saline	30	30	—	—	—	286
Glucose 4%, sodium chloride, 0.18%, potassium chloride 0.3%	Dextrose saline + KCl	30	70	40	—	—	366
Glucose 4%, sodium chloride 0.18%, potassium chloride 0.15%	Dextrose saline + KCl	30	50	20	—	—	326
Sodium chloride 0.45%	Half normal saline	75	75	—	—	—	150
Sodium chloride 1.8%	Twice normal saline	300	300	—	—	—	600
Sodium bicarbonate 8.4%	—	1000	—	—	1000	—	2000
Sodium bicarbonate 1.4%	—	167	—	—	167	—	334

this is infused into a patient most will stay in the ECF, which is of similar osmolality, and because the ICF osmolality is similar there is little movement into the cells. Conversely a patient losing water and electrolytes together (e.g. severe diarrhoea) loses fluid from the ECF and very little from the ICF.

Three aspects of prescribing fluids need to be considered: maintenance, continuing abnormal losses above maintenance requirements and the correction of pre-existing dehydration.

Fluids for maintenance

A patient who is temporarily unable to take fluid by mouth will need a basic intravenous maintenance regimen. In temperate climes adults need 1.5 l of water per m^2 surface area or 30–40 ml/kg in 24 h. Children need relatively more water as set out in Table 27.12.

Basic electrolyte requirements are sodium 1 mmol/kg/day and potassium 1 mmol/kg/day. Humans can be very efficient at conserving sodium and can manage with much lower sodium intakes but there are obligatory losses of potassium and patients not given potassium will soon become depleted.

Looking at the crystalloid solutions available (Table 27.11) we can see that there are a number of ways of supplying the basal requirements. Normal saline, 5% glucose and dextrose saline are the most commonly used. Although potassium (supplied as ampoules containing 20 mmol) was traditionally added to the bags it is much safer to use preparations already containing potassium. Table 27.13 gives two basic regimens for a 70-kg patient. Potassium can cause fatal arrhythmias and must never be given as a bolus. There have been a number of tragedies reported to the defence societies in which potassium chloride was mistakenly used as flush. Hyperkalaemia can also occur if potassium is given to anuric patients. Safe rules for giving potassium are: (1) urine output at least 40 ml/h; (2) not more than 40 mmol added to 1 l; and (3) no faster than 40 mmol/h. During surgery it should be remembered that stored blood can have a high potassium and suxamethonium can raise potassium, albeit briefly. It is rarely necessary to give potassium during routine surgery but where it is the above rules apply.

TABLE 27.12 Water requirements for children

WEIGHT (kg)	WATER REQUIREMENTS
0–10	100 ml/kg
10–20	1000 ml + 50 ml/kg for each kg >10
>20	1500 ml + 25 ml/kg for each kg >20

TABLE 27.13 Basal daily water and electrolyte regimens for a 70-kg patient on iv fluids

SOLUTION	VOLUME (ml)	Na^+ mmol	K^+ mmol
5% glucose + KCl 0.3%	2000	—	80
Saline 0.9%	500	75	—
Dextrose saline + KCl 0.3%	2500	75	100

Not all the crystalloid solutions are of neutral pH. Five per cent dextrose and dextrose saline have a pH range 3.5–5.5, depending on the age of the solution, and Hartmann's has a pH 5–7. In the normal patient with a large buffering capacity this is not significant but it may well be in the acidotic patient.

Continuing losses

Extra fluid for continuing losses should, of course, resemble as closely as possible the fluid that has been lost. The electrolyte content of common body fluids is shown in Table 27.14. The only hypotonic secretions are saliva and sweat. Gastric secretion, though having a sodium content of 50 mmol/l, is isotonic with ECF because of the hydrogen ions that it contains. From this it can be seen that all bowel losses must be replaced with saline and potassium. If bowel fluid (Na^+ 140 mmol/l) is replaced with dextrose saline (Na^+ 30 mmol/l) or, even worse, 5% dextrose, hyponatraemia will ensue. Where the losses are from the stomach it might be thought necessary to provide hydrogen ions. In fact, the kidney compensates by retaining hydrogen and excreting sodium and bicarbonate ions so that the net effect is loss of sodium and chloride. Normal saline with potassium should therefore be used in rehydration.

Correction of existing dehydration

The problem here is to identify the compartments from which fluid has been lost and the extent of the losses. Once this has been done the principles of replacement are as stated above, namely to use fluid of similar composition and volume to that which has been lost. Clinical history and examination are important here but one may also be assisted by the measurement of changes in electrolytes, haematocrit and plasma protein. It is important to realize that when ECF is lost (e.g. in a bowel obstruction) sodium and water are lost together so that the sodium concentration in the remaining ECF does not change. However, protein and red cells are not lost so that when ECF is lost both albumin concentration and haematocrit will rise. This can be used to quantify the loss if the starting level of albumin is known or can be estimated. If plasma is lost only the haematocrit will rise. This is illustrated in Fig. 27.4 which shows that when ECF is lost (A) both albumin and haematocrit are concentrated, but when only plasma is lost (B) only the haematocrit rises.

$$\% \text{ fall in ECF volume} = (1 - Pr_1/Pr_2) \times 100$$

where Pr_1 and Pr_2 are the albumin concentrations before and after dehydration. Thus, if the albumin concentration rises from 35 to 45 g/l the fall in ECF volume will be:

$$\% \text{ fall in ECF volume} = (1 - 35/45) \times 100 = 22\%$$

TABLE 27.14 Electrolyte content and daily volume of body secretions

	Na^+ (mmol)	K^+ (mmol)	Cl^- (mmol)	VOLUME (l/day)
Saliva	15	19	40	1.5
Stomach	50	15	140	2.5
Bile, pancreas, small bowel	130–145	5–12	70–100	4.2
Insensible sweat	12	10	12	0.6
Heat-induced sweat	50	10	50	varies

Intraoperative fluid balance

During an operation several things are going on at the same time. The patient has usually starved for 6–12 h, there may be blood loss, plasma loss, ECF loss and evaporation from exposed bowel. It is generally recommended that Hartmann's solution 5 ml/kg up to a maximum of 2 l is given during abdominal surgery to compensate for these losses as well as any blood or colloid that may be necessary.

PARENTERAL NUTRITION

Parenteral nutrition is indicated where the normal use of the bowel is restricted and is likely to remain so for more than several days. Parenteral nutrition is not without complication and therefore should not be undertaken lightly. There are several broad categories of indications for parenteral nutritional support but the presence of adequately functioning bowel is an absolute contraindication.

Preoperative nutritional support

Nutritional support for the malnourished preoperative patient is of proven benefit but at least 14 days are required to see this benefit.

Postoperative nutritional support

Parenteral nutrition in the immediate postoperative period is of no value for the majority of patients and indeed can increase morbidity. Return of bowel function is usually swift in these patients unless there are postoperative complications such as high gastrointestinal fistulae or prolonged ileus.

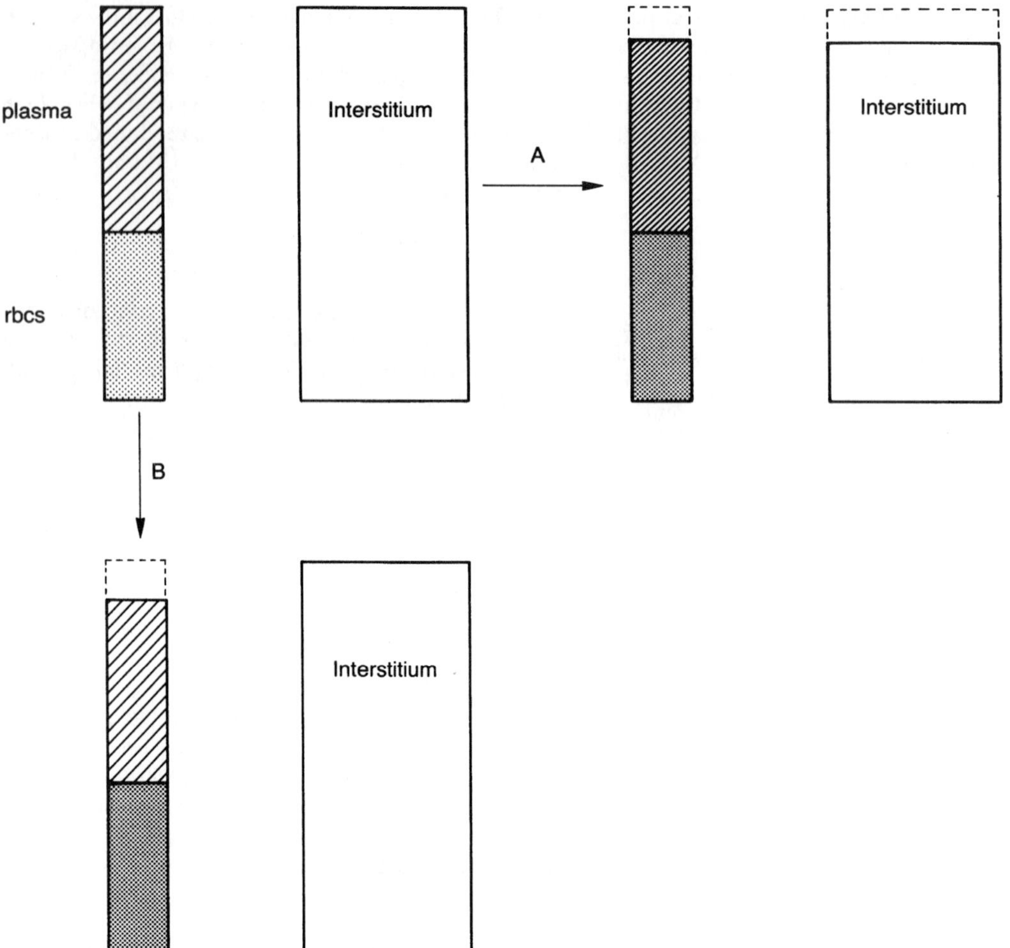

FIGURE 27.4 Changes in volume and composition of extracellular fluid (ECF). (A) Fluid is lost from the whole ECF; albumin and haematocrit are concentrated. (B) Plasma alone is lost and haematocrit rises (see text).

Medical indications

In medical patients, disturbance of bowel function is usually partial rather than complete. Parenteral nutrition may be of benefit to supplement oral or enteral feeding and rarely to replace oral or enteral feeding in malabsorption states, chronic intestinal obstruction (e.g. radiation enteritis), short bowel syndrome or wasting diarrhoeal diseases (e.g. ulcerative colitis or Crohn's disease).

Hypercatabolic patients

Burns, trauma and sepsis fit into this category. These patients may have limited bowel function due to ileus or severe diarrhoea yet have high metabolic requirements. On the one hand supplementing oral or enteral nutrition is undoubtedly useful but on the other, the ability to utilize exogenous nutrients in these hypercatabolic states is severely limited.

Nitrogen source

Since the bowel is bypassed, intravenous nutrition requires that the protein source has been broken down either by hydrolysis or by the provision of synthetic amino acid solutions. Amino acids exist as both laevo (L) and dextro (D) isomers although the body can only utilize L-amino acids with the exception of small quantities of D-methionine and D-phenylalanine. Protein hydrolysates always contain a significant amount of peptides, which are often poorly utilized and have been blamed for allergic reactions. Synthetic amino acid solutions are preferred. Plasma and albumin solutions are poor nitrogen sources since they must be broken down to their constituent amino acids prior to utilization.

There are differences between the amino acid contents of the various available amino acid preparations (Table 27.15). Some solutions are incomplete lacking aspartate, glutamate, cystine, serine or tyrosine.

Table 27.16 shows the amino acids found in man. Essential amino acids cannot be synthesized by man

TABLE 27.15 Amino acid content (g/l) of intravenous feeding solutions (essential amino acids in bold)

	AMINOFUSIN FORTE	AMINOPLASMAL L3	AMINOPLASMAL L5	AMINOPLASMAL L10	AMINOPLEX 5	AMINOPLEX 12	AMINOPLEX 14	AMINOPLEX 24	AMINOVEN 12	HEPANUTRIN	PERIFUSIN	SYNTHAMIN 9	SYNTHAMIN 14	SYNTHAMIN 17	VAMIN 9	VAMIN 14	VAMIN 18
Ala	12.0	4.1	6.9	13.7	4.0	10.0	14.8	20.0	10.0	9.2	4.0	11.4	17.6	20.8	3.0	12.0	16.0
Arg	8.0	2.8	4.6	9.2	3.7	9.2	9.2	18.4	9.2	9.6	2.6	5.7	8.8	10.4	3.3	8.4	11.3
Asp	0.0	0.4	0.7	1.3	*0.8	*2.0	*2.0	*4.0	*2.0	0.0	0.0	0.0	0.0	0.0	4.1	2.5	3.4
Cys	0.0	0.2	0.4	0.7	0.0	0.0	0.0	0.0	0.0	0.0	0.0	0.0	0.0	0.0	1.4	0.4	0.6
Glu	18.0	1.4	2.3	4.6	0.8	2.0	0.0	4.0	2.0	0.0	5.9	0.0	0.0	0.0	9.0	4.2	5.6
Gly	20.0	2.4	4.0	7.9	1.8	4.4	12.0	8.8	4.4	11.0	6.6	11.4	17.6	20.8	2.1	5.9	7.9
His	2.0	1.6	2.6	5.2	0.9	2.2	2.8	4.4	2.2	3.0	0.7	2.4	3.7	4.4	2.4	5.1	6.8
Ileu	3.1	1.6	2.6	5.1	1.5	3.8	3.2	7.6	3.8	11.1	1.1	2.6	4.1	4.8	3.9	4.2	5.6
Leu	4.4	2.7	4.5	8.9	2.3	5.8	4.4	11.6	5.8	13.5	1.5	3.4	5.3	6.2	5.3	5.9	7.9
Lys	5.0	2.1	3.5	7.0	2.2	5.4	8.5	10.9	5.4	7.5	1.7	3.2	4.9	5.8	3.9	6.8	9.0
Met	4.2	1.2	1.9	3.8	1.9	4.8	6.4	9.6	4.8	1.2	1.4	3.2	4.9	5.8	1.9	4.2	5.6
Phe	4.4	1.6	2.6	5.1	2.8	6.9	4.4	13.8	6.9	1.2	1.5	3.4	5.3	6.2	5.5	5.9	7.9
Pro	14.0	2.7	4.5	8.9	4.8	12.0	4.0	24.0	12.0	9.8	4.6	2.3	3.6	4.2	8.1	5.1	6.8
Ser	0.0	0.7	1.2	2.4	1.0	2.4	0.0	4.8	2.4	6.1	0.0	0.0	0.0	0.0	7.5	3.4	4.5
Thr	2.0	1.3	2.1	4.1	1.3	3.2	3.2	6.4	3.2	5.6	0.7	2.3	3.6	4.2	3.0	4.2	5.6
Try	0.9	0.6	0.9	1.8	0.6	1.4	1.6	2.8	1.4	0.8	0.4	1.0	1.5	1.8	1.0	1.4	1.9
Tyr	0.0	0.4	0.7	1.5	0.0	0.0	0.0	0.0	0.0	0.0	0.0	0.2	0.3	0.4	0.5	0.2	0.2
Val	3.0	1.5	2.4	4.8	1.8	4.5	5.2	9.0	4.5	10.4	1.0	2.5	3.9	4.6	4.3	5.5	7.3
Nitrogen	15.2	4.8	8.0	16.0	5.0	12.4	13.4	24.9	12.5	15.6	5.0	9.3	14.3	16.9	9.4	13.5	18.0

*as L-ornithine-L-aspartate.

TABLE 27.16 Amino acid profile of man

ESSENTIAL	SEMI-ESSENTIAL	NON-ESSENTIAL
Isoleucine	Arginine	Alanine
Leucine	Histidine	Aspartic acid
Lysine		Citrulline
Methionine		Cysteine-cystine
Phenylalanine		Glutamic acid
Threonine		Glycine
Tryptophan		Ornithine
Valine		Proline
		Serine
		Taurine
		Tyrosine

and are necessary for protein synthesis. Arginine and histidine are considered semi-essential since the ability to synthesize them is limited. Ten further amino acids found in man can be synthesized but are generally provided in balanced amino acid solutions. The transamination reactions, which provide the non-essential amino acids, require functioning enzyme systems which cannot be relied upon in malnourished and ill patients and synthesis of certain non-essential amino acids requires larger quantities of essential amino acids. Essential amino acids should constitute at least 30–40% of the total.

Of the non-essential amino acids alanine, proline and glutamic acid improve amino acid utilization compared with glycine. Glycine rich amino acid solutions that are deficient in proline and glutamic acid are associated with a high urinary excretion of glycine. Such a urinary loss of amino acid is not found when patients are given glutamic acid-rich solutions.

Interest has focused recently on the use of solutions (e.g. Hepanutrin) rich in branched chain amino acids (valine, leucine and isoleucine) with low levels of aromatic amino acids (phenylalanine and tyrosine) and methionine. Branched chain amino acids are not metabolized in the liver and patients with sepsis, trauma and hepatic failure all have plasma amino acid profiles which are rich in aromatic amino acids and methionine. Although such solutions may offer a physiologically appropriate amino acid profile for sepsis, trauma or hepatic failure there is currently little evidence of major benefit.

Solutions with a high glycine content can lead to hyperammonaemia. An excess of the cationic amino acids lysine, arginine and histidine may lead to metabolic acidosis. Furthermore, the hypertonic nature of the amino acid solutions can contribute to metabolic acidosis. Generally, however, the buffering capacity of amino acid solutions offsets any metabolic acidosis.

Parenteral amino acid solutions are strongly hypertonic. Intravenous infusion bypasses osmotic control systems in the liver and may be responsible for oliguria, oedema and electrolyte disturbances. Hypertonic infusions with an acid pH cause thrombophlebitis if infused peripherally.

Energy source

As with nitrogen, energy has to be provided in a form that is equivalent to digestion of carbohydrates and fats. In modern parenteral nutrition energy is usually provided as a balanced combination of glucose and fat emulsion.

Amino acids have a calorific value of about 4 cal/g but a non-nitrogen energy source is required to ensure optimal utilization of infused amino acids and to reduce catabolism of tissue proteins. Although there is considerable individual variation approximately 125–175 cal/g nitrogen/day is required as non-protein energy. Some of the amino acid solutions contain an added non-nitrogen energy source (Table 27.17).

Carbohydrate

At least 400 cal are required per day as carbohydrate to prevent ketosis and to exert a nitrogen-sparing effect. However, carbohydrate is not ideal as the sole energy source since the low calorific value of carbohydrates (4.1 cal/g for glucose) would require extremely large volumes of isotonic fluid or an extremely hypertonic solution. For isotonic (5%) glucose 2000 cal would require an infusion of 10 000 ml whereas for 50% glucose 2000 cal is provided in 1000 ml but with an osmolality of 3800 mOsmol/kg.

It is now almost universal to use glucose as the carbohydrate energy source. It has the metabolic advantages of being utilizable by all tissues, it is obligatory to some tissues such as the central nervous system and red blood cells and it can still be metabolized under anaerobic conditions. Alternative carbohydrate sources provided the advantage of metabolism independent of insulin, the function of which is reduced by excessive secretion of catecholamines and steroids in ill patients. Modern practice allows careful insulin supplementation, avoidance of excessive glucose infusion rates and the use of fat emulsions to provide some of the energy requirement. The following carbohydrate energy sources have largely been abandoned.

Fructose

Metabolized rapidly in the liver by phosphorylation. Further intracellular metabolism forms glucose and

TABLE 27.17 Energy content of amino acid solutions per litre

	AMINOPLEX 5	VAMIN 9 GLUCOSE
Glucose (g)	—	100
Sorbitol (g)	125	—
Ethanol (g)	50	—
Non-nitrogen energy (cal)	868	400

lactate. Thus the use of fructose was a common cause of lactic acidosis and hypophosphataemia.

Sorbitol

Initial metabolism is in the liver where sorbitol forms fructose. Thereafter the disadvantages are the same as for fructose.

Xylitol

Metabolized via the pentose phosphate and glucose-6-phosphate pathways to glucose and lactate. Disadvantages are similar to fructose with the addition of greater uric acid production.

Ethanol

The advantage of the high calorific value of ethanol (7 cal/g) is offset by the risks of intoxication and lactic acidosis.

Fat

Glucose utilization is reduced after surgery and trauma whereas fat utilization and blood fat clearance is increased. Fat has an energy value of 9.3 cal/g and is not water soluble. The provision of large amounts of energy can therefore be accomplished by infusing a small volume of an isotonic emulsion. The most commonly used preparation of intravenous fat emulsion is Intralipid (Table 27.18), a 20% solution providing 2000 cal in 1000 ml with an osmolality of 250 mOsmol/kg.

Intralipid is prepared from fractionated soybean oil to provide 85% unsaturated and polyunsaturated triglycerides. Egg phosphatides are used as emulsifers and glycerol is used to render the water phase isotonic. The emulsion particle size in an Intralipid emulsion resembles the size of chylomicrons. Intralipid is thus cleared in the same way as chylomicrons but lipaemia may occur rarely. This is more likely if fat emulsions are infused rapidly as part of an intermittent infusion regimen.

Fat emulsion infusion is necessary to cover the daily requirement for essential fatty acids, phosphate and fat-soluble vitamins. Essential fatty acids form a necessary and considerable part of cell membrane phospholipids and are precursors of prostaglandins and thromboxanes. The parent essential fatty acids (linoleic and linolenic acids) can only be synthesized by plants although their further metabolism to polyunsaturated derivatives and prostaglandins can only be accomplished by animals. Certain animals, although not man, cannot accomplish the synthesis of the derivatives and are therefore obligatory carnivores.

Adverse effects of fat emulsion infusion are now rare. Older preparations were not cleared as efficiently as modern preparations relying heavily on reticuloendothelial system uptake. Side-effects associated with prolonged use of fat emulsions included reticuloendothelial system dysfunction. Prolonged infusion of Intralipid has been associated rarely with reticuloendothelial system uptake.

TABLE 27.18 Percentage fatty acid composition of Intralipid

Linoleic acid	54
Oleic acid	26
Palmitic acid	9
Linolenic acid	8
Stearic acid	3

Water, electrolytes and minerals

While water requirement may be high in certain conditions of excessive loss, it is more common that the amount of water required to give infusion solutions a reasonable osmolality is high.

The electrolyte and mineral contents of common supplement solutions are shown in Table 27.19. Sodium and potassium balance are best managed with reference to baseline daily requirements adjusted according to individual clinical conditions. It must be remembered that at least 5 mmol potassium is required for utilization of 1 g nitrogen in the form of amino acids. Calcium and magnesium are similarly given according to daily requirements adjusted according to clinical conditions.

Inorganic phosphate requirements are increased in illness and where carbohydrates are metabolized in great quantity or in states of insulin excess. Hypophosphataemia is a common sequel of parenteral nutrition, particularly in patients receiving L-amino acid solutions and carbohydrates alone.

Trace elements are necessary as cofactors for enzyme systems. In man it is known that chromium, cobalt, copper, fluoride, iodine, iron, manganese, molybdenum, selenium and zinc are essential minerals. Deficiency states have been described for each but are only likely in prolonged parenteral nutrition.

Vitamins

Table 27.20 shows the vitamin contents of commonly used supplemental preparations. None of the vitamin preparations can provide the whole of the basal daily requirement alone. A combination of Solivito N and Vitlipid N covers daily requirements for a normal man, the apparent deficiency of vitamin E being covered by its presence in Intralipid. In disease states vitamin requirements can increase dramatically requiring

TABLE 27.19 Electrolyte and mineral content of supplement solutions

	RECOMMENDED	ADDAMEL 10 ml	ADDITRACE 10 ml	ADDIPHOS 20 ml
Na^+	70–220 mmol	—	—	30 mmol
K^+	60–120 mmol	—	—	30 mmol
Ca^{2+}	5–10 mmol	5 mmol	—	—
Mg^{2+}	5 20 mmol	1.5 mmol	—	—
Fe^{3+}	20 µmol	50 µmol	20 µmol	—
Zn^{2+}	100 µmol	20 µmol	100 µmol	—
Mn^{2+}	5 µmol	40 µmol	5 µmol	—
Cu^{2+}	20 µmol	5 µmol	20 µmol	—
Cr^{3+}	0.2 µmol	—	0.2 µmol	—
Se^{4+}	0.4 µmol	—	0.4 µmol	—
Mo^{6+}	0.2 µmol	—	0.2 µmol	—
PO^{4-}	20–40 mmol	—	—	40 mmol
F^-	50 µmol	50 µmol	50 µmol	—
I^-	1 µmol	1 µmol	1 µmol	—
Cl^-	70–220 mmol	13.3 mmol	—	—

TABLE 27.20 Vitamin contents of supplement solutions

	RECOMMENDED BASAL	SOLIVITO N 1 VIAL	MULTIBIONTA 10 ml	VITLIPID N 10 ml	PARENTEROVITE IVHP 10 ml
Retinol (vitamin A)	700 µg	—	5.9 mg	990 µg	—
Thiamine (vitamin B_1)	1.4 mg	3 mg	50 mg	—	250 mg
Riboflavine (vitamin B_2)	2.1 mg	3.6 mg	10 mg	—	4 mg
Nicotinamide	14 mg	40 mg	100 mg	—	160 mg
Pyridoxine (vitamin B_6)	2.1 mg	4 mg	15 mg	—	50 mg
Pantothenic acid	14 mg	15.3 mg	25 mg	—	—
Biotin	350 µg	60 µg	—	—	—
Cyanocobalamin (vitamin B_{12})	2.1 µg	5 µg	—	—	—
Folic acid	210 µg	400 mg	—	—	—
Ascorbic acid (vitamin C)	35 mg	100 mg	50 mg	—	500 mg
Ergocalciferol (vitamin D_2)	2.8 µg	—	—	5 µg	—
dl-α-tocopherol (vitamin E)	32 mg	—	5 mg	9.1 mg	—
Phytomenadione (vitamin K_1)	140 µg	—	—	150 µg	—

supplementation with other less complete but more concentrated preparations.

The vitamin preparations should generally be infused in the fat emulsion since the B group vitamins are light sensitive. Alternatively protection from light can be achieved by a light-proof bag.

Complications of parenteral nutrition

Many of the metabolic complications of parenteral nutrition have been mentioned with reference to the individual nutrient sources above. With modern solutions and parenteral feeding techniques, complications of parenteral nutrition are more commonly related to choice of delivery system and intravenous route. Infusion of the hyperosmolar solutions required to provide adequate nutrients for all but short-term parenteral nutrition requires central venous access. In addition to the possibility of catheter misplacement, damage to adjacent structures and venous thrombosis, the most common catheter-related problem remains infection. Parenteral nutrition solutions provide ideal conditions for bacterial growth when infused at room temperature over a 24-h period. Strict asepsis is therefore required both with respect to care of the catheter and to care of the infusion system. There should be no break of the infusion system at any time other than to connect the next container of feed. Thus there should be no addition of drugs to the parenteral feed once it has been connected and there should be no monitoring or blood sampling through the central venous catheter. Modern parenteral nutrition solutions can be compounded such that all nutrients can be infused from a single large flexible container. Compounding is either done at manufacture or in specially designed sterile pharmacy suites with a laminar flow hood. Manufacturers of parenteral nutrition solutions are listed in Table 27.21.

TABLE 27.21 Manufacturers of parenteral nutrition solutions

B Braun Medical Ltd	Aminoplasmal L3 Aminoplasmal L5 Aminoplasmal L10
Bencard	Parenterovite IVHP
E Merck Ltd	Aminofusin Forte Multibionta Perifusin
Geistlich Sons Ltd	Aminoplex 5 Aminoplex 12 Aminoplex 14 Aminoplex 24 Hepanutrin
Kabi Vitrum Ltd	Addamel Addiphos Additrace Intralipid 10% Intralipid 20% Solivito N Vamin 9 Vamin 9 glucose Vamin 14 Vamin 18 Vitlipid N
MCP Pharmaceuticals Ltd	Aminoven 12
Travenol Laboratories Ltd	Synthamin 9 Synthamin 14 Synthamin 17

FURTHER READING

Edelman LS, Leibman J. Anatomy of body water and electrolytes. *American Journal of Medicine* 1969; **27**: 256.

Karren SJ, Alberti KGMM. *Practical nutritional support.* London: Pitman, 1980.

Mishler JM. Synthetic plasma volume expanders—their pharmacology, safety and clinical efficacy. *Clinical Haematology* 1984 **13** (1): 75–92.

Robarts WM, Parkin JV, Hobsley M. A simple clinical approach to quantifying loss from the extracellular and plasma compartments. *Annals of the Royal College of Surgeons of England* 1979; **61**: 142–5.

Shenkin A, Fell GS, Halls DJ, Dunbar PM, Holbrook IB, Irving MH. Essential trace element provision to patients receiving home IVN in the United Kingdom. *Human Nutrition, Clinical Nutrition* 1986; **5**: 91–7.

Webb AR. The physical properties of plasma substitutes. *Clinical Intensive Care* 1990; **1**: 58–61.

Woolfson AMJ. Intravenous feeding – a review of current practice. *Clinical Nutrition* 1981; **4**: 187–94.

Vitamin and trace element recommendations during intravenous nutrition: theory and practice. *Proceedings of the Nutrition Society* 1986; **45**: 383–90.

28

Kidneys

PART I RENAL FUNCTION AND DRUGS

KM Erbeck, GR Aronoff

INTRODUCTION

Patients with renal disease are difficult management problems. Uraemia affects every organ system in the body. Platelet dysfunction, poor wound healing, anaemia, and volume excess state are challenges in the perioperative period. In addition, changes in the absorption, distribution, metabolism and excretion of drugs must be taken into account when dosing patients with renal disease. The problems of end-stage renal disease are often superimposed on underlying hypertension, diabetes and heart disease, compounding the complexity of management.

The kidney is the major regulator of the internal fluid environment. Therefore, the physiological changes associated with renal disease can be expected to have pronounced effects on the pharmacology of many drugs. Physicians caring for patients during the perioperative period must possess a basic understanding of the biochemical and physiological effects of drugs in patients with the inability to excrete waste products, excess salt and water, and drugs. This chapter deals with these problems, and offers suggestions on how to deal effectively with the patient with impaired renal function.

INITIAL PATIENT ASSESSMENT

Knowledge of previous medication history, drug-related allergy or toxicity, and concurrent medicines is important in the initial evaluation of patients with renal disease undergoing anaesthesia. Estimating extracellular fluid volume is necessary to determine the distribution volume of anaesthetics and analgesics that might be used. Measurements of body height and weight are needed to individualize the drug regimen. For obese patients, ideal body weight (IBW) should be calculated. For men, IBW is 50 kg plus 2.3 kg for each inch over five feet. For women, IBW is 45.5 kg plus 2.3 kg for each inch over five feet. Many clinicians use the average of the measured body weight and the ideal body weight as the value on which to base drug doses.[1]

Evaluating functional impairment of other excretory organs is also important. The failure of other organs limits the possibilities for alternate pathways of drug and metabolite elimination. For instance, the stigmata of liver disease suggest the potential need to further substantially alter drug dosages in patients with impaired renal function.

Reviewing the possibility of drug interactions before choosing anaesthetic agents reduces potentially adverse drug effects. Focusing therapy on specific diagnoses allows the clinician to limit the number of drugs the patient is taking prior to surgery and lessens the chances of untoward drug interactions.

MEASURING RENAL FUNCTION

The rate of drug and metabolite elimination by the kidneys is proportional to the glomerular filtration rate. Before surgery, renal function can be estimated from the Cockcroft and Gault expression:[2]

$$Cl_{\mathrm{cr}} = \frac{(140 - \text{age}) \times (\text{IBW in kg})}{72 \times (S_{\mathrm{cr}} \text{ in mg/dl})} \times (0.85 \text{ if female})$$

where Cl_{cr} is the creatinine clearance, IBW is the ideal body weight and S_{cr} is the serum creatinine concentration. In patients with unstable renal function, the serum creatinine does not reflect the true clearance rate. Therefore, renal function should be estimated by timed urine collection before surgery. The midpoint serum creatinine should be used when calculating creatinine clearance for the collection period. If the patient is oliguric, creatinine clearance can be assumed to be less than 5 ml/min.

The serum creatinine reflects muscle mass, as well as glomerular filtration rate. Serum creatinine measurements within the normal range are frequently used to establish the presence of 'normal' renal function. This erroneous assumption may cause serious overdose and resultant toxic drug or metabolite accumulation in elderly or debilitated patients with decreased muscle mass.

PHYSIOLOGICAL EFFECTS OF DECREASED RENAL FUNCTION

The major determinant of extracellular fluid (ECF) volume is sodium. As the glomerular filtration rate decreases to less than 25% of normal, the ability of the kidney to respond to changes in sodium is limited.[3] Therefore, ECF volume expansion is a common problem in the patient with chronic renal failure. Signs of ECF volume excess include peripheral oedema, pulmonary oedema, and hypertension.

The patient with evidence of fluid overload should be diuresed or dialysed to normal ECF volume prior to surgery if possible. On the other hand, patients with renal insufficiency due to polycystic kidney disease or pyelonephritis accompanied by salt wasting with hypovolaemia are at risk for hypotension due to vasodilatation at the time of induction of anaesthesia.[4] Invasive monitoring with Swan Ganz catheterization or central venous pressure monitoring may be helpful in determining the volume status.

Disorders of potassium in patients with renal disease, particularly hyperkalaemia, may be exacerbated during perioperative management. Tissue trauma, anaesthetic agents such as succinylcholine, and transfusion of packed red blood cells may all contribute to hyperkalaemia.

The severity of hyperkalaemia dictates management. In general, ECG changes rarely occur with potassium levels less than 6 mmol/l. Any elevation of potassium greater than 6 mmol/l with or without ECG changes such as peaked T waves, QRS widening, or loss of P waves should be treated. Treatment includes calcium gluconate to stabilize cardiac membranes, and bicarbonate, glucose, and insulin to shift potassium into cells. These temporary therapies do not alter the total body stores of potassium. Therefore, sodium/potassium exchange resins or dialysis must be employed to permanently remove potassium from the body. Immediately postoperative potassium levels should be measured to assess the need for intervention.

Although unusual, hypokalaemia may occur in patients with chronic renal failure in the presence of diarrhoea, biliary fistulae, or continuous nasogastric suction. The replacement of potassium must be cautious in these patients with frequent repeat levels after supplementation.

Hypocalcaemia is often asymptomatic in patients with chronic renal failure despite levels below 7.5 mg/dl (1.88 mmol/l). The ionized calcium may be normal when corrected for hypoalbuminaemia (0.8 mg/dl (0.2 mmol/l) for every 1 g below normal albumin). Also, the acidaemia of renal failure results in a higher ionized calcium. Therefore, restoration of normal pH may precipitate symptomatic hypocalcaemia with tetany, laryngeal stridor, seizures and cardiac instability.[5] Transfusion of blood containing citrate may also result in symptomatic hypocalcaemia.

The inability of the diseased kidney to produce ammonia for titration of acid leads to chronic metabolic acidosis, characterized by the presence of an abnormally increased anion gap. The resulting acidaemia causes depression of myocardial contractility with serum bicarbonate levels less than 20 mEq/l. Associated hyperkalaemia adds to the risk of cardiac arrhythmia. Preoperatively, the blood pH should be greater than 7.25 to lessen these complications. Acidaemia may be treated with exogenous bicarbonate or dialysis.

Haematological derangements such as chronic anaemia and platelet dysfunction are common in patients with renal disease. Transfusion is rarely necessary prior to surgery if the haematocrit is above 25%. The decision to transfuse must take into account the volume and potassium accompanying the cells. It may be advisable to transfuse patients with renal failure while on dialysis to avoid these complications. The use of erythropoietin has diminished the need for transfusion in patients with end-stage renal disease.

Although the pathology of platelet dysfunction in uraemic patients is not well defined, elevation of the bleeding time despite a normal platelet count is common. Approaches to treatment have included haemodialysis, deamino 8-D arginine vasopressin (DDAVP), cryoprecipitate, and conjugated oestrogens. The administration of 0.3 μg/kg DDAVP immediately preoperatively can shorten the bleeding time. This effect may last up to 4 h.[6] When longer duration of action is needed, conjugated oestrogens may have an extra benefit, with the effects lasting up to 14 days.[7] However, the onset of action may be as long as 6 h. The dosage of conjugated oestrogens is 1–3 mg/kg intravenously or orally. Haemodialysis does not completely correct the bleeding time in patients with severe renal failure.

The neurological sequelae of chronic renal disease include peripheral and autonomic neuropathy. The peripheral neuropathy of end-stage renal disease is both sensory and motor. Uraemic neuropathy may present with decreased deep tendon reflexes and diminished sensation in the lower extremities. Nerve conduction velocity is slowed. Autonomic neuropathy prevents the normal sympathetic response to hypotension, particularly important at the time of induction of anaesthesia.

Hypertension seen in patients with chronic renal disease is often the result of volume excess. This effect may be prevented with diuretics, dialysis and antihypertensive medications. A variety of antihypertensive drugs may be used when intravascular volume is normal and patients remain hypertensive.

Blood pressure may be labile when patients present with hypertension and volume excess requiring the removal of large amounts of fluid. In order to prevent hypotension on haemodialysis, antihypertensive treatment must be cautious. High plasma renin levels are present in a portion of dialysis patients, identified by hypertension refractory to volume control and antihypertensive medication. The dialytic removal of volume from these individuals may result in a higher blood pressure rather than the desired effect.

EFFECTS OF URAEMIA ON DRUG DISPOSITION

Bioavailability

The amount of a drug that enters the general circulation and the rate at which it appears are called bioavailability. Drugs given intravenously enter the venous circulation directly and generally demonstrate rapid onset of action. Drugs given by other routes must first traverse a series of membranes and may need to pass through important organs of elimination before entering the systemic circulation. Only a fraction of the administered dose may reach the site of drug action. Even drugs given intravenously and by inhalation must pass through the lungs before reaching arterial blood flow. Like other organs, the lungs may remove substantial amounts of the agents.

For drugs given orally, the rate and extent of gastrointestinal absorption are important considerations. Once an orally administered drug is absorbed into the portal circulation, it must pass through the liver. Therefore, the bioavailability of an orally administered drug is also dependent on the extent of its metabolism during its first pass through the liver.

Generally, gastrointestinal absorption of drugs is decreased in patients with uraemia. Gastrointestinal symptoms are common in uraemia, but little specific information about bowel function is available in patients with renal failure. When urea accumulates in the plasma, the salivary concentration of urea increases as well. In the presence of gastric urease, ammonia is formed which buffers gastric acid and increases gastric pH. The ammonia is absorbed and converted to urea again by the liver. the gastric alkalinizing effect of his internal urea–ammonia cycle has been suspected to decrease the absorption of drugs that are best absorbed in an acidic environment.[8] In addition, the dissolution of many tablet dosage forms requires the acid environment normally found in the stomach. Absorption of these products may be incomplete and may occur more slowly in an alkaline environment.

The ingestion of multivalent cations frequently used in antacids may also diminish drug absorption.[9] Patients with renal impairment often ingest large quantities of antacids to bind dietary phosphate. Chelation and the formation of non-absorbable complexes reduce bioavailability of some drugs by as much as 80%.

Impaired gastrointestinal absorptive function has also been demonstrated. Craig and colleagues showed that the absorption of the simple sugar, D-xylose is reduced in patients with renal failure.[10] Gastroparesis, commonly observed in diabetic patients with renal failure, may prolong gastric emptying and delay drug absorption. Similarly, diarrhoea may decrease gut transit time and diminish drug absorption by the small bowel.

First-pass hepatic metabolism may be altered in uraemia. Decreased biotransformation may lead to the appearance of increased amounts of active drug in the systemic circulation and enhanced bioavailability of some drugs. Conversely, impaired protein binding may allow more free drug to be available at the site of hepatic metabolism, thereby increasing the amount of drug removed during the hepatic first pass. With the complex interaction of absorption and first-pass hepatic metabolism, it is not surprising that drug bioavailability is more variable in patients with renal impairment than in patients with normal renal function.

Distribution

After a drug is administered, it is dispersed throughout the body at a given rate. At equilibrium, the apparent volume of distribution is calculated by dividing the amount of the drug in the body by its plasma concentration. This apparent volume of distribution does not correspond to a specific anatomical space but rather is a mathematical construct used to estimate the dose of a drug to be given in order to achieve a therapeutic plasma concentration. Agents that are highly protein bound, or those that are water soluble, tend to be restricted to the ECF space and have small volumes of distribution. On the other hand, drugs that are highly lipid soluble penetrate body tissues and exhibit large volumes of distribution.

Renal insufficiency frequently alters drug distribution volume. Oedema and ascites may increase the apparent volume of distribution of highly water-soluble or protein-bound drugs. Usual doses of such drugs given to oedematous patients may result in inadequate, low plasma levels. Conversely, dehydration or muscle wasting tend to decrease the volume of distribution. In these cases, usual doses may result in unexpectedly high plasma concentrations.

The alteration of plasma-protein binding in patients with renal insufficiency is an important factor affecting eventual drug action. The volume of distribution of a drug, the quantity of free drug available for action, and the degree to which the agent can be eliminated by hepatic or renal excretion are all influenced by protein binding. Drugs that are protein bound attach reversibly either to albumin or glycoprotein in plasma. Organic acids are thought to bind to a single binding site, while organic bases probably have multiple sites of attachment.[11]

The binding of many acidic drugs is decreased in renal failure.[12] Organic bases, on the other hand, are less affected by altered protein binding. Reduced protein binding has generally been attributed to a combination of decreased serum albumin concentration and a reduction in albumin affinity for the drug. Even when the plasma albumin concentration is normal, the protein-binding defect of some drugs correlates with the level of azotaemia.[13,14] As illustrated in Fig. 28.1, affinity may be influenced by uraemia-induced changes in the structural orientation of the albumin molecule or by the accumulation of endogenous inhibitors of protein binding which compete with drugs for their binding sites.

The consequences of impaired plasma protein binding in uraemia are important since the unbound fraction of several acidic drugs may be substantially increased. Serious toxicity can occur if the total plasma concentration of these drugs is pushed into the therapeutic range by increasing the dose. For such drugs, total and unbound plasma concentrations should be measured.

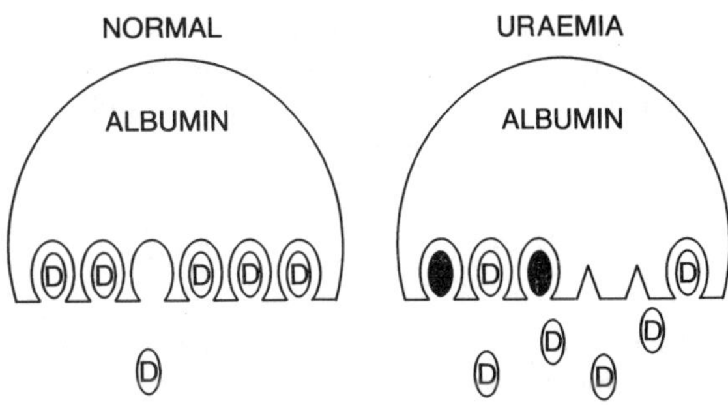

FIGURE 28.1 Protein binding defect in uraemia. Displacement of drug (D) from its binding site by the accumulation of undefined uraemic toxin or a uraemia-induced conformational change in the binding site geometry results in more free drug in plasma.

Predicting the clinical consequences of altered protein binding in uraemia is difficult. Although decreased binding results in more free drug being available at the site of drug action or toxicity, the distribution volume may be increased, resulting in lower plasma concentrations after a given dose. In addition, since more unbound drug is available for metabolism and excretion, the half-life of the drug in the body may be decreased.

Metabolism

Renal failure substantially affects drug biotransformation. The rate of reduction and hydrolysis reactions is generally slowed. For example, peptide and ester hydrolysis are substantially reduced. Glucuronidation, sulphate conjugation and microsomal oxidation usually occur at normal rates in patients with uraemia.[15]

The production of active or toxic metabolites is an important aspect of drug metabolism in patients with renal failure. Many of these metabolites depend on the kidneys for their removal from the body. The high incidence of adverse drug reactions seen in renal failure may be explained in part by the accumulation of active metabolites.

CALCULATING DRUG DOSES

The goal of the initial drug dose is to rapidly achieve therapeutic drug concentrations. A loading dose equivalent to the dose given to a patient with normal renal function should be given to patients with renal impairment, if the physical examination suggests normal ECF volume. If the loading dose of a drug is not known, it can be calculated from the following expression:

$$\text{Loading dose} = V_d \times \text{IBW} \times C_p$$

where V_d is the drug's volume of distribution in l/kg, IBW is the patient's ideal body weight in kg, and C_p is the desired steady-state plasma drug concentration.

Several methods can be used to determine subsequent drug doses. The fraction of the normal dose recommended for a patient with renal insufficiency can be calculated as follows:

$$D_f = F_u \times \left[\left(\frac{Cl_{cr}}{120}\right) - 1\right] + 1$$

where D_f is the fraction of the normal dose to be given, F_u is the fraction of the drug excreted unchanged in the urine, and Cl_{cr} is the creatinine clearance. When the fraction of the drug excreted unchanged in the urine is not known, the ratio of the drug's half-life in patients with normal renal function ($t_{\frac{1}{2}}$ normal) to that measured in patients with renal failure ($t_{\frac{1}{2}}$ renal) may be substituted as follows:

$$D_f = (t_{\frac{1}{2}}\ \text{normal} \div t_{\frac{1}{2}}\ \text{renal}) \times [(Cl_{cr} \div 120) - 1] + 1$$

To maintain the normal dose interval in patients with renal impairment, the amount of each dose, following the loading dose, can be determine from the following relationship:

$$\text{Dose in renal impairment} = \text{Normal dose} \times D_f$$

The resulting dose is usually given at the same dose interval as that for patients with normal renal function. This method is effective for drugs with a narrow therapeutic range and a short plasma half-life. Figure 28.2 illustrates plasma concentrations following an initial loading dose and reduction of the individual doses.

Prolonging the dose interval in patients with impaired renal function is frequently a convenient method to reduce drug dosage. This method is particularly useful for drugs with a broad therapeutic range and long plasma half-life. If prolonging the dose interval, rather than decreasing the individual doses, is desirable, the dose interval in renal impairment can be estimated from the following expression:

$$\text{Dose interval in renal impairment} = \text{Normal dose interval} \div D_f$$

If the range between therapeutic and toxic levels is too narrow, either potentially toxic or subtherapeutic plasma concentrations may result. The resulting plasma concentrations from prolonging the dose interval in an individual with impaired renal function are shown in Fig. 28.3.

A combined approach using both the dose reduction and interval prolongation methods is often practical. The dosage is modified by multiplying the usual daily maintenance dose by the dose fraction. Once the average daily dose is calculated, it can be divided into convenient dosing intervals. The decision to extend the dosing interval beyond a 24-h period should be based on the need to maintain therapeutic peak or trough levels. The dosing interval may be prolonged if the peak level is most important. When the minimum

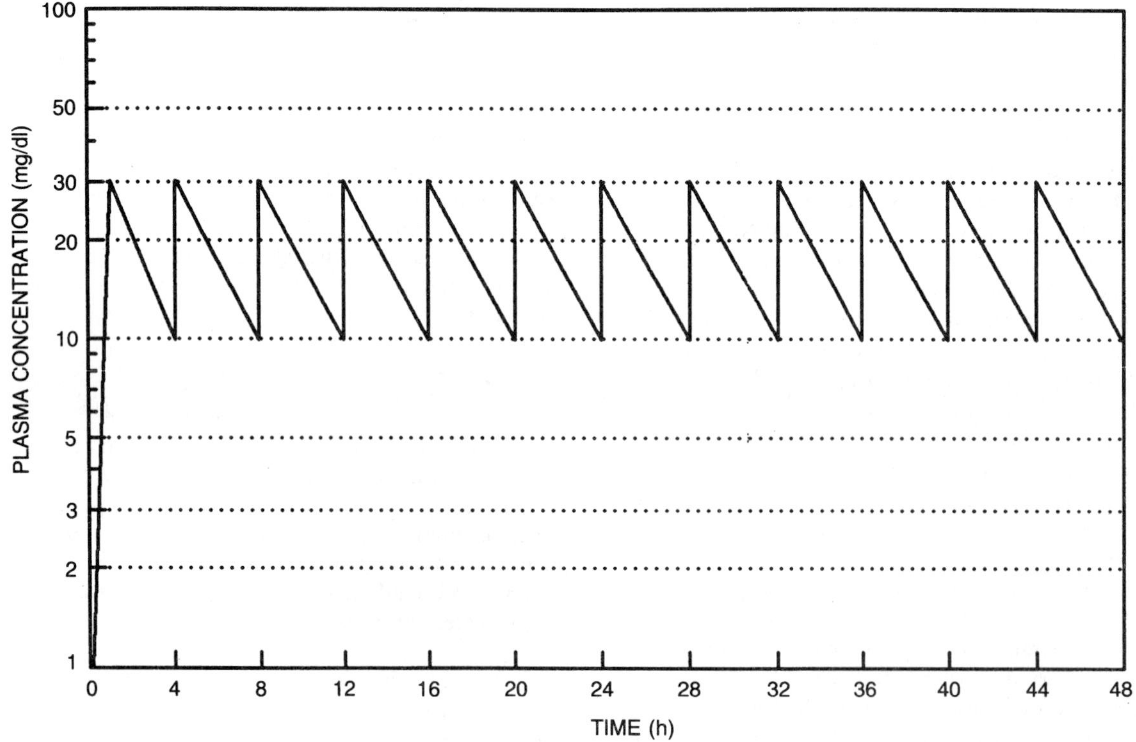

FIGURE 28.2 Plasma concentrations following a normal loading dose and reduced maintenance doses. This approach avoids high peak and low trough concentrations and is best for drugs with a narrow range between the therapeutic and toxic concentrations.

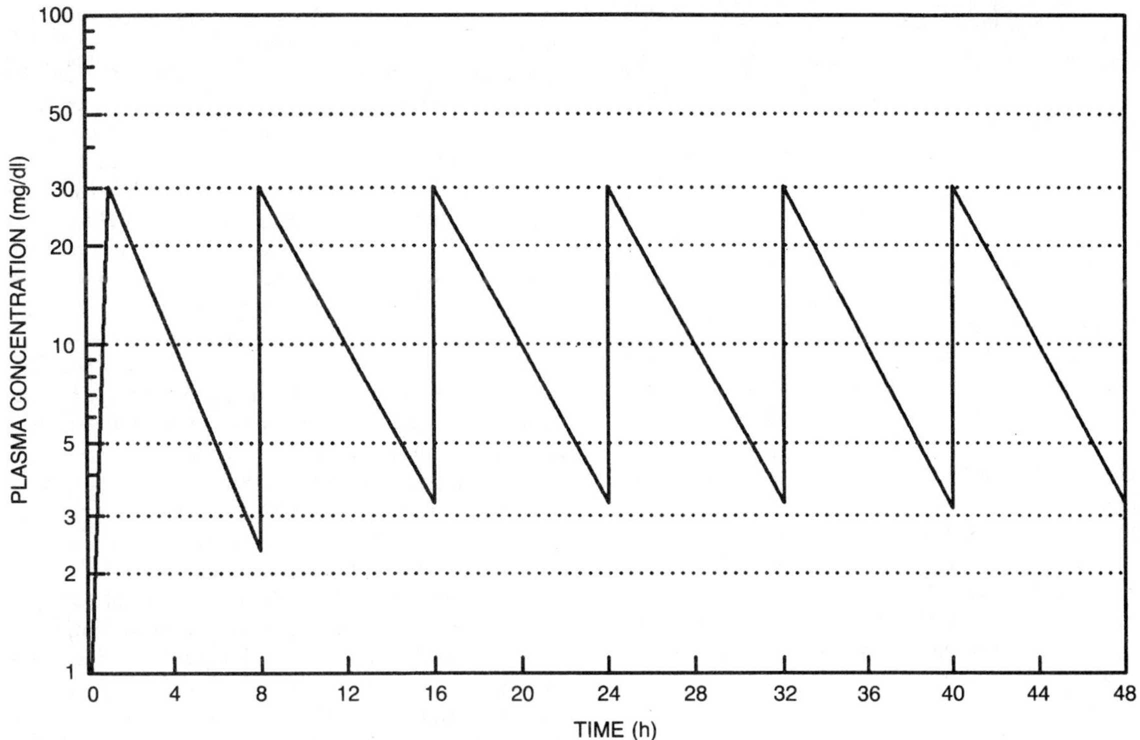

FIGURE 28.3 Plasma concentrations following a normal loading dose and repeated normal doses at a prolonged dose interval. Higher peak and lower trough concentrations result.

trough level must be maintained, it may be preferable to modify the individual dose or utilize a combination of dose and interval methods to determine the correct dosing strategy.

DRUG-LEVEL MONITORING

Measurement of plasma drug concentrations may be helpful in assessing a particular dosage regimen when the relationship between drug levels and efficacy or toxicity has been established. These measurements are clearly most important for drugs with a narrow therapeutic range or difficult to measure pharmacological effects.

Serum levels may be determined after an appropriate loading dose has been given. In the absence of a loading dose, three or four doses of the drug should be administered before serum levels are measured. This ensures that a steady-state serum concentration has been established. For some drugs, both maximum and minimum concentrations are relevant. Peak levels are most meaningful when measured after rapid drug distribution has occurred. Conversely, minimum concentrations are usually measured just before giving the next scheduled dose. A practical schema for drug prescribing in patients with renal impairment is shown in Fig. 28.4.

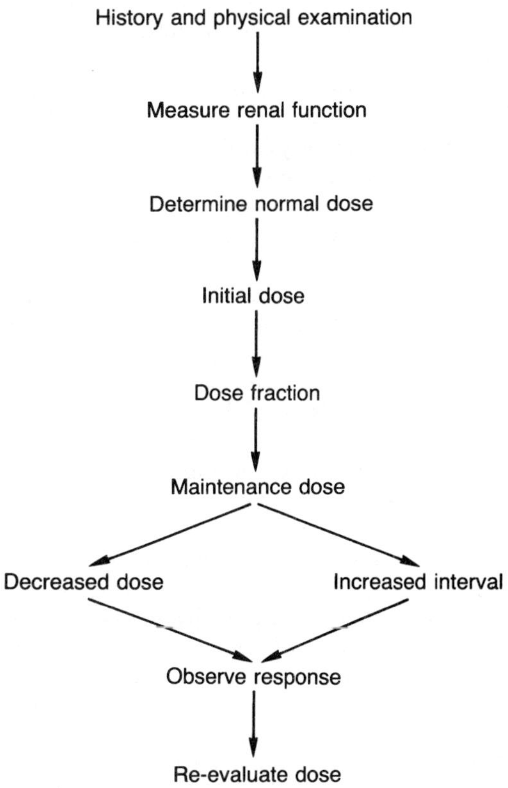

FIGURE 28.4 A practical schema for drug dosing in patients with impaired renal function.

DRUG SELECTION IN RENAL IMPAIRMENT

The choice of medication in the patient with renal dysfunction depends in part upon the severity of renal disease. In the patient with renal insufficiency, it is essential to avoid those drugs that are potentially nephrotoxic. Decreased dosage of those drugs metabolized or excreted by the kidneys is also prudent.

Despite the hepatic metabolism of narcotics, their effects are prolonged in the patient with renal disease. For example, the clearance of glucuronide metabolites of morphine is impaired. Therefore, the effect of morphine is the sum of the parent compound and its metabolites.[16] The uraemic patient is more susceptible to respiratory depression due to decreased plasma protein binding.

This effect occurs especially in hypoalbuminaemic patients. As mentioned previously, the accumulation of normeperidine, the metabolite of meperidine, produces seizures in patients with renal failure. Meperidine should be avoided in patients who cannot excrete the potentially toxic metabolite.

Fentanyl is excreted in the urine after biotransformation in the liver. Only a small percentage is excreted unchanged by the kidney.[17]

Benzodiazepines are widely used for preoperative medication. Like narcotics, they may cause excessive sedation and encephalopathy in patients with renal disease due to the formation of active metabolites, decreased protein binding, and increased volume of distribution.

The alkaloids, atropine and hyoscyamine, should be avoided in the patient with severe renal insufficiency and patients requiring dialysis. These drugs may cause prolonged neurological effects. Psychiatric disturbances and seizures have been reported.[18] Scopolamine should be administered cautiously to these patients.

When barbiturates are used in patients with renal impairment, drugs with a short half-life and metabolized by the liver should be chosen. Thiopental is metabolized by the liver, and has a half-life of 6–18 h in patients with renal disease. This compares with a half-life of 117–160 h for pentobarbital in the same patients.[19] However, changes in protein binding may enhance the effect of thiopental and increase its toxicity. Twice as much thiopental is unbound in patients with severe renal insufficiency as in patients with normal renal function.[20]

The kidneys excrete most of the neuromuscular-blocking drugs. Decreased cholinesterase levels in chronic renal disease may result in prolongation of the effects of these agents. Thirty to forty per cent of *d*-tubocurare is normally excreted by the kidneys. However, more of the drug can be eliminated by the liver in patients with renal failure.[21] This drug is preferred over pancuronium, which has the same renal excretion, but has an active metabolite that accumulates in uraemic patients and may be responsible for the inability to reverse its effect.[22]

Succinylcholine produces a transient rise in the serum potassium, and should be avoided in patients with impaired ability to excrete potassium. Gallamine and decamethonium should not be used in patients with renal disease. The kidneys excrete 85–100% of the dose of these drugs. Their half-life in renal failure is nearly 6 h. Prolonged paralysis has been reported with metocurine, which is excreted unchanged in the urine.

The newer non-depolarizing neuromuscular-blocking agents are not dependent on renal excretion, and are therefore preferable in the patient with renal disease. Vecuronium is predominantly excreted in bile. Its action is not prolonged in patients with renal failure. The metabolite of the neuromuscular-blocking agent, atracurium, has no activity other than stimulation of the central nervous system. Atracurium is broken down by Hofmann elimination and ester hydrolysis.

A phenomenon known as recurarization occurs after neuromuscular blockade. Recurrence of paralysis occurs after the surgical procedure has been completed. Initially, this observation was thought to be due to the decreasing effects of apparently satisfactory reversal with neostigmine. However, studies have demonstrated that the renal excretion of neostigmine, like *d*-tubocurare, is decreased in patients with renal disease, which should theoretically lead to prolongation of the effect.[23] The event is now thought to be a combination of rewarming after hypothermia with reactivation of the neuromuscular blocker, acidaemia and electrolyte imbalance. All contribute to the prolonged residual muscle relaxation.

The inhalation agents used in patients with renal disease were limited in the past due to their nephrotoxicity. Methoxyflurane is nephrotoxic and should not be used in patients with pre-existing renal disease. The metabolism of methoxyflurane results in deposition of oxalate in the kidney. Inorganic fluoride is toxic to the proximal tubular cells. Enflurane is also nephrotoxic.[24]

Halothane does not depend on renal excretion. However, the idiosyncratic hepatotoxicity occurring on subsequent exposure to halothane makes this drug less attractive. The combination of nitrous oxide, a narcotic and a neuromuscular blocking agent for induction requires a fairly high concentration of nitrous oxide, thereby limiting the oxygen delivery. This effect may be significant in patients with chronic anaemia whose oxygen-carrying capacity is limited. Isoflurane is considered safe for patients with renal disease.

Regional blockade is an attractive alternative to general anaesthesia in the patient with renal disease. Brachial plexus blockade is beneficial in the creation of an arteriovenous fistula due to the sympathetic blockade with subsequent peripheral vasodilatation. Slower nerve conduction in uraemic patients results in increased sensitivity to the effect of the local anaesthetic agent. Also, the decreased protein binding of local anaesthetics leads to increased availability to the tissues. Despite these factors, the duration of regional anaesthetic effects is shorter because of the higher cardiac index with resultant rapid venous removal of the drug.

CONCLUSION

Despite careful consideration of uraemia-induced changes in drug disposition, adverse drug responses remain common in patients with impaired renal function. Some toxicity can be eliminated by avoiding drugs known to cause adverse events as a result of direct toxicity of the drug or its metabolites, poor efficacy of the drug in decreased renal function, or production of an increased metabolic load that diseased kidneys cannot excrete.

The heterogeneity of renal disease makes responses to drug therapy quite variable. Dosage nomograms, drug tables, and computer-assisted dosing recommendations provide guidelines for deriving an initial approach to drug administration in patients with decreased renal function. Continuing evaluation of therapeutic response and modification of the regimen individualized for each patient and each clinical situation ensure effective clinical management of patients with impaired renal function.

REFERENCES

1 Aronoff GR, Abel SR. Principles of administering drugs to patients with renal failure. In: Bennett WM, McCarron DA, Brenner BM, Stein JH eds. *Contemporary issues in nephrology. Pharmacotherapy of renal diseases and hypertension.* New York: Churchill Livingstone, 1987: 1.

2 Cockcroft DW, Gault MH. Prediction of creatinine clearance from serum creatinine. *Nephron* 1976; **16**: 31–4.

3 Epstein FH, Merrill JP. Chronic renal failure. In: Harrison TR ed. *Principles of internal medicine.* New York: McGraw Hill, 1972: 1373–83.

4 Burke JF, Francos GC. Surgery in the patient with acute or chronic renal failure. *Medical Clinics of North America* 1987; **79**: 489–97.

5 Gilbert PL, Stein R. Preoperative evaluation of the patient with chronic renal disease. *Mount Sinai Journal of Medicine* 1991; **58** (1): 69–74.

6 Mannucci PM, Remuzzi G, Pusineri F. Deamino-8-D-arginine vasopressin shortens the bleeding time in uremia. *New England Journal of Medicine* 1986; **315**: 731–5.

7 Livio M, Mannucci PM, Marchiaro G. Conjugated estrogens for the management of bleeding associated with renal failure. *New England Journal of Medicine* 1986; **315**: 736.

8 Anderson RJ, Gambertoglio JG, Schrier RW. *Clinical use of drugs in renal failure.* Springfield, IL: Charles C. Thomas, 1976.

9 Hurwitz A. Antacid therapy and drug kinetics. *Clinical Pharmacokinetics* 1977; **2**: 269–80.

10 Craig RM, Murphy P, Gibson TP, Quintanilla A. Kinetic analysis of D-xylose absorption in normal subjects and in patients with chronic renal failure. *Journal of Laboratory and Clinical Medicine.* 1983; **101**: 496–506.

11 Reidenberg MN. The binding of drugs to plasma proteins and the interpretation of measurements of plasma concentration of drugs in patients with poor renal function. *American Journal of Medicine* 1977; **62**: 482–5.

12 Dromgoole SH. The binding capacity of albumin and renal disease. *Journal of Pharmacology and Experimental Therapeutics.* 1974; **191**: 318–23.

13 Reidenberg MM, Affrime M. Influence of disease on binding of drugs to plasma proteins. *Annals of the New York Academy of Sciences.* 1973; **226**: 115–26.

14 Reidenberg MM, Odar-Cederlof I, Von Bahr C, Borga O, Sjoquist I. Protein binding of diphenylhydantoin and desmethylimipramine in plasma from patients with poor renal function. *New England Journal of Medicine* 1971; **285**: 264–7.

15 Reidenberg MN. The biotransformation of drugs in renal failure. *American Journal of Medicine* 1977; **62**: 482–5.

16 Sear JW, Hand CW, Moore RA, McQuay HJ. Studies on morphine disposition: influence of renal failure on the kinetics of morphine and its metabolites. *British Journal of Anesthesiology* 1989; **62**: 28–32.

17 Linke CL. Anesthesia considerations for renal transplantation. *Contemporary Anesthesia Practice* 1987; **10**: 183–231.

18 Richet G, Lopez de Novales E, Verroust P. Drug intoxication and neurological episodes in chronic renal failure. *British Medical Journal* 1970; **2**: 394–5.

19 Bennett WM, Aronoff GR, Golper TA, Morrison G, Singer I, Brater DC. *Drug prescribing in renal failure: dosing guidelines for adults.* Philadelphia: American College of Physicians, 1991.

20 Ghoneim MM, Pandya H. Plasma protein binding of thiopental in patients with impaired renal or hepatic function. *Anesthesiology* 1975; **42**: 545–9.

21 Cohen EN, Brewer HW, Smith D. The metabolism and elimination of d-tubocurarine-H^3. *Anesthesiology* 1967; **28**: 309–17.

22 Abrams RE, Hornbein RF. Inability to reverse pancuronium blockade in a patient with renal failure and hepatic disease. *Anesthesiology* 1975; **42**: 362–4.

23 Cronnelly R, Stanski DR, Miller RD. Renal function and the pharmacokinetics of neostigmine in anesthetized man. *Anesthesiology* 1979; **51**: 222–6.

24 Loehning RW, Mazze RI. Possible nephrotoxicity from enflurane in a patient with severe renal disease. *Anesthesiology* 1984; **40**: 203–5.

PART II DIURETIC DRUGS

AF Lant

INTRODUCTION

Diuretics were among the first synthetic drugs introduced into modern medicine. They remain among the most widely used in management of cardiovascular disease. Although initially introduced for the management of congestive cardiac failure, their application to the treatment of hypertension has expanded remarkably such that by the mid-1980s 118 million prescriptions were being issued per anum for diuretics in the USA alone.[1] Despite the advent of exciting newer vasodilators such as the angiotensin-converting enzyme (ACE) inhibitors, calcium-channel blockers and the selective α-blockers, diuretics have retained their primacy of position as first-line therapies in initial management of hypertension in both the USA[2] and the UK.[3] The effective partnership that diuretics form in combined use with ACE inhibitors in management of cardiac failure has not only offered dramatic relief of symptoms but has encouraged a preventative approach to be adopted that has also significantly improved prognosis in this highly lethal condition.[4]

At the same time as these clinical applications of diuretics have become firmly established, availability of these drugs has offered the investigational scientist powerful tools with which to explore the intricacies of renal function and also of ion transport mechanisms in a variety of non-renal tissues.[5,6]

CLASSIFICATION OF DIURETICS

The chemical characteristics of diuretics are heterogeneous; all share the common property of inhibiting renal sodium reabsorption and thereby inducing diuresis. A convenient classification with clinical relevance is that based on the maximal amount of filtered sodium chloride that is rejected by the kidney after diuretic administration; this inevitably reflects the selectivity of certain diuretics to inhibit specific sodium transporting mechanisms that are spatially separated within discrete segments of the nephron (Fig. 28.5).

Four major sites of action for diuretics have been identified. Site I corresponds to the proximal tubule; site II includes the medullary and cortical portions of the thick ascending limb of Henle's loop (TALH); site III is localized to the early portion of the distal tubule, while site IV includes the later portions of the distal tubule and cortical collecting tubule. In some instances, evidence has been obtained for diuretics operating at more than one segment of the nephron as, for example, some of the sulphonamide loop diuretics such as frusemide which also have actions in the proximal tubule, or some 'thiazide-like' agents such as metolazone which appear to act at both sites II and III. Although initially it was thought that the most powerful diuretics would be those whose actions were localized to the proximal tubule, it was soon realized that this was not the case because sodium chloride losses created by rejection proximally were mostly compensated for by increased sodium chloride reabsorption in more distal nephron segments, notably the loop of Henle, whose major contribution to renal sodium chloride reabsorption in man was underestimated for many years.

CHEMICAL INTERRELATIONSHIPS

Within the heterogeneous assembly of available diuretic agents a number of clearly defined chemical families can be identified (Table 28.1).

Phenoxyacetic acid analogues

The starting point for this group of diuretics was the organomercurial compound, merbaphen, tried as an antisyphilitic drug and found fortuitously to cause diuresis as an adverse effect.[7]

The systematic search for non-mercurial phenoxyacetic acid derivatives culminated in the development of ethacrynic acid as well as in the uricosuric diuretics, tienilic acid and indacrinone (Fig. 28.6). The latter drug has particularly interesting features in possessing an asymmetric carbon atom at the 2 position, which results in there being two optical isomers. The (+) isomer has the more powerful uricosuric properties while the (−) isomer is the more effective diuretic, acting predominantly in the ascending limb of Henle's loop.[8,9] Unfortunately, neither of these uricosuric diuretics is available for general clinical use.

Sulphamoyl-containing diuretics

Evolution of the sulphamoyl-containing diuretics also owes its origin to the fortuitous discovery of diuresis as an adverse effect, this time of sulphanilamide, a sulphonamide analogue that was being used clinically for its antimicrobial properties just before the Second World War. The occurrence of a mild alkaline diuresis coupled with a metabolic acidosis was soon followed by a realization that the inhibition of renal carbonic anhydrase was the responsible mechanism. The way was ready for the creation of an organized synthetic programme in which large numbers of sulphamoyl-

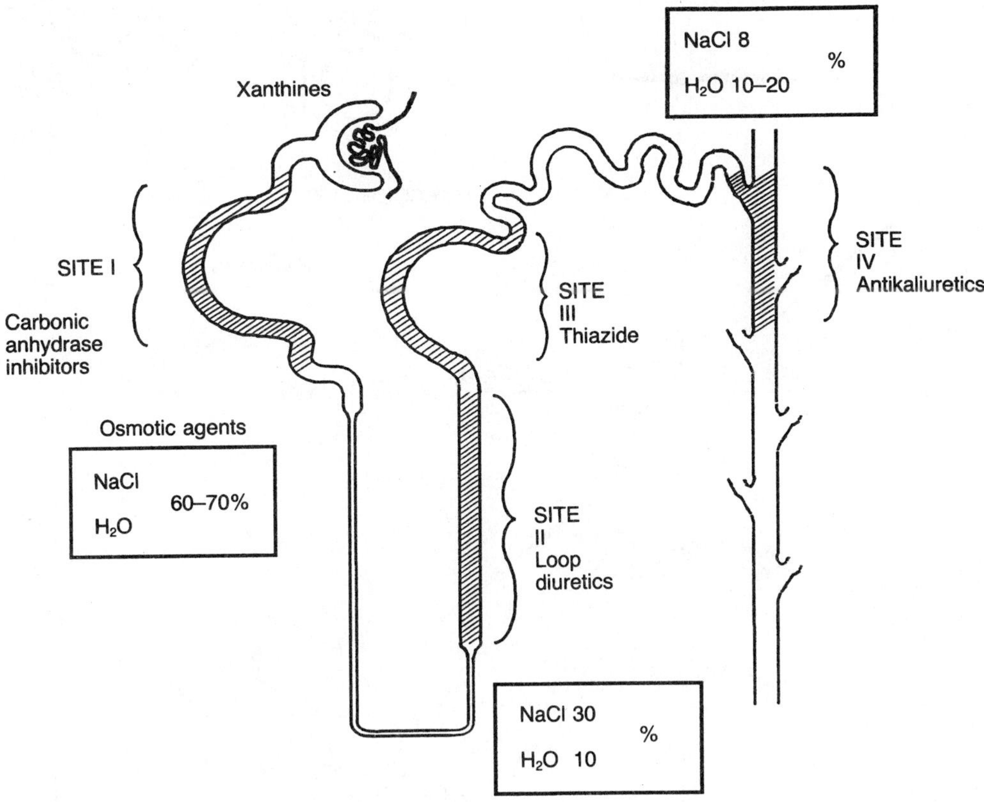

FIGURE 28.5 Diagrammatic representation of the major sites of action of diuretic agents within the nephron. Also shown are the relative proportions of the filtered load of sodium and water reabsorbed proximally, in the loop of Henle and in the distal segments of the nephron.

TABLE 28.1 Classification and principal sites of actions of diuretics. Percentages in parentheses are the drug-induced maximal fractional excretions of sodium chloride expressed as percentage of the filtered load of sodium chloride

High efficacy

(> 15% (thick ascending limb; site II))

Organomercurials

Mersalyl

Phenoxyacetic acids

Ethacrynic acid

Sulphamoyl benzoates

Frusemide

Bumetanide

Piretanide

Pyridine-sulphonylureas

Torasemide

Medium efficacy

(5–10% (early distal nephron; site III))

Chlorothiazide and thiazide family

Includes a large number of heterocyclic variants of the benzothiadiazine structure

Adjunct or weak diuretics

(< 5% (variable sites in nephron))

Xanthines (glomerular arteriolar dilators)

Mannitol (osmotic agent acting on site I, proximal tubule)

Potassium-sparing agents (distal nephron/collecting duct; site IV)

Aldosterone antagonists

Spironolactone

Canrenoate

Sodium-channel blockers

Triamterene

Amiloride

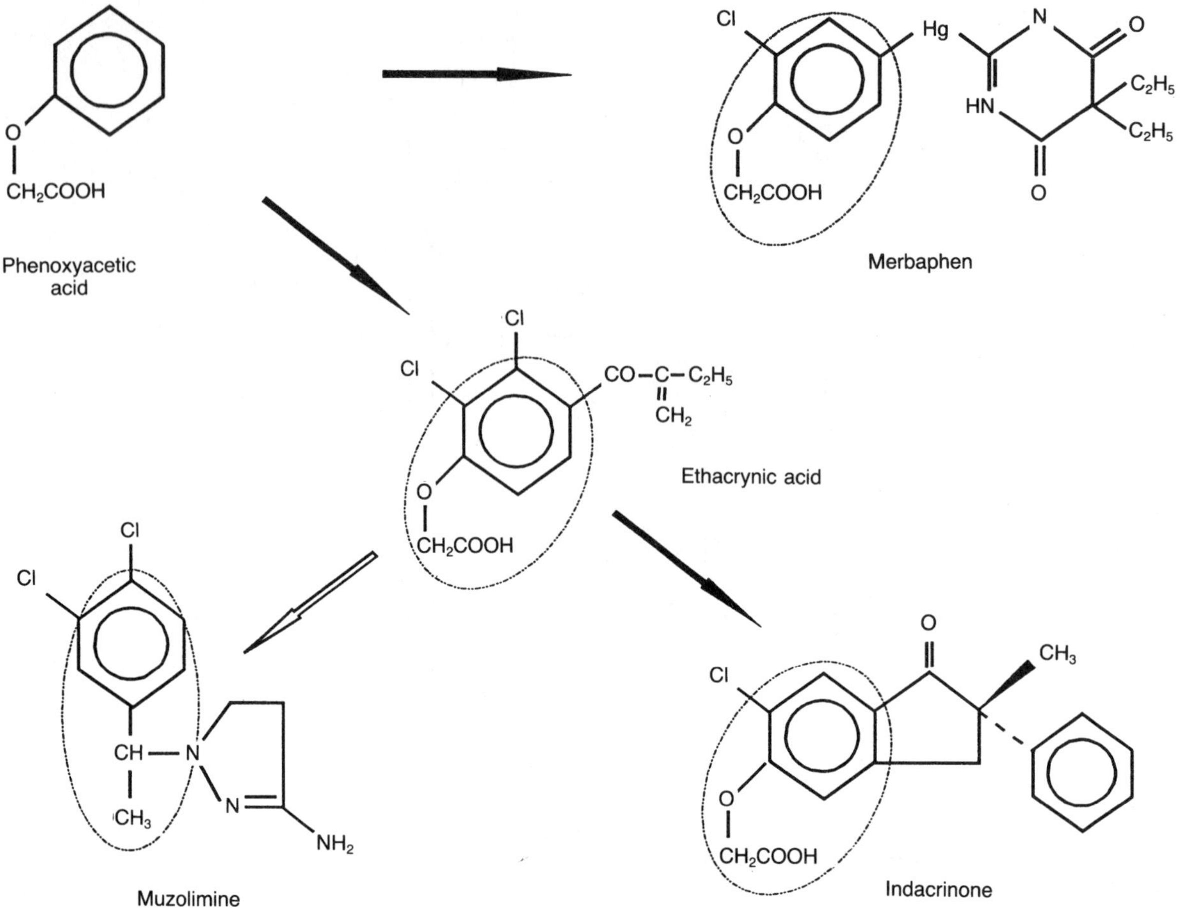

FIGURE 28.6 Structural evolution of the phenoxyacetic acid-based diuretics. Indacrinone has both laevo- and dextrorotatory isomers based on a chiral centre at position 2 of the indanone ring.

containing compounds were screened for both carbonic anhydrase inhibitors and associated diuretic activities. A major breakthrough occurred in 1958 when the benzothiadazine (or 'thiazide') heterocycle was synthesized and found to cause predominant renal loss of sodium chloride rather than sodium bicarbonate.[10] Reversion to a single substituted benzene ring structure shortly afterwards produced a striking change in characteristics of diuresis with the emergence of frusemide (furosemide) as the prototype of the family of sulphamoylbenzoate 'high ceiling' diuretics,[11] which also includes bumetanide and piretanide (Fig. 28.7). An unrelated substituted sulphonylurea derivative, torasemide, possesses an anionic group and a secondary amine in its structure (Fig. 28.8).

The largest group of sulphonamide diuretics is undoubtedly the 'thiazide' family which includes a number of monocyclic or heterocyclic sulphamoyl derivatives all possessing either a halogen (Cl) or pseudohalogen (CF_3) substituent adjacent to the SO_2NH_2 radical. The heterocyclic variants include phthalimidines such as chlorthalidone; quinazolinones, such as quiethazone and metolazone; the monocyclic variants include benzene-sulphonamides such as mefruside; and chlorobenzamides such as xipamide and indapamide.

All thiazide-like agents show parallel dose–response relationships and their maximal saliuretic efficacy is about 5–10% of the filtered load in keeping with their inhibitory action on salt reabsorption localized within the early portion of the distal tubule.

'Prodrug' loop diuretics

A number of loop diuretics exist that do not in their own right inhibit sodium chloride transport in the loop of Henle when tested experimentally as, for example, in single isolated perfused cortical segments of rabbit TALH. However, these compounds are effective loop diuretics when tested *in vivo* using conventional clearance methodology.[12]

Three classes of drug can thus be identified where the diuretic activity resides in a metabolite or in metabolites rather than in the parent drug. First, the *thiazolidone group* that lacks either a benzene ring or a sulphamoyl group in the molecule; etozoline with its asymmetrical carbon at position 4 is metabolized to the 2-methylene carboxylic acid, ozolinone and only the (−) enantiomer is active as a diuretic.

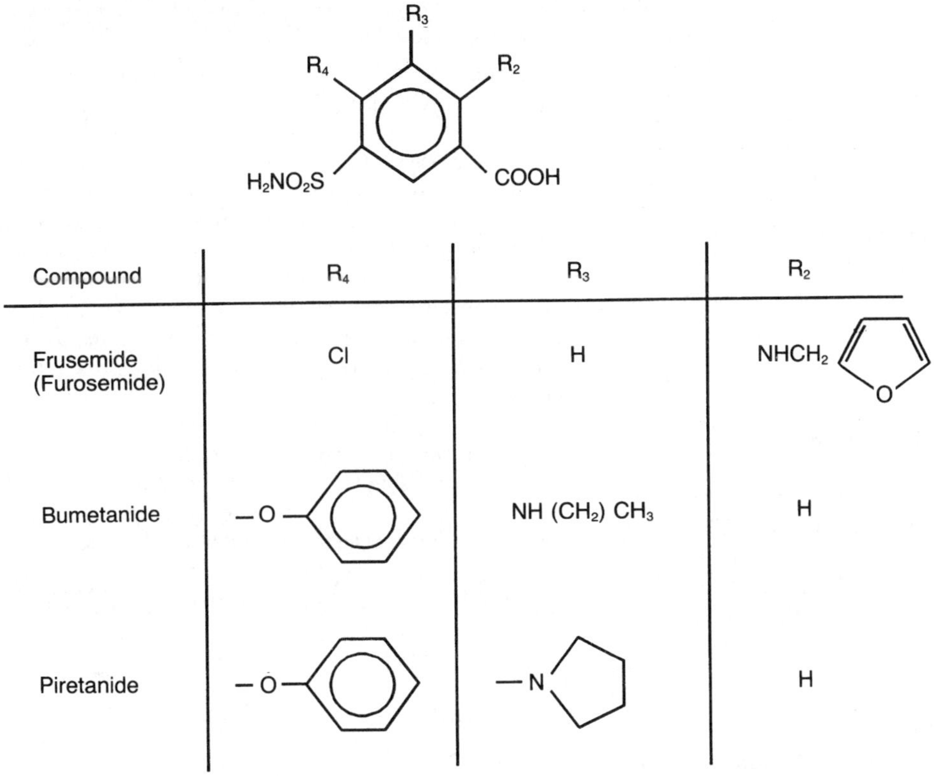

R3
R4
R2
H2NO2S
COOH
Compound
R4
R3
R2
Frusemide (Furosemide)
Cl
H
NHCH2
O
Bumetanide
—O
NH (CH2) CH3
H
Piretanide
—O
—N
H

FIGURE 28.7 Structural relationships of three sulphamoylbenzoate analogues with high-ceiling diuretic activity and with a principal site of action in the ascending limb of the loop of Henle.

R
CH3
Torasemide [25%]
R
CH3
OH
M3 [3%]
R
CH2OH
M1 [11%]
R
COOH
M5 [44%]
R =
N
SO2 · NH · C · NH · CH (CH3)2
O
NH

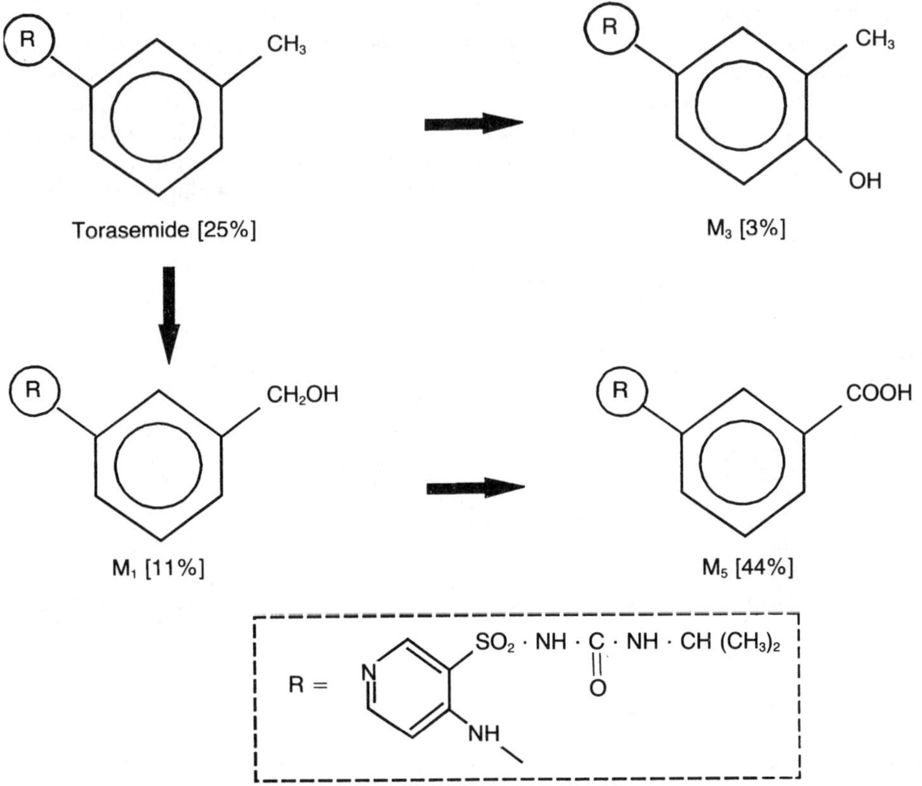

FIGURE 28.8 The metabolic fate of torasemide, a loop diuretic of substituted sulphonylurea structure. The percentages in parentheses indicate the relative percentages of an intravenous dose of the drug that appear in the urine.

Second, the *aminopyrazolinone group*, which includes muzolimine, a compound that has a dichlorobenzene ring in common with ethacrynic acid, but lacks a sulphamoyl substituent or carboxylic acid residue (Fig. 28.6). A muzolimine metabolite that is secreted into the tubular urine by a probenecid-sensitive mechanism is probably responsible for the *in vivo* diuretic activity.[13]

Third, the *amino-methylphenols*, which again lack a sulphamoyl substituent or carboxylic radical and are represented by the compound MK 447 that also behaves *in vivo* as a loop diuretic.

Potassium-sparing diuretics

These diuretics act in the last half of the distal nephron – that is, in the connecting and initial collecting tubule plus the cortical collecting tubule (site IV). Since at most only 5% of the filtered load of sodium chloride is normally reabsorbed by these tubular segments, potassium-sparing diuretics exhibit only weak natriuretic properties.

Chemically, they divide into three distinct groups. The first group is based on the 5-membered ring synthetic steroid structure necessary for antimineralocorticoid action and includes spironolactone and its major metabolite, potassium canrenoate. The second group consists of a triaminopteridine family of drugs with structural resemblance to folic acid, and represented by the diuretic, triamterene. The third group consists of pyrazine carboxamides exemplified by amiloride which shares an amino-substituted pyrazine ring and also three unsubstituted amino groups with triamterene (Fig. 28.9). Whereas triamterene is extensively metabolized, amiloride is excreted unchanged in the urine.

SUBCELLULAR MECHANISMS OF ACTION

Clearance methodology has been widely applied to the study of diuretic drugs in man. Using such techniques, important evidence has been obtained of the likely sites of action of these drugs within the nephron. However, apart from the one group with an obvious enzyme target for action, the carbonic anhydrase inhibitors, it has been virtually impossible to rely on the 'global' study of whole kidney function as a means of determining the intricate cellular and subcellular mechanisms of diuretic action. To this end, micropuncture and use of isolated tubular perfusion techniques have been developed as have electrophysiological approaches using renal epithelial as well as other isolated tissue cell or membrane preparations. Study of diuretic drug action using a variety of techniques in both renal and non-renal transporting tissues has identified discrete cellular targets for different diuretic classes implying the localization of specific membrane receptors in different segments of the nephron (Fig. 28.10).

Loop diuretics and $Na^+K^+2Cl^-$ cotransport

It has been clearly established that the predominant mode of entry of sodium chloride ion into the TALH cell is via the $Na^+K^+2Cl^-$ cotransporter which is present in the apical cell membrane and is highly sensitive to inhibitors of one of the Cl^--binding sites by sulphamoyl benzoate diuretics. The NaK, ATPase in the basolateral membrane provides the driving force for operation of the luminal $Na^+K^+2Cl^-$ cotransporter. Structure activity studies have shown that the molecular requirements for reversible binding to the Na^+K^+

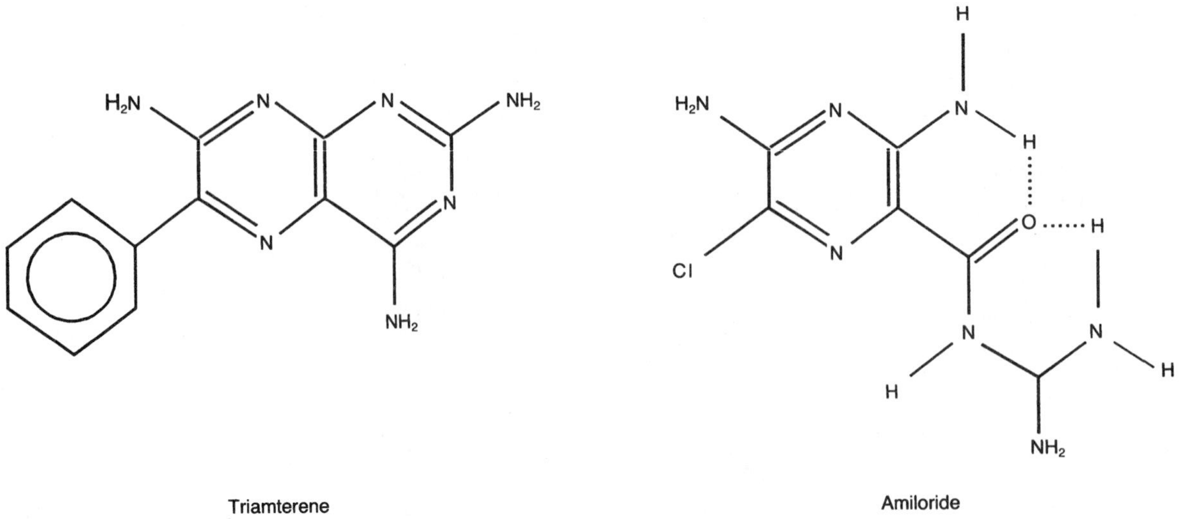

FIGURE 28.9 The structures of triamterene and amiloride. Both drugs contain a common substituted amino-pyrazine ring present on the left-hand part of each molecule.

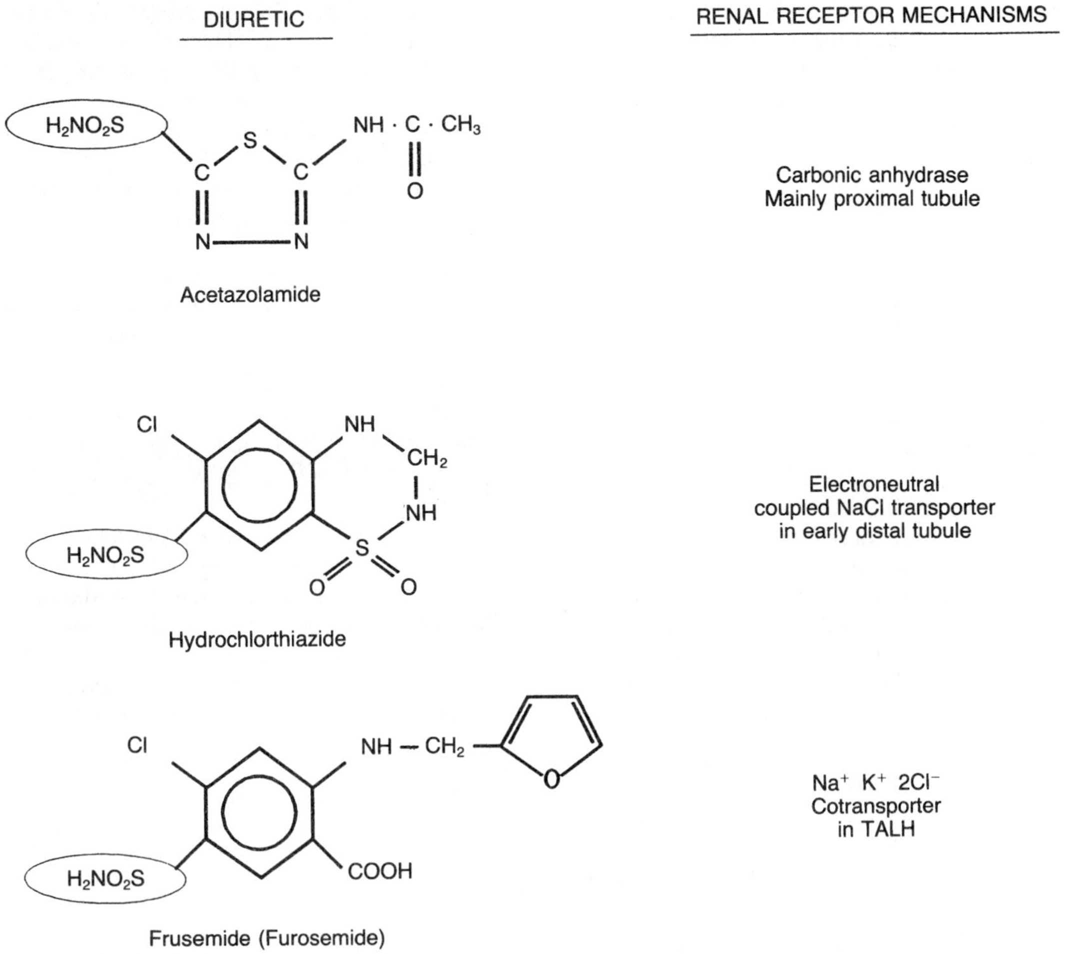

DIURETIC	RENAL RECEPTOR MECHANISMS
Acetazolamide	Carbonic anhydrase Mainly proximal tubule
Hydrochlorthiazide	Electroneutral coupled NaCl transporter in early distal tubule
Frusemide (Furosemide)	Na^+ K^+ $2Cl^-$ Cotransporter in TALH

FIGURE 28.10 Three examples of sulphamoyl ($—SO_2—NH_2$) substituted compounds with diuretic activity, each possessing an unique specialized sodium-transporting receptor within the nephron. TALH, thick ascending limb of Henle's loop.

$2Cl^-$ cotransporter are from an amino group such as a carboxylic sulphonic or sulphonylurea group with a secondary (as in frusemide and torasemide) or tertiary (as in piritenide) amine in an adjacent position. Though there have been a number of suggestions that the $Na^+K^+2Cl^-$ cotransporter may be identical with the Tamm–Horsfall protein found in the TALH, this is not a universally held view. There are also uncertainties as to whether phenoxyacetic acid diuretics also bind exclusively to the $Na^+K^+2Cl^-$ cotransporter.

Loop diuretics and chloride channels

The sulphamoyl benzoates have structural similarities with a number of chemicals that are highly effective inhibitors of chloride channels in the basolateral membrane of the TALH. However, whereas diuretics like frusemide lower cell chloride activity and secondarily alter membrane voltage and resistance, the primary effect of chloride-channel blockers is to hyperpolarize the basolateral membrane and increase its resistance so that cell chloride activity rises secondarily because of continued activity of the uninhibited $Na^+K^+2Cl^-$ cotransporter. Torasemide has an affinity for the $Na^+K^+2Cl^-$ carrier that is approximately 100-fold higher than that for the chloride channel.[14]

Thiazide diuretics and a distal electroneutral NaCl cotransporter

The original development of the benzothiadazine or thiazide diuretics was an offshoot of a systematized synthetic programme aimed at improving the diuretic efficacy of carbonic anhydrase inhibitors.[15] As soon as it was apparent that the major anion accompanying sodium with actions of the thiazides was chloride and not bicarbonate it was clear that the mechanism of action must be different from classic carbonic anhydrase inhibitors.

The nature of the thiazide renal receptor has proved difficult to unravel even though it has been known for some time that these drugs localize their effects to the cortical diluting segment, namely, the early water impermeable part of the distal tubule. It now seems clear that benzothiadiazine and related diuretics inhibit a coupled, electrically silent NaCl transport system in the luminal membrane of the early distal tubule by a mechanism that is similar if not identical to that found in a number of other types of epithelia such as the flounder bladder and Amphiuma.[16,17]

Potassium-sparing diuretics and sodium channels

Spironolactone and its active metabolites bind competitively to a cytoplasmic receptor protein in aldosterone-responsive cells in the distal nephron; this leads to enhanced transcription of mRNA and the production of new cation-transporting proteins such as Na,K ATPase in the basolateral membrane.[18]

Shortly after their synthesis, both triamterene and amiloride were found to reversibly inhibit sodium transport across frog skin and toad urinary bladder (Fig. 28.11). These particular epithelia have since been studied as models of high resistance or 'tight' epithelia. These potassium-sparing drugs do not have any effect on the basolateral Na,K ATPase, but are limited primarily to those portions of the late distal tubule and cortical collecting tubule that possess sodium-selective channels. The antikaliuresis that occurs with such diuretics is not due to an inhibition of selective potassium channels but due to decrease in the electrochemical driving force that favours apical potassium movement through these channels. This indirect effect occurs by hyperpolarization of the apical plasma membrane, thereby favouring downhill potassium movement via potassium-selective channels.[19]

PHARMACOKINETIC CONSIDERATIONS (Table 28.2)

It was appreciated already in the early 1970s by the use of isolated perfused tubule preparations that the majority of diuretics achieve their effects on the luminal surface of the tubule.[20] Since diuretics are very substantially bound to plasma protein, it is only possible for diuretics to reach the tubular lumen after being carried by the vasa secta to the organic acid transport

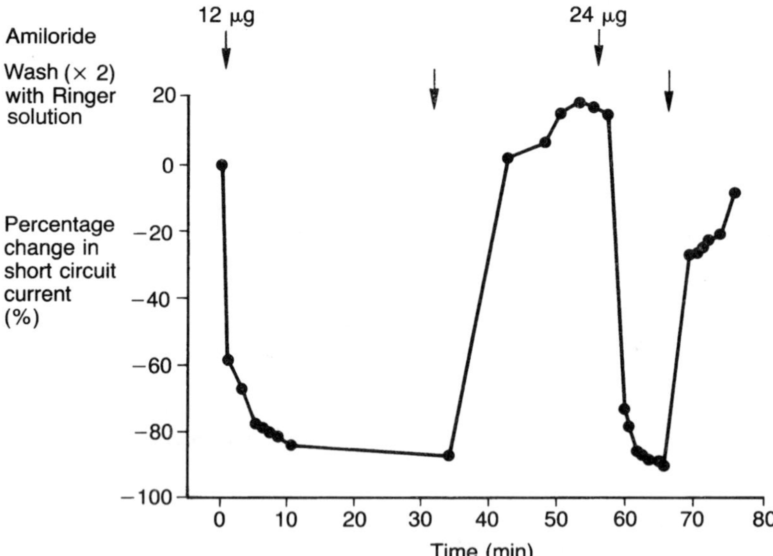

FIGURE 28.11 Effect of amiloride in increasing dosage (4.5×10^{-9} M; 9.0×10^{-8} M) on short-circuit current across isolated frog skin. The drug was added to the outside bathing solution of an Ussing and Zerahn chamber for 30-min periods and removed by changing the bathing solution to fresh Ringer-solution as marked by the arrows. (Adapted from Baba *et al.*[104])

TABLE 28.2 Pharmacokinetic characteristics of four major representatives of the sulphonamide series of loop diuretics

	FRUSEMIDE	BUMETANIDE	PIRETANIDE	TORASEMIDE
Equipotent oral dose (mg)	40	1	6	20
Bioavailability (%)	50	80	100	80
Volume of distribution (l/kg)	0.16	0.17	0.25	0.16
Clearance (ml/min/kg)	2.2	2.6	3.2	0.8
Half-life (h)	1.0	1.2	0.9	3.0
Fraction of dose (iv) excreted unchanged (%)	60	65	44	20
Reference	102	103	22	105

pumps located in the proximal tubule. By use of the classic inhibitor of the organic acid transport pathway, probenecid, it has been possible to confirm that secretion of diuretics into the lumen of the proximal tubule is a prerequisite for expressions of the diuresis.[12,21]

The determinants of the overall renal response to a diuretic link pharmacokinetic behaviour with phamacodynamic actions. Thus, the time course of entry of diuretic into the urine and the relationships between the urinary excretions of diuretic and sodium chloride all appear to be critical. The magnitude of the amount of diuretic delivered to the kidney after intravenous administration appears to be related directly to the state of hydration.[22]

Interpretation of kinetic responses to diuretics after pretreatment with probenecid may be complicated by the fact that not only may this inhibitor of weak acid transport block renal tubular excretion of a diuretic but it may at the same time also interfere with extrarenal handling at other tissue sites including for example the biliary tract.

Renal insufficiency results in a reduced delivery of active diuretics to its site of action in the nephron. In the case of frusemide, reduced renal function not only lowers the renal clearance of the drugs but also its nonrenal clearance by possible reduction in renal glucuronidation; the result is a prolongation of the elimination half-life. With the other loop diuretics, non-renal clearance appears to occur via the cytochrome P-450-dependent hepatic microsomal systems and because this is unaffected by diminished kidney function, elimination half-lives are not prolonged in renal insufficiency.[23] In severe renal insufficiency, maintenance of an effective concentration of diuretic at the site of action in the nephron for a more prolonged period by administration of a continuous intravenous infusion, may increase the global sodium excretory response.[24]

CLINICAL USE OF DIURETICS

Diuretics maintain a key role in cardiovascular therapy. They continue to represent one of the first-line treatments for oedematous states, notably congestive cardiac failure, which was of course the original disease state for which they were designed. The incidental discovery that the benzothiadiazines also lowered blood pressure in non-oedematous hypertensive subjects soon after the discovery of the thiazides paved the way for general application of these agents to the treatment of essential hypertension. Every one of the fourteen major clinical trials of treatment of hypertension published up to 1990 employed a thiazide diuretic as a first-line therapy choice.[25]

Acute left ventricular failure

Treatment of acute pulmonary oedema has been transformed by the availability of loop diuretics. In addition to this rapid saliuretic effect, loop diuretics have been shown to exert a direct venodilator action within the first few minutes of intravenous administration leading to increased venous capacitance and a rapid reduction in pulmonary pressure. It remains uncertain whether this venous 'pooling' effect occurs independently[26] or not of renally induced salt and water loss.[27]

Congestive heart failure

The beneficial effects of chronic diuretic therapy in congestive cardiac failure are well established. The major causes of heart failure today are coronary artery disease and raised arterial pressure. Before the development of diuretic drugs, digitalis glycosides were the only agents available for treating heart failure. Awareness that mercury salts could induce a diuresis led to their use as a standard means of treating failure, already well documented about 150 years ago;[28] this subsequently evolved first to the combined use of digitalis and mercury (Guy's Hospital pills) and then to the development of the organomercurials at the end of the First World War.[10]

Current management strategies for management of cardiac failure incorporate three main drug approaches.

Drugs possessing positive isotropic activity

Many have viewed the major defect in chronic heart failure as defective cardiac contractility and have sought to correct this by use of drugs possessing positive isotropic activity. Use of some of the agents introduced, such as the cAMP phosphodiesterase inhibitors or the partial β_1-agonist, xamoterol, has resulted in shortened survival and has cast serious doubts on the merits of this approach in management.[29]

The β_1-selective agonist, dobutamine, and the dopaminergic precursor of noradrenaline, dopamine, are used as short-term parenteral inotropes. The latter at low dosage (< 5 mg/kg/min) selectively dilates renal arterioles and thereby improves renal perfusion.

Controversy has continued to surround the use of oral digoxin though several recent trials have re-evaluated its position in very positive terms.[30,31] The major indication for digoxin use has been to control ventricular response in atrial fibrillation associated with congestive cardiac failure. Recent studies have also shown clear benefit where digoxin has been used in conjunction with diuretics and ACE inhibitors in patients with chronic heart failure and impaired systolic function who are in sinus rhythm.[32]

Diuretics

Diuretics improve cardiac performance by relieving pulmonary congestion with reduction in right atrial, right ventricular and pulmonary artery wedge pressure. Increased diuresis leads to reduction in pulmonary water with increased pulmonary compliance and diminution in resistance to airflow.[33] Decreased oxygen consumption by respiratory muscles is accompanied by a redistribution of blood flow away from the muscles of the thoracic and abdominal walls in favour of other important systemic vascular systems. The result is a reduction in the key symptoms of heart failure – breathlessness and fatigue – as exercise tolerance improves.

In the early stages of heart failure use of moderate dosage of a thiazide-like agent on 2–3 days per week may be sufficient to give symptomatic relief in most heart failure patients. Continued progression of myocardial dysfunction may require the introduction of a loop diuretic on a daily basis.

Activity of the renin–angiotensin–aldosterone (RAA) system is enhanced in most patients with congestive cardiac failure. Excessive retention of sodium and water is encouraged by this means and also through stimulation of arginine vasopressin production. These neurohormonal mechanisms may be further activated if excessive diuretic treatment is given too early in the progression of clinical heart failure. One way of diminishing the secondary wastage of renal potassium in this situation is by the addition of a potassium-sparing diuretic such as triamterene, amiloride or spironolactone as a combination regime with thiazide or loop diuretic therapy. An alternative approach that has rapidly become standard clinical practice in recent years is to introduce ACE inhibitor thereby attenuating the compensatory stimulation of the RAA system brought about by the syndrome of heart failure and the consequences of diuretic therapy (see below).

Vasodilator therapy

The concept that *vasodilator therapy* might benefit the prognosis of chronic heart failure received major impetus in the mid-1980s with publication of the first of two vasodilator-heart failure (V-HeFT I) trials.[34] This showed that survival improved in patients with moderately severe heart failure when the combination of hydralazine and isosorbide dinitrate was added to standard treatment with digoxin and diuretics. The V-HeFT II study, which was published in 1991, compared enalapril with the combination of hydralazine and isosorbide dinitrate in patients with mild to moderate heart failure who were already receiving standard digoxin/diuretic therapy.[35] Mortality after 2 years was significantly lower in the enalapril arm of the study (18%) than in the patients treated with hydralazine/isosorbide dinitrate (25%). In between these two major trials, the CONSENSUS trial reported in 1987 on the beneficial effects of adding enalapril to existing therapy with digoxin and diuretics in patients with severe congestive heart failure [NYHA functional class IV; n = 253]. This trial was terminated prematurely when it was shown that mortality at 1 year had been reduced by addition of enalapril by 31% when compared with addition of placebo. Two subsequent clinical trials have reported the striking benefits of ACE inhibition in preventing the occurrence of heart failure by attenuating the progression of asymptomatic and symptomatic left ventricular dysfunction [SAVE trial, 1992; SOLVD trial, 1992]. When, however, the effect of initiating enalapril within the first 24 h after myocardial infarction was tested to see whether the process of cardiac remodelling could be arrested before left ventricular dilatation had occurred, no survival benefit of this early intervention was found [CONSENSUS II trial, 1992].

The realization that drug therapy with ACE inhibitors can dramatically modify the progression of left ventricular dysfunction as well as significantly improve mortality in established heart failure has meant that traditional reliance on digoxin and diuretic therapy as the mainstay drugs for managing heart failure has had to be challenged.[36]

An additional benefit that has occurred from the partnership between ACE inhibitors and diuretics in managing more severe forms of heart failure has been the ability of this combined approach to improve myocardial function while at the same time correcting hyponatraemia, a not uncommon complication of class III/IV congestive heart failure.[37,38] (See Hyponatraemia, later.)

Other types of vasodilator that have been found efficacious in treating congestive heart failure include orally active dopamine agonists such as fenoldopam and ibopamine.[39] Flosequinan, a quinolone derivative that vasodilates by inhibiting both protein kinase C and inositol triphosphate production in smooth muscle, was found to give symptomatic relief in heart failure and offered an alternative therapy choice in patients who were not responsive or were intolerant of ACE-inhibitors. Unfortunately, its use was associated with increased mortality and the drug was withdrawn from clinical use in 1993.

Diminished responsiveness to diuretics in heart failure

Patients in severe heart failure can become refractory to the action of oral loop diuretics. This may relate to poor gastrointestinal absorption of agents such as frusemide with relatively low bioavailability; substitution of frusemide by bumetanide or torasemide may restore diuretic responsiveness. Alternatively, the loop diuretic can be given intravenously with occurrence of an effective saliuretic response since it is clear that diuretic delivery to the active site of action in the nephron remains unimpaired in oedematous states.[40]

Another phenomenon that may contribute to diminished responsiveness to diuretics in chronic heart failure is enhanced renal tubular reabsorption of sodium both proximally and distally even in the presence of significant amounts of loop diuretic in the tubular lumen. The cause of this 'braking' effect is unclear but may result from down-regulation of the tubular receptors for diuretic action or hypertrophy of the distal tubular epithelium following long-term exposure to persistently increased distal salt delivery.[41]

Such hypertrophied and hyperfunctional distal nephron cells may readily reabsorb a substantial amount of sodium rejected through diuretic action on the loop of Henle. Addition of thiazide diuretic or the drug metolazone may in these circumstances provoke a supra-additive effect with particularly powerful diuresis in an otherwise non-responsive patient.[42]

Hypertension

Thiazide diuretics have remained at the forefront of treatment for hypertension since their original introduction into clinical medicine in 1957. A meta-analysis of the fourteen major randomized trials of antihypertensive treatment undertaken up to 1990 showed a mean length of treatment of 3–5 years with a decrease in diastolic blood pressure (DBP) of 5–6 mmHg.[25] All these trials involved the use of a diuretic and a mean reduction of 42% was noted in stroke deaths; this was in broad agreement with observational estimates indicating the likelihood of 35–40% in stroke deaths. By contrast, epidemiological data suggested that this reduction in DBP should decrease coronary heart disease (CHD) events by about 20–25% while the meta-analysis showed a reduction, even though significant, of only 14%. This shortfall in CHD benefit has been much discussed in the literature. One of the main reasons is probably the relatively short duration of the hypertension trials but this explanation has been overshadowed by the argument that metabolic changes induced by diuretic therapy are likely to be responsible.[43,44]

A major impetus for this concern that diuretic therapy may actually increase cardiovascular risk came from the Multiple Risk Factor Intervention Trial (MRFIT) in the United States.[45] In this trial, a subgroup of patients in the Special Intervention (SI) group with abnormal resting electrocardiograms who were treated with relatively high doses of diuretics, either chlorothiazide or chlorthalidone, had a higher death rate than expected when compared with another group of usual care (UC) patients who were treated with less intensive management. The hypothesis was propounded that diuretic-induced hypokalaemia and hypomagnesaemia is likely to have led to dysrhythmias and an increase in sudden death.[46] The fact that the findings on which this hypothesis was based had emanated from a retrospective subgroup analysis of data, was largely overlooked and encouraged a very substantial literature to accumulate that implied that therapy with thiazide diuretics was cardiotoxic. The published literature has been reviewed critically on several occasions and no support has been found for the view that long-term use of thiazide diuretics adversely affects cardiovascular risk.[47,48] What has emerged quite clearly is a relation between potential cardiac toxicity with diuretics and dose.

Dose–response relationship in hypertension

There have been several well-conducted studies that have shown that the dose–response curve for thiazide action in hypertension was relatively flat and that no further antihypertensive benefit occurred with progressive increase in dosage once the plateau had been reached.[49–51] Curiously, this knowledge failed to be taken into account when the majority of major clinical trials of hypertension were planned up until the execution of the European Working Party for Hypertension in the Elderly (EWPHE) trial that was published in 1985.[52] This trial was unusual in not only using a low-dose thiazide but in combining this with a potassium-sparing agent, triamterene, and studying the antihypertensive effects in an elderly population; a beneficial effect of diuretic treatment on mortality from CHD was shown (Table 28.3). A population-based case control study in North America has shown that both the dose of thiazide and the addition of a potassium-sparing agent influence the risk of primary cardiac arrest in patients with hypertension. Patients prescribed thiazide diuretics and potassium-sparing diuretics together were less likely to have cardiac arrest than those prescribed thiazides alone (odds ratio: 0.3); the risk for cardiac arrest increased with thiazide dose.[53] Low-dose thiazide therapy is not only as effective as more conventional dosage in lowering blood pressure in hypertensive patients but it produces no adverse metabolic effects – in particular no deleterious effects on either peripheral or hepatic insulin action.[54]

Mechanism of antihypertensive effect of diuretics

Another important contributory factor to the continued use of unnecessarily high doses of diuretics when treating hypertension was the lack of appreciation that prolonged powerful saliuresis was not needed for maintenance of the antihypertensive effect.[10,55]

The initial and long-term blood pressure lowering effects of diuretics differ. The initial response is that of negative sodium and fluid balance with shrinkage of plasma volume and cardiac output.[56] After this, over subsequent months, a substantial reduction in peripheral vascular and renal resistance occurs while cardiac output returns to normal but there remains a small persistent reduction in plasma volume.[57]

Why and how the vasodilatory response is maintained is still unclear despite the fact that diuretics

TABLE 28.3 Diuretic choices and dosages in major hypertension studies. Comparison of first-line drug choices and dosages in major clinical trials following the Medical Research Council Trial (MRC - 1).[93] All these studies employed a thiazide diuretic on its own (hydrochlorothiazide, HCTZ), a thiazide-like drug (chlorthalidone) or a mixture of thiazide and potassium-sparing agent, in consistently lower dosage than the 10 mg dose of bendrofluazide (BFZ) used in the MRC - 1 trial.[93]

STUDY	AGE RANGE	PATIENT NUMBER	BLOOD PRESSURE (mmHg)	FIRST-LINE DRUGS AND DOSAGE
MRC - 1[93]	35–60	17 354	DBP 90–109	BFZ 10 mg propranolol 240 mg
EWPHE[52]	>60	940	DBP 90–119	HCTZ 25 mg plus triamterene 50 mg (Dyazide)
STOP[80]	78–84	1627	SBP 180–230 or DBP 105–120	Atenolol 50 mg *or* HCTZ 50 mg *or* HCTZ 50 mg plus amiloride 2.5 mg *or* metoprolol 100 mg *or* pindolol 5 mg
SHEP[79]	>60	4736	SBP 160–219 DBP <90	Chlorthalidone 12.5–25 mg
MRC - 2[81]	65–74	4736	SBP 160–209 DBP <115	HCTZ 25–50 mg plus amiloride 2.5–5 mg
TOMHS[66]	45–69	902	DBP <100	Chlorthalidone 15 mg *or* acebutolol 400 mg *or* doxazosin 1–2 mg *or* amlodipine 5 mg *or* enalapril 5 mg

DBP, diastolic blood pressure; SBP, systolic blood pressure.

have had such a dominant role in antihypertensive therapy for almost 40 years. Two main explanations exist for the undoubted correct observation that sustained antihypertensive effects occur with continued doses of diuretic that are subsaliuretic. First, there may be significant changes in the sodium and fluid content of the arterial wall that would affect vascular smooth muscle reactivity especially to adrenergic stimuli.[58] Second, there may be a reversed autoregulatory response to the persistent small reduction in plasma volume that elicits a vasodilatory response through a mixture of local metabolic or humoral mechanisms.[59]

Diuretics as first-line treatment for hypertension

It has become increasingly apparent in recent years that high blood pressure, although an independent risk factor for adverse clinical events, commonly exists as part of a syndrome of associated vascular and metabolic abnormalities such as disturbed glucose tolerance, left ventricular hypertrophy, dyslipidaemia and obesity.[60] It is thus clear that besides a careful assessment of blood pressure on several occasions, it is important in each patient to determine the presence of other vascular risk factors. A number of these associated with reduced tissue insulin sensitivity, such as upper body obesity and glucose intolerance, can be effectively tackled by non-pharmacological methods.[61]

For a long time, emphasis with respect to morbidity and mortality in hypertension focused mainly on diastolic blood pressure. It is now evident that at every level of diastolic blood pressure, risks are greater with higher levels of systolic blood pressure. In middle-aged and elderly patients, there has been a growing realization that increases in vascular disease are associated with elevated systolic blood pressure, not only when diastolic blood pressure is also high but also when the latter is normal, emphasizing the distinct entity of isolated systolic hypertension or ISH.[62]

The realization that even modest elevations of blood pressure that are sustained have a major impact on vascular risk has led to greater emphasis of the term 'high-normal' blood pressure in preference to the older terms of 'mild' or 'moderate'. This means that all stages of hypertension are associated with increased risk of non-fatal and fatal vascular events including renal damage. The higher the blood pressure, the greater the risk.[2]

Traditional stepped-care management of hypertension as determined by a WHO expert committee in 1978[63] advocated a first choice of antihypertensive treatment of either a diuretic or a β-blocker; the second step was an association of the two and then the addition of a representative of the then-available vasodilator agents such as methyldopa or hydralazine. The subsequent years to date have witnessed two very important changes. First, the development of at least three groups of 'new generation' vasodilator drugs capable of being given on their own in monotherapy without causing reflex tachycardia: ACE inhibitors, calcium-channel blockers and selective α-blockers. Second, through availability of a choice of effective drugs, it became possible for the first time to allow the physician to select first-line drug therapy on an individual basis, attempting to match the choice of drug to the needs and clinical profile of each particular patient.[64]

Thus in JNC IV, 1988,[65] as well as considering demographic profiles and metabolic aspects of individual patients in helping determine the first-line choice of antihypertensive drug therapy, individualization of drug choices was offered from four classes of agent: diuretics, β-blocker, calcium antagonist or ACE inhibitor. JNC V (1993)[2] promotes diuretics and β-blockers *only* as the optimal first steps in treatment, with the other drugs to be used in specific cases or in situations where diuretics and β-blockers are not tolerated or have failed. The reason for this more restrictive approach to first-line options, which is also propounded by the British Hypertension Society Management Guidelines (1993),[3] is that the only controlled outcome studies in which antihypertensive treatment has been shown to effectively reduce stroke and other cardiovascular end points have been based on the clinical trials of diuretics and β-blockers. The WHO/ISH Guidelines[61] list available drugs in order of proven benefit based on mortality and morbidity studies; first, diuretics; second, β-blocking drugs; third, ACE inhibitors, calcium antagonists and α-adrenoceptor-blocking drugs. The TOHM study, which included a representative from each class of drug in a 4-year study in combination with a nutritional–hygienic intervention as baseline, also concluded that its findings agreed with the view that diuretics and β-blockers are preferred initial drug therapy for most hypertensive patients unless contraindicated.[66]

The one domain where serious concern has been expressed about diuretic use has been in diabetes where a retrospective study from the Joslin Clinic showed excess mortality in a group of diabetic patients with severe retinopathy who had received diuretics as antihypertensive therapy.[67] As has been discussed in respect of the MRFIT study, the findings of such investigations relate to use of diuretics at inappropriately large dosage with all the attendant metabolic sequelae thereby distorting the interpretation of morbidity and mortality data.[68] The place of low or very-low diuretic therapy in the management of diabetic hypertension has not been defined.

Available evidence shows unique protective qualities of ACE inhibition, independent of the capacity to effectively control hypertension on the progression of renal damage in diabetes.[69] Thus, in the management of diabetic hypertension ACE inhibitors would appear to be the first-line choice in preference to diuretics. The question of whether diuretics can significantly reduce left ventricular hypertrophy as compared with other antihypertensive agents has been the subject of much discussion, especially as left ventricular hypertrophy has been identified as a major independent risk factor for cardiovascular morbidity in hypertension.[70] A number of studies have shown that there is clear reduction in left ventricular mass with diuretic therapy and that the reason this has not always been consistently detected may have related to short duration of therapy and excessive diuretic dosage.[71] Whether diuretics are as efficacious in reversing left ventricular hypertrophy in hypertension as other antihypertensive agents will require longer-term prospective and comparative investigations like the TOHM study.

Other oedematous states

Renal insufficiency

In renal failure, the number of intact nephrons is reduced, leading to a fall in glomerular filtration rate. Endogenous organic acids accumulate and may block the active secretion of diuretic agents by the proximal tubule into the lumen. For both these reasons, the amount of an administered diuretic that reaches the tubular urine is significantly decreased and saliuretic efficacy is diminished.

Thus, in defining an optimal therapeutic strategy for using diuretic therapy in renal disease, it is important that allowance is made for sufficiently high dosage to ensure that adequate amounts are delivered to the active tubular reabsorptive sites for sodium chloride. Because of their greater capacity to reject a substantial portion of filtered sodium chloride, loop diuretics are predominantly used in renal failure.

The relationship between the amount of diuretic reaching the tubular lumen and the natriuretic response is defined by a sigmoid curve and the therapeutic aim is to administer sufficient drug to activate the steep portion of the dose response curve.

At very reduced glomerular filtration rate of around 15 ml/min, the renal clearance of frusemide is about one-fifth of normal and hence a dosage of five times normal may be required to achieve the same saliuretic response as in a subject with normal glomerular filtration.[23] Continuous infusion of a loop diuretic in severe renal insufficiency may lead to persistently effective concentrations of diuretic in the tubular lumen with increase in overall saliuretic response when compared with bolus injections.[24]

The pharmacodynamics of loop diuretics are not usually disturbed in renal failure. In nephrotic syndrome, however, with preserved glomerular filtration rate, renal clearance of loop diuretics is normal and the total amount of drug reaching the tubular lumen may be the same as in normal subjects. However, because of the presence of substantial amounts of protein in the urine, the amount of 'unbound' or 'free' diuretic able to act at the luminal surface is diminished. It is difficult to estimate the extent of this binding effect upon the critical availability of diuretic at the ascending limb of the loop of Henle but an approximate guideline of increasing intravenous doses of frusemide or bumetamide three-fold in these circumstances seems reasonable.[72] If these drugs are being administered orally, allowance has to be made for approximately 50% bioavailability of frusemide or 80%, in the case of bumetanide. Torasemide (Fig. 28.9) is unusual in having a substantial hepatic metabolism so its total clearance and length of action are determined by hepatic rather than by renal function.[73]

In nephrotic syndrome, tubular responsiveness to diuretic action may be abnormal even allowing for the luminal binding effects of protein leak. A number of possible explanations exist for this including enhanced proximal and distal sodium reabsorption that may be humorally dictated, for example by activation of the renin–angiotensin aldosterone system, vasopressin, prostaglandins and the sympathetic nervous system.[74] These additional factors may explain why diuretic compounds with mixed tubular sites of action, such as metolazone, may be particularly useful in treating patients with nephrotic syndrome.

Hepatic cirrhosis with ascites

The mechanisms involved in the abnormal salt and water handling characteristic of advanced liver cirrhosis are complex. A key factor is decreased effective arterial blood volume which results from transudation of lymph into the peritoneal cavity, hypoalbuminaemia, and splanchnic venous pooling. The reduced blood volume in turn results in a compensatory increase in overall salt and water reabsorption by the kidney. Increased portal venous pressure and activation of the renin–angiotensin aldosterone system also feature with an associated non-osmotic stimulation of vasopressin release.[75]

In mild cases of hepatic ascites, bed rest and significant sodium restriction (25 mmol Na/day) may suffice. Where patients become unresponsive, spironolactone up to 400 mg/day can be used as the initial diuretic, in the presence of normal renal function low doses of a loop diuretic may be added in from 20 mg frusemide upwards until an adequate diuresis is achieved. In some patients, a refractory state develops to such combined regimens, probably due to avid reabsorption of sodium at tubular sites not affected by spironolactone or the loop diuretics. In this situation, addition of 'hybrid' diuretics like metolazone may be effective in restoring an effective saliuresis as was noted above in management of the nephrotic syndrome.

Careful balancing between the magnitude of the induced diuresis and the extent of blood volume contraction and associated organ hypoperfusion is essential to prevent the development of the major electrolyte disturbances and the hepatorenal syndrome which carry such serious prognostic consequences in these patients.

ADVERSE EFFECTS OF DIURETICS

Diuretics have formed the cornerstone for treatment for heart failure and hypertension for close on 40 years. Their overall safety profile has been good considering, as we have seen from the discussion of their clinical pharmacology, that fundamental misunderstandings of the dose–response relationships of these drugs with respect to kidney and vascular tissue led to continued unnecessary use of excessively high doses worldwide for many years. Appreciation that many of the metabolic sequelae of chronic diuretic therapy are dose-related has now been carefully documented.[51,54,76]

It has also become clear that multiple risk factors exist in ischaemic heart disease and hypertension even before any diuretic therapy has been given. This is especially time for disturbances in insulin sensitivity and lipoprotein metabolism.[77,78] With greater awareness of the clustering of risk factors in cardiovascular disease and the need to take into account the clear dose-related metabolic effects of diuretics at the planning stages of large-scale trials involving diuretic therapy, it has been possible to identify clinical usage of diuretics in situations of multiple risk such as the elderly hypertensive where not only has there been a beneficial effect on mortality from stroke but also from coronary heart disease (Table 28.3).[79–81]

It is important, therefore, that any discussion of the adverse effects of diuretics is viewed with these perspectives in mind and taking into account the fact that most of the published data are of a historical nature dating back to the era of clinical 'overdosage' highlighted by the Multiple Risk Factor Intervention Trial (1982).[45]

METABOLIC COMPLICATIONS

The various metabolic complications of diuretic therapy are listed in Table 28.4.

Hyponatraemia

All diuretics produce a natriuresis capable of causing a degree of extracellular fluid volume contraction dependent on the extent of renal sodium loss. Even though the induced decrease in effective plasma volume may not be easily detectable clinically, it is sufficient to interfere with the renal capacity to excrete water.[82] A number of mechanisms participate in this process, notably diminution in glomerular filtration rate (GFR), increase in proximal salt reabsorption with decreased delivery of fluid of the diluting segments of the nephron, and non-osmotic release of arginine vasopressin (AVP) leading to increased thirst and increased water intake.

TABLE 28.4 Metabolic complications of diuretic therapy

Hyponatraemia	Hyperuricaemia
Hypo- and hyperkalaemia	Hyperglycaemia
Hypomagnesaemia	Disturbed lipid metabolism
Hypo- and hypercalcaemia	

Diuretic-induced hyponatraemia can be particularly troublesome in the elderly, more often in women over the age of 65 years and triggered by a benzothiadiazine or thiazide-like diuretic, though some reports show a relationship also with frusemide therapy.[83] The incidence of hyponatraemia is increased in conditions associated with high circulating AVP, such as congestive cardiac failure, or hepatic cirrhosis, and it is in these situations that plasma sodium requires careful monitoring when treatment with diuretics has been instituted.

Once hyponatraemia has developed, treatment may require cessation of diuretic therapy, water restriction, and replacement of any sodium deficit present, which can be complex when an underlying salt-retaining state is present in the first place.

Hypokalaemia and hypomagnesaemia

Because low plasma concentrations of potassium and magnesium in patients with cardiac disease can be associated with a higher incidence of dysrhythmias, especially after myocardial infarction, there has been considerable interest in the relationship between disturbances in these ions in the circulation and diuretic therapy.[84]

The two main reasons for potassium and magnesium wastage by the kidney with use of diuretics are first, the increased delivery of sodium and water to the distal nephron and second, increased circulating mineralocorticoid concentrations. The magnitude of the decreases in plasma K and Mg is related to both the dose and duration of action of the diuretic being used. Loop diuretics tend on the whole to cause less perturbation of ionic balance because their action is over by 6 h and the compensatory postsaliuretic retention period allows for decrease in urinary K and Mg excretion to, or even below, baseline levels. With long-acting thiazide-like drugs such as chlorthalidone, lowering significantly the dose of drug may leave the antihypertensive efficacy unaltered but diminish markedly the extent of potassium wastage.[85]

The simultaneous administration of two potassium-wasting diuretics, acting at different sites in the nephron, can cause a dramatic degree of urinary potassium (and magnesium) loss with severe hypokalaemia and hypomagnesaemia. This can happen, for example, by combining frusemide and metolazone therapy. Some of these cation losses can be offset by maintaining adequate dietary intake of foods rich in potassium and magnesium, but the most efficient way of retaining potassium and magnesium is by concurrent use of a potassium-sparing diuretic.[86]

Although the literature abounds with papers discussing the potential increase in cardiovascular risk caused by diuretic-induced changes in circulating potassium and magnesium, it must not be forgotten that these are primarily intracellular cations and the relationship between plasma and intracellular concentrations remains unclear.[87] Furthermore, much of the evidence for cardiotoxicity comes from the many years of diuretic overdosage in common clinical use such that critical review of the subject has concluded that diuretic-induced hypokalaemia and hypomagnesaemia do not increase the incidence of dysrhythmia and sudden death.[88] Any risk that may exist would be reduced by employing low-dosage and combining thiazides with a potassium-sparing agent.[53]

Hyperkalaemia

The potassium-sparing diuretics are all capable of causing hyperkalaemia and are more likely to do so where there is pre-existing renal insufficiency as in normal ageing, concurrent administration of other K-relating substances such as ACE inhibitors, or in the presence of diabetes. The simultaneous use of non-steroidal anti-inflammatory drugs (NSAIDs) and K-sparing diuretics can precipitate acute renal failure and should be avoided (see Interactions below).

Altered calcium balance

Alterations in sodium reabsorption within the proximal convoluted tubule and the loop of Henle tend to cause parallel changes in calcium reabsorption. Approximately 10% of filtered calcium is reabsorbed distally. This means that diuretics can affect renal calcium handling in paradoxical ways. Thus, loop diuretics produce an acute hypercalciuria by reducing the lumen-positive transepithelial potential difference that drives passive calcium reabsorption in this tubular segment. Hypocalcaemia does not usually arise in these circumstances because of compensatory mechanisms, such as increased reabsorption of calcium from the loop by action of parathyroid hormone. However, in hypoparathyroid patients, the risk of symptomatic hypocalcaemia after a loop diuretic is much increased.

By contrast, thiazide diuretics markedly *reduce* urinary calcium excretion and have been usefully applied to the treatment of hypercalciuric nephrolithiasis. Reduction of hip fracture has been reported and a case argued for the need to study formally the potential clinical benefit of thiazides in preventing osteoporosis.[89]

Hyperuricaemia

Although acutely, diuretics may cause an initial rise in urate excretion, chronic therapy, particularly with thiazides, invariably leads to decreased urate clearance with a rise in plasma urate. Volume depletion is the primary cause of the hyperuricaemia and so the effect is clearly dose related.[51] In the absence of overt gout, the increase in plasma urate does not require any treatment.

Hyperglycaemia

Impairment of glucose tolerance and precipitation of overt diabetes and, in the elderly, of hyperglycaemic hyperosmolar coma, have all been described with chronic diuretic therapy especially when long-acting thiazides or thiazide analogues have been used.

The hyperglycaemic effects can be seen early in therapy, in normal people as well as in those with impaired glucose tolerance. The effect is more marked with increasing age, with decreased plasma potassium concentrations, and is usually reversible in stopping diuretic therapy.[90]

Hyperglycaemia is less common with loop diuretics and the potassium-sparing diuretics leave carbohydrate tolerance undisturbed.

The question of whether thiazide-induced changes in glucose tolerance matter in the context of increasing the risk of coronary artery disease remains unanswered. Certainly, at low-dose the evidence is clear that the impact on glucose tolerance is trivial.[51] The large-scale trials of such low-dosage formulations in hypertension in the elderly where one would expect age-related diminution in carbohydrate tolerance, show that coronary events were significantly *reduced* by as much as 25% in SHEP[79] and by 44% in MRC-2.[81] The dosage issue must significantly feature as an explanation for the excess mortality reported by Warram *et al.*[67] when diuretic therapy had been studied retrospectively in a cohort of diabetes with advanced retinopathy. No dosages are given in this study but in view of its historical overview, it would of necessity have studied patients treated with diuretics, for whatever reason, in high dosage.

Hyperlipidaemia

Thiazide diuretics and loop diuretics raise low-density lipid (LDL)-cholesterol, high-density lipid (HDL), while leaving HDL-cholesterol and its major apoproteins A_1 and A_2, unchanged. The ratios LDL/HDL-cholesterol and total cholesterol/HDL usually are increased.

Premenopausal women do not show these changes suggesting that oestrogens exert their protective effect in preventing diuretic-induced alterations in lipids.[19]

Dyslipidaemia, as with other metabolic sequelae of diuretic therapy, is dose related. Thus the thiazide-like compound, indapamide, which has been marketed as an antihypertensive at subdiuretic dosage, does not cause disturbances in lipid metabolism.[92]

The clinical significance of the effects of diuretics on lipids in the long term is also unclear since many studies again employed large doses of thiazides when it was generally fashionable to do so. The consensus of opinion is that it seems unlikely that the diuretic-induced lipid changes could explain the shortfall in ischaemic heart disease benefit as compared with stroke reduction encountered in earlier hypertension trials.[48]

NON-METABOLIC ADVERSE EFFECTS

Some of the non-specific side-effects encountered with diuretics, such as lethargy and dizziness, may relate directly to the hypotensive actions of these agents. Acute hypotension with hypovolaemia and sudden accumulation of large volumes of urine within the bladder may precipitate acute urinary retention in elderly male patients with prostatism. In the MRC-1 trial,[93] a prominent subjective symptom that was responsible for about twenty withdrawals from thiazide treatment per 1000 patient years was impotence; this study, as has been noted before, employed the high dose of 10 mg bendrofluazide per day. In the dose–response study reported by Carlsen *et al.*,[51] also employing bendrofluazide, the incidence of subjective side-effects was identical to placebo, up to a dosage of 5 mg/day, with the incidence doubling to twenty-four out of fifty-two patients at the 10 mg dose.

Hypersensitivity reactions such as blood dyscrasias, or skin reactions, pancreatitis or intestinal can occur but are rare.[94] Ultra-high dosage of loop diuretics can be associated with deafness of a sensorineural nature, which is usually a transitory phenomenon but can be permanent. This effect is probably due to diuretic effects on cation exchange within the middle ear affecting endolymph constituents and cochlear membrane potentials.

Acetazolamine, which cannot really be regarded as a clinically relevant diuretic today, was however one of the important precursor drugs to the thiazides and through its carbonic anhydrase inhibitory actions, is still used widely in the management of glaucoma. The drug causes a significant metabolic acidosis and produces a marked reduction in urinary citrate excretion; this increases urinary calcium excretion and may increase the incidence of renal stone formation in susceptible patients.[95]

Another diuretic capable of causing nephrolithiasis is triamterene, the potassium-sparing agent; this is a relatively rare event with an estimated incidence of only 1 per 15 000 per annum of patients taking triamterene. It is probably best to avoid this drug in patients with a previous history of renal stone.[96]

Gynaecomastia in male patients is a relatively common occurrence with continued use of spironolactone; the mechanism probably involves competitive inhibition of the binding of testosterone to androgen receptors.[97]

DRUG INTERACTIONS

NSAIDs interfere with the antihypertensive and renal actions of loop diuretics and thiazides, emphasizing the important role that increase in renal prostaglandins plays in both the blood pressure lowering and saliuretic activities of diuretics. Changes in intrarenal haemodynamics may feature in the mechanism of this interaction[98] as well as possibly a NSAID-induced enhancement of the renal actions of arginine vasopressin.[99] Co-administration of indomethacin with triamterene may precipitate acute renal failure.[100]

Diuretic-induced hypokalaemia and hypomagnesaemia have been known for many years to potentiate the actions of cardiac glycosides and predispose to increased incidence of cardiac dysrhythmias.[101] The patients who are at greatest risk of dangerous ventricular dysrhythmias are those with underlying ischaemic heart disease and those with a previous history of cardiac rhythm disturbances.[84] Diuretic-induced hypokalaemia may also interfere with neuromuscular conduction, but this effect may also be related to a reduction in serum magnesium and calcium. Consequently the dose of non-depolarizing muscular relaxants should be reduced or their effects are likely to be prolonged.

Important pharmacokinetic interactions involving diuretics relate to probenicid and lithium. Probenecid is a uricosuric agent which competitively inhibits the proximal renal secretory pathway for weak acids and prevents the access of loop diuretics and thiazides to their tubular sites of action.[98] Both loop diuretics and thiazides may enhance the proximal reabsorption of lithium in chronic therapy by a mechanism parallel to that responsible for the hyperuricaemia seen after diuretic therapy – namely, by stimulation of proximal tubular sodium reabsorption secondary to diuretic-induced contraction of intravascular volume.[6]

REFERENCES

1 Gross TP, Wise RP, Knapp DE. Antihypertensive drug use. Trends in the United States from 1973 to 1985. *Hypertension* 1989; **13** (Suppl 1): I113–I118.

2 Joint National Committee. Fifth report on the Joint National Committee in detection, evaluation and treatment of high blood pressure (JNCV). *Archives of Internal Medicine* 1993; **153**: 154–82.

3 British Hypertension Society. Management guidelines in essential hypertension: report of the Second Working Party. Sever P, Beevers G, Bulpitt C, Lever A, *et al. British Medical Journal* 1993; **306**: 983–7.

4 Cohn JN. The prevention of heart failure – a new agenda. *New England Journal of Medicine* 1992; **327**: 725–7.

5 Benos DJ. Amiloride: a molecular probe of sodium transport in tissue and cells. *American Journal of Physiology* 1982; **242**: C131–C145.

6 Lant A. Diuretics: Clinical pharmacology and therapeutic use. Part II. *Drugs* 1985; **29**: 162–88.

7 Vogl A. The discovery of the organic mercurial diuretics. *American Heart Journal* 1950; **39**: 881–3.

8 Brooks BA, Lant AF, McNabb WR, Noormohamed FH. Renal actions of a uricosuric diuretic, racemic indacrinone, in man: Comparison with ethacrynic acid and hydrochlorothiazide. *British Journal of Clinical Pharmacology* 1984; **17**: 497–512.

9 Brooks BA, Lant AF, McNabb WR, Noormohamed FH. Stereospecificity of diuretic receptors in the nephron – a study of the enantiomers of indacrinone (MK196) in man. *Renal Physiology* 1984; **7**: 304–10.

10 Lant AF. Evolution of diuretics and ACE inhibitors, their renal and antihypertensive actions – parallels and contrasts. *British Journal of Clinical Pharmacology* 1987; **23**: 27s–41s.

11 McNabb WR, Noormohamed FH, Brooks BA, Lant AF. Renal actions of piretamide and three other loop diuretics in man. *Clinical Pharmacology and Therapeutics* 1984; **35**: 328–37.

12 Noormohamed FH, Lant AF. Analysis of natriuretic action of a loop diuretic, piretanide, in man. *British Journal of Clinical Pharmacology* 1991; **31**: 463–9.

13 Wangemann P, Braitsch R, Greger R. The diuretic effect of muzolimine. *Pflügers Archives* 1987; **410**: 674–6.

14 Wittner M, DiStefano A, Schlatter E, Delarge J, Greger R. Torasemide inhibits NaCl reabsorption in the thick ascending limb of Henle. *Pflügers Archives* 1986; **407**: 611–14.

15 Beyer KH. Chlorothiazide. How the thiazides evolved as antihypertensive therapy. *Hypertension* 1993; **22**: 388–91.

16 Ellison DH, Velazquez H, Wright FS. Thiazide-sensitive sodium chloride cotransport in early distal tubule. *American Journal of Physiology* 1987; **253**: F546–F554.

17 Gesek FA, Friedman PA. Mechanism of calcium transport stimulated by chlorothiazide in mouse convoluted tubules cells. *Journal of Clinical Investigation* 1992; **90**: 429–38.

18 Fanestil DD. Mechanism of aldosterone blockers. *Seminars in Nephrology* 1988; **8**: 249–63.

19 Giebisch G, Wang W. Properties of renal potassium channels and their regulation. In: Puschett JB, Greenberg A eds. *Diuretics IV: Chemistry, pharmacology and clinical applications*. Amsterdam: Excerpta Medica: 791–800.

20 Burg M, Stoner L, Cardinal J, Green N. Furosemide effect on isolated perfused tubules. *American Journal of Physiology* 1973; **225**: 119–24.

21 Brater DC. Pharmacodynamic considerations in the use of diuretics. *Annual Reviews in Pharmacology and Toxicology* 1983; **23**: 45–62.

22 Noormohamed FH, McNabb WR, Dixey JJ, Lant AF. Renal responses to and pharmacokinetics of piretanide in humans: effect of route of administration, state of hydration and probenecid pretreatment. *Journal of Pharmacology and Experimental Therapeutics* 1990; **254**: 992–9.

23 Voelker JR, Brown-Cartwright D, Anderson S. Comparison of loop diuretics in patients with chronic renal insufficiency: mechanism of difference in response. *Kidney International* 1987; **32**: 572–8.

24 Rudy DW, Voelker JR, Greene PK, Esparanza FA, Brater DC. Loop diuretics for chronic renal insufficiency. A continuous infusion is more efficacious than bolus therapy. *Annals of Internal Medicine* 1991; **115**: 360–6.

25 Collins R, Peto R, MacMohan S, Hebert P, *et al.* Blood pressure, stroke and coronary heart disease. Part 2. Short-term reductions in blood pressure: Overview of randomised clinical trials in their epidemiological context. *Lancet* **335**: 827–38.

26 Dikshit K, Vyden JK, Forrester JS, Chatterjee K, Prakash R, Swann HJC. Renal and extrarenal hemodynamic effects of furosemide in congestive cardiac failure after acute myocardial infarction. *New England Journal of Medicine* 1973; **288**: 1087–90.

27 Hasenfuss G, Holubarsch C, Herzog C, Knauf H, Spahn H. Influence of cardiac function on the diuretic and hemodynamic effects of the loop diuretic, piretanide. *Clinical Cardiology* 1987; **10**: 83–8.

28 Stokes W. *The diseases of the heart and the aorta.* Dublin: Hodges & Smith, 1854; 354–5.

29 Packer M. The search for the ideal positive inotropic agent. *New England Journal of Medicine* 1993; **329**: 201–2.

30 Marcus FI. The use of digitalis for the treatment of congestive cardiac failure: a tale of decline and resurrection. *Cardiovascular Drug Therapy* 1989; **3**: 473–6.

31 Smith TW. Digoxin in heart failure. *New England Journal of Medicine* 1993; **329**: 51–3.

32 Packer M, Gheorghiade M, Young JB, Costantini PJ, *et al.* Withdrawal of digoxin for patients with chronic heart failure treated with angiotensin-converting-enzyme inhibitors. *New England Journal of Medicine* 1993; **329**: 1–7.

33 Mathur PNB, Puglsey SC, Powles P, McEwan MP, Campbell JM. Effect of diuretics on cardiopulmonary performance in severe chronic airway obstruction. *Archives of Internal Medicine* 1984; **144**: 2154–7.

34 Cohn JN, Archibald DG, Zeische S, *et al.* Effect of vasodilator therapy on mortality in chronic congestive heart failure: results of a Veterans Administration Cooperative Study. *New England Journal of Medicine* 1986; **314**: 1547–52.

35 Cohn JN, Johnson G, Ziesche S, Cobb F, Francis G, Tristani F, Smith R, Dunkman WB, Loeb H, Wong M. A comparison of enalapril with hydralazine-isosorbide dinitrate in the treatment of chronic congestive cardiac failure (Veterans Administration Co-operative Vasodilator Heart Failure Trial II: V-HeFT II). *New England Journal of Medicine* 1991; **325**: 303–10

36 Dargie HJ, Murray JJV. Diagnosis and management of heart failure. *British Medical Journal* 1994; **308**: 321–8.

37 Dzau VD, Hollenberg NK. Renal responses to captopril in severe heart failure: Role of furosemide in natriuresis and reversal of hyponatremia. *Annals of Internal Medicine* 1984; **100**: 777–82.

38 Packer M, Medina N, Yushak M. Correction of dilutional hyponatremia in severe chronic heart failure by converting-enzyme inhibition. *Annals of Internal Medicine* 1984; **100**: 782–9

39 Opie LH. Pharmacologic profile of ibopamine and related dopamine-like modulators. *Cardiovascular Drugs and Therapy* 1989; **3**: 1041–54.

40 Brater DC, Seiwell R, Anderson S, Burdette A, Dehmer GI, Chennavasin P. Absorption and disposition of furosemide in congestive heart failure. *Kidney International* 1982; **22**: 171–6.

41 Stanton BA, Kaissling B. Adaptation of distal tubule and collecting duct to increased Na delivery II. Na^+ and K^+ transport. *American Journal of Physiology* 1988; **255**: F1269–F1275.

42 Kiyinji A, Field MJ, Pawsey CC. Metolazone in treatment of severe refractory congestive cardiac failure. *Lancet* 1990; **335**: 29–31.

43 Lant A. Diuretic drugs. Progress in clinical pharmacology. *Drugs* 1986; **31**: (Suppl 4): 40–55.

44 Moser M. The diuretic dilemma and the management of mild hypertension. *Drugs* 1986; **31** (Suppl 4): 57–67.

45 Multiple Risk Factor Intervention Trial. Risk factor changes and mortality results. *Journal of American Medical Association* 1982; **248**: 1465–77.

46 Kolata G. Heart study produces a surprise result. A massive study of heart disease that seems to contradict conventional wisdom may have been skewed by drug toxicity. *Science* 1982; **218**: 31–2.

47 Freis ED. The cardiotoxicity of thiazide diuretics: a review of the evidence. *Journal of Hypertension* 1990; **8** (Suppl 2): s23–s32.

48 Moser M. Diuretics and cardiovascular risk factors. *European Heart Journal* 1992; **13** (Suppl G): 72–80.

49 Cranston WI, Juel-Jensen BE, Semmence AM, Handfield-Jones RPC, Forbes JA, Mutch LMM. Effect of oral diuretics on raised arterial pressure. *Lancet* 1963; **ii**: 966–70.

50 Macgregor GA, Banks RA, Markandu ND, Roulston J. Xipamide and cyclopenthiazide in essential hypertension – Comparative effects on blood pressure. *British Journal of Clinical Pharmacology* 1982; **13**: 859–63.

51 Carlsen JE, Kober L, Torp-Pederson C, Johansen P. Relation between dose of bendrofluazide, antihypertensive effect, and adverse biochemical effects. *British Medical Journal* 1990; **300**: 975–8.

52 European Working Party on High Blood Pressure in the Elderly. Mortality and morbidity results from the European Working Party on High Blood Pressure in the Elderly. *Lancet* 1985; **i**: **1349–54.**

53 Siscovick DS, Raghunathan TE, Psaty BM, Koepsell TD, Wicklund KG, Lin X, Cobb L, Rautaharju PM, Copass MK, Wagner EH. Diuretic therapy for hypertension and the risk of primary cardiac arrest. *New England Journal of Medicine* 1994; **330**: 1952–7.

54 Harper R, Ennis CN, Sheridan B, Atkinson AB, et al. Effects of low dose versus conventional dose thiazide diuretic on insulin action in essential hypertension. *British Medical Journal* 1994; **309**: 226–30.

55 Birkenhager WH. Diuretics and blood pressure reduction: physiologic aspects. *Journal of Hypertension* 1990; 8 (Suppl 2): s3–s7.

56 Frohlich ED, Schnaper WH, Wilson IM, Freis ED. Hemodynamic alterations in hypertensive patients due to chlorothiazide. *New England Journal of Medicine* 1960; **262**: 1261–3.

57 Van Brummelen P, Man In't Veld AJ, Schalekamp MADH. Hemodynamic changes during long-term thiazide treatment of essential hypertension in responders and non-responders. *Clinical Pharmacology and Therapeutics* 1980; **27**: 328–36.

58 Tobian L. How sodium and the kidney relate to the hypertensive arteriole. *Federation Proceedings* 1974; **33**: 138–42.

59 Struyker-Boudier HAJ, Smits JFM, Kleinjans JCS, Van Essen H. Hemodynamic actions of diuretic agents. *Clinical and Experimental Hypertension* 1993; **A5**(2): 209–23.

60 Kaplan NM. The deadly quartet: upper body obesity, glucose intolerance, hypertriglyceridemia and hypertension. *Annals of Internal Medicine* 1989; **149**: 1514–20.

61 WHO/ISH Guidelines Committee. Prevention of hypertension and associated cardiovascular disease: a 1991 Statement. *Clinical and Experimental Hypertension* 1992; **14**: 333–41.

62 Staessen J, Amery A, Fagard R. Isolated systolic hypertension in the elderly. *Journal of Hypertension* 1990; **8**: 393–405.

63 WHO Expert Committee. *Arterial hypertension. WHO Technical Report Series* **No. 628**. Geneva: WHO, 1978.

64 Brunner HR, Menard J, Weaber B, Burnier M, *et al.* (1990). Treating the individual hypertensive patient: Considerations on dose sequential monotherapy and drug combinations. *Journal of Hypertension* **8**: 3–11.

65 The 1988 report of the Joint National Committee on Detection, Evaluation and Treatment of High Blood Pressure (JNC IV). *Archives of Internal Medicine* 1988; **148**, 1023–38.

66 Neaton JD, Grimm RH, Prineas RJ, Stamler J, Grandits GA, Elmer PJ, Cutler JA, Flack JM, Schoenberger JA, McDonald R, Lewis CE, Liebson PR. Treatment of mild hypertension study. *Journal of the American Medical Association* 1993; **270**, 713–24.

67 Warram JH, Laffel LMB, Valsania P, Christlieb AR, Krolewski AS. Excess mortality associated with diuretic therapy in diabetes mellitus. *Archives of Internal Medicine* 1991; **151**: 1350–6.

68 Lant AF. Challenges facing the choice of diuretics as first-line treatment for hypertension. *Cardiovascular Risk Factors Journal* 1991; **1**: 480–2.

69 Lewis EJ, Hunsicker LG, Bain RP, Rohde RD. The effect of angiotensin-converting-enzyme inhibition on diabetic nephropathy. *New England Journal of Medicine* 1993; **329**: 1456–62.

70 Moser M, Setaro JF. Antihypertensive drug therapy and regression of left ventricular hypertrophy: a review with a focus on diuretics. *European Heart Journal* 1991; **12**: 1034–9.

71 Massie BM. Effect of diuretic therapy on hypotensive left ventricular hypertrophy. *European Heart Journal* 1992; **13** (Suppl G): 53–60.

72 Brater DC. Use of diuretics in chronic renal insufficiency and nephrotic syndrome. *Seminars in Nephrology* 1988; **8**: 333–41.

73 Knauf H, Spahn H, Mutschler E. The loop diuretic torasemide in chronic renal failure. Pharmacokinetics and pharmacodynamics. *Drugs* 1991; **41** (Suppl 3): 23–34.

74 Schrier RW. Pathogenesis of sodium and water retention in high-output and low-output cardiac failure, nephrotic syndrome, cirrhosis and pregnancy. *New England Journal of Medicine* 1988; **319**: 1065–72.

75 Better OS, Schrier RW. Disturbed volume homeostasis in cirrhosis of the liver. *Kidney International* 1983; **23**: 303–11.

76 McVeigh G, Galloway D, Johnston D. The case for low dose diuretics in hypertension: comparison of low and conventional doses of cyclopenthiazide. *British Medical Journal* 1988; **297**: 95–8.

77 Modan M, Halkin H, Almog S, Lusky A, *et al.* Hyperinsulinemia: a link between hypertension, obesity and glucose tolerance. *Journal of Clinical Investigation* 1985; **75**: 809–17.

78 Smith U. Gudbjornsdottir S, Landin K. Hypertension as a metabolic disorder – an overview. *Journal of Internal Medicine* 1991; **229** (Suppl 2): 1–7.

79 SHEP Cooperative Research Group. Prevention of stroke by antihypertensive drug treatment in older patients with isolated systolic hypertension: final results of Systolic Hypertension in the Elderly Program (SHEP). *Journal of the American Medical Association* 1991; **265**: 3255–64.

80 Dahlof B, Lindholm LH, Hansson L, Schersten B, Ekbom T, Webster PO. Morbidity and mortality in the Swedish trial in old patients with hypertension (STOP-Hypertension). *Lancet* 1991; **338**, 1291–5

81 MRC - 2. MRC Working Party. Medical Research Council trial for treatment of hypertension in older adults: principal results. *British Medical Journal* 1992; **304**: 405–12.

82 Chung HM, Kluge R, Schrier RW, Anderson RJ. Clinical assessment of extracellular fluid volume in hyponatremia. *American Journal of Medicine* 1987; **83**: 905–8.

83 Sunderam SG, Mankikar GD. Hyponatremia in the elderly. *Age and Aging* 1983; **12**: 79–80.

84 Caralis PV, Perez-Stable E. Electrolyte abnormalities and ventricular arrhythmias. *Drugs* 1986; **31** (Suppl 4): 85–100.

85 Grimm RH Jr, Neaton JD, McDonald M, Case J, McGill E, Allen R, Bailey-Hoffman G, Kousch D, Childs J, Hulley SB. Beneficial effects from systematic dosage reduction of the diuretic, chlorthalidone: a randomized study within a clinical trial. *American Heart Journal* 1985; **109**: 858–64.

86 Schnaper HW, Freis ED, Friedman RG, *et al.* Potassium restoration in hypertensive patients made hypokalemic by hydrochlorothiazide. *Archives of Internal Medicine* 1989; **149**: 2677–81.

87 Wills MR. Magnesium and potassium inter-relationship in cardiac disorders. *Drugs* 1986; **31** (Suppl 4): 121–31.

88 McInnes GT, Yeo WW, Ramsay LE, Moser M. Cardiotoxicity and diuretics: much speculation – little substance. *Journal of Hypertension* 1992; **10**: 317–35.

89 Ray WA. Thiazide diuretics and osteoporosis: time for a clinical trial? *Annals of Internal Medicine* 1991; **115**: 64–5.

90 Ramsay LE, Yeo WW, Jackson PR. Diabetes, impaired glucose tolerance and insulin resistance with diuretics. *European Heart Journal* 1992; **13** (Suppl G): 68–71.

91 Boehringer K, Weidmann P, Mordasini R, Schiff H, Bachmann C, Riesen W. Menopause-dependent plasma lipoprotein alterations in diuretic-treated women. *Annals of Internal Medicine* 1982; **97**: 206–9.

92 Weidmann P, De Courten M, Ferrari P. Effect of diuretics on plasma lipid profile. *European Heart Journal* 1992; **13** (Suppl G): 61–7.

93 MRC Working Party. Medical Research Council trial of treatment of mild hypertension: principal results. *British Medical Journal* 1985; **291**, 97–104.

94 Prichard BN, Owens CW, Woolf AS. Adverse reactions to diuretics. *European Heart Journal* 1992; **13** (Suppl G): 96–103.

95 Sutton RAL, Dewer J, Walker VR, *et al.* Renal calculi and acetazolamide (ACZ) therapy. *Kidney International* 1983; **23**: 137 (abs).

96 Editorial. Triamterene and the kidney. *Lancet* 1986; i: 424.

97 Lant A. Diuretics: Clinical pharmacology and therapeutic use. Part 1. *Drugs* 1985; **29**: 57–87.

98 Dixey JJ, Noormohamed FH, Pawa JS, Lant AF, Brewerton DA. The influence of nonsteroidal anti-inflammatory drugs and probenecid on the renal response to and kinetics of piretanide in man. *Clinical Pharmacology and Therapeutics* 1988; **44**: 531–9.

99 Dixey JJ, Williams TD, Lightman SL, Lant AF, Brewerton DA. The effect of indomethacin on the renal

response to arginine vasopressin in man. *Clinical Science* 1986; **70**: 409–16.

100 Favre L, Glasson P, Riondel A, Vallotton MB. Interaction of diuretics and non-steroidal anti-inflammatory drugs in man. *Clinical Science* 1983; **64**: 407–15.

101 Seller RK. The role of magnesium in digitalis toxicity. *American Heart Journal* 1971; **82**: 551–6.

102 Beermann B, Groschinsky-Grind M. Clinical pharmacokinetics of diuretics. *Clinical Pharmacokinetics* 1980; **5**: 221–45.

103 Rudy DW, Brater DC. Pharmacokinetics and pharmacodynamics of bumetanide. In: Lant AF ed. *Bumetanide. The diuretic agents*. Vol 1. Carnforth: Marius Press, 1990: 31–57.

104 Baba WI, Lant AF, Smith AJ, Townshend MM, Wilson GM. Pharmacological effects in animals and normal human subjects of the diuretic amiloride hydrochloride (MK870). *Clinical Pharmacology and Therapeutics* 1968; **9**: 318–27.

105 Brater DC, Leinfielder J, Anderson S. Clinical pharmacology of torasemide, a new loop diuretic. *Clinical Pharmacology and Therapeutics* 1987; **42**: 187–92.

29

Gastrointestinal Tract and Liver

PART I DRUGS AFFECTING THE GASTROINTESTINAL TRACT

JC Foreman

INTRODUCTION

The greater part of this chapter will concentrate on those areas of gastrointestinal pharmacology where there are new developments that are relevant to the practice of anaesthesia and will focus on a review of the mechanisms of action. For completeness, other relevant aspects of this area of pharmacology are dealt with, but in less detail. Table 29.1 gives a general classification of drugs acting on the gastrointestinal tract.

Very considerable advances have been made in gastrointestinal pharmacology within the last 20 years and these advances are having great impact upon clinical pharmacology in anaesthesia.

Prior to the early 1970s, the control of gastric acid secretion by pharmacological means was essentially limited to the use of muscarinic cholinergic antagonists, such as atropine, which were non-selective and gave rise to numerous problems with adverse side-effects. These side-effects were largely related to the principal action of the drugs at muscarinic cholinergic receptors and hence it was not easy to see a way forward for improvement of these drugs. The discovery by Black and colleagues[1] of compounds that could act as antagonists of the H_2 receptor for histamine, revolutionized the pharmacological control of gastric acid secretion but other novel mechanisms for the control of gastric acid secretion have been developed and include inhibitors of the parietal cell H^+/K^+ ATPase, selective muscarinic antagonists and analogues of the E prostaglandins.

Another field of major advance has been in the control of emesis where the early drugs, antagonists of the dopamine D_2 receptors such as the phenothiazines and butyrophenones, suffered from the disadvantage of producing extrapyramidal motor side-effects. More recently, dopamine D_2 antagonists,

TABLE 29.1 Classification of gastrointestinal drugs

GASTRIC SECRETION	
Neutralization	Antacids: soluble e.g. sodium bicarbonate insoluble e.g. magnesium trisilicate
Inhibition	Muscarinic M_1 antagonists e.g. pirenzepine Histamine H_2 antagonists e.g. ranitidne H^+ Pump inhibitors e.g. omeprazole PGE analogues e.g. enprostil
Stimulation	Gastrin analogue e.g. pentagastrin
VOMITING	
Stimulation	Local irritant e.g. ipecachuanha Central effect e.g. apomorphine
Inhibition	Dopamine D_2 antagonists e.g. domperidone 5-HT_3 antagonists e.g. ondansetron Histamine H_1 antagonists e.g. cyclizine Muscarinic antagonists e.g. hyoscine Cannabinoids e.g. nabilone
GASTROINTESTINAL MOTILITY	
Inhibition	Muscarinic antagonists e.g. propantheline Opiate agonists e.g. codeine, diphenoxylate, loperamide
Stimulation	Muscarinic agonists e.g. bethanechol Domperidone Metoclopramide Stimulant purgatives e.g. senna, bisacodyl

which do not cross the blood–brain barrier, have been developed and these drugs, such as domperidone, are anti-emetic without having major extrapyramidal side-effects. Moreover, research on the mechanism of action of metoclopramide indicated that antagonists at the 5-hydroxytryptamine (5-HT_3) receptor could have anti-emetic action and this has indeed turned out to the case, with the development of a series of anti- emetic drugs that are selective 5-HT_3 receptor antagonists.

PHARMACOLOGY OF GASTRIC SECRETION

Antacids

Antacids do nothing to reduce gastric acid secretion and may even increase it. Furthermore, they are not effective in promoting the healing of peptic ulcers, unless used at doses and frequencies that cause a maintained elevation of gastric pH. Generally, patients find it impossible to comply with the amounts and dosing frequency of antacids necessary to promote peptic ulcer healing. Nevertheless, antacids do provide symptomatic relief of the pain associated with hyperacidity.

Insoluble compounds of magnesium and aluminium, such as hydroxides, carbonates, silicates and phosphates, have a slow, sustained action, in contrast to water-soluble sodium bicarbonate which has a rapid, transient action. Examples include aluminium hydroxide, magnesium trisilicate and magnesium carbonate. The mechanism of action is neutralization of acid. They may also adsorb pepsin and the metal ions can inactivate pepsin.

Large doses given over a long period can lead to several problems. Sodium bicarbonate can give rise to systemic alkalosis, magnesium compounds produce a laxative action and several of the antacids can interfere with the absorption of other drugs.

Calcium- and bismuth-containing antacids should be avoided because of the potential toxicity of the metal ion if it is absorbed in sufficient quantities.

Some preparations of antacids contain alginates to give mucosal protection or antifoaming agents (e.g. dimethicone, gaviscon).

Histamine H_2 receptor antagonists

The antagonists of the H_2 receptor for histamine are an example of the rational development of drugs with the specific aim of suppressing the secretion of gastric acid, and the first drug with this mechanism of action to be introduced into routine clinical practice was cimetidine (Fig. 29.1). Subsequently, several other H_2 receptor antagonists have been introduced and, in terms of their pharmacological mechanism of action, they offer nothing new. The newer H_2 receptor antagonists include ranitidine, famotidine, tiotidine, oxmetidine, nizatidine and roxatidine (Fig. 29.1). The development of these new H_2 receptor antagonists has brought changes in potency, pharmacokinetics and side-effects compared with cimetidine. It is often difficult to compare the various drugs when the clinical trials of them

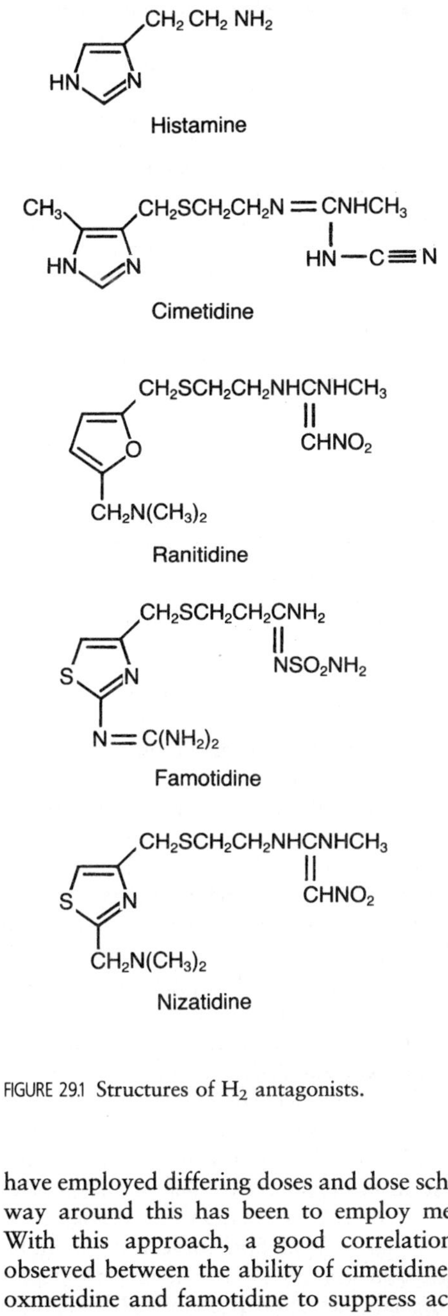

$CH_2CH_2NH_2$

HN N

Histamine

CH_3 $CH_2SCH_2CH_2N{=}CNHCH_3$

HN N $HN{-}C{\equiv}N$

Cimetidine

$CH_2SCH_2CH_2NHCNHCH_3$

O $CHNO_2$

$CH_2N(CH_3)_2$

Ranitidine

$CH_2SCH_2CH_2CNH_2$

S N NSO_2NH_2

$N{=}C(NH_2)_2$

Famotidine

$CH_2SCH_2CH_2NHCNHCH_3$

S N $CHNO_2$

$CH_2N(CH_3)_2$

Nizatidine

FIGURE 29.1 Structures of H_2 antagonists.

have employed differing doses and dose schedules. One way around this has been to employ meta-analysis. With this approach, a good correlation has been observed between the ability of cimetidine, ranitidine, oxmetidine and famotidine to suppress acid secretion and the ability to produce healing of duodenal ulcers in 4 weeks.[2] Different doses and dose schedules were compared in this analysis. It seems, therefore, that with respect to the healing of duodenal ulcers, the drugs differ in potency and pharmacokinetics but, providing an adequate dose is given at the appropriate interval, the degree of suppression of acid secretion by blockade of the H_2 receptor is what determines the clinical effect.

Unwanted effects

After the introduction of cimetidine, two important side-effects became apparent. First, the drug inhibits cytochrome P-450 oxidative metabolism of foreign compounds in the liver which gives rise to significant drug interactions between cimetidine and other drugs. Imidazole has been shown to inhibit microsomal drug metabolism[3] by interacting with the haem iron atom of cytochrome P-450 and cimetidine, of course, has an imidazole ring in its structure (Fig. 29.2). Both imidazole and cimetidine bind avidly to rat hepatic cytochrome P-450 and inhibit aminopyrine demethylation. Second, cimetidine was found to have an anti-androgen effect with loss of libido, gynaecomastia and impotence in some patients.[4] Cimetidine binds to androgen receptors and displaces dihydrotestosterone from these receptors.[5] Cimetidine lowers the sperm count in man, raises serum follicle stimulating hormone levels and increases plasma testosterone levels in both rat and man.

The newer H_2 receptor antagonists developed subsequently to cimetidine do not appear to suffer from these unwanted effects on drug metabolism and gonadal function – at least not to the same extent. Most of the newer drugs do not possess an imidazole ring in their structure and it is possible, though not entirely clear, that the side-effects of cimetidine are related to its imidazole ring. Famotidine and ranitidine have been found not to prolong antipyrine metabolism or hexobarbital sleeping time in rats, whereas cimetidine prolonged both of these parameters. Also, famotidine and ranitidine showed little or no interaction with cytochrome P-450 *in vitro* and no evidence of alteration of microsomal drug metabolism *in vivo*. Similarly, nizatidine shows no binding to cytochrome P-450 and does not alter drug metabolism *in vivo*. On the other hand, oxmetidine, which does have an imidazole ring, binds to cytochrome P-450 and also inhibits microsomal drug-metabolizing enzymes *in vitro* but tiotidine, which has no imidazole ring, also binds to cytochrome P-450. However, *in vitro* binding of drugs to cytochrome P-450 does not necessarily imply an *in vivo* alteration of drug metabolism because tiotidine,

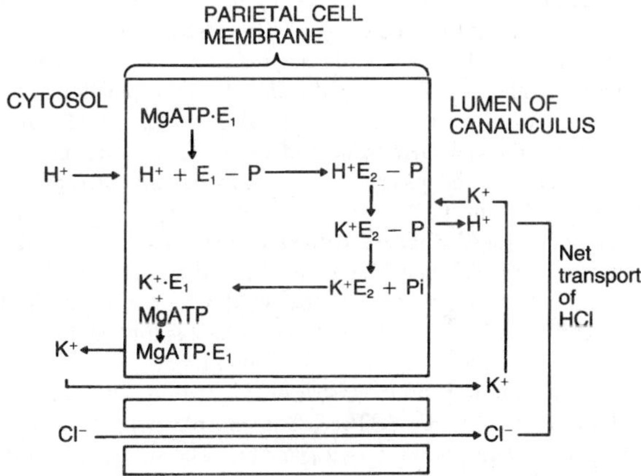

FIGURE 29.2 The molecular mechanism for the generation of gastric acid by operation of the H^+/K^+ ATPase. E_1 and E_2 represent two states of the catalytic subunit of the ATPase.

which binds to cytochrome P-450, did not, like ranitidine, inhibit oxidative drug metabolism *in vitro*. Interestingly, *in vivo*, nizatidine inhibited neither caffeine nor aminopyrine metabolism but tiotidine inhibited caffeine metabolism, as did ranitidine, whereas it did not inhibit aminopyrine metabolism. Thus, although drugs like cimetidine and tiotidine bind to cytochrome P-450, tiotidine shows less inhibition of oxidative drug metabolism that cimetidine.

Ranitidine, famotidine, nizatidine and roxatidine appear to have no effect on gonadal function in man. Nizatidine has been demonstrated not to reduce sperm counts[6] and famotidine and ranitidine do not increase serum testosterone.[7]

Inhibitors of H^+/K^+ ATPase

Histamine plays a major role in the normal physiology of gastric acid secretion and the H_2 receptor antagonists have permitted a clear demonstration of this. Apart from histamine, gastric acid secretion is under the control of acetylcholine and gastrin but histamine appears to be required for the full expression of the response to either of these other stimuli. How histamine interacts with gastrin and acetylcholine is unclear but there are two models, or indeed a combination of them, that are used to explain the role of histamine: these are the transmissive and the permissive models.[8] Intuitively, however, one would expect a drug that prevented the actual secretion of H^+ ions from the parietal cell to be more effective than a drug that blocked the action of one of the stimuli to the parietal cell and this appears to be the case. Omeprazole is an inhibitor of the parietal cell H^+ pump which is able to produce almost total inhibition of 24-h intragastric acidity.[9]

The proton pump of the parietal cell is responsible for the generation of gastric acid and the pump is molecularly an H^+/K^+ ATPase enzyme which has several similarities to the uniquitous Na^+/K^+ ATPase of mammalian cells. The H^+/K^+ ATPase is located in the tubulovesicles of the resting parietal cell but the signal transducers cyclic AMP (for histamine) and intracellular free calcium $[Ca]_1$ (for gastrin and acetylcholine) cause translocation of the enzyme to the microvilli of the parietal cell's secretory canaliculus. In this position, the enzyme causes an electrically neutral exchange of H^+ and K^+ across the cell membrane and at the same time, there is an increase in the passive permeability of the membrane, allowing K^+ and Cl^- to leave the cell. In other words, H^+ is actively moved from the cytosol of the parietal cell to the exterior of the cell in exchange for inward movement of K^+. K^+ and Cl^- then move out of the cell down an electrical and concentration gradient so that the net effect is the secretion of H^+ and Cl^-. Figure 29.3 shows diagrammatically how the pump operates to produce gastric acid secretion. The catalytic subunit of the H^+/K^+ ATPase, E is phosphorylated by ATP and has two conformations, E_1 and E_2. The transported ion binds to E_1 and the E_2 form releases the ion to bind the counterion which in turn is released from the E_2. K^+ increases the sensitivity of the magnesium ATPase by up to thirty times so that when K^+ is present on the luminal surface of the cell the phosphoenzyme E-P is hydrolysed and ATPase activity is stimulated.

Gastric acid secretion may be blocked by inhibiting the pump or by inhibiting the passive Cl^- and K^+ permeabilities necessary for its operation. This membrane ion transport system is similar to many others in mammalian cells but its special location in an acid environment and certain other specific properties have enabled the development of specific inhibitors.[10]

The substituted benzimidazole, omeprazole, is converted in the acid environment of the lumen of the parietal cell canaliculus to a protonated derivative that binds to the H^+/K^+ ATPase. The drug forms a disulphide linkage with the phosphoenzyme. In the formation of the active intermediate, the sulphinyl moiety of the parent compound is converted to sulphanic acid and sulphenamide derivatives and it is these that interact with the luminal sector of the ATPase.

Pharmacokinetics

Depending on the route of administration and species, omeprazole has been shown to be several times more potent than cimetidine at inhibiting gastric acid secretion *in vivo*.

Because it is a weak base (pKa = 4), omeprazole ionizes in the parietal cell canaliculus and becomes trapped. This leads to extracellular concentration of the drug at its site of action on the luminal membrane of the parietal cell and the drug therefore has a long duration of action. Only about 15% of the drug is absorbed after oral dosing but about 75% is absorbed with intraduodenal dosing. With oral administration of a single daily dose, the maximum inhibition of gastric acid secretion by omeprazole is expressed in 3–4 days and thereafter remains stable. Raising the dose above the single daily level of 30 mg produces virtually no increase in the inhibition of acid secretion.

Any absorbed drug binds to plasma protein (95% binding) but the mean elimination half-life is about 1 h. There is no relationship between plasma level and the effect on gastric acid secretion, and although plasma levels fall rapidly, the effect of the drug persists because of its sequestration in the canaliculus of the parietal cell. However, there is a relationship between the area under the plasma level–time curve and the inhibition of gastric acid secretion.[11] The action of omeprazole on gastric acid secretion is completely reversible within 14 days of the last dose.

Basic pharmacology

More important than the modestly greater potency of omeprazole compared with cimetidine is its inhibition of gastric secretion by all stimuli. Omeprazole inhibits basal gastric acid secretion, secretion induced by sham-feeding and pentagastrin infusion, and also secretion induced by histamine and betazole. However, the drug fails completely to inhibit gastric acid secretion over a 24-h period although it persists at its site of action. This may reflect resynthesis by the parietal cell of new H^+/K^+ ATPase.

Clinical studies

In clinical trials, omeprazole has been shown to promote the healing of duodenal ulcers and erosive oesophageal lesions.[12,13] It also provides relief of symptoms in patients with these conditions and in the therapy of duodenal ulcer and reflux oesophagitis, omeprazole is significantly more efficacious than either of the H_2 receptor antagonists cimetidine and ranitidine. Omeprazole was also shown to be a superior treatment for Zollinger–Ellison syndrome in a 4-year international trial.

Side-effects

Omeprazole is well tolerated in human studies and the various reported side-effects appear unrelated to the main action of the drug. A therapeutic index achieved by comparing the LD_{50} in rat to the ED_{50} in man is of the order of 10^4. Drugs that suppress gastric acid secretion, with the exception of some analogues of prostaglandin E (see below), may produce hypergastrinaemia because acid in the stomach is one of the regulatory controls of gastrin secretion. Raised gastrin levels are able to produce hyperplasia of the oxyntic mucosa and also of enterochromaffin cells. In animal studies, omeprazole has been shown to have these effects and chronic dosing of rats with the drug causes the development of gastrin-secreting carcinoid tumours.

Prostaglandin analogues

Mechanism of action

Prostaglandins are local hormones derived from the metabolism of arachidonic and other fatty acids and they have widespread effects that are important in the present context because of their potential to generate unwanted side-effects. The E prostaglandins have been shown to inhibit the secretion of gastric acid by a mechanism that appears to be mediated by a decrease in the intracellular level of cyclic AMP in the parietal cell.[14] Inhibition of prostaglandin synthesis increases the secretion of acid in response to several different stimuli[15] which raises the interesting question of whether the normal physiological regulation of gastric secretion involves prostaglandin synthesis within the gastric mucosa (Fig. 29.3).

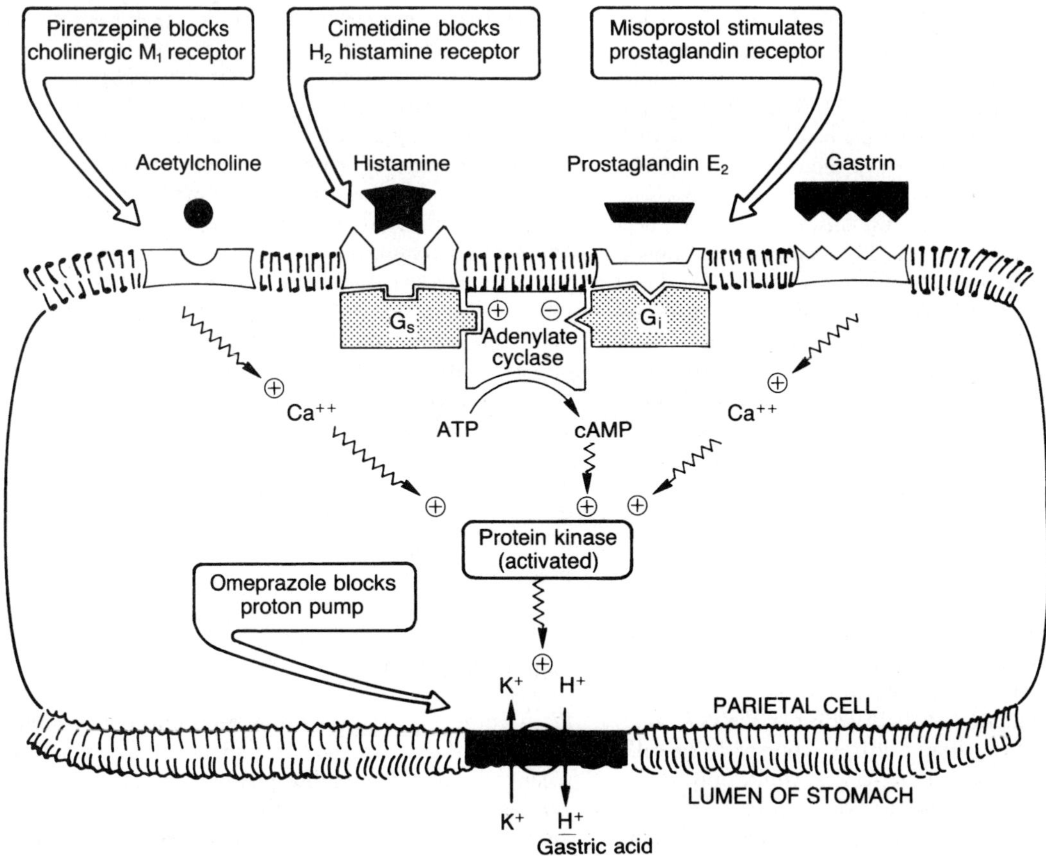

FIGURE 29.3 Effects of acetylcholine, histamine, prostaglandin E_2 and gastrin on gastric acid secretion of the parietal cell of the stomach; G_s and G_i are membrane proteins that mediate the stimulatory or inhibitory effect of receptor binding to adenylate cyclase. (From Lippincotts Illustrated Reviews 'Pharmacology' 1992).

In addition to the ability of prostaglandin E (PGE) to inhibit gastric acid secretion, it has what is described as a 'cytoprotective' effect on the gastric mucosa. Essentially, this means that in the presence of PGE, the gastric mucosa appears more resistant to the damaging effects of various noxious stimuli such as ethanol and aspirin. 'Cytoprotection' is probably not a single effect of PGE but a result of combined actions which include: (1) increased mucosal blood; (2) increased mucus and bicarbonate secretion; (3) strengthening of the mucosal barrier;[16] and (4) increased repair processes.[17]

Clinical pharmacology

Natural PGE is unsuitable for clinical use because of rapid metabolism after oral administration and so a number of different analogues of PGE have been introduced. Those for which there is an already large literature include: enprostil ((+)-4,5-didehydro-16-phenoxy-ω-tetranor-prostaglandin E_2), rioprostil (16-methyl-1,11-1 16 (RS)-trihydroxyprostaglandin E_1), arbaprostil (15(R)-15 methylprostaglandin E_2), trimoprostil (11(R)-16, 16-trimethylprostaglandin E_2) and misoprostol ((+) (16RS)-15-deoxy-16-hydroxy-16-methylprostaglandin E_1).

With the exception of enprostil, these PGE analogues have relatively short half-lives, requiring that multiple daily doses are given to achieve a therapeutic effect: usually four times a day. All of the PGE analogues have been shown to inhibit basal and stimulated gastric acid secretion, and all of them produce significant increased healing of peptic ulcers in comparison with a placebo. Enprostil and misoprostil have been shown to be as effective as H_2 receptor antagonists in promoting the healing of peptic ulcers.[18] The PGE analogues protect against aspirin-induced damage to the mucosa of the upper gastrointestinal tract[19] and there are various pieces of evidence confirming a 'cytoprotective' effect of these compounds. Trimoprostil and misoprostil increase duodenal bicarbonate production and rioprostil and trimoprostil increase mucus production.

Side-effects

In contrast to the H_2 receptor antagonists and omeprazole, some PGE analogues, notably enprostil, reduce rather than increase serum gastrin levels.

The principal unwanted side-effect of the PGE analogues is diarrhoea, though this is reported to be self-limiting in most cases and in clinical trials, only about 1% or less of the patients withdrew because of diarrhoea. The diarrhoea may be accompanied by abdominal pain, flatulence, nausea and vomiting. The incidence of diarrhoea with the use of these compounds may, however, approach 40% of the patients. As might be expected from the vasodilator action of natural E prostaglandins, some patients report headache when treated with the analogues. A further potential problem is the risk of abortion. Prostaglandins E are known to cause contraction of the pregnant uterus and there is some evidence that misoprostil has this action in pregnant women.

Muscarinic antagonists

It is well established that the classical muscarinic antagonist, atropine, is able to inhibit gastric acid secretion. However, the ability of atropine to inhibit gastric acid secretion is dependent upon the stimulus to the secretion (Fig. 29.3), and the presence of muscarinic receptors in many tissues other than the gastric mucosa means that the control of gastric secretion with non-selective muscarinic antagonists is limited by numerous side-effects.

Basic pharmacology

Muscarinic receptors are heterogeneous and multiple subtypes (M_1, M_2, M_3, etc.) have been identified by pharmacological and molecular biological techniques. M_1 and M_3 muscarinic receptors are the subtypes involved in gastric acid secretion, and it has been possible to synthesize compounds with selectivity for M_1 receptors. Pirenzepine is such a selective M_1 receptor antagonist, being about fifty times more potent at M_1 receptors compared with M_2 receptors. In contrast, atropine is only about three times more potent at M_1 receptors compared with M_2 receptors. Synthesis of compounds related to pirenzepine in an attempt to improve selectivity and potency has yielded telenzepine[20] which is ten times more potent than pirenzepine. Although more potent than pirenzepine, telenzepine has an affinity for M_1 receptors that is only twenty times greater than its affinity for M_2 receptors. However, telenzepine exists as (+) and (−) enantiomers with the (+) enantiometric potency ratio being about 400 at M_1 receptors. Thus, if the (+) enantiomer were to be used, telenzepine would offer considerable potency and selectivity improvements over pirenzepine.

Clinical pharmacology

Pirenzepine has been shown to be as effective as cimetidine in the treatment of patients with duodenal ulcer.[21] Telenzepine inhibits peptone-stimulated gastric acid secretion in healthy volunteers in a dose-dependent manner and was found to be about twenty-five times more potent than pirenzepine in this respect. Telenzepine has also been shown to reduce oesophageal reflux time and the maximum duration of reflux in the supine position.

Even at lower doses, telenzepine has been found to reduce salivary secretion and subjects given the drug report dry mouth. Neither pirenzepine nor telenzepine have been found to change near point vision at the doses used to suppress gastric acid secretion though both drugs were found to *reduce* heart rate. No effect of either telenzepine or pirenzepine has been observed on basal or stimulated gastrin release.

PHARMACOLOGY OF ANTI-EMETICS

Dopamine antagonists

Activation of dopamine D_2 receptors in the chemoreceptor trigger zone in the floor of the IVth ventricle is associated with emesis and the use of dopamine antagonists as anti-emetics is commonplace. Examples of such drugs are prochlorperazine, chlorpromazine, trifluoperazine and thiethylperazine. These drugs, which cross the blood–brain barrier, cause the side-effects of sedation and extrapyramidal dystonia to varying degrees (see Chapter 22). Generally it is possible to use a dose that is sufficient to have an effective anti-emetic action but is too low to produce significant unwanted effects.

More recently, dopamine D_2 receptor antagonists, which do not cross the blood–brain barrier, have been developed. Since the chemoreceptor trigger zone lies outside the functional blood–brain barrier, these compounds are effective anti-emetics but do not produce the same degree of side-effects associated with those drugs that do cross the blood–brain barrier. Domperidone is an example of a dopamine D_2 receptor antagonist that does not cross the blood–brain barrier and it has been found to be effective against postoperative emesis, the emesis induced by cytotoxic therapy and L-DOPA-induced emesis.[22] In addition to its action on D_2 receptors in the chemoreceptor trigger zone, domperidone has been shown to accelerate gastric emptying by increasing the motility of the upper gastrointestinal tract. It appears that this effect is also brought about by D_2 receptor antagonism since dopamine released from neurones within the wall of the gastrointestinal tract normally suppresses motility. There is some evidence that this action of domperidone is of value in the treatment of reflux oesophagitis.

5-Hydroxytryptamine antagonists

5-Hydroxytryptamine (5-HT) is a neurotransmitter of both the central and peripheral nervous systems. The amine is also present in the enterochromaffin cells of the gastrointestinal tract and in blood platelets. Classification of the receptors for 5-HT has been hampered by the paucity of selective agonists and antagonists but recent advances have expanded the first classification of M and D receptors into a much more elaborate scheme. The classification is still not definitive but comprises: 5-HT_1 (further divided into subtypes A–F), 5-HT (subtypes A–C)$_2$, 5-HT_3, 5-HT_4, 5-HT_5, 5-HT_6 and 5-HT_7. From the original classification, D corresponds to 5-HT_2 and M to 5-HT_3(see Chapter 20).

One of the explanations for the anti-emetic effect of metoclopramide is that the drug antagonizes 5-HT receptors and this led to a search for more selective 5-HT antagonists with an anti-emetic action. A number of selective 5-HT_3 receptor antagonists have now been synthesized and have been shown to have anti-emetic action. The drugs include ondansetron, granisetron and zacopride.

Basic pharmacology

The *in vitro* pharmacology of ondansetron demonstrates a high degree of selectivity for 5-HT_3 receptors. Ondansetron was found to be a very potent antagonist of the 5-HT_3 receptor-mediated depolarization of either the rat vagus nerve or superior cervical ganglion, with an affinity for the 5-HT_3 receptor of between 1 and 10 nM. Ondansetron had no effect at 5-HT receptors mediating relaxation of cat saphenous vein (5-HT_1) or on the receptors mediating contraction of the dog saphenous vein (5-HT_1) and rabbit aorta (5-HT_2), even at concentrations about three orders of magnitude larger than those at which 5-HT_3 receptors were blocked. The data were also consistent with ondansetron being a competitive 5-HT_3 receptor antagonist.

The *in vivo* preclinical pharmacology of ondansetron confirmed the selectivity. Stimulation of the Bezold–Jarisch reflex in the anaesthetized cat with the selective 5-HT_3 agonist, 2-methyl-5-HT was inhibited by ondansetron with an ED_{50} (intravenous) of 0.4 μg/kg. Even at doses up to 5 mg/kg, ondansetron had no activity against the cardiovascular actions of histamine, adrenaline and acetylcholine, and at doses up to 1 mg/kg the drug had no effect on the vascular responses or on the central action of dopamine.

Ondansetron has potent anti-emetic action over the intravenous dose range of 0.01–1 mg/kg when tested against cisplatin-induced emesis in the ferret. In this model it is about 200 times more potent than metoclopramide. In other animal models, ondansetron has also been reported to have antipsychotic and anxiolytic effects without sedation. Zacopride is also active against cisplatin-induced emesis in the cat. However, it is interesting that the anti-emetic effect of zacopride is a property of the R enantiomer: the S enantiomer having an emetic action.

Clinical pharmacology

The anti-emetic 5-HT_3 antagonists are active by the oral route in man, and clinical trials have shown them to be effective against the emesis caused by cytotoxic drugs. Ondansetron is anti-emetic in adults and children receiving a variety of cytotoxic drugs, including cisplatin.[24] Zacopride is also effective against radiation-induced emesis as well as the emesis caused by cytotoxic drugs but it does not prevent emesis induced by apomorphine or copper sulphate.[25,26]

PHARMACOLOGY OF GASTROINTESTINAL MOTILITY

Muscarinic agonists and antagonists

The motility of the gastrointestinal tract is principally under the control of the autonomic nervous system. Parasympathetic activity through cholinergic muscarinic receptors increases the motility and sympathetic activity through adrenoceptors decreases activity. Muscarinic antagonists may be employed as antispasmodics, for example dicyclomine and propantheline. Muscarinic agonists can be used to increase gastrointestinal motility but are rarely used for this purpose because metoclopramide (see below) is superior and has fewer side-effects on other systems. Adrenoceptor agonists and antagonists are not used to control gastrointestinal motility because of widespread effects on other organs.

Metoclopramide

Mechanisms of action

The exact mechanism of action of metoclopramide in man is unknown but it has a distinct ability to produce co-ordinated increase of gastrointestinal motility with an increase in the rate of emptying of the upper gastrointestinal tract. Its actions are different from those of non-specific muscarinic receptor activation and appear to be complex. Like the other dopamine D_2 receptor antagonists described above, metoclopramide acts on the chemoreceptor trigger zone dopamine receptors and this may account for its anti-emetic action. The ability of metoclopramide to enhance gastric emptying is blocked by antimuscarinic drugs but it is not abolished by vagotomy[27] and it has been suggested that it acts by increasing the release of acetylcholine from the postganglionic, intramural cholinergic neurones. The drug may also sensitize the postjunctional tissue to the action of acetylcholine. It is possible that some of the modulation of the cholinergic system by metoclopramide results from its action at peripheral dopamine receptors that regulate cholinergic transmission.[28] However, a drug that is structurally related to metoclopramide, cisapride, does not have dopamine antagonist action but it does increase gastrointestinal motility by increasing acetylcholine release from the neurones of the intramural plexus.

Pharmacokinetics

Metoclopramide can be given orally, when it is well absorbed, but it is usual to give it intravenously or intramuscularly. It has a half-life of 4 h and hence a sustained action may require infusion. Most of the drug (80%) is excreted unchanged in the urine within 24 h. Cisapride has a half-life of 10 h and is largely inactivated by first-pass metabolism, hence the oral route may be inappropriate.

Clinical pharmacology

Metoclopramide has been shown to be of value in a number of clinical situations. It is effective in reducing the symptoms of gastrointestinal reflux and appears to increase the resting tone of the lower oesophageal sphincter.

The drug increases gastric emptying and has been found to reduce gastric stasis and its associated symptoms after gastric surgery. The evidence that it is effective in diabetic gastroparesis is less strong.

Metoclopramide is an effective anti-emetic drug and its effectiveness and spectrum of activity against nausea and vomiting arising from various causes appears comparable to that of other dopamine D_2 antagonists.

The action of metoclopramide on gastrointestinal motility is also utilized to promote the passage of barium sulphate in diagnostic radiology and of small bowel biopsy capsules. The detail of the clinical trials of the various clinical uses of metoclopramide has been thoroughly reviewed.

Unwanted effects

Single or short-term dosing with the drug produces little in the way of side-effects. The most frequent side-effect is drowsiness. Although not common, extrapyramidal dystonia can occur and, as would be expected, is increased if the patient is also receiving other dopamine antagonists. The extrapyramidal effects are reduced by muscarinic antagonists but, as has already been pointed out, these drugs also block the effect of metoclopramide on gastrointestinal motility.

Metoclopramide has the potential to interact with a large variety of drugs from different classes, though this may not be of great importance in the context of single or short-term dosing that is encountered in anaesthetic practice. Centrally acting drugs which may increase the likelihood of metoclopramide-induced extrapyramidal dystonia are those that may give rise to significant interaction.

REFERENCES

1 Black JW, Duncan WAM, Durant CJ, Ganellin CR, Parsons ME. Definition and antagonism of histamine H_2-receptors. *Nature* 1972; **236**: 385–90.
2 Jones DB, Howden CW, Burget BW, Kerr GD, Hunt RH. Acid suppression in duodenal ulcer: a meta-analysis to define optimal dosing with antisecretory drugs. *Gut* 1987; **28**: 1120–7.
3 Hajeck KK, Cook NI, Novak RF. Mechanism of inhibition of microsomal drug metabolism by imidazole. *Journal*

of Pharmacology and Expimental Therapeutics 1982; **223**: 97–104.

4 Van Thiel DH, Gavaler JS, Smith WI, Paul G. Hypothalamic–pituitary–gonadal dysfunction in men using cimetidine. *New England Journal of Medicine* 1979; **300**: 1012–15.

5 Funder JW, Mercer JE. Cimetidine occupies androgen receptors. *Journal of Clinical Endocrinology and Metabolism* 1979; **48**: 189–91.

6 Van Thiel DH, Gavaler JS, Heyl A, Susen B. An evaluation of the anti-androgen effects associated with H_2 antagonist therapy. *Scand. J. Gastroenterol* 1987; **136** (Suppl): 24–8.

7 Peden NR, Boyd EJS, Browning MCK, Saunders JHB, Wormsley KG. Effects of two histamine H_2-receptor blocking drugs on basal levels of gonadotrophins, prolactin, testosterone and oestradiol-17 during treatment on duodenal ulcer in male patients. *Acta Endocrinologica* 1981; **96**: 564–8.

8 Black JW, Shankley NP. How does gastrin act to stimulate oxyntic cell secretion. *Trends in Pharmacological Sciences* 1987; **8**: 486–90.

9 Lind T, Cederberg C, Ekenved G, Olbe L. Inhibition of basal and betazole- and sham-feeding-induced acid secretion by omeprazole in man. *Scandinavian Journal of Gastroenterology* 1986; **21**: 1004–10.

10 Sachs G, Carlsson E, Lindberg P, Wallmark B. Gastric H,K-ATPase as therapeutic target. *Annual Review of Pharmacology and Toxicology* 1988; **28**: 269–84.

11 Cederberg C, Ekenved G, Lind T, Olbe L. Acid inhibitory characteristics of omeprazole in man. *Scandinavian Journal of Gastroenterology* 1985; **20** (Suppl 108): 105–12.

12 Lauritsen K, Rune SJ, Bytzer P. Effect of omeprazole and cimetidine on duodenal ulcer. *New England Journal of Medicine* 1985; **312**: 958–61.

13 Sandmark S, Carlsson R, Fausa O, Lundell L. Omeprazole or ranitidine in the treatment of reflux oesophagitis. *Scandinavian Journal of Gastroenterology* 1988; **23**: 625–32.

14 Malinowska DM, Sachs G. Cellular mechanisms of acid secretion. *Clinics in Gastroenterology* 1985; **13**: 309–26.

15 Levine RA, Schwartzel EH. Effect of indomethacin on basal and histamine stimulated human gastric acid secretion. *Gut* 1984; **25**: 718–22.

16 Miller TA. Protective effect of prostaglandins against gastric mucosal damage: current knowledge and proposed mechanisms. *American Journal of Physiology* 1983; **245**: 601–23.

17 Hawkey CJ, Rampton DS. Prostaglandins and the gastrointestinal mucosa: are they important in its function, disease or treatment? *Gastroenterology* 1985; **89**: 1162–88.

18 Sontag SJ, Prostaglandins in peptic ulcer disease: an overview of current status and future directions. *Drugs* 1986; **32**: 445–57.

19 Hawkey CJ, Daneshmend TK. The clinical pharmacology of prostaglandins in the human gastrointestinal tract. *Recent Advances in Clinical Pharmacology and Toxicology* 1989; **4**: 57–73.

20 Eltze M, Gonne S, Riedel R, Schlotke B, Schudt C, Simon WA. Pharmacological evidence for the selective inhibition of gastric acid secretion by telenzepine, a new antimuscarinic drug. *European Journal of Pharmacology* 1985; **112**: 211–24.

21 Carmine AA, Pakes GE, Brogden RN, Heel RC, Speight TM, Avery GS. Pirenzepine. A review of its pharmacology and therapeutic use in peptic ulcer disease and other allied diseases. *Drugs* 1985; **30**: 85–126.

22 Towse G. Progress with domperidone. *Royal Society of Medicine International Congress* 1981; **36**: 1–110.

23 Zifa E, Fillion G. 5-Hydroxytryptamine receptors. *Pharmacological Reviews* 1992; **44**: 401–58.

24 Cunningham D, Pople A, Ford HT, Hawthorn J, Gazet J-C, Challoner T. Prevention of emesis in patients receiving cytotoxic drugs by GR38032F, a selective 5-HT_3 receptor antagonist. *Lancet* 1987; i: 1461–3.

25 Bunce K, Tyers MB, Berebek P. Clinical evaluation of 5-HT_3 receptor antagonists as anti-emetics. *Trends in Pharmacological Sciences* 1991; **12**: 46–8.

26 Smith WL, Alphin RS, Jackson CB, Sancillo LF. The anti-emetic profile of zacopride. *Journal of Pharmacy and Pharmacology* 1989; **41**: 101–5.

27 Stadaas J, Aune S. The effect of metoclopramide (Primperan) on gastric motility before and after vagotomy in man. *Scandinavian Journal of Gastroenterology* 1971; **6**: 17–21.

28 Alibibi R, McCallum RW. Metoclopramide: pharmacology and clinical application. *Annals of Internal Medicine* 1983; **98**: 86–95.

PART II LIVER FUNCTION AND DRUGS

S Cottam, SJ Milroy, C Beard

INTRODUCTION

Traditionally pharmacologists use a strictly defined model to assess pharmacokinetic and pharmacodynamic characteristics of a drug. As information accumulates, attention may be diverted to study the effects of a stable chronic disease on the drug handling and metabolism. Such studies are usually performed under controlled conditions in isolated animal and human models which undeniably provide useful information, and form the basis for safe and effective drug administration. However, the practising anaesthetist rarely administers a single drug in isolation and never under totally controlled and predictable circumstances. More commonly, drugs are given in combination to a patient whose physiological response may be rapidly changing. The combination of dynamic physiological conditions and underlying chronic disease may at first seem daunting. It is possible however to make a limited prediction as to the effects of liver disease on drug handling. This is reliant on a basic understanding of normal liver physiology, the pathophysiology of the various disease processes and of the additional effects of surgery and anaesthesia.

REVIEW OF NORMAL HEPATIC ANATOMY AND PHYSIOLOGY

Knowledge of the normal structure and function of the liver is fundamental to understanding the changes induced by disease states, anaesthesia and surgery. This subject has been well reviewed elsewhere.[1–4]

The size, position and metabolic requirements of the liver are unique, and they reflect its pivotal role in many homeostatic mechanisms. These include: overall regulation of intermediate metabolism, regulation of metabolic rate and rate of growth, vitamin and mineral metabolism, and biotransformation and elimination of xenobiotics and drugs. Intermediate metabolism refers to the homeostasis of carbohydrates and related energy substrates which require that the liver is able to synthesize, store, biotransform and eliminate a wide variety of biologically active compounds. (see Table 29.2)

Hepatic blood supply

The liver possesses a dual blood supply, which is derived from the hepatic artery and the portal vein. Total blood flow to the liver is 1100–1800 ml/min (100 ml/100 g liver tissue/min), approximately 25% of the resting cardiac output. This flow reflects the high hepatic oxygen consumption in the face of the reduced oxygen saturation of portal venous blood. Although the hepatic artery carries only 30% of the total blood flow, it supplies 40–50% of hepatic oxygen requirements. Flow into the portal vein is controlled by arterioles in the splanchnic bed. Portal pressure (normally 7–10 mmHg) is determined by the resistance to flow of the portal vasculature within the liver. Precapillary (presinusoidal) sphincters act to produce a uniform distribution of the portal flow throughout the liver, although it appears that the dominant site of intrahepatic venous resistance is post sinusoidal. Smooth muscle in the walls of the hepatic venules responds to sympathetic innervation mediated via α-receptors. Myogenic and metabolic intrin-

TABLE 29.2 Principal liver functions important in homeostasis

STORAGE	SYNTHESIS	BIOTRANSFORMATION	ELIMINATION
Glycogen	Albumin	*Endogenous compounds*	*Vascular filter* Immune complexes
Proteins	Globulins α e.g. caeruloplasmin β e.g. ferritin	e.g. Ammonia to urea	Bacteria and endotoxins
Vitamins A,D,B12,K		*Exogenous compounds*	Encephalopathic toxins
Iron	All clotting factors including protein C + S fibrinogen	Xenobiotics or drugs to compounds with altered activity or differing pathways for elimination	*Biliary* Bilirubin
Copper	Triglycerides		Organic ions
	Lipoproteins		Steroids e.g. cholesterol
	Cholesterol		Intermediate sized lipophilic molecules

sic regulation appear to exert little or no effect on portal vascular resistance.

In contrast, the major site of resistance in the hepatic artery is the arteriole, which appears to respond to local or intrinsic mechanisms. These adjust hepatic arterial flow to compensate for changes in portal flow (the so-called arterial buffer response), provided that the systolic blood pressure exceeds 80 mmHg. The mediator of this response is probably adenosine which is generated within the liver when portal blood flow decreases. This mechanism serves to preserve hepatic oxygen delivery in the case of decreased portal flow. The portal venous system appears to be unable to increase its flow in response to a decrease in arterial supply.

Hepatic blood flow in health can vary widely, predominantly reflecting changes in portal flow. Increased portal flow will be seen on lying supine and following a meal which initiates an increase in splanchnic blood flow. Portal blood flow will decrease during exercise due to splanchnic vasoconstriction. This decrease is offset by increased hepatic arterial flow and oxygen extraction. The liver acts as a vascular reservoir and contains approximately 20–30 ml of blood per 100 g of tissue (almost 15% of total blood volume). Half of this can be mobilized under conditions of increased sympathetic drive and can enter the circulation.

Anaesthesia and surgery are responsible for acute changes in hepatic haemodynamics whereas chronic drug therapy has long-term effects. Both general and regional anaesthesia may alter splanchnic blood flow and cardiac output, as may laparotomy and surgical haemorrhage. β-Antagonists such as propranolol, which are commonly prescribed for the treatment of portal hypertension, may reduce markedly the clearance of other drugs which are reliant on hepatic blood flow for their clearance. Similar effects have been described with H_2-receptor antagonists, such as cimetidine (see above). This is probably mediated by enzyme inhibition, rather than by a direct action on the hepatic vasculature, since ranitidine and famotidine seem devoid of this effect. Chronic therapy with agents such as phenobarbitone, which causes enzyme induction, may in contrast produce an increase in hepatic blood flow, presumably by increasing metabolic demand. These changes are summarized in Table 29.3.

TABLE 29.3 Factors influencing hepatic blood flow

INCREASE LIVER BLOOD FLOW	DECREASE LIVER BLOOD FLOW
Hypercapnia	IPPV and PEEP
	Surgery (laparotomy)
	Hypocapnia, hypoxia
Supine position	Upright posture
Food	
Drugs:	Drugs
β-Agonists	α-Agonists
Phenobarbitone	β-Antagonists
Other enzyme inducers	Ganglion blockers
	H_2 antagonists
	Vasopressin, somatostatin
	Anaesthetics
	Volatile agents
	Intravenous agents

IPPV, intermittent positive pressure ventilation; PEEP, positive end-expiratory pressure.

Liver structure

Structural concepts of liver architecture have been developing since the 17th century. The classical 'lobule' is 0.7–2 mm in size and has at its centre a hepatic venule, with several portal tracts, containing branches of the hepatic artery, vein and bile duct, around its periphery. This anatomical description was largely discarded in the 1950s by Rappaport who described liver micro-architecture in a more functional way. In this more useful concept, the 'acinus' centres on the portal tract, with venules at the periphery. Hepatocytes can be grouped into three 'zones' depending on their distance from the portal inflow tract (Fig. 29.4), which supplies blood with the greatest oxygen saturation and nutrient supply. Branches of the hepatic artery and portal vein radiate from the portal tract, with blood flowing towards the hepatic veins. In terms of oxygen supply, three arbitrary 'zones' are described.

Zone I hepatocytes have a lavish blood supply and are richly furnished with rough endoplasmic reticulum. They are the major site for enzyme, plasma protein and glycogen synthesis, and also for glycogenolysis. Some enzymes synthesized by *zone I* hepatocytes are involved in drug biotransformation, which is achieved by conjugation with some of the readily available local products of metabolism. Drug biotransformation by conjugation is called a 'phase II' reaction. *Zone I* is the last area to develop necrosis following a reduction in hepatic blood supply and the first to regenerate. *Zone III* is at the greatest distance from the nutrient vessels, and hepatocytes here are the least resistant to hepatotoxins or reductions in oxygen delivery. They contain smooth endoplasmic reticulum which contains the greatest concentration of cytochrome enzymes. Finally, *zone II* is concerned with oxygen delivery and functions intermediate between the other two zones.

Liver cells

The sinusoids within the liver are larger and more variable in diameter than typical capillaries. Their walls are lined with two distinct cell types, endothelial cells and Kupffer cells. Kupffer cells are fixed macrophages and are the largest such group in the body. Their role is to endocytose bacterial endotoxins and damaged erythrocytes from the blood. The endothelial cells possess wide fenestrations which enable large molecules such as drug–plasma-protein complexes to diffuse passively into the perisinusoidal space (of Disse). There, they come into direct contact with the hepatocyte cell membrane, facilitating diffusion or active transport of free drug into the hepatocyte. Hepatocytes constitute 78% of liver volume and have an enormous capacity to regenerate.

BIOTRANSFORMATION ENZYME SYSTEMS

The majority of biologically 'active' drugs are fat soluble, or possess lipophilic properties, without which they could not be absorbed from the gastrointestinal tract. Once a drug is absorbed (or after parenteral injection), its fat solubility facilitates penetration of cell membranes and enables the site of action to be reached.

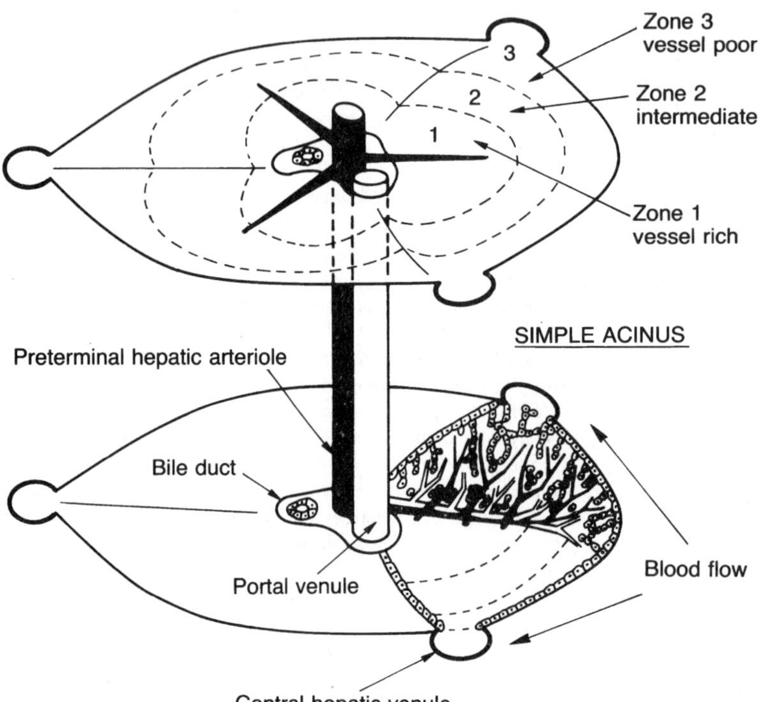

FIGURE 29.4 Functional hepatic anatomy.

Lipophilic drugs bind to plasma proteins and redistribute among fat stores, so their renal excretion will be predictably poor. Before renal excretion of such drugs can take place, they must be rendered water soluble. Enzyme systems capable of increasing the water solubility of lipophilic drugs are widely distributed throughout the body, but by far the greatest concentrations are to be found in the liver. Both the strategic positioning and the microscopic architecture of the liver lend it a pivotal role in drug biotransformation. Historically, the elucidation of the main pathways of drug biotransformation started in the post-war period, when it became possible to extract subcellular fractions from homogenized liver tissue obtained by differential centrifugation. Rough and smooth endoplasmic reticulum could not at that stage be isolated as discrete structures, but fractions of membrane vesicles called microsomes, which had a reddish brown colour, were obtained. In the early 1950s, it was found that this microsomal fraction in the presence of reduced nicotinamide-adenine dinucleotide phosphate (NADPH) was capable of catalysing the majority of drug transformations known to occur in the liver. Over the next decade the myriad of possible reactions catalysed by these microsomes were divided into two groups. These were either phase I (*oxidative*) reactions, where an oxygen atom is inserted into the drug (usually as a hydroxyl group); or phase II *conjugation* reactions, where a drug or its metabolite was covalently bonded to a water-soluble ligand, such as sulphate or glucuronate (see Chapter 3).

Phase I enzyme systems

During the early 1960s, study of microsomal pigment fraction revealed considerable similarity between it and the haem proteins (cytochromes) known to be present in mitochondria. Cytochrome pigments bind oxygen which can be displaced by carbon monoxide (CO). In the presence of CO, cytochromes strongly absorb light with a wavelength of 450 nm and hence have been dubbed 'cytochrome P-450'.[5] (Recent changes in nomenclature have resulted in the prefix 'CYP' when referring to members of the P-450 family of enzymes and '*CYP*' when referring to the gene responsible for that enzyme.)[6] Carbon monoxide, by binding avidly to cytochromes, inhibits oxidative reactions, an effect that can be reversed by exposure to intense light with a wavelength of 450 nm, which causes the CO–cytochrome bond to dissociate. By the 1970s it became apparent that a single enzyme was unlikely to be responsible for the growing number of oxidative reactions that were being described. Agents such as 3-methylchloanthrene were found to increase or 'induce' cytochrome activity in rats, but the cytochrome had a different affinity for various substrates. Currently, over twenty different cytochromes have been identified from human liver, with the greatest concentrations in smooth endoplasmic reticulum where they are responsible for oxidation reactions.[5] Other phase I enzymes are found in the cytoplasm and are capable of reduction and hydrolysis reactions. Overall, cytochromes are found in greater abundance in pericentral hepatocytes – that is, in *zone III*.

Phase II enzyme systems

Phase II or enzymes of 'conjugation' are found in greatest concentration in the rough endoplasmic reticulum. Their overall distribution in the liver is more uniform, although higher concentrations are found in periportal hepatocytes (*zone I*). The varying distribution of these enzyme systems may go some way towards explaining the variable effects of liver disease on drug handling. Phase I reactions can produce drug metabolites that are more reactive than their precursors. While phase I reactions can increase water solubility, this is not invariable, so phase I products may have to undergo secondary phase II conjugation to complete the process. Indeed, in some instances, the phase I reaction is a necessary precursor to enable the phase II reactions to occur. Phase II reactions usually involve the attachment of a hydrophilic group to the pre-existing or newly formed —OH, —COOH, —NH_2 or —SH groups. The most common reaction is glucuronidation, mediated by a family of uridine diphosphate (UDP)-glucuronyl-transferase enzymes.

The genetics of the cytochrome system

The amino acid sequences of a number of cytochrome enzymes have been determined[7] and it is evident that apart from similarities in a few key areas, there are marked structural differences between groups. All cytochrome enzymes seem to be expressions of similar genes which are widely distributed among different chromosomes, and have probably evolved from a common precursor. At least ten distinct human cytochrome gene families have been identified to date.[8] Different gene families appear to have evolved different roles in drug metabolism, and are induced by different substrates (see Table 29.4).

In man, the CYP1A subfamily appears to be produced by two genes, only one of which (*CYP1A2*) is consistently expressed. CYP1A2 is induced by cigarette smoking and consumption of charcoal-grilled foods. The CYP2 family is the largest group identified in man, and individual members are induced by different agents, for example CYP2E1 is induced by ethanol and isoniazid, but not by phenobarbitone.

The CYP3 family is perhaps the most interesting, as members are produced by four closely related genes whose expression may be regulated developmentally. The major CYP3A7 cytochrome present in fetal livers was thought to be absent in adults until recently. It has now been identified in human placenta and endometrium, with levels being much greater in samples from pregnant women. The presence of CYP3A7 in these tissues may play a role in protection of the fetus from the toxic effects of endogenous steroids and foreign substrates.[9] Certain members of this group are expressed in only 25% of the population[5] (CYP3A5). This may explain why some changes in phase I metabolism are seen during development, and why differences can occur between individuals, a situation analogous to differences in acetylator status (a non-cytochrome enzyme). The levels and activities of CYP enzymes are also influenced by dietary factors, which may affect drug handling. For example narangerin, present in grapefruit juice, inhibits CYP3A4. This may explain the observation that drinking 200ml of grapefruit juice can markedly inhibit the oxidation of nifedipine, and will also influence cyclosporin levels via the same cytochrome system.[10]

TABLE 29.4 Human hepatic cytochrome families – inducers and substrates

GENE FAMILY	PROBABLE INDUCERS	DRUG SUBSTRATES
IA2	Cigarette smoke Charcoal-grilled food	Caffeine Theophylline Paracetamol
IIC	None identified	Diazepam Tolbutamide Phenylbutazone
IID	None identified	Metoprolol Perhexiline Amitriptyline Codeine
IIE1	Ethanol Isoniazid	Paracetamol Ethanol
IIIA	Rifampicin Dexamethasone Cortisol Carbamazepine Phenytoin Phenobarbitone Phenylbutazone	Erythromycin Nifedipine Cyclosporin Steroids Ketaconazole Oestrogens Midazolam Lignocaine

The original concept of a 'mixed function' oxidase system is now being challenged. It appears that each cytochrome enzyme embedded in the endoplasmic reticulum has a specific binding site, which may be capable of binding to a number of different, but not all, drugs. Many drugs, however, are reliant on specific cytochromes for their metabolism. Furthermore, two drugs may compete for the same cytochrome-binding site, a concept that may explain drug interactions previously thought to be idiosyncratic.

In order for differences in cytochrome genetic activity to contribute to the altered pharmacokinetic effect of a drug, there must be a 'rate limiting step' in the drugs' metabolism. Cyclosporin and Tacrolimus (FK506) are examples of such drugs. The daily dose of cyclosporin required to achieve a particular drug level can vary as much as 10-fold. This has implications due to the risks associated with toxicity and immunosuppression. CYP3A4 is the major enzyme responsible for the metabolism of cyclosporin and FK506. Its levels show genetic polymorphism. This may explain wide variations in dosage regimes used for individual patients when administering cyclosporin. It is possible to determine CYP3A activity non-invasively using an erythromycin breath test. Enzyme levels appear to predict oral clearance of cyclosporin, certainly for renal transplant patients.[11,12] A similar approach has recently been employed in liver transplant recipients using intravenous midazolam (known to be another CYP3A substrate) as a probe to investigate CYP3A activity.[13] This type of work has relevance in the field of anaesthesia.

The discovery that midazolam is metabolised by at least three different cytochrome systems[14] which may exhibit genetic polymorphism and be influenced by concurrent drug administration may go some way to explaining the wide variation in patients handling of midazolam, particularly demonstrated in the intensive care setting. This type of work paves the way for the day when simple non-invasive tests of specific liver enzyme activity are available, and the information used to develop target drug dosages for the individual patient.

LIVER DISEASE

Syndrome of acute liver failure

'*Acute liver failure*' (ALF) can be defined as the onset of severe hepatic dysfunction, manifesting itself as either encephalopathy or coagulopathy with an interval of between 8 and 28 days from jaundice to encephalopathy. These patients have a high incidence of cerebral oedema, and often have a very poor prognosis without liver transplantation. '*Hyperacute liver failure*' is the suggested term used for patients where liver failure occurs within 7 days of the onset of jaundice. This group includes the sizeable cohort, likely to survive with medical management, despite the high incidence of cerebral oedema. Finally, the term *subacute liver failure* is reserved for those patients with encephalopathy which develops within 5 to 12 weeks of the onset of jaundice. These patients are characterised by a low incidence of cerebral oedema, but have a poor prognosis. These terms were suggested in 1993,[15] in an attempt to standardise definitions to enable outcome predictions and comparison of clinical trials between different centres. Previously, different centres had used differing criteria for the terms acute liver failure and fulminant liver failure. In the UK the most common cause of FHF is paracetamol overdose (50%), followed by viral hepatitis. On a worldwide basis viral hepatitis (especially hepatitis B) is the more common. A third group comprises idiosyncratic reaction to drugs which include: halothane, isoniazid, monoamine oxidase inhibitors, non-steroidal anti-inflammatory drugs, gold, sodium valproate, phenytoin, co-trimoxazole, sulphonamides, ketoconazole, various herbal remedies, mushrooms and 'ecstasy' (3,4-methylenedioxymetamphetamine, MDMA).[16,17] (for summary see Table 29.5).

Paracetamol provides an interesting example of how biotransformation enzyme systems may lead to liver damage. Paracetamol contains a hydroxyl group and therefore does not normally require phase I oxidation prior to conjugation with glucuronide or sulphate. Normally less than 5% of a therapeutic dose of paracetamol is metabolized by the cytochrome system. If the total dose exceeds 15 g (in the average adult),

TABLE 29.5 Causes of acute liver damage

CAUSATIVE AGENTS	COMMENTS
Infective – vital	
Hepatitis A	Predominantly hepatocellular with prodromal 'Flu-like' illness
B	
Non-A Non-B	
Epstein–Barr Virus	Infectious mononucleosis, mild hepatitis in 15%
Cytomegalovirus	
Herpes simplex	Rare unless patient immunosuppressed
Herpes zoster	
Infective – bacterial	
Septicaemia	Liver abscesses and intrahepatic cholestasis
Mycotoxins	
Amanita phalloides	Severe gastrointestinal symptoms, frequently fatal.
Aflatoxins	Hepatocellular damage (carcinogenic in animals)
Drugs	An almost unlimited number (see text) Various patterns e.g. paracetamol – hepatocellular necrosis, hepatitis with antituberculous drugs, cholestasis with chlorpromazine
Chemicals	
Alcohol	Fatty changes sometimes marked cholestasis
Carbon tetrachloride	Marked fatty change, centrilobular necrosis
Trichlorethylene	
Iron	Periportal necrosis
Miscellaneous	
Heart failure	Intrahepatic cholestasis, centrilobular necrosis

the total dose exceeds 15g (in the average adult), phase II pathways become saturated, and large amounts of the drug are metabolized by the cytochrome system (specifically CYP2E1) with production of the electrophilic metabolite N-acetyl-*p*-benzoquinone imine (NAPQI) (The pathway is shown in Fig. 3.3). This highly reactive metabolite can cause tissue damage and in small amounts is rapidly conjugated with glutathione. In paracetamol overdose, the hepatic glutathione pool is rapidly depleted resulting in direct hepatotoxicity. Treatment of paracetamol overdose with agents such as acetylcysteine (N-acetyl-L-cysteine, NAC) is effective. NAC, and in particular its thiol metabolites L-cysteine, and reduced glutathione are effective antioxidants and reducing agents.[18] NAC is used rather than antioxidants and reducing agents. NAC is used instead of glutathione itself, as NAC, unlike glutathione, can cross cell membranes. Chronic alcohol ingestion tends to induce CYP2E1 and decrease levels of hepatic glutathione. This leads to increased formation of the toxic paracetamol metabolite NAPQI. Acute alcohol ingestion at the same time as paracetamol, however, tends to reduce NAPQI formation, as the two drugs compete for metabolism by the same cytochrome.[19]

Treatment of patients with syndromes of acute liver failure should be confined to specialized units with facilities for emergency hepatic transplantation. The clinical manifestations of ALF are numerous and include neurological, acid-base, cardiovascular, renal and haematological abnormalities. The use of *all* sedative drugs in patients with ALF should be avoided, except perhaps in the context of elective intubation and ventilation on the advice of a specialist liver failure unit prior to transfer.

Chronic liver disease

Chronic liver disease can present a confusing picture due to the vast number of possible aetiologies. Patients may present with complications of cirrhosis, such as bleeding oesophageal varices or hepatic encephalopathy. More frequently patients will present with either stable chronic liver disease or with abnormal liver function tests, which have been found on preoperative screening. Occasionally, underlying liver function may be completely normal despite evidence of liver damage, for example in the patient with isolated deposits from a hepatocellular carcinoma.

If liver function is impaired, then the impairment may affect one particular aspect of liver function, such as synthesis, storage, biotransformation or elimination. This is especially true in the early course of the disease, whereas in the final stages, all specificity may be lost. Table 29.6 classifies causes of liver disease along the lines of predominant dysfunction.

Patients with cholestatic disease generally manifest signs or symptoms relating to failure of excretory function while retaining the synthetic, biotransformation and storage aspects until late in the disease process. Thus a patient with obstructive jaundice, although unable to adequately excrete drugs in the bile, would still retain the ability to biotransform and inactivate them until late in the disease. Similarly, vitamin K is reliant on unobstructed biliary flow for its absorption, but hepatic stores are maintained and adequate synthesis of plasma proteins and clotting factors continue until late in the obstructive process. In contrast, patients with predominantly hepatocellular disease manifest defects related to failure of hepatic synthesis, storage and biotransformation, at a much earlier stage.

Phase I reactions, especially the CYP mediated oxidative reactions, are most affected by conditions such as acute viral hepatitis and alcoholic liver disease, which predominantly affect the 'centrilobular' hepatocytes. These *zone III* hepatocytes have the highest concentration of CYP. Diseases with a predominantly 'periportal' distribution, such as primary biliary cirrhosis and chronic hepatitis (in the absence of cirrhosis), have few effects upon the cytochrome system. Although phase II reactions occur more commonly in periportal

TABLE 29.6 Causes of chronic liver disease. Classified by nature of predominant dysfunction

PATIENT GROUP	CHOLESTATIC GROUP	HEPATOCELLULAR DISEASES	OTHER DISEASES
Paediatric patients	Biliary atresia Bylers syndrome Alagille's syndrome	α_1-Antitrypsin deficiency Chronic active hepatitis Cryptogenic cirrhosis Neonatal hepatitis Wilson's disease Tyrosinaemia Glycogen storage diseases	Hepatoma
Adult patients	Primary biliary cirrhosis Sclerosing cholangitis Biliary obstruction[†]	Cirrhosis* Wilson's disease Tyrosinaemia α_1-antitrypsin deficiency Haemochromatosis	Caroli's disease Hepatoma Secondary biliary cirrhosis

* Includes viral hepatitis, alcoholic cirrhosis, cryptogenic cirrhosis, chronic active hepatitis, and cirrhosis complicating acute liver damage.

† Most commonly due to biliary disease, cholelithiasis, cholangitis or carcinoma of the biliary tract or pancreas.

hepatocytes, their distribution throughout the liver is much more even than those involved in phase I reactions. To summarize, phase II reactions,[20] such as glucuronidation, are well preserved in both acute and chronic liver disease. This may be due to the wide distribution of capable hepatocytes, or to factors such as their predominantly intracellular nature. Alternatively, there may also exist extrahepatic glucuronidation sites in the kidney and gut. The aetiology of the disease will also enable a prediction of the likely effects on the liver architecture, and consequently the probable effects on drug handling. The associated signs of portal hypertension warn of the existence of intra- and extrahepatic shunts. Liver disease is once again the subject of numerous excellent reviews.[21,22]

Laboratory tests of liver function

Most clinical biochemistry laboratories offer packages of biochemical tests that include measurement of serum bilirubin, alkaline phosphatase, alanine-aminotransferase, γ-glutamyltranspeptidase and serum albumin estimations. While these estimations are of value in monitoring specific diseases, in the differential diagnosis of obstructive jaundice, or in the detection of drug-induced hepatotoxicity, they are only of limited value in predicting how patients will handle a particular drug.[23] Bilirubin and albumin concentrations, while they may reflect hepatocellular function, are affected by factors such as haemolysis and nutritional state. Elevated transaminase levels may indicate hepatocellular damage but are non-specific. Massive increases in transaminase levels may accompany a mild viral hepatitis, while levels may remain within the normal range in patients with advanced cirrhosis. Alternative tests of liver function are becoming available. Dynamic tests such as the ^{13}C-aminopyrine demethylation breath test quantitatively assess hepatic microsomal metabolism. The erythromycin breath test[5] has already been mentioned as an example of a test which can be used to assess the activity of a specific cytochrome enzyme. Information obtained from such tests, when combined with measurements of hepatic blood flow such as indocyanine green clearance or ^{133}Xe uptake, may in the future make it possible to adjust drug doses in patients with liver disease in a similar manner to adjustments made in patients with renal disease on the basis of alterations in creatinine clearance.[12] Pending the development and widespread application of newer tests of hepatic function, clinicians must use the 'conventional' liver function tests in combination with a detailed knowledge of the particular patient and rely on the results of published studies on the effects of liver diseases on drug handling.

TABLE 29.7 Child–Pugh scoring. Risk grading by score

	SCORE 1	SCORE 2	SCORE 3
Encephalopathy	None	Grade 1–2	Grade 3–4
Ascites	Absent	Slight	Moderate
Bilirubin (mmol/l)	<25	25–40	>40
Albumin (g/l)	> 35	28–35	<28
Prothrombin time	Prolongation <4 s	4–6	>6

<6, good; 6–8, moderate; >10 high risk.

RISK FACTORS IN PATIENTS WITH LIVER DISEASE

Numerous studies have shown that patients with advanced parenchymal liver disease are a high surgical risk.[24] They tend to have the most profound disturbances in hepatic blood flow and microsomal function, and handle drugs abnormally. The scoring system originally described by Child and later modified by Pugh (Table 29.7) can identify such high-risk patients. While originally used in patients with cirrhosis undergoing portocaval shunt surgery, it is useful in the assessment of patients for other forms of surgery. Recently, scoring systems have been devised to assess disease severity and survival following major abdominal surgery[25] or liver transplantation. All of these systems rely on a combination of physical signs and of simple laboratory investigations. Many of the poor prognostic factors identified in these systems are themselves indicators of poor drug handling, for example encephalopathy, low serum albumin, high bilirubin concentrations, ascites with poor nutrition and co-existing renal impairment. Other factors, such as coagulopathy, although not directly linked to drug handling are sensitive and easily determined markers of poor hepatocellular function.

PHARMACOKINETICS

The study of pharmacokinetics involves drug absorption, distribution and elimination. The two main variables are the nature of the drug and the characteristics of the patient receiving it. The first is perhaps the simplest as it is constant and easy to determine. Important drug variables are: its lipid solubility, ionization (reflected in the pKa), charge and molecular size. The importance of this is in predicting the drug's likely volume of distribution, and its principal mode of elimination (see Chapter 2). Highly ionized drugs tend to have a small volume of distribution and are renally excreted, whereas uncharged molecules will have large volumes of distributions and require biotransformation by the liver prior to elimination in either the bile or urine.[26]

Pharmacokinetic data on the way patients with particular diseases handle drugs are now becoming available. While renal physicians are able to adjust dosages of drugs given to patients with renal impairment on the basis of tests such as the creatinine clearance, the situation is a little more complex in the case of advanced liver disease. There is, as yet, no definitive single test to estimate the degree of organ damage due to the variations in damage produced by differing diseases, which affect drug handling in a complex way by alterations in drug distribution, transformation and elimination. Despite these problems, the clinician can make limited predictions of the effects of drugs on this group of patients.[26]

Volume of distribution

The apparent volume of distribution of a drug (V_d) is the *theoretical* volume to which a drug distributes at equilibrium, assuming that the drug is distributed throughout the body in the same concentration as it is in the plasma.

$$V_d = \frac{\text{Amount of drug in the body}}{\text{Plasma concentration (prior to elimination)}}$$

or

$$V_d = \frac{D}{C_0}$$

where D is the drug, and C_0 is plasma concentration at administration.

C_0 is usually calculated by extrapolation of the curve of intravenous concentration against time back to the vertical axis.[27] Volume of distribution may be altered in liver disease due to altered plasma-protein concentration,[28] or by the displacement of drugs from their carrier proteins, for example by raised plasma bilirubin levels. Protein binding, if decreased, results in a higher free-drug concentration in the plasma and more drug is available for redistribution to the tissues. In this way, the apparent volume of distribution may be increased. This effect is variable, depending on effects on tissue drug binding. Finally, the sizes of the various fluid compartments may be changed. Patients with cirrhosis have an altered circulating volume and the development of ascites may vastly increase the apparent volume of distribution. One example is propranolol, whose volume of distribution doubles in patients with ascites irrespective of changes in protein binding.

Protein binding

Protein binding refers to the rapidly achieved equilibrium obtained between free drug and that bound to circulating plasma proteins such as albumin, globulin, α_1-acid glycoprotein, ceruloplasmin, lipoproteins and transferrin. Acidic drugs bind to specific anionic receptors on serum albumin, whereas basic drugs may bind to non-ionic albumin-binding sites and to α_1-acid glycoprotein. Only unbound drugs are available to evoke a response at the drug receptor. Changes in binding may therefore alter the pharmacological response. Variation in binding may also modify the drugs distribution and elimination. If binding is decreased, then more unbound drug is available to cross biological membranes (increasing volume of distribution), and becomes available for hepatic elimination. The plasma or serum drug concentration used in the calculation of the volume of distribution is usually the *total* drug concentration. This may cause confusion, as obviously changes in distribution associated with changes in protein binding may be masked by measurement of unbound volumes of distribution. Cirrhosis may alter drug protein binding by decreasing serum albumin concentration or by the production of structurally abnormal proteins. The high serum bilirubin levels seen in diseases such as primary biliary cirrhosis may avidly bind to albumin and displace some acidic drugs. Changes in protein binding may be important for some of the highly protein-bound drugs, but in the chronic situation will be offset by an increase in elimination. Fortunately, changes in distribution are as a rule slight when compared with those seen in drug elimination. This topic is widely discussed in reviews by Wood[29] and Keiding.[20]

Elimination

Elimination is the removal of a drug from the plasma by metabolism or excretion. It is often expressed using clearance (Cl) or by use of the elimination half-life ($t_{\frac{1}{2}}$.) The latter term may be confusing when data on drug elimination are presented.

The elimination half-life is the time taken for the plasma concentration to fall by half and is calculated using the following formula:

$$t_{\frac{1}{2}} = \frac{0.693 V_d}{Cl}$$

As can be seen, the $t_{\frac{1}{2}}$ depends on the volume of distribution of the drug in addition to the clearance. The volume of distribution of a drug in liver disease may alter, so that changes in elimination half-life are confusing, unless it is known that the volume of distribution is unchanged.[27] A frequently quoted example is that of lorazepam whose increased $t_{\frac{1}{2}}$ in liver disease is due to an increase in volume of distribution rather than due to any change in elimination.

Total clearance

Clearance of a drug may be defined as irreversible loss of the drug from the site of measurement, and hence includes that lost by metabolism and excretion. The term does not imply a specific mechanism of elimination – merely the volume of plasma completely cleared of a drug per unit time. It comes as no surprise to consider total elimination as the sum of individual organ clearances.[27] Therefore, for a drug excreted by both the liver and the kidney:

$$Cl_{total} = Cl_{hepatic} + Cl_{renal}$$

In the case of a lipid-soluble drug, the renal component will be so small as to be insignificant and hepatic clearance will be dependent on the rate at which the drug is presented to the liver (the hepatic blood flow (Q)), and on the amount of drug extracted by the liver (the hepatic extraction ratio (E)).[30] Hence:

$$Cl_{hepatic} = Q\,E$$

The hepatic extraction ratio is a useful concept and is defined as:

$$E = \frac{(C_{\text{portal circulation}} - C_{\text{hepatic vein}})}{C_{\text{portal circulation}}}$$

where C is the concentration of drug.

Hepatic clearance

This is dependent on three factors: the fraction of free drug in the plasma, the rate at which the drug is presented to the liver and the ability of the hepatic enzyme systems to irreversibly remove unbound drug (often confusingly termed the intrinsic clearance). All of these factors can be altered individually by liver disease. It is possible, however, to make distinctions between groups of drugs on the basis of their hepatic extraction. Drugs with a low hepatic extraction ratio (< 0.3) are metabolized slowly by the liver – hepatic enzymatic activity becomes the rate-limiting step in their clearance. Clearance is independent of hepatic blood flow, and they are termed 'capacity limited'. In contrast, drugs with a high hepatic extraction ratio (> 0.7) are rapidly metabolized by the liver. The rate-limiting step in their clearance is the rate of presentation of the drug to the liver (the hepatic blood flow). Such drugs are termed 'flow limited'.

It is now possible to start to predict the effects of anaesthesia and liver diseases on the elimination of drugs based on knowledge of hepatic extraction and protein binding.

Flow-limited drugs

	Extraction ratio	Protein binding (%)
Labetalol	0.85	40
Lignocaine	0.6	65
Morphine	0.75	35
Propranolol	0.65	95
Verapamil	0.8	92

This class of drugs is metabolized very rapidly by the liver, hence the effects of disease and anaesthesia on hepatic blood flow will be the major determinants in clearance. Any alterations in free drug concentration due to altered protein binding are rapidly offset by increasing hepatic elimination. This group has a low bioavailability when administered orally due to the 'first-pass effect', as they are rapidly cleared from the portal blood flow before reaching the systemic circulation. Liver disease may, however, disturb normal hepatic blood flow. Patients with cirrhosis may handle this class of drugs as if they were capacity limited,[31] due to a combination of intra- and extrahepatic effects. The normal sinusoidal architecture is disturbed with collagen building up in the space of Disse. This tends to interfere with rapid drug transfer. In addition, intrahepatic shunting may allow drugs to be routed around functioning hepatocytes. Disruption of the normal anatomy further disturbs hepatic blood flow, and increasing intrahepatic resistance leads to portal hypertension and the production of extrahepatic shunting. Not only may the portal contribution to hepatic blood flow be reduced, but the compensatory shunting, either via oesophageal, rectal or abdominal wall communication will increase the bioavailability of this class of drugs when administered orally.

The elimination of flow-limited drugs may be further disturbed by the administration of drugs either chronically or acutely, which affect cardiac output and/or hepatic blood flow. In the chronic situation, propranolol administered for the treatment of portal hypertension will reduce cardiac output and portal blood flow. During anaesthesia and surgery, hepatic blood flow is reduced and may fluctuate widely with haemorrhage, surgical manipulation of abdominal viscera or by the creation of a portosystemic shunt. While these factors are often difficult to predict or control, they serve to illustrate the importance of selecting an anaesthetic technique that will best maintain baseline cardiac output and hepatic blood flow.

Capacity-limited drugs

	Extraction ratio	Protein binding (%)
Chlordiazepoxide	0.02	96
Diazepam	0.02	97
Warfarin	0.005	99
Theophylline	0.05	62
Caffeine	0.04	31
Antipyrine	0.05	10

This class of drugs has a low hepatic extraction ratio and hence is only slowly metabolized by the liver. Clearance is almost completely independent of hepatic blood flow, and on oral administration there is an inconsequential 'first-pass' effect. The effects of liver disease will depend on changes in the capacity for metabolism due to changes in biotransformation enzymes and protein binding.

Highly protein-bound 'capacity-limited' drugs will have their clearance most affected by the changes in protein binding induced by liver disease, whereas those with less extensive protein binding will not be significantly affected.

Flow and capacity-limited drugs

A large group of drugs exist whose properties are such that their elimination is dependent on changes in all the previously described factors. Examples include pethidine, methohexitone, chlorpromazine and ranitidine. These drugs have hepatic extraction ratios of approximately 0.3, and the rate-limiting step in their elimination may depend on individual disturbances in either hepatic blood flow or hepatic enzymatic activity.

PHARMACODYNAMIC PRINCIPLES

Liver disease may have important effects on the actions of drugs on the body. Drug toxicity may occur at plasma concentrations normally considered therapeutic. Examples of this were first seen in the effects of morphine and chlorpromazine on patients with liver disease and previous hepatic encephalopathy. Increased sedative effects of these drugs were ascribed to an increased 'cerebral sensitivity'. Further work in this area concentrated on the effects of benzodiazepine (BDZ) drugs on patients with a history of encephalopathy.[32] Measurable levels of endogenous compounds with BDZ-receptor-binding and BDZ-immunoreactive properties were subsequently demonstrated. These endogenous compounds have been implicated in the pathogenesis of hepatic encephalopathy, and their effects seem to be reversed by the BDZ antagonist, flumazenil.[33] These BDZ receptor ligands have been identified more recently as diazepam and *N*-desmethyldiazepam, present in patients with stage 4 encephalopathy who have not been exposed to pharmaceutical BDZs. Work in this field continues to contribute towards understanding of the pathogenesis of hepatic encephalopathy.[34]

Patients with advanced liver disease are more susceptible to the cerebral-depressant effects of drugs such as BDZ and barbiturates whose effects are mediated through BDZ receptors.

A second explanation for abnormal pharmacodynamic effects has been alluded to. This proposes an increased amount of 'free' drug as a result of abnormal pharmacokinetics. Examples of this are the increased bioavailability of drugs such as propranolol, with high hepatic extraction ratios on oral administration, and the effects of abnormal protein binding and decreased metabolic capacity on capacity-limited drugs.

EFFECTS OF ANAESTHESIA AND SURGERY

Anaesthesia and surgery will have additional effects on hepatic function and drug handling. Patients may have pre-existing cardiovascular abnormalities. A decreased systemic vascular resistance with increased resting cardiac output is typical of advanced hepatic disease,[35] although oxygen delivery exceeds extraction, possibly due to arteriovenous shunting. Anaesthetic agents causing additional peripheral vasodilatation and/or reduction in cardiac output may produce profound hypotension below the limits of autoregulation for flow. Organs are often unable to increase oxygen extraction in response to demand, resulting in a lactic acidosis despite normal oxygen delivery. Tissue hypoxia may result which, in the liver, will affect the precarious cytochrome enzymes located in the functional '*zone III*' involved in phase I drug metabolism. As phase I enzymes may already be affected by the underlying liver disease, it is prudent to avoid drugs reliant on phase I activity for deactivation. Volatile agents may produce a decrease in hepatic blood flow. This effect may be slightly offset by a tendency to decrease hepatic oxygen requirements. Furthermore, if endogenous catecholamine levels are high due to inadequate anaesthesia, hepatic blood flow will fall dramatically, and the argument becomes rather academic. Overall, the effects of anaesthesia are transient, and are often insignificant when compared with the long-standing alterations produced by the surgical procedure. Portosystemic shunts performed to treat patients with portal hypertension (a patient group with a decreased hepatic blood flow preoperatively) are an obvious example. More recently, the development of interventional radiology techniques has allowed transjugular intrahepatic portosystemic shunt (TIPS) placement under local anaesthesia. The place of this technique for treatment of the complications of portal hypertension to prevent recurrent bleeding is still being evaluated.[36] Although it avoids the need for general anaesthesia (with its inevitable effects on hepatic blood flow), encephalopathy can worsen after the procedure as with conventional surgery. This is not unexpected, as the procedure increases the portosystemic shunt fraction.[37]

This new technique has the great benefit of being much less invasive than traditional surgical procedures, and is useful in reducing the likelihood of recurrent variceal haemorrhage, particularly in patients awaiting liver transplantation.

It seems reasonable to accept that since some form of anaesthesia will be required for a surgical procedure, it is best to try and maintain cardiac output and hepatic blood flow as near baseline as possible, while obtunding the response to surgical stimulation. Anaesthetic regimes for major hepatic surgery are chosen in accordance with these aims and are well described.[38] The major variable in altered drug handling will be the surgical procedure, its duration and associated haemodynamic and metabolic disturbances. Surgical haemorrhage is variable depending on the procedure and technique, but may have major effects. Massive blood replacement is associated with a metabolic acidosis and especially in patients with poor liver function, ionic hypocalcaemia. Hypothermia is an almost inevitable consequence of massive transfusion. The effects on drug kinetics are difficult to predict for an individual patient, as on the one hand there will be 'washout' effects, which will be important for drugs with a small volume of distribution. In contrast, drugs reliant on enzymatic inactivation will be potentiated in conditions of hypothermia and acidosis, as may atracurium whose non-enzymatic breakdown is markedly reduced. Highly protein-bound drugs may also be affected by changes in pH and temperature.

Drug handling during liver transplantation

Liver transplantation involves patients with either syndromes of acute liver failure or with end-stage chronic liver disease. The patient groups are distinctly different. Patients with acute liver failure (including the '*hyper*', '*acute*', and '*subacute*' forms) often have no stigmata of chronic liver disease, although they may have developed acute renal failure and cerebral oedema as a result of their disease. The patients with end-stage chronic liver disease will often be in a poor nutritional state with signs of portal hypertension and severe ascites. The anaesthetic and surgical aspects of liver transplantation have been the subject of numerous reviews.[35,38] A brief outline discussion allows application of some of the principles discussed in this chapter. The operation for both groups consists of three distinct 'phases'. The dissection phase, where the recipient's diseased liver is skeletonized in preparation for removal, the 'anhepatic' phase, in which the recipient's liver is excluded from the circulation and the donor liver is anastomosed with the suprahepatic and infrahepatic vena cava, the portal vein and the hepatic artery, and the 'Neohepatic' phase in which the donor liver is reperfused and the biliary anastomosis completed. The dissection phase can be prolonged, especially in patients with chronic hepatic failure who have frequently undergone previous surgery and who may have numerous adhesions and portal hypertension. This, combined with the haemostatic defects which accompany liver disease, may lead to considerable haemorrhage. Both groups of patients may present in a high cardiac output, vasodilated state. In patients with chronic liver disease the drainage of large volumes of ascites may have profound haemodynamic effects. Since the liver is to be removed, the maintenance of the patient's general condition is perhaps more important than preservation of hepatic function. Changes seen in the anhepatic phase are dependent on whether an extracorporeal circuit is used to maintain venous return while the vena cava and the portal vein are clamped. In the simpler situation often used in children, no bypass circuit is used. While the vena cava and portal vein are clamped and the liver removed there is obviously no route for hepatic drug elimination. In addition, however, the renal perfusion pressure is decreased as a result of a decreased cardiac output (reduced venous return) and due to increased caval pressures. Therefore, renal elimination of drugs is also reduced. Drug elimination may still occur as a result of haemorrhage. Blood loss may be excessive, due to increased pressures in the splanchnic bed. In the situation where an extracorporeal circuit is used, the inferior caval and portal venous blood is diverted via a pump to the superior vena cava. This situation tends to preserve venous return and consequently cardiac output. By decompressing the venous system renal perfusion is maintained and blood loss in this phase may be reduced. The additional volume of the bypass circuit (approximately 800 ml) will, of course, alter the distribution volume of the drugs but this will have a relatively unimportant effect. Numerous authors have attempted to utilize the anhepatic period for studies of drug metabolism. Studies of propofol metabolism during the anhepatic phase support the existence of an extrahepatic site of metabolism.[39] Other results so far have proved difficult to interpret as numbers are small, and the studies are complicated by the varying use of veno venous bypass techniques and the effects of transfusion. There is obviously a potential for cumulation and toxicity of drugs administered at this stage. Reperfusion of the donor liver may again be accompanied by considerable haemorrhage. Since the donor liver has been subjected to a harvesting procedure, cold storage and a reperfusion injury, it is not surprising that immediate function is not completely restored. In reality, metabolic function in a successful graft seems to return fairly rapidly. Attention is paid to haemostasis and the preservation of liver blood flow. With a successful graft, the recipient normally shows an increase in oxygen consumption by the end of the surgical procedure and preoperative cardiovascular abnormalities correct themselves within 24 h. The speed with which the drug handling of the patient returns to normal is uncertain. The patients will normally recover consciousness quickly on the cessation of sedation. This is particularly so where techniques involving propofol are used. This effect may, however, be due to a combination of redistribution and extrahepatic elimination. Analgesic requirements are within the normal range, although some cumulative effects may be seen with morphine and on occasion with fentanyl infusions.

ANAESTHETIC DRUGS

The following section is not intended to be comprehensive. The drugs are chosen to illustrate general principles or because they are commonly used in patients with hepatic disease.

Premedication – benzodiazepines

The need for anaesthetic premedication in patients with liver disease is debatable. As already discussed, there is evidence for an increased pharmacodynamic effect (and in some cases with advanced encephalopathy endogenous production) of the BDZ drugs in patients with cirrhosis and previous encephalopathy.[34] However, in patients with compensated cirrhosis, BDZ drugs are widely used for sedation during endoscopic procedures and for anaesthetic premedication. The pharmacodynamics of orally administered BDZ sedatives in patients with cirrhosis have been extensively studied by Hoyumpa,[40] who demonstrated an increased elimination half-life for diazepam in patients with cirrhosis, acute viral hepatitis and chronic active hepatitis. This was attributed to both an increase in the steady-state volume of distribution and a decreased clearance. Since diazepam is highly protein bound (99%), then small changes in protein binding will account for the increased volume of distribution. The clearance of diazepam was also found to be decreased. Diazepam, with low hepatic extraction (0.02), is sensitive to changes in activity of the biotransformation enzymes. Its metabolism is two stage, requiring demethylation to desmethyldiazepam followed by hydroxylation to oxazepam, which is then conjugated with glucuronic acid to form an inactive metabolite. It is probably the early phase I reactions that serve as the rate-limiting step in its elimination. Drugs such as temazepam and oxazepam, which rely on conjugation for their deactivation, have clearances largely unaffected by chronic stable liver disease. Lorazepam is metabolized by conjugation and has a normal clearance in cirrhotic patients. However, due to an increased volume of distribution, it may exhibit a prolonged elimination half-life in patients with cirrhosis.[28] The elimination of BDZ drugs reliant on phase I enzymes can be further reduced by cimetidine, due to inhibition of the cytochrome (CYP2C) responsible for their mutual metabolism.

Midazolam, a widely used drug both orally and intravenously, seems initially not to fit this pattern.[40] The drug is metabolized to α-hydroxymidazolam by hydroxylation, and then conjugated to form inactive metabolites excreted in the urine. In patients with mild cirrhosis, the pharmacokinetic profile is unchanged from that of healthy volunteers. Only in patients with severe cirrhosis are the pharmacokinetics disturbed. Although midazolam undergoes predominantly phase I metabolism, this reaction is not inhibited by cimetidine. The work of Watkins suggests that this is due to the drugs being substrates for different cytochrome enzymes, midazolam being metabolised by CYP3A4 as opposed to CYP2C. The CYP3A system may be better preserved in liver disease. Alternatively, since midazolam metabolites have been detected in patients given midazolam in the anhepatic phase of liver transplantation,[41] it seems likely that cytochrome systems at extrahepatic sites may also be involved. The gut wall and the kidney have been proposed as likely sites. These findings are supported by more recent work suggesting that midazolam is metabolised by at least three different cytochrome enzymes. (CYP3A3, CYP3A4 and CYP3A5.)[14] This finding may also provide a possible explanation for the 'first-pass' effect seen when midazolam is administered orally.

Intravenous induction agents

Thiopentone

Thiopentone is a highly lipid-soluble molecule that cannot be renally excreted without oxidative hydroxylation and desulphuration (phase I) metabolism. Its hepatic extraction ratio is approximately 0.2, hence its elimination would be predicted to be reliant on hepatic enzymatic function and prolonged in hepatic disease. Pandele, studying patients with mild alcoholic cirrhosis, found that the patients with cirrhosis had a lower (but statistically insignificant) intrinsic clearance and unbound volume of distribution, and that the free fraction of thiopentone in the plasma was higher as a result of lower serum albumin concentrations. On the basis of this he concluded that a prolonged response to a single dose of thiopentone was unlikely, although there was an increased risk of acute toxic effects during induction due to the increased free fraction.[42]

Recovery of consciousness following a single dose of an induction agent is due to redistribution. In the case of thiopentone, the volume of distribution is very large and the rate-limiting step in its elimination is not hepatic metabolism, but the slow reuptake of the drug from fat stores. Patients with early alcoholic liver disease often require larger doses than the normal population. This is unlikely to be due to enzyme induction and is more likely to be due to obesity and an increased resting cardiac output, allowing more rapid redistribution.[27] A degree of central nervous system 'tolerance' to sedatives may also be a factor due to chronic alcohol ingestion in this group of patients.

Methohexitone

Following a bolus injection, recovery from this agent is due to redistribution. Studies on patients with acute viral hepatitis have revealed similar results to the thiopentone data and the induction dose is again unchanged although the rate of administration should be reduced.

Propofol

The effects of liver disease on this drug are of great interest as it has a high hepatic extraction ratio, and rapid hepatic metabolism. Forty per cent of an administered dose is eventually recovered in the urine as propofol glucuronide. Its clearance is expected to be dependent on hepatic blood flow, but has been measured as exceeding hepatic blood flow, suggesting the presence of extrahepatic metabolism. This has been cofirmed by Gray by studies using radiolabelled propofol administered during the anhepatic phase of liver transplantation.[39] The high hepatic extraction ratio also indicates that its pharmacokinetics will not be greatly altered by changes in protein binding.

Recovery is again by redistribution following a bolus dose. Propofol is being increasingly used by continuous infusion for maintenance of anaesthesia. A study by Servin *et al.*[43] showed that patients with cirrhosis both lost consciousness at a similar time to normal controls following a loading infusion of propofol, and regained consciousness at similar blood concentrations. The elimination half-life was unaltered. Most interestingly, the time to recover following cessation of the infusion was prolonged in two patients who had undergone the formation of a portocaval shunt with its associated reduction in hepatic blood flow. These results therefore seem to support the predictions made for the drug on the basis of its pharmacokinetic profile and to suggest that in this group of patients there is no increased pharmacodynamic response in mild to moderate cirrhosis.

Opiate analgesics

Morphine

Morphine has been extensively studied in patients with liver disease.[44] It is a drug with a high (0.75) hepatic extraction ratio and hence extensive first-pass effects on oral administration. It is metabolised by glucuronidation to morphine-3-glucuronide and morphine-6-glucuronide. The latter compound also demonstrates analgesic properties. Both metabolites are principally renally excreted. It is not extensively protein bound (35%). Armed with this information, it is reasonable to deduce that morphine when administered intravenously to patients with liver disease will be handled fairly normally. Abnormalities would be expected if hepatic blood flow were to be disturbed by anaesthetic or surgical procedures, and in the presence of renal impairment. If the drug is administered orally to patients with portal hypertension then bioavailability is increased. Most authors recommend no alteration of dosage in chronic liver disease, but suggest that morphine is best avoided in severe liver disease, possibly on the grounds that if hepatic blood flow is severely reduced the drug may behave as a capacity-limited drug and cumulation could occur. Additionally with severe liver disease a degree of hepatorenal impairment is almost universal.

Fentanyl

A study in anaesthetized cirrhotic patients receiving a single bolus dose of fentanyl revealed no alteration in the pharmacokinetics of fentanyl (5 μg/kg) when compared with healthy controls.[45] Fentanyl has a high hepatic extraction ratio (0.8) and volume of distribution. The long elimination half-life of fentanyl in both normal and cirrhotic patients probably reflects its slow release from fat deposits. While bolus injection appears to be safe, there are limited reports of cumulation in patients with liver disease following continuous infusions. Explanations for these observations are speculative, but may reflect alterations in hepatic blood flow or impaired phase I amide hydrolysis.

Alfentanil

In contrast to morphine and fentanyl, the hepatic extraction ratio for alfentanil has been estimated at between 0.3 and 0.6. Alfentanil is almost exclusively metabolized in the liver by oxidative N-dealkylation to inactive metabolites. Although it is extensively protein bound, it is carried principally by α_1-glycoprotein. It therefore belongs in the category of flow/capacity sensitive drugs and changes in hepatic blood flow and enzymatic activity will combine to produce pharmacokinetic changes in patients with liver disease. Ferrier *et al.* have demonstrated a prolonged elimination half-life in cirrhotic patients, who had higher free fractions of alfentanil, and when kinetic parameters were corrected for protein binding the unbound volume of distribution and the free drug clearance were decreased.[46] Following a single dose these changes are likely to be relatively insignificant due to redistribution of the drug. However, cumulation is to be expected following a large bolus, multiple boluses or especially following a continuous infusion.

Muscle relaxants

Suxamethonium

Although the production of plasma cholinesterase may be reduced in advanced liver disease, and a small but clinically insignificant prolongation in action is to be expected, this alone is not a contraindication to its use in liver diseases.

Competitive neuromuscular-blocking drugs

With the use of a peripheral nerve stimulator, the duration of action of competitive neuromuscular-blocking drugs can be monitored. This simplifies their use in clinical practice. As long ago as 1953 apparent resistance to curare was reported. Proposed explanations included increased binding to plasma globulin, sequestration in an enlarged liver or spleen and an increased volume of distribution. The competitive neuromuscular-blocking drugs are not extensively protein bound, and would not be expected to be susceptible to changes in protein binding. Increases in the volumes of distribution have been subsequently described for drugs such as pancuronium, vecuronium and rocuronium.[49-51] Pancuronium has a low hepatic extraction ratio and is primarily metabolized by phase I ester hydrolysis, so a decreased hepatic clearance would be expected in patients with liver disease. Vecuronium has a somewhat higher hepatic extraction ratio and the majority of the drug is excreted unchanged in the bile. Both drugs therefore have a potential for accumulation when used in repeated doses or by continuous infusion. Rocuronium onset time and recovery time are increased in cirrhosis.[51] Pipecuronium shows a similar pharmacokinetic and pharmacodynamic profile in patients with cirrhosis when compared with normal subjects.[52] The pharmacokinetics of atracurium are also unaltered in patients with hepatic failure,[53] although some authors have expressed concern over possible accumulation of its potentially neurotoxic metabolite laudanosine and the acrylate metabolites, which appear to be hepatotoxic in rats. These concerns may theoretically be less with the recent introduction of a commercially available form of the 'cis'-isomer of atracurium besylate. This preparation is said to result in much lower levels of laudanosine formation and histamine release.[54]

Mivacurium

A solution of mivacurium hydrochloride contains three stereoisomers.

The pharmacokinetics of mivacurium has been studied in a limited number of patients with hepatic cirrhosis. Onset and recovery from neuromuscular block are slower in patients with hepatic cirrhosis, and it has been found to have reduced clearance (halved) and a prolonged elimination half life for two of the three stereoisomers.[47] The reduction in clearance is related to its metabolism by plasma cholinesterase,[48] and would be an expected finding in cirrhotic patients, who often have low serum levels of cholinesterase. The volume of distribution remained unchanged.

Volatile anaesthetic agents

The literature concerning the effects of volatile anaesthetic agents on liver function is extensive, almost universally concentrating on the effects of these agents on patients with normal preoperative hepatic function. All volatile agents in current use have been associated with hepatotoxicity.[55] Anaesthesia and surgery are almost inevitably associated with a deterioration in hepatic function, the extent of which is most dependent on the duration and extent of the surgical procedure. It is prudent to chose an anaesthetic technique that maintains hepatic blood flow and oxygen delivery to as near baseline values as possible, not only to 'preserve' hepatic function, but also to maintain the elimination pathways for other drugs administered concurrently. If a volatile agent is used, then isoflurane (at up to 1 mean alveolar concentration (MAC)) appears to best preserve hepatic blood flow.[56] Of the newer volatile agents, desflurane has been administered to patients with chronic liver disease with little change from preoperative values for liver function tests.[57] Theoretical concerns over the use of sevoflurane for such patients exists, due to its potential to increase serum fluoride ion levels.[58]

Nitrous oxide

The use of nitrous oxide is declining, certainly during major hepatic surgery. The reasons for this are mainly to avoid gaseous visceral distension and the exacerbation of any air emboli produced during hepatic dissection. Also, concerns about the effect of nitrous oxide on bone marrow function may become more than theoretical due to the prolonged nature of hepatobiliary surgery. There is also evidence that nitrous oxide is potentially hepatotoxic (in a hypoxic rat model), and that it may cause a decrease in hepatic blood flow (in greyhounds). There is published evidence to support these findings in man.

Local anaesthetics

Local anaesthetic pharmacology has not been studied in depth in patients with liver disease. Data exist for lignocaine, mainly when used as an anti-arrhythmic drug.[59] Local anaesthetics have a high hepatic extraction ratio, and are flow limited in their elimination. Care must be exercised in low cardiac output states (as may occur during cardiac arrhythmias) or in patients receiving β-blocking drugs, as hepatic clearance will be reduced. Bupivacaine has a lower hepatic extraction ratio than lignocaine, and its clearance is more dependent on hepatic enzymatic activity.[60] However, it is more extensively bound to α_1-acid-glycoprotein, an acute phase protein which is often elevated in liver disease and following liver transplantation. It *may*, therefore, be preferable in patients with low serum albumin concentrations in order to minimize the potentially toxic effects of increased levels of free drug. Local anaesthetic techniques are not widely used in patients with liver disease, due to the adverse effects of sympathetic blockade on hepatic blood flow and the co-existing coagulopathy. They are increasingly being used in selected patients to provide postoperative analgesia following liver transplantation[61] and seem to be well tolerated in conventional doses. However, care is advised in their use in patients with chronic liver disease pending the results of further studies.

CONCLUSIONS

The changes in drug metabolism induced by liver disease are complex, and have been described briefly. The exact disturbances produced will depend on the particular disease, its secondary complications and on the clinical situation. The liver has a huge regenerative and reserve capacity that enables it to compensate for mild to moderate disease. Most new drugs are now tested at an early stage in their development on groups of patients with stable chronic liver disease. This, combined with the introduction of newer, non-invasive dynamic tests of liver function, provide information that will eventually lead to rational drug dosing in patients with specific diseases in specific clinical situations. At present, sensible drug administration is reliant on a detailed knowledge of the drug itself and the patient to whom it is administered. Fortunately, there are many anaesthetic agents available that are tolerated even by patients with advanced disease. The effects of liver disease on some of the commonly used anaesthetic drugs have been discussed, and are summarized in the Appendix.

REFERENCES

1 Maze M. Hepatic physiology. In: Miller RD ed. *Anaesthesia.* New York: Churchill Livingstone, 1986; **2:** 1199–221.

2 Sear JW. Hepatic physiology. *Current Anaesthesia and Critical Care* 1990; **1:** 196–203.

3 Reilly CS. The role of the liver and red blood cell. In: Nimmo WS, Smith G eds. *Anaesthesia.* London: Blackwell Scientific, 1989; **1:** 231–47.

4 Parks DA, Gelham S. Normal liver function and the hepatic circulation. In: Park GR, Kang Y eds. *Anesthesia and intensive care for patients with liver disease.* Boston: butterworth-Heinemann, 1995, 3–12.

5 Watkins PB, Role of cytochromes P450 in drug metabolism and hepatotoxicity. *Seminars in Liver disease* 1990; **10:** 235–47.

6 Nebert DW, Nelson DR, Coon RW, *et al.* The P450 superfamily: update on new sequences, gene mapping, and recommended nomenclature. *DNA and Cell Biology* **10:** 1–14.

7 Guengerich FP. Characterization of human cytochrome P450 enzymes. *FASEB Journal* 1992 **6:** 745–48.

8 Coon MJ, Ding X, Pernecky SJ, Vaz AND. Cytochrome P450: progress and predictions. *FASEB Journal* 1992, **6:** 669–73.

9 Schuetz JD, Kauma S, Guzelian PS. Identification of the fetal liver cytochrome CYP3A7 in human endometrium and placenta. *Journal of Clinical Investigation* 1993; **92:** 1018–24.

10 Yang C, Brady JF, Hong J. Dietary effects on cytochromes P450, xenobiotic metabolism, and toxicity. *FASEB Journal* 1992; **6:** 737-44.

11 Cakaloglu Y, Tredger JM, Devlin J, Williams R. Importance of cytochrome P450 IIIA activity in determining dosage and blood levels of FK506 and cyclosporine in liver transplant recipients. *Hepatology* 1994; **20:** 309–16.

12 Reichen J. Assessment of hepatic function with xenobiotics. *Seminars in Liver Disease.* 1995; **15:** 189–201

13 Thummel KE, Shen DD, Podoll TD, *et al.* Use of midazolam as a human cytochrome P450 3A probe: II. Characterization of inter- and intraindividual hepatic CYP3A variability after liver transplantation. *Journal of Pharmacology and Experimental Therapeutics* 1994; **271:** 549–56.

14 Wandel C, Böcker R, Böhrer H, *et al.* Midazolam is metabolised by at least three different cytochrome P450 enzymes. *British Journal of Anaesthesia* 1994; **73:** 658–61.

15 O'Grady JG, Schalm SW, Williams R. Acute liver failure: redefining the syndromes. *Lancet* 1993; **342:** 273–5.

16 Larrey D, Pageaux P. Hepatotoxicity of herbal remedies and mushrooms. *Seminars in Liver disease* 1995; **15 (3):** 183–8.

17 Henry JA, Jeffreys KJ, Dawling S. Toxicity and deaths from 3,4-methylenedioxymetamphetamine. ('ecstasy'). *Lancet* 1992; **340:** 384–7.

18 Deleve LD, Kaplowitz N. Importance and regulation of hepatic glutathione. *Seminars in Liver Disease* 1990; **10:** 251–62.

19 Nelson S. Molecular mechanisms of the hepatotoxicity caused by acetaminophen. *Seminars in Liver disease* 1990; **10 (4):** 267–76.

20 Keiding S. Drug administration to liver patients: Aspects of liver pathophysiology. *Seminars in Liver Disease* 1995; **15 (3):** 268–82

21 Strunin L. Liver disease. In: Vickers MD, Jones RM eds. *Medicine for anaesthetists.* London: Blackwell Scientific, 1989: 196–223.

22 Strunin L, Eagle CJ. Liver diseases. In: Katz J, Benumof J, Kadis LB eds. *Anesthesia and uncommon diseases.* Philadelphia: WB Saunders, 1990: 512–36.

23 Laker MF. Liver function tests. *British Medical Journal* 1990; **301:** 250–1.

24 Garrison RN, Cryer HM, Howard DA, Polk HC. Clarification of risk factors for abdominal operations in patients with hepatic cirrhosis. *Annals of Surgery* 1984; **199:** 648–55.

25 Shaw BW Jr, Wood RP, Stratta RJ, Pillen TJ, Langnas AN. Stratifying the cause of death in liver transplant recipients. An approach to improving survival. *Archives of Surgery* 1989; **124(8):** 895–900.

26 Bass NM, Williams RL. Guide to drug dosage in hepatic disease. *Clinical Pharmacokinetics* 1988; **15:** 396–420.

27 Eagle CJ, Strunin L. Drug metabolism in liver disease. *Current Anaesthesia and Critical Care* 1990; **1:** 204–12.

28 Kraus JW, Desmond PV, Marshall JP, Johnson RF, Schenker S. Wilkinson GR. Effects of ageing and liver disease on disposition of lorazepam. *Clinical Pharmacology and Therapeutics* 1978; **24:** 411–19.

29 Wood M. Plasma drug binding: implications for anesthesiologists. *Anesthesia and Analgesia* 1986; **65:** 786–804.

30 Howden CW, Birnie GC, Brodie MJ. Drug metabolism in liver disease. *Pharmacology and Therapeutics* 1989; **40:** 439–74.

31 Secor JW, Schenker S. Drug metabolism in patients with liver disease. *Advances in Internal Medicine* 1987; **32:** 379–406.

32 Basile AS, Jones EA, Skolnick P. The pathogenesis and treatment of hepatic encephalopathy: evidence for the involvement of benzodiazepine receptor ligands. *Pharmacological Reviews* 1991; **43:** 27–71.

33 Pomier-Layrargues G, Giguère JF, Lavoie J, Perney P, Gagon S, *et al.* Flumazenil in cirrhotic patients in hepatic coma: A randomised double-blind placebo-controlled crossover trial. *Hepatology* 1994. **19(1):** 32–7.

34 Basile AS, Harrison PM, Hughes RD, Gu Z, Pannell L, Mckinney A, Jones EA, Williams R. Relationship between plasma benzodiazepine receptor ligand concentrations and

severity of hepatic encephalopathy. *Hepatology* 1994; **19 (1)**: 112–21.

35 Ginsburg R, Peachey T. Anaesthesia for liver transplantation (1). In: Kaufman L. ed. *Anaesthesia review* 7. London: Churchill Livingstone, 1990: 133–45.

36 Azoulay D, Castaing D, Dennison A, Martino W, Eyraud D, Bismuth H. Transjugular intrahepatic portosystemic shunt worsens the hyperdynamic circulatory state of the cirrhotic patient: preliminary report of a prospective study. *Hepatology* 1994: **19 (1)**: 129–32.

37 Sanyal AJ, Freedman AM, Schiffman ML, Purdam PP (3rd), Luketic VA, Cheatham AK. Portosystemic encephalopathy after transjugular intrahepatic portosystemic shunt: results of a prospective controlled study. *Hepatology* 1994; **20(1, Pt 1)**: 46–55.

38 Eason J, Potter D. Anaesthesia for liver transplantation (2). In: Kaufman L ed. *Anaesthesia review* 7. London: Churchill Livingstone, 1990: 147–60.

39 Gray PA, Park GR, Cockshott ID, Douglas EJ, Shuker B, Simons PJ. Propofol metabolism in man during the anhepatic and reperfusion phases of liver transplantation. *Xenobiotica* 1992: **22(1)**: 105–14.

40 Hoyumpa AM. Disposition and elimination of minor tranquilisers in the aged and in patients with liver disease. *Southern Medical Journal* 1978; **71** (Suppl 2): 23–8.

41 Shelly MP, Dixon JS, Park GR. The pharmacokinetics of midazolam following orthotopic liver transplantation. *British Journal of Clinical Pharmacology* 1989; **27**(5): 629–33.

42 Pandele G, Chaux F, Salvadori C, Farinotti M, Duvaldestin P. Thiopental pharmacokinetics in patients with cirrhosis. *Anesthesiology* 1983; **59**: 123–6.

43 Servin F, Cockshott ID, Farinotti R, Harberer JP, Winckler C, Desmonts JM. Pharmacokinetics of propofol infusions in patients with cirrhosis. *Anesthesiology* 1990; **65**: 177–83.

44 Patwardhan RV, Johnson RF, Hoyumpa A, Sheehan JJ, Desmond PV, Wilkinson GR, Branch R, Schenker S. Morphine metabolism in cirrhosis. *Gastroenterology* 1982; **81**: 1006–11.

45 Harberer JP, Schoeffler P, Courec E, Dulvaldestin P. Fentanyl pharmacokinetics in anaesthetized patients with cirrhosis. *British Journal of Anaesthesia* 1992; **54**: 1267–70.

46 Ferrier C, Marty J, Bouffard Y, Harberer JP, Levron JC, Duvaldestin P. Alfentanil pharmacokinetics in patients with cirrhosis. *Anesthesiology* 1985; **62**: 480–4.

47 Head-Rapson AD, Devlin JC, Parker CJR, Hunter JM. Pharmacokinetics of the three isomers of mivacurium and pharmacodynamics of the chiral mixture in hepatic cirrhosis. *British Journal of Anaesthesia* 1994; **73**: 613–18.

48 Sockalingham I, Green DW. Mivacurium-induced prolonged neuromuscular block. *British Journal of Anaesthesia* 1995; **74**: 234–6.

49 Duvaldestin P, Saada J, Berger JL, D'Hollander AA, Desmonts JM. Pharmacokinetics, pharmacodynamics and dose–response relationship of pancuronium in control and elderly subjects. *Anesthesiology* 1982; **56**: 36–40.

50 Lebrault C, Berger JL, D'Hollander AA, Gomeni R, Henzel D, Duvaldestin P. Pharmacokinetics and pharmacodynamics of vecuronium [ORG NC45] in patients with cirrhosis. *Anesthesiology* 1985; **62**: 501–5.

51 Khalil M, D'Honneur G, Duvaldestin P, Slavov V, De-Hys C, Gomeni R. Pharmacokinetics and phamacodynamics of rocuronium in patients with cirrhosis. *Anesthesiology* 1994; **80 (6)**: 1241–7.

52 D'Honneur G, Khalil M, Domenique C, Haberer JP, Kleef UW, Duvaldestin P. Phamacokinetics and pharmacodynamics of pipecuronium in patients with cirrhosis. *Anesthesia and Analgesia* 1993; **77(6)**: 1203–6.

53 Ward S, Neill EAM. Pharmacokinetics of atracurium in acute hepatic failure (with renal failure). *British Journal of Anaesthesia* 1993; **55**: 1169–71.

54 Konstadt SN, Reich DL, Stanley III TE, DePerio M, Chuey C, Schwartzbach C, Abou-Donia M. A two-center comparison of the cardiovascular effects of cisatracurium (Nimbex™) and vecuronium in patients with coronary artery disease. *Anesthesia and Analgesia* 1995; **81**: 1010–4.

55 Stoelting RK. Editorial – Isoflurane and postoperative hepatic dysfunction. *Canadian Journal of Anaesthesia* 1987; **34**: 223–6.

56 Goldfarb G, Debaene B, Roulot D, Jolis P, Lebrec D. Hepatic blood flow in humans during isoflurane N_2O and halothane N_2O anesthesia. *Anesthesia and Analgesia* 1990; **71**: 349–53.

57 Zaleski L, Abello D, Gold MI. Desflurane versus isoflurane in patients with chronic hepatic and renal disease. *Anesthesia and Analgesia* 1993; **76 (2)**: 353–6.

58 Newman PJ, Quinn AC, Hall GM, Grounds RM. Circulating fluoride changes and hepatorenal function following sevoflurane anaesthesia. *Anaesthesia* 1994; **49 (11)**: 936–9

59 Mann DE. Antiarrhythmic drugs. In: Schrier RW, Gambertoglio JG eds. *Handbook of drug therapy in liver and kidney disease.* Boston: Little, Brown, 1991; 107–26.

60 Tucker GT. Pharmacokinetics of local anaesthetics. *British Journal of Anaesthesia* 1986; **58**: 717–31.

61 Bodenham A, Park GR. Plasma concentrations of bupivacaine after intercostal nerve block in patients after orthotopic liver transplantation. *British Journal of Anaesthesia* 1990; **64**: 436–41.

APPENDIX SOME COMMONLY USED ANAESTHETIC DRUGS

DRUG	VOLUME OF DISTRIBUTION (l/kg)	PROTEIN BINDING (%)	ELIMINATION HALF-LIFE [NORMAL] (h)	ELIMINATION HALF-LIFE IN LIVER DISEASE (h)	METABOLISM AND ELIMINATION [E = HEPATIC EXTRACTION RATIO]	RECOMMENDATIONS FOR USE IN PATIENTS WITH LIVER DISEASE [PATENTERAL DOSAGE UNLESS STATED]
Induction agents						
Etomidate	3–6	71–75	2–5	?	Ester hydrolysis	Induction dose unchanged, decrease rate as unbound fraction increases with decreasing serum albumin
Methohexitone	4–6	73	2	3.6	90% hepatic, oxidative hydroxylation [E = 0.53]	Bolus dose unchanged, decrease rate of administration
Propofol	5–6	>99	4	5.1	E is high, glucuronidation at hepatic and ? extrahepatic sites	Dosage unchanged for both bolus doses and for continuous infusions, providing hepatic blood flow maintained
Thiopentone	2.3	85	9	11	E is low, metabolism 99% hepatic by oxidative hydroxylation and desulphuration	Bolus dose unchanged, if a continuous infusion is used expect a prolonged effect
Analgesics						
Non-steroidal	—	—	—	—	—	Relatively contraindicated, due to increased risk of bleeding and renal impairment
Paracetamol	0.9–1	20	1.9–2.5	4.2	Hepatic conjugation oxidated metabolites are hepatotoxic	Appears to be well tolerated in cirrhotics ? hepatotoxicity more common with pre-existing disease
Alfentanil	0.28	90	1.5	3.2	99% hepatic, by oxidative N-dealkylation	Decrease dose by 50% and avoid a continuous infusion – effects pronounced and prolonged in cirrhotics
Fentanyl	3.5	80	4	5	E is high metabolism 92% hepatic by amide hydrolysis	Dosage unaltered, cumulation reported after prolonged infusion
Morphine	3.3	35	2–3	2–3 (variable)	E = 0.75 metabolism 90% by conjugation in liver and ? gut wall	Does unchanged in 'mild disease', excessive sedation may occur in patients with a history of encephalopathy or co-existing renal impairment. Best avoided in advanced disease. Reduce oral dose by 50%
Pethidine	4.5	65	4.5	6–7	E = 0.5, hepatic hydrolysis and conjugation produces an active metabolite – norpethidine, which is renally excreted	Unpredictable and best avoided. Reduce oral dose by 50%
Sufentanil	4	90	3.5	4.1	E is high, metabolism 95% hepatic by oxidative N-dealkylation	Pharmacokinetics appear unchanged following a single bolus dose in uncomplicated cirrhosis
Muscle relaxants						
Suxamethonium	—	—	0.1	0.1–0.2	Plasma pseudocholinesterase	Dosage unchanged, expect a slight prolongation of action. Observe normal contraindications
Atracurium	0.16	—	0.33	0.33	Hofmann degradation	Dosage unaltered, ? care with long-term infusions. Probably the relaxant of choice
Vecuronium	0.18	30	0.9	0.9	E is high, majority of drug is excreted unchanged in the bile	Dosage unchanged, beware of cumulation of multiple doses or a continuous infusion, elimination will be prolonged if hepatic blood flow is reduced
Pancuronium	0.27	11–29	1.91	3.47	E is low, predominantly hepatic ester hydrolysis	Some patients may show resistance to competitive neuromuscular blocking agents, but elimination is prolonged, use with caution

APPENDIX (Cont'd)

DRUG	VOLUME OF DISTRIBUTION (l/kg)	PROTEIN BINDING (%)	ELIMINATION HALF-LIFE [NORMAL] (h)	ELIMINATION HALF-LIFE IN LIVER DISEASE (h)	METABOLISM AND ELIMINATION [E = HEPATIC EXTRACTION RATIO]	RECOMMENDATIONS FOR USE IN PATIENTS WITH LIVER DISEASE [PATENTERAL DOSAGE UNLESS STATED]
Sedative and hypnotic						
Chlormethiazole	8	70	6.6	8.7	E is high	Reduce oral dose by 50% due to increased bioavailability
Diazepam	1.1–1.8	99	20–77	66–145	E is low, reliant on hydroxylation and conjugation for deactivation	Best avoided as reliant on phase I reactions for elimination, if used decrease dose by 50%
Lorazepam	0.8–2	90	8–24	22–41	Extensive hepatic glucuronide conjugation	Increase in volume of distribution may account for prolongation of elimination half-life (in some studies)
Midazolam	1.3	—	1.6	3.9	Hydroxylation and conjugation	Despite reliance on hydroxylation seems to be well tolerated in mild cirrhosis, reduce dose by 50% in advanced disease
Temazepam	1.3–1.5	96–98	10–15	13	Conjugation to inactive metabolites	No change in dosage, beware of increased effects in patients with previous encephalopathy
Local anaesthetics						
Lignocaine	1.7	50–70	1.5–1.8	5	E = 0.6. To an extent flow limited, metabolism by amide hydrolysis and N-dealkylation	Reduce dose by 50% in cirrhotics, care if cardiac output is decreased. Antiarrhythmic maintenance dose 2 mg/kg max [large decrease in intrinsic clearance]
Bupivacaine	1.5	95	2.7	?	E is lower than lignocaine, although metabolism similar	Reduce dose. Extensive protein binding to α_1-acid glycoprotein
Cardiovascular drugs						
Amiodarone	66	>95	25–52 (days)	—	Extensive hepatic metabolism to desmethylamiodarone [active]	Use with care especially if plasma proteins low ? decrease dose
Atenolol	1.2	<5	5–6	6.5	Renal 75% hepatic 10%	Dose unchanged, beware of decreased cardiac output decreasing clearance of flow-limited drugs
Digoxin	6	30	36–44	36–44	Excretion 30% hepatic, 70% renal	No change in dose, care with co-existing renal impairment
Hydralazine	1.5	87	1	?	Metabolism 75% hepatic, elimination dependent on acetylator status	Decrease dose
Nifedipine	1.2	98	2–4	7	100% hepatic	Decrease dose
Nitrates (iv)	—	—	—	—	E is high ? some extrahepatic metabolism	Dose unchanged
Isosorbide mononitrate	0.66	—	4.5	4.5		
Labetalol	11.5	50	3	3	E > 0.85 metabolism 95% hepatic	Dose unchanged but be cautious of cardiovascular effects and on the clearance of other flow-limited drugs
Verapamil	3.2–6.2	90	2.7–5.8	14	E = 0.8	Decrease oral dose by 80%, decrease iv dose by 50%

APPENDIX (Cont'd)

DRUG	VOLUME OF DISTRIBUTION (kg)	PROTEIN BINDING (%)	ELIMINATION HALF-LIFE [NORMAL] (h)	ELIMINATION HALF-LIFE IN LIVER DISEASE (h)	METABOLISM AND ELIMINATION [E = HEPATIC EXTRACTION RATIO]	RECOMMENDATIONS FOR USE IN PATIENTS WITH LIVER DISEASE [PATENTERAL DOSAGE UNLESS STATED]
Miscellaneous						
Cimetidine	0.9–1.1	20	1.5	2.9–4.0	40% hepatic	Associated with confusion especially in alcoholics, inhibitor of cytochromes, and reduces hepatic blood flow therefore avoid
Ranitidine	0.8–1.2	15	1.4–2.7	1.7–2.8	70% excreted unchanged, some hepatic metabolism	Dosage unchanged, less of an effect on hepatic blood flow
Cyclosporin	3.5	>96	6–13	20	—	Clearance dependent on hepatic function monitor levels to avoid toxicity
Frusemide	0.11	95	0.5–1	0.9–1.4	Renal 67%	Slight dose reduction, beware of electrolyte imbalances
Naloxone	2–3	54	1–1.5	Unchanged	Rapid N-dealkylation and glucuronide conjugation	Dose unchanged
Phenytoin	0.5–0.7	89–95	10–30	Unchanged	90% hepatic, 5% excreted unchanged	Beware of interactions with cyclosporin, measure levels
Theophylline	0.3–0.7	56	3–12	10–59	Hepatic	Decrease dose by 50% or more, measure levels

SECTION NINE

Drugs Affecting the Endocrine System

30

Hypothalamo–Pituitary Function

G Clarke

INTRODUCTION

Although most of the homeostatic and visceral systems of the body operate primarily under local and reflex control, the majority if not all are also regulated by the hypothalamus. This modulatory influence, which is sometimes global and sometimes selective, takes the form of both hormonal and neuronal messages. The hormonal or endocrine component is directed through and amplified by the pituitary gland, whereas the neuronal outflow is predominantly through the autonomic nervous sytem to influence visceral structures. This is not exclusive, however, for many behavioural responses that complement homeostatic function, such as feeding, drinking and sleeping, are also under the influence of the hypothalamus. As more has been learnt about neuronal pathways within the brain it has become apparent that these two routes of control, the endocrine and the autonomic, are linked. Thus the same hypothalamic peptides that regulate the pituitary gland also act as neurotransmitters in hypothalamic projections to a variety of other brain regions.

As the hypothalamus has such a central role in the co-ordination of homeostatic mechanisms, it follows that a knowledge of how drugs act within this region would be invaluable clinically. Defining these effects, however, is not as straightforward as might be anticipated, since many pharmacological experiments have generated opposing results. An explanation for such contradictions can be found by considering the way the hypothalamus is organized and functions. The majority of homeostatic changes are achieved through a multifaceted response involving a variety of peripheral organs and tissues, and the outflow of command signals is often via several routes which may or may not interact. Similarly, in order to make appropriate decisions as to the most effective and advantageous way to operate the systems of the body, the hypothalamus needs information and thus receives an unprecedented number of afferent fibres from other parts of the nervous system. These afferent inputs are complemented by humoral blood-borne signals which the hypothalamic neurones are exquisitely organized to sample, for several areas of the hypothalamus and adjacent diencephalic regions have a blood–brain barrier that is much more leaky than in other areas of the brain. This further complicates predicting pharmacological actions. Thus it may not be possible to know for certain what action a drug will have and the outcome of its administration will have to be estimated by considering many interacting influences. The circumstances of the patient will also need to be addressed for the relevance of different signals alters with changing conditions. For example, peripheral baroreceptors may be indicating a need to reduce blood pressure, yet a stressful incident may override the commands and drive the pressure higher. Similarly, low plasma osmolality may require a reduction in vasopressin secretion but a sudden fall in blood pressure will cause additional hormone to be released. A thorough knowledge of the appropriate neural pathways and their neurotransmitters is therefore required in order to make a realistic prediction of a drug's action. Thus, it may excite one system while inhibiting a parallel and related system and the end result will depend on the interplay of the two, or more, component parts.

HYPOTHALAMO–PITUITARY AXIS

Anatomy and physiology

The neuroendocrine neurones of the hypothalamus are essentially similar to other central neurones. They are depolarized and hyperpolarized by synaptic input from other neurones, they generate action potentials which depolarize the terminals, which in turn initiates a calcium-mediated exocytosis of the secretory product. Two features are unique to these hypothalamic neurosecretory neurones. First, the majority synthesize and release peptides as their primary secretory product, though dopamine and γ-aminobutyric acid (GABA) containing tubero-infundibular neurones are notable exceptions. The second difference is that though these neurones may well form conventional synaptic connections through collateral branches, the main function is neurosecretion into the vasculature. These neurones terminate on capillary networks at one of two sites. The axons of the so-called magnocellular neurones (some would argue that there is no clear division between parvocellular and magnocellular groups) pass through the internal zone of the median eminence, continue down the infundibulum (pituitary stalk) to terminate in the neurohypophysis (posterior pituitary). Over 95% of the terminals in the neurohypophysis have been shown to contain either oxytocin or vasopressin (antidiuretic hormone), which, when released, circulate in the plasma to act directly on their target tissues the mammary glands and uterus, and the kidneys and vasculature, respectively. The remaining neurosecretory cells terminate on capillaries in the median eminence, from where their secretory products are transported down the portal vessels on the surface of the infundibulum to bathe and thus influence the non-neuronal secretory cells of the adenohypophysis (anterior pituitary).

The cell bodies of neurones staining for vasopressin, oxytocin or the related neurophysins (peptide components derived from the propeptide precursor) are located predominantly in the supraoptic and paraventricular nuclei of the hypothalamus, though up to 50% may be dispersed in accessory nuclei in the adjacent regions of the anterior hypothalamus. The supraoptic nucleus consists almost entirely of magnocellular neurones projecting to the neurohypophysis. A more heterogeneous population of both magnocellular and parvocellular neurones is found in the paraventricular nucleus, with the magnocellular neurones being located more laterally and ventrally.

Five distinct secretory cell types can be distinguished in the adenohypophysis. The most numerous cells are the somatotropes, which synthesize and release growth hormone, and which account for approximately 50% of the total cells. The lactotropes, or prolactin cells, though not as abundant are still fairly numerous (approximately 20%). Corticotropes synthesize the propeptide pro-opiomelanocortin (POMC), which in turn can be processed to yield a variety of peptide hormones, the major products being adrenocorticotrophic hormone (ACTH), β-lipotropin and endorphins. The gonadotropes similarly produce more than one product, in this case follicle stimulating hormone (FSH) and luteinizing hormone (LH). The least numerous of the secretory cells in the human adenohypophysis are the thyrotropes, which release thyrotropin (TSH).

The original concept proposed by Harris nearly half a century ago was that releasing factors originating in the hypothalamus stimulated the pituitary cells to release their products. Although subsequent knowledge has substantiated this hypothesis it has also revealed the complexity of the system. Thus more than one stimulatory influence may operate on any one secretory cell, such as occurs with corticotropin-releasing hormone (CRH) and vasopressin on the corticotropes. Conversely, the adenohypophysial cell may be exposed to conflicting excitatory and inhibitory signals, as occurs with the lactotropes. Dual functions are also apparent; thyrotropin-releasing hormone (TRH) has its primary action on thyrotropes to secrete TSH, yet it also stimulates lactotropes to release prolactin. This interaction of hypothalamic signals in regulating the pituitary is fairly complex but the story is further exacerbated by signals from peripheral target tissues feeding back to influence further secretion. One only has to consider the action of the gonadal steroids, which can exert both positive and negative feedback, and which can act at pituitary, hypothalamic and extrahypothalamic sites, to appreciate the full diversity of these modulatory systems.

INDIVIDUAL PITUITARY HORMONES

Growth hormone

Regulatory control

Physiological factors

Growth hormone (GH) is released in an episodic fashion with the secretory peaks occurring every 3–4 h. The largest peaks occur during sleep and this relates to the electroencephalographic state rather than the nocturnal phase of a circadian rhythm. Sleep deprivation or inversion of the sleep–wake cycle cause an immediate corresponding shift in GH secretion. Other stimuli for secretion of GH are hypoglycaemia and consumption of a high-protein meal. A fall in plasma glucose levels is a reliable stimulus for GH release, and conversely elevated levels will inhibit GH release. The increase in GH secretion following protein ingestion appears to be a response to the amino acids, in particular arginine and leucine. In contrast, an increase in serum free fatty acids suppresses GH secretion (see Table 30.1).

Somatotropes are influenced by both a growth-hormone releasing hormone (GHRH) and a growth-hormone release inhibiting factor. GHRH is a forty-four amino acid peptide; almost complete activity, however, is displayed by the N-terminal twenty-nine amino acids. The peptide acts selectively on somatotropes to stimulate both the synthesis and secretion of GH, the latter acting through a cAMP-mediated mechanism. GHRH belongs to the glucagon-secreting family of

TABLE 30.1 Summary of the stimuli and chemcial modulators that influence the release of growth hormone, prolactin and ACTH from the pituitary

	GROWTH HORMONE	PROLACTIN	ACHT
Release	Episodic/pulsatile (every 3–4 h)	Episodic/pulsatile (intermittent about 10 pulses/day)	Episodic/pulsatile (every 2–3 h)
Rythmicity	Highest levels during sleep	Highest levels during sleep. Higher in post-pubertal females than in males or children; with a mid-cycle high.	Circadian; highest levels late night–early morning.
Stimuli for release	Hypoglycaemia High protein meal Exercise Stress; psychological and physical	Hypoglycaemia Exercise Stress; psychological and physical Trauma Anaesthesia	Hypoglycaemia Exercise Stress; psychological and physical Trauma Infection
Suppression of release	Hyperglycaemia High serum levels of free fatty acids	Water loading	Elevated serum levels of glucocorticoids
Pregnancy and lactation	—	Levels elevated during pregnancy but fall at birth Episodes of suckling induce an acute rise	Elevated in pregnancy
Secretagogues	GHRH (VIP) (GIP) (Oestrogens)	VIP (TRH) (Oestrogens)	CRF-41 Vasopressin (Angiotensin-11) (VIP) (Adrenaline)
Secretion-suppressors	Somatostatin Growth hormone Insulin-like growth factor	Dopamine Prolactin (GABA)	Glucocorticoids (Somatostatin) (Substance-P)

gastrointestinal peptides which includes vasoactive intestinal polypeptide (VIP) and gastric inhibitory peptide (GIP). Both peptides potentiate the secretory action of GHRH and high levels of VIP have been found in hypophysial portal blood.

The structure of somatostatin, the GH release inhibiting factor, has been known for rather longer than GHRH. In the hypothalamus the predominant form of the peptide has fourteen amino acids. Somatostatin cell bodies are found fairly widely both within the hypothalamus and elsewhere in the brain. It seems that the majority of the neurones projecting to the median eminence originate from the preoptic-anterior hypothalamus, in particular from periventricular sites. Somatotropes have a high-affinity receptor for somatostatin, and the peptide is capable of powerfully inhibiting growth hormone release to most secretogogues including cAMP.

Like most of the regulatory systems controlling the adenohypophysis, the GH system is subject to modulatory feedback. GH will suppress the activity of the somatotropes to prevent the release of more hormone. This action has been attributed to an activation of the somatostatin pathways; this can be considered as a short loop feedback. A second form of inhibitory feedback (long loop) involves the production of somatomedins, produced particularly by the liver, which mediate some of the actions of GH. They have been found to stimulate somatostatin release and also to have a direct action on somatotropes.

Neuropharmacology

The neurotransmitters most clearly implicated in the regulation of GH secretion are the monoamines. The strongest evidence indicates a stimulatory role for noradrenaline, though a similar action is attributed to both dopamine and serotonin (5-hydroxytryptamine) (5-HT). Centrally acting adrenergic stimulants, such as clonidine and guanfacine, induce GH secretion. Further evidence for an α-adrenoceptor action is provided by antagonists such as phentolamine, which block not only pharmacologically induced release but also the GH response to exercise, stress, hypoglycaemia and arginine. In contrast, the sleep-induced rise in GH is unaffected by α-adrenoceptor antagonists. As is often the case, β-adrenoceptors appear to have the reverse effect, for in the presence of propranolol many GH-releasing stimuli are enhanced. It has been suggested that the β-adrenergic inhibitory action may result from stimulation of somatostatin release. These effects are summarized in Table 30.2.

L-DOPA (dihydroxyphenylalanine) increases GH secretion and though this has been ascribed to an increase in noradrenaline synthesis, other evidence suggests that dopamine itself may be significant in regulat-

TABLE 30.2 Summary of the neurotransmitter influences acting to influence pituitary hormone release

	GROWTH HORMONE	PROLACTIN	ACTH	VASOPRESSIN	OXYTOCIN
Acetylcholine	⇧	×	(⇧)	⇧	⇧
Noradrenaline					
α	⇧	(⇩)	⇧	⇧	⇧
β	⇩	×	⇩	(⇩)	⇩
Dopamine	(⇧)	⇩	(⇧)	(⇧)	⇧
5-hydroxytryptamine	⇧	⇧	⇧		(⇩⇧)
GABA	⇧	(⇩)	⇩	?	(⇩)
Opioids	⇧	⇧	⇩	(⇩)	⇩

The information shown is a generalisation, for, as stated in the text, some neurotransmitters do not interact with all types of stimuli and others have multiple involvement within neural pathways. Symbols: ⇑ elevation in hormone levels following neurotransmitter activation; ⇓ decrease in level; X no change; symbols in brackets indicate contradictions in the literature or species variations.

ing GH. Apomorphine, bromocriptine, lergotrile and piribedil all provoke GH secretion and the effects can be blocked by pimozide.

The monoamine serotonin is also a candidate for a regulatory role. Certainly, serotonin, L-tryptophan and 5-hydroxytryptophan (5-HTP) cause GH release in man, and the GH response to hypoglycaemia is blocked by the antagonists, methysergide and cyproheptadine. The latter drug has also been shown to prevent the sleep-associated GH surge, though others claim the reverse effect. This contradiction illustrates the difficulties of unravelling hypothalamic function where the same transmitter may be performing fundamentally different actions on adjacent neurones.

Acetylcholine has increased in importance as a possible candidate for a transmitter role involved in regulating GH. Cholinomimetics and drugs that block acetylcholinesterase increase circulating levels of GH in man. Muscarinic antagonists prevent this elevation and also the rise in GH in response to many of the stimuli described above. The most significant difference between the adrenergic and cholinergic antagonists, however, is the ability of the latter to also prevent the sleep-induced rise in GH.

Surprisingly, GABA stimulates GH secretion. The most likely explanation is that it suppresses somatostatin secretion and thus removes a tonic inhibitory influence from the somatotropes. When administered acutely, muscimol and baclofen similarly stimulate GH release though, curiously, chronic treatment with baclofen leads to a blunted GH response to hypoglycaemia and arginine. Again this conflict probably reflects the ubiquitous nature of GABA as a transmitter in the hypothalamus and the presence of different GABA receptor subtypes.

Opioids also stimulate GH secretion and this action can be effectively blocked using the antagonist naloxone. In contrast to GABA, the effect is not mediated by an action on somatostatin. The more likely route of action is through the cholinergic system, for the GH rise induced by synthetic met-enkephalin analogues is blocked both by naloxone and by muscarinic antagonists. It is doubtful whether opioids have a major physiological role in regulating GH, for though naloxone has been reported to suppress stress-induced GH secretion it has little effect on basal secretion or hypoglycaemia-induced release.

Mechanism of action

The principal form of human GH is a single chain, 191 amino acid protein although a variety of peptides are formed as a single gene product encoded on chromosome 17. There is also considerable similarity between GH, prolactin and placental lactogen though human homology is less than for other species. As the name implies, GH influences growth of most tissues though skeletal structures are most profoundly affected; action is predominantly by increasing cell number rather than cell size. Although over a prolonged duration the effect of elevated GH secretion is increased tissue formation, the main acute response is on metabolism. In conjunction with insulin, GH acts as an anabolic influence; however, in a fasting situation when insulin levels are low GH further depresses carbohydrate metabolism and promotes fat mobilization. Conversely, when GH is deficient, insulin acts unopposed to utilize carbohydrate and generate fat and as a result fat is not mobilized for fuel.

Although GH stimulates some cells directly it usually acts through intermediate agents or somatomedins. These are now more commonly known as insulin-like growth factors of which two main proteins are recognized IGF-1 and IGF-2. Both peptides have approximately 50% homology with pro-insulin; the former is the more dependent on GH and appears to be the principal mediator of its action. Many tissues generate IGF in response to GH but the liver appears to be the main source of circulating peptide.

Therapy

Insufficiency of GH secretion can result in short stature though limited growth can of course result from a variety of other causes. Nevertheless, 65% of the growth between 4 and 12 years can be attributed to the secretion of GH. As a result GH has been used as a replacement therapy for children of short stature in whom a deficiency of endogenous hormone is suspected. Low efficacy and high immunoreactivity of animal GH led to the use of human GH extracted from cadaveric pituitaries. However, the transmission, in a few cases, of prions resulting in the fatal neurodegenerative disorder Creutzfeldt–Jacob disease terminated this approach. The availability of recombinant DNA techniques now provides biosynthetic peptide for therapeutic use. Hypothyroidism has been reported in children undergoing treatment but in part this may result from the primary hypopituitarism rather than the therapy. Subcutaneous injection may lead to lipodystrophy. Antibody production may be a problem but can be overcome by increased dosage or the use of an alternative preparation.

The use of IGF-1 has proved less effective than GH for promoting growth and the insulin-like action of this material gives rise to hypoglycaemic problems. More recently, GHRH has been used but effective therapy relies on a frequent pulsatile injection regime which is rather impractical. Modulation of endogenous GHRH has been attempted using DOPA, bromocriptine and clonidine; however, the effects have been modest or equivocal.

Hypersecretion of GH (acromegaly) most commonly results from GH-secreting adenomas. Patients present with characteristic skeletal changes – typically enlarged hands and feet. Thickening of the tongue and enlargement of the nose and mandible are also common, which may cause practical problems for the anaesthetist. Excessive GH can give rise to insulin resistance and glucose intolerance and also retention of sodium and potassium ions. Respiratory, vascular and cardiac problems are also common.

Three approaches are currently used for the treatment of acromegaly – surgical intervention, irradiation and drug therapy. Curiously in acromegalic patients dopamine analogues suppress GH secretion (cf. the stimulation of GH by dopamine in normal patients) and bromocriptine has had a valuable role in their treatment. Other approaches have involved the use of antagonists to serotonin and to α-adrenoceptors. Not all individuals respond, however, and a more recent approach has been the use of somatostatin or its analogues. Intravenous somatostatin suppresses GH secretion but rebound hypersecretion follows after cessation of the infusion. The somatostatin analogue, octreotride, has proved of value as it provides a long-lasting inhibition of GH without rebound yet has only a transient effect on insulin secretion. It can be administered subcutaneously on a thrice-daily regimen. Side-effects are mostly mild and consist of transient abdominal discomfort and increased postprandial glucose levels resulting from decreased insulin secretion.

Prolactin

Regulatory control

Physiology

Prolactin, like other anterior pituitary hormones, is secreted in an episodic manner. Approximately ten peaks occur each day, but they are irregular in amplitude, duration and frequency. As with GH, the major release is during periods of sleep, though the increase is delayed compared with GH. Serum levels of prolactin are considerably higher in postpubertal females than in men and children, though the variation in individual levels is considerable. Most women show a small midcycle rise followed by a decrease in basal levels in the luteal phase. In pregnancy the serum concentration rises 10–20-fold by term, yet the episodic pattern and sleep-associated maxima are still retained. Prolactin concentration falls dramatically during labour, though a second peak occurs about 2 h postpartum. In both nursing and non-nursing mothers basal prolactin returns to the prepregnant level about 4 weeks after birth; the stimulus of suckling, however, produces an acute eight-fold increase in serum concentration, lasting about 2 h. These changes during different reproductive states are attributable, in part, to oestrogen, a major positive modulatory factor in the secretion of prolactin. Several sites and mechanisms of action have been ascribed to the steroid, including increasing transcription of the prolactin gene, stimulation of the number of prolactin-producing cells, and suppression of hypothalamic inhibitory control (see Table 30.1).

The other major stimulus for prolactin release is stress. Anaesthesia, surgery, hypoglycaemia, exercise and psychogenic stress have all been shown to be powerful triggers for elevating serum prolactin. Basal levels are elevated by up to five-fold, and the increase in women is significantly greater than in men. The degree of hyperprolactinaemia following surgery relates to the level of physical trauma, but normal levels usually return within 24 h. Following thoracotomy or mastectomy, high prolactin levels may remain for months probably as a result of nerve stimulation mimicking the suckling stimulus.

The hypothalamic control of prolactin secretion is not entirely understood, but it is clear that the pituitary is under the influence of both prolactin-releasing factors (PRFs) and prolactin-inhibiting factors (PIFs). Prolactin synthesis and secretion is maintained and even enhanced when the pituitary is isolated from the hypothalamus. This has fostered the belief that the hypothalamus has a predominantly inhibitory influence on the lactotropes. Dopamine is established as the major inhibitory influence acting to suppress prolactin. The catecholamine acts directly on the pituitary through D_2 receptors to cause a reduction in cAMP production. Prolactin can also act as its own inhibiting factor by means of short-loop feedback, for it stimulates synthesis and turnover of dopamine in neurones, located in the arcuate nucleus, that project to the median eminence. Another neurotransmitter located in arcuate neurones that has been postulated to be a PIF is the amino acid GABA. In the rat, GABA is present in hypophyseal blood and has an inhibitory action directly on lactotropes, and in this respect GABA differs in action in the control of GH and prolactin. Evidence for a similar action in the human is less conclusive and it is unlikely that the amino acid represents a major PIF.

Experiments involving suckling-induced prolactin release have demonstrated that suppression of inhibitory influences cannot adequately account for the elevation of hormone concentration observed; thus there must also be some stimulatory releasing factors. The two most likely candidates as PRFs are TRH and VIP. There are abundant TRH terminals in the median eminence though their exact origin is not known. VIP-containing neurones, with projections to the median eminence, are found in the paraventricular and suprachiasmatic nuclei. Both peptides are present in the hypophysial portal blood and both are stimulators of prolactin secretion. During suckling there is no elevation of TSH, which argues against TRH being the mediator of the suckling-induced rise, and VIP is currently favoured. Of other possible candidates for a role as PRFs, the suckling-induced peptide oxytocin has some support, as does PHM-27 a peptide closely related to VIP.

Neuropharmacology

As with GH, the major regulatory influence is provided by the monoamines. However, in the case of prolactin it is dopamine, rather than noradrenaline, that has the major influence. As described above, dopamine provides a tonic inhibition which suppresses hormone release. Synthetic drugs with agonist activity at dopamine receptors, such as bromocriptine, piribedil, lisuride and lergotrile, or the precursor L-DOPA, all lower prolactin levels. Conversely, drugs that interfere with dopamine neurotransmission, either by blocking receptors, inhibiting synthesis or depleting stored transmitter, cause a rise in prolactin level. Thus phenothiazines, butyrophenones, pimozide, metoclopramide and sulpiride all cause hyperprolactinaemia, and if therapy is prolonged hypogonadism and galactorrhoea may result. Conversely, clinical hyperprolactinaemia, particularly in microadenoma, is readily reversed by dopamine agonists such as bromocriptine (Table 30.2).

There is little evidence to suggest that noradrenaline in the human has any major role in regulating prolactin. Some stimuli that release prolactin, such as hypoglycaemia, may be less effective in the presence of α-adrenergic agonists, suggesting the possibility of an adrenergic inhibitory pathway. Unlike noradrenaline, there is good evidence to support the view that serotonin is a primary neurotransmitter regulating prolactin. Administration of the serotonin precursors 5-HTP or L-tryptophan results in a marked increase in prolactin secretion. This effect is not a direct one on the pituitary, nor is it likely that TRH is involved for TSH levels do not rise. Current opinion favours serotonin acting through VIP release, a view substantiated by the fact that the elevation in prolactin level induced by suckling (VIP-mediated) is impaired by the serotonin antagonist, methysergide. Serotonin may also have an inhibitory action on arcuate dopamine neurones.

There is no convincing evidence for a physiological role for acetylcholine in the regulation of prolactin. In animals a dual role has been postulated for GABA, both stimulating prolactin secretion by inhibiting dopamine neurones and inhibiting secretion by a direct action on the lactotropes. No conclusive evidence is available for humans. Opioids, on the other hand, are potent stimulators of prolactin secretion. The opioids do not act as PIFs, however, as they are without effect on lactotropes *in vitro*. An interaction with dopamine neurones seems the most likely mechanism as opioids decrease the turnover and release of dopamine in the median eminence. Opioids are also ineffective if a maximal dose of a dopamine antagonist has already been administered. By analogy with other catecholamine systems it is assumed that the opioid action is a presynaptic one. Although the opioids are potent prolactin secretagogues, it appears that endogenous opioid systems are not tonically active as the opioid antagonist naloxone is without effect on basal or stimulated prolactin secretion.

Mechanism of action

Prolactin is secreted as a monomeric protein of 198 amino acid residues, though dimers and oligomers can be detected. A proportion (10–20%) occurs as glycosolated hormone which only has about 25% the potency of unmodified peptide though this form is more stable. Plasma concentration is variable and 'normal' concentrations may differ considerably between individuals; adult human levels are about 5–10 ng/ml. Cell-surface receptors for prolactin are widely distributed and have a similarity to GH receptors. Both GH and human placental lactogen bind to prolactin receptors and are lactogenic but prolactin does not act at GH receptors and is without somatotrophic activity. The major target organs for prolactin are the mammary gland and gonads. Physiologically, prolactin has its most significant effect on breast tissue during pregnancy and lactation. As the level of the hormone rises it causes proliferation and differentiation of the mammary tissue, particularly the ducts and alveolar tissue. Simultaneously, there is increased induction and synthesis of milk proteins and synthetic enzymes for lactose. Full development only occurs when prolactin is working in conjunction with other hormonal changes associated with pregnancy; the hormones of the adrenal cortex, thyroid and gonads all participate in association with insulin and GH. Nevertheless, even in non-pregnant women, men and children, galactorrhoea can occur as a result of hyperprolactinaemia. Elevated levels of prolactin have a suppressive effect on reproductive function, both by inhibiting the secretion of gonadotrophins and also by a direct action. In lactation this provides a natural, but unpredictable and unreliable, form of contraception. Similarly, prolactin-secreting tumours often give rise to amenorrhoea and anovulation in women and to loss of libido and impotence in men.

Pathology

A deficiency of prolactin can result from anterior pituitary hypofunction but is of little significance, particularly compared with the loss of other pituitary hormones. Conversely, hyperprolactinaemia invariably results in reduced sexual function and/or galactorrhoea and these are common reasons for the patient presenting. The first consideration in cases of hyperprolactinaemia should always be that of complicating factors of concomitant drug therapy (see below). Of the natural causes micro- and macroprolactinomas are the most frequent pituitary adenomas which usually, but not always, result in extremely high levels of prolactin (>200 ng/ml). Other conditions leading to hyperprolactinaemia include chronic renal failure, cirrhosis of the liver, hypothyroidism, polycystic ovary syndrome and pseudocyesis (phantom pregnancy). In 30% of patients with kidney failure prolactin is high, and this rises to 80% of those needing dialysis. Ectopic tumours in the lung or kidney may secrete prolactin but these conditions are rarely seen.

Therapeutic considerations

Prolactin is not used therapeutically. A variety of drugs can stimulate the release of prolactin and, if treatment is prolonged, can give rise to hyperprolactinaemia. These are predominantly drugs that interfere with dopamine's inhibitory action or are direct secretagogues. Dopamine antagonists such as the neuroleptics (phenothiazines, butyrophenones and substituted benzamides) and agents interrupting transmission in catecholaminergic neurones, for example reserpine and methyldopa, all elevate plasma prolactin. High doses of oestrogens stimulate prolactin release, and though hyperprolactinaemia is not common with the use of oral contraceptives, it has been reported. The increase in TRH that accompanies hypothyroidism can also give rise to high circulating levels of prolactin.

Treatment of hyperprolactinaemia resulting from pituitary tumours can be surgery, irradiation or drug therapy, all of which may be combined. The drug therapy consists of dopamine agonists, most commonly bromocriptine. Not all patients respond well but in those that do the effect is long lasting and a single daily dose can be effective (usual therapy consists of two to three doses daily). Depot preparations utilizing an intramuscular injection can keep hormone levels low for up to 1 month. Side-effects to bromocriptine are usually only a problem initially and may consist of nausea, vomiting and postural hypotension.

Hypothalamo–Pituitary–Adrenal Axis

Regulatory control

Physiological factors

Adrenocorticotrophic hormone (ACTH) is the main regulatory influence acting on the adrenal cortex. It induces a rapid increase in corticosteroid secretion and also has a trophic action on adrenal mass. Lack of ACTH results in atrophy of the adrenals and reduced synthesis of steroid. ACTH is derived from the precursor peptide POMC which can also give rise to the peptide hormones β-endorphin and melanotrophins. Secretion of ACTH, like that of growth hormone, is episodic and shows a nocturnal peak. The secretion of the two hormones differs, however, in so far as ACTH is not related to sleep but shows a true circadian rhythm peaking in the latter part of the sleep cycle or soon after awakening. The secretion of ACTH is also profoundly enhanced by all forms of stress, ranging from psychological threat to physical damage resulting from trauma or infection (Table 30.1).

It has been known for many years that the hypothalamus regulates the release of ACTH from the pituitary, and initially a single corticotrophin-releasing factor (CRF) was suspected. Progressive evidence has confirmed, however, that CRF is probably a multifactorial component, consisting of several peptides. A forty-one amino acid peptide CRF-41, located particularly in parvocellular neurones in the paraventricular nucleus of the hypothalamus, appears to be the most potent stimulus for ACTH secretion and synthesis. The other clearly identified CRF is the peptide vasopressin (AVP), in this case released from terminals in the median eminence, rather than the posterior pituitary, whose cell bodies are again found predominantly in the parvocellular part of the paraventricular nucleus (see Fig. 30.1). Other less potent hypothalamic secretogogues include angiotensin II, VIP and bombesin-like peptides. Two hypothalamic peptides may also have inhibitory regulatory roles, for it has been shown *in vitro* that both somatostatin and substance-P suppress ACTH secretion.

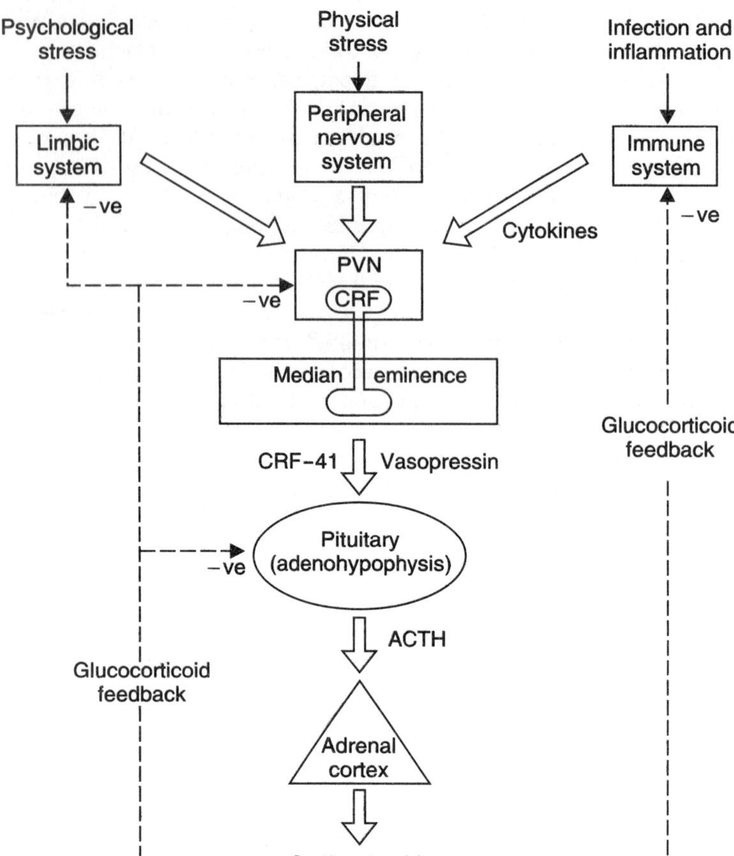

FIGURE 30.1 Schematic outline of the hypothalamo–pituitary–adrenal axis showing the stages leading from stimulation to the release of corticosteroids, also the negative feedback role of glucocorticoids.

Feedback control is a particularly powerful regulatory mechanism in ACTH secretion. The major inhibitory influence on ACTH synthesis and hence release is that exerted by circulating corticosteroids on the corticotropes. Negative feedback by peripherally released steroids also occurs at the level of the hypothalamus to suppress CRF release, and at other brain sites. Not only are there various sites of steroid feedback but the nature of the responses is also variable. More than one type of corticosteroid receptor has been postulated on the basis of binding and pharmacological studies. The corticosteroid-preferring variety are referred to as type I, or 'CR', receptors, whereas type II, 'GR', receptors are glucocorticoid-preferring. Under normal conditions occupancy of CRs is almost 100%, and thus it is likely that negative feedback is due to increased occupancy of the GR sites. Both types of corticosteroid receptor are found in the hippocampus, septal nuclei, amygdala, some brain stem nuclei and the hypothalamus. In the last region the GRs predominate and there is a strong correlation between receptor distribution and CRH immunoreactivity in the parvocellular paraventricular nucleus (PVN). Second, the inhibition of the hypothalamo–pituitary–adrenal axis (HPA) can be separated into at least two categories on the basis of time-course, for both 'fast-feedback' and 'delayed' inhibition can be demonstrated. The fast-feedback inhibition is immediate and is believed to involve membrane-bound receptors which cause a rapid decrease in the excitability of hypothalamic neurones and corticotropes. The delayed feedback results from entry of the steroid into cells and translocation of the hormone–receptor complex to the nucleus. The subsequent genomic actions lead to a reduction in synthesis of secretory product and a change in cell-surface receptors to a variety of neurotransmitters. This occurs in both hypothalamic neurones and adenohypophyseal corticotropes (Fig. 30.1).

Thus corticosteroids have a profound inhibitory effect on the HPA; however, major secretory stimuli such as fear, pain, trauma, fever and hypoglycaemia can override this normal inhibitory feedback. In pathological conditions of steroid hypersecretion, or in prolonged therapy with high doses of corticosteroids, ACHT secretion is suppressed leading to atrophy of the adrenals.

Circulating catecholamines of peripheral origin have also been implicated as regulators of ACTH release, and thus as providing feedback control. Inhibitory actions have been described but the better documented effect is of a catecholamine-mediated stimulation of secretion. It is unclear whether the catecholamines act directly or indirectly on the corticotropes.

Neuropharmacology

Evidence for the involvement of catecholamines in the control of CRH neurones is contradictory. The weight of opinion favours a stimulatory action of noradrenaline, via α-adrenoceptors, and a suppressive action via β-adrenoceptors. The role of dopamine is even less clear and is probably negligible. Administration of serotonin precursors leads to an increase in ACTH secretion, whereas serotonin antagonists cause a reduction in basal release, disrupt the circadian rhythms, and prevent insulin-stimulated secretion.

In experimental animals considerable evidence favours a stimulatory action for acetylcholine, both muscarinic and nicotinic receptors being implicated. In man the exact physiological role of acetylcholine is unclear but it seems that it may be significant, possibly acting through serotonergic neurones. The amino acid GABA has a powerful inhibitory effect on many central neurones and the CRH neurones are no doubt similarly affected. The convulsive action of GABA antagonists prevents any meaningful studies being performed in humans. GABA analogues have been tried; however, muscimol was without effect but baclofen induced a decrease in plasma cortisol under both basal and stimulated conditions (Table 30.2).

It is generally agreed that opioids have a suppressive effect on ACTH release, though a few authors have also suggested a stimulatory role. The pharmacological profile of the responses and the need for high doses of naloxone to reverse the suppressive effect suggests that κ-opioid receptors are involved. It is possible that this opioid action is mediated through catecholamine neurones. However opioids do not influence all ACTH-releasing stimuli. It appears that there is an endogenous opioid tone present throughout the day, but it is not part of the circadian rhythm.

Mechanism of action of ACTH

ACTH acts on the adrenal cortex to stimulate the secretion of steroids, which are either corticosteroids or androgens. This stimulatory action is essential as corticosteroids are not stored in the adrenal tissue and therefore biosynthesis equates to secretion. The peptide acts through adenyl cyclase stimulation to increase cAMP, which causes both increased steroidogenesis and trophic effects, particularly the induction of steroidogenic enzymes but also an increase in cell number and size. The predominant effect is on the production of cortisol and corticosterone (glucocorticoids) rather than on aldosterone (mineralocorticoid), and following removal of the adenohypophysis glucocorticoid secretion diminishes whereas mineralocorticoid levels stay about the same. In the atrophy of the adrenal gland that follows this hypophysectomy, the zona glomerulosa (site of mineralocorticoid synthesis) is least affected. In the same way it is the glucocorticoids that provide the feedback inhibition of ACTH secretion, exerted by steroids. Nevertheless, ACTH does stimulate aldosterone secretion and in its absence there is a reduced response to sodium depletion.

Adrenal corticosteroids

Although the corticosteroids represent a family of related steroids which share activity to a greater or lesser extent, it is normal to subdivide the corticosteroids into those that primarily influence metabolic activity, the glucocorticoids, and those that influence electrolyte and water balance, the mineralocorticoids. It should always be borne in mind, however, that whatever category a steroid is placed in it has the potential to exert the alternative action at some concentration. Cortisol, corticosterone, aldosterone and desoxycorticosterone are the main corticosteroids secreted in the human. Desoxycorticosterone is considered to be the prototypic mineralocorticoid with potent actions on the kidney but with almost no effect on carbohydrate metabolism. In functional terms, however, it has only a minor role in comparison to aldosterone, for though similar quantities of the two steroids are secreted by the adrenals, aldosterone is considerably more potent. Aldosterone is almost as potent as corticosterone in terms of carbohydrate metabolism; however, it has no significant role in this regard as the rate of aldosterone secretion is appreciably less than that of the glucocorticoids. Thus, under normal conditions, the main influence on carbohydrate metabolism is from cortisol and corticosterone. Although aldosterone is the primary influence on the kidney because of its greater potency, cortisol and corticosterone are contributory because of their higher concentrations in the plasma.

Mode of action

Corticosteroids, like other steroids, act within the cell by binding to specific steroid hormone receptors in the cytoplasm. When bound the receptor–steroid complex can enter the nucleus and bind to chromatin to regulate transcription. In most cells transcription is promoted and specific mRNA formed, an exception is the suppression of the transcription of POMC which forms ACTH. Glucocorticoids are also believed to bind to cell surface receptors on neurones in the hypothalamus to provide fast feedback inhibition.

By binding to type I (mineralocorticoid) receptors, corticosteroids increase the reabsorption of sodium in the distal tubules of the kidney and other secretory tissues. Sodium ions are exchanged for potassium ions and hydrogen ions. Thus a deficiency of corticosteroids (hypocorticism) gives rise to hyponatraemia, hyperkalaemia and contraction of the extracellular fluid volume. Conversely, excess hormone activity increases sodium uptake but this is compensated for by increased fluid, thus plasma sodium is close to normal but extracellular fluid volume is increased; hypokalaemia and alkalosis are also present.

Corticosteroids produce a variety of effects on intermediary and lipid metabolism. The major effects are increased gluconeogenesis, formation of glycogen in the liver and protein metabolism. As such, the action opposes the effect of insulin and appears to be a protective one to ensure adequate glucose for cerebral function. In the absence of glucocorticoids the individual can survive provided regular food is available; if fasting occurs hypoglycaemia develops rapidly. The steroids also facilitate lipolysis in adipose tissue.

Correct concentrations of mineralo- and glucocorticoids are essential for effective cardiovascular function. A deficiency of corticosteroids results in hypotension, reduced cardiac efficiency and impaired arteriolar tone. In part this results from the reduced plasma volume due to increased sodium excretion but glucocorticoids also seem to have a direct facilitatory action on the tissues. Conversely, elevated corticosteroid concentration in plasma results in hypertension and hypokalaemia. Similarly, skeletal muscle function is impaired by perturbation of corticosteroid concentration, low levels cause weakness through poor blood supply and high levels cause weakness because of the hypokalaemia.

The ability of glucocorticoids to act as anti-inflammatory agents and immunosuppressants is covered in detail in Chapter 24. In brief, they exert a variety of actions on leucocytes, particularly by preventing the formation or action of a constellation of chemical mediators. These include prostaglandins and leucotrienes, platelet-activating factor, tumour necrosis factor and interleukins.

Pathology

Primary adrenal insufficiency (Addison's disease) is a consequence of adrenal damage and results in hyposecretion of corticosteroids. Hypoglycaemia, weight loss, hyponatraemia, hyperkalaemia, muscle wasting and pigmentation are characteristic changes. The pigmentation is due to hyperproduction and secretion of POMC derivatives as a result of non-existent negative feedback. Secondary adrenal insufficiency results from the failure to secrete adequate quantities of ACTH. Causes may be either malfunction or damage at the pituitary level or hypothalamic dysfunction preventing CRF release. Signs and symptoms are usually less dramatic than with primary dysfunction, and since ACTH has greater effect upon glucocorticoids, hypoglycaemia is most common.

Inappropriately elevated corticosteroid levels (Cushing's disease) can arise for several reasons. The most common pathological cause is hypersecretion of ACTH either from the pituitary or from ectopic sites. The elevated peptide concentration leads to bilateral adrenal hyperplasia and hypersecretion of cortisol and adrenal androgens. Less common are autonomous cortisol-secreting adenomas or carcinomas. In this case the hypersecretion of cortisol suppresses ACTH release, leading to atrophy of the contralateral adrenal. Characteristic manifestations are change in body form (moon face, truncal obesity) and hypertension, hyperglycaemia and psychiatric symptoms are particularly common.

Therapeutic use of ACTH

ACTH is mainly used as a diagnostic agent to determine the presence of adrenal insufficiency. It is rapidly absorbed following parenteral administration but only has a short half-life (about 15 min) in plasma due to hydrolysis. The peptide has been used therapeutically in cases of secondary adrenocortical insufficiency instead of glucocorticoid therapy. It should be recognized, however, that the two are not similar and the use of ACTH will also stimulate mineralocorticoid and androgen secretion. Conventionally, ACTH has been obtained from animal pituitaries but a synthetic peptide consisting of amino acids 1–24 (cosyntropin) is also available. This synthetic peptide, though truncated, has full activity and has the benefit of not being contaminated with vasopressin.

Therapeutic use of glucocorticoids

In cases of adrenal insufficiency cortisol (hydrocortisone) is the most appropriate therapy. Most patients will also require mineralocorticoid therapy though some individuals can be controlled on cortisol and a high salt diet. In severe acute cases initial therapy will need to address the life-threatening problems of distorted ion balance and cardiovascular dysfunction. Drug regime will depend upon the underlying pathology and if irreversible damage has occurred to the adrenals replacement therapy will need to be tailored to the patient's daily need for the rest of life, typical dosage 20–30 mg/day. Cortisol has a serum half-life of about 100 min with more than 90% being reversibly protein bound. Actions are long lasting, however, and it is usual to divide treatment into two daily doses, sometimes with a higher morning dose to simulate diurnal fluctuation.

Glucocorticoid-deficient patients have a greatly reduced ability to cope with stress and this should be considered with regard to trauma and surgery. Substantial steroid therapy should be commenced prior to the operation and continued postoperatively (suggested dose range is 100–200 mg hydrocortisone/70 kg body weight/day). In normal patients cortisol may remain high for over 72 h after a major operation. Pretreatment with a mineralocorticoid may also be required, particularly if hyperkalaemia is present.

Glucocorticoids have a wide range of therapeutic uses as well as their role in substitution therapy. These steroids and their synthetic analogues have a unique and valuable role therapeutically. Used acutely, these agents are relatively non-toxic and in life-threatening situations large doses can justifiably be administered, and indeed may be the only effective short-term remedy. The anti-inflammatory and immunosuppressive actions of glucocorticoids also make them a popular choice for chronic treatment of many conditions. Dosage in such cases tends to be empirical, prolonged and in some cases poorly monitored, which results in adaptive changes to pituitary–adrenal function. Two scenarios can occur: (1) glucocorticoid overdosage, for conditions such as asthma, arthritis and allergies, gives rise to Cushing's syndrome; and (2) abrupt withdrawal of steroids from patients receiving chronic glucocorticoid therapy leads to adrenal insufficiency. This arises from the glucocorticoids causing inhibition of ACTH and subsequent atrophy of the adrenals, which cannot then respond to challenge. Effects can be long lasting and steroid cover, in times of stress, may be necessary up to 2 years later. At physiological replacement doses (hydrocortisone 20–30 mg/day) this does not appear to be a problem, nor with acute high-dose therapy.

Several drugs are known to interfere with glucocorticoid production and secretion and some have been used successfully for the treatment of Cushing's disease. All are capable of causing hypoadrenalism. Aminoglutethimide blocks steroid synthesis at the initial stage of conversion of cholesterol, thus all adrenal steroids are affected. Ketoconazole is primarily an antifungal agent but at higher doses has a similar action to aminoglutethimide. Metyrapone also impairs synthesis but predominantly by preventing the final stage conversion to cortisol and thus has a fairly specific profile. As cortisol is the main influence in terms of inhibitory feedback, metyrapone is used as a diagnostic challenge of pituitary function; in a normal individual increased secretion of ACTH should follow its administration. Each of these drugs is used in the treatment of Cushing's disease, sometimes together. Etomidate is another imidazole that has significant inhibitory effects on steroid synthesis. Its significance is that it is used as a short-acting general anaesthetic. Severity of effect relates to duration of administration but even after a single induction dose adrenal function may be compromised for over 24 h. It is recommended that patients who received etomidate and who show signs of adrenal insufficiency, for example hypotension, hyponatraemia and hypokalaemia, should receive cortisol 100 mg every 12 h.

Vaspressin and oxytocin

Regulatory control

Physiology

Vasopressin and oxytocin are two related nonapeptide hormones differing in structure by just two amino acids. They are synthesized in separate neurones from two specific yet related propeptides. A variety of other peptides have been reported to co-exist within oxytocin and vasopressin neurones. By far the most abundant are the two neurophysins, which are cosynthesized from the two propeptides; they differ from each other but show a high degree of homology. The neurophysins have no known physiological actions once released from the neurones. Of the other co-existing peptides the most important may be the opioids, for these have a profound effect on the release of vasopressin and oxytocin. Proenkephalin derivatives are present in the oxytocin cells and prodynorphin derivatives in the vasopressin neurones.

The main stimuli for vasopressin release are hypertonicity and hypotension. Raised plasma osmolality (>280 mOsm/kg) activates osmoreceptors both directly through raised plasma ion concentration and indirectly through angiotensin II, a potent vasopressin secretagogue. Sudden and precipitous reductions in blood pressure or more prolonged changes associated with hypovolaemia result in vasopressin secretion as a result of baroreceptor stimulation. Other stimuli for release include pain, nausea, emesis, stress, intestinal traction, abdominal compression and hypoglycaemia. Vasopressin is therefore considered by many to be a stress hormone. Factors which suppress the release of vasopressin tend to be the converse of the above, the most influential being an increase in vascular pressure.

Oxytocin is fundamental to maternal behaviour. In many species oxytocin secretion facilitates birth by contracting the uterus, thereby aiding expulsion of the fetus and placenta. Release of the hormone is initiated by dilatation of the cervix and birth canal. Postpartum, the release of oxytocin is essential during lactation for the effective ejection of milk during suckling. The stimulus for secretion during nursing is provided by the sucking of the young on the nipples. Centrally projecting oxytocin-containing neurones are believed to be important both for maintenance of the milk-ejection reflex and for the expression of maternal behaviour. The hormone may also have physiological roles at other times in the life of the female, and generally in the male. Osmotic stimuli are potent at releasing oxytocin and in some species the hormone may have a natriuretic action; such a function has not been demonstrated in the human. Oxytocin is also released by stress but this response declines during pregnancy and lactation.

Neuropharmacology

There is substantial evidence that noradrenaline stimulates the release of both vasopressin and oxytocin. This action is blocked in both cases by α-adrenoceptor antagonists. A stimulatory dopamine system may also be present. Catecholamines also have an inhibitory role in some species, the β-adrenoceptor mediated suppression of oxytocin in the rat is particularly potent. Whether this is a direct action on the oxytocin neurones or indirect and acting through opioid systems (see below) is unresolved at present. Whether a similar effect occurs in the human is also unknown. The action of serotonin on vasopressin and oxytocin secretion is complex; in some situations a facilitation of release occurs, in others secretion is suppressed. Again this contradiction probably reflects serotonin acting at several sites, and the involvement of different serotonergic receptors.

Acetylcholine is significantly involved in the neural pathways that regulate the release of oxytocin and vasopressin. Nicotinic receptors of the ganglionic type are involved in neuronal projections relaying from the brain stem, for both suckling-induced oxytocin secretion and cardiovascular-stimulated vasopressin release. Conversely, osmotic stimulation, which operates through forebrain circumventricular organs, utilizes muscarinic cholinoceptors.

As with many hypothalamic peptides, opioids exert a powerful influence over the secretion of oxytocin; their action on vasopressin secretion is less clear. Oxytocin secretion in response to suckling can be prevented by opioids at several sites. To date, an action has been demonstrated on the afferent pathway in the spinal cord, on the oxytocin cell bodies in the hypothalamus, and on the nerve terminals in the neurohypophysis. The last site is of particular interest in so far as dynorphin, which is coreleased with vasopressin during osmotic stimulation, may act on the adjacent oxytocin terminals to suppress release. Certainly, subjects given insulin (to produce hypoglycaemia) or nicotine (in the form of a strong cigarette) show an increase in plasma vasopressin, but their oxytocin levels remain low unless naloxone is given concurrently. This opioid inhibition of oxytocin would be expected to have a significant effect during childbirth. At such times endogenous opioid tone may be high, particularly if the patient is stressed, and opioid analgesics are often administered. Evidence suggests that opioid receptor numbers may fall just prior to the onset of parturition; nevertheless, an effective opioid-mediated suppression of oxytocin can still occur. Failure to suckle successfully, and thus to eject milk, may also be attributable to opioids, particularly in patients who are stressed.

In contrast to oxytocin, the action of opioids on vasopressin secretion is equivocal. Established texts state that following the intravenous injection of an opioid, vasopressin levels are elevated. This probably results from vasodilatation or from an effect on baroreceptors causing a reflex release of the hormone. Experiments in animals have only revealed inhibitory actions directly on the vasopressin neurones. Of particular interest is the κ-opioid mediated suppression of vasopressin secretion which is responsible in part for the profound diuresis observed with κ-opioid agonists. Opioid receptors appear to be influenced by gonadal steroids and thus there are sex differences in responsiveness. Similarly, efficacy of opioids varies at different times of the reproductive cycle. Human studies have been less conclusive and opioids may be less significant in the regulation of human vasopressin.

Mechanism of action

Vasopressin, or antidiuretic hormone, as its names imply has both a potent pressor action on vessels and a urine-concentrating action on the kidney. The latter renal effect occurs, however, at a much lower concentration. The difference in potency results from the existence of at least two types of receptors, V_1 and V_2, with the latter having a much greater affinity for the peptide. Activation of the V_2 receptors on the collecting ducts of the kidney results in increased resorption of water. Failure to secrete adequate vasopressin (hypothalamic diabetes insipidus) causes a profound polyuria. Conversely, excess (inappropriate) secretion of the hormone gives rise to dilutional hyponatraemia. Although large doses, in physiological terms, are required to produce a direct pressor response (through V_1 receptors) it is now considered that vasopressin at subpressor levels may act in conjunction with angiotensin and other peptides to augment the pressor effect of noradrenaline. Other actions of vasopressin include a corticotrophin-releasing action on the pituitary to stimulate ACTH secretion (see above), a variety of actions within the brain, and an action on the liver to induce hyperglycaemia. Vasopressin stimulates uterine smooth muscle and mammary myoepithelial cells to contract but has less than 20% of the potency of oxytocin. For the effects of vasopressin on clotting see Chapter 27, part I.

Oxytocin contracts uterine smooth muscle but the effects are oestrogen dependent. Sensitivity to the peptide increases considerably towards the end of pregnancy. The hormone similarly contracts myoepithelial cells in the mammary gland to force milk from the alveoli into the teat ducts. This contractile action on both the uterus and the mammary tissue is inhibited by catecholamines through β-adrenoceptors. Circulating adrenaline may well contribute to failure to eject milk during nursing when under psychological or emotional stress. Other actions of the peptide include a weak natriuretic and antidiuretic effect and a weak relaxing action on vasculature; this can be more marked in deeply anaesthetized patients. Interestingly, oxytocin is a powerful constrictor of umbilical arteries and veins and may play a role in their closure at birth.

Pathology

Polyuria is defined as the production of excessive hypotonic urine and results from one of three causes all relating to vasopressin. Primary polydipsia arises when individuals drink large volumes in excess of requirements – the resultant reduction in plasma osmolality then suppresses vasopressin secretion. Cranial diabetes insipidus results from a failure to secrete vasopressin in response to the normal osmotic stimuli. Primary causes can be idiopathic or genetic in origin, secondary causes are trauma, resulting from neoplasia, infections or vascular accidents. Treatment is in the form of replacement hormone or an analogue. Nephrogenic diabetes insipidus, in contrast, results from a failure of the kidney to respond adequately to circulating vasopressin. The condition often arises as a secondary consequence of metabolic disturbance, particularly resulting when hypercalcaemia or hypokalaemia is present. Therapeutic use of lithium can also give rise to nephrogenic diabetes insipidus (>30% of patients) even at normal therapeutic concentrations.

SIADH (syndrome of inappropriate antidiuretic hormone) is a condition in which excessive secretion of vasopressin occurs and is unrelated to serum osmolality. This results in fluid retention and hyponatraemia, which in turn can lead to brain oedema, weakness, lethargy and mental confusion and, if the condition progresses, to convulsions and coma. The cause may be due to a hypothalamic or pituitary tumour or an ectopic vasopressin-secreting tumour. A variety of drugs can also stimulate release including nicotine, opioids, chlorpropamide, vincristine, vinblastine and cyclophosphamide. Treatment usually involves removal of the tumour or cessation of the drug regime. No specific inhibitors of release are currently used although interest is increasing in relation to κ-receptor selective opioid ligands. Drugs that desensitize the kidney to vasopressin are used (see below) and the search for more selective vasopressin antagonists is on-going.

Therapeutic considerations

Vasopressin is used to compensate for the lack of endogenous peptide in cases of vasopressin-sensitive diabetes insipidus. Major limitations are the need to give it parenterally and its short half-life in the circulation of 10–20 min. These problems have been overcome by the use of nasal sprays, depot intramuscular injections, or by the use of the potent V_2-selective and long-lasting analogue desmopressin (dDAVP). Using the latter drug, normal urine volume can be maintained with doses of 2–20 μg twice daily intranasally. Drugs such as chlorpropamide, acetaminophen (paracetamol) and indomethacin sensitize the kidney to vasopressin. Conversely, the antibiotic demeclocycline antagonizes the action of vasopressin, as does lithium. Replacement therapy is of course useless in cases of nephrogenic diabetes insipidus where the kidney is unresponsive to the hormone. In these cases thiazide diuretics or amiloride are used. Vasopressin is not often administered for its vasopressor action because of its potent constrictor effect on cardiac vessels; the exception is its use to control bleeding in the gastrointestinal tract.

The main use of oxytocin is for induction of labour. Strategies for administration vary, but in general weak solutions are infused intravenously starting from 1 mU/min and increasing slowly until labour commences. Steady-state concentrations require some time to achieve as the peptide has a short half-life (5–10 min) in the circulation; the kidney and liver are mainly responsible for its removal. Oxytocin has also been used in the form of a nasal spray to induce milk ejection. High doses of oxytocin, particularly when given in conjunction with electrolyte-free solutions, can cause overhydration and hyponatraemia leading to headache, convulsions and coma.

CONCLUDING REMARKS

The nature of the hypothalamo–pituitary axis, the one part neuronal the other secretory tissue, is significant in relation to anaesthesia. The activity of the regulatory hypothalamic neurones will be suppressed by anaesthetics whereas the secretory functions of the pituitary cells will be more resistant. Thus pituitary secretions will tend to 'free-run', in some cases such as prolactin this will result in elevated hormone levels, in others the hormone level will fall. Furthermore, the pituitary cells may well be exposed to unopposed peripheral feedback which could give rise to exaggerated responses.

Many of the neurosecretory nerve terminals in the median eminence are inhibited by opioids and thus the use of narcotic analgesics will invariably interfere with hypothalamo–pituitary function. The combination of anaesthetic and analgesic will often compound these suppressive actions. When dopamine antagonists are also involved, as in neurolept-analgesia, the effects on hormones such as prolactin and growth hormone are quite considerable.

In the context of the clinical use of anaesthetics and analgesics, the potential benefits invariably outweigh the acute disruption to the endocrine systems. An awareness of the potential problems, however, should prove providential both for the management of the patient during operations and in the recovery phase. Perhaps the most significant influence on the patient, irrespective of drug treatment, is the stress to which they are exposed. All forms of stress, whether they be noxious, metabolic or emotional, are potent modulators of hormone secretion, which are often capable of overriding inhibitory control. Thus all stress should be minimized, and of the many stressors that individuals may be exposed to, emotional or psychological stress appears to be the most pernicious in terms of endocrine disruption.

FURTHER READING

Clinical endocrinology, Grossman A ed. London: Blackwell Scientific, 1992.

The physiology of reproduction Vol. 2, 2nd Edn, Knobil E, Nei JD eds. New York: Raven Press, 1994.

Williams textbook of endocrinology 8th Edn, Wilson JD, Foster DW eds. Philadelphia: WB Sanders, 1992.

31

The Thyroid: Drugs Used in Thyrotoxic and Hypothyroid States

AB Kurtz

INTRODUCTION

Historical descriptions have left us with many eponymous thyroid disorders and an international cast. Graves (Ireland 1797–1853) and Basedow (Germany 1799–1854) both described thyrotoxicosis of the type now known to have an autoimmune aetiology; Plummer (USA 1874–1936) described toxic nodular goitre; Gull (Great Britain 1816–1890) described hypothyroidism; Hashimoto (Japan 1881–1934) described autoimmune thyroiditis and de Quervain (Switzerland 1868–1940) subacute thyroiditis.

THE THYROID

The thyroid is an endodermal structure containing thyrocytes arranged in follicles. In the adult it weighs approximately 20 g. The thyrocytes actively take up iodide from the circulation and in several stages convert inorganic iodide to thyronines contained in thyroglobulin which is stored in the follicles. This pool of iodinated protein contains approximately 8 mg of iodine. Stimulation of thyrocytes causes reabsorption of thyroglobulin followed by hydrolysis and release of the thyronines thyroxine (T_4) and triiodothyronine (T_3) into the circulation.

These functions of the thyroid are controlled by thyrotrophin (thyroid-stimulating hormone or TSH) secreted from the anterior pituitary; secretion of thyrotrophin is controlled in part by thyrotrophin-releasing hormone (TRH) which is produced in the supraoptic and paraventricular nuclei of the hypothalamus, stored in the median eminence and released into the hypophyseal portal circulation. Thyrotrophin is a glycoprotein composed of α- and β-subunits, as are the gonadotrophins, while TRH is a tripeptide – pyroglutamyl-histidyl-proline amide. The synthesis and secretion of thyrotrophin is inhibited by thyroid hormones – that is, there is negative feedback control.

Iodide is actively transported into thyrocytes; the first step in the synthesis of thyroid hormones (Fig. 31.1). The only other tissues to actively take up iodide from the circulation are salivary glands and placenta. The second step is the oxidation of iodide by peroxidase with iodination of tyrosyl residues in thyroglobulin. The products of this step are sequentially 3-monoiodotyrosine and 3,5-diiodotyrosine. The third step, which is also mediated by peroxidase, occurs within the thyroglobulin molecule and is the coupling of iodotyrosines to yield iodothyronines. The final step is hydrolysis of thyroglobulin with release into the circulation of thyroxine and triiodothyronine and re-utilization of uncoupled iodotyrosines.

A daily intake of 250–500 μg of iodine is sufficient for health; an intake of less than 100 μg of iodine is not. Deficiency of dietary iodine remains a major problem in many parts of the world. With low iodine

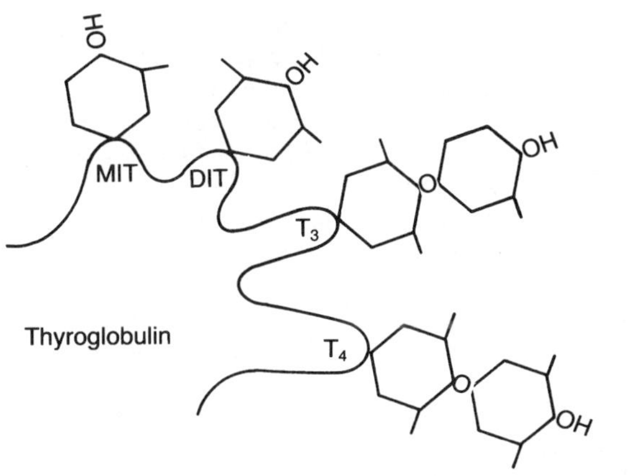

FIGURE 31.1 Thyroglobulin containing monoiodothyrosine (MIT), diiodothyrosine (DIT), triiodothyronine (T_3) and thyroxine (T_4).

intakes compensatory changes ensue. Increased secretion of thyrotrophin causes thyroid enlargement and more avid trapping of iodide. In iodine-deficient areas goitre is common and adults are usually able to achieve metabolic normality. Scarcity of iodide limits the formation of diiodotyrosine; the consequent production of triiodothyronine rather than thyroxine allows more efficient use of available iodine. However, iodine deficiency causes major problems of fetal neurological development; so called endemic cretinism.

THYROID HORMONES

The major thyroid hormones are thyroxine (L-3,5,3′,5′-tetraiodothyronine) and triiodothyronine (L-3,5,3′triiodothyronine) often referred to as T_4 and T_3 (Fig. 31.2). In health the principal product of thyroid secretion is thyroxine; a small amount of triiodothyronine is also directly secreted. The ratio of thyroxine to triiodothyronine for both production and secretion is approximately 10 : 1. Thyroxine is largely an inactive prohormone which is deiodinated in extrathyroidal sites to either active triiodothyronine or inactive reverse triiodothyronine (L-3,3′5′-triiodothyronine). This step of activation or deactivation is carefully controlled in line with metabolic requirements. Following trauma, severe illness or starvation 5- rather than 5′-monodeiodination of thyroxine in liver and kidney causes production of large amounts of reverse triiodothyronine with little or no active triiodothyronine. Glucocorticoids, propranolol and propylthiouracil also reduce peripheral triiodothyronine production.

In the circulation both thyroxine and triiodothyronine are largely bound to proteins. Thyroxine-binding globulin (TBG) binds both thyroxine and triiodothyronine as does albumin, while thyroxine-binding pre-albumin (TBPA) just binds thyroxine. The concentrations of total thyroxine (60–160 nmol/l) and triiodothyronine (0.8–2.7 nmol/l) are much greater than those

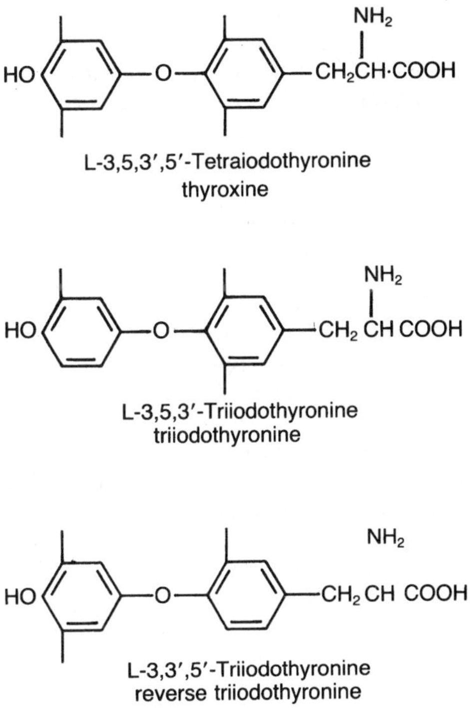

L-3,5,3′,5′-Tetraiodothyronine
thyroxine

L-3,5,3′-Triiodothyronine
triiodothyronine

L-3,3′,5′-Triiodothyronine
reverse triiodothyronine

FIGURE 31.2 The structures of thyroid hormones.

of free thyroxine (9.4–24 pmol/l) and triiodothyronine (3–8 pmol/l) with which they are in equilibrium. The concentrations of the binding proteins can alter under a number of different situations with large changes in total thyroid hormone concentration; however, it is the concentration of free hormone that matters physiologically and thyroid status is best determined by reference to free thyroid hormone and thyrotrophin concentrations.

Thyroid hormones act at the cell nucleus in a similar way to steroid hormones and vitamin D. After gaining access to cells, thyroid hormones bind to a receptor protein in the cytosol. This protein has a separate DNA-binding domain containing ‘zinc fingers’. Binding of the thyroid hormone receptor complex to DNA – possibly as a protein dimer – causes synthesis of new messenger RNA and new protein. Thyroid hormones are transcriptional enhancers promoting synthesis of enzyme proteins; their biological effects are therefore not immediate but require several hours to become manifest. Whether thyroxine can act in this way without intracellular conversion to triiodothyronine is not certain; intracellular activation to triiodothyronine does occur in some tissues, for example the pituitary, but most tissues respond only to triiodothyronine from the circulation.

THYROTOXICOSIS

Excessive production of thyroid hormones occurs in Graves’ disease where thyroid stimulation is caused by an immunoglobulin G binding to the thyrotrophin receptors on thyrocytes. The other common causes of thyrotoxicosis are toxic multinodular goitre and toxic (follicular) adenoma; in both the secretion of thyroid hormone is autonomous rather than stimulated. The hallmark of thyrotoxicosis is elevation of the circulating concentration of free triiodothyronine with suppression of TSH secretion. The effects of thyroid hormones are wide ranging with stimulation of protein, carbohydrate and lipid metabolism, and calorigenesis.

The principal choices in the management of thyrotoxicosis are between drug therapy, radioactive ^{131}I and surgery; where thyrotoxicosis is severe drug therapy would be used in conjunction with ^{131}I or surgery.

Thyroid crisis is a rarely seen medical emergency. It occurs where severe thyrotoxicosis, usually undiagnosed, is complicated by a major stress such as pneumonia, trauma, diabetic ketoacidosis or childbirth. It is characterized by tachycardia, pyrexia, circulatory collapse, coma and death. Treatment is with parenteral iodide, glucocorticoid, and β-adrenergic antagonists; and with circulatory support with fluids.

THIOAMIDES

The simplest compound in this group is thiourea which does have an antithyroid effect inhibiting the formation of thyroid hormones by blocking the organification of iodine. There are three drugs in this group: carbimazole, methimazole and propylthiouracil (Fig. 31.3). The most frequently used drug in the UK is carbimazole. Carbimazole and methimazole are very similar; indeed carbimazole is hydrolysed to methimazole which is the active drug. All three drugs are rapidly absorbed after oral administration. The drugs are actively taken up by the thyroid and the intrathyroidal half-life is considerably longer than the half-life in the circulation, the latter being about 6 h for carbimazole and methimazole and 2 h for propylthiouracil. The thioamides exert their effect by interfering with several of the steps involved in the incorporation of iodide into thyronines: all of these steps require peroxidase. In order of descending sensitivity the drugs block the coupling of iodotyrosines to thyroxine and triiodothyronine, the iodination of monoiodotyrosine to diiodotyrosine and the iodination of tyrosine to monoiodotyrosine.

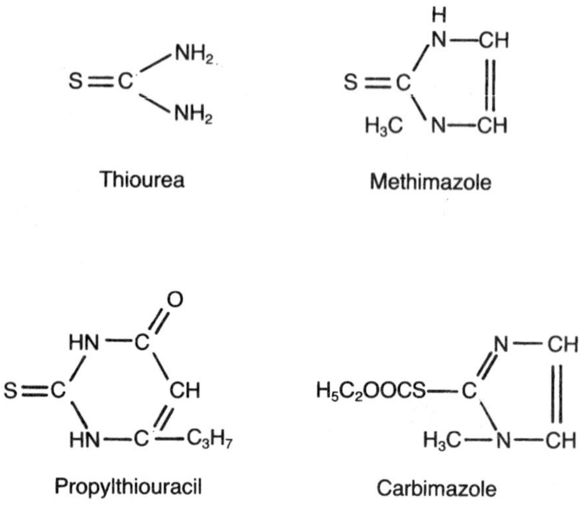

Thiourea

Methimazole

Propylthiouracil

Carbimazole

FIGURE 31.3 The structures of thioamides.

There are two main ways in which these drugs are used. Either as a long course – typically 18 months – with a large initial dose for 1–2 months followed by a reduced maintenance dose or as a shorter course – typically 9 months – with a large dose throughout plus added thyroxine after 1–2 months (so called 'block-replace regimen'). The range of dosage for carbimazole/methimazole is 5–60 mg daily and for propylthiouracil 50–450 mg daily. The enzyme block caused by thioamides is reversible and in 50% of patients with Graves' disease the autoimmune disorder will abate during therapy to a sufficient extent that the thyrotoxicosis does not recur when the drugs are stopped. It is thought that thioamides exert a locally immunosuppressive effect in the thyroid. With autonomous thyrotoxicosis – toxic adenoma and toxic multinodular goitre – recurrence of thyrotoxicosis is to be expected with withdrawal of thioamides so that prolonged drug treatment is not the usual treatment of choice.

Propylthiouracil has a separate effect not shared by the other thioamides; it blocks the extrathyroidal conversion of thyroxine to triiodothyronine. It is therefore the drug producing the most rapid resolution of severe thyrotoxicosis. In order to make use of the extrathyroidal effect 6-hourly dosage is required.

The thioamides cross the placenta and can affect the fetal thyroid; thyroid stimulating immunoglobulin also crosses the placenta and can cause fetal and neonatal thyrotoxicosis. Graves' disease in the fetus can therefore be treated to a certain extent by giving the mother antithyroid drugs.

Thioamides are secreted in breast milk, but breast feeding is not precluded provided that the dose of thioamide is low and neonatal development monitored.

Adverse effects

The most obvious adverse effect is overtreatment. This causes hypothyroidism with thyroid enlargement as a consequence of elevated TSH. During late pregnancy high doses can cause fetal goitre and hypothyroidism.

The most serious adverse effect is agranulocytosis; the incidence is $<1\%$ and when it does occur it usually occurs early in the course of treatment. Agranulocytosis usually resolves provided that the thioamide is discontinued promptly; otherwise the problem can be fatal. Skin rashes can occur and in a proportion of patients a switch to a different thioamide may be possible with clearing of the rash. All patients should be made aware of these two adverse effects before initiating treatment. Other adverse effects do occur but are very rare.

IODIDE

Iodide in pharmacological doses (50–100 mg daily compared with a physiological intake of 500 μg) has several effects on the thyroid. First, it inhibits the peroxidase responsible for the oxidation of iodide and its incorporation into iodotyrosines: this is the 'Wolff–Chaikoff' effect.

Second, iodide directly inhibits the hydrolysis of thyroglobulin and release of thyroid hormones into the circulation. High doses of glucocorticoid also inhibit the release of thyroid hormones. This is the only step where therapeutic intervention can produce a near immediate response and intravenous administration of sodium iodide is effective in thyroid crisis.

Finally, iodide reduces the hypervascularity of the thyroid seen in Graves' disease and it has been much used prior to thyroid surgery usually in conjunction with thioamides. The usual preparation is Lugol's iodine which is a solution of elemental iodine (5%) in aqueous potassium iodide (10%) taken orally; the timing of administration is for 10–15 days before surgery by which time the effect has reached its maximum.

RADIOACTIVE IODINE

Tracer doses of radioactive iodine can be used to assess the extent to which the thyroid takes up iodide and also, using a γ-camera, to provide an anatomical representation of uptake – a thyroid scan. The radionuclides available include ^{123}I, ^{125}I, ^{131}I and the anion pertechnetate (99mTc).

^{131}Iodide is used for therapy. Concentration of iodide in the thyroid allows a high local dose of β-emission to cause radiation damage limited to the thyrocytes. The usual dose is in the range 5–15 mCi (185–555 MBq) given orally. In order to ensure maximum uptake of the radioactive iodine into the thyroid thioamides should be discontinued 5–7 days before treatment and not resumed until 5 days after treatment. It takes some weeks or months for thyroid activity to fall and in the long term the majority of patients with Graves' disease treated with radioactive iodine will become hypothyroid; hence the need for post-treatment surveillance.

Adverse effects

Patients should be on reliable contraception or known not to be pregnant. Radioactive iodine can seriously damage a fetus and treatment must never be given during pregnancy. Otherwise radioactive iodine is remarkably free from adverse effects. Its use is not associated with any risk of malignancy. Very rarely, uptake of radioactive iodine by salivary glands can cause sialadenitis. The risk of developing hypothyroidism is so high that it is not so much an adverse outcome as an expected one.

PROPRANOLOL

During the initial phase of treatment of thyrotoxicosis a β-adrenergic antagonist can be used to provide relief from symptoms such as tachycardia, palpitation and tremor. A low dose of a non-selective β-blocker such as propranolol is usually used, typically 20 mg three times daily. A potential advantage of the use of such an agent is propranolol's ability to inhibit to some degree the 5′-monodeiodinase involved in the conversion of thyroxine to triiodothyronine. Treatment of thyrotoxicosis with propranolol alone prior to surgery may achieve sufficient 'control' to allow a partial thyroidectomy to be undertaken with safety. A further use of propranolol is in thyroid crisis; in this situation it should be given intravenously at a rate of 1 mg/min up to a dose of 5 mg.

Adverse effects

In the context of thyrotoxicosis the principal adverse effect is the precipitation of heart failure. Thyrotoxicosis increases the cardiac work load; the basal metabolic rate is increased, the demand for oxygen delivery to tissues is increased, cardiac output is increased and the pulse rate is increased. Particularly if there is underlying cardiac disease, for example, ischaemic heart disease in the elderly, a non-selective β-antagonist can precipitate heart failure.

PERCHLORATE

A group of anions competitively inhibit the uptake of iodide by the thyroid – they are ionic inhibitors. Thiocyanate, perchlorate and pertechnetate belong to this group. Potassium perchlorate is used therapeutically; the dose required to achieve inhibition of iodide uptake is in the range 100–800 mg per day. This drug is seldom used for the treatment of thyrotoxicosis as it has a relatively high incidence of side-effects including aplastic anaemia. As it is a competitive inhibitor of iodide uptake it should never be used in conjunction with pharmacological doses of iodide.

Perchlorate is also used to test for enzyme defects limiting organification of iodide, a rare inherited cause of hypothyroidism. The test, called the 'perchlorate discharge test' involves the administration of perchlorate a short time after the administration of a tracer dose of radioactive iodine. Iodide that has been trapped but not organified is displaced from the thyroid by perchlorate; organified iodine is not displaced.

THYROTROPHIN-RELEASING HORMONE

TRH has been used as a test for assessing the ability of the pituitary to secrete TSH. Circulating concentrations of thyrotrophin are measured at intervals over 1 h following the intravenous administration of 200 μg of TRH. In thyrotoxicosis, thyrotrophin secretion is suppressed and in pituitary or hypothalamic disease it may well be compromised. With the introduction of highly sensitive assays for thyrotrophin the suppression of basal thyrotrophin concentrations in thyrotoxicosis can be easily demonstrated rendering the 'TRH test' largely obsolete.

HYPOTHYROIDISM

Hypothyroidism occurs as an autoimmune disorder where cell-mediated autoimmunity causes destruction of the thyroid; rarely a humoral antibody blocks the TSH receptor. Hypothyroidism is also a common sequel to treatment of thyrotoxicosis, either surgically or with radioactive iodine, and is also commonly seen in Hashimoto's thyroiditis. Destructive lesions of the hypothalamus or anterior pituitary can cause hypothyroidism too, often in association with deficiency of other pituitary hormones. Congenital hypothyroidism, for which all babies in the UK are screened shortly after birth, has an incidence of approximately 1:5000. Congenital enzyme defects causing hypothyroidism, and goitre, may well present somewhat later in life. Hypothyroidism of whatever aetiology requires treatment with thyroxine.

THYROXINE

The treatment of hypothyroidism with thyroxine is from all points of view an ideal 'replacement' treatment. It is the principal product of thyroid secretion. Thyroxine is rapidly absorbed after oral administration. The presence of binding proteins in the circulation provides a large reservoir of hormone so that once-daily treatment provides a steady concentration of free thyroxine. The enzymes responsible for 5- and 5′-monodeiodination of thyroxine function normally to provide the 'right' amount of triiodothyronine. Fine tuning of the replacement dose of thyroxine is not needed as long as enough thyroxine is taken to keep the free thyroxine in the high normal range and the TSH concentration in the normal range or below. For an adult the usual maintenance replacement dose is from 0.1 to 0.15 mg of thyroxine daily.

In the elderly, the reduced metabolic rate in hypothyroidism may protect the patient from symptoms of underlying ischaemic heart disease. Indeed ischaemic heart disease may have been worsened by the hypercholesterolaemia associated with hypothyroidism. The symptoms of ischaemic heart disease may become manifest as the metabolic derangement of hypothyroidism is corrected by thyroxine. Treatment should be initiated with a small dose of thyroxine – 25 μg daily – and then increased rather slowly to a full maintenance dose.

There seems little reason to consider using triiodothyronine for thyroid replacement. As the protein-bound pool of triiodothyronine is quite small it must be taken three times per day to give a stable concentration in the circulation. As triiodothyronine is biologically active, rather than a prohormone, overtreatment can easily occur and fine tuning of the dose, which is difficult to achieve, is needed.

Adverse effects

For thyroxine there are no adverse effects with doses up to 0.2 mg or so; overtreatment – exemplified by an elevated free triiodothyronine concentration – virtually never occurs. With triiodothyronine, overtreatment is not uncommon and clinical signs and symptoms of thyrotoxicosis can occur; rarely patients become 'thyroid addicts', a problem seen in the past with thyroid extract that contains both thyroxine and triiodothyronine, but never seen with thyroxine.

FURTHER READING

Becker DV. Choice of therapy for Graves' hyperthyroidism. *New England Journal of Medicine* 1984; **311**: 464–6.

Braverman LE, Utiger RD eds. *The thyroid: a fundamental and clinical text*, 6th edn. Philadelphia: JB Lippincott, 1991.

Burman KD, Baker JR. Immune mechanisms in Graves' disease. *Endocrine Reviews* 1985; **6**: 183–232.

Cooper DS. Which antithyroid drug? *American Journal of Medicine* 1986; **80**: 1165–8.

Oppenheimer JH, Schwarz HL, Mariash CN, Kinlaw WB, Wong NC, Freake HL. Advances in our understanding of thyroid hormone action at the cellular level. *Endocrine Reviews* 1987; **8**: 288–308.

Ross DS. Subclinical hypothyroidism: possible danger of overzealous thyroxine replacement therapy. *Mayo Clinic Proceedings* 1988; **63**: 1223–9.

Utiger RD. Treatment of Graves' ophthalmology. *New England Journal of Medicine* 1989; **316**: 44–5.

Wilson JD, Foster DW eds. *Williams textbook of endocrinology*, 8th edn. Philadelphia: WB Saunders, 1992.

32

The Reproductive Systems

GCL Lachelin

INTRODUCTION

There has been an enormous increase in the understanding of the pathophysiology of the reproductive systems and, in particular, of the hypothalamic pituitary gonadal axes, in the last 30 years. This has been due to the development of the ability to measure very small quantities of circulating hormones by radioimmunoassay and newer techniques, to the elucidation of the structure of many of the hormones involved and to the synthesis of many hormones and drugs which modify the activity of the hypothalamic pituitary gonadal axes.

HYPOTHALAMIC HORMONES

Luteinizing hormone releasing hormone

The hypothalamic hormone most involved in the control of reproductive function is luteinizing hormone releasing hormone (LHRH) otherwise known as gonadotrophin-releasing hormone (GnRH).

LHRH is a decapeptide which was isolated and synthesized in the USA in the early 1970s. Its structure is shown in Fig. 32.1. It is secreted down the axons of neurones whose cell bodies are in the arcuate nucleus of the hypothalamus. It is released from their axon terminals, which lie in the median eminence, into the portal circulation, in a pulsatile manner. It binds to specific receptors on the gonadotrophs in the anterior pituitary and stimulates production and release of both luteinizing hormone (LH) and follicle-stimulating hormone (FSH). It induces its own receptors when delivered in pulsatile fashion, but continuous occupation of the receptors results in decreased production and release of gonadotrophins, a phenomenon that has been termed down-regulation or desensitization.

The half-life of LHRH is only a few minutes. Several analogues have been produced that have a longer half-life and much greater receptor-binding affinity than natural LHRH. The continuous administration of LHRH or of an LHRH agonist analogue causes an initial stimulation of gonadotrophin secretion and then a reduction of gonadotrophin secretion, because of down-regulation.

Clinical uses of LHRH

Synthetic LHRH can be administered subcutaneously (or less commonly intravenously) in pulsatile fashion, every 90 min, using a small portable pump, to induce ovulation in some anovulatory women. It can also be

pyro—Glu—His—Trp—Ser—Tyr—Gly—Leu—Arg—Pro—Gly—NH_2

FIGURE 32.1 Structure of LHRH.

used, less commonly, to induce testicular function in boys and men with deficient LHRH production (as in Kallmann's syndrome).

LHRH analogues are used to suppress ovarian function in various clinical situations such as endometriosis, fibroids, the polycystic ovary syndrome, menorrhagia, the premenstrual syndrome, precocious puberty and in some women prior to ovulation induction therapy with gonadotrophins. They are also used to suppress testicular function in men with prostatic carcinoma. They can be given intranasally, subcutaneously or by depot injection.

GONADOTROPHINS

The two pituitary gonadotrophins (LH and FSH) and the placental gonadotrophin (human chorionic gonadotrophin – hCG) are of great importance in reproductive physiology. Like thyroid-stimulating hormone, they are glycoproteins, which consist of α- and β-subunits. The α-subunits are very similar and biological specificity resides in the β-subunits, which share many of the same amino acids but which contain different carbohydrate residues. The molecular weight of the α-subunits is approximately 14 000. The half-lives of the gonadotrophins are related to their sialic acid content; that of hCG (10% sialic acid) is approximately 6–12 h, that of FSH (5%) 3–4 h and that of LH (2%) 20–30 min.

LH and FSH are produced by the pituitary gonadotrophs, which lie in the pars distalis of the adenohypophysis. LH and FSH synthesis and release are stimulated by the pulsatile discharge of LHRH from the hypothalamus. Alterations in the frequency and amplitude of LHRH pulses during the cycle are thought to be related to changes in oestrogen and progesterone levels. The differential control of LH and FSH appears to be related to the action of inhibin, which is a glycoprotein consisting of two dissimilar disulphide-linked subunits (α and β), produced by the gonads.

LH and FSH levels are low in childhood and begin to increase prior to the onset of puberty. In women in the reproductive age group, plasma concentrations of LH and FSH vary according to the phase of the menstrual cycle (Fig. 32.2). After the menopause and in women with untreated primary or premature ovarian failure, gonadotrophin levels are markedly increased.

FSH acts on the ovary to initiate follicular development and oestradiol production by the granulosa cells of the developing follicles. Increasing levels of oestradiol act, by a time- and dose-dependent effect, to initiate the LH surge. This causes ovulation from a then ripe dominant follicle, measuring approximately 20 mm in diameter. Following ovulation, a corpus luteum is formed; this produces increasing amounts of progesterone, as well as oestradiol. In the absence of implantation, oestradiol and progesterone levels begin to fall and menstruation ensues. The luteal phase of the cycle normally lasts for between 10 and 14 days. If implantation occurs, the corpus luteum is maintained by hCG produced by the conceptus, and oestradiol and progesterone levels increase. Their production is subsequently taken over by the developing placenta.

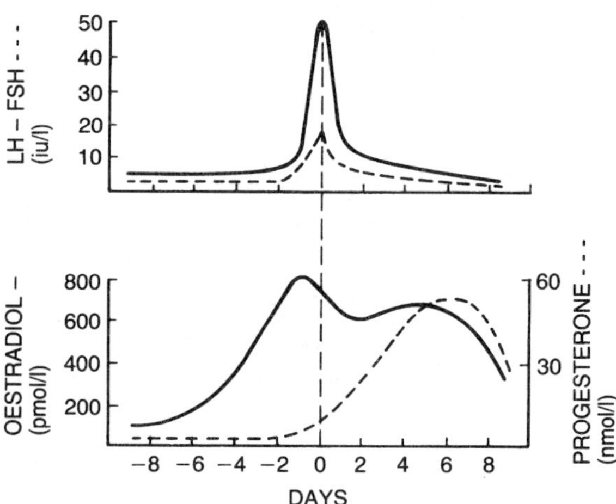

FIGURE 32.2 Diagrammatic representation of hormonal changes of the menstrual cycle, related to the LH peak.

In men, testicular function is regulated by LH and FSH. In response to stimulation by LH the Leydig cells produce testosterone which diffuses locally into the seminiferous tubules as well as entering the bloodstream. Under the influence of FSH the Sertoli cells produce inhibin, which reduces FSH secretion by the pituitary, and also androgen-binding protein, which binds testosterone. FSH also acts with testosterone to stimulate spermatogenesis. Damage to the Sertoli cells results in decreased inhibin production and raised FSH levels.

Clinical uses of gonadotrophins

FSH can be given to induce ovulation in some anovulatory women who fail to respond to clomiphene. It can also be used in women and men with pituitary failure. It is available combined with LH in a preparation derived from menopausal urine, and more recently in a preparation that contains almost no LH. It is important that these drugs are only used in centres with experience of their use, and with ultrasound and steroid radioimmunoassay monitoring facilities, in order to decrease the likelihood of multiple pregnancy and of the ovarian hyperstimulation syndrome which can be life-threatening.

Human chorionic gonadotrophin

hCG is produced by the syncytiotrophoblast following implantation, which occurs approximately 7 days after fertilization. It can be detected by radioimmunoassay before a period is missed. Levels rise rapidly in early pregnancy, with an initial doubling time of 1–4 days, and reach a peak about 8 weeks after fertilization. hCG acts to maintain steroid production by the corpus luteum, until this function is taken over by the placenta.

Clinical uses of hCG

Because of its similarity to LH, hCG can be used therapeutically to mimic the LH surge in the management of some anovulatory women and in assisted conception programmes. hCG is also sometimes used in boys with delayed puberty to stimulate testosterone production by the testes.

STEROID HORMONES

Progestogens are C_{21} steroid hormones which can be converted to androgens (C_{19} compounds) which can in turn be converted to oestrogens (C_{18} compounds). Conversion in the opposite direction does not occur.

Some important sex steroid hormone pathways are shown in Fig. 32.3.

Testosterone

Testosterone is bound in the blood to the carrier protein sex hormone binding globulin (SHBG). It is converted to the potent androgen dihydrotestosterone by the action of the enzyme 5α-reductase in target tissues.

In men, testosterone is produced by the Leydig cells of the testes. It is necessary for the development of male secondary sexual characteristics and for sexual function.

In women, testosterone is mainly produced in the ovaries and by peripheral conversion of other androgens. Total testosterone levels are increased in women with the polycystic ovary syndrome and in the presence of an androgen-secreting tumour. Free testosterone levels are increased when SHBG levels are decreased (in the polycystic ovary syndrome, obesity and hypothyroidism). Increased testosterone levels lead to the development of hirsutism and acne, and to virilism

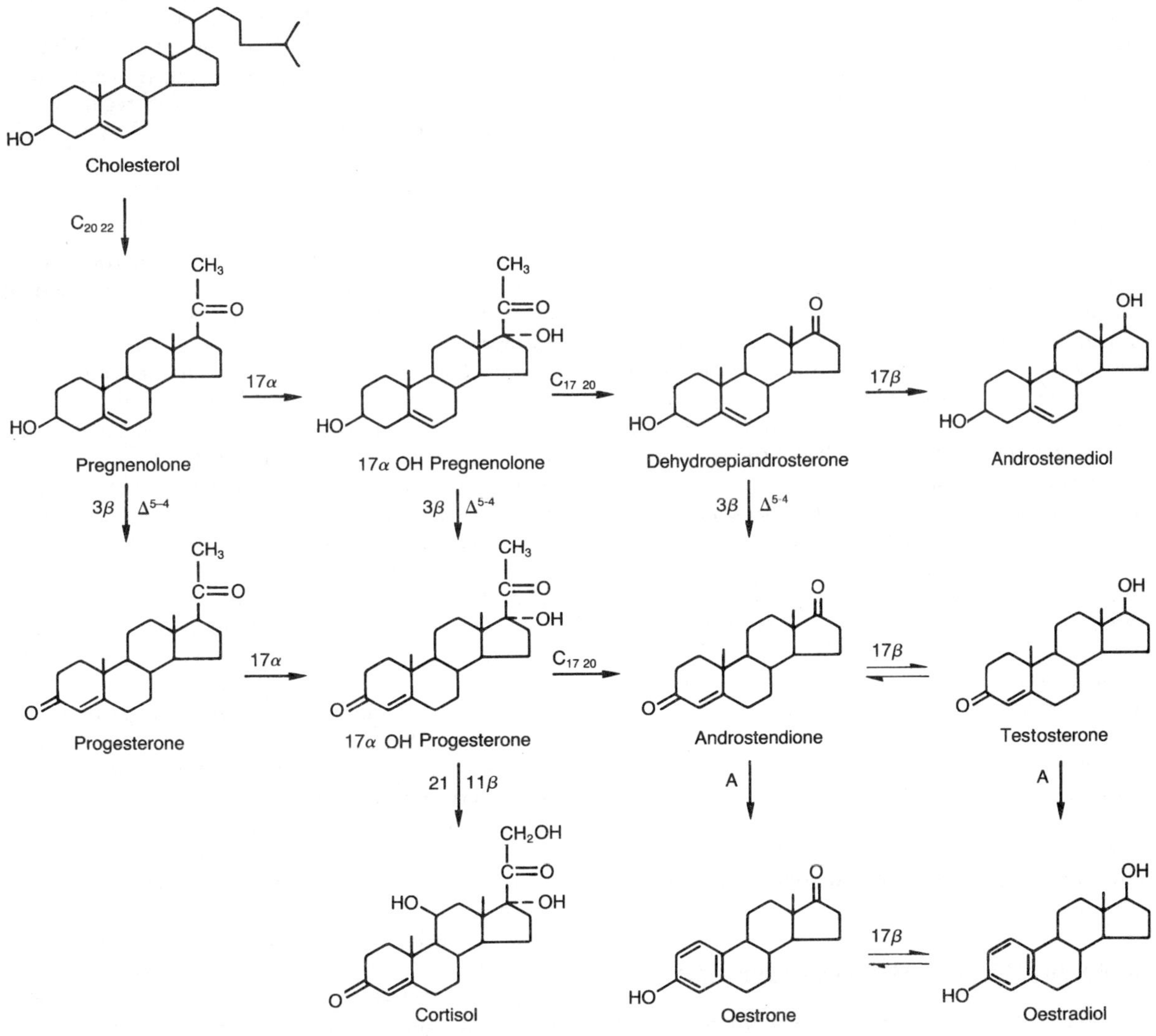

FIGURE 32.3 Steroid pathways. $C_{20.22}$, $C_{20.22}$-desmolase; $C_{17.20}$, $C_{17.20}$-desmolase; 3β, 3β-ol-dehydrogenase; 11β, 11β-hydroxylase; 21, 21-hydroxylase; 17α, 17α-hydroxylase; 17β, 17β-reductase; A, aromatase; Δ^{5-4}, Δ^{5-4} isomerase.

with clitoromegaly and deepening of the voice if the levels are markedly increased.

Clinical uses of testosterone

Testosterone administration is mainly indicated in boys with delayed puberty and men with hypogonadism. In cases of hypopituitarism, testosterone can restore normal sexual development and potency but has little effect on fertility where hCG is usually employed. Testosterone is also used as a secondary line of treatment in breast cancer.

Progesterone

Progesterone is produced in large amounts by the corpus luteum and by the placenta. In the menstrual cycle it transforms the proliferative endometrium of the follicular phase into secretory endometrium, into which a developing blastocyst can implant. It also causes an increase in the basal body temperature in the luteal phase. In pregnancy, progesterone acts to maintain uterine quiescence. It also increases the sensitivity of the respiratory centre to the partial pressure of CO_2 and thus causes hyperventilation.

Oestrogens

Oestrogens are necessary for the development of female secondary sexual characteristics.

Oestrone and oestradiol are produced by the ovary and also from androgens by peripheral conversion, which is increased in obese women. Following the menopause oestrogen levels fall and symptoms of oestrogen deficiency, such as hot flushes and vaginal dryness and discomfort, may occur; in the long term there is an increasing likelihood of osteoporosis.

Oestriol is a pregnancy hormone formed by interaction between the fetus and the placenta. The fetal adrenal gland has a fetal zone unique to pregnancy. This produces large amounts of dehydroepiandrosterone sulphate ($DHEASO_4$). Some of this is converted by the placenta into oestrone and oestradiol and some is converted to $16\alpha DHEASO_4$ in the fetal liver, before reaching the placenta; this is then desulphated, by placental sulphatase, and converted to oestriol in the placenta.

Levels of the three oestrogens and of progesterone rise markedly in pregnancy. The actions of oestrogens on the myometrium are to promote gap junction formation and the production of oxytocin receptors and prostaglandins, whereas progesterone has the opposite effects.

Clinical uses of oestrogens and progestogens

Oestrogen and progestogen combinations are widely used for postmenopausal hormone replacement therapy and for contraception.

Hormone replacement therapy

Hormone replacement therapy is indicated in the management of women with primary gonadal failure or secondary premature ovarian failure and in those with menopausal symptoms due to oestrogen deficiency. It is also given prophylactically to many perimenopausal and postmenopausal women.

Oestrogens can be given orally, by implant or using skin patches; they can also be given vaginally for a local effect but it must be appreciated that systemic absorption takes place from the vagina. First-pass metabolism in the intestine and the liver occurs with oral medication. The other routes of administration do not have this disadvantage.

In other than very short courses oestrogen should only be given in combination with a progestogen, as continuous unopposed oestrogen administration causes endometrial hyperplasia which can progress to endometrial carcinoma.

In most hormone replacement therapy regimens oestrogen is administered continuously and a progestogen is given for 10–14 days each month. Symptoms due to the progestogen are common and withdrawal bleeding occurs following progestogen withdrawal. Continuous oestrogen and progestogen regimens are being evaluated to see if these problems can be safely overcome.

Combined oral contraception

Oral contraception is most effectively provided by a combined oral contraceptive preparation containing an oestrogen and a progestogen. Combined oral contraceptive pills act by preventing follicular maturation and the LH surge; they also alter endometrial development and decrease the penetrability of cervical mucus. In general, the preparation chosen should be the one with the lowest concentration of oestrogen and progestogen which gives good cycle control and causes minimal side-effects. Most combined oral contraceptive pills today contain less than 50 μg oestrogen.

Combined oral contraceptive pills are usually taken once daily for 21 days followed by 7 pill-free days during which withdrawal bleeding occurs. Side-effects include a small but increased risk of thromboembolic and cardiovascular disorders; the risk increases with age, cigarette smoking, obesity and other predisposing conditions. Hypertension may develop on therapy; when it is due to oral contraception the blood pressure will revert to normal on cessation of treatment. Other side-effects of combined oral contraception include nausea, vomiting, headaches, breast tenderness, weight gain, depression, breakthrough bleeding and amenorrhoea.

Combined oral contraception should be discontinued (and adequate contraceptive precautions taken) 4 weeks before elective major surgery and before surgery to the legs, and it should not be recommenced until at least 2 weeks after surgery. It is not thought to be necessary to discontinue oral contraception before minor surgery with a short duration of anaesthesia, such as laparoscopic sterilization.

Progestogen-only contraception

Progestogens can be given orally on their own on a continuous daily basis (or by depot injection) for contraception when there is a contraindication to combined oestrogen and progestogen therapy, as in women who are breast feeding and those with risk factors for thromboembolism. Oral progestogen-only contraception has a higher failure rate than combined oral contraception. It is very important that the medication is taken at the same time every day or there will be further loss of efficacy. Another disadvantage is that progestogen-only medication does not result in the good cycle control that is associated with oestrogen/progestogen combinations.

Other indications for progestogen therapy

Progestogens are also used in the management of anovulatory bleeding, for which they are very effective, and of ovulatory menorrhagia for which they are less effective. A progestogen can be given in combination with an oestrogen in the form of a combined oral contraceptive pill or on its own. Norethisterone is commonly given from day 12 or 15 to 25, or from day 5 to 25 of the cycle, in a dose of 5–20 mg.

Alternative treatment for the management of menorrhagia includes danazol, given continuously in a dose of 200 mg/day. Danazol (Fig. 32.4) is more commonly used in the treatment of endometriosis, in a dose of 400–800 mg/day. Treatment must be commenced on the first day of a period and pregnancy must be prevented, as masculinization of a female fetus can occur if danazol is taken during pregnancy. Side-effects of danazol include bloating, weight gain, acne, hirsutism and hot flushes. It markedly decreases levels of SHBG and of thyroxine-binding globulin and it is important that an erroneous diagnosis of hypothyroidism is not made in a woman taking danazol. Gestrinone can also be used for the treatment of endometriosis. It is given in a dose of 2.5 mg twice a week. Side-effects are similar to those experienced with danazol and adequate contraceptive precautions must be used.

Non-hormonal treatment of menorrhagia includes the use of prostaglandin synthetase inhibitors such as mefenamic acid (500 mg tds after food) from the onset of bleeding. Ethamsylate and antifibrinolytic agents such as tranexamic acid are also used occasionally.

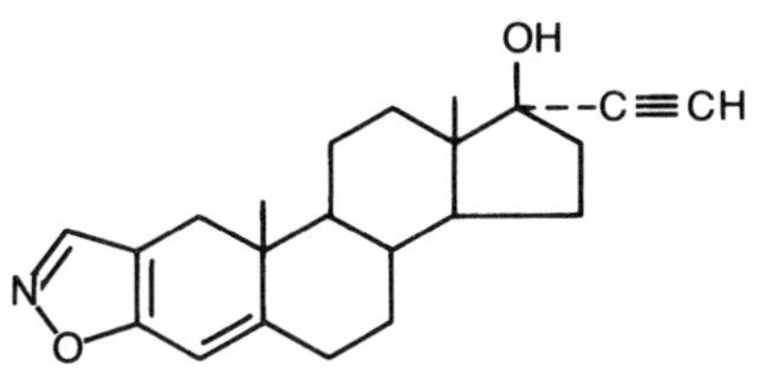

Progesterone (pessaries) and progestogens such as dydrogesterone are also used in the management of the premenstrual syndrome and of dysmenorrhoea. There is no evidence that progesterone pessaries are of value in the prevention of miscarriage.

FIGURE 32.4 Structure of danazol.

Malignant disease

Oestrogens and progestogens are also used in the management of some forms of malignant disease such as breast cancer and carcinoma of the prostate.

SEX HORMONE ANTAGONISTS

These include anti-oestrogens, anti-androgens and antiprogesterones. Antihormones are compounds which bind to specific receptors but which do not activate intracellular events in the way in which the relevant hormone would, but instead block the action of the hormone.

ANTI-OESTROGENS

The anti-oestrogens that are prescribed most frequently are clomiphene and tamoxifen. Clomiphene is mainly used for ovulation induction whereas although tamoxifen can also be used for this purpose its main indication is in the management of breast cancer.

Clomiphene citrate

Clomiphene (Fig. 32.5) is a triphenylethylene derivative, which was synthesized in 1956 and introduced for clinical trial in 1960. It is a mixture of two isomers – zuclomiphene and enclomiphene – of which the former appears to be the effective isomer for ovulation induction.

Clomiphene acts both as an oestrogen agonist and an anti-oestrogen. It has been shown to occupy oestrogen receptors for a prolonged period of time; in one study clomiphene or its metabolites were found in the circulation for 1–2 weeks or more after the last dose, in some women. It acts at hypothalamic–pituitary level, as well as on oestrogen receptors in other tissues; it causes an increase in LH and FSH levels in association with an increase in pulse frequency.

Clinical uses of clomiphene

Clomiphene has been used in clinical practice for more than 30 years, mainly to stimulate follicular development. Some of the indications for its use in the management of subfertility are shown in Table 32.1

In some anovulatory women treated with clomiphene there is stimulation of follicular development,

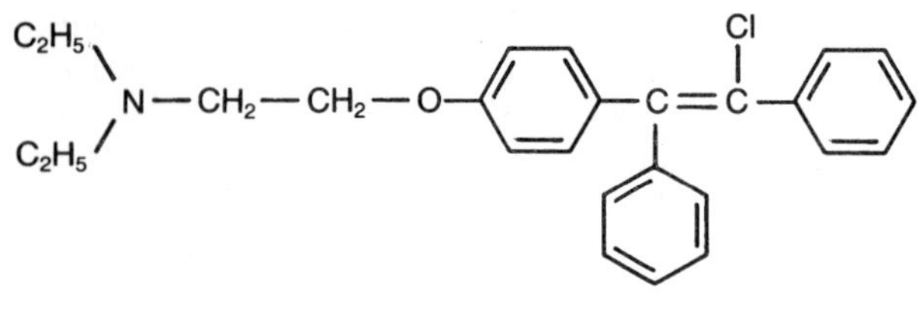

FIGURE 32.5 Structure of clomiphene.

but failure of the LH surge. In such cases ovulation can be induced, when a follicle has been shown to have reached 18–20 mm diameter on ultrasound, by the administration of 5000 or 10 000 units hCG, because of its similarity to LH.

Severe side-effects are unusual with clomiphene. The commonest side-effects are discomfort due to ovarian enlargement, hot flushes and an increased incidence of twin pregnancy. Visual symptoms, such as blurring, spots or flashes are less common, but are an indication for stopping treatment. Massive ovarian hyperstimulation is uncommon with clomiphene treatment, but it can occur unexpectedly, particularly in women with polycystic ovaries or hypothyroidism.

In a series of 2369 pregnancies, the incidence of multiple pregnancy following spontaneous conception was increased to approximately 8% in women treated with clomiphene. Fortunately, most of these were twin pregnancies, and a higher multiple pregnancy occurred in less than 1% (0.5% triplets, 0.3% quadruplets, 0.13% quintuplets) of these pregnancies.

Tamoxifen citrate

Tamoxifen is another anti-oestrogen which can be used for ovulation induction and for treatment of a luteal phase defect in the same way as clomiphene. It is mainly used, however, in the management of breast cancer, for which clomiphene is not appropriate because of its toxicity when used for a prolonged period of time.

ANTI-ANDROGENS

Cyproterone acetate (Fig. 32.6)

Cyproterone acetate has been in clinical use for about 20 years. It is both an anti-androgen and a progestogen. It acts by reducing androgen action at cellular level, by blocking androgen receptors and by decreasing 5α-reductase activity, and by reducing LH secretion.

It was originally prescribed for the treatment of hirsutism in a reverse sequential regimen devised to ensure adequate contraception and regular withdrawal bleeding; cyproterone acetate (100 mg/day) was given from day 5 to 15 of the menstrual cycle with ethinyl oestradiol 50 μg/day from day 5 to 25. The contraceptive pill Diane (cyproterone acetate 2 mg and ethinyl oestradiol 50 μg, taken from day 5 to 25 of the cycle) was subsequently introduced and has now been replaced by Dianette (cyproterone acetate 2 mg and ethinyl oestradiol 35 μg). Cyproterone acetate and ethinyl oestradiol both decrease LH output by the pituitary and therefore reduce androgen production by the ovary. Ethinyl oestradiol also increases circulating levels of SHBG and thus reduces free (biologically available) levels of testosterone. These effects combine to reduce androgen availability for action at cellular level, where cyproterone acetate acts as an anti-androgen.

Clinical uses of cyproterone acetate

A combination of cyproterone acetate and ethinyl oestradiol can be used in the management of women with hirsutism and acne, either in the form of Dianette or in a higher dose as described above.

Cyproterone acetate is also used in the treatment of severe hypersexuality and sexual deviation in boys and men and in the treatment of carcinoma of the prostate. It has also been used in the management of precocious puberty.

TABLE 32.1 Some indications for the use of clomiphene citrate in the management of subfertility

Hypothalamic (eugonadotrophic euprolactinaemic) amenorrhoea
Long cycles
Polycystic ovary syndrome
Luteal phase defect
Assisted conception programmes

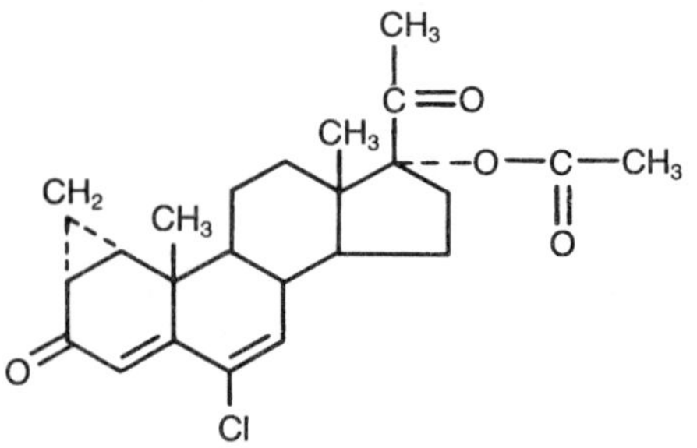

FIGURE 32.6 Structure of cyproterone acetate.

ANTIPROGESTERONE

Mifepristone

A product licence has recently been obtained for the antiprogesterone mifepristone (RU 486). Mifepristone (Fig. 32.7) is a derivative of norethisterone. It has an affinity for progesterone receptors about three times that of progesterone and for glucocorticoid receptors about twice that of dexamethasone. Fortunately, the antiglucocorticoid activity has not been found to be important in clinical practice when it is given, as at the present time, in a single dose of 600 mg.

Clinical uses of mifepristone

The main indication for mifepristone is in the medical termination of early pregnancy. When used alone, complete abortion occurs in about 85% of cases up to 6 weeks gestation but in only about 60% up to 8 weeks gestation. When mifepristone is used in combination with a prostaglandin pessary, given 48 h later, complete abortion occurs in about 95% of women up to 8 weeks gestation. It has also been found that the administration of mifepristone prior to extra-amniotic infusion, or vaginal administration, of prostaglandins for termination of second trimester pregnancies reduces the induction/abortion interval and also the total dose of prostaglandin required. Mifepristone has also been used in the management of women with an intrauterine fetal death.

DRUGS THAT ALTER UTERINE ACTIVITY

Spread of excitation through the uterus is facilitated by the presence of gap junctions between myometrial cells. There is a marked increase in the number of gap junctions in late pregnancy and there is also an increase in the number of oxytocin receptors and in prostaglandin synthesis. It is thought that these changes are enhanced by oestrogens and opposed by progesterone.

The administration of drugs that stimulate uterine contractions and those that relax the uterus (tocolytics) may be indicated in pregnancy.

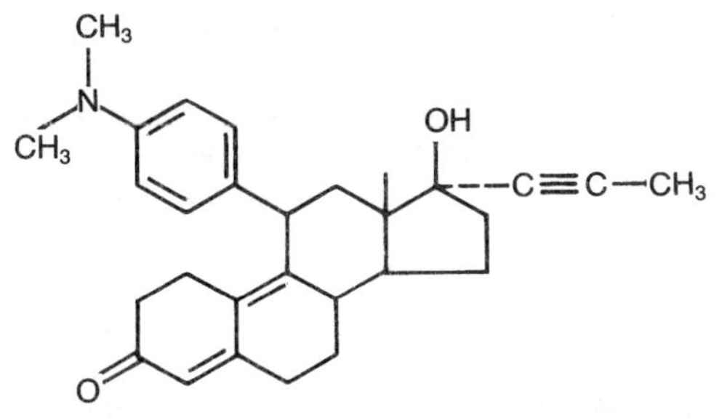

FIGURE 32.7 Structure of mifepristone.

DRUGS THAT STIMULATE UTERINE ACTIVITY

The drugs used to cause uterine contractions include prostaglandin E_2 and $F_{2\alpha}$, oxytocin and ergometrine.

Prostaglandins

The prostaglandins PGE_2 and $PGF_{2\alpha}$ are used to induce cervical ripening and to promote uterine contractions.

Clinical uses of prostaglandins

Termination of pregnancy

Prostaglandin E_2 pessaries can be given prior to surgical termination of pregnancy by dilatation and evacuation, to soften the cervix and to reduce the likelihood of cervical damage. Prostaglandins are also used to induce abortion. They can be given either as pessaries, or extra-amniotically or intra-amniotically. The intravenous route is not often used because of the high incidence of side-effects that include nausea, vomiting, diarrhoea, flushing, shivering, headache, dizziness and pyrexia. In addition a local tissue reaction may occur with intravenous administration.

Induction of labour

PGE_2 is frequently given vaginally for the induction of labour. It acts to soften the cervix and to cause uterine contractions. It can be given as tablets, pessaries or gel, which are not bioequivalent and are given in different doses. The main danger is tonic contraction of the uterus which can lead to fetal hypoxia and to uterine rupture.

Postpartum haemorrhage

Prostaglandins (Carboprost) have also been used for the control of postpartum haemorrhage which does not respond to ergometrine and oxytocin but the best preparation, dose and route of administration have not yet been established.

Prostaglandin synthetase inhibitors

Indomethacin has been given in an attempt to prevent preterm labour but there is concern about its use because it can cause constriction of the ductus arteriosus and other fetal effects, including reduced urine output which leads to oligohydramnios.

Other prostaglandin synthetase inhibitors, such as mefenamic acid, are used in the treatment of primary dysmenorrhoea and menorrhagia. It is thought that menorrhagia is sometimes due to an imbalance between prostaglandins that cause vasoconstriction and those that cause vasodilatation.

Oxytocin

Oxytocin is a nonapeptide differing from vasopressin in only two of its nine amino acid residues. It is secreted down the axons of neurones whose cell bodies lie in the supraoptic and paraventricular nuclei and it is then released into the peripheral circulation. Its half-life is approximately 10 min. Oxytocin stimulates myometrial contractions and also causes milk ejection by causing contraction of the myoepithelial cells in the breast in response to suckling, by a neurogenic reflex transmitted to the hypothalamus via the spinal cord. It also has an antidiuretic action which is of clinical importance when it is given with large volumes of fluid, as water intoxication can occur. Oxytocin release is suppressed by ethanol and this is why ethanol is sometimes used as a tocolytic agent.

Clinical uses of oxytocin

Oxytocin is used to increase the frequency and force of uterine contractions. The uterus is relatively insensitive to oxytocin in early pregnancy but becomes increasingly sensitive in the last few weeks of pregnancy, in association with the increase in oxytocin receptors which is probably related to the increasing oestrogen dominance that occurs in late pregnancy.

Induction and augmentation of labour

Oxytocin is most effective in the induction of labour when the membranes have ruptured and it is mainly used for this indication following either spontaneous or artificial rupture of the membranes. It is also used for augmentation of labour when spontaneous uterine activity diminishes in an otherwise straightforward labour. It is given by carefully controlled intravenous infusion.

The main dangers of oxytocin infusion are fetal hypoxia and uterine rupture and it is essential to monitor uterine contractions and the fetal heart rate during oxytocin infusion. If the resting uterine tone is increased or the contractions become too frequent or too forceful, or there are signs of fetal distress, the infusion must be immediately discontinued. Particular care must be taken with women of high parity and those who have had a previous Caesarean section.

Care must also be taken to avoid fluid overload.

Third stage of labour

Syntometrine is a combination of syntocinon (5 units) and ergometrine (0.5 mg); it is commonly given with delivery of the anterior shoulder, with the aim of decreasing blood loss following delivery. An oxytocin infusion (10–20 units/500 ml) can be given prophylactically postpartum (e.g. following delivery of twins) or as part of the treatment of uterine atony.

Oxytocin antagonist

An oxytocin receptor antagonist has been produced and its use in the inhibition of uterine contractions in preterm labour is being evaluated.

Ergometrine

Ergometrine causes sustained contraction of the uterus and it is therefore unsuitable for use in labour.

Clinical uses of ergometrine

Ergometrine is used to cause contraction of the uterus either in relation to abortion, or postpartum to control uterine bleeding. When it is given intravenously (0.1–0.5 mg) it acts in less than a minute. Side-effects include nausea, vomiting, vasoconstriction and hypertension. Its use should be avoided in women with raised blood pressure.

TOCOLYTIC DRUGS

In spite of major advances in neonatal care, preterm birth is the most important single determinant of adverse outcome in terms of both the chances and the quality of survival.

Preterm labour is often difficult to diagnose other than in retrospect and this makes evaluation of the efficacy of tocolytic drugs extremely difficult. Contractions will cease in many women admitted in what is thought to be preterm labour, without treatment. In addition it is important in each case to weigh up the benefits and risks of prolonging the pregnancy, of treatment and of delivery. Contraindications to the use of a tocolytic include antepartum haemorrhage and rupture of the membranes. Some of the drugs that are widely used (such as salbutamol) have not been tested against no active treatment in preterm labour.

Betamimetic drugs

These include ritodrine, salbutamol and isoxsuprine. They stimulate β-receptors in the uterus and in other organs throughout the body. They are usually given by infusion in an attempt to stop preterm labour or occasionally to counteract uterine overactivity. They are sometimes given to relax the uterus prior to external cephalic version. There is no evidence that long-term oral administration of betamimetic drugs is effective in the prevention of preterm labour.

Side-effects include nausea, vomiting, flushing, sweating, tremor, tachycardia, nervousness, palpitations, hypokalaemia and hyperglycaemia. Pulmonary oedema has occurred, usually in association with overhydration and sometimes in association with the administration of corticosteroids and other drugs. The use of betamimetics is contraindicated in women with hypertension, diabetes, cardiac disease or hyperthyroidism.

PRE-ECLAMPSIA

Pre-eclampsia is one of the commonest complications of pregnancy. Its progress can be reversed by delivery, but it may be in the interests of the fetus to prolong the pregnancy for some days or weeks.

Until recently the emphasis has been on the treatment of established pre-eclampsia, rather than prophylaxis, but several trials are in progress to determine the efficacy of low-dose aspirin (75 mg od) in the prevention and treatment of pre-eclampsia and intrauterine growth retardation.

The management of established pre-eclampsia is aimed at decreasing the incidence of complications. In some cases the use of antihypertensive and anticonvulsant drugs may be indicated. Magnesium sulphate has been used in the United States for many years and has been introduced in several centres in the United Kingdom. It is given by intravenous infusion using a syringe pump; very close clinical and biochemical monitoring (including magnesium levels) is mandatory.

ANTIHYPERTENSIVE DRUGS

The aim of treatment is to keep the blood pressure below 170/110. It must be remembered, however, that control of the blood pressure may reduce placental perfusion and that even if the blood pressure is controlled, other changes that occur in pre-eclampsia such as abnormalities of coagulation and renal function may not be improved.

Oral methyldopa is the most widely used antihypertensive agent in pregnancy and it is given when it is thought desirable for the pregnancy to continue for some days. Hydralazine has been the preferred antihypertensive agent in the management of acute severe pre-eclampsia. It can be given intravenously by infusion or slow bolus injection. Side-effects include headache, tachycardia, restlessness and hyperreflexia. More recently labetalol and diazoxide have been used. Maternal labetalol administration has been found to be associated with fetal and neonatal α-adrenergic blockade resulting in severe and long-lasting bradycardia. Diazoxide may provoke a precipitous fall in maternal blood pressure, leading to a reduction in uteroplacental perfusion especially in women with severe pre-eclampsia in whom placental blood flow is already compromised. Neonatal hyperglycaemia has been reported following maternal treatment with diazoxide.

ANTICONVULSANTS

The aim of management of a woman who has an eclamptic fit is to protect the maternal airway, to control convulsions, to control the blood pressure and to expedite delivery.

Diazepam and chlormethiazole have both been widely used as anticonvulsants in the management of severe pre-eclampsia and eclampsia. Diazepam (10 mg) can be given intravenously and can be repeated if necessary. It crosses the placenta and causes loss of beat to beat variability in the fetal heart rate and may also cause neonatal respiratory depression, hypotonia, poor sucking and hypothermia. Neonatal depression may last for several days because of the long half-life of diazepam in the neonate. Chlormethiazole (0.8% solution) is given by intravenous infusion with a loading dose of 30–50 ml, at a rate of 4 ml/min, (up to 40–100 ml over 5–10 min in eclampsia) and a maintenance dose of up to 60 ml/h, titrated to keep the woman drowsy but easily rousable. Very close supervision is essential to prevent overdosage. Chlormethiazole can cause neonatal as well as maternal respiratory depression but it is excreted rapidly by the fetus. Other maternal side-effects include hypotension, related to the rate of infusion, conjunctival irritation, headaches and thrombophlebitis.

FURTHER READING

Altura BM, Altura BT. Actions of vasopressin, oxytocin and synthetic analogs on vascular smooth muscle. *Federation Proceedings* 1984; **43**: 80–6.

Chalmers I, Enkin M, Keirse M. *Effective care in pregnancy and childbirth*. Oxford: Oxford University Press, 1989.

Conn PM, Crowley WF. Gonadotrophin-releasing hormone and its analogues. *New England Journal of Medicine* 1991; **324**: 93–103.

de Swiet M ed. *Medical disorders in obstetric practice*, 2nd edn. Oxford: Blackwell Scientific, 1989.

Drife JO. New developments in contraception. *Progress in Obstetrics and Gynaecology* 1989; **7**: 245–61.

Filshie M, Guillebaud J. *Contraception: Science and practice*. London: Butterworths, 1989.

Kruse J. Oxytocin: pharmacology and clinical application. *Journal of Family Practice* 1986; **23**: 473–9.

Lachelin GCL. *Introduction to clinical reproductive endocrinology*. Oxford: Butterworth Heinemann, 1991.

Mooradian AD, Morley JE, Korenman SG. Biological actions of androgens. *Endocrine Reviews* 1987; **8**: 1–28.

Namer M. Clinical applications of antiandrogens. *Journal of Steroidal Biochemistry*. 1988; **31**: 719–29.

Segal SJ. Mifepristone (RU 486). *New England Journal of Medicine* 1990; **322**: 691–3.

33

The Endocrine Pancreas: Drugs used in Diabetes and Obesity

PV Taberner

INTRODUCTION

The endocrine function of the pancreas in controlling the blood sugar level was first demonstrated by the classical experiments of Minkowski and von Mering in 1889. They showed that the removal of the pancreas in dogs produced symptoms that closely resembled those observed in diabetic patients. That this was due to an endocrine secretion was shown by ligating the pancreatic ducts which empty into the duodenum. Following this operation, the digestive (exocrine) functions of the pancreas were impaired, but the control of blood sugar level remained intact.

Over the subsequent 40 years a number of attempts were made to treat the symptoms of diabetes by the administration of pancreatic extracts. These were largely unsuccessful since, as we now know, the extraction procedure causes release of proteases from the exocrine tissue which destroy any insulin present in the extract. In 1922, Banting and Best made two major advances which made it possible to obtain active extracts from pancreas. First, they produced a selective atrophy of the exocrine pancreatic acini by ligation of the pancreatic ducts; then the intact islets were removed, and the active principle extracted by precipitation with 90% alcohol. This extract, although fairly crude, was spectacularly successful in producing remission of the hyperglycaemia and ketosis in juvenile diabetics. The specific activity of crystalline insulin, first prepared in 1926, has gradually increased over the years to the point where pure insulin is now available.

Ironically, although the discovery of insulin has improved the prognosis for the juvenile diabetic such that their life expectancy has increased enormously, this has resulted in a growing population of surviving diabetics, and has revealed a number of hitherto unsuspected cardiovascular, renal and neuropathological complications in the long-term diabetic patient.

THE ENDOCRINE PANCREAS

The internal secretions of the pancreas originate from the islets of Langerhans. These discrete bodies, ranging from 20 to 300 μm in diameter, number about 2 million in a normal pancreas and represent about 1% of the total tissue weight.

Immunostaining has revealed four types of granulated cell in the islet. Their relative proportions and secretory products are summarized in Table 33.1.

TABLE 33.1 Cells in the islets of Langerhans

CELL TYPE	PROPORTION OF TOTAL CELL MASS	SECRETORY PRODUCTS
A(α)	0.20	Proglucagon Glucagon
B(β)	0.70	Pro-insulin Insulin C-peptide
D(δ)	0.05–0.1	Somatostatin
F (PP)	0.01–0.02	Pancreatic polypeptide (PP)

The β-cells, concentrated in the middle of the islet, contain spherical darkly staining granules in which insulin is stored as a crystalline hexamer with Zn^{2+}. The α-cells contain glucagon and are concentrated in the outer regions of the islet. The less well known cell types (D(δ) and F) contain somatostatin and pancreatic polypeptide respectively and have close physical connections with the α- and β-cells. Somatostatin acts on both α- and β-cells to regulate the release of glucagon and insulin. Several analogues of somatostatin are currently under investigation as potential drugs for the treatment of diabetes and other endocrine disorders.

Pancreatic polypeptide is released in response to feeding, but the detailed physiological function of this hormone has not yet been convincingly demonstrated and it has no clinical applications.

THE PANCREATIC HORMONES

Insulin

Insulin was the first protein ever to be completely sequenced, and the first to be chemically synthesized. Also, the insulin gene was one of the first human genes to be cloned. In recent years, recombinant DNA technology has made it possible to produce human insulin on a commercial scale so that it is now available for clinical use. Previously, it was necessary to prepare insulin from porcine or bovine pancreas and express the activity in terms of standard units, determined by bioassay. Pure insulin has an activity of 28 units/mg.

Insulin consists of two peptide chains (A and B) linked by disulphide bridges. It is synthesized as a folded single chain precursor (preproinsulin) which is then acted upon by a specific protease to remove a section of the peptide chain to leave an eighty-six amino acid peptide, pro-insulin. This single chain has a molecular weight of about 8000 Da. A specific protease excises a thirty-five amino acid peptide (C-peptide) from the chain, leaving active insulin, which consists of a twenty-one amino acid A chain and a thirty amino acid B chain linked by two disulphide bridges. It has a molecular weight of 5808 Da. There are slight species differences in the amino acid sequence of mammalian insulin, but both bovine and porcine insulin are sufficiently similar to the human hormone to be active in man, and to cross-react in radioimmunoassays for human insulin. Pro-insulin is without biological activity, but it nevertheless can induce the production of anti-insulin antibodies in patients. It used to be a significant contaminant of insulin preparations, but recent advances in purification techniques have improved the homogeneity of the product.

Insulin secretion and metabolism

Insulin secretion is the single most important factor in the control of glucose homoeostasis. The primary stimulus for secretion is the blood glucose level. Glucose acts to close an ATPase-sensitive K^+ channel in the β-cell membrane. This, in turn, leads to the opening of a voltage-sensitive Ca^{2+} channel (Fig. 33.1). The consequent influx of Ca^{2+} activates a number of intracellu-

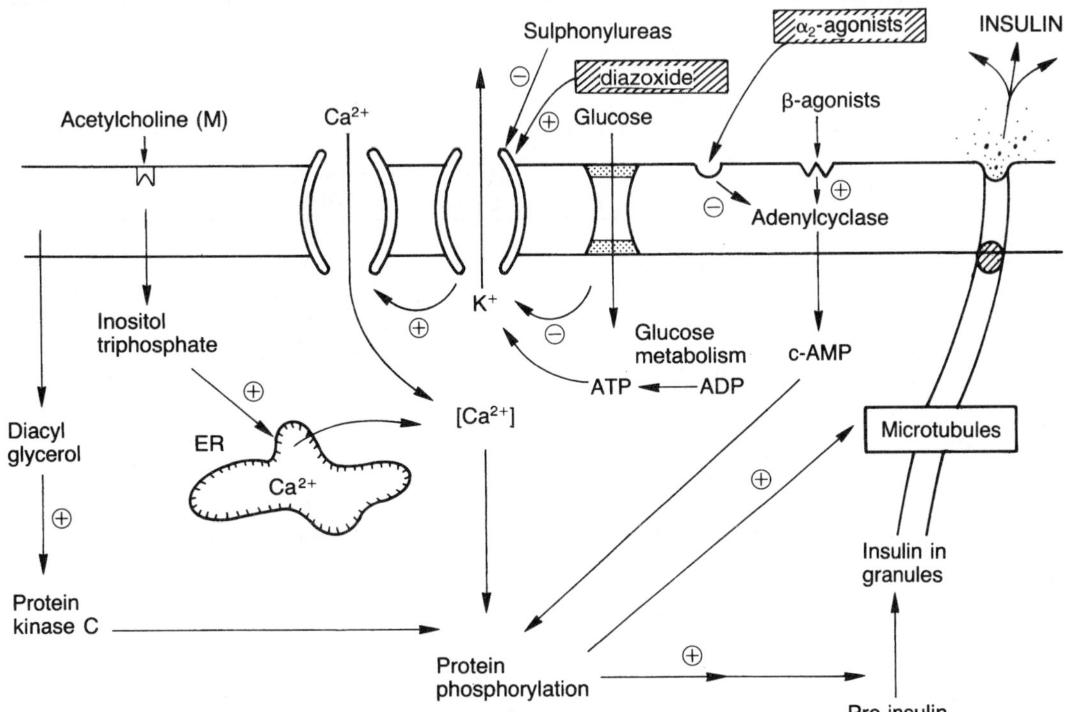

FIGURE 33.1 Control of insulin secretion.

lar proteins which result in the mobilization and release of insulin from its storage granules. Insulin secretion in response to a glucose load is biphasic: an initial brief surge is followed by a slower, more sustained, output. It has recently been recognized that the hypoglycaemic sulphonylureas stimulate insulin secretion by closing K^+ channels. Conversely, the hyperglycaemic drug diazoxide acts to open K^+ channels.

Insulin exerts its metabolic effects through insulin receptors situated on the plasma membranes, particularly of the liver, muscle and adipose tissue. These actions of insulin are summarized in Table 33.2. The overall effect is to remove glucose from the bloodstream and into the tissues. Insulin acts similarly on muscle and adipose tissue to increase glucose breakdown and glycogen synthesis. In the liver the situation is more complicated, since there is a fine balance between glucose breakdown and synthesis. In adipose tissue and liver, insulin also acts to increase fatty acid synthesis.

After binding to the receptor, the insulin molecule is endocytosed into the cell where it is destroyed by two enzymes, present in most peripheral tissues: insulin-glutathione transhydrogenase, which breaks disulphide bridges thereby separating the A and B chains; and an insulin protease which cleaves the peptide bonds in the intact molecule. The latter enzyme is thought to be the more important under physiological conditions. Although insulin has to be taken up into cells to be inactivated, the half-life of injected insulin is only about 10 min, reflecting the normally rapid turnover of the hormone.

A very large number of preparations of insulin are available, and these will be discussed below, in relation to the control of the blood sugar in diabetes.

Glucagon

Human glucagon consists of a single polypeptide chain of twenty-nine amino acids with a molecular weight of 3485 Da. It is stored in the α(A) cell granules as an oligomer, but at its normal physiological plasma concentration (10^{-10}M) it is thought to exist as the monomer, with a half-life of about 5 min. Glucagon for injection is usually in the form of a lyophilized powder of the hydrochloride salt together with lactose. It is relatively insoluble in water and is prepared for injection by adding a diluent containing glycerol (1.6%) and phenol (0.2%) as a preservative. One unit of activity is equivalent to 1.09 mg of the salt.

The principal physiological role of glucagon is to prevent hypoglycaemia during the postabsorptive phase, and to mobilize fatty acids and ketones during starvation. Its actions are generally antagonistic to those of insulin (see Table 33.2). Its release is stimulated by hypoglycaemia, noradrenaline, and a number of gastrointestinal peptide hormones. Glucagon release is inhibited by hyperglycaemia, high fatty acid levels, ketone bodies and somatostatin.

Clinical use of glucagon

Glucagon is employed in the acute treatment of hypoglycaemic coma. It can be given by subcutaneous, intramuscular, or intravenous injection at a dose of 0.5–1.0 units. It is particularly effective in counteracting insulin-induced coma following accidental overdosage. Since glucagon acts to raise the blood glucose

TABLE 33.2 The metabolic effects of insulin and glucagon

SITE OF ACTION	TISSUE	EFFECT	
		INSULIN	GLUCAGON
Carbohydrate metabolism			
Glucose active transport	Muscle, liver, adipose tissue	Increased	—
Gluconeogenesis	Liver	Reduced	Increased
Glycolysis	Liver, muscle, adipose tissue	Increased	Reduced
Glycogen synthesis	Liver, muscle	Increased	Reduced
Glycogenolysis	Liver, muscle	Reduced	Increased
Lipid metabolism			
Lipolysis (mobilization of FFAs)	Adipose tissue	Reduced	Increased
Lipogenesis	Liver, adipose tissue	Increased	Reduced
Ketogenesis	Liver	Reduced	Increased
Utilization of dietary lipid	Liver, adipose tissue	Increased	—
Protein metabolism			
Amino acid transport	Liver, muscle, adipose tissue	Increased	—
Protein synthesis	Liver, muscle, adipose tissue	Increased	Reduced
Proteolysis	Liver, muscle	Reduced	Increased

The effects of insulin on glucose and amino acid transport are rapid; the effects on carbohydrate and lipid metabolism take longer; the effects on cell growth and cell division are long term.
FFAs, free fatty acids.

level primarily through the stimulation of hepatic glycolysis, it will be ineffective in chronic hypoglycaemia, or in hypoglycaemia associated with starvation or adrenal insufficiency. Glucagon is fairly short acting (10–20 min), and intravenous infusion of glucose may also be necessary if recovery does not occur within 5 min of the injection. The principal side-effects of glucagon are nausea and vomiting.

Somatostatin

Somatostatin is synthesized from a large precursor (prosomatostatin) and stored in the δ-cells of the islets. It consists of a cyclic peptide of fourteen amino acids. It is released in response to the same signals as insulin and acts to regulate both the endocrine and exocrine functions of the pancreas. At the islet level it inhibits the release of both insulin and glucagon, and therefore appears to be part of a local feedback control loop.

Somatostatin is also found in other tissues including the CNS, where it inhibits release of growth hormone and thyrotrophin from the anterior pituitary. The half-life of somatostatin following intravenous injection is only 2–3 min, due to its rapid inactivation by plasma peptidases.

Clinical use of somatostatin

Infusion of somatostatin in normal subjects produces a fall of up to 50% in the blood glucose level by the inhibition of glucagon release. In diabetic subjects it has been found to prevent the ketoacidosis following withdrawal from insulin. Although somatostatin itself is of limited practical use due to its lack of specificity and short half-life, a number of stable analogues (e.g. the octapeptide octreotide) are now being introduced in an attempt to find an α-cell selective peptide that could control glucagon release α cell carcinoma (glucagonoma). Other potential applications include the control of gastric bleeding, and the inhibition of hormone release from a variety of endocrine tumours.

C-peptide

C-peptide, the side product of insulin synthesis, is co-released on an equimolar basis with insulin. It has no biological activity, but is present in the plasma at about five times the concentration of insulin. This is because it has a longer half-life than insulin, being largely cleared through the kidney. The assay of circulating levels of C-peptide rather than insulin is a useful diagnostic test for the origin of hypoglycaemia in diabetics, since its plasma concentration provides an index of the rate of release of endogenous insulin and is not influenced by the administration of exogenous insulin. It is therefore possible to distinguish between improved insulin output and insulin overdosage.

DIABETES

Diabetes mellitus is the most important disorder involving the endocrine pancreas. It is currently thought to affect between 1 and 2% of the population of North America and Europe. Diabetes almost certainly represents a number of different diseases, their common feature being an inability to control the blood glucose level in response to the fluctuating demands of dietary intake and energy expenditure.

Spontaneous juvenile onset (type I) diabetes is characterized by a rapid onset, usually before the age of 30 years, destruction of β-cells, lack of insulin, circulating antibodies to β-cells, a tendency to ketoacidosis, and loss of weight. These patients are entirely reliant on injections of insulin for survival; consequently, it is also referred to as insulin-dependent diabetes mellitus (IDDM). The precipitating factor is an autoimmune mechanism in which autoantibodies to β-cells appear. The autoantigen has recently been identified as the γ-aminobutyric acid (GABA)-synthesizing enzyme, glutamate decarboxylase, which is present in β-cells. IDDM can also occur in response to a viral infection in subjects who have a genetic defect on chromosome six which predisposes them to β-cell destruction. During normal pregnancy there is an increased production of hormonal antagonists to insulin, and this can result in a temporary gestational diabetes in patients with a genetic susceptibility to β-cell insufficiency.

Non-insulin-dependent diabetes (type II, NIDDM), in contrast, occurs later in life (maturity onset) and is characterized by a gradual onset, mild to severe obesity, the presence of normal or elevated levels of circulating insulin, and no β-cell antibodies. These patients, about 75–80% of all diabetics, rarely experience ketoacidosis and may remain undiagnosed for years. Their treatment consists of dietary control, supplemented by oral hypoglycaemic drugs where appropriate.

A minority of cases of diabetes result from pancreatic disease, such as alcoholic pancreatitis, pancreatic tumours of the α- or δ-cells, or secondary to drug treatment or chemical toxicity. The use of growth hormone in acromegaly often produces diabetes, and corticosteroids and thiazide diuretics also have a diabetogenic action. The pancreatic toxins, alloxan and streptozotocin, which are used experimentally to produce insulin-dependent diabetes, selectively destroy the β-cells following systemic administration. It has been suggested that some similarly acting toxins present in the environment may be responsible for some of the instances of IDDM.

The rarer forms of diabetes, pituitary (cranial) diabetes insipidus and nephrogenic diabetes insipidus, are due to defects in antidiuretic hormone (ADH, vasopressin) production and function respectively. In these situations treatment requires the use of analogues of vasopressin such as lypressin or desmopressin (see p. 561).

Control of blood glucose in diabetes

The inability of all diabetics to respond adequately to the demands of a large glucose load means that dietary control is a primary objective of the treatment regime. The type I diabetic will respond to insulin, although the insulin requirement may fluctuate. The avoidance of insulin hypoglycaemia is also an important objective. In the obese, type II diabetic dietary control will have the added advantage of reducing body weight. The insulin resistance of these diabetics can be attributed to a reduction in the number of insulin receptors on the target organs (down-regulation), which occurs in response to the high circulating levels of insulin released in response to the hyperglycaemia. The oral hypoglycaemic drugs currently in use require functioning β-cells in order to be effective, consequently, their use is limited to the treatment of type II NIDDM.

To summarize, the blood glucose in type I IDDM is normally controlled by diet and regular insulin injections; in type II NIDDM the blood glucose is controlled by diet, oral hypoglycaemics, and occasionally acute insulin to manage hyperglycaemic crises. Alternative treatments for NIDDM associated with obesity include the reduction of carbohydrate absorption, the suppression of appetite by centrally acting drugs, or the inhibition of fatty acid oxidation (see below).

Preparations of insulin

A confusingly large number of insulin preparations are commercially available; they differ in their source of origin, their purity and concentration, and their rate of onset and duration of action. Although the administration of insulin may be seen as a hormone replacement therapy, the regular injection of insulin cannot possibly replace the constantly fluctuating insulin output of the normal pancreas in response to periods of feeding or fasting. Insulin infusion systems that respond to signals from implanted glucose sensors are currently being developed to overcome this problem but, at present, the insulin requirement of each patient has to be individually assessed. Once a dosing regime has been established, the insulin requirement may still vary as a consequence of dietary changes, exercise, pregnancy, infection, drug treatment or surgery. The widely varying needs of individual patients are reflected in the large range of insulins available.

In terms of their pharmacokinetics, three principal preparations of insulin are used:

- Short-acting soluble crystalline zinc insulin, which has a rapid onset of action. This is the only form which can be given by intravenous injection or infusion. It is mainly used for the acute treatment of ketoacidosis.
- Intermediate-acting, in which amorphous insulin is in a turbid suspension with zinc in acetate buffer at a neutral pH (semilente, lente, ultralente), or with protamine (isophane insulin).
- Long-acting, in which insulin is combined with protamine and zinc in a phosphate buffer (protamine zinc insulin) which has a slow onset and a very long duration.

In addition, a number of biphasic (mixed) insulins are available containing differing proportions of soluble and isophane insulins. The traditional practice of mixing soluble insulin with protamine zinc insulin in a single syringe has been discontinued.

The properties of the most widely used preparations are summarized in Table 33.3. The variations in onset and duration are achieved by combining different proportions of crystalline pork zinc insulin (which dissolves quickly), and crystalline beef zinc insulin (which dissolves more slowly). A combination of semilente and ultralente insulins will produce a fast onset and a long duration. Increasing the dose of insulin also tends to increase the duration of action. The current view is that a basal insulin level is best maintained by a once or twice daily injection of a long-acting preparation. This can then be supplemented, when appropriate, with a short-acting soluble insulin to mimic the postabsorptive burst of insulin output that would occur in a normal subject in response to a meal.

Species of insulin

Pork insulin differs from human insulin by only one amino acid (residue 30 on the B chain, where alanine replaces threonine). In beef insulin, alanine replaces threonine at A_8 and B_{30}, and valine replaces isoleucine at A_{10}. Beef insulin is more antigenic than pork insulin in humans, but the relatively lower solubility of the crystals renders it more suitable for the longer-acting preparations. The most widely used preparations in the USA consist of 70% beef and 30% pork insulin. Human insulin, not unexpectedly, is the least antigenic of the three. It is prepared either semisynthetically from pork insulin (the alanine at B_{30} is replaced by threonine), or by recombinant DNA technology. The appropriate mRNAs for the A and B chains are expressed in *E. coli* cells from which they can be extracted and linked using sulphydryl reagents to yield purified human insulin. Human pro-insulin has also been produced by the same means. It has less biological activity *in vivo*, but has the advantage of a plasma half-life of about 1 h. The presence of pro-insulin as a contaminant in the early preparations was a contributory factor to the induction of antibodies in patients. Improved purification procedures have yielded monocomponent insulins that are less antigenic.

TABLE 33.3 Preparations of insulin

	ROUTE OF ADMINISTRATION	ONSET (min)	PEAK ACTION (h)	DURATION OF ACTION (h)
Rapid acting				
Soluble (neutral) insulin	sc	30–60	2–4	6–8
(human, porcine, bovine)	im			
(e.g. Actrapid)	iv	2–5	—	0.5
(Given as required in diabetic emergencies (e.g. ketoacidosis) and preoperatively)				

		PEAK ACTION (h)	DURATION OF ACTION (h)	FREQUENCY OF DOSING
Intermediate (Onset: 1–2 h)				
Amorphous insulin zinc suspension (semi-lente)	sc	5–10	12–16	Twice daily
Isophane insulin suspension (lente) human, porcine, bovine	sc	7–15	12–24	Twice daily
Biphasic insulin (mixtures of neutral and crystalline or isophane human or porcine insulins)	sc	3–8	16–24	Once daily
Long acting (Onset 1–2 h)				
Crystalline insulin zinc suspension (ultra lente)	sc	10–24	30–36	Once daily
Protamine zinc insulin suspension	sc	12–24	24–36	Once daily
Biphasic insulin (mixtures of amorphous and crystalline bovine or porcine insulin)	sc	6–18	18–30	Once daily

The above preparations are only a representative list, but in the UK most preparations of insulin are now genetically engineered (ge). The preparations may come in vials, as cartridges or preloaded pens. In the UK from April 1995 some insulins have been discontinued to avoid confusion.

Protamine insulin is rarely used. Rapid-acting insulin is available as Human Actrapid, while intermediate insulin is given in the form of Human Isophane insulin or Human Monotard (human insulin zinc suspension). Long-acting insulin may be given as Human Ultratard (insulin zinc suspension). Human Mixtard 30 ge contains a mixture of human insulin (30%) and biphasic isophane insulin (70%).

The lower antigenicity of human insulin might be expected to provide a clear clinical advantage. However, a number of independent reports have indicated that a proportion of patients experience unexpected hypoglycaemic crises after switching from porcine to human insulin. The problem appears to be due to a diminution in the patient's awareness of impending hypoglycaemia. Either the warning signs change in character or become less severe. There is no functional reason why glycaemic control should be impaired when using human insulin, but it is a potential risk which should be explained to patients when any change in insulin species is made.

Routes of administration

With the exception of soluble insulin, which can be given iv, most insulins are administered subcutaneously either by injection or by means of an infusion pump. An intranasal formulation of insulin has recently been developed which would avoid some of the problems associated with insulin injections (see below).

Adverse reactions to insulin

Apart from the immediate risk of hypoglycaemia (seen most frequently when patients are transferred from porcine to human monocomponent insulin), the commonest problem is that of lipodystrophy; the proliferation or, occasionally, loss of subcutaneous fat at the site of injection. This is a local allergic reaction (see Chapter 38) which can be a cosmetic problem in female patients. More severe allergic responses occur indirectly in response to the protamine moiety or to the presence of other proteins, possibly pro-insulin, in the preparations. The use of highly purified monocomponent insulin has reduced this problem.

ORAL HYPOGLYCAEMIC AGENTS

The earliest drugs used as oral hypoglycaemics were guanidine and ethanol (at one time the British Medical Association actually endorsed a 'Diabetes' whisky for diabetics!). Guanidine proved too toxic for clinical use, but it ultimately led to the development of the biguanides, notably metformin and phenformin, which were introduced in 1957. These drugs have now been withdrawn in the USA. The hypoglycaemic properties of sulphonylurea compounds were first observed in 1942, in typhoid patients being treated with sulphonamide antibiotics, but it was not until tolbutamide was introduced in 1955 that a sufficiently safe drug became available for the chronic treatment of diabetes. Apart from the unacceptable toxicity associated with many sulphonamide sulphonylureas during long-term use, it was also important to have a drug devoid of antibiotic activity in order to avoid the spread of bacterial drug resistance. The structures of some widely used sulphonylureas are shown in Fig. 33.2.

Sulphonylureas

The so-called first-generation sulphonylureas (tolbutamide, aceto-hexamide, chlorpropamide, tolazolide) have a relatively lower potency than the more recently introduced drugs (glibenclamide, glipizide, gliclazide), although their mechanism of action is the same. They all act to stimulate insulin release from β-cells by closing ATPase sensitive K^+ channels in the cell membrane. For this reason they are ineffective in type I (insulin-dependent) diabetes, and in experimental diabetes produced by destruction of the β-cells. There is some evidence that they can potentiate the peripheral actions of insulin at the receptor level by increasing the number of insulin receptors (up-regulation), and it has also been suggested that glucagon secretion becomes suppressed during long-term treatment with sulphonylureas. In some patients a degree of tolerance may develop, such that the drugs eventually cease to be effective and additional insulin becomes necessary to control the blood glucose level. The basis of this reaction has not yet been established. A summary of the pharmacological properties of the sulphonylureas is given in Table 33.4.

Chlorpropamide has the longest duration of action, since a large proportion of the drug is excreted unchanged. In contrast, *tolbutamide* is rapidly metabolized by the liver, but because the principal metabolite also has hypoglycaemic activity the duration of action is longer than might be expected. Tolbutamide is also highly plasma protein bound and can be displaced by other drugs possessing a high affinity for the binding sites. *Dicoumarol* for example not only displaces tolbutamide, thereby increasing its free plasma concentration, but also prolongs the half-life of the drug. Other vitamin K antagonists appear to be less interactive. However, care should be taken when hypoglycaemic and anticoagulant therapy is combined with regular monitoring of the blood glucose level. *Tolazamide* and *acetohexamide* have similar half-lives but, as with tolbutamide, there are active metabolites which prolong their action. Acetohexamide is rapidly converted to an active metabolite 75% of which is

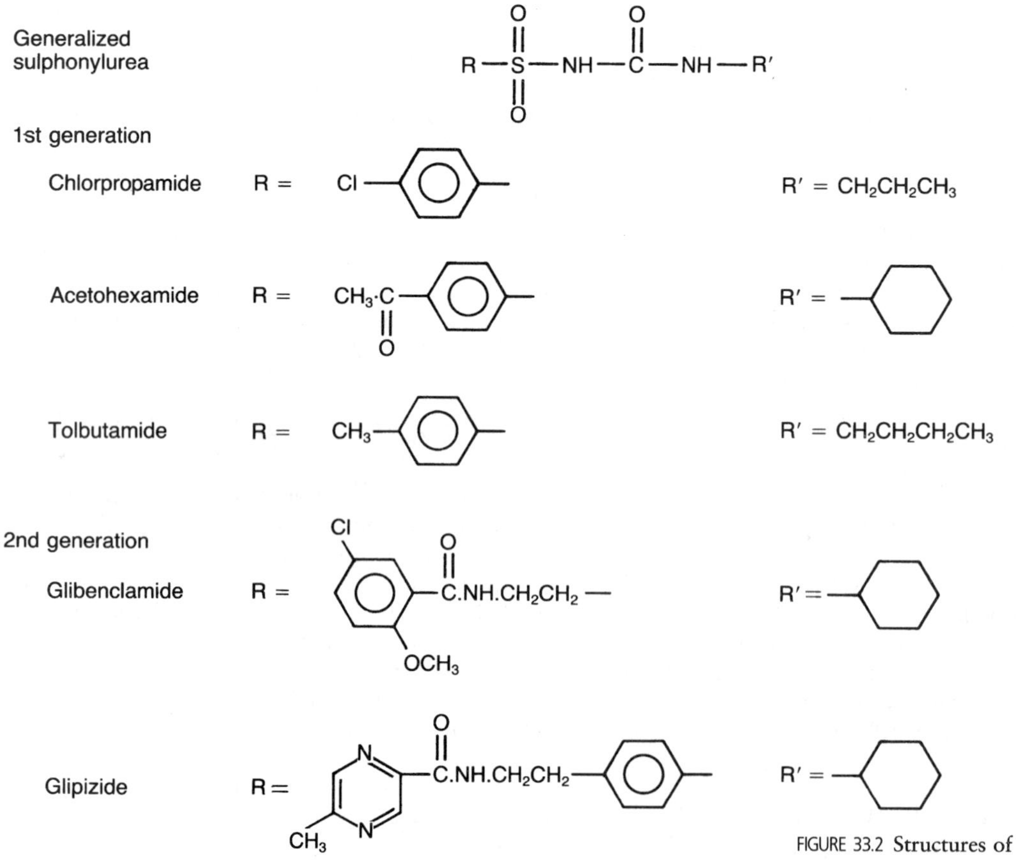

Generalized sulphonylurea: R—S(=O)(=O)—NH—C(=O)—NH—R′

1st generation

Chlorpropamide R = Cl–C_6H_4– R′ = $CH_2CH_2CH_3$

Acetohexamide R = CH_3·C(=O)–C_6H_4– R′ = cyclohexyl

Tolbutamide R = CH_3–C_6H_4– R′ = $CH_2CH_2CH_2CH_3$

2nd generation

Glibenclamide R = (Cl, OCH_3)C_6H_3–C(=O).NH.CH_2CH_2– R′ = cyclohexyl

Glipizide R = (CH_3-pyrazinyl)–C(=O).NH.CH_2CH_2–C_6H_4– R′ = cyclohexyl

FIGURE 33.2 Structures of sulphonylureas.

TABLE 33.4 Pharmacokinetic properties of the sulphonylureas

SULPHONYLUREA	DAILY DOSE	RATE OF ONSET	DURATION (h)	$t_{\frac{1}{2}}$ (h)	PROPORTION METABOLIZED (%)
Tolbutamide (ORINASE, USP)	0.5–2 g (divided)	Rapid	6–12	6	100
Tolazamide (TOLINASE, USP)	0.1–1.5 g	Slow	10–14	7	100
Acetohexamide (DYMELOR, USP)	0.25–1.5 g	Moderate	12–14	2 (48 for active metabolite)	100 25
Chlorpropamide (DIABINESE, USP)	0.1–0.5 g	Moderate	48–60	24–40	70
Glibenclamide (Glyburide, US)	2.5–10 mg	Rapid	10–24	6–12	25
Glipizide (GLUCOTROL, USP)	15–40 mg	Rapid	10–24	2–6	90

excreted unchanged, so that it is contraindicated in patients with renal impairment. Tolazamide is more slowly absorbed than the other first-generation sulphonylureas and there can be a delay of several hours before any hypoglycaemic effect is seen.

The 100-fold greater potency of the newer sulphonylureas led initially to a tendency for overdosage, resulting in cases of prolonged hypoglycaemia. However, it is now recognized that at the correct dosage they produce fewer adverse reactions than the earlier drugs. *Glibenclamide* (glyburide) is metabolized to inactive products in the liver, but its effects are relatively long-lasting. *Glipizide*, in contrast, has a short half-life due to 90% inactivation by liver enzymes, the remaining 10% being excreted unchanged. For these reasons its effects will be potentiated and prolonged in patients with hepatic or renal impairment. *Gliquidone* and *gliclazide* are short-acting and usually given in divided doses. Since they are almost completely inactivated by the liver, they can be used in patients with impaired renal function.

Biguanides

The biguanides phenformin, metformin and buformin share the same basic chemical structure (see Fig. 33.3). They act by a different mechanism from the sulphonylureas which does not involve stimulation of insulin release. They appear to lower the blood glucose concentration by suppressing hepatic gluconeogenesis and increasing glucose uptake in peripheral tissues. These actions require the presence of insulin, but are not dependent upon insulin sensitivity. The fasting blood glucose level is unaffected by the biguanides (particularly in normal non-diabetic subjects), but the postprandial rise in blood glucose is attenuated. In other words, glucose tolerance is improved. One metabolic consequence of the increase in glucose utilization is that blood lactate levels increase. This can be a problem, particularly in cases of renal insufficiency and, in the case of phenformin, the high incidence of lactic acidosis was responsible for its withdrawal from the

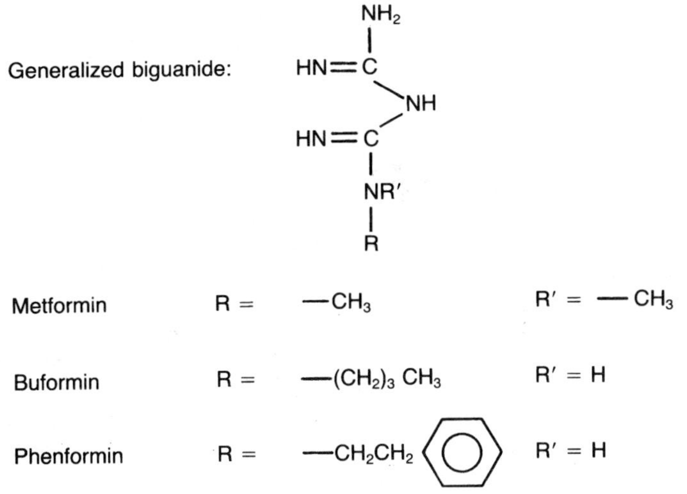

Generalized biguanide:

$$\begin{array}{l} \quad\;\; NH_2 \\ \quad\;\;\; | \\ HN{=}C \\ \qquad\;\; \diagdown NH \\ \qquad\;\; \diagup \\ HN{=}C \\ \quad\;\;\; | \\ \quad\;\; NR' \\ \quad\;\;\; | \\ \quad\;\;\; R \end{array}$$

Metformin	R = $-CH_3$	R′ = $-CH_3$
Buformin	R = $-(CH_2)_3CH_3$	R′ = H
Phenformin	R = $-CH_2CH_2C_6H_5$ (phenyl ring)	R′ = H

FIGURE 33.3 Structures of biguanides.

market. Metformin and buformin are still in clinical use outside the USA, principally in overweight patients with NIDDM whose symptoms have proved refractory to sulphonylureas, and in the absence of contraindications.

Metformin is the least toxic of the biguanides with the lowest incidence of lactic acidosis. It is not metabolized to any significant extent and is excreted unchanged; the plasma half-life is 3–4 h. In a few cases it has been found to reduce vitamin B_{12} absorption.

Adverse reactions to oral hypoglycaemics

In addition to the obvious risk of hypoglycaemia resulting from overdosage or pharmacokinetic interactions, a number of side-effects are associated with the chronic use of these drugs. *Chlorpropamide* stimulates vasopressin secretion and therefore has an antidiuretic action which can lead to water and sodium retention. In contrast, acetohexamide, glibenclamide, and tolazamide have diuretic properties.

In subjects with a genetic predisposition to alcohol intolerance, chlorpropamide in particular can produce a disulfiram-like reaction. Although many sulphonylureas are highly plasma-protein bound, and can be displaced by other drugs competing for the binding sites, this interaction is transient and has little clinical significance. More important are the effects of diuretics, which will tend to reduce the effectiveness of the poorly metabolized hypoglycaemics, and competitors for oxidative metabolism in the liver (e.g. ethanol, dicoumarol, phenylbutazone and sulphonamides) which will tend to potentiate the highly metabolized sulphonylureas (see Table 33.4). Ethanol has hypoglycaemic properties in its own right which can be potentiated by oral hypoglycaemics. Acute reactive hypoglycaemia is a significant risk in the diabetic who drinks alcohol to excess.

The hypertensive diabetic also presents a more complicated problem, particularly if renal function is impaired due to nephropathy. The angiotensin-converting enzyme (ACE) inhibitors such as captopril have been shown to be effective in helping to preserve renal function in this situation.

Immunosuppression in diabetes

The presence of circulating antibodies to pancreatic β-cells in a proportion of patients with clinical diabetes has led to a number of clinical trials with immunosuppressive agents. Their limited success is probably due to the inability of the residual intact β-cells to maintain euglycaemia. Nevertheless, studies with *cyclosporin* in newly diagnosed type I diabetics have proved promising, and the use of *azathioprine* and *prednisone* in combination has also proved encouraging in that remission of the diabetes persists beyond the course of treatment.

DRUG TREATMENT OF DIABETIC COMPLICATIONS

Anorectic drugs

Obesity is a frequent problem in type II diabetes mellitus, and the control of body weight by dieting tends to improve glucose tolerance. If a reduction in weight cannot be achieved by this means then appetite suppressant (anorectic) drugs can be used. In the past, many of these drugs, such as the amphetamine derivatives diethylpropion and phentermine, lost favour because of the undesirable stimulant effects resulting from their general sympathomimetic activity. There is also a potential for abuse in drugs of this type. The benefit of these drugs in obese diabetics is unproven.

More recently, non-stimulant anorectic agents have been developed which act more selectively than the amphetamines. *Fenfluramine* specifically stimulates the release of 5-hydroxytryptamine (5-HT) from nerve terminals in the ventromedial hypothalamus which have an input into the satiety centre. The end result is a decrease in appetite. *Fluoxetine* and *sertraline*, originally developed as antidepressants, have recently been shown to suppress appetite and promote weight loss. These drugs act by inhibiting the neuronal re-uptake system responsible for terminating the transmitter action of 5-HT (see Chapter 20). Early clinical trials have indicated that fluoxetine can improve the control of the blood glucose level, as evidenced by a decrease in glycosylated haemoglobin levels in diabetic patients.

Thermogenic drugs

It has long been recognized that the administration of adrenergic agonists, indirectly acting sympathomimetics, or thyroxine can increase the basal metabolic rate (BMR) and cause weight loss. The increase in metabolic rate is due, in part, to the stimulation of uncoupled oxidative phosphorylation (thermogenesis) in brown adipose tissue. Under normal circumstances the catabolic activity of brown adipose tissue is insulin sensitive and under the control of the sympathetic nervous system through β-adrenergic and, to a lesser extent, α-adrenergic receptors. Recent evidence suggests that in obesity there is an inability of brown adipose tissue to respond to circulating glucose and lipids. Lipolysis is reduced, and excess calories in the diet are used to increase body mass.

Drugs such as *amphetamine*, *fenfluramine*, and *mazindol* all stimulate thermogenesis indirectly through their central actions. The use of peripherally acting β-adrenergic agonists to stimulate thermogenesis has been limited by their widespread effects on the cardiovascular and respiratory systems. However, the β-receptor on brown adipose tissue has recently been found to be a discrete protein structure, distinguishable from the β_1- and β_2-receptors found on other tissues. A number of selective agonists for this receptor (β_3) have been developed and are at the clinical trial stage in obese diabetic patients. Two of them (BRL 26380A and ZD 2079) appear to be effective at doses that have no CNS stimulant or cardiovascular effects. The ability of drugs of this type to reduce obesity in humans suggests that brown adipose tissue may play a more important role in regulating energy balance than had previously been thought. This has important implications for the future drug treatment of obese diabetics.

Aldose reductase inhibitors

Many of the complications associated with diabetes, such as cataract formation, microvascular changes (retinopathy and nephropathy) and the neuropathies, are thought to be due to the accumulation of sorbitol and galactilol, produced from glucose and galactose by the action of the enzyme aldose reductase. The tissues most at risk – the peripheral nerves, the lens and retina, the kidney and the blood vessels – are tissues in which glucose transport does not depend upon insulin, so the intracellular concentration of glucose closely reflects the high extracellular levels. Aldose reductase catalyses the NADPH-dependent reduction of glucose to sorbitol and, under normal circumstances, this is subsequently oxidized to fructose. High levels of both sorbitol and fructose have been found in tissue biopsies from type II diabetics.

The earliest aldose reductase inhibitor (alrestatin) proved disappointing in clinical trials, but the later compounds (sorbinil, statil, and tolrestat) have been shown to improve nerve conduction in asymptotic patients. Long-term diabetic complications will require long-term treatment studies in order to evaluate fully the effectiveness of these drugs.

Inhibitors of carbohydrate absorption

The systemic absorption of glucose from carbohydrates present in the diet is dependent upon the action of α-glucosidase enzymes in the gastrointestinal tract. Several drugs have been developed that competitively inhibit these enzymes and therefore reduce or delay the entry of glucose into the bloodstream.The first of these inhibitors, acarbose, was found to be of benefit in controlling the postprandial rise in the blood glucose level of diabetics who could not be controlled by diet alone. Since these drugs are acting within the intestinal endothelium, systemic absorption is not necessary. The systemic availability of acarbose for example is only 0.5–1.7%, although subsequent absorption of metabolites does occur. The main side-effect of acarbose is flatulence. It is contraindicated in patients with inflammatory bowel disease or colonic ulceration.

The various therapeutic strategies that have been employed in the treatment of the insulin resistance particularly associated with type II diabetes are summarized in Table 33.5. It should be pointed out that, although all the treatments listed have undergone clinical trials, insulin-like growth factors, inhibitors

TABLE 33.5 Therapeutic approaches to insulin resistance

THERAPY	EXAMPLES	MECHANISM OF ACTION
Diet and exercise		Improve energy balance
α-glucosidase inhibitors	Acarbose Miglitol	Delay carbohydrate absorption from gut lumen
5-HT uptake blockers	D-fenfluramine Fluoxetine	Appetite suppression: evoke satiety via ventromedial hypothalamus
Sulphonylureas	Glipizide Tolbutamide Gliclazide etc.	Stimulate insulin release from β-cells of islets (K^+ channel block)
Biguanides	Metformin*	Potentiate peripheral actions of insulin, especially glucose uptake
Insulin-like growth factors	IGF-1*	Receptor mechanism similar to insulin itself
Inhibitors of fatty acid oxidation	Etomoxir*	Inhibits carnitine-palmitoyl transferase; reduces substrate availability for hepatic glucose synthesis
ACE inhibitors	Captopril	Increase insulin sensitivity (?)
Atypical β_3-adrenoceptor agonists	BRL 35135 ZD 2079	Stimulation of brown adipose tissue thermogenesis

*Indicates drugs that have been used in severe insulin resistance.
5-HT, 5 hydroxytryptamine; ACE, angiotensin-converting enzyme; IGF, insulin-like growth factor.

of fatty oxidation, and the atypical β_3-adrenoceptor agonists are still in the experimental stage of development.

Hyperglycaemic drugs

Apart from glucagon, which has already been mentioned, the only drug currently in use as a hyperglycaemic agent is diazoxide, although a number of other unrelated drugs, notably the corticosteroids, have hyperglycaemic side-effects. *Diazoxide* suppresses insulin secretion by opening ATP-ase sensitive K^+ channels on β-cells. It is of no value in the acute hypoglycaemia resulting from insulin overdose and is normally used for treating the chronic hypoglycaemia associated with overproduction of insulin. The principal side-effects are anorexia, hypotension, cardiac arrhythmias and hyperuricaemia.

FURTHER READING

Alford FP, Best JD. The aetiology of type 2 diabetes. In: Nattrass M ed. *Recent advances in diabetes*, 2. Edinburgh: Churchill Livingstone, 1986: 1–22.

Arner P. Adrenergic receptor function in fat cells. *American Journal of Clinical Nutrition* 1992; **55**: 228S–236S.

Balfour JA, McTavish D. Acarbose. An update of its pharmacology and therapeutic use in diabetes mellitus. *Drugs* 1993; **46**: 1025–54.

Binder C, Lauritzen T, Faber O, Pramming S. Insulin pharmacokinetics. *Diabetes Care* 1984; 7: 188.

Bougneres PF, Carel JC, Castano L, Boitard C, Gardin JP, Landais, P, Hors J, Mihatsch MJ, Paillard M, Chaussain JL, Bach JF. Factors associated with early remission of Type I diabetes in children treated wth cyclosporin. *New England Journal of Medicine* 1988; **318**: 663–70.

Carpenter MA, Bodansky HJ. Drug treatment of obesity in type 2 diabetes mellitus. *Diabetic Medicine* 1990; **7**: 99–104.

Espinal J. *Understanding insulin action: principles and molecular mechanisms*. Chichester: Ellis Horwood, 1989.

Everett J, Kerr D. Changing from porcine to human insulin. *Drugs* 1994; **47**: 286–96.

Greene DA, Lattimer SA, Sima AAF. Sorbitol, phosphoinositides, and sodium-potassium-ATPase in the pathogenesis of diabetic complications. *New England Journal of Medicine* 1987; **316**: 599–606.

Huupponen R. Significance of insulin receptors in the action of sulphonylurea drugs. *Annals of Clinical Research* 1988; **20**: 373–9.

Jackson JE, Bressler R. Clinical pharmacology of sulphonylurea hypoglycaemic agents. *Drugs* 1981; **22**: 211–45.

Lonnqvist F, Krief S, Strosberg AD, Nyberg B, Emorine LJ, Arner P. Evidence for a functional β_3-adrenoceptor in man. *British Journal of Pharmacology* 1993; **110**: 929–36.

MacPherson JN, Feely J. Diabetes I: Insulins. *British Medical Journal* 1983; **286**: 1502–4.

Palmer KJ, Brogden RN. Gliclazide. An update of its pharmacological properties and therapeutic efficacy in non-insulin dependent diabetes mellitus. *Drugs* 1993; **46**: 92–125.

Ruffolo RR, Nichols AJ, Stadel JM, Hieble JP. Pharmacologic and therapeutic applications of α_2-adrenoceptor subtypes. *Annual Review of Pharmacology and Toxicology* 1993; **32**: 243–79.

Seltzer HS. Efficacy and safety of oral hypoglycaemic agents. *Annual Review of Medicine* 1980; **31**: 261–72.

SECTION TEN

Chemotherapeutic Drugs

34

Use of Drugs against Micro-organisms

GMS Scott

INTRODUCTION

Antimicrobial agents interfere with specific chemical pathways that do not form a part of the host's metabolism. In this way they inhibit the growth of microbes without inhibiting that of host cells. Most antimicrobials inhibit the growth of genera restricted by structure or metabolism. Although the cell walls of different species of bacteria are individually different, they retain sufficient specific similarities to allow an acceptable breadth of action. Agents active against the bacterial cell wall do not inhibit the growth of mammalian cells, viruses or fungi. This phenomenon is known as selective toxicity. The toxic properties of antimicrobial agents to the host are therefore not usually due to the specific inhibitory properties for which the agents are used, but rather to some other unwanted pharmacological property or to allergy.

Because viruses employ host cell metabolic processes for replication, the likelihood that an antiviral agent will actually inhibit host cell protein or nucleic synthesis is much greater than for antibacterial agents, which act on metabolic pathways not present in eukaryotic cells. This applies even to interferon, a protein secreted by nucleated cells in higher animals in response to viral infection, which renders other cells resistant to virus infection.

The interferon response is rapid and innate, in that it does not require prior exposure to the virus, yet is responsible for switching off host cell protein synthesis and causing considerable toxicity (e.g. the febrile symptoms and leucopenia associated with influenza). The short-lived interferon response with negative feedback is critical to limiting the spread of infection and the short-term toxicity is acceptable for the species to ensure survival. Compared with many other antivirals that suppress the bone marrow, the lack of toxicity of acyclovir reflects the need for phosphorylation of this molecule to make it active, a process that can only happen in herpes simplex virus infected cells.

Antimicrobials were discovered by the serendipitous observation of the inhibition of growth of micro-organisms exposed to extracts of others. Two approaches have yielded new agents: first, a systematic examination of 'soups' from the culture of many different fungi and bacteria; and latterly the chemical modification of existing molecules to improve antimicrobial activity to counteract resistance mechanisms or to improve pharmacological properties. Antiviral drugs have been discovered by testing novel chemical structures in virus–cell tissue culture.

Although a chronological classification is interesting in many respects, the best classification for antimicrobials is broadly according to their sites of action (Table 34.1). We may then consider some important compounds within the families of antimicrobials and search for those properties that are of particular

TABLE 34.1 Mechanisms of antibiotic action

DNA	*Mitomycin* (C): causes abnormal cross-linkage: non-specific antitumour agent. Not used clinically
	Quinolones (e.g. ciprofloxacin): inhibit DNA topoisomerase which is responsible for splicing DNA during supercoiling and uncoiling
	Proflavine (S): binds to DNA by intercalation; interferes with DNA function; mutagenic; used topically
	Sulphonamides (S): inhibit bacterial dihydropterate synthetase and *trimethoprim* (S) inhibits dihydrofolate reductase in the synthesis of folate
mRNA Transcription	*Actinomycin D* (C): H-bonds with guanine: inhibits synthesis of mRNA by occupying binding site of DNA-dependent RNA polymerase; non-specific antitumour agent. Not used as an antimicrobial agent
	Rifamycins (e.g. rifampicin) (C): bind to DNA-dependent RNA polymerase; inhibit initiation
	Metronidazole: inhibits RNA polymerase under reducing conditions, mutagenic
Translation	*Puromycin* (S): binds to end of growing polypeptide chain causing 'abortion'. Not used clinically
	Streptomycin (C): binds to the P10 protein of free 30S ribosome preventing attachment of mRNA
	Other aminoglycosides (C): causes misreading ('ambiguity') usually to a connected codon; can inhibit all stages of protein synthesis, i.e. *initiation*, elongation, termination
	Chloramphenicol (S): binds to 50S ribosomal fraction; prevents completion of polypeptide chain by blocking transfer to AA from tRNA/AA complex, i.e. the peptidyl transferase. Stabilizes on RNA on ribosome. No binding to 30S. Also prevents binding of mRNA to free ribosome
	Erythromycin (C): binds at similar sites to chloramphenicol, inhibits translocation, i.e. the passage of the ribosome along the mRNA
	Tetracycline (S): prevents binding of tRNA/AA complex
	Mupirocin (C): inhibits isoleucyl tRNA synthetase
	Fusidic acid (C): inhibits elongation factor 'G' and protein chain synthesis
Cell membrane	*Gramicidin tyrocidin* (C): inhibit energy producing reactions, not used clinically
	Polymyxins (C): attach to anionic binding sites (PO_4) causing detergent action, immediate release of intracellular contents, *toxic* therefore only used topically
	Polyenes (e.g. nystatin, amphotericin): bind to specific sterol groups of fungal cell membrane: no effect on prokaryocytes
	Imidazoles (e.g. fluconazole), triazoles (e.g. itraconazole): bind to different sites in the fungal cell membrane causing increased permeability
Cell wall	*Cycloserine:* blocks catalysis of L-alanine to D-alanine
	Glycopeptides: (e.g. vancomycin, teicoplanin): bind to *d*Ala-*d*Ala, stearically hinder the transpeptidase that brings about elongation of the peptidoglycan. *Bacitracin*: acts at a very similar position. Only used topically
	β-Lactams: (penicillins, cephalosporins, monobactams, carbapenems, etc): block cross-linkage of pentapeptide chains between D-ala and D-lys or D-APA

S, bacteriostatic; C, bacteriocidal; AA, amino acids.

interest to the anaesthetist in operating theatre and intensive care unit (ICU). Antimicrobial resistance, drug toxicity and dose modification in systems failure are of major importance in the anaesthetist's practice.

PHARMACOLOGY OF ANTIMICROBIALS

Important considerations in the use of any antimicrobial are as follows:

- The compound must be active against the microbial agent(s) causing the disease.
- It must not be inactivated by enzymes produced by the target organisms (or by *others in the vicinity*).
- The pharmacokinetics must be such that the antimicrobial achieves a concentration in the vicinity of the infecting organism that exceeds the minimal inhibitory concentration (MIC) for sufficiently long to inhibit the growth or kill the micro-organism.
- It is important to know whether the antimicrobial is 'static' (inhibits growth) or 'cidal' (kills) to the micro-organism. Residual inhibitory activity after removal of an antibiotic, the 'postantibiotic effect', may be advantageous in prolonging the activity of an agent.
- The pharmacokinetic properties of importance are: 1 *Absorption*. Some drugs may be well absorbed but unpalatable (e.g. chloramphenicol). The absorption of antimicrobials may be significantly affected by food (e.g. rifampicin, tetracycline) or stomach pH (e.g. benzyl penicillin). Unabsorbed active antibiotics (e.g. ampicillin, tetracycline) affect gut flora resulting in diarrhoea.

2 *Protein binding*. There is controversy over the requirement for protein binding. Reversibility of this binding is important. High binding often leads to a longer half-life of a compound in the plasma but bound compound may not be bioavailable to kill micro-organisms. Protein binding may prevent diffusion but may also act as a biological pool from which active drug is leached slowly. Protein binding may be saturable so dependent on the concentration of the compound. Enormous variations in protein binding are exhibited by different penicillins and cephalosporins.
3 *Distribution*. Excretion curves after peak plasma concentrations are achieved indicate the volume of distribution, plasma half-life and excretion. These parameters may be different in healthy volunteers and sick patients. There is no guarantee that antimicrobials will home in on the site of infection – indeed the distribution is dependent on chemical properties other than antimicrobial action.
4 *Cell penetration*. Organisms such as *Salmonella*, *Listeria*, *Mycobacteria* and *Brucella* reside and even replicate intracellularly, particularly in macrophages and the success of therapy is dependent on intracellular penetration by antimicrobials.
5 *Excretion*. Knowledge of excretion patterns is necessary to prevent unnecessarily high concentrations of an agent and unwanted toxicity in disease states. Furthermore, these properties can be put to good use in treating biliary or urinary infections.

- Drug interactions between antimicrobials may lead to reduced activity. This is known as antagonism and may, for example, be seen with some protein synthesis inhibitors and cell wall active antibiotics. (Typically, penicillin and chloramphenicol are antagonistic in the treatment of *Streptococcus pneumoniae*.)
- Without an intact immune system, the antimicrobial is much less likely to cure a patient, although the infection may be kept under control until the immune system recovers.
- Toxicity, allergy and drug interactions may limit the usefulness of an antibiotic in an individual.
- Micro-organisms have an enormous capacity to adapt to the inhibitory effect of antimicrobials. Breeding multiply resistant organisms is very easy, and new drug development needs to keep one step ahead of resistance problems.

ANTIBACTERIAL AGENTS

The term 'antibiotic' used to be reserved for antibacterial agents derived from micro-organisms but this semantic differentiation from artificial or chemically modified (semi-synthetic) compounds ('antimicrobials') has fallen out of fashion.

Mechanisms of antibiotic action (Table 34.1)

Most bacteria have a specialized cell wall structure that is quite unlike that of eukaryotic cells. Although no two bacterial species have exactly the same cell wall there is enough similarity throughout the bacterial kingdom for antibiotics that act on the cell wall to have enormous breadth of activity. Those antibiotics acting on the cell wall include the β-lactams (penicillins, cephalosporins, monobactams, carbapenems), glycopeptides (vancomycin and teicoplanin) and various less important compounds such as cycloserine.

Bacteria may have an outer cell membrane. These organisms stain Gram-negative and in order for cell wall (and protein) inhibitors to act they have first to pass through this membrane. Specialized porin proteins allow the passage of materials depending on their molecular weight and charge. Organisms may produce β-lactamases which are present in sufficient quantity in the periplasmic space to inactivate antibiotics after they have crossed the outer membrane but before they reach their target site. These organisms may appear *not* to be resistant *in vitro*. Polymyxins act as a detergent and are able to disrupt the outer cell membrane. They are only active against Gram-negative organisms but are too toxic to be used systemically.

The second major targets for antibiotics are protein synthesis mechanisms which, although in principle are similar in all species, have some specialized components specific to bacterial species. A broad-spectrum protein synthesis inhibitor such as puromycin is an excellent antibiotic but also inhibits mammalian protein synthesis so is too toxic to be used clinically. Useful specific bacterial protein synthesis inhibitors include aminoglycosides, macrolides, lincosamines, tetracyclines and chloramphenicol.

The third broad group of mechanisms of action involves interference with DNA structure, function and replication. Sulphonamides and trimethoprim inhibit critical enzymes in the pathways of folic acid metabolism. Another important target is the topoisomerase responsible for super-coiling DNA (see below) inhibited by quinolones. Nitroimidazoles, such as metronidazole, cause DNA breakages, but only under reducing (anaerobic) conditions. Rifamycins, such as rifampicin, bind to the DNA-dependent RNA polymerase and inhibit the formation of mRNA.

Antibiotic resistance

Some organisms are constitutively resistant to certain antibiotics. This may be because the antibiotic cannot get to the site of action (e.g. vancomycin in Gram-negative organisms) or that the particular target enzyme system is not present in that species (e.g. mycoplasmas do not have a peptidoglycan cell wall) or that the organism produces an inactivating enzyme (e.g. *Klebsiella* spp. produce β-lactamases which inactivate penicillin and ampicillin).

Alternatively, these characteristics can be acquired. The widespread use of antibiotics exerts a profound selective pressure on the development of antibiotic resistance. The selection of resistant organisms is seen frequently on ICUs, particularly when attempts are made to treat bacteria at heavily colonized preferred sites. In this situation the organism is intermittently exposed to a fraction of the minimal inhibitory concentration of the antibiotic mimicking an effective way of selecting resistance *in vitro*. The most common problems arise with troublesome saprophytes such as *Pseudomonas aeruginosa* in the respiratory tract, in the catheterized urinary tract and in the damaged gut. These organisms are not usually virulent in the immunocompetent host.

Antibiotic resistance may be constitutive or acquired and is coded on chromosomes or separate small strands of DNA called plasmids. This plasmid or chromosomal resistant DNA codes for altered structure (such as a change in the porins in Gram-negative bacteria), for altered target site enzymes or for the production of antibiotic-inactivating enzymes. Plasmids replicate with the bacteria and are transferable between bacteria even of different species. The source of most plasmid-mediated resistance is the food chain. The pressure to develop resistance is applied in farm animals given excessive antibiotics (previously for growth promotion and now for 'mass treatment' of suspected infections). These organisms are the source of plasmids which can be transferred to troublesome organisms that cause nosocomial infections (e.g. *Pseudomonas*, *Klebsiella*, *Enterobacter*). The resistance is not stable and the plasmid may be a disadvantage to these organisms so the exhibition of antibiotics is necessary to maintain their presence. Such pressure occurs perpetually in ICU settings.

One important form of chromosomally mediated resistance is that inducible in many species of *Pseudomonas* and *Enterobacter*. The best inducers are some penicillins (e.g. benzyl penicillin, ampicillin), clavulanic acid, and some cephalosporins (e.g. cefoxitin) and carbapenems (e.g. imipenem). This β-lactamase will hydrolyse many powerful β-lactam antibiotics to which the organism may well appear sensitive *in vitro* at the start of therapy.

The incidence of novel β-lactamases increases in response to antibiotic pressure. For example, organisms bearing cefotaximase are now common in areas where cefotaxime is widely used.

Alternatively, an organism may acquire resistance which is stable and not detrimental to growth and replication. Examples would be *Staphylococcus aureus* resistant to penicillin and multiply resistant *Salmonella* spp. and *Vibrio cholerae*. The antibiotic-resistant gene may be associated with a virulence factor as in the case of invasive *Salmonella typhimurium*, which is causing a pandemic of infection across Asia and North Africa.

Virtually all *S. aureus* was exquisitely sensitive to penicillin when this antibiotic was first introduced widely in the 1940s. By the early 1950s resistance had emerged and fewer than 5% of strains now isolated are sensitive to penicillin. Tiny doses of penicillin appeared to be clinically effective in the early days but the organism became relatively more resistant and virulent through the 1950s and remains the prime cause of postsurgical sepsis.

Many organisms develop multiple mechanisms of resistance to antibiotics. A good example is *Neisseria gonorrhoeae* which may have altered permeability of the outer membrane to penicillin, have altered penicillin-binding proteins or produce β-lactamase. Each exerts an increasing degree of resistance to penicillin, manifest as gradually increasing MIC.

The development of new antibiotics is done to fill some perceived gap not filled by the clinically available compounds. New agents should have improved activity and spectrum with better pharmacokinetics and should get over existing problems of resistance. However, there has, unfortunately, been no new antibiotic that does not carry with it further 'unexpected' problems of resistance. All new antibiotics are strikingly more expensive than the existing ones and should be used only if they have significant advantages.

INHIBITORS OF CELL WALL SYNTHESIS

The bacterial cell wall peptidoglycan consists of a backbone of alternating units of N-acetyl glucosamine (NAG) and N-acetyl muramic acid (NAMA). Five amino acids are linked to the latter and cross-linking between these amino acids gives the structure rigidity. The third amino acid in the pentapeptide chain differs slightly between Gram-positive (L-ala, D-glu, L-lys) and Gram-negative organisms (L-ala, D-glu, diaminopimelic acid). The terminal amino acids are two D-alanine residues which are covalently linked by an enzyme that may be blocked by cycloserine.

The NAG-NAMA-pentapeptide is transiently attached to phospholipid which is to form part of the internal lipid membrane. This pathway is blocked by glycopeptide antibiotics. Finally, cross-linking is catalysed by transpeptidases and carboxypeptidases ('penicillin-binding proteins' (PBP)) which are the targets of the β-lactam antibiotics. These form the most useful and largest family of antibiotics available for clinical use.

These may be divided into the penicillins, cephalosporins, monobactams and carbapenems. β-Lactamase inhibitors (e.g. clavulanic acid, sulbactam) have similar structures and block inactivating enzymes without in themselves having significant antibacterial activity.

The original penicillins and cephalosporins and clavulanic acid were derived from various fungi and the molecules have been extensively modified to broaden their spectrum of activity, to reduce the susceptibility to β-lactamases and to improve pharmacokinetics.

Penicillins

The penicillins are based on the penam ring substituted at several positions. The first penicillin to be developed was benzylpenicillin (penicillin G) and it remains valuable for the treatment of many life-threatening infections (e.g. by streptococci, *Neisseria meningitidis* and *Clostridium perfringens*) where resistance has not become a major problem.

Pharmacology

Benzyl penicillin is acid labile so not bioavailable when given orally. Intramuscular administration is painful but yields excellent pharmacokinetics and activity because of slow release from the intramuscular depot. Intravenous bolus doses of benzyl penicillin give rise to rapid high peak serum concentrations that fall rapidly as the drug is excreted rapidly through the kidney, giving a serum half-life of only some 30 min. Hence the need to give large bolus doses frequently to maintain blood levels and a high concentration gradient into tissue or CSF. There used to be a vogue for giving continuous intravenous infusions of penicillin to maintain a high blood level but there is some (insubstantial) evidence that this is less efficient at killing organisms *in vivo*. Cell wall inhibitors do not work unless the cell is actively metabolizing or dividing. Combinations of protein synthesis inhibitors and cell wall inhibitors may under certain conditions be antagonistic (e.g. penicillin and chloramphenicol vs. *S. pneumoniae*). Theoretically, intermittent exposure of an organism to a cell wall inhibitor will be more effective at killing the organism than continuous exposure. Eagle and Musselman[1] described a peculiar *in vitro* phenomenon in which certain bacteria were less well inhibited by higher concentrations of antibiotics but the relevance of this to clinical practice was not clearly demonstrated. Controversy exists over the optimal dose for patients with life-threatening infections. A dose of 1.2 g (2 mega units (MU)) given 4- or 6-hourly seems effective but 0.6 g given 6-hourly may not be effective because of rapid clearance. There used to be controversy over whether it was better to give penicillin by continuous infusion but intermittent treatment is now favoured.

A dose over 14 g (24 MU) per day in an adult (and proportionally less in a child) may cause irritability and epileptic convulsions and this risk is increased when the glomerular filtration rate (GFR) falls below 3 ml/min. Although more closely related to CSF levels, fits occur with blood levels over approximately 90 mg/l. Fits may also be induced by intrathecal administration and this is no longer recommended.

A young adult with pneumococcal meningitis and encephalitis was treated with 24 MU benzyl penicillin daily. He went into oliguric renal failure and began to have generalized convulsions. The clinicians were convinced that the convulsions were due to encephalopathy caused by the infection and that to reduce the dose of penicillin would be a great risk. Blood levels of penicillin were found to be 350 mg/l and the organism had an MIC of 0.006 mg/l penicillin. Thus some 40 000-fold the MIC was present in the blood. The fits eventually ceased when the penicillin was reduced.

High doses given for a prolonged period are also more likely to sensitize a patient. Although true type I hypersensitivity is relatively rare, urticarial rashes due to penicillin are common. Non-urticarial macular–papular erythematous rashes due to ampicillin during viral infections are often mistakenly used as evidence for *not* choosing a penicillin. Skin tests may be performed to test for true allergy.

Other rare toxicity problems of benzyl penicillin include interstitial nephritis, hypokalaemia and hypernatraemia, haemolytic anaemia and leucopenia.

The excretion of penicillins is inhibited by the uricosuric agent, probenecid, which competes in the active excretion of penicillin in the renal tubule and this still has a role to play in the improvement of the serum level of oral penicillins.

Semi-synthetic penicillins: acid-stable orally active penicillins

Phenoxymethyl penicillin (penicillin V) is acid stable and better absorbed than benzyl penicillin. Nevertheless, it is not consistently or well absorbed and should be given 30 min before food. It has limited usefulness for the treatment of streptococcal tonsillitis (most effectively following a single intramuscular injection of benzyl penicillin) or prevention of pneumococcal sepsis in a splenectomized patient. Anaphylaxis may occur in a patient with type I hypersensitivity to penicillin. Other allergic rashes occasionally occur but, apart from minor gastrointestinal disturbance, side-effects are rare.

Long-acting penicillins

Procaine, benethamine and benzathine penicillins may be administered intramuscularly and because they are relatively insoluble, they have longer plasma half-lives than benzyl penicillin or phenoxymethyl penicillin. These drugs are often combined to give a continued high level of penicillin in the serum from the start of therapy over many days. They are now used perhaps only in the treatment of syphilis.

Semi-synthetic penicillins: broadening the spectrum

The widespread use of penicillin stimulated the emergence of penicillinase (β-lactamase) producing *S. aureus* and there was a perceived need to manufacture derivatives of the 6-amino penicillinic acid that were stable to staphylococcal β-lactamase. The breakthrough was the discovery of methicillin whose side-chain protects the β-lactam ring from hydrolysis.

Methicillin is resistant to staphylococcal penicillinase but not necessarily to those of other (e.g. Gram-negative) bacterial species. It is, however, less active than penicillin against organisms that do not produce penicillinase. Extensive use of analogues of the drug has selected for the emergence of methicillin-resistant *S. aureus* (MRSA), which has the unfortunate property of often being resistant to many other antibiotics. It is thought that such strains originated by the transfer of plasmid DNA coding for resistance from coagulase-negative *Staphylococcus*. Some MRSA strains are endowed with 'spreadability' and patients shedding the organism are usually placed in source isolation. MRSA strains are not more virulent than methicillin-sensitive *S. aureus*. Resistance to methicillin is mediated by complex changes in target enzymes, in particular the development of a novel penicillin-binding protein (PBP 2a). Methicillin has the (probably unfounded) reputation for being more toxic than penicillin in terms of neutropenia and nephritis, and it is not in clinical use.

Semi-synthetic penicillins resistant to penicillinase and acid

Other similar derivatives include oxacillin, cloxacillin and flucloxacillin (isoxazolyl penicillins) which are also acid resistant. Flucloxacillin is in common usage and, like cloxacillin, is 4–8-fold more active than methicillin against *S. aureus*. It is well absorbed given orally but highly protein bound (95%) and more slowly excreted than oxacillin. The amount of free active flucloxacillin is greater than a similar dose of oxacillin but the two drugs have never been formally compared in a proper clinical trial.

Flucloxacillin causes gastritis, which is dose-related, and patients are often unable to tolerate oral doses greater than 500 mg q6h. Parenteral preparations must not be mixed with any proteinaceous infusion or with an aminoglycoside. Doses need be modified only in very severe renal failure (GFR <10 ml/min), and because of protein binding, flucloxacillin is not removed by dialysis. Very large doses (e.g. 2 g q4h or q6h) are recommended for the initial treatment of septicaemic patients or those with staphylococcal endocarditis. Flucloxacillin is synergistic with aminoglycosides against staphylococci. Toxicity is similar to that of the other penicillins. Interstitial nephritis is of particular interest and may be dose related but seems to be rare.

Semi-synthetic penicillins with broader spectrum and acid resistance

Whereas penicillin and methicillin are relatively inactive, ampicillin (α-amino benzyl penicillin) and the closely related amoxycillin are 4–8-fold more active against many Gram-negative organisms. These include *Haemophilus* and most Enterobacteriaceae but exclude most *Klebsiella*, *Enterobacter*, *Serratia* spp. and all *Pseudomonas* spp. which are constitutively resistant. They sacrifice some activity against Gram-positive organisms (such as *Streptococcus pneumoniae*) and are not resistant to staphylococcal β-lactamase.

The absorption of ampicillin is poor and is reduced by food. The proportion absorbed is not dependent on the dose given. Amoxycillin is better absorbed than ampicillin, giving approximately twice peak levels in the blood after an equivalent dose and food does not interfere with absorption. Oral amoxycillin is therefore preferred to oral ampicillin. Both antibiotics have low protein binding (~20%) and are excreted rapidly through the kidney. However, significant concentrations of the antibiotics also appear in the bile. Ampicillin accumulates in amniotic fluid and penetrates the inflamed blood–brain barrier. Amoxycillin is more active than ampicillin at killing *E. coli*, both *in vitro* and *in vivo*.

Ampicillin (and probably amoxycillin) is associated with maculopapular rash in 5–10% of recipients. This side-effect is particularly seen in Epstein–Barr virus associated infectious mononucleosis and is not a contraindication to the future use of penicillin (or even ampicillin) in patients who warrant this treatment. The other common side-effects relate to the gastrointestinal tract. Amoxycillin is more likely to cause nausea and ampicillin to cause diarrhoea, a reflection of their relative rapidity and degree of absorption.

Ampicillin and amoxycillin have gradually become less valuable for the treatment of urinary infection both in hospital and at home, because about one-half of urinary isolates now have reduced sensitivity. This is mostly due to an increase in the number of isolates that produce β-lactamase. Because it is better absorbed than penicillin, amoxycillin is often prescribed for tonsillitis or pneumonia but Group A *Streptococcus* and *S. pneumoniae* are slightly less sensitive to the latter. This does not seem to matter in clinical practice but the gastrointestinal toxicity and induction of candidosis may be more common with ampicillin and amoxycillin.

Ampicillin esters

To improve the absorption of ampicillin, several esters have been manufactured. These are well absorbed and rapidly hydrolysed to active ampicillin in blood and tissue. Blood levels are 2–3-fold those achieved after the equivalent dose of ampicillin. Talampicillin, bacampicillin and pivampicillin are available.

Absorption is generally not influenced by food and there is a reduced incidence of lower gastrointestinal side-effects compared with ampicillin. However, there is little to choose between these esters and amoxycillin itself.

Penicillins active against *Pseudomonas*

Carbenicillin (α-carboxy benzyl penicillin), the first useful antipseudomonal penicillin, was superseded by the four-fold more active ticarcillin (α-carboxy-3-thienyl methyl penicillin). Both are sensitive to β-lactamases and may be inactive against certain strains of Enterobacteriaceae, particularly *Klebsiella* and *Enterobacter*. There are minor differences in protein binding (50% for carbenicillin vs. 65% for ticarcillin) and ticarcillin penetrates less well into tissues. Both are excreted in the kidney but ticarcillin is in part broken down to penicilloic acid. Very large doses are required for *Pseudomonas* infections and at these doses platelet dysfunction may occur. (This adverse effect was subsequently also found in moxolactam but ureidopenicillins (see below) do not appear to have this problem.)

Three ureidopenicillins have been developed and are in common use. Azlocillin and mezlocillin have similar activities against Enterobacteriaceae but the latter is slightly less active against *Pseudomonas*. They may be active in strains of *Pseudomonas* that are resistant to ticarcillin, yet they are not in themselves resistant to β-lactamase hydrolysis. Therefore, they have limited use in the treatment of *Pseudomonas* infections in preferred sites from which the organism is not rapidly eradicated (e.g. the respiratory tract or the catheterized urinary tract). Selection for resistance in these circumstances is very common. There is a wide discrepancy for many strains between the inhibitory (minimal inhibitory concentration, MIC) and the killing (minimal bactericidal concentration, MBC) concentrations of these antibiotics. They could be considered to have only static activity against these strains, so in severe infections it would seem wise to combine them with an aminoglycoside. Piperacillin has similar activity to azlocillin and mezlocillin and resistance is, to a certain extent, shared between these closely related antibiotics.

In treatment, these drugs need to be given in high doses (6–20 g/day), have half-lives of about 1 h increasing to 6 h in oliguric renal failure, are modestly protein bound (piperacillin and mezlocillin 16%, azlocillin 30%) and about 20% is excreted in the bile. None is stable to staphylococcal β-lactamase so they are not active against common strains of *S. aureus* or *S. epidermidis*. They retain activity against *Streptococcus* and *Enterococcus* spp. although piperacillin is the least active against the latter.

Azlocillin and piperacillin have been used extensively, usually in combination with an aminoglycoside, in the treatment of Gram-negative infections in neutropenic patients with considerable success. However, antipseudomonal cephalosporins (see ceftazidime below) are more stable to the β-lactamases which are manufactured by *Pseudomonas* and Enterobacteriaceae. Perhaps the main usefulness of ureidopenicillins is in the prophylaxis or short-term treatment of polymicrobial infections (such as in the biliary tract) which often include enterococci.

Amidinopenicillin

6-β-Amidinopenicillins (e.g. mecillinam and its absorbable prodrug ester pivmecillinam) have good activity against Enterobacteriaceae but not *Pseudomonas* and not Gram-positive organisms. Mecillinam causes ballooning of the bacterial cells and is synergistic with ampicillin. Five to ten per cent is protein bound and the half-life is about 1 h. MIC values for common Enterobacteriaceae are usually below 0.1 mg/l. It was developed as a treatment for urinary infections and, although more stable to β-lactamases than ampicillin and active against some *Klebsiella*, *Enterobacter* and *Serratia*, it is not in common use.

β-Lactamase inhibitors

Three compounds similar to penicillin that bind avidly to β-lactamases but are not bacteriologically active have been developed to extend the spectrum of ampicillin, amoxycillin or ticarcillin. Clavulanic acid (orally or parenterally) and sulbactam (parenterally) have similar pharmacokinetics to amoxycillin and ampicillin, the antibiotics with which they have been combined. They inhibit β-lactamases from *S. aureus*, *Klebsiella*, *Proteus*, *Haemophilus* and *Neisseria* spp. but not those produced by *Proteus* (indole positive), *Serratia*, *Enterobacter* or *Pseudomonas* spp. They are active against many anaerobes. However, it is difficult to measure the *in vitro* sensitivity of an organism to antibiotics combined with β-lactamase inhibitors. These agents will not overcome other forms of resistance (e.g. permeability or changes in PBP). Clavulanic acid has been combined with ticarcillin ('Timetin') to improve the spectrum to include *Pseudomonas* and β-lactamase-producing Gram-positive organisms. β-Lactam/β-lactamase inhibitors are one alternative for surgical prophylaxis and may be used in treatment of documented Gram-negative infections. Clavulanate may induce β-lactamases in *Klebsiella*, *Enterobacter* and *Pseudomonas*, so these drugs are not recommended for prolonged therapy of infections in privileged sites.

The most recent combination to be marketed is piptazobactam, a combination of piperacillin and tazobactam, a penicillinase- and cephalosporinase-inhibitor of broad spectrum with little inherent antimicrobial activity. The combination extends the usefulness of piperacillin to include β-lactamase-producing *S. aureus*, *H. influenzae* and many Enterobacteriaceae, but does not significantly improve the activity against *Pseudomonas* spp.

Cephalosporins

The cephalosporin nucleus incorporates a six- rather than a five-membered ring adjacent to the β-lactam ring. This allows one further set of substitutions to be made to improve activity or stability to β-lactamases. Earliest cephalosporins studied (cephalothin and cephaloridine) seemed very active against Enterobacteriaceae and stable to *S. aureus* β-lactamase. Unfortunately, they did not hold up to the promise of being particularly effective in penicillinase-producing *S. aureus* infections.

Further developments in the molecule have resulted in agents that are progressively more active against Gram-negative organisms, eventually including activity against *Pseudomonas*. This has been achieved to the detriment of activity against Gram-positive species. It has become traditional to discuss cephalosporins in terms of 'generation'. There have been very large numbers of cephalosporins developed but most hospitals exercise a restrictive policy in pharmacy that allows only a limited choice of antibiotics within each 'generation' and it is necessary to know only about those. Within each 'generation', the drugs are very similar.

1st generation: orally active including activity against Gram-positives

Cephalothin (in the USA) and cephaloridine (in the UK) were developed from cephalosporin C, the original prototype from a mixture of seven antibiotics derived from *Cephalosporium acremonium* mould. Cephaloridine is more active against Gram-positives than cephalothin, which is degraded to the inactive desacetyl derivative, but cephaloridine proved to cause proximal renal tubular necrosis. This is a general property of many cephalosporins but was first identified in patients treated with cephaloridine, which was therefore removed from the formulary. Delays in identifying this side-effect probably arose because of the multifactorial nature of renal failure in seriously ill patients and the tendency to give such patients excessive doses of the drugs.

Cephalothin may be given orally, intramuscularly (though it is painful) or intravenously. It is 70% protein bound and reduced by esterases in the plasma. For this reason there is no increase in plasma half-life in renal failure. Cephacetrile and cephapirin have similar structure and properties but have not been developed.

Useful 1st generation derivatives include cephalexin, cephradine, cefaclor and cefadroxil. They are well absorbed. Each is 15% protein bound, has a half-life of 1 h, prolonged in renal failure of 20 h (except for cefaclor (only 3 h, because it is partly metabolized)). The activity against *S. aureus* is retained and there is some resistance to some β-lactamases of Enterobacteriaceae and *Haemophilus influenzae*. However, they are less active than ampicillin against those strains that are sensitive. They are also significantly less active against streptococci and pneumococci than cephaloridine. None penetrates the CSF well enough for the treatment of meningitis. Cross-hypersensitivity occurs in 9% of patients who are sensitive to penicillin. In general, oral cephalosporins should not be used for serious infection but should be restricted to the treatment of urinary infections with organisms that have been shown to be sensitive. There is little to choose between the four examples given.

2nd generation: parenterally administered, β-lactamase stable

These are not absorbed when given orally. They are more stable to Gram-negative β-lactamases than 1st generation compounds so are generally more active against Enterobacteriaceae including *Klebsiella* and *Proteus*. Examples include cephamandole, cefoxitin and cefuroxime.

Cefuroxime is active against most species of Enterobacteriaceae and retains activity against penicillin-resistant *S. aureus* and *S. pneumoniae*. It is very active against *Neisseria* spp. and *Haemophilus influenzae*. It is very stable to most β-lactamases. It is 33% bound with a half-life of 1.5 h and most is excreted in the urine over 8 h. Cefoxitin is, strictly speaking, a cephamycin. It is much less active than cephaloridine against Gram-positives but is highly active against many Gram-negatives producing β-lactamases, and is not hydrolysed at all. However, it is an excellent inducer of chromosomal β-lactamase in *Klebsiella*, *Enterobacter* and *Serratia* spp. and is not active against certain *Enterobacter* spp.

Cefuroxime axetil is an orally active ester of cefuroxime. It is best absorbed after food, yet it is not consistently absorbed and should not be used for serious infections. Cefixime is a new orally active 2nd–3rd generation cephalosporin that has recently been introduced in a once-daily dosage formulation. Cefixime is well absorbed giving peak levels of 1 mg/l after 50 mg and 4 mg/l after 400 mg. It has a serum half-life of 3 h but only 19% of a dose is excreted in the urine in 24 h. Currently it is recommended for respiratory infections in general practice and may also be useful for certain resistant urinary infections. The drug has good stability against a range of β-lactamases and may offer a valuable improvement on 1st generation cephalosporins in areas where there is a significant problem with resistance. It is not particularly active against staphylococci and is generally less active than ceftizoxime, a closely related parenteral drug. It has been associated with considerable gastrointestinal symptoms and there is no good evidence yet that this treatment is significantly better than other currently available antibiotics for the empirical therapy of upper respiratory infections for which it has been recommended.

3rd generation parenteral, high activity against Enterobacteriaceae, some against *Pseudomonas*, β-lactamase stable

These agents (cefotaxime, ceftazidime, cefoperazone, ceftizoxime, ceftriaxone) are 10- to 100-fold more active than 2nd generation cephalosporins against Gram-negative organisms, have excellent stability against β-lactamases and some (ceftazidime) have the added property of consistent activity against *Pseudomonas*. Some penetrate the CSF well (cefotaxime, ceftazidime) so are useful in neonatal meningitis or as an alternative to penicillin and chloramphenicol in childhood meningitis. They are not active against *S. aureus* strains which produce β-lactamase, or against enterococci.

Cefotaxime is given iv or im, is about 40% protein bound, has a half-life of 1 h, and is metabolized to the desacetyl derivative which is less active (see also cephalothin) but this does not seem to be a disadvantage in terms of therapeutic usefulness.

Ceftazidime has the advantage of good stability against β-lactamases and activity against *Pseudomonas aeruginosa*. It is not orally active and is uncomfortable given intramuscularly. It is more convenient to administer the drug intravenously. It is 15% protein bound, is excreted entirely by glomerular filtration giving a serum half-life of about 2 h. In renal failure, the dose must be reduced and the dosage interval increased. Ceftazidime has been shown to have *in vitro* activity against Gram-positive organisms including methicillin-sensitive *S. epidermidis*, *S. aureus* and *S. pneumoniae*. Clinical experience suggests that it is not particulary active *in vivo*. Ceftazidime usage selects for the emergence of *E. faecalis* and related species as the dominant nosocomial pathogen. The antibiotic has its main value in the management of severe Gram-negative sepsis, particularly in neutropenic patients. Its general use in a unit does lead to infections with resistant psychrophiles (*Acinetobacter*, *Agrobacterium* spp., *Stenotrophomonas maltophila*, etc.) and *Enterococcus* spp.

Ceftriaxone has been used very widely in the USA for many years and has recently been licensed for a broad range of infections in the UK. It has similar activity to ceftazidime, and is similarly hydrolysed by some chromosomal cephalosporins of *Enterobacter* spp. and is not active against enterococci. An advantage lies in the pharmacokinetics: it has a longer half-life (5.5–11 h) than ceftazidime (0.9 h) possibly explained by the high degree of protein binding of the former. Ceftriaxone is recommended at a once-daily dosage (or twice-daily in serious infections). Both these antibiotics penetrate the CSF but this is very dependent on meningeal inflammation.

Monobactams

Aztreonam is an interesting compound containing only the core of the β-lactam nucleus and is strangely only active against Gram-negative organisms. It should be given intravenously for severe documented Gram-negative infections and can spare the clinical use of aminoglycosides. It does not induce β-lactamase production (as do penicillin, clavulanate, cefoxitin and imipenem) but may be hydrolysed by certain (rare) β-lactamases. It does not affect the normal gut anaerobic flora. However, though broadly active against most Enterobacteriaceae and *Pseudomonas*, it is not uniquely active and has not found a specific role. Occasionally, resistant isolates in the laboratory may be tested for sensitivity to aztreonam, but most isolates resistant to ceftazidime or imipenem (see below) are also resistant to aztreonam. The drug is 56% protein bound, has a half-life of 1.7 h, is excreted in the kidneys over 12 h and the dose must be reduced in renal failure.

The volume of injection restricts the method of administration to intravenous infusion. The drug is not compatible with metronidazole and may cause local thrombophlebitis. Perhaps the most valuable indication for aztreonam is in the patient with true hypersensitivity to penicillin, as there appears to be little cross-hypersensitivity between these two classes of drugs. Aztreonam has no effect on coagulation or platelet function. Test doses should be given if alternative drugs (e.g. aminoglycosides, quinolones) prove to be ineffective. Although many minor side-effects have been reported from extensive clinical trials they occur at low frequency, several may be unrelated to the use of the drug and the drug is considered to be safe. Nevertheless, it is not now available in the UK.

Carbapenems

Substitution of carbon for the sulphur of the penam ring yields a new family of antibiotics, the first to be developed being imipenem (thienamycin). This is hydrolysed by dehydropeptidase-1 in the proximal renal tubule so the drug must be given with a dehydropeptidase inhibitor, cilastatin, which has similar pharmacokinetics to the active compound. A new compound, meropenem, has similar activity but resists hydrolysis by dehydropeptidase-1. Imipenem has the broadest spectrum of activity against bacteria of any antibiotic licensed. The spectrum includes activity against most anaerobic organisms. It is stable to bacterial β-lactamase yet is an effective inducer of chromosomal β-lactamase in *Klebsiella*, *Enterobacter* and *Pseudomonas*. These organisms are still killed by imipenem *in vitro* but resistant *Pseudomonas* may be selected in preferred sites. Enterococci, some other streptococci, methicillin-resistant *S. aureus* and *Stenotrophomonas* (*Xanthomonas*) *maltophila* are usually resistant to imipenem. Slight reductions in dosage are made in renal failure but the drug is not recommended in oliguric renal failure unless haemodialysis is just about to begin.

The most important side-effect is a tendency to central nervous system irritability and epileptic convulsions at high dosage or in renal failure. Imipenem may share the hypersensitivity of other β-lactam antibiotics. Minor adverse effects in liver and renal function have been reported.

Imipenem has a very broad spectrum of action but it has yet to establish a unique role in the treatment of any condition. It is less active against *Enterococcus*, so it does not show a particular advantage over 3rd generation cephalosporins in this respect and may actually select for troublesome nosocomial enterococcal infections. Though active against, for example, methicillin-sensitive *S. aureus* and *S. pyogenes*, it would be an extravagant drug to use for these conditions. It is likely to be valuable for the blind treatment of febrile neutropenic episodes because of the low risk of resistance but the more widespread introduction of the drug will in itself cause novel problems of resistance. Selection of β-lactamase (type 1 cephalosporinase) production in *Klebsiella*, *Enterobacter* and *Pseudomonas* is theoretically not of immediate relevance to an individual because the organisms remain sensitive to imipenem. However, it is not difficult to select *in vivo* for *Pseudomonas* spp. that are resistant probably due to a permeability change. These organisms are usually resistant to many other antibiotics.

Toxicity of β-lactams

Nine per cent of penicillin-allergic patients will probably develop similar reactions to one or more cephalosporins. Cephaloridine and perhaps some other cephalosporins have the disadvantage of causing renal tubular necrosis at high dose levels. Those agents with a methyltetrazolethiomethyl side-chain at C3 are associated with hypoprothrombinaemia and platelet toxicity and bleeding. These include the cephalosporins, cephamandole, cefotetan, cefmenoxime and cefoperazone, and the oxacefem, moxalactam. The latter molecule has oxygen substituted for sulphur in the six-membered chain. Though each of these drugs has certain advantages, none is sufficient to warrant their inclusion in the hospital formulary. Otherwise the penicillins and cephalosporins are remarkably free of side-effects.

GLYCOPEPTIDES

This useful group of naturally derived large complex molecules bind to D-Ala-D-Ala residues of the peptidoglycan chain and prevent cross-linkages and polymerization. They are inactive against Gram-negative organisms.

Vancomycin

Vancomycin, a family of molecules derived from *Streptomyces orientalis* in 1956, has a well-founded reputation for being difficult to administer and toxic, though dangers of ototoxicity and renal toxicity have been exaggerated. Vancomycin is not absorbed from the gastrointestinal tract but is useful given orally for the treatment of pseudomembranous colitis associated with *C. difficile*. It must be given by slow intravenous infusion to reduce the risk of excessive histamine-like activity which results in the 'red man' syndrome. Because the drug is retained in renal failure and the levels are not predictable on the basis of body mass, serum levels are measured at trough (just before a dose) and peak (2 h after commencing the infusion which usually lasts for 1 h). Trough levels of 5–10 mg/l and peak levels of 25–30 mg/l are regarded as satisfactory. MIC for vancomycin against *S. pyogenes*. *S. aureus*, *E. faecalis* and *Clostridium* spp. range from 0.1 to 4 mg/l. Although the trend has been to give less frequent doses, dosing should be started at 6-hourly intervals in neutropenic patients with serious Gram-positive infections. Conventional starting doses are 500 mg q6h or 1 g q12h. Patients in renal failure may be given a single dose of 1–2 g and high serum levels will be maintained for many days. The drug cannot be removed by dialysis. Vancomycin does not penetrate into the CSF but may be given intraventricularly for Gram-positive shunt associated ventriculitis.

Immediate reactions to vancomycin are dependent on the concentration of histamine released and occur in 50–90% of healthy volunteers. True anaphylactoid reactions (e.g. hypotension without rash) may occur on first dose and repeated dosing may lead to allergic reactions that are not dependent on histamine release. Early theories that reactions were dependent on impurities in the vancomycin preparations have not been confirmed by observing fewer reactions with very pure preparations. Vancomycin has an unfounded reputation of causing deafness and renal failure. Used alone, and with appropriate drug monitoring, these side-effects are very rare. However, co-administration with aminoglycosides (e.g. as in the treatment of *S. epidermidis* endocarditis) is highly likely to result in renal failure. Side-effects are potentiated by aminoglycosides and any degree of renal failure (e.g. creatinine clearance <50 ml/min).

Teicoplanin

This new glycopeptide antibiotic derived from *Actinomyces teichomyceticus* is very similar to vancomycin in activity but has several striking advantages. First it has a longer half-life and may be administered once daily. Secondly, because it does not induce histamine release, immediate toxicity is much less common and the drug can be given by iv bolus or even by im injection, though the latter is poorly tolerated.

Protein binding is 90% and the terminal phase half-life is 20–70 h (doubling in anuric patients). However, once-daily dosing does not lead to significant accumulation. Modifications of dosage are recommended in renal failure. Tissue distribution is excellent but penetration into the CSF is not predictable. About 50% of a dose is excreted in the urine. The recommended dose of teicoplanin of 400 mg at first followed by 200 mg daily probably should be doubled for neutropenic patients with severe infections.

Ototoxicity is a rare complication of teicoplanin therapy, occurring in 1/340 patients, which is as often as might be expected in ill hospitalized patients. As with vancomycin, combination with aminoglycosides may be more likely to cause ototoxicity or renal toxicity. There is no simple method for measuring serum teicoplanin as for vancomycin, except by high performance liquid chromatography (HPLC) or biological plate assay. However, teicoplanin levels need only be measured in renal failure and serious infections (e.g. endocarditis). Trough levels of 15–20 mg/l are acceptable in most cases although levels above 20 mg/l with peaks of 40 mg/l should be aimed for in staphylococcal endocarditis.

One significant disadvantage of teicoplanin over vancomycin is that certain strains of coagulase negative staphylococci (in particular *S. haemolyticus*) are resistant and nosocomial infections with such strains may be selected where teicoplanin is heavily used.

Glycopeptide resistance

Apart from constitutive resistance of *S. haemolyticus* to teicoplanin, some rare organisms (e.g. *Leuconostoc* sp.) and some common commensals such as *Lactobacillus acidophilus* are also resistant to vancomycin but they rarely cause human infections. Of more concern is the emergence of glycopeptide-resistant *Enterococcus faecium*. This was first described in a renal unit where all infections were treated with ceftazidime (which would be expected to select for enterococci) and vancomycin. The resistance was multiple and many strains are also resistant to gentamicin. The resistance is coded for on plasmids and could be transferred into recipient strains. There is, at present, no antibiotic regimen effective against such infections.

PROTEIN SYNTHESIS INHIBITORS

Aminoglycosides

The clinically useful aminoglycosidic aminocyclitols (referred to below as aminoglycosides) may be divided into those containing streptidine (streptomycin, the first antibiotic to be discovered by the systematic examination of fungal soups) or 2-deoxystreptamine substituted at the 4,5 sites (neomycin family and paromomycin) or the 4,6 sites (kanamycin, tobramycin, gentamicin, netilmicin). There is one pure aminocyclitol, spectinomycin, whose value is restricted to the second line treatment of gonorrhoea. There are many other examples that are either not clinically useful or are currently in development.

All aminoglycosides have a variety of properties in common. They bind to a protein in the 30S ribosomal subunit causing defective reading of certain codons and the production of faulty proteins. Theoretically, they also interfere with protein synthesis initiation. A secondary effect of protein synthesis inhibition is cell membrane damage (which can be abolished by chloramphenicol). The defective proteins contribute to defects in the cell membrane increasing permeability, particularly to the aminoglycoside itself. The result is potent bactericidal activity. This may account for the cidal activity of aminoglycosides compared with the other protein synthesis inhibitors.

They are soluble but not orally active, have similar pharmacokinetic properties and are toxic to hearing (VIII cranial nerve) and kidney function. This toxicity varies between different compounds and is sometimes so potent (e.g. as with neomycin) as to preclude all but topical clinical use. In terms of antimicrobial spectra, most examples are active against *S. aureus* and Enterobacteriaceae, and some (tobramycin, gentamicin, netilmicin and amikacin) are also useful against *Pseudomonas*. Activity against streptococci is generally poor though aminoglycosides synergize with penicillin in this respect. Streptomycin, kanamycin, amikacin and capreomycin are also active against *Myobacterium tuberculosis*.

Spectinomycin was discovered in 1961 and is a pure aminocyclitol. Not being particularly active against most bacteria and being regarded as bacteristatic rather than bactericidal, it was surprising to find that MIC and MBC for *N. gonorrhoeae* strains were the same and within achievable limits (2–16 mg/l) after a single large dose. However, clinical success in treating gonorrhoea with spectinomycin is not closely related to MIC of the isolate. Restriction of the use of the antibiotic (2 g as a single dose) for this indication has been very successful. Cure is achievable in over 90% of infected men and women with urethritis but this drug is ineffective in gonococcal pharyngitis. Resistance is still relatively rare.

Streptomycin

Streptomycin is now recommended only for the treatment of tuberculosis. Paradoxically, the fact of requiring parenteral administration is sometimes of value in severely ill patients on ICU. The antibiotic has a broad spectrum of activity, being bactericidal against many Enterobacteriaceae, *Neisseria* and *S. aureus* but not streptococci. *In vitro*, it has greater activity against *M. tuberculosis* than any of these organisms.

Streptomycin sulphate is very soluble, slightly acid and causes moderate discomfort on im injection. By contrast, streptomycin itself is alkaline and causes much discomfort. Conventionally, in the treatment of tuberculosis, a single daily dose (500 mg–1 g) is given and trough levels are monitored, because excretion is not at all predictable on weight and renal function alone. Trough levels of <3 mg/l and peaks of 25 mg/l are acceptable and should be checked weekly or more often if there is any sign of renal function deterioration. Plasma half-life is very variable and is higher in the infant and older adult. Local pain after injection can be reduced by concomitant procaine. Perioral paraesthesiae, vertigo, ataxia, headaches and lassitude are common within the first hours after injection. A dose of 2 g per day will consistently cause vestibular damage manifest as vertigo and nystagmus but the likelihood of toxicity is dependent on the total dose. Persistent symptoms represent permanent damage to the sensory cells of the labyrinth. Deafness is less common than vertigo in adults but damage may occur to the fetus of a woman undergoing treatment for tuberculosis.

Curare-like neuromuscular blockade may occur but the effect is <0.01% that of tubocurarine. However, note that relatively high doses of streptomycin would be used. Other rare toxicities include aplasia or bleeding due to a factor V antagonist.

Resistance to streptomycin

Ten per cent of strains of *M. tuberculosis* isolated from the Far East are resistant to streptomycin or isoniazid. The drug is still extensively used in the developing world, usually as part of an initial supervised month or two of therapy.

The advantages are cheapness and assurance that the treatment has been administered. However, regimens containing streptomycin but not rifampicin are less effective and need to be continued for longer. Drug manufactured in the third world may be impure and of low potency. Streptomycin is sometimes used as part of an intensive five-drug regimen in which the total course of treatment is reduced to 4 months. The failure rate of this regimen is unacceptably high.

Resistance arises as a unique single step mutation to a change in the ribosomal structure reducing the binding avidity for streptomycin. Moderate resistance may be due to a permeability change. Organisms may also produce inactivating enzymes. (Paradoxically, some coliform organisms may be totally dependent on streptomycin for growth.)

Neomycin

This family of deoxystreptamine aminoglycosides consists of several related compounds that are too toxic to be given systemically. Neomycin B is available for topical treatment and is not absorbed after oral administration unless very large doses are given or in exceptional medical circumstances. Neomycin B may be absorbed from visci and after oral or bladder administration in sufficient quantity to cause deafness and renal failure so is no longer recommended.

A patient with a longstanding empyema was treated by decortication of the lungs and at the time of the operation, 10 g of neomycin was instilled into the thoracic cavity. The patient became irreversibly deaf and developed acute renal failure which recovered over a period of several months. There was also a suggestion of persistent curare-like effect in this patient, neomycin being more potent than streptomycin in this respect.

Neomycin is available in a number of topical preparations for use on skin and in the ear. This is also to be discouraged because of sensitization of the patient not only to neomycin but also to other more important aminoglycosides such as gentamicin. Short courses of intranasal neomycin will reduce carriage of staphylococci but this treatment has now been superseded by mupirocin (see below).

The drug is also included in proprietary preparations for the treatment of diarrhoea. This use is disputed. Similarly, neomycin was often recommended for gut decontamination preoperatively or in liver failure but has no effect on anaerobic flora. This latter observation makes neomycin a popular component of selective digestive decontamination, used in some ICU to reduce the risk of nosocomial pneumonia.

Paromomycin is very similar to neomycin and, interestingly, has some activity against pathogenic amoebae, *Leishmania* and *Taenia* spp. Like neomycin, the major side-effect is deafness.

Kanamycin group

The kanamycin group of antibiotics derived from *S. kanamyceticus* is modified to give gentamicin and amikacin. Tobramycin is a naturally occurring antibiotic of very similar structure though derived from a different fungal species. Tobramycin is slightly more active against *Pseudomonas* than gentamicin but otherwise has remarkably similar properties. Sissomicin is modified to give netilmicin, which is possibly less toxic than gentamicin and stable to some aminoglycosidases. Kanamycin behaves like neomycin but is more active against *M. tuberculosis* and some *Proteus* spp. The drug is ototoxic like neomycin and may be sufficiently absorbed after long-term oral administration to cause this side-effect. Its use is restricted to the second-line treatment of tuberculosis.

Gentamicin

Gentamicin is the most important of the aminoglycosides in practical terms because of its useful broad spectrum against Enterobacteriaceae and *Pseudomonas*. It is soluble, may be given intramuscularly or intravenously and has a half-life of 2 h. There is a postantibiotic effect, that is, a tendency to continue to kill bacteria after the antibiotic has been removed from culture, lasting 3–5 h. The drug is 20–30% protein bound. The drug crosses the placenta and achieves levels one-third of those in the maternal circulation. Aminoglycosides do not penetrate the intact blood–brain barrier in sufficient concentration to treat meningitis.

For a patient with normal renal function a dose of 4–5 mg/kg/day may be given in three divided doses. Conventionally, a loading dose of 40 mg greater than the 8-hourly dose is given to ensure more rapid filling of the extravascular compartments. Steady-state serum peaks and trough levels are achieved 3 days after starting treatment in those with normal renal function. Patients vary enormously in their ability to handle gentamicin and the peak level achieved after equivalent doses based on body mass. Because gentamicin is distributed in extracellular water, obese people require proportionately smaller doses. Several mathematical nomograms have been devised to adjust dose for mass and creatine clearance. However, the variables involved cannot all be encompassed in a mathematical equation, so they are not entirely reliable. They have been superseded by making serum level measurements more easily available. Any degree of renal impairment will lead to retention of the drug and this will increase further the risk of nephrotoxicity. The drug is usually restricted for the treatment of seriously ill patients, but because such patients are highly likely to develop renal failure following their illness complicated by sepsis, it is critical to modify the dose according to serum levels of gentamicin. Often retention of gentamicin will be the first sign of renal dysfunction, preceding the first detectable rise in creatinine. Current recommendations are that gentamicin levels are measured around the fourth dose if there is no known renal impairment. If there is any impairment, a simple approach is to give a generous loading dose according to body weight and measure one level 8 or 12 h afterwards. Further doses may then be administered with daily monitoring. We measure gentamicin levels every day on patients treated in ICU. The temptation for the clinician is to give *less* gentamicin than necessary because of its toxicity, but this often leads to undertreatment which may be fatal, particularly in the case of *Klebsiella* and *Pseudomonas* septicaemia.

Recent work has suggested that aminoglycosides such as gentamicin can be given as a single daily dose with the same clinical benefit. Monitoring of serum levels, particularly at trough, is still very important.[2]

Modern measurement techniques can be done with very small volumes of serum. Take blood immediately before the next due dose (trough) and exactly 1 h later (peak). The trough level should be below 2 mg/l. If it is above this level (e.g. 2–4 mg/l), the dose *interval* must be increased and further trough levels checked. The 'peak' level must be taken at a consistent time because the results are otherwise uninterpretable. One hour after a dose, the level should be well on the way towards the second phase of the excretion curve. A level of up to 7 mg/l at this time would be optimal and the *dose* should be modified if the peak is too high or too low. Increasing the dose because of a low peak level will inevitably have some effect on trough levels when steady state is re-established about 3 days later. Relatively low doses (80 mg q12h) are given to patients with endocarditis when gentamicin is used as synergistic therapy with a penicillin.

Haemodialysis removes gentamicin at a rate of 60% of that of the creatine clearance but peritoneal dialysis is much less effective. Aminoglycosides are commonly used to treat peritonitis associated with peritoneal dialysis. In this situation gentamicin is introduced into the dialysis bags at 4–8 mg/l which eventually equilibrates with the serum and has proved remarkably free of ototoxicity.

Ototoxicity occurs only significantly in those with impaired renal function. This occurs at extremes of age and associated with other illness. The toxicity of gentamicin on the auditory–vestibular apparatus is directly on the hair cells which form the sensory organs of hearing or balance. When the ear drum is perforated, topical gentamicin (or neomycin) ear drops can be ototoxic. In the kidney, aminoglycosides accumulate in the renal tubular cells and cause concentration-related necrosis. This effect is usually reversible but auditory–vestibular damage often persists.

The relationship between peak or trough levels and the likelihood of toxicity is not absolute, there being considerable variation in individual patient tolerance. Some have related the risk of toxicity to the area under the curve and it is likely that the length of treatment is a critical factor.

A 50-year-old patient with culture-negative endocarditis was treated with penicillin and gentamicin for 4 weeks. Regular trough levels were within acceptable limits but the patient nevertheless developed a disorder of balance that was irreversible.

A more serious risk occurs when patients are not monitored properly.

A patient undergoing a urological procedure received ampicillin and gentamicin prophylaxis perioperatively. Because the operation had been long and complex and because the patient was febrile postoperatively, these antibiotics were continued postoperatively. A weekend intervened with change of staff and the first gentamicin level was not done until 5 days after the start of treatment. The trough level at this time was 8 mg/l. The patient was in mild renal failure which showed some resolution later.

Renal toxicity is much more likely to occur if aminoglycosides are combined with other potentially nephrotoxic drugs such as vancomycin. Gentamicin plus vancomycin is a useful combination for resistant *S. epidermidis* endocarditis but as many as 75% of patients will develop renal failure despite maintenance of levels of the drugs within 'safe' limits. Similarly, toxicity is increased with loop diuretics such as frusemide. Like other aminoglycosides, gentamicin may potentiate the effects of curare-like drugs.

Organisms of all species may be resistant to gentamicin. This resistance is generally mediated by plasmids which confer the ability to produce aminoglycoside inactivating enzymes that are more or less specific. In addition, some organisms may become impermeable to gentamicin, and this may confer resistance to a wide range of aminoglycosides. Organisms can be bred in the laboratory which are paradoxically more sensitive to gentamicin.

Netilimicin

Netilmicin is the n-ethyl derivative of sissomycin, a naturally occurring derivative of gentamicin C with similar activity to gentamicin against Enterobacteriaceae and slightly less activity against *Pseudomonas*. Netilmicin is active against some gentamicin resistant strains because it is not inactivated by nucleotidyl transferase 2″. The advantage of netilmicin seems to be that it is slightly less ototoxic and nephrotoxic than gentamicin in animal models. For this reason it has been adopted in some hospitals as a substitute for gentamicin as the first-line aminoglycoside.

Like other aminoglycosides it is bactericidal, has improved activity in alkaline conditions and synergizes with β-lactam antibiotics. The pharmacokinetics are similar to gentamicin with serum half-life of 2.2 h, expected peaks of 5–10 mg/l and troughs of <2 mg/l.

Amikacin

Amikacin is a derivative of kanamycin whose advantage is that it may be active against some strains of Enterobacteriaceae and *Pseudomonas* which are resistant to gentamicin and tobramycin by virtue of specific inactivating enzymes. However, the latter antibiotics are more active against strains that are sensitive, so there is no advantage in choosing amikacin as the first-line aminoglycoside unless gentamicin resistance is prevalent.

Amikacin is not protein bound, has a similar serum half-life to gentamicin (2 h) extended to 2.8 h after intramuscular injection. Peak serum levels of around 25 mg/l after a dose of 500 mg and trough levels of 5–10 mg/l are acceptable.

Conventionally amikacin is given q12h compared with gentamicin q8h. At these dosage frequencies, amikacin tends not to accumulate whereas gentamicin does. Most amikacin is excreted through the kidneys, and as for the other aminoglycosides, care must be taken in the patient with renal impairment. The toxicity of amikacin is similar to that of gentamicin but no comparative trials have been done. Formal testing reveals high tone deafness in many patients receiving amikacin. Noticeable deafness is detected in 1–2%, vestibular damage in 1–2% and impaired renal function in 4% of treated patients. Toxicity is more likely to occur with prolonged treatment and in those with trough levels exceeding 10 mg/l.

The value of amikacin is in the treatment of resistant Gram-negative infections and it may be of value in the second-line treatment of tuberculosis as a substitute for streptomycin.

Tobramycin

Tobramycin is one of the nebramycins derived from a *Streptomyces* sp., which is closely related to kanamycin. It has very similar properties to gentamicin and its advantage seems to be in having slightly better activity against *Pseudomonas*. However, there is less activity against some *Serratia* and *Proteus* spp. and *S. aureus*. The pharmacokinetics are almost exactly the same as gentamicin with similar trough and peak levels being acceptable. The drug is thought to be slightly less toxic than gentamicin to the auditory–vestibular apparatus but this is not proven in man and there is insufficient evidence to warrant general use in preference to gentamicin. Aminoglycoside-inactivating enzymes that destroy gentamicin may also destroy tobramycin. The drug is mostly reserved for the treatment of severe documented *Pseudomonas* infections, for example, ecthyma gangrenosum in febrile neutropenic patients.

Use of aminoglycosides

Aminoglycosides should be reserved for treating severe infections in hospitalized patients. It is not wise to use these drugs in general practice because of serious difficulties monitoring levels and because of the high risk of toxic levels developing insidiously in the sort of patients who may benefit from this treatment (e.g. the elderly catheterized patient with a multiply resistant organism in the urine).

Severe infections include Gram-negative sepsis and endocarditis. In the former, aminoglycosides are often combined with a broad-spectrum penicillin or cephalosporin. Treatment should be modified with the results of blood or other cultures. Synergy with penicillins or glycopeptides against streptococci and staphylococci make these combinations the treatment of choice for the treatment of endocarditis guided by culture results. Culture negative endocarditis should be treated with penicillin and gentamicin. Low doses of aminoglycoside may be used in this situation (e.g. gentamicin 80 mg q12h) but treatment will need to be continued for a long period. The patient must be warned about the risks of toxicity. If minor vestibular or auditory disturbance occurs, the drug must be stopped and not restarted.

Streptomycin, kanamycin, amikacin and capreomycin (not discussed above) are sometimes used in the second-line treatment of tuberculosis. In poorer countries, streptomycin forms part of the routine therapy of tuberculosis. If used without rifampicin, chemotherapy regimens starting with streptomycin (for, say, 2 months) must continue for 18 months. If used as part of a four or five drug initial 2-month regimen for tuberculosis, a continuation phase of rifampicin and isoniazid need only be continued for a further 2 or 4 months to achieve an acceptable cure rate.

Macrolides

These comprise many drugs derived from fungi consisting of a large lactone cyclic ring to which various sugars are attached. Various examples have been used clinically (e.g. oleandomycin, rosaramycin, spiramycin) but only erythromycin is in common use in the UK. Recently, new macrolides (e.g. azithromycin, clarithromycin) have been developed with better pharmacokinetics than erythromycin.

Macrolides interfere with translocation in bacterial protein synthesis. They are bacteriostatic in general but may be cidal at high concentrations and with prolonged exposure. They are most active against Gram-positive organisms but have some useful activity against *B. pertussis* and *Brucella* spp., and also *H. influenzae* and *Neisseria* spp. although erythromycin is not the first drug of choice for these latter two infections. Macrolides are also active against *Chlamydia, Mycoplasma pneumoniae*, *Legionella* and some rickettsiae and have activity against atypical mycobacteria and *Plasmodium*.

Erythromycin

This is the most important of the macrolides available for clinical use. Erythromycin base is acid labile. Early experiments with enteric coating showed inconsistent and incomplete absorption and various esters and salts were developed. Erythromycin stearate is acid resistant but broken down to erythromycin base in the small intestine. Erythromycin estolate is broken down to and absorbed as the propionyl ester which is inactive and must be hydrolysed after absorption. Hydrolysis occurs at a fairly constant rate so the ratio between active base and ester remains constant. However, it is difficult to assay active material in serum because of continuing hydrolysis of the ester. A fine particle preparation in an enteric coat is now available and shows excellent and consistent absorption kinetics.

Absorption is generally less reliable in women than men. Furthermore, the drug is less well absorbed in pregnancy. Continued dosing leads to accumulation of the drug and high levels are achieved in the urine. Intravenous preparations are available, the gluceptate and lactobionate giving rise to high levels of active drug in the serum. The half-life is reduced from 2–5 h to 1–2 h, so paradoxically larger doses are given intravenously.

Protein binding of the base is about 75%. The drug distributes through body water and achieves half serum levels in otitis media exudate and aqueous humour. However, erythromycin does not penetrate the blood–brain barrier at all. Relatively little drug gets into the amniotic fluid and less into the fetal circulation, but it is concentrated in fetal liver tissue.

Most erythromycin is degraded, a small proportion appearing in the urine being filtered and possibly partially reabsorbed. Levels 4–30-fold the serum levels are achieved in bile but this represents excretion of only 1.5% of a dose of base in 8 h.

Erythromycin *estolate* may cause hepatitis which is reversible. A component of the damage may be allergy because eosinophils are sometimes found in the peripheral circulation at this time. Hepatitis is not a major feature of other erythromycin esters and salts, but has been reported with the free base and stearate. Transient rises in transaminases are common. Otherwise the drug is relatively free of side-effects. Nausea and vomiting, with some myalgia, are not uncommon at high dose levels. Transient deafness may occur rarely.

Even though the fate of erythromycin is not absolutely clear, sufficient drug is excreted through the liver to suggest caution when giving the drug to a patient with liver disease. Erythromycin also decreases the rate of degradation of digoxin, warfarin, carbamazepine and theophylline, potentiating their effects.

A topical solution of erythromycin base is available for the treatment of acne.

Clarithromycin

Clarithromycin is a new fourteen-membered macrolide with slightly better activity than erythromycin against a number of important pathogens that cause pneumonia: these include *S. pneumoniae*, *L. pneumophila*, and probably *Chlamydia pneumoniae*. Again the agent is not particularly active against *H. influenzae*.

Clarithromycin is rapidly absorbed, is acid stable and absorption is not affected by food. The drug is hydrolysed to an active 14-hydroxy derivative which is cleared at a lower rate (4.7–7.2 h, depending on the dose) than the parent compound (3.5–4.9 h). The dosage frequency recommended is twice daily. Renal clearance is important, half-lives increasing to >30 h at creatinine clearance rates of <30 ml/min. In liver disease, less clarithromycin is hydrolysed and the clearance is that of the parent drug. Dosage needs be modified in renal but not hepatic impairment. The drug is concentrated in tissues at levels several-fold those in the serum.

Good activity has been shown in pneumonia due to the agents mentioned above (with the exception of *H. influenzae*). Gastrointestinal side-effects occur less commonly than with erythromycin. Comparison with roxithromycin, a similar compound with a half-life of 13 h, although not stringent, shows the two drugs to be comparable in efficacy and side-effects. Comparison with penicillin V in the treatment of streptococcal tonsillitis and with ampicillin in the treatment of exacerbations of chronic bronchitis shows no major differences between these treatments.

Clarithromycin has an important indication in the prevention and treatment of *Mycobacterium avium* infection in AIDS.

Azithromycin

This prototype azolide has a methyl substituted nitrogen in the erythromycin molecule. This substitution increases activity of the drug against Gram-positives and particularly against Gram-negatives including *Neisseria*, *Haemophilus* and *Klebsiella*. It is slightly less active *in vitro* against *Chlamydia* but has fewer side-effects and more attractive pharmacokinetics compared with erythromycin. In the first 8 h after exposure to susceptible bacteria it is bacteriostatic; later it appears to be bactericidal. The drug is acid resistant, about 40% orally bioavailable and protein binding is concentration dependent ranging from 50 to 20%. It is concentrated in tissues to concentrations up to 30-fold those in the serum. This applies to bronchial mucosa and to alveolar macrophages.

The half-life of azithromycin in tissue is 2–3 days. Continuing dosing after initial loading leads to very prolonged levels in the tissue of around 3 mg/l which are probably bactericidal. Elimination is not log-linear but dependent on time after dosing. Preliminary clinical results using once-daily regimens suggest equal efficacy to erythromycin in respiratory and genital infections with fewer side-effects. Saturation of tissue compartments occurs by three days of treatment. High intracellular concentrations correlate with good activity against *Chlamydia* and *Legionella*. However, there has been disappointment in the treatment of chronic bronchitis exacerbations associated with *H. influenzae*.

Lincosamines

Lincomycin was derived from *Streptomyces lincolnensis* and modified to form clindamycin (7-chloro-7-deoxy-lincomycin) which is more active and has excellent pharmacokinetics. Lincosamines have a novel structure and although they are very similar in activity to macrolides, are not active against Gram-negative aerobic organisms. Organisms resistant to erythromycin may have plasmid-mediated inducible resistance to lincosamines.

Clindamycin

Three different preparations of clindamycin are available: capsules which contain (bitter) hydrochloride, a syrup of palmitate and injection of phosphate. The palmitate is inactive but hydrolysed to active compound in the gut before absorption. The phosphate is hydrolysed over several hours after injection. Equivalent doses give very similar peak serum levels (1.5–4 mg/l) with half-life ranging from 1.5 to 4 h. Clindamycin is 90% protein bound but distributed well within the tissue as prodrug, active drug and more or less active metabolites. The penetration into CSF is poor but clindamycin does penetrate into the placenta and cord blood, a useful observation as the drug is very useful for perinatal infections. Of note is the penetration into bone and clindamycin is particularly useful for treating osteomyelitis. A small proportion of clindamycin is excreted in the kidneys and is reduced in moderate to severe renal failure. Whereas this hardly affects the serum levels, the half-life is doubled in liver failure. The drug also accumulates at higher levels in bile and gall bladder.

Clindamycin is highly active against many anaerobes so is useful in mixed Gram-positive aerobic plus anaerobic infections. One example in such mixed infections in ICU would be inhalation pneumonitis. Clindamycin reduces the activity of gentamicin against Enterobacteriaceae yet the combination is useful in puerperal sepsis, covering many of the potential pathogens. Clindamycin is not consistently effective in endocarditis.

The use of clindamycin for the treatment of any but the more serious infections has been tempered by the observation of pseudomembranous colitis associated with toxin-producing *C. difficile*. This is a rare, but often fatal, condition that may occur with almost any antibiotic treatment. However, it does occur more commonly with clindamycin than with ampicillin and particularly affects elderly, sick, hospitalized patients who are at high risk of being colonized with toxigenic *C. difficile*. Well-documented nosocomial outbreaks of *C. difficile* colonization have been described. Mild diarrhoea is much more common than pseudomembranous colitis, affecting as many as 10% of those treated with any antibiotic. Other rare side-effects of clindamycin include reversible neuromuscular weakness precipitated by postsynaptic block, through a different mechanism than that of aminoglycosides. Minor changes in hepatic transaminases are not uncommon but of little consequence.

Clindamycin should therefore be restricted to moderate or severe infections of bone, lung and genitourinary tract and (as for all antibiotics) stopped if the patient develops diarrhoea.

Chloramphenicol

Chloramphenicol was isolated from *Streptomyces venezuelae* but is manufactured synthetically. It was the first broad-spectrum antibiotic with useful activity against life-threatening conditions ranging from pneumonia through meningitis to typhoid. Its usefulness has only been gradually and recently eroded by the emergence of some resistant strains but the use of the drug in the developed world has been tempered by awareness of the possibility of a rare fatal aplastic anaemia.

Thiamphenicol, a closely related derivative of chloramphenicol, has better pharmacokinetic properties, is supposed not to cause aplasia yet has not been developed in many countries.

Chloramphenicol is bactericidal against some staphylococci, *Haemophilus* and *Neisseria* spp. but only static against coliforms. Nevertheless, the drug is very effective in enteric (typhoid) fever, probably a result of intracellular penetration. Chloramphenicol inhibits peptidyl transferase at the 70S ribosomes. This prevents peptide bond formation. Resistance arises by the production of one of several chloramphenicol acetyl transferases. There has been a gradual increase in chloramphenicol resistance in *H. influenzae*. For several years, there have been major outbreaks of typhoid due to organisms which are constitutively resistant. Resistance is classically selected by heavy usage, and in hospital practice, restriction of antibiotic use has been shown to reduce the prevalence of resistance in troublesome organisms such as *S. aureus*.

Chloramphenicol is bitter so is usually given orally as the inactive palmitate hydrolysed to active drug in the gut. Palmitate and stearate esters both exist in two different forms, one of which is much better absorbed than the other. The formulation is also important to ensure dispersability and proper hydrolysis in the gut. Chloramphenicol sodium succinate may be given intravenously (or intramuscularly). Again, it is not active until hydrolysed to active antibiotic in the tissues. Peak levels of drug are often lower than after oral administration but are rather variable.

Chloramphenicol may be measured in serum relatively easily but this should be done solely to monitor the dose requirements in children under 6 months of age. In these children hydrolysis and absorption are even less consistent than later in life. High doses of chloramphenicol lead to a shock reaction called 'grey baby' syndrome, which is now exceedingly rare. The excretion half-life of chloramphenicol in the adult is 2–5 h and in the neonate 24 h.

Protein binding is 60% but reduced in neonates and the drug distributes freely into all tissue including CSF, the fetus, the eye and any serous exudate. The drug is conjugated or reduced in the liver and this process is reduced in liver disease. Chloramphenicol will reduce the clearance of warfarin and tolbutamide. The inactive glucuronide is excreted in the urine but 10% of the active drug is excreted unchanged. Clearance is reduced linearly with falling renal function but serum levels of the active drug rise only marginally and inactive metabolites accumulate.

Chloramphenicol causes consistent depression of the bone marrow resulting in low total circulating white blood cell counts. This effect is dose dependent, rapid and reversible. More sinister is irreversible aplastic anaemia, which occurs 2 to 3 weeks (or more) after commencing therapy – that is, usually when therapy has been completed. The risk of fatal aplastic anaemia is probably very low (relative risk increased from 2 to 26 per million population). The side-effect is thought to arise from an inhibitory effect on protein synthesis in mitochondria in eukaryocytic cells – the mechanism being more like bacterial protein synthesis than that in the cytoplasm.

Tetracyclines

Chlortetracycline was derived from *Streptomyces aureofaciens* in 1948 and there have been several variants on the basic molecule developed with different pharmacological properties.

Tetracyclines are concentrated inside sensitive bacteria by an active transport system. They bind to the 30S ribosome subunit interfering with the attachment of aminoacyl transfer RNA. This inhibits protein synthesis but bacterial inhibition is static rather than cidal. Resistance is mainly due to inhibition of the active transport of the antibiotic into the cell and there is virtually complete cross-resistance between different tetracyclines.

Tetracylines have a very wide spectrum of activity which includes many of the causes of atypical pneumonia (e.g. *Mycoplasma pneumoniae*, *Chlamydia* spp.) in addition to common Gram-negative and Gram-positive organisms. Some hospital-associated strains of *S. aureus* and Enterobacteriaceae began to show resistance through the 1960s, so the drug fell into disfavour as a general broad-spectrum antibiotic. With its use restricted to the treatment of specific conditions (e.g. chlamydial infections, brucellosis), the level of resistance is now considerably reduced. The antibiotic is a cheap, useful choice in the treatment of exacerbations of chronic bronchitis.

Tetracycline is poorly absorbed from the gut but constant levels of around 5 mg/l are achieved with continuous dosing at 500 mg q6h. Solubility is reduced in non-acidic conditions. Absorption is inhibited by antacids, by milk (tetracyclines chelating calcium) and by ferrous sulphate. The drug is excreted both through the bile and kidneys and is retained in renal failure. Doxycycline, however, does not accumulate in renal failure.

Minocycline and doxycycline have longer decay half-lives than tetracycline so should be given twice and once per day respectively. The maintenance of serum levels is in part achieved by resorption of active compound from the gut after biliary excretion.

Tetracyclines are widely distributed in tissues, particularly bone, and achieve levels in the CSF around 15% of the serum levels. Biliary concentrations of tetracycline are 5–20-fold higher than serum levels, doxycycline achieving the highest levels. Minocycline achieves higher levels in bronchial secretions in bronchiectasis than oxytetracycline or doxycycline.

Common side-effects include nausea, vomiting and diarrhoea. Pseudomembranous colitis occurs less commonly than with clindamycin and ampicillin.

Overgrowth of candida in mouth, vagina and gut is common. Tetracyclines are deposited in bone and developing teeth. Staining of teeth and degree of hypoplasia depend on the total dose given and the variety of tetracycline. This effect will be seen at any age from after 5 months of gestation until the age of 7 years when the final molars are laid down.

Early studies suggested that tetracyclines could exacerbate renal failure. Doxycycline does not accumulate in renal failure in part passively diffusing into and being chelated in the gut. Tetracycline should be given with care parenterally and during pregnancy, being implicated in fatty degeneration of the liver.

Tetracyclines are now reserved for the treatment of respiratory infections and specific infections with *Rickettsia*, *Coxiella*, *Mycoplasma*, *Chlamydia* and *Brucella* spp. Resistance in pneumococci has risen gradually. Tetracyclines (except doxycycline) are useful in acne vulgaris. Demeclocycline was found to precipitate nephrogenic diabetes insipidus and may be used to treat inappropriate antidiuretic hormone secretion.

Fusidanes

Fusidic acid is the only useful fusidane. It has a steroid-like structure and inhibits protein chain synthesis by interfering with elongation 'factor G', a translocase. It exhibits no postantibiotic effect and may reduce the postantibiotic effect of potential co-administered antibiotics like teicoplanin. It is active against Gram-positive and Gram-negative cocci, many anaerobes and *Nocardia asteroides*. It also has activity against some *Corynebacteria* and *M. tuberculosis* although these properties are not used clinically. The only important use of fusidic acid is in the treatment of *S. aureus* infection. Selection of resistant isolates is easy *in vitro* but there is controversy about the rate at which this occurs *in vivo*.

Sodium fusidate is well absorbed given orally but absorption is delayed by milk. Less of a suspension is absorbed than capsule form but areas under the curves suggest that the capsule form is as bioavailable as the same dose of an intravenous preparation. Peak levels of 20, 30 and 40 mg/l are achieved after 500 mg doses of suspension, capsule and infusion respectively. The drug is about 95% protein bound. The antibiotic distributes widely in tissues including bone but not into the CSF. Antibiotic concentrations in bone range from 2 to 15 mg/g on a dose of 1.5 g/day and this range is not significantly changed by doubling the dose. The drug is excreted in the bile, mostly in conjugated form. Little active antibiotic appears in urine or faeces.

Side-effects after oral dosing are mild, consisting of nausea and vomiting. Rapid infusion causes vasospasm. The most important side-effect is hepatotoxicity, which is a particular property of the intravenous preparation and is therefore likely to be seen in severely ill patients treated for staphylococcal infection in ICUs.

Resistance to fusidic acid arises as a one-step chromosomal mutation which may be easily selected *in vitro* and is due to a change in the target enzyme. Resistant organisms are less robust than their sensitive counterparts and tend to revert to full sensitivity on culture in the absence of fusidic acid. There is also plasmid-mediated resistance which is probably due to a permeability block seen in strains from patients who have not been exposed to fusidic acid.

Resistance has been shown to arise in strains from between 3 and 7% of patients treated for 3–10 days. This is much more likely if the drug is used alone, if the patient has chronic or severe ineradicable infection (e.g. burns, chronic osteomyelitis). Fusidic acid is therefore usually combined with an antistaphylococcal penicillin (penicillin or flucloxacillin, depending on the sensitivity of the organism) in severe infections. Fusidic acid has no postantibiotic effect and actually decreases the postantibiotic effect seen with glycopeptides. Fusidic acid and flucloxacillin are not clearly synergistic against *S. aureus in vitro*. Some combinations of concentrations appear antagonistic and there is considerable doubt as to the value of adding fusidic acid to flucloxacillin in the treatment of endocarditis. Nevertheless, fusidic acid does penetrate into bone and pus in therapeutic concentrations and is favoured as an important component in the treatment of osteomyelitis.

Pseudomonic acid, mupirocin

This unique drug derived from *Pseudomonas fluorescens* is highly active against staphylococci. It is toxic given parenterally but is extraordinarily effective when used topically against *S. aureus* colonization of the nose and much more so than topical neomycin. It is also recommended for the topical treatment of supposed infected eczema, wounds or ulcers. However, resistance may emerge and has been seen in methicillin-resistant *S. aureus*. The drug acts by reversible inhibition of isoleucyl tRNA synthetase.

DNA SYNTHESIS INHIBITORS

Sulphonamides and trimethoprim inhibit two different enzymes on the folate synthesis pathway – dihydropteroic acid synthetase and dihydrofolate reductase (DHFR) respectively. Although mammalian cells are unable to synthesize folate, they do possess similar enzymes that have a very low affinity for these antibiotics.

Sulphonamides

The sulphonamides were derived from prontosil, a red dye found to be active against streptococcal infections in mice and men in 1930s. The first derivative, sulphanilamide, was modified to produce many molecules to improve pharmacological properties and reduce toxicity. Poorly absorbed molecules and others have been used in the treatment of ulcerative colitis and have been used for gut decontamination. Others have been developed for topical treatment of burns. Although less useful as broad-spectrum agents for the treatment of urinary, respiratory and CNS infection because of the gradual increase in resistance, the sulphonamides remain extremely useful in some specific cases. Combined with trimethoprim, as co-trimoxazole, they are still the most widely prescribed drug for urinary and respiratory infections. There are, however, few indications for sulphonamide alone in the ICU.

Most sulphonamides are well absorbed from the gut achieving peak serum levels of over 100 mg/l around 3 h of a dose of 1–2 g. Protein binding varies from 45% (sulphadiazine) to 99% (sulphadimethoxine) but the influence of this on therapeutic activity is not known. Only unbound sulphonamide can penetrate the cells or the CSF. Commonly, 60–80% of plasma levels are found in the CSF, and sulphonamides also cross the placenta.

Sulphonamides may be displaced from albumin by drugs such as phenylbutazone, but in turn they may displace bilirubin from albumin and this may predispose to kernicterus in newborns. Sulphonamides therefore should not be given in the last 3 months of pregnancy and during breastfeeding, or to newborns.

Sulphadimidine and sulphadiazine may be given intravenously as well as orally. Plasma half-lives vary between compounds from 7 h (sulphadimidine) or less, through 11 h (sulphamethoxazole, commonly presented with trimethoprim) to 150 h (sulfadoxine, a component of Fansidar used in prophylaxis or treatment of chloroquine-resistant malaria). Sulfametopyrazine has a half-life of 65 h due to tubular reabsorption. Although this may be given weekly, low levels are achieved in the urine and severe side-effects are more common.

The most important side-effect is hypersensitivity, manifesting as skin reactions which may occasionally be fatal. Stevens–Johnson syndrome was particularly associated with long-acting compounds. Blood dyscrasias may also occur, again more commonly with the long-acting compounds. Sulphonamides may precipitate haemolysis in glucose-6-phosphate dehydrogenase deficiency. Minor effects include nausea, headaches and transient rashes. Certain compounds may be precipitated in the renal tubules.

Increasing antibiotic resistance has curtailed the usefulness of sulphonamides. For sensitive meningococci, they are effective in eradicating carriage. They remain the primary choice for nocardiasis which may be a problem in immunosuppressed patients. Sulphasalazine has a specific usefulness in ulcerative colitis. Topical sulphonamides, such as silver sulphadiazine, are often used in burns but are associated with inevitable problems of selection of resistant organisms.

Trimethoprim

Trimethoprim is a synthetic diaminopyrimidine originally released only in combination with sulphamethoxazole (as co-trimoxazole). Later it became available alone. The combination was supposed to offer synergistic activity, two consecutive enzymes in the folic acid pathway being inhibited. However, this can only be demonstrated *in vitro* with suboptimal combinations of the two agents. Furthermore the combination was proposed to reduce the likelihood of resistance to sulphonamide developing in an individual. There has been little change in the rate of sulphonamide resistance emerging since the combination was in use. Like sulphonamide, trimethoprim is generally bacteristatic or slowly cidal but in some strains it appears to be rapidly bactericidal.

Trimethoprim is absorbed orally to give levels between 0.9 and 3.2 mg/l after doses of 100–250 mg. About half is protein bound and plasma half-life is around 9 h. In order to monitor the absorption and pharmacokinetics of cotrimoxazole, it is conventional to measure the sulpha component. Trimethoprim is distributed in a volume exceeding body water but sulphamethoxazole only within a volume corresponding to extracellular fluid. The ratio by weight in the mixture of the drugs is 5 : 1 but by concentration is 20 : 1 in the serum. Trimethoprim is excreted in the urine giving very high concentrations in this site.

Resistance to trimethoprim is easily selected in the laboratory. Mutants are thymine dependent – thymine providing a substrate that bypasses the action of DHFR. Resistance may be transferred on plasmids that code for a modified DHRF enzyme.

Trimethoprim alone is useful for treating urinary infections and respiratory infections providing the causative organism is sensitive. More than half of *S. pneumoniae* isolates appear to be trimethoprim resistant *in vitro* but the relevance of this in clinical usage has not been demonstrated. Trimethoprim alone remains a useful urinary antibiotic, and combined with rifampicin is excellent second-line treatment for *S. aureus* infections. The main advantage of trimethoprim over co-trimoxazole is the reduction in side-effects. However, some severe rashes have been observed occasionally on trimethoprim alone.

Co-trimoxazole in high dose is the treatment of choice for *Pneumocystis carinii* infection. It may be given intravenously in severely ill patients who cannot tolerate the oral form. However, the intravenous infusion may cause phlebitis. Levels (of the sulphonamide component) may be measured to ensure therapeutic levels (200 mg/l) or in order to adjust the dose if there is any renal failure.

Pyrimethamine

Pyrimethamine also inhibits DHFR and is active against the mammalian enzyme in the high therapeutic concentrations necessary for a therapeutic effect against protozoa. It is useful in malaria prophylaxis combined with sulphone or sulphonamide but not alone. It is also used to treat active toxoplasmosis.

Rifamycins

The most important antibiotic of a large group derived from *Streptomyces mediterranei* is rifampicin, but two other agents (rifapentin and rifabutin) with more favourable pharmacokinetics for the treatment of tuberculosis have been developed. Rifampicin is the most active agent known against *S. aureus*, and it is also active against *Chlamydia*. Mutation to resistance in *S. aureus* is prevented by combination with trimethoprim and in *M. tuberculosis* by combination with isoniazid or other antituberculous agents. Rifampicin acts by binding to the reverse transcriptase which synthesizes RNA from DNA. The antibiotic is bactericidal and has a postantibiotic effect of about 3.5 h. Resistance arises by mutations of the target enzyme.

Rifampicin is well absorbed on an empty stomach. The drug should be given 30 min before food. Peak levels after 600 mg should be >5 mg/l and the drug is 70% protein bound with a plasma half-life of 3 h. A parenteral preparation is available. The antibiotic is excreted mainly in the bile, metabolized to the inactive desacetyl form with any excess appearing in the urine. This is not important in renal failure but increases in biliary obstruction.

The major toxicity is hepatitis but minor gastrointestinal effects also occur. High-dose intermittent therapy often causes fever and influenza-like symptoms. Rifampicin is a powerful hepatic microsomal enzyme inducer, reducing the efficacy of many drugs including warfarin, sulphonylureas and the contraceptive pill (which must be doubled in dose). Rifampicin is an important part of antituberculosis regimens, allowing a very significant reduction in the period needed for therapy compared with regimens where rifampicin is not available or cannot be used because of toxicity. Rifampicin is useful for eradicating meningococci and *H. influenzae* from the respiratory tract in carriers and has taken over in this role from sulphonamides.

Quinolones

Several compounds with heterocyclic nuclei were developed from the late 1950s. Nalidixic acid was the most successful and was slightly improved upon by oxolinic acid, cinoxacin and flumequine. They are poorly active against Gram-positive organisms. These drugs have now been eclipsed by substitution of fluorine and piperazine into the quinolone nucleus. The new generation of fluoroquinolones (e.g. norfloxacin, ciprofloxacin, enoxacin, ofloxacin) have a broader spectrum of activity, are more active in general and have some novel advantages over previous antimicrobials. Quinolones act by inhibiting DNA gyrase, a topoisomerase enzyme that is responsible for supercoiling or unwinding tight coils of DNA to allow compaction or replication. The specific site of action may be interference with joining of the DNA strands that are to be resealed by the topoisomerase. In addition to this mechanism present in all quinolones, the fluorinated 4-quinolones exert some other cidal effect on bacteria, perhaps on the membrane, that is not yet fully elucidated. So far as has been established, there is no plasmid-mediated resistance to quinolones but chromosomal resistance can emerge by mutation of the enzyme substrate. Organisms resistant to nalidixic acid may well be sensitive to the fluoroquinolones.

The two types of antibiotics that will be discussed are nalidixic acid and ciprofloxacin. There are many new fluoroquinolones to come, a proliferation of compounds that will mirror the vast number of cephalosporins available.

Nalidixic acid

This compound is active against Gram-negative organisms alone but not *P. aeruginosa*. It is well absorbed giving rather variable peak serum levels. Better absorption is achieved in the presence of alkali which increases solubility. Serum levels are irrelevant to clinical practice because nalidixic acid does not diffuse well into tissues, but is protein bound and is excreted rapidly through the kidneys, partly in metabolized form. The serum half-life is 1–2 h. Its main indication, therefore, is the treatment of urinary infections with sensitive Enterobacteriaceae. Gram-positive organisms are resistant. Renal failure does not significantly increase serum levels of active compound but there is an accumulation of inactive metabolites. However, probenecid prolongs the serum half-life of active compound.

Nalidixic acid is not without side-effects. Nausea is common. Central nervous system disturbance includes hallucinations, seizures and visual disturbances. Skin rashes may or may not be associated with photosensitivity.

Ciprofloxacin

Ciprofloxacin was one of the first to be licensed of the new generation of fluorinated 4-quinolones. This and other similar compounds (ofloxacin, norfloxacin) now represent 10% of the world antibiotic market. These agents have a broader spectrum of activity than nalidixic acid (including superior activity against staphylococci and some streptococci) and have a lower likelihood of resistance. They have specific clinical advantages that include activity against *Pseudomonas aeruginosa* after oral administration, the eradication of *Salmonella typhi* in carrier states and the effective single dose oral treatment of penicillin-resistant gonorrhoea.

All fluoroquinolones are rapidly absorbed after oral dosing, being 80–90% bioavailable. Peak serum concentrations occur at 1–2 h. For a single 250-mg dose of ciprofloxacin this peak is around 1 mg/l and the half-life is about 4 h. Thirty to sixty per cent of the active antibiotic and 10% as metabolite are excreted in the urine and 15–20% appears in the faeces. Biliary concentrations 2–8-fold the serum concentration are achieved. Ciprofloxacin is 35% protein bound.

Very similar pharmacokinetics are seen with ofloxacin but the maximum concentration is slightly higher, the half-life slightly longer and more is excreted in the urine as parent compound.

Urine concentrations of active drugs remain above MIC for common urinary pathogens for as long as 48 h after a single dose. Partial tubular secretion of most quinolones can be blocked by probenecid.

Antacids containing magnesium or aluminium chelate and drastically reduce the absorption of ciprofloxacin and also reduce the activity of the drug *in vitro* and *in vivo*. Ferric and ferrous ions but not calcium also interfere with antibacterial activity *in vitro*. Food and H_2 antagonists delay the peak serum levels of fluoroquinolones. Peak titres of quinolones are reduced in sick patients.

Protein synthesis inhibitors (chloramphenicol, tetracycline, erythromycin) in combination with quinolones are antagonistic. β-Lactam antibiotics do not affect bactericidal activity of quinolones but aminoglycosides potentiate the activity.

There is less ciprofloxacin excreted in the urine after an oral dose compared with an iv dose and a proportionate increase in metabolites. This suggests a first-pass effect after oral administration.

Excretion half-life in serum is approximately doubled in anuria. High concentrations of antibiotic are achieved in the urine by tubular secretion. Ofloxacin by comparison has a very prolonged half-life (40–50 h) in oliguric renal failure. Thus the dose interval should be increased for ofloxacin but need not be for ciprofloxacin and norfloxacin. Similarly, liver failure results in only a slight prolongation in half-lives of the latter two drugs.

There is an important interaction between enoxacin and theophylline, the excretion of the two drugs being mutually delayed. Ciprofloxacin and ofloxacin have little effect but occasionally elevated theophylline levels have been shown. An interaction with non-steroid anti-inflammatory drugs has led in some cases to CNS disturbance and convulsions.

Extravascular penetration is good, ciprofloxacin achieving levels in lymph some 70% of those in serum. CSF levels are relatively poor (5–10% of serum levels) unless the meninges are inflamed when levels of 40–90% of serum levels are achieved. Ciprofloxacin is active against intracellular bacteria such as *S. typhi*.

Ciprofloxacin has proved valuable in the treatment of severe Gram-negative sepsis, of typhoid, gonorrhoea, and of urinary, bilary and respiratory sepsis. Combination therapy (with a β-lactam or aminoglycoside) is preferred in febrile neutropenic episodes.

Phlebitis may occur at the site of infection and high doses cause nausea and other upper gastrointestinal symptoms. Rare side-effects include myalgia, arthralgia, dizziness and confusion and myoclonic seizures. Very high doses interfere with the synthesis of cartilage in the ends of long bones of growing beagle pups so quinolones are contraindicated in children.

Use of the drug as prophylaxis in neutropenics is valuable to prevent sepsis but selects for resistance. Similarly, the intensive promotion and widespread uncontrolled use has inevitably been associated with the emergence of resistance even in *S. typhi* and *N. gonorrhoeae*. Cross-resistance between quinolones is the rule. Mutations affect interaction with target enzyme or transport through the cell membrane.

Antibiotic treatment of acute gastroenteritis is discouraged on the grounds of dubious efficacy and selecting for prolonged carriage. However, studies with ciprofloxacin suggest that the illness can be shortened. This treatment does not, however, eradicate the causative organism. Similarly, ciprofloxacin prophylaxis, like co-trimoxazole and tetracycline, is effective in reducing the risk of traveller's diarrhoea. Oral ciprofloxacin compares favourably with intraperitoneal antibiotics in the management of continuous ambulatory peritoneal dialysis (CAPD) associated peritonitis. However, high doses are required and nausea may result.

Useful activity against Gram-positive infections is much less secure.

Nitroimidazoles

The most important antibiotic in this large group is metronidazole which is highly active against most anaerobic bacteria and various important protozoal pathogens including *Giardia intestinalis*, *Entamoeba histolytica* and *Trichomonas vaginalis*. Metronidazole is also a valuable radiation sensitizer. Metronidazole is reduced intracellularly in conditions of low eH to an active metabolite that induces strand fracture of DNA.

Metronidazole is well absorbed orally, achieving peak levels averaging 7 mg/l at 1.5 h with a half-life of 8 h. Metronidazole may also be given per rectum or intravenously. Some of the antibacterial activity in the serum is due to active metabolites. The drug is about 50% protein bound and 70% is excreted in the urine giving rise to very high concentrations. In renal failure the half-life of metronidazole remains the same but the metabolites accumulate.

Metronidazole causes nausea, a metallic taste in the mouth and a furred tongue. It interacts with alcohol to cause vomiting. Rashes and angioedema, transient leucopenia, dark urine and central nervous system disturbance are relatively uncommon. Prolonged treatment at high doses (as in the case of radiation sensitization) may cause painful peripheral neuritis, that may sometimes be irreversible. The drug is carcinogenic in rats and mutagenic in bacteria but there is no evidence that these effects occur in man. Because so many women have been treated with metronidazole, evidence for a minor effect on the subsequent likelihood of developing cancer would be difficult to find.

Metronidazole is cleared by hepatic oxidation and clearance is impaired in severe hepatic damage. Cumulation occurs in hepatic encephalopathy and may contribute to the symptoms. Warfarin levels may be increased.

Resistance in anaerobic flora is exceedingly rare but may be selected in the faeces of patients on intensive care receiving the drug for a very prolonged period.

ANTIFUNGAL AGENTS

The commonest fungal infections involve the skin and nails. *Candida albicans* infects the mucous membranes. Some respiratory organisms excite hypersensitivity classically of the Arthus type (e.g. bronchopulmonary aspergillosis). Fungi may invade and cause systemic granulomatous disease or fungaemia with meningitis.

Invasive fungal infections of man are relatively rare. Certain fungi have a propensity to invade (e.g. *Histoplasma capsulatum* and *Coccidioides imitis*) but these are rarely seen in temperate latitudes. More importantly, immunosuppressed patients may develop invasive disease with benign organisms including *Candida* spp. *Cryptococcus neoformans* and *Aspergillus* spp. or *Mucor* spp. Virtually any fungus may invade the severely immunosuppressed including those with AIDS and transplants.

Control of fungal infections seems to require intact antibody production (deficient in patients with cryptococcal meningitis), cell-mediated immunity and macrophage function (deficient in AIDS) and neutrophils (deficient in neutropenic patients susceptible to *Aspergillus* infections).

Invasive disease is best managed using amphotericin B, which is toxic, or the newer azole agents which are less so. Flucytosine is active against *Candida*, and is a useful adjuvant to amphotericin treatment. Antibacterial agents usually have no activity. Problems in therapy of fungal infections include serious difficulties with the diagnosis of deep infection, toxicity of systemic regimens and the need for long-term treatment of nailbed infections. Problems with drug development include difficulties performing *in vitro* sensitivity tests and performing critical controlled trials to establish efficacy.

Polyenes

These constitute a very large naturally occurring complex of macrocyclic antibiotics that act by interfering with the cholesterol metabolism of the fungal cell membrane. The large ring contains, on one side, a series of unsaturated bonds and on the other a series of hydroxyl groups. Thus one side is hydrophilic and the other hydrophobic. Fungi, but not yeasts, contain a chitinous outer cell wall that may prevent access of the antifungal and will prevent rapid dissolution of the mould when the membrane is damaged. The cause of fungal death is not clearly understood but is presumed to arise from the loss of vital nutrients from the cell.

The main problem in the clinical use of polyenes is not in their activity, which is generally satisfactory, but in their toxicity. Nystatin is not soluble and is too toxic to be given systemically. Only amphotericin B is acceptable but in the face of consistent effects on tubular function.

Nystatin

Nystatin was the original polyene antifungal discovered in 1950. It is not soluble so is presented as pessaries or suspension. It is useful for oral and gastrointestinal candidiasis and may form part of a regimen for selective digestive decontamination. Topical nystatin was for many years the mainstay of treatment of vaginal thrush.

Amphotericin B

This is one of two polyenes derived from *Streptomyces nodosus*. It has a broad spectrum against yeasts and filamentous fungi. Although early studies suggested that large oral doses of amphotericin (and nystatin) had some effect on systemic disease, the drugs are regarded as insufficiently absorbed from the gastrointestinal tract and amphotericin must be given intravenously to systemically infected patients.

Dose is limited by consistent renal toxicity to 1.2 mg/kg/day. This achieves blood levels of between 0.5 and 3.5 mg/l and such levels are maintained in the blood for 24 h. A slow elimination half-life suggests that alternate day treatment ought to be satisfactory. Amphotericin methyl ester is better absorbed but may cause ototoxicity, so it has not been developed. The most recent advance in formulation has been the incorporation of amphotericin B into liposomes. Larger doses can be given with less fear of renal toxicity – indeed tubular damage and raised creatinine levels return to normal when conventional amphotericin B is switched to the liposomal form in higher dosage. There are anxieties about the bioavailability of liposomal amphotericin B. Although ideal for liver infection, it is less certain whether this formulation is as effective against pulmonary fungus as the conventional drug. Liposomal amphotericin B is less effective than the parent compound against oral thrush.

The drug is given as ascending doses to the maximum over 3–4 days. Fever, nausea and thrombophlebitis are common. Corticosteroids and opiates (e.g. pethidine) given shortly before the infusion may reduce toxicity. Creatinine levels rise and patients become hypokalaemic. When prolonged treatment is anticipated, alternate day dosing should be adopted so that the patient has the best chance of cure before receiving the maximum recommended total dose of 2–3 g.

Azoles

Development of clotrimazole and micronazole, which were useful for topical treatment, resulted in the discovery of ketoconazole and more recently fluconazole and itraconazole, which are well tolerated and orally active in systemic mycoses. Ketoconazole was associated with idiosyncratic hepatic necrosis so has fallen out of favour in preference to the newer agents, except for specific syndromes such as chronic mucocutaneous candidiasis which reflects a T-cell defect. A topical formulation is also useful against pityrosporum yeasts thought to be aetiological agents in the seborrheic dermatitis of AIDS.

Itraconazole and fluconazole

These are triazole antifungal agents initially introduced for the treatment of superficial infections but also proving extremely effective in deep and life-threatening infection. Both are bioavailable orally. Both are active against yeasts but itraconazole is also active against common skin dermatophytes causing tinea and against some *Aspergillus* spp. *Candida glabrata* is often resistant to fluconazole.

Itraconazole is lipophilic and absorbed better with food, but in individuals the peak serum levels are rather variable. Peak blood levels are slowly achieved and low (200-mg dose gives 0.3 mg/l), but there is some accumulation (to 0.5 mg/l) on repeated dosing, the half-life being >20 h. The drug is concentrated in tissues but not in CSF. Itraconazole suspension is much better absorbed.

Fluconazole is more consistently absorbed than itraconazole resulting in concentrations of 1 mg/l after 50 mg, levels not affected by the presence or absence of food in the stomach. The half-life is 24 h. Ketoconazole and itraconazole are virtually all protein bound but only 12% fluconazole is bound. Fluconazole penetrates the CSF moderately well, perhaps better in those with cryptococcal meningitis.

Uniquely, fluconazole is excreted in the urine, so dose modification is needed in renal failure. There were early fears for the safety of azoles following the occasional severe hepatotoxicity in those treated with systemic ketoconazole. However, this does not seem to be a problem with miconazole, fluconazole or itraconazole.

Fluconazole is a useful alternative to amphotericin (usually given with flucytosine) in the treatment of cryptococcal meningitis in AIDS patients. However, patients on maintenance therapy with fluconazole may develop recrudescent infections either because of a decrease in perfusion across the blood–brain barrier or because of poor compliance. It is clear that this type of failure is sometimes due to drug resistance.

5-Fluorocytosine (flucytosine)

In practice, flucytosine is only active against yeasts. It is therefore useful in the treatment of systemic candidiasis and cryptococcosis. Resistance develops rapidly, so that unless a very short course of treatment is envisaged, it should be combined with amphotericin. Combinations with azoles (and indeed polyenes with azoles) are possibly antagonistic *in vitro*. Flucytosine is converted into 5-fluorouracil (5-FU) and uptake is proportional to candicidal activity. 5-FU is incorporated into DNA interfering with protein synthesis. The MIC for *Cryptococcus neoformans* is up to 4 mg/l and MBC up to 16 mg/l. Resistance in *Cryptococcus* and *Candida* is not uncommon.

Large doses are required to achieve optimal peak serum levels of 75 mg/l and troughs of 35 mg/l. Serum monitoring is required and dose interval modified according to the degree of renal failure.

Toxicity resembles those of other antimetabolites and includes bone marrow suppression, diarrhoea and abnormal liver function tests.

ANTIVIRAL AGENTS

Compared with the enormous number of antibacterial drugs, there are relatively few antiviral agents available. This is despite an enormous amount of research in the pursuit of active molecules, not the least a cure for the common cold. Viral agents reproduce by employing host cell nucleic acid and protein synthetic mechanisms. It is likely, therefore, that antiviral agents that inhibit metabolic steps in viral synthesis are likely to be toxic to the host. Most antiviral agents have been found by testing new compounds (either any novel molecule or those derived from known active agents) in cell culture systems challenged with appropriate viruses. It is conventional to test the concentration of the agent that will kill the cells as well as the antiviral activity, in order to assess the therapeutic ratio.

Nucleoside analogues and related compounds

A very wide range of drugs has been tested. The first in general use against herpes simplex and varicella zoster (idoxuridine) was effective topically in the eye and on skin lesions if combined with dimethylsulphoxide (which enhanced cutaneous penetration), but was too toxic to be given systemically. Trifluorothymidine is also a potent antiherpetic agent used in eye disease but acyclovir topically is now the preferred drug. Adenine arabinoside was established in excellent controlled trials as effective in biopsy-proven herpes simplex encephalitis. As monophosphate, it also has activity in chronic hepatitis B virus infection. It is toxic to the bone marrow and causes peripheral neuropathy. Cytosine arabinoside is one of the most potent antiherpetic agents available but it is considered too toxic for this indication. It is used as an antimetabolite in the management of neoplasia but also rather specifically for the treatment of polyomavirus related progressive multifocal leucoencephalopathy.

Acyclovir

This modified guanosine molecule lacking the complete cyclic sugar ring was found by serendipity to be active against herpes simplex virus in tissue culture. It is not active until phosphorylated by herpes simplex thymidine kinase within infected cells. It then inhibits virus DNA polymerase and acts as a DNA chain terminator. Some herpes virus mutants lack the thymidine kinase enzyme necessary for phosphorylation, and these are resistant to the drug. In practice, little clinical resistance has emerged. This may be because most clinical disease arises from reactivation of herpes viruses latent in sensory ganglia. Acyclovir is active though much less so against varicella-zoster virus.

Acyclovir is only 20% bioavailable when given orally. Very large oral doses are therefore necessary to achieve therapeutic levels against varicella zoster. For therapy in hospital, it is conventional to give the drug by slow intravenous infusion. Rapid injection in a dehydrated patient leads to precipitation of the drug in the renal tubules leading to transitory renal impairment. The drug is toxic locally if the infusion extravasates. Minor reversible side-effects include central nervous system disturbance, nausea, occasional and unpredictable bone marrow suppression and changes in liver enzymes.

The drug is effective topically in herpes simplex corneal ulceration but there is considerable doubt about topical therapy in cutaneous infections. Oral acyclovir is very effective in preventing recurrences of genital herpes simplex but this does not affect latency. A course of 1 month's treatment does not affect subsequent likelihood of getting recurrences. Some patients are therefore on long-term prophylactic therapy and, so far, no untoward effects have been demonstrated. Oral prophylaxis is also useful for preventing shingles (herpes zoster) in Hodgkin's disease and bone marrow transplant recipients.

Acyclovir reduces the severity and length of illness in early shingles and severe chicken pox particularly in immunocompromised patients but only if the drug is given early. Where possible, intravenous administration should be used. Acyclovir is also active against Epstein–Barr virus but has no effect on the course of glandular fever.

Recent additions to the formulary include valaciclovir, the L-valyl ester of aciclovir, a prodrug with much better absorption, and famciclovir, a prodrug of penciclovir which is another guanine analogue.

Ganciclovir

This close relative of acyclovir is more active against cytomegalovirus. It is phosphorylated by mammalian thymidine kinase and is therefore more toxic than acyclovir. Cytomegalovirus is a very common infection in healthy subjects who do not often manifest any disease: a glandular fever syndrome occasionally occurs. However, immunosuppressed patients do get severe ulcerative disease of mucous membranes, hepatitis or retinitis. This is a particular problem in patients with advanced AIDS and it is in this group that ganciclovir has found a major indication.

Zidovudine

The drug inhibits the DNA polymerase of human immunodeficiency virus (HIV). This enzyme is essential for the conversion of the single strand of RNA – the form in which the virus exists outside cells – into double-stranded DNA which will be incorporated into host cell chromosomes. It is 50–70% bioavailable orally, crosses the blood–brain barrier and has a plasma half-life of about 1 h. The drug is metabolized intracellularly and in the liver to glucuronide. It is excreted in the urine partly as drug and partly as metabolite.

Zidovudine is used for the treatment of AIDS and has been shown to delay death and reduce the risk of opportunistic infections. The use of the drug for asymptomatic HIV-infected individuals is controversial. There is some evidence for the delay in progression of disease but it is uncertain whether this treatment results in prolongation of life. One major anxiety is the selection of zidovudine-resistant virus in the patient under treatment. The clinical implication of this observation is not yet clear. Combination with another nucleoside analogue di-deoxyinosine prolongs disease-free survival.

Zidovudine is toxic to the bone marrow, resulting in consistent falls in haemoglobin concentrations and macrocytosis. Blood transfusion may be necessary. General side-effects of nausea, malaise and myalgia led to discontinuation of the drug in 15% of healthy subjects given the drug after needlestick accidents. Nail discoloration may occur. Transient alterations in liver function tests may occur but it is not certain whether these are due to the drug or intercurrent illness.

Ribavirin

Ribavirin is a broad-spectrum agent active against many RNA and DNA viruses *in vitro*. In volunteer studies, inhaled ribavirin has activity against experimental influenza and respiratory syncytial virus (RSV) infections. Its main indication appears to be in the management of severe RSV bronchiolitis in infants. For this indication, the drug is administered by aerosol from a special nebulizer. Given in large doses in this way, the drug is remarkably free of toxic effects.

Systemic ribavirin may be used in Lassa fever.

Amantadine

During tests for this drug in the prophylaxis of influenza in elderly subjects, it was noted in some patients that the symptoms of Parkinsonism were markedly improved. Amantadine was then developed for this indication (see Chapter 23). However, it does also have very good activity against influenza A, particularly in the prophylaxis of disease in institutions early on in an outbreak but also reducing the symptoms in those with early disease. Given in doses of 100 mg or 200 mg per day, the risk of symptomatic infection is reduced by 60–80%.

Amantadine inhibits uncoating of the RNA virus in the cytoplasm of the infected cell. It is well absorbed given orally, achieves high concentrations in respiratory secretions and is excreted through the kidneys. Side-effects, in particular, on the central nervous system (irritability, insomnia, blurred vision and convulsions) gave the drug a poor reputation in early days. The lower dose of 100 mg per day is very well tolerated.

Interferons

Several interferon preparations are available for therapeutic use. These include natural and recombinant α-interferons and recombinant γ-interferons. α-Interferon is a mixture of several closely related proteins derived from buffy coat leucocytes for transfusion, or from continuous lymphoblastoid cell lines; β-interferon is from fibroblasts and γ-interferon is from T-lymphocytes. The latter is induced by antigen or mitogen, the former two varieties by viruses or dsRNA. Any variety may be made by recombinant DNA technology.

Despite a vast amount of work in many fields, interferons seem only to be indicated for a small number of chronic virus infections (e.g. hepatitis B virus and papillomavirus) and certain sensitive tumours (e.g. hairy cell leukaemia, other myeloproliferative diseases and AIDS-associated Kaposi sarcoma). γ-Interferon is effective in reducing the infective complications of chronic granulomatous disease. Although α- and β-interferon were shown to be active in several herpes virus infections, treatment of these is usually by acyclovir. Synergy between acyclovir (and other nucleoside analogues) and α-interferon was shown in herpes simplex keratitis. This approach has not been pursued.

For the treatment of chronic hepatitis B virus infection, interferon is given im or sc at a dose of 3–10 million units either daily or three times per week. This treatment is associated with fever and influenza-like symptoms. After repeated doses, the patient may develop fatigue, malaise and myalgia.

Some patients may develop binding or even neutralizing antibody to rDNA-derived interferon and even to components of the natural interferon preparation. When this occurs it is usually possible to find another preparation that is active.

A response in terms of significant and permanent reduction of viral replication is noted in 30–40% of patients, and is marked by a rise in hepatic transaminases which should have occurred with 3 months of starting treatment.

USE OF ANTIBIOTICS IN ICU

Most patients in the ICU will be treated empirically with antibiotics for presumed and unidentified infections. Rarely will the identity of an infecting organism be known at this time. The exceptions are patients admitted with severe community-acquired infections such as pneumonia, meningitis or endocarditis. In these conditions, there are clear antibiotic choices to be made, and although problems may arise with unusual or resistant organisms, these can be resolved with microbiological help.

Most patients are in the ICU recovering from some iatrogenic insult. Many are ventilated and thereby have a compromised respiratory tract susceptible to nosocomial infection. Abnormal colonization of the intubated respiratory tract and catheterized bladder are inevitable. Most intravenous lines eventually become colonized with coagulase negative staphylococci. Abdominal sepis with multiple organisms will often precipitate ICU admission. Use of any antibiotic will select for resistance. Decisions as to whether to treat a patient empirically must be based on the suspicion of sepsis (principally manifesting as fever, leucocytosis and hypotension) and knowledge of the likely site and source, the likely organism and the local resistance pattern. A strict policy for empirical therapy should be followed.

The choice of antibiotic will vary between units, depending on local resistance patterns and personal experience of antibiotics. Regimens for supposed Gram-negative sepsis could either be monotherapy with an aminoglycoside, β-lactam or fluoroquinolone. Each of these would be bactericidal but better killing would theoretically be achieved by the combination of the aminoglycoside with either the β-lactam or the fluoroquinolone. For good measure, it is usual to add an anti-anaerobic agent such as metronidazole, but this is unnecessary if the β-lactam chosen is a carbapenem or a β-lactam/β-lactamase inhibitor combination which have excellent anti-anaerobe activity. The β-lactam choice to cover the possibility of coliform or pseudomonal infection will be a ureidopenicillin (e.g. piperacillin) or an advanced cephalosporin (e.g. ceftazidime) or a carbapenem (e.g. imipenem). There is no hard evidence that one is better than another in the specific situation exhibited by an individual patient. For respiratory infections (fever, increased purulent respiratory secretions with chest X-ray changes), empirical therapy is usually the best that can be offered and microbiological results on sputum are usually noncontributory or at worst misleading. *Pseudomonas* spp. or coliform colonization of the upper respiratory tract may be a pointer but it is exceedingly difficult to prove their role in the pathogenesis of pneumonia.

Rationalization of antibiotic use after a period of empirical therapy requires more deliberation than that required to start the antibiotics. There is an irresistible temptation to continue antibiotics for 'a little longer' just in case infection is lurking somewhere. Strangely, stopping antibiotics does not appear to be very dangerous: certainly if the patient shows no sign of recovery from the presumed sepsis, then the antibiotics which were chosen are inappropriate either because the organisms are resistant, or because there is no infection or because there is a deep-seated abscess that requires draining. Stopping antibiotics, then taking further microbiological cultures is the best approach.

Persistence with antibiotics unnecessarily in chronically ventilated patients will inevitably result in colonization with resistant organisms. These will arise by mutation or be introduced on the hands of the medical staff from other patients or from the environment. Changing the antibiotics in response to this new flora will simply result in colonization by more and more troublesome organisms. Alternatively, constitutively resistant endogenous flora such as *Candida albicans* will appear in the mouth, groin, urine and on intravenous lines.

LABORATORY MONITORING OF ANTIMICROBIALS

Several drugs can and should be assayed regularly in the laboratory to check that sufficient drug is being administered for therapeutic activity or that toxic levels are not reached. The most obvious example is the aminoglycosides where auditory–vestibular or renal toxicity are less likely to occur if serum levels are strictly monitored. In the ICU, retention of an aminoglycoside may be the first indication of renal failure and may be detected before a rise in creatinine. If a drug is started in the ICU in an unconscious patient, the potential long-term side-effects must be explained to the relatives. Recent case histories suggest that compensation may be due to a patient with long-term sequelae from a drug started while they were unconscious.

TABLE 34.2 Representative concentrations in serum of antimicrobial agents

	CONCENTRATION	
	TROUGH (mg/l)	PEAK (mg/l)
Aminoglycosides		
Gentamicin	< 2	4–8
Amikacin	< 5	15–25
Netilmicin	< 2	5–12
Tobramycin	< 2.5	4–8
Streptomycin	< 3	25
Others		
Vancomycin	5–10	18–26
Teicoplanin	10–20	20–40
Sulphamethoxazole	NE	200
Fluconazole	15	25
5-Fluorocytosine (flucytosine)	NE	30–80
Ciprofloxacin	1–2	3–5
Chloramphenicol	5–10	25

All peak levels should be taken 1 h after the dose except for vancomycin (2 h after starting the infusion) and chloramphenicol (2 h after dose). The high concentration of sulphamethoxazole supports the use of cotrimoxazole in *Pneumocystic carinii* pneumonia. Chloramphenicol is only measured in babies under 6 months of age because of the risk of toxicity in this age group.
NE, trough not relevant.

Table 34.2 gives suggested serum levels which may vary from laboratory to laboratory. Assuming that a reasonable dose has been started depending on the patient's body mass, a high trough level suggests decreased excretion and indicates prolongation of the interval between doses. A high peak suggests that each dose is too large.

Antibiotics administered to patients with chronic ambulatory peritoneal dialysis are often given into the peritoneum directly by incorporation into the bags of dialysate (Table 34.3). This is an efficient method of treatment and is surprisingly not associated with much overt toxicity even though toxic drugs are recommended, the antibiotics equilibrate with the serum and the patients have complete renal failure. The choice of antibiotic is guided by culture results but blind treatment of possible peritonitis is often started with vancomycin and gentamicin.

TABLE 34.3 Suggested concentrations of antibiotics (mg/l) for incorporation into peritoneal dialysis fluid. All are stable in fluid for 24 h or more

Ampicillin	125	Amikacin	25
Azlocillin	250	Cefuroxime	125
Gentamicin	4–8	Ceftazidime	125
Tobramycin	4–8	Vancomycin	25
Netilmicin	4–8		

ANTIBIOTIC PROPHYLAXIS

Surgical antibiotic prophylaxis

The anaesthetist may be asked by the surgeon to administer antibiotics during the course of an operation. This situation will usually arise when the surgeon encounters infection unexpectedly or has delayed treatment so that intraoperative specimens can be taken for culture. It behoves the anaesthetist, therefore, to make sure that the patient is not allergic to any antibiotics before the anaesthetic, and to ensure that adequate specimens have been taken for microbiological examination. Intravenous antibiotic should then be given to prevent the severe sequelae of bacteraemia. This is technically not prophylaxis but treatment guided towards the most likely infecting organism.

Surgical operations predispose the patient to wound sepsis, bacteraemia (if the surgical field is heavily contaminated), to intravenous and bladder catheter infections and to pulmonary atelectasis (particularly if the patient has a viral respiratory infection at the time of surgery).

Prevention of postsurgical sepsis is achieved by providing a properly ventilated operating theatre, using sterile instruments, proper skin preparation of the patient and the hygiene, discipline and operating technique of the surgical team.

The principles of antibiotic prophylaxis are as follows:

- The operation should be attended by such a risk that giving antibiotics will significantly reduce that risk. For example, there is no point in giving antibiotics before uterine curettage because such patients almost never develop infection. There is, however, excellent justification for giving antibiotic prophylaxis before gut or vaginal surgery.
- The antibiotic should be active against the organisms likely to cause infection.
- The antibiotic should be present in high concentrations in the tissue and the serum at the time of surgery. Pharmacokinetic principles suggest that the first dose should be given at an appropriate interval before the operation and the second dose should be given intraoperatively if the operation is prolonged. Intravenous administration of prophylactic antibiotics at induction of anaesthesia is ideal.
- The prophylaxis should not be continued unless infection was encountered.

Most trials of antibiotic prophylaxis are able to show benefit over placebo but then fail to demonstrate superiority of one regimen over another because insufficient patients are entered and insensitive tests are used to measure outcomes. The measurement of infection is only achieved by using a realistic scoring system that encompasses all aspects of the pathology and morbidity of the infection. This requires dedicated staff and is extremely time consuming and expensive to accomplish.

An important principle of routine prophylaxis is that large numbers of patients will receive unnecessary antibiotics. Thus if abdominal hysterectomy results in an abdominal wound infection rate of 16%, reduced to 8% by appropriate prophylaxis, 92 out of every 100 women so treated will receive unnecessary antibiotics and, of these, eight will get infection despite prophylaxis. The implications for drug toxicity, allergy, cost and impact on the environmental flora are immense. These must be balanced against the beneficial effect on the eight who were prevented from getting wound sepsis.

Selective digestive decontamination

The troublesome organisms most likely to cause sepsis in intensive care are *Pseudomonas* and coliforms. Colonization of the upper respiratory tract precedes pneumonia which may be life-threatening. It is likely that organisms find their way into the respiratory tract from the oropharynx where colonization is likely in recumbent patients on antacids and on broad-spectrum antibiotics. Coliforms are not normally found in the mouth of healthy subjects but will appear within a few days of starting a broad-spectrum antibiotic and will take weeks to disappear when the antibiotic is stopped. The aim of selective digestive decontamination (SDD), a special form of antibiotic prophylaxis, is to reduce colonization of the upper respiratory tract by using oral non-absorbable antibiotics and antifungals. The latter prevent the overgrowth of *Candida*. An important principle is that antibiotics should not interfere with the anaerobic gut flora which is in itself theoretically protective. Aminoglycosides are ideal in this respect but care should be taken because of the risk of auditory–vestibular toxicity. An appropriate regimen would be FRACON (neomycin, colistin and nystatin). Several well-conducted trials of SDD in ICU patients have been performed. Some have incorporated routine administration of an injectable cephalosporin for 2 days as part of the primary prevention of Gram-negative sepsis but this rather goes against the overall concept. Interestingly, in one trial there was a real increase in the number of patients with documented anaerobic bacteraemia when this regimen was used. The trials have shown reduction in infection morbidity particularly in those with mid-range Apache II scores. This group is presumed to be the most vulnerable to a bad outcome if infected, more seriously ill patients having a poor prognosis anyway and less ill patients being far less likely to develop Gram-negative pneumonia. The apparent advantage of these regimens has to be balanced against considerable cost.

ADJUVANT THERAPY

Septic shock arises as a result of a cascade reaction of cytokines resulting in loss of the integrity of the vascular endothelium and arteriolar dilatation. There is inability to maintain blood pressure by colloid replacement and by inotropic support; indeed, most patients are in a high-output state. Fluid leakage from the vascular compartment will particularly compromise respiratory function. The cascade is set off by a number of rather different stimuli but the most potent stimulus of all is lipopolysaccharide of Gram-negative organisms, also known as endotoxin. Mediators involved early in the cascade are tumour necrosis factor (TNF), interleukins-1 and -6 and endothelin but the true relationship between these is not known. It is proposed that prevention of cascade activation can be achieved by giving antibody to one or more early components. To this end a number of candidate molecules have been made and tested in animal models and man. Recently, three trials of antibodies to the core of endotoxin have been published. The first is a polyclonal antibody, the second a murine monoclonal antibody and finally a humanized monoclonal antibody. There is a considerable controversy about the applicability of these molecules in clinical practice. Theoretically, if septic shock is established, switching off the stimulus should not affect the cascade. Administration of antibody before shock in those who might be susceptible (e.g. arbitrarily to all patients requiring intensive care for more than 3 days) has not been tested.

However, preliminary trial results suggest that, although the endotoxin monoclonal antibodies do not affect 28-day mortality in the whole group with sepsis when compared with placebo, subsets of individuals seem to do rather better. The problem is that different subsets were identified between the effects of two monoclonal antibodies tested in almost identical circumstances. Both had an effect in those with subsequently proven Gram-negative bacteraemia. With one antibody, the group that did well had established shock; with the other, the group that did not have established shock did better. The problem with retrospective subset analysis is that statistically significant observations may occur at random. Furthermore, to be clinically useful it is necessary to identify the subset *before treatment* in order to make optimal use of these drugs. At present, there is no simple way to do this. The antibodies are well tolerated with no side-effects and do not appear to have any pharmacological action. There would be a reluctance to give a murine antibody on more than one occasion because of the risk of serum sickness. It is not known whether repeated doses of a 'humanized' antibody would be a risk for subsequent autoimmune disease. We may see a proliferation of such molecules – an antibody to TNF is already under study. Unless a very profound effect on survival is observed and is repeatable in several studies, it will be agonizingly difficult to make decisions in ICU as to whether and when to give these exciting but expensive compounds.

THE FUTURE

In the last 50 years man has succeeded in harvesting the antimicrobial potential of micro-organisms, developing a range of drugs with different sites of action, and chemically modifying the molecules to enhance activity and overcome resistance problems. In parallel, invasive medicine has increased and with it the risk of nosocomial infection. The use of antibiotics has led to the emergence of antibiotic resistance in many organisms which is now at a level that seriously threatens the value of antibiotics in the management of diseases which were successfully treated. It is possible to envisage a time when there are no candidates available for the satisfactory treatment of typhoid fever when the organism is resistant to ampicillin, chloramphenicol, co-trimoxazole and ciprofloxacin. In ICU, we can easily select for *Pesudomonas* spp. that are resistant to *every* appropriate antibiotic in the formulary. The emergence of untreatable *Enterococcus faecium* is a very real threat.

There is no doubt that resistance will be a prime reason to develop new and more powerful antibiotics but these will inevitably be more expensive than the generation that preceded them. Antibiotics do save lives but they are used too freely and a very high proportion of patients are treated unnecessarily or inappropriately. Governments have addressed (rather ineffectually) the issue of antibiotics selecting for resistant organisms by widespread use in farming. Yet doctors seem to be quite unable to control the abuse of antibiotics in clinical practice.

Antibiotic policies are in place in most institutions. A restricted list of antibiotics in the pharmacy prevents much misuse. Surveys of antibiotic prescriptions by pharmacists and microbiologists may reveal strange combinations, non-recommended dose regimens and ensure drug monitoring where necessary.

Areas with high antibiotic use should write didactic policies for prophylaxis or treatment. Finally, on-going rationalisation, case reviews, reviews of the application of antibiotics and alternative therapies and infection prevention strategies are important components of continuing postgraudate learning. Staff in ICU should have a close working relationship with the clinical microbiologist.

REFERENCES

1 Eagle H. Musselman AD. The rate of bactericidal activity in vitro as a function of its concentration and its paradoxically reduced activity at high concentrations against certain organisms. *Journal of Experimental Medicine* 1948; **88:** 99–131.

2 Nicolau DP, Freeman CD, Belliveau PP, Nightingale CH, Ross JW, Quintiliani R. Experience with a once-daily aminoglycoside program administered to 2,184 adult

patients. *Antimicrobial Agents and Chemotherapy* 1995; **39**: 650–5.

FURTHER READING

General reading and reference

Greenwood D. *Antimicrobial chemotherapy* 3rd edn. Oxford: Oxford University Press, 1995.

Kucers A, Bennett NMcK. *The use of antibiotics* 4th edn. Heinemann, 1987.

Lambert HP, O'Grady FW. *Antibiotic and chemotherapy* 6th edn. Edinburgh: Churchill Livingstone, 1992.

New drugs

Felmingham DF. Antibiotic resistance: Do we need new therapeutic approaches? *Chest* 1995; **108**: 70S–8S.

Finch RG, Neu H, DeClercq E. Antimicrobial agents. *Current Opinions in Infectious Diseases* 1989; **2**: 347–423.

Mehtar S, Drabu YJ, Blakemore PH. The in vitro activity of piperacillin/tazobactum, ciprofloxacin, ceftazidime and imipenem against multiple resistant Gram-negative bacteria. *Journal of Antimicrobial Chemotherapy* 1990; **25**: 915–19.

Rolan P. Pharmacokinetics of new antiherpetic agents. *Clinical Pharmacokinetics* 1995; **29**: 333–40.

Rubenstein E(ed). Second International Symposium on New Quinolones. *Reviews of Infectious Disease* 1989; **11**: S897–S1410.

Intensive care

Bergamini TM, Polk HC Jr. The importance of tissue antibiotic activity in the prevention of operative wound infection. *Journal of Antimicrobial Chemotherapy* 1989; **23**: 301–13.

Cotterill S. Antimicrobial prescibing in patients on haemofiltration. *Journal of Antimicrobial Chemotherapy* 1995; **36**: 773–80.

DiNubile MJ. Treatment of endocarditis caused by relatively resistant non-enterococcal: Is penicillin enough? *Reviews of Infectious Disease* 1990; **12**: 112–17.

Gruneberg RN, Wilson APR. Anti-infective trreatment in intensive care: the role of glycopeptides. *Intensive Care Medicine* 1994; **20**: S17–S22.

Wilson APR, Ridgway GL. Intensive therapy units. In: Taylor EW ed. *Infection in surgical practice.* Oxford: Oxford University Press, 1992; 292–9.

35

Chemotherapy of Neoplastic Disease

HM Earl

INTRODUCTION

This chapter deals with commonly administered chemotherapeutic agents in terms of pharmacokinetics, metabolism and common toxicities, and in the second section, attempts to make this as relevant as possible to the practising anaesthetist. Clearly this cannot be a comprehensive guide, but common problems that have clinical relevance for the anaesthetist involved in intra-, postoperative or intensive care of cancer patients have been included. It is important that anaesthetists are aware of the possible side-effects associated with cancer chemotherapy prior to anaesthetic induction in cancer patients requiring surgery. They need information on the chemotherapy that the patient has received, and the interval since the last course so that an assessment can be made of the potential problems during and after anaesthesia. Knowledge of the side-effects and interactions of the more commonly used chemotherapeutic agents will allow the anaesthetist to carry out a rational preoperative assessment, which will lead to safe and effective intra- and postoperative management of the cancer patient.

CHEMOTHERAPEUTIC AGENTS USED IN THE TREATMENT OF NEOPLASTIC DISEASE

Plant alkaloids

These chemotherapeutic drugs were first developed from the periwinkle plant, *Catharanthus roseus* (or *Vinca rosea*). The commonly used plant alkaloids include vincristine, vinblastine, VP-16 and VM-26. These drugs bind to tubulin, a constituent protein of the microtubules, the assembly and function of which during metaphase are essential for mitotic cell division. Exposure of the cell to plant alkaloids produces rapid disappearance of microtubules and failure of cell division. Epipodophyllotoxins bind to one site of tubulin, while the other vinca aklaloids bind to another. Microtubules are involved in axonal transport, and vinca alkaloids have predictable neurotoxicity. They also inhibit synthesis of DNA and RNA by unknown mechanisms. Resistance to vinca alkaloids may develop from mutations in tubulin, and pleiotropic drug resistance, with amplification of P-170 membrane glycoprotein, which appears to function as an efflux channel and remove vinca alkaloids and other natural products from cells.

Vincristine is administered intravenously at a dose of 1.5 mg/m^2 (maximum 2 mg) and can be repeated weekly in some instances. After iv injection the drug has three phases of elimination from the plasma, with half-lives of 4 min, 1 h and 16 h. The vincristine remains tissue bound for many days and most of the drug is still in the body 6 days later, and is then metabolized in the liver and excreted in the bile. In patients with impaired hepatic function there is an increased incidence of toxic reactions. The main side-effects are neurological with peripheral sensory and motor neuropathy, loss of reflexes, and autonomic neuropathy which may produce a paralytic ileus. Myelosuppression is mild, and indeed the drug may produce thrombocytosis by endoreduplication in megakaryocytes. Alopecia is unknown. A syndrome of inappropriate antidiuretic hormone (ADH) secretion has been occasionally reported.

Vinblastine has very similar pharmacokinetics and excretion to vincristine, but its major metabolite deacetylvinblastine is more active on a weight basis than the parent compound. Vinblastine is more myelosuppressive and less neurotoxic than vincristine. Doses of 6 mg/m^2 iv can be given weekly as a single agent. Vindesine is a newly introduced semisynthetic plant alkaloid that has similar pharmacokinetics to the other vinca alkaloids and causes both myelosuppression and neurotoxicity.

Epipodophyllotoxins

Podophyllotoxin is an extract of the mandrake root, and has been used since Medieval times for the treatment of parasites, warts and poisonings. The glycosidic derivatives in clinical use, VP-16 and VM-26, have important activities in lymphomas, small cell carcinoma of the lung and testicular cancer. Activity is by inhibition of topoisomerase-II and possibly the formation of free-radical derivatives of the parent compound. Resistance may develop through amplification of P-170 glycoprotein, and alterations in formation or repair of strand breaks.

Detailed pharmacokinetic studies of VP-16 have been carried out following both iv and oral administration. Bioavailability by the oral route varies from 30 to 100% and shows both inter- and intrapatient variation. The activity of the drug is schedule dependent as shown by Slevin in clinical studies in small-cell lung cancer.[1] Approximately 45% of the administered dose is excreted in the urine either as the parent compound or a metabolite, and the doses administered should be reduced in renal impairment. Plasma half-life is 6 h. Side-effects include moderate myelosuppression, mild nausea and vomiting, alopecia, mucositis and peripheral neuropathy.

Antitumour antibiotics

Anthracyclines are part of a large group of highly coloured bacterial products, rhodomycins, which have a wide range of biologic activities including antibacterial and antitumour effects. Daunomycin and doxorubicin, the first anthracyclines in clinical use, were produced from the *Streptomyces* species. These agents show exceptionally wide clinical usefulness in leukaemias, lymphomas, carcinomas and sarcomas. They have a planar anthraquinone nucleus attached to an amino-sugar, and over 500 analogues have now been isolated and synthesized. Anthracyclines intercalate in DNA and block DNA replication, and RNA and protein synthesis. However, these effects may happen at drug levels far in excess of those achieved clinically, and the activity of these anthraquinones probably relies more on topoisomerase-II mediated antitumour effects and the formation of drug free-radicals.

The pharmacokinetics of doxorubicin are complex, but its disappearance from plasma fits a three-compartment model with half-lives of 11 min, 3 h and 25–28 h.[2] Renal clearance is minor, and doxorubicin is metabolized in the liver so that drug doses must be modified in the presence of impaired hepatic function. Doxorubicin is administered at doses of 50–75 mg/m^2 by iv bolus injection into the bung of a fast-running drip. It is given every 3 weeks, produces a marked myelosuppressive effect, with complete alopecia, mucositis and cardiomyopathy. Analogues of doxorubicin have been developed in attempts to lessen toxicities while preserving antitumour activity – that is, epirubicin, esorubicin and idarubicin. *Mitoxantrone* does not appear to produce free-radical damage, but actually blocks doxorubicin-induced free-radical injury.[3] It does, however, produce topoisomerase-II-mediated DNA damage.

Mitomycin C is another commonly used antitumour antibiotic. There are at least three reactive centres of this compound: the C1 carbon of the mitosane ring, the quinone ring structure which can form reactive species, and the urethane group which can open to form an alkylating site. Mitomycin C is activated by cytochrome C reductase, xanthine oxidase or cytochrome P-450 reductase, and this metabolic reaction appears to occur in all tissues. Activated drug produces alkylation and cross-linking of DNA,[4] which leads to cell death. Administration is iv, by bolus into a fast-running drip at 6 mg/m^2 every 3 weeks, or 10–12 mg/m^2 every 6 weeks. Metabolism is ubiquitous and drug clearance is rapid. However, renal clearance is minor, and the role of the liver is poorly defined. Primary half-life is 54 min. The drug produces marked myelosuppression that may be delayed and cumulative, leading to leucocyte and platelet nadirs between 4 and 6 weeks. Mitomycin C has been implicated in the production of micro-angiopathic haemolytic anaemia, which was partly responsible for deaths in the adjuvant chemotherapy study of the British Stomach Cancer Group.[5] Mitomycin may produce interstitial pneumonitis and cardiomyopathy.

Actinomycin D is an antitumour antibiotic which was also isolated from the *Streptomyces* species. It is effective in Wilm's tumour, Ewing's sarcoma, embryonal rhabdomyosarcoma and choriocarcinoma. This antibiotic binds to DNA by intercalation, and at low concentrations inhibits RNA synthesis, but at high concentrations inhibits both RNA and DNA synthesis.[6,7] It also produces single strand breaks.[8] Actinomycin is not significantly metabolized and excretion of the unchanged drug occurs in both bile and urine. Plasma clearance is rapid, but is followed by a slow phase of excretion with a plasma half-life of 36 h. Doses of 0.6 mg/m^2 may be given by bolus injection into a fast-running drip, daily for 5 consecutive days every 3–4 weeks. It produces marked myelosuppression, with alopecia and mucositis.

Bleomycin, a commonly used antitumour antibiotic, is a mixture of small molecular weight peptides isolated from the fungus *Streptomyces verticullus*. Bleomycin produces single and double strand breaks in DNA,[9] and produces superoxide or hydroxyl radicals. Bleomycin can be administered by subcutaneous, intramuscular or iv injection, has a two-phase clearance with half-lives of 24 min, and 2–4 h, and is excreted unchanged in the urine. Dose reductions are necessary in patients with impaired renal function. Bleomycin may be injected into pleural or peritoneal spaces to control malignant effusions, and about 50% of the dose will enter the systemic circulation. Bleomycin does not have a significant myelosuppressive effect except in single doses >25 mg/m^2. The most serious toxicity of bleomycin is interstitial pneumonitis which is progressive, cumulative and relates to the total dose given and renal function. A maximum total dose of 300 mg is usually advised. Bleomycin commonly produces fever, rigors, and occasional hypersensitivity reactions that can be prevented with prior use of antihistamines and hydrocortisone. Bleomycin often produces erythema, induration, thickening and peeling of the skin on fingers, palms and extremity joints. Most patients develop hyperpigmentation in skin creases and scars, and also generalized skin darkening.

Alkylating agents

Alkylating agents have the ability to form covalent bonds with nucleic acids, which interfere with the integrity and function of DNA, causing misreading of the DNA code, cross-linking of DNA, and single- and double-strand breaks. Alkylation occurs preferentially at sites of active DNA transcription. The intracellular action of alkylating agents is inhibited by conjugation to glutathione, and increased intracellular glutathione is a general mechanism of resistance to this group of compounds.[10,11]

Cyclophosphamide is an alkylating agent used widely in the treatment of lymphomas, carcinomas and soft tissue sarcomas. Cyclophosphamide is metabolized to 4-OH cyclophosphamide in hepatic microsomes, and is then converted peripherally to aldophosphamide and ultimately to phosphoramide mustard (believed to be the active product) and acrolein. Acrolein is capable of depleting glutathione and causing single strand alkylation of DNA. It is also responsible for the haemorrhagic cystitis which is a complication of cyclophosphamide therapy. Cyclophosphamide is given iv, 500–1500 mg/m^2 every 3 weeks, or daily by mouth in doses of 100 mg/m^2, daily for 2 weeks. Cyclophosphamide has a 90% bioavailability after oral administration. It produces myelosuppression, nausea, vomiting, alopecia, haemorrhagic cystitis at high dose and occasionally the syndrome of inappropriate ADH secretion. Systemic administration of sodium-2-mercapto-ethano sulfarate (Mesna) will bind acrolein in the urine and prevent haemorrhagic cystitis. The half-life of cyclophosphamide is 5.3 h, and that of 4-OH cyclophosphamide is 1.5–6 h but is primarily a function of its rate of production in the liver.[12] In both renal and hepatic failure, the half-life of cyclophosphamide is prolonged with increased myelosuppression.

Ifosfamide is closely related to cyclophosphamide, but more often causes dose-limiting haemorrhagic cystitis. Plasma half-life is 5–6 h, after oral or iv administration and there is 100% oral bioavailability. Ifosfamide produces myelosuppression, alopecia, nausea and vomiting, cystitis and disturbed mental state sometimes progressing to seizures, coma and death. The development of ifosfamide encephalopathy is particularly common in patients with pelvic malignancy, who have a low serum albumin, and impaired renal function. A useful nomogram has been developed in Birmingham[13] to predict the likelihood of ifosfamide encephalopathy in an individual patient.

Melphalan is a phenylalanine derivative that enters cells by active transport, via the high affinity carrier—the 'L' amino acid transport system. After iv administration the drug has a half-life of 1–2 h. Fifteen per cent of the drug is excreted intact in the urine. Bioavailability after oral administration is variable, and food slows the absorption of melphalan considerably. Melphalan produces myelosuppression and alopecia. It has been used at high dose either as a single agent[14] or in combination with other cytotoxics, often followed by autologous bone marrow transplantation.[15] At high dose it produces profound neutropenia and thrombocytopenia, and may also produce severe generalized gastrointestinal mucositis. Because of its short half-life, when used alone in high dose, non-cryopreserved bone marrow can be used. Unfortunately, melphalan appears to be more carcinogenic than cyclophosphamide, and the incidence of acute leukaemia in women with ovarian cancer treated with melphalan, is 93-fold increased compared with an age-matched population.

Chlorambucil is an alkylating agent that has structural similarities to melphalan and is administered orally. Its pharmacokinetics are poorly understood. It produces myelosuppression, and has been implicated in the production of acute myeloid leukaemia (AML)[16] and pulmonary fibrosis.[17]

Cis*(II)platinum diaminedichloride* (*cis*-DDP) is a heavy metal compound, and has been found to be effective in the treatment of testicular tumours, ovarian, bladder and lung cancer. Activated cisplatinum interacts with nucleophilic sites on DNA, RNA or proteins to form bifunctional covalent links analogous to alkylating agents. The consequences of cisplatinum on DNA include changes in DNA conformation and inhibition of DNA synthesis.[18] The formation of cross-links is a slow process that continues for hours after drug exposure and is opposed by enzymatic repair mechanisms that excise and rebuild damaged DNA segments.[19]

Cisplatinum has a high rate of covalent binding to protein. The first phase of clearance of plasma cisplatinum occurs rapidly in the first 2 h after iv injection, but the second phase of excretion is slower because of covalent binding of the drug to serum proteins.[20]

Unbound cisplatinum has a half-life of 30–40 min.[21] By 24 h, 20–75% of cisplatinum is excreted in the urine, and the remainder is bound to tissues or plasma proteins.[22] Excretion is in the urine, by glomerular filtration of unbound platinum complexes, and there is also evidence of tubular reabsorption and secretion.[23] Cisplatinum is given at a dose of 50–100 mg/m^2 every 3 weeks. Initially it was found to be profoundly nephrotoxic, and the pathological findings include coagulative necrosis of the distal tubular epithelium and collecting ducts.[24] There is also a rapid reduction in renal blood flow and glomerular filtration rate which occurs within a few hours, and changes in tubular function including magnesium and potassium loss and excretion of high molecular weight proteins occurs.[25,26] Nausea and vomiting are very severe with cisplatinum chemotherapy, and are an indication for the use of the new 5-HT_3 (5-hydroxytryptamine) antagonists. Myelosuppression is not usually severe. Renal toxicity has been considerably reduced with adequate hydration and diuresis with mannitol and frusemide, but magnesium and potassium loss remains a problem. Peripheral neuropathy and ototoxicity are seen and are discussed below. Cisplatinum analogues have been successfully developed with the aim of reducing renal and neurotoxicity.

Antimetabolites

Methotrexate competitively inhibits dihydrofolate reductase, the enzyme that reduces dihydrofolate to tetrahydrofolate in the presence of NADPH. Tetrahydrofolate is responsible for one-carbon transfer reactions involved in the synthesis of thymidylate, purines, methionine and glycine which leads to inhibition of DNA, RNA and protein synthesis.

Methotrexate can be administered by mouth or by intravenous, intra-arterial or intrathecal injection. At low doses oral absorption is efficient but at high doses less so. Methotrexate is excreted as unchanged drug by the kidney by combined glomerular filtration and active tubular transport.[27] At an acid pH, high levels of methotrexate will crystallize in the renal tubules and produce profound tubular damage. To avoid this the urine is maintained alkaline during the administration of high-dose methotrexate. This is traditionally managed by the administration of oral or iv bicarbonate, but urinary alkalinization can be produced more effectively by acetazolamide.[28] Most of the drug excreted into the bile is reabsorbed. The pharmacokinetics of methotrexate are complex. The plasma disappearance curve is triphasic, with half-lives of 0.75, 3.5 and 27 h. Long-term retention of methotrexate is seen in kidney and liver. The drug may be slowly released from ascites or a pleural effusion which produces a third-space effect. Toxicity from methotrexate depends on the duration of inhibitory levels, so it is important to be aware of the complex pharmacokinetics of the drug. When given at high dose, methotrexate needs to be followed by folinic acid rescue to prevent fatal toxicity, and the dose of rescue is calculated from the plasma methotrexate levels at 24 and 48 h. Unexpected toxicity may be seen after low-dose administration when there is a significant pleural effusion or ascites, and methotrexate is probably best avoided in these circumstances. Toxicity from methotrexate depends on the dose given and the adequacy of folinic acid rescue. With adequate rescue even when given in high dose, there is no bone marrow toxicity. If folinic acid rescue is inadequate, toxicity includes profound myelosuppression, oral and generalized gastrointestinal mucositis, and widespread erythroderma.

6-Mercaptopurine (6-MP) produces inhibition of purine synthesis but the drug inhibits many different reactions depending on the tumour cell type involved. 6-MP is given orally despite incomplete and variable absorption in the gastrointestinal tract. The drug is 20% protein bound, and the half-life in children is 21 min, while in adults it is 47 min. The drug is extensively metabolized and excreted in the urine. Use of the xanthine oxidase inhibitor, allopurinol, to prevent hyperuricaemia and tumour lysis syndrome will also prevent metabolism of 6-MP to one of its inactive metabolites, so if used in conjunction the dose of 6-MP needs to be reduced to one-quarter or one-third of the normal dose. Side-effects include myelosuppression and occasional nausea and vomiting.

5-Fluorouracil (5-FU) is a fluorine-substituted analogue of uracil which inhibits DNA synthesis. The primary mechanism for this effect is through thymidylate synthetase inhibition. It is usually administered intravenously, because gastrointestinal tract absorption is incomplete and unpredictable. 5-FU can also be administered intra-arterially, directly into body cavities, and topically. After iv administration plasma half-life is 10–20 min, and after intracavitary injection 5-FU remains in the cavity for 12 h. 5-FU is metabolized predominantly in the liver, and only 15% is excreted in the urine as unchanged drug. Recently the addition of folinic acid to 5-FU has increased its effectiveness as a single agent. Toxicity includes nausea, vomiting, anorexia and diarrhoea. Myelosuppression can occur manifest as leucopenia, and there may be thinning of the skin, nail changes, photosensitivity and mild alopecia. Very rarely an acute cerebellar syndrome is seen which usually recovers within 6 weeks.

Cytosine arabinoside (Ara-C) inhibits mammalian DNA polymerases and is an S-phase-specific cytotoxic drug. Only 20% is absorbed orally, and so it is routinely administered intravenously or subcutaneously. After iv injection there is a biphasic excretion with half-lives of 12 min and 2 h. About 80% of the administered dose can be recovered in the urine within 24 h, 8% as the parent compound and the rest as metabolites. Entry of this drug into the CSF is reasonably efficient and with constant intravenous infusion CSF levels are about 40% of plasma levels. Ara-C can be given intrathecally and the half-life in the CSF after injection is about 2 h. Toxicities include myelosuppression, nausea, vomiting, and diarrhoea.

CANCER CHEMOTHERAPY AND ANAESTHESIA

Cardiac toxicity

Anthracycline antibiotics are the antineoplastic drugs most frequently associated with cardiotoxicity. Doxorubicin is the most commonly used anthracycline, and produces both acute and delayed effects on the heart. The acute effects are most often reversible, and rarely of clinical significance. Acute rhythm disturbances include atrial and ventricular ectopics, and occasionally supraventricular and ventricular tachycardias. Prolongation of the QT interval, non-specific ST–T wave changes, and T-wave abnormalities have been described immediately following bolus injection of doxorubicin. Rarely myocardial infarction, and life-threatening ventricular dysrhythmias have been documented in adults and children.[29] A case report of peri-operative cardiovascular collapse, 2 months following completion of doxorubicin chemotherapy at a cumulative dose of 460 mg/m^2 has been published.[30] Of more concern is the development of dose-dependent dilated cardiomyopathy which has a mortality rate of 30–70%.[31,32] Maximum cumulative doxorubicin doses of 550 mg/m^2 when given on a 3-weekly basis are advised.[32] Slow infusion of anthracyclines over 24 h, and weekly drug scheduling, have both been shown to protect against the risk of cardiotoxicity.[33] Synergistically cardiotoxic drugs should be avoided in combination with anthracyclines. It has been suggested that patients who have received a dose of greater than 250 mg/m^2 of doxorubicin, and are undergoing general anaesthesia should have a cardiological assessment by ECG, chest x-ray (CXR), Doppler echocardiography and nuclear cardiac scanning if indicated.[29] Anaesthesia is difficult in patients with cumulative cardiotoxicity and has proved fatal on occasion.[29] Perioperative doxorubicin should be avoided if possible.

Pulmonary toxicity

Pulmonary toxicity severe enough to interfere with general anaesthesia may occur with a number of drugs. The commonest are bleomycin, mitomycin C, busulphan, 1,3-bis(2-chloroethyl)-1-nitrosourea (BCNU), chlorambucil, cyclophosphamide, methotrexate and melphalan. Table 35.1 shows different common pulmonary toxicities, the commonest being interstitial pneumonitis and pulmonary fibrosis. Rarer pulmonary toxicity includes pleural effusion reported with methotrexate and interleukin-2 (IL-2),[41,49] pleuritis reported with methotrexate,[50] bronchospasm with IL-2, vindesine and methotrexate,[49–51] pulmonary nodules with bleomycin,[52] pulmonary veno-occlusive disease with carmustine,[54] and bronchiolitis obliterans organizing pneumonia with bleomycin.[55] Table 35.2 shows the incidence of interstitial pneumonitis and pulmonary fibrosis with different cytotoxics. In addition chlorambucil,[58] and cyclophosphamide[59] have been reported to cause this problem in less than 1% of patients treated. Mitomycin-C can cause interstitial pneumonitis and pulmonary fibrosis in 3–12%, and methotrexate may cause a lymphocytic alveolitis (with eosinophilia in 40%) not related to total dose.[41,60] Restrictive ventilatory defects and decrease in carbon monoxide transfer factor (DLCO) are sensitive indicators of interstitial pneumonitis and can be reduced in the presymptomatic phase. Clinical presentations are usually with dyspnoea on exertion and a non-productive cough. Stopping the cytotoxic drug is essential and oral corticosteroids may be helpful in reversing interstitial pneumonitis, particularly that seen with bleomycin, mitomycin C, chlorambucil and methotrexate. It has been suggested that high inspired oxygen concentration may accelerate pulmonary damage caused by bleomycin, so that during anaesthesia inspired oxygen of 30% is advised with monitoring of arterial blood gases.

TABLE 35.1 Pulmonary toxicities associated with cytotoxics

RESPONSE OF LUNG	DRUGS
Interstitial pneumonitis/pulmonary fibrosis	Bleomycin[34] Mitomycin-C[35] Busulphan[36] Carmustine[37] Chlorambucil[38] Cyclophosphamide[39] Melphalan[40] Methotrexate[41]
Hypersensitivity reaction	Bleomycin[42] Methotrexate[41] Procarbazine[43]
Noncardiogenic pulmonary oedema	Methotrexate[44] Cyclophosphamide[45] Ara-C[46] Teniposide[47] Mitomycin-C[48]

TABLE 35.2 Incidence of interstitial pneumonitis/pulmonary fibrosis with cytotoxics

DRUG	% WITH TOXICITY	COMMENT
Bleomycin	5 10	Total dose <450 mg[34] Total dose >450 mg
Busulphan	4	Pathological changes[56] in 46% treated patients
Carmustine	15–23	Dose-dependent risk[57] 50% at dose >1500 mg

Neurotoxicity

Neurotoxicity is a well-recognized feature of cytotoxic chemotherapy. *Vincristine* was one of the first drugs to be shown to commonly produce a peripheral sensory and sometimes motor neuropathy. This toxicity seems to be due to the effect of the drug on axonal transport and has been reported to be progressive during the time of treatment. The most common symptom is glove and stocking parasthesiae and numbness, with problems with fine movements of the hands. The commonest physical finding is diminished or absent deep tendon reflexes which is almost universal among patients on treatment. Vincristine-induced sensory peripheral neuropathies seem to be short lived and recovery usually occurs over a few months after completing treatment.[61] Vincristine-induced motor neuropathies are uncommon, but seem to be less readily reversible. Acute toxicities of vincristine include painful paralytic ileus, and limb and jaw muscle pain. Accidental intrathecal injection of vincristine produces progressive paralysis, coma and death, although vigorous CSF washout via the intraventricular route has recently proved successful in preventing death, and reducing neurological damage in one patient (see below).[62]

Cisplatin is also frequently neurotoxic, producing a peripheral sensory and sometimes motor neuropathy. This drug also produces ototoxicity which appears to be both peripheral and central in nature.[63] Physical signs include diminished or absent deep tendon reflexes and vibration sense impairment, sometimes progressing to a sensory ataxia. An interesting but uncommon symptom is the development of L'Hermitte's sign which suggests damage to the central nervous system. The pathological damage to the peripheral nerves is in the dorsal root ganglion, with destruction of the largest and longest fibres first. A recent study at the Middlesex Hospital shows considerable neurophysiological abnormality in sensory conduction and vibration perception thresholds in adolescents and young adults treated with cisplatinum for bone and soft tissue sarcomas.[61] The degree of neurotoxicity relates to the cumulative dose of cisplatin administered, to the intensity of treatment delivery, and to the age of the patient, neurotoxicity being more common in patients with ovarian cancer than in those with testicular teratomas or osteosarcomas who are much younger. WR2721[64] and an adrenocorticotrophic hormone (ACTH) analogue[65] have both been reported to be successful in preventing or actually reversing neuropathy. Cisplatin does not appear to produce documented autonomic neuropathy. Cisplatin can also produce renal tubular wasting of magnesium and calcium. Marked hypomagnesaemia may produce exaggerated deep tendon reflexes, muscular weakness, tremulousness, peripheral parasthesiae, tetany and personality changes. Hypomagnesaemia may be severe enough to produce generalized seizures.

Ifosfamide may produce encephalopathy with drowsiness, coma, fits and sometimes death. High dose *methotrexate*, particularly when combined with CNS irradiation, as in the treatment of childhood leukaemia may rarely lead to a necrotizing leukoencephalopathy.

Renal toxicity

Renal toxicity may be seen with a number of chemotherapeutic agents. Cisplatin is nephrotoxic and this side-effect may be dose limiting. This agent produces tubular dysfunction with magnesium wasting, hypomagnesaemia and hypokalaemia. The site of the renal tubular defect in these conditions is uncertain, but evidence suggests that renal tubular active transport systems are disrupted. The glomerular filtration rate (GFR) is diminished following cisplatinum chemotherapy. The tubular damage seen with cisplatinum chemotherapy is reversible although it may take several months to resolve, but the decrease in GFR is often permanent. Similar nephrotoxicity is seen with carboplatin although with a much lower frequency than with the parent compound.

High-dose methotrexate may be associated with acute and life-threatening renal toxicity, whose pathogenesis is multiple. Methotrexate is insoluble at an acid pH and if the urine is acidic methotrexate will precipitate in the renal tubules and produce obstruction and damage. Methotrexate seems to have a direct effect on renal tubular cells, altering regeneration of epithelial cells, anion secretory channels, and other metabolic processes which produces a secondary feedback decrease in GFR. Methotrexate seems also to have a direct effect on the afferent blood supply to the glomerulus with a decrease in the GFR.

Mitomycin-C has been reported to produce the haemolytic–uraemic syndrome, and has now been described in over 50 cases.[66] It presents with a microangiopathic haemolytic anaemia, thrombocytopenia and renal failure and is often fatal. The pathophysiology is thought to be vascular endothelial damage. Histopathology of the kidney shows mesangial proliferative glomerulonephritis with partial thickening and splitting of the basement membrane.

Bone marrow toxicity

Bone marrow toxicity is the commonest toxicity seen with antineoplastic chemotherapy. It is almost universal with the notable exceptions of vincristine, bleomycin and methotrexate (if used with folinic acid rescue). Cytotoxic drugs affect rapidly dividing bone marrow stem cells and the maximum effect on the peripheral blood count is generally seen between 7 and 14 days after chemotherapy. BCNU, 1-(2-chloroethyl)-3-cyclohexyl-1-nitrosourea (CCNU), and mitomycin C produce a blood count nadir at 4–5 weeks, and so these drugs are usually given with a 6-week interval. Carboplatin, a widely used platinum analogue, produces a white count and platelet nadir at 3 weeks, and is usually given with a 4-week interval. Patients treated with intermittent chemotherapy in this way are at risk from infection during the nadir of the white cell count, but the chemotherapy does not appear to produce increased risk of infection throughout the 3 weeks. It is important to treat patients for infection promptly during this period, and to avoid surgical procedures and general anaesthetics if possible, until the white count has recovered. Sometimes this is not possible, and emergency surgery is required during periods of neutropenia. If surgery cannot be avoided, appropriate prophylactic antibiotics need to be given. However, patients receiving weekly intensive programmes of chemotherapy will be at risk from infection over many weeks and in most circumstances need to receive prophylactic antibiotics, including prophylaxis against pneumocystis pneumonia.

Gastrointestinal and hepatotoxicity

The majority of chemotherapeutic agents will produce nausea and vomiting particularly cisplatinum. The advent of high-dose metoclopramide and more recently the 5-HT_3 antagonists has seen increasing success at controlling the nausea and vomiting induced by chemotherapy treatment. Oral mucositis is a common side-effect of chemotherapy. Hepatotoxicity may be seen with busulfan, cyclophosphamide, dacarbazine and 6-MP. High-dose methotrexate may cause an acute rise in liver enzymes suggesting an inflammatory process, and chronic low-dose oral methotrexate may be associated with liver fibrosis or cirrhosis.

Metabolic disturbances and anaesthesia

A number of chemotherapeutic agents may cause acute metabolic problems which need to be taken into account if a general anaesthetic has to be administered during or immediately after chemotherapy. A syndrome of inappropriate ADH secretion (SIADH) has been reported with a number of agents and may produce important electrolyte disturbances during anaesthesia. Vincristine and cyclophosphamide are the agents in which SIADH has been well described. Acute renal toxicity may be seen with platinum drugs, high-dose methotrexate, interferon and mitomycin C. Acute hepatic impairment may be seen with busulphan, cyclophosphamide, dacarbazine, methotrexate and thiopurines (azathioprine, 6-mercaptopurine and 6-thiouracil).

Specific interactions with anaesthetic agents

There are some anaesthetic drugs that have specific interactions with cytotoxic chemotherapy. This will only be of relevance if the patient undergoing general anaesthesia is actually receiving chemotherapy at the time of anaesthesia, which is rarely the case.

Cyclophosphamide inhibits synthesis of plasma cholinesterase and may result in a prolonged response to succinylcholine chloride.[67] A recent animal study has shown that mice exposed to halothane have an increased sensitivity to the lethal effects of cyclophosphamide. The study suggests that the increased toxicity is only present when cyclophosphamide and halothane are given simultaneously. How this relates to the human situation is as yet uncertain, but it is probably best to avoid the simultaneous administration of these two agents. High-dose methotrexate may produce transient impairment of hepatic function and if hydration and urinary alkalinization is inadequate it may lead to acute renal failure. These complications are of obvious importance in the face of anaesthesia. Plant alkaloids may produce neurotoxicity and if this is the case the use of succinylcholine may induce a hyperkalaemic state and therefore should be used only if essential.

Anthracycline antibiotics may produce cardiotoxicity and patients presenting for general anaesthetic should have a detailed cardiological screen before anaesthesia. Thorne[68] has suggested that doxorubicin-exposed patients preserve their cardiac function best with an anaesthetic technique that maintains a low systemic vascular resistance. Bleomycin may produce pulmonary toxicity and it has been suggested that high inspired oxygen concentration administered during anaesthesia may worsen the pulmonary toxicity.[69] It is therefore recommended that inspired oxygen concentration should be limited to 30% so long as this maintains adequate arterial oxygen saturation, which clearly has to be monitored during surgery.[70–72]

Intrathecal administration

There are very few cytostatic or cytotoxic drugs which it is safe to administer intrathecally. Methotrexate can be given, and there are specific intrathecal preparations which must be used. The dose is usually 12.5–15 mg by slow intrathecal injection. In the past, intrathecal injections have sometimes been associated with neurotoxicity. The vast majority of these side-effects were thought to be due to the benzyl alcohol or its derivatives which were used as preservatives in the intrathecal preparations. Now that these preservatives are no longer used, toxic effects of intrathecal treatment rarely occur. The only situation in which they are likely is when craniospinal irradiation has also been given, when nerve root damage and necrotizing leucoencephalopathy may occur. Because of this further i.t. methotrexate is usually avoided following craniospinal irradiation. Sometimes acute, transient neuropathy is seen.[72]

Cytosine arabinoside is the only other antineoplastic drug that is commonly given i.t., usually at a dose of 50–100 mg. This has been associated with the same problems as i.t. methotrexate in the past due to the same factors. Hydrocortisone may be combined with other i.t. agents, particularly in the treatment of leukaemias and lymphomas.

The accidental i.t. injection of other cytotoxic substances constitutes an emergency and the drug must be removed as soon as possible. Occasionally, vincristine has been injected accidentally and has resulted in ascending paralysis, coma and death in all cases reported to the manufacturers. Recently, however, a report was made in one adult in whom ascending paralysis was arrested with some subsequent recovery, when the following treatment was initiated immediately.[62] Removal of as much CSF as was safely possible by re-insertion of a lumbar puncture needle. Immediate flushing of CSF with lactated Ringer's solution by continuous infusion at 150 ml/h through a catheter inserted into a cerebral lateral ventricle, and removal via lumbar access until fresh frozen plasma (FFP) became available. Then 25 ml of FFP was diluted in 1l of lactated Ringer's and infused at 75 ml/h. The rate of infusion was adjusted to a spinal fluid protein of 1.5 g/l. The above management is therefore advised in patients with accidental i.t. administration of vincristine and should probably be extended to all patients who have had accidental i.t. administration of cytotoxic drugs that are vesicant or neurotoxic.

Septic shock

Septic shock is an important cause of death in cancer patients treated with intensive chemotherapy. The usual cause of the syndrome is Gram-negative septicaemia, but it is also seen in Gram-positive and fungal infections. In spite of our increasing understanding of the processes and pharmacological advances, mortality rates of 57% and greater are reported in patients with septic shock.[73–75] Septic shock produces cardiac insufficiency with depression of myocardial contractility and ventricular dilatation,[76–81] with a marked decrease in systemic vascular resistance, generalized blood flow maldistribution, and endothelial damage.[73,82–84] The results of these changes are multi-organ failure and a high mortality. The initial treatment of septic shock in the non-neutropenic patient is volume loading in order to correct volume depletion and increase cardiac output, with the addition of dopamine to raise the mean arterial pressure to 60 mmHg. When the dose of dopamine exceeds 20 μg/kg/min, another vasopressor, typically noradrenaline, is added. In non-neutropenic patients, if vigorous volume loading results in fluid overload, interstitial pulmonary oedema and inadequate oxygenation, mechanical ventilation can be instituted. In the immunosuppressed group, however, mechanical ventilation is usually associated with mortality. In the Bloomsbury Transplant Group, thirty patients have required ventilation over the past 24 months[85] and none has survived. Whether the use of assisted ventilation is cause or effect is difficult to determine, but these patients are certainly at particular risk from nocosomial infection and bleeding. This experience led us to examine earlier pharmacological intervention with vasopressors and inotropes in septic shock to support the circulation, while avoiding over-vigorous volume loading.

In a pilot study of early pharmacological intervention in neutropenic patients with septic shock carried out at the University College and Middlesex School of Medicine, we used noradrenaline (NA) as the vasopressor, and enoximone (EN) as the inotrope. The use of NA is safe[86–88] and the drug has been shown to increase mean arterial pressure (MAP), systemic vascular resistance index (SVRI), cardiac index (CI), together with O_2 delivery (Do_2) and oxygen consumption (Vo_2).[89] Reluctance to use NA is based on its possible contribution to renal insufficiency, splanchnic ischaemia and its proarrhythmic effects. However, in clinical studies in patients with septic shock there was no evidence of deterioration of renal function, and renal performance improved with the use of NA.[86] We have combined the early use of NA with EN, one of the new group of type IV phosphodiesterase inhibitors which exert both positive inotropic and vasodilating effects.[90] Recent studies have confirmed the inotropic effects of EN, and have also shown that EN potentiates the response of the myocardium to vasopressor catecholamines.[91] This may be of particular importance when there is down-grading of the adrenergic receptors as a result of the high circulating endogenous or exogenous catecholamines. This potentiating effect of EN means that lower doses of possibly toxic vasopressor substances may be used to obtain the same effect. It can be argued that EN would also reduce central venous pressure (CVP) and pulmonary artery wedge pressure (PAWP) through direct venodilatation, and therefore reduce the risk of pulmonary oedema and adult respiratory distress syndrome (ARDS). The fall of CVP in septic shock has been found to be an independent predictor of survival.[82] Any adverse effects of arterial dilatation on MAP produced by EN would in theory be offset by NA, whose vasopressor effect on the systemic circulation is more prominent than in the pulmonary circulation.

The preliminary results of these studies have been reported,[92] and are supported by some interesting intensive care data which include information on SVR, CI and PAWP.[93] So far we have treated six patients all of whom survived the septic episode, having had a calculated individual hospital mortality of 52–82%.[94] Clearly these small pilot studies are exciting but must be extended with more detailed monitoring of haemodynamic effects to assess this combination of NA and EN in septic shock. Before clinical studies have demonstrated clear improvement in haemodynamic parameters and outcome, this combination cannot be recommended outside the clinical trial setting.

In septic shock endotoxins and exotoxins are released and produce a severe host inflammatory response by stimulating the production of tumour necrosis factor-α (TNFα), interleukins and other cytokines, the levels of which are directly related to prognosis. There has been recent development in the production and use of human monoclonal antibodies to endotoxin, which may be useful in the treatment of patients with septic shock due to Gram-negative organisms. However, in a recently reported study when patients were selected on clinical criteria in a randomized trial, overall survival of the treated group was not improved, when compared with the control group.[95] There is as yet no rapid test to confirm the diagnosis of Gram-negative septicaemia so at present there is no mechanism for deciding which patients will benefit. Patients who were subsequently confirmed to have Gram-negative septicaemia did benefit from the monoclonal antibody treatment, but the group as a whole did not. This suggests that the treatment may be doing definite harm to patients who received it but who did not have Gram-negative septicaemia. In development at present are monoclonal antibodies to other molecules in the cytokine cascade, and their development for clinical use is awaited with some interest.

REFERENCES

1 Slevin ML. The clinical pharmacology of etoposide. *Cancer* 1991; **67** (Suppl 1): 319–29.

2 Benjamin RS. Pharmacokinetics of adriamycin in patients with sarcomas. *Cancer Chemotherapy Reports* 1974; **58**: 271–3.

3 Sinha BK, Motten AD, Hanck K. The electrochemical reduction of 1,4-bis-(2-hydroxyethyl)-amino-(ethylamino)-anthracenedione and daunomycin: Biochemical significance of superoxide formation. *Chemico-Biological Interactions* 1983; **43**: 371–7.

4 Dorr RT, Bowdan GT, Alberts DS *et al.* Interactions of Mitomycin-C with mammalian DNA detected by alkaline elution. *Cancer Research* 1985; **4**: 3510–16.

5 Allum W, Hallisey M, Kelly K, *et al.* Five year follow-up of the first British Stomach Cancer Group Study. *Lancet* 1989; 571–4.

6 Sobell HM, Jain SC, Sakere TD *et al.* Stereochemistry of actinomycin-DNA binding. *Nature* 1971; **231**: 200–5.

7 Reich E, Franklin RM, Shatkin AJ, *et al.* Action of actinomycin-D on animal cells and viruses. *Proceedings of the National Academy of Science* 1962; **48**: 1238–45.

8 Ross WE, Glaubiger DL, Kohn KW; Quantitation and qualitative aspects of intercalator induced DNA damage. *Biochemica Biophysica Acta.* 1979; **562**: 41–50.

9 Takeshita M, Grollman AP, Ohtsubo E *et al.* Interaction of bleomycin with DNA. *Proceedings of the National Academy of Science Biochemica Biophysica Acta* 1978; **75**: 5983–7.

10 Wang AL, Tew KD. Increased glutathione-S-transferase activity in a cell line with acquired resistance to nitrogen mustard. *Cancer Treatment Reports* 1985; **69**: 677–82.

11 Crook TR, Souhami RL, Whyman GD, *et al.* Glutathione depletion as a determinant of sensitivity of human leukaemia cells to cyclophosphamide. *Cancer Research* 1986; **46**: 5035–8.

12 Sladek NE, Powers JF, Grage GM. Half life of oxazophosphorins in biological fluids. *Drug Metabolism Disposition* 1984; **12**: 553–9.

13 Meanwell CA, Blake AE, Kelly KA, Honisberger L, Blackledge G. Prediction of ifosfamide/mesna associated encephalopathy. *European Journal of Cancer and Clinical Oncology* 1986; **22**: 815–19.

14 McElwain TJ, Hedley DW, Burton G, *et al.* Marrow autotransplantation accelerates haematological recovery in patients with malignant melanoma treated with melphalan. *British Journal of Cancer* 1979; **40**: 72–80.

15 Gribben JG, Goldstone AH, Linch DC, *et al.* Effectiveness of high-dose combination chemotherapy and autologous bone marrow transplantation for patients with non-Hodgkin's lymphomas who are still responsive to conventional dose therapy. *Journal of Clinical Oncology* 1989; **7**: 1621–9.

16 Kaldor JM, Day NE, Pettersson F, *et al.* Leukaemia following chemotherapy for ovarian cancer. *New England Journal of Medicine* 1990; **322**: 1–6.

17 Cole SR, Myers TJ, Klatsky AU. Pulmonary disease with chlorambucil therapy. *Cancer Research* 1978; **46**: 5035–8.

18 Cohen GL, Bauer WR, Barton JK, Lippard SJ. Binding of *cis*- and *trans*-dichlordiamineplatinum (II) to DNA: Evidence for unwinding and shortening of the double helix. *Science* 1979; **203**: 1014–16.

19 Meyn RE, Jenkins SF, Thompson LH. Defective removal of DNA cross-links in a repair deficient mutant of chinese hanster cells. *Cancer Research* 1982; **42**: 3106–11.

20 Litterst CL, LeRoy AF, Guarino AM. The disposition and distribution of platinum following parenteral administration of *cis*-dichlorodiamineplatinum (II). *Cancer Treatment Reports* 1979; **63**: 1485–92.

21 Vermorken JB, Van der Vijgh WJF, Klein I *et al.* Pharmacokinetics of free and total platinum species after short-term infusion of cisplatin. *Cancer Treatment Reports* 1984; **68**: 505–13.

22 Patton TF, Himmelstein KJ, Belt R *et al.* Plasma levels and urinary excretion of filterable platinum species following bolus injection and i.v. infusion of *cis*-dichlorodiamineplatinum (II) in man. *Cancer Treatment Reports* 1979; **63**: 1359–61.

23 Jacobs C, Kalman SM, Tretton M *et al.* Renal handling of *cis*-diamineplatinum (II). *Cancer Treatment Reports* 1980; **64**: 1223–6.

24 Madias NE, Harrington JT: Platinum nephrotoxicity. *American Journal of Medicine* 1978; **65**: 307–14.

25 Schisky RL, Anderson T. Hypomagnesaemia and renal magnesium wasting in patients receiving *cis*-platin. *Annals of Internal Medicine* 1979; **90**: 929–31.

26 Jones B, Mladek J, Bhalla R, *et al.* Enzymuria and beta-2-microglobulinuria as a sensitive index of cis-platinum nephrotoxicity. *Proceedings of the American Society of Clinical Oncology* 1979; **20**: 336.

27 Liegler DG, Henderson ES, Hahn MA, Oliverio VT. The effects of organic acids on renal clearance of methotrexate

in man. *Clinical Pharmacology and Therapeutics* 1969; **10**: 849.

28 Shamash J, Earl HM, Souhami RL. Acetazolamide for alkalinisation of urine in patients receiving high dose methotrexate. *Cancer Chemotherapy Pharmacology* 1991; **28**: 150–7.

29 McQuillan P, Morgan B, Ramwell J. Adriamycin cardiomyopathy. *Anaesthesia* 1988; **43**: 301–4.

30 Borgeat A, Chiolero R, Baylon P, Freeman J, Neff R. Perioperative cardiovascular collapse in a patient previously treated with doxorubicin. *Anesthesia and Analgesia* 1988; **67**: 1189–91.

31 Porembka D, Lowder J, Orlowski J, Bastulli J, Lockrem J. Etiology and management of doxorubicin cardiotoxicity. *Critical Care Medicine* 1989; **17**(6): 569–72.

32 Von Hoff D, Layard M, Basa P, *et al.* Risk factors for doxorubicin-induced congestive heart failure. *Annals of Internal Medicine* 1979; **91**: 710–17.

33 Beiling P, Winkler K, Bielack S, *et al.* Continuous infusion versus short term infusion of doxorubicin in osteosarcoma. *Proceedings of the American Society of Clinical Oncology* 1991; A1079.

34 Blum RH, Carter SK, Agre K. A clinical review of bleomycin – a new antineoplastic agent. *Cancer* 1973; **31**: 903–14.

35 Gunstream SR, Seidenfeld JJ, Sobonya RE. McMahon LJ. Mitomycin associated lung disease. *Cancer Treatment Reports* 1983; **67**: 301–4.

36 Burns WA, McFarland W, Mathews MJ. Busulphan induced pulmonary disease. Report of a case and review of the literature. *American Review of Respiratory Disease* 1970; **101**: 408–13.

37 Durrant JR, Norgard MJ, Murad TM, Bartolucci AA, Langford KH. Pulmonary toxicity associated with bischloroethylnitrosourea (BCNU). *Annals of Internal Medicine* 1979; **90**(2), 191–4.

38 Godard P, Marty JP, Michel FB. Interstitial pneumonia and chlorambucil. *Chest* 1979; **76**: 471–3.

39 Gould VE, Miller J. Sclerosing alveolitis induced by cyclophosphamide: ultrastructural observations on alveolar damage and repair. *American Journal of Pathology* 1975; **81**: 513–30.

40 Taetle R, Dickman PS, Feldman PS. Pulmonary histopathological changes associated with melphalan therapy. *Cancer* 1978; **42**: 1239–45.

41 Sostman HD, Matthay RA, Putman CE. Cytotoxic induced lung damage. *American Journal of Medicine* 1977; **62**: 608–15.

42 Holoye PY, Luna MA, MacKay B, Bedrossian CWM. Bleomycin hypersensitivity pneumonitis. *Annals of Internal Medicine* 1978; **88**: 47–9.

43 Jones SE, Moore M, Blank N, Casellino RA. Hypersensitivity to procarbazine manifested by fever and pleuropulmonary reaction. *Cancer* 1972; **29**: 498–500.

44 Hamous JE, Guffy M, Aschenbrener CA. Fatal acute respiratory failure following intrathecal methotrexate administration. *Cancer Treatment Reports* 1983; **67**: 1025–6.

45 Maxwell I. Reversible pulmonary oedema following cyclophosphamide treatment. *Journal of the American Medical Association* 1974; **229**: 137–8.

46 Haupt HM, Hutchins GM, Moore GW. Ara-C lung: noncardiogenic pulmonary oedema complicating cytosine arabinoside therapy of leukaemia. *American Journal of Medicine* 1981; 70: 256–61.

47 Commers JR, Foley JF. Pulmonary hyaline membrane disease occurring in the course of VM-26 therapy. *Cancer Treatment Reports* 1979; **63** (11–12): 2093–5.

48 Jolivert J, Giroux L, Laurin S, *et al.* Microangiopathic haemolytic anaemia, renal failure, and noncardiogenic pulmonary oedema: a chemotherapy induced syndrome: *Cancer Treatment Reports* 1983; **67**: 429–34.

49 Rosenberg SA, Lotze MT, Mule JJ. New approaches to the immunotherapy of cancer. *Annals of Internal Medicine* 1988; **108**: 853–64.

50 Walden PAM, Mitchell-Hegg PF, Coppin C, *et al.* Pleurisy and methotrexate treatment. *British Medical Journal* 1977; **2**: 867.

51 Luedke D, McLaughlin TT, Daughaday C, *et al.* Mitomycin-C and vindesine associated pulmonary toxicity with variable expression. *Cancer* 1985; **55**: 542–5.

52 Jones G, Mierins E, Karsh J. Methotrexate-induced asthma. *American Review of Respiratory Disease* 1991; **143**: 179–81.

53 Zucker KP, Khouri NF, Rosenshein NB. Bleomycin-induced pulmonary nodules: a rare variant of bleomycin pulmonary toxicity. *Gynaecologic Oncology* 1987; **28**: 284–91.

54 Lombard CM, Churg A, Winokur S. Pulmonary veno-occlusive disease following therapy for malignant neoplasms. *Chest* 1987; **92**: 871–6.

55 Santrach PJ, Askin FB, Wells RJ, Azizkhan RJ, Merten DF. Nodular form of bleomycin-related pulmonary injury in patients with osteosarcoma. *Cancer* 1989; **64**: 806–11.

56 Heard BE, Cooke RA. Busulphan lung. *Thorax* 1968; **23**: 187–93.

57 Aronin PA, Mahaley MS, Rudnick SA, *et al.* Prediction of BCNU pulmonary toxicity in patients with malignant gliomas. *New England Journal of Medicine* 1980; **303**: 183–8.

58 Rubio FA. Possible pulmonary effects of alkylating agents. *New England Journal of Medicine* 1972; **287**: 1150–1.

59 Abdel Karim FW, Ayash RE, Allam C, Sallem PA. Pulmonary fibrosis after prolonged treatment with low-dose cyclophosphamide. A case report. *Oncology* 1983; **40**: 174–6.

60 White DA, Rankin JA, Stover DE, Gellene RA, Gupta S. Methotrexate pneumonitis: Bronchoalveolar lavage findings suggest an immunological disorder. *American Review of Respiratory Disease* 1989; **139**: 13–21.

61 Earl HM, Latoufis C, Connelly S, Eagle K, Ash CM, Souhami RL. Long-term toxicity of chemotherapy in adolescents and young adults with sarcomas. In preparation.

62 Data Sheet Compendium, 1990–1991.

63 Hansen SW, Helweg-Larson S, Trojaborg W. Long-term neurotoxicity in patients treated with cisplatin, vinblastine and bleomycin for metastatic germ cell cancer. *Journal of Clinical Oncology* 1989; **7**: 1457–61.

64 Mollman JE, Glover DJ, Hogan WM, *et al.* Cisplatin neuropathy risk factors, prognosis and protection by WR-2721. *Cancer* 1988; **61**: 2192–5.

65 Van der Hoop RG, Vecht CJ, van der Burg ME, *et al.* Prevention of cisplatin neurotoxicity with an ACTH (4–9) analogue in patients with ovarian cancer. *New England Journal of Medicine* 1990; **322** (2): 89–94.

66 Mackintosh J, Tattersal M. Mitomycin-C induced haemolytic–uraemic syndrome. *Australian and New Zealand Journal of Medicine* 1988; **18**: 182.

67 Zsigmond EK, Robins G. The effects of a seies of anticancer drugs on plasmacholinesterase activity. *Canadian Journal of Anaesthesia* 1972; **19**: 75–82.

68 Thorne AC, Shah NK, Matarazzo D. Isoflurane or fentanyl for patients with adriamycin-induced cardiomyopathy? *Anesthesiology* 1988; A58.

69 Sogal RN, Gottlieb AA, Boutros R, *et al.* Effect of oxygen on bleomycin-induced lung damage. *Cleveland Clinical Journal of Medicine.* 1987; **54**(4), 503–8.

70 Toledo CH, Ross WE, Hood CI, Block CI. Potentiation of bleomycin toxicity by oxygen. *Cancer Treatment Reports* 1982; **66** (2): 359–62.

71 Goldiner PL, Carlon GC, Cvitkovic E, *et al.* Factors influencing postoperative morbidity and mortality in patients treated with bleomycin. *British Medical Journal* 1978; **1**: 1664–7.

72 Dunkelman H, Earl HM, Twelves C. Acute reversible neurological deficit following intrathecal chemotherapy. *Cancer Chemotherapy Pharmacology* 1991; **27**: 329–33.

73 Parillo JE, Parker MM, Natanson C, Suffredini AF, Danner RL, Cunnion RE, Ognibene FP. Septic shock in humans: Advances in the understanding of the pathogenesis, cardiovascular dysfunction and therapy. *Annals of Internal Medicine* 1990; **113**: 227–42.

74 Li TC, Phillips MC, Shaw L, *et al.* Onsite physician staffing a community hospital intensive care unit. *Journal of the American Medical Association* 1984; **252**: 2023–73.

75 Reynolds HN, Haupt MT, Hill-Baharozian MC, Carlson RW. Impact of critical care physician staffing on patients with septic shock in a university hospital intensive care unit. *Journal of the American Medical Association* 1988; **260**: 3446–50.

76 Parker MM, Shelhamer JH, Bacharach SL, *et al.* Profound but reversible myocardial depression in patients with septic shock. *Annals of Internal Medicine* 1984; **100**: 483–90.

77 Parker MM, Suffredini AF, Natanson C, *et al.* Responses of left ventricular function in survivors and non-survivors of septic shock. *Journal of Critical Care* 1989; **4**: 19–25.

78 Schremmer B, Dhainaut J-F. Heart failure in septic shock: Effects of inotropic support. *Critical Care Medicine* 1990; **18**: S49–55.

79 Vincent J-L, Van Der Linden P. Septic shock: Particular type of acute circulatory failure. *Critical Care Medicine* 1990; **18**: S70–4.

80 Parker MM, McCarthy KE, Ognibebe FP, Parillo JE. Right ventricular dysfunction and dilation, similar to left ventricular changes characterise the cardiac depression of septic shock in humans. *Chest* 1990; **97**: 126–31.

81 Cunnion RE, Parillo JE. Myocardial dysfunction in sepsis. Recent insights. *Chest* 1989; **95**: 941–5.

82 Parker MM, Shelhamer JH, Natanson C, Alling DW, Parrillo JE. Serial cardiovascular variables in survivors and non-survivors of human septic shock: heart rate as an early predictor of prognosis. *Critical Care Medicine* 1987; **15**: 923–39.

83 Wilson RF, Thal AP, Kindling PH, *et al.* Hemodynamic measurements in septic shock. *Archives of Surgery* 1965; **91**: 121–9.

84 Winslow EJ, Loeb HS, Rahimtoola SH, Kamath S, Gunnar RM. Haemodynamic studies and results of therapy in 50 patients with bacteraemic shock. *American Journal of Medicine* 1973; **54**: 421–32.

85 Personal communication, Dr Raj Chopra.

86 Mathru MM, Dries DJ. Is levophed lethal? *Chest* 1989; **95**: 1177–8.

87 Schreuder WO, Schnieder AJ, Groeneveld ABJ, Thijs LG. Effect of dopamine vs. noradrenaline on haemodynamics in septic shock. Emphasis on right ventricular performance. *Chest* 1989; **95**: 1282–8.

88 Desjars P, Pinaud M, Potel G, Tasseau F, Touze MD. Reappraisal of norepinephrine therapy in human septic shock. Emphasis on right ventricular performance. *Critical Care Medicine* 1987; **15**: 134–7.

89 Edwards JD. Practical application of oxygen transport principles. *Critical Care Medicine* 1990; **18**: S45–48.

90 Kariya T, Wille LJ, Dage RC. Biochemical studies on the mechanism of the cardiotoxic action of MDL17043. *Journal of Cardiovascular Pharmacology* 1982; **4**: 509–14.

91 Hall JA, Latimer M. Enoximone potentiates the positive inotropic effect of B1 and B2 adrenoceptor stimulation in human atrial myocardium. *Cardiology* 1990; 77 (Suppl 3): 14–20.

92 Shamash J, Earl HM, Souhami RL, Chopra R. The successful management of neutropenic patients with septic shock using a novel combination of noradrenaline and enoximone. *European Society of Medical Oncology* Dec 1990.

93 Kox W, Brydon C. The effect of enoximone and adrenaline on oxygen delivery and consumption; a cross over study. *Intensive Care Medicine* 1990; **16**: A481.

94 Knaus WA, Draper EA, Wagner DP, Zimmerman JE. APACHE II. A severity of disease classification system. *Critical Care Medicine* 1985; **13**(10): 818–24.

95 Ziegler EJ, Fisher CJ, Sprung CL, *et al.* Treatment of Gram-negative bacteraemia and septic shock with HA-IA human monoclonal antibody against endotoxin. *New England Journal of Medicine* 1991; **324**: 429–36.

SECTION ELEVEN

Sterilization

36

Sterilization and Disinfection

GMS Scott

Sterilization implies the complete destruction of all 'living' or transmissible agents. In practice, this means rendering vegetative and sporing bacteria, fungi, protozoa and viruses non-infectious. Whereas most viruses are inactivated by processes that kill bacteria, some agents (e.g. the prion responsible for Creutzfeld–Jacob disease) appear capable of withstanding the extremes of moist heat that would normally kill bacterial spores. Disinfection implies the killing of vegetative organisms, reducing bacterial contamination to safe levels. In the past, disinfection referred exclusively to treatment of inanimate objects but has now come into general use to include treatment of skin and mucous membranes. An antiseptic is a non-irritant disinfectant that can be safely applied to the skin and even more sensitive tissues. Most disinfectants are chemical solutions or compounds but there is a small number of such solutions called sterilants that will kill bacterial spores under favourable conditions and these include activated glutaraldehyde.

The first principle of decontamination is thorough cleaning. The removal of excessive bacteria and biological materials such as mucus is a prerequisite for effective disinfection or sterilization. Sterilization conditions in autoclaves designed for clean instruments would not be expected to kill all the organisms in, say, a sample of soil.

Sterilization is reliably achieved by:

- moist heat
- dry heat
- low temperature steam and formaldehyde vapour
- ethylene oxide gas
- gamma irradiation
- chemical 'sterilization'

METHODS OF STERILIZATION

Moist heat

The principle of moist heat sterilization is that exposure of cold instruments to steam results in flash condensation and evaporation which transiently releases enormous amounts of free latent energy locally. Protein and DNA is denatured by coagulation. Autoclaves provide steam under pressure which must not be contaminated by air. The partial pressure of any air present will contribute to the overall pressure in the system resulting in a reduced temperature in the vessel. Furthermore, air acts as an insulator.

Two types of autoclaves are in common use. High vacuum autoclaves employ pumps to remove air and are generally supplied by quality controlled steam from a remote source. In a high vacuum autoclave, steam effectively penetrates porous paper and materials that are used to wrap sets of surgical instruments, and the process yields dry packs. A more simple machine ('bowl and instrument' type) employs either steam from a remote source or from an internal water boiler. Air is removed by downward displacement and is presumed to have been removed when the temperature at the chamber drain in the floor of the machine (the coolest part) has reached a preset level. This type of machine sometimes incorporates a water boiler and may be used in clinical areas. Wrapped instruments must not be placed in these machines but they must be laid out in perforated racks in such a way that steam can flow freely around them. The instruments will come out wet reflecting the water of condensation on to cold objects.

High vacuum autoclaves are used in central sterile supply departments and some operating theatre units. They are regularly maintained and checked daily for efficiency of air removal by the Bowie–Dick or equivalent test, and for appropriate function by continuous chart recordings of pressure and/or temperature. Quality assurance of the contents of the packs is achieved by knowing that the instruments were cleaned and that the autoclave was functioning properly according to a planned preventive maintenance programme when that pack was processed. The probability of a non-sterile pack arising if it was contaminated with 10^6 organisms before autoclaving should be in the order of 10^{-6}. Therefore quality control cannot be performed by testing random packs for contamination. Each pack should have a quality-control docket attached (often a computer-generated punch card) which can be traced back to the autoclave used and specific cycle. It behoves theatre staff who use these packs to stick these dockets somewhere in the patient's anaesthetic record during an operation. This may provide vital evidence in a subsequent charge of negligence arising from a postoperative wound infection.

Bowl and instrument autoclaves are used in small theatre sterile supply units for preparing trays of instruments for immediate use. All hospital autoclaves should be maintained to similar mechanical standards but problems arise with stand-alone small autoclaves used in clinical areas. Quality assurance of the process in autoclaving an instrument from one of these machines is by no means guaranteed, particularly if attention has not been paid to the diligent cleaning of the instruments. Recent Department of Health guidelines suggest that the operators of autoclaves should be professionally trained. Nevertheless, stand-alone autoclave units are enormously preferable to boiling water baths, which require long periods of immersion to achieve disinfection, cannot be regarded as sterilizers and have many disadvantages. They should be removed from all clinical areas.

Dry heat

Comparison of the kill curves (Fig. 36.1) of a prototype heat-resistant organism (e.g. 10^8 *Bacillus stearothermophilus*) by moist and dry heat indicates the relative inefficiency of oxidation by dry heat. At 180°C, paper will char and very prolonged incubations at lower temperatures are necessary to guarantee sterilization. Hot air ovens must be fan assisted to ensure uniform heating, and to protect the operator they must have door interlocks so that they cannot be opened at temperatures above 60°C. Hot air ovens are used only in highly specialized areas such as laboratories and are used mainly for sterilizing clean glassware. Having said this, most microbiology laboratories have now dispensed with glassware altogether because of the risks of breakages and inoculation accidents causing infection of staff.

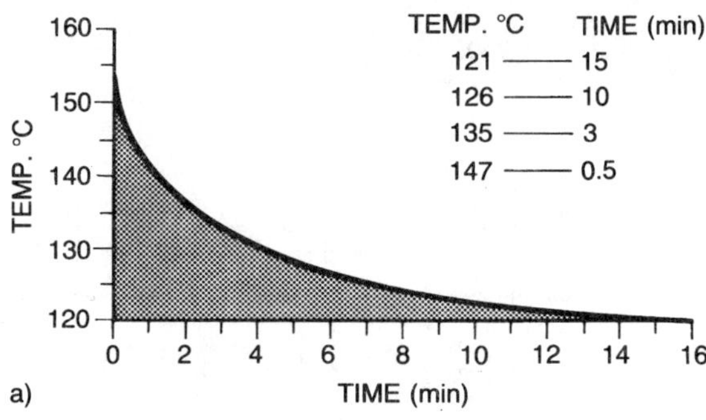

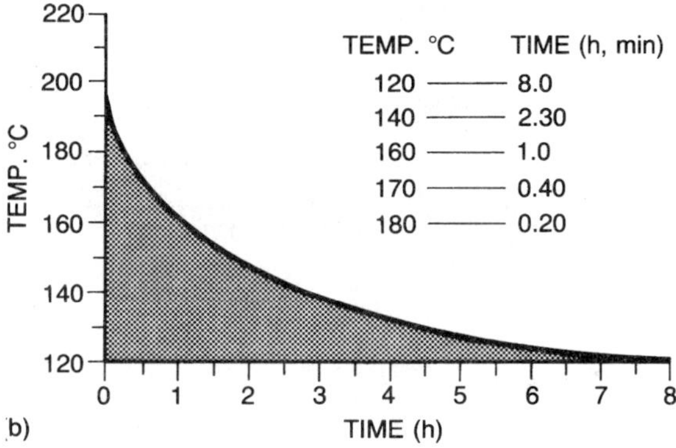

FIGURE 36.1 Killing of a standard inoculum of a typical heat-resistant spore forming bacterium in (a) moist and (b) dry heat, under different time-temperature conditions. Note the differences in the scales of the abscissae.

Low temperature steam and formaldehyde

This is a convenient method for decontaminating heat-sensitive electronic and bulky equipment such as anaesthetic machines and reusable tubing, ventilators and baby incubators. This equipment is cleaned and dried, then placed in the aseptor. A dose of formalin, often with ballasted steam at 70°C, is boiled off for a hold time characteristically of 3 h. The formalin is neutralized by an exact dose of ammonia and the decontaminated equipment returned to service. Excess ammonia will result in deposition of an ammonium salt on all equipment. Equipment should be decontaminated on a regular basis according to set protocols.

Ethylene oxide

Ethylene oxide is a highly effective, penetrating sterilizing gas that is ideal for sterilizing heat-sensitive equipment with fine bore channels. There are several disadvantages. The gas is expensive, poisonous and explosive. Ethylene oxide is usually ballasted with steam at 70°C. The only reliable quality control for the process is exposure of cultures laden with resistant bacterial spores. This spore strip is placed at the end of a long spiral attached to the machine. A negative culture at 5 days indicates that the process was satisfactory, but equipment cannot be released until then. This is a fundamental disadvantage of this method of sterilization. In the early days of endoscopy on patients with HIV, it was considered that ethylene oxide was the only safe method for decontamination before reuse. However, the expense and long interval before release makes this an unacceptable process, and chemical decontamination with glutaraldehyde is now relied upon.

Patent ethylene oxide decontaminators are available for local use with sachets that release doses of the gas and simple colour change indicators to control the process. These units are dangerous, cannot be relied upon to sterilize equipment, and should be removed from service.

Gamma irradiation

Irradiation sterilization is used for radiation resistant single-use items such as needle, syringes and catheters. The standard sterilization dose is 2.5 Mrads. A suitable radiation source is cumbersome and may require several hours of exposure and considerable heat is generated. When single-use items have been removed from their packets and used, they must not be reused. If an end-user does elect to decontaminate and reuse such equipment, he then takes 'product liability' for the product, which potentially carries unlimited liability for compensation in the event of successful prosecution after an accident.

Chemical 'sterilization'

Activated glutaraldehyde is the most commonly used chemical sterilant. Once activated it remains stable for 2 weeks. It is active against bacterial spores and mycobacteria but only after relatively prolonged exposure, and is commonly used to decontaminate endoscopes between patients. Several problems are observed: glutaraldehyde is irritant and causes upper respiratory symptoms in those working permanently in the presence of the vapour. Some patent endoscopic washers tend to dilute the aldehyde beyond its effective concentration and this must be monitored. The Control of Substances Hazardous to Health (CoSHH) Act has made it a condition of managers that employees experience the least exposure possible to potentially toxic compounds. Alternatives to glutaraldehyde include Dettol endoscopic disinfectant with alcohol or peracetic acid but neither is as well evaluated as glutaraldehyde. The best solution to this problem is to introduce proper extraction equipment in designated endoscopy units until suitable alternatives are available.

DISINFECTION

The process of disinfection is initiated by thorough cleaning with water and detergent. Drying is also important because water-borne organisms of low virulence such as *Pseudomonas* spp. will replicate on moist or damp surfaces.

Pasteurization

Disinfection by heat implies pasteurization, a process of short exposure of liquids to high temperature (e.g. 62.8–65.8°C for 30 min or 71.5°C for 15 s). Alternatively, surgical objects may be placed in a boiling water bath. Although water at 100°C is likely to kill vegetative organisms, the instruments must be clean and must be left submerged for an undefined period of time. Often they are then removed by non-sterile Cheatle's forceps which may themselves be heavily contaminated – indeed they are often kept in old disinfectant solutions. Apart from the major disadvantage of unreliability of the boiling water bath as a means of decontamination and the obvious dangers of burns and scalds to staff, instruments become coated with scale and become impossible to clean properly.

Biocides

Certain chemical disinfectants are particularly used to decontaminate water supplies either for drinking or to reduce the risk of legionellosis for water used in wet condensors. Dosing water reservoirs with, for example, chlorine-releasing agents on an intermittent basis may transiently increase the number of bacteria present in the water by releasing the biofilm from underwater surfaces. It should be noted that chlorination of potable water supplies is not efficient at killing *Giardia intestinalis* or *Cryptosporidium* spp.

Chemical disinfection

Chemical disinfectants are compounds that kill vegetative organisms and many viruses but cannot be relied upon to kill bacterial spores. The killing power of a disinfectant is difficult to measure precisely because, in order to check how many organisms have survived, they have somehow to be separated from the inhibitory compound. Several methods of achieving this are possible, including dilution beyond the minimal effective dose or repeated washing and centrifugation. The methods are not important but they do reveal that killing is dependent on concentration, time, conditions (e.g. heat) and the presence of biological contamination (e.g. mucus) and possible inactivating substances (e.g. rubber or cork). *In vitro* assays often suggest a high degree of activity belied by the killing power in practical clinical situations. Furthermore, 'in-use' tests made by examining directly pots of diluted disinfectants in clinical areas often show that they support the growth of difficult hospital organisms such as pseudomonads.

Disinfectants are characterized by their mode of action, their practical usefulness and disadvantages, preparations available and cost. Organisms such as tuberculosis, hepatitis B virus and multiresistant coliforms have been shown to be transmitted from patient to patient by equipment (e.g. fibreoptic endoscopes) that was not properly decontaminated.

The important disinfectants and their properties useful in hospital practice are listed in Table 36.1. Membrane active disinfectants include phenolics, biguanides, alcohols and quaternary ammonium compounds (QAC). Halogen-based disinfectants kill by oxidation and aldehydes by fixation.

Gram-negative organisms have an outer bilipid membrane which makes them 5–200 fold more resistant to surface-acting disinfectants than Gram-positive organisms. This outer membrane is more complex in the case of *Pseudomonas* and related species, which are 20–40-fold more resistant than *E. coli*. Mycobacteria have a hydrophobic waxy outer membrane consisting of multiple sheets of peptidoglycan covered by peptidoglycolipids linked to mycolic acid. Bacterial spores are thick walled and the cytoplasm has lost water. They resist drying and chemical attack. Mycobacteria and spores are resistant to killing by surface acting disinfectants.

Factors affecting efficacy of disinfectants

Concentration

For most disinfectants, increased concentration leads to increased killing efficacy. This is not so for alcohols, which perform best when mixed with water in a concentration of 60–80%.

Temperature

Although disinfectants do act at room temperature, for most, increasing the temperature reduces the time needed for a given reduction in bacterial viable counts. The temperature coefficient for a disinfectant reflects this increased activity and is the ratio of the time taken to kill at a given temperature to the time to kill 10°C over that temperature.

Examples of approximate temperature coefficients are:

Formaldehyde	2
Ethylene oxide	3
Glutaraldehyde	4
Phenolics	4
Alcohols	40

pH

The pH of a solution may have a profound effect on the activity of disinfectants. Increasing pH decreases the activity of phenolics, enhances the activity of halogens, chlorhexidine and quaternary ammonium compounds. Chlorhexidine is active over a wide range (5.5–8.0) but is more active in the alkaline region.

Formulation

Alterations in formulation may influence activity. For example, water added to alcohols improves activity and phenolics contain detergents to aid solubility. Skin preparations often contain conditioners to reduce inflammatory and drying effects. Compatible disinfectants may be combined to enhance activity (e.g. alcohols with chlorhexidine or iodophors). In general, though, disinfectants are more likely to antagonize each other so must not be combined.

Interfering substances

Organic matter, especially blood pus and mucus, acts as a mechanical barrier to disinfectants. Hypochlorite and potassium permanganate coagulate and precipitate proteins, protecting micro-organisms from effective contact.

Cork inactivates chlorhexidine, rubber phenols and diguanides and plastics inactivate the phenolics. Hard water reduces the activity of phenolics and, to a lesser extent, hypochlorite. Anionic soaps inactivate cationic diguanides (chlorhexidine) which in turn may inactivate phenolics and hypochlorites.

Families of disinfectants

Phenolics

Phenolics and their derivatives from the distillation of coal tar have been known to have disinfectant properties since the early 1800s and were used by Lister in his classic development of antiseptic method in operating theatres. The distillation of coal tar yields a range of antibacterial fractions. Those with highest boiling points have greatest antibacterial activity and are least toxic to tissue but are least soluble in water. Formulation is therefore of importance and the insoluble agents are taken up into soap solutions either in solution (black fluids) or as an emulsion (white fluids). Many phenols and their derivatives are now made synthetically.

They are now unpopular in hospital practice. They are relatively cheap and in the past were used extensively for cleaning surfaces such as floors. It has been recognized that simple cleaning by detergents is quite satisfactory for most hospital hard surfaces and this has led at least to a reduction in the awful institutional smell of most units. Certain phenolics were used as hand and skin antiseptics (e.g. chloroxylenol – castor oil developed in 1930s for midwifery practice) but have been superseded by chlorhexidine and betadine preparations.

TABLE 36.1 Some disinfectants in clinical use

CHEMICAL GROUP	EXAMPLE	MODE OF ACTION	ADVANTAGES	DISADVANTAGES	RECOMMENDED USAGE
Alcohols	Ethyl Isopropyl	Membrane	Highly effective at reducing skin colonization. Non-toxic for skin application	Inflammable. Transient effect after topical application. Denatures some plastics	Skin disinfection. Clean hard surfaces (e.g. trolley tops)
Biguanides	Chlorhexidine	Membrane	Relatively non-toxic in topical application. True allergy very rare	Limited range of activity. Very much inactivated by organic matter. Not cheap. Minor skin irritation	Skin disinfectant, patients' wounds, clinical hand decontamination
Quaternary ammonium compounds	Cetrimide	Membrane	Cheap, good detergent action, little smell, pleasant to use. Non-toxic	Very limited range of antibacterial activity. Very much inactivated by organic matter. Totally inactivated by soap. Support growth of *Pseudomonas*	General cleaning of wounds; used as a detergent rather than a disinfectant
Halogens	Chloorine-releasing agents (hypochlorite, dichloroisocyanurate)	Oxidation	Wide range of antibacterial activity, rapid action, little smell, mostly cheap	Very much inactivated by organic matter. May need to be mixed with detergent. May corrode some metals. Released chlorine is toxic in high concentrations	Suitable for items that come in contact with food. Used to decontaminate high-risk blood and body fluids
	Iodophors		Wide range of antibacterial activity, rapid action, pleasant smell	Very much inactivated by organic matter. Stains clothes. Not cheap. Allergy may occur	Skin disinfection. Wound irrigation
Aldehydes	Glutaraldehyde	Fixation	Broad-spectrum effective microbicidal activity	Fumes cause irritation in users. Requires proper ventilation. May be ineffective if organic matter present	A chemical 'sterilant' for equipment that cannot be autoclaved
	Formaldehyde		Highly active in vapour form	Irritating. Possibly carcinogenic	Decontamination of fume cupboards. Use in controlled 'aseptors' sometimes with steam (70°C), then neutralized with ammonia, for large or electronic equipment
Xylenols	'Dettol'	Chemical denaturation of DNA	Clean smell	Very limited range of antibacterial activity. Inactivated by organic materials	Dettol endoscope disinfectant with alcohol may be an alternative to glutaraldehyde for decontaminating endoscopes
Phenolics	Black (Jeyes)	Membrane	Wide range of antibacterial activity. Not much inactivated by organic matter. Cheap	Messy, strong smelling	Lavatories and drains in high-risk areas
	White (Izal)		Wide range of antibacterial activity. Not much inactivated by organic matter. Cheap	Strong smell, may be inactivated by plastics	Lavatories and drains in high-risk areas
	Clear (Hycolin)		Wide range of antibacterial activity. Not much inactivated by organic matter. Less smell than other phenolics	Not cheap except 'Sudol'. May be inactivated by plastics	Laboratory discard, general sanitation. Treating infected stools and urine before washing. Disinfecting hard surfaces
Synthetic phenolics	Hexachlorophane	Membrane	Little local irritation. Good antistaphylococcal activity	Less active against Gram-negatives. Toxic in babies if absorbed. Insoluble. Dissociation in alkaline conditions	Dusting powders, e.g. for umbilici, staphylococcal carriage
Hydrogen peroxide		Oxidation	Potent oxidant. Sometimes used for cleaning wounds	Requires fresh solution	Some specific chlorine-resistant parasites (e.g. *Cryptosporidium*)

Phenolics (e.g. lysol or hycolin) are used in the microbiology laboratory for disinfecting heavily contaminated items. (All of this discard should anyway be autoclaved before removal from the laboratory for incineration.) They may be recommended for decontaminating hard surfaces after cleaning in clinical areas where patients shedding certain virulent or resistant organisms (e.g. *S. pyogenes*, methicillin-resistant *S. aureus* (MRSA) have been nursed.

Pine disinfectants (deodorants)

These products of distillation of pine needles or wood smell pleasant enough and are associated in the mind with cleanliness but are relatively free of any antimicrobial activity. Addition of certain pine oil distillates to chloroxylenols may add activity against some, but not all, bacteria. There is no place for these compounds in hospitals or in the home, or anywhere.

Bis-phenols

Several useful hydroxy-halogenated derivatives of diphenol compounds linked by a methyl group, sulphur or oxygen atom have been developed. They include hexachlorophane, which is still a valuable antiseptic powder or cream for reducing *Staphylococcus aureus* carriage in axillae and perineum. It is insoluble and much less active against Gram-negative organisms. Although it used to be a popular constituent of surgical scrubs and cosmetics, it caused systemic toxicity in neonates and has since been the subject of an order limiting its concentration in such preparations and forbidding its use in children.

Triclosan is the most widely used phenolic compound active against *S. aureus* and some *E. coli* but relatively inactive against *P. aeruginosa*. Several preparations are available. Although not soluble in water it is taken up in alkalis and organic solvents and may be present in some 'medicated' soaps. These are of limited value in hospital practice.

Acids

Acids are best in their non-ionized form and are therefore pH dependent. They act as uncoupling agents by preventing the uptake of essential substrates dependent on a protonmotive force. Acetic acid has been used as a pickling agent and as a dressing where *Pseudomonas* was involved.

Various acids (e.g. undecenoic, benzoic, salicylic) may be applied to the skin to treat mycoses.

Esters of parahydroxybenzoic acid

These may be found as preservatives in topical solutions such as eye drops. They are less active against *P. aeruginosa* than against other important bacteria and indeed, the former bacteria were found to be able to utilize the dilute parabens esters as a carbon source.

Halogens

Chlorine-releasing agents are some of the most useful and powerful disinfectants for inactivating infective material. However, free chlorine is toxic and damages metal and many dyed materials. It is reliable for inactivating high-risk viral agents and may be presented as granules of dichloroisocyanurate (which is more stable than hypochlorite) which can be sprinkled on to a spillage of blood. Solutions of chlorine-releasing agents should be made up fresh.

Iodophors are effective antiseptics that are relatively non-toxic. Activity is improved by mixing with alcohol. As surgical scrub and skin preparation for patients, iodophor and chlorhexidine compete well. Iodophors can be applied on tampons in the vagina to reduce bacterial colonization pre-operatively and can be used to irrigate deep-seated infected cavities including peritoneum, subphrenic space or mediastinum.

Biguanides

Biguanides are cationic and bind strongly to bacterial cell surfaces changing the surface charge and allowing leakage of the cytoplasmic contents. This stops when the chemical enters the cell and precipitates the cytoplasm. Chlorhexidine arose from screening of many compounds at ICI. The gluconate is freely soluble and other preparations (dihydrochloride and diacelatate) are much less so. As an antiseptic it may be combined with a quaternary ammonium compound or alcohol. Chlorhexidine is active against many bacteria including *M. tuberculosis* (but not cidal, and not sporicidal). It is cationic, and activity is reduced in the presence of anionic soaps. It is inactivated by organic material. It will be precipitated in the presence of phosphate and many other salts. It is very useful as a skin disinfectant (particularly in an alcoholic solution), and a hand wash often presented with skin conditioners to reduce drying and chapping.

HAND DISINFECTION

Qualitative measurement of colonization of hands is extremely difficult. Resident bacteria exist within microcolonies firmly adherent to squamous cells. Methods to reveal bacterial carriage include streaking fingers on agar or washing in a nutrient broth and making colony counts from the broth. Neither are particularly sensitive tests yet they give some idea of the number of organisms that could be liberated during clinical practice. The organisms adherent to skin scales, those detached in clumps or those floating individually have different susceptibilities to applied disinfectants. A relevant test is to apply a wash, then contaminate the hands with a known number of pathogenic organisms and observe the recovery of these organisms from control hands and those washed with various soaps or disinfectants.[1]

Diligent hand washing with anionic soap can reduce the transient flora of bacteria but not the resident more adherent flora. Prolonged scrubbing with soap can actually increase the number of organisms recoverable from the hands presumably by traumatizing the skin and allowing more prolific growth, say, within surgical gloves. It is critical to dry the hands very carefully.

Preoperative surgical skin preparation is best performed with a detergent and antiseptic such as chlorhexidine or any iodophor. Scrubbing the skin should be reduced to a minimum. Repeated use of chlorhexidine leads to apparent residual activity and very low recoverable bacterial counts. Rinsing hands in chlorhexidine with alcohol also has a very useful residual disinfectant effect. After thorough washing with chlorhexidine, staff may use chlorhexidine with alcohol to reduce skin colorization between patients.[2] However, if hands become overtly contaminated they should be washed again.

Skin cleaning and disinfection

It is important to ensure that aseptic precautions are taken when doing minimally invasive procedures in theatre and ICU. The sites of drips inserted in emergency situations in casualty almost always become infected within 48 h.

Anaesthetists who perform invasive procedures should attempt to perform these with as full aseptic precautions as possible. The air supply to the ICU is often not cleaned to theatre standard but this is no reason not to take precautions in other directions.

TABLE 36. ICU handwashing standard

At each WHB, there will be Hibiscrub and liquid soap in proper dispensers.
At each patient, there will be Hibisol in a proper dispenser.
No wrist watches, sleeves rolled to the elbow.

1. At the beginning of a session (ie on starting work or after a break), proper surgical **WASH IN HIBISCRUB for 2 minutes***
   *There will then be residual disinfectant activity
2. Wear a new pair of GLOVES **before** breaking a drip line or attending to a drip site or touching a wound. Wear gloves during suction and when you are likely to touch blood or body fluids. Wash hands in liquid soap or use Hibisol *after removing gloves.*
3. Do as many procedures as possible using a non-touch technique.
4. Wash hands in Hibiscrub **after accidental soiling** with any body secretions (saliva, tracheal secretions, urine, faeces, etc).
5. Use Hibisol (or wash with liquid soap) if moving from one bed to another, or if moving to the patient from the telephone.

If a container of Hibiscrub/Hibisol or soap runs out when you use it, *you* must ensure it is replaced.
Wipe pens, stethoscope head and controls of all machines with alcohol at the beginning of each shift.
Do not suck pencils/pens. Wipe them with an alcohol wipe if they fall on the floor.

Techniques

Techniques should be aimed at reducing the transmission of micro-organisms from the operator or from other patients. The most important of these is proper handwashing. This will reduce the burden of transient organisms on the hands and should be done before touching any patient. A standard should be set (see example Table 36.2) against which practices can be measured. Washing the hands with chlorhexidine or betadine is more efficient than with soap. Use of chlorhexidine with alcohol hand rub is also extremely efficient at reducing recoverable bacteria on the hands and gives persistent or residual activity. This is no substitute for handwashing but is a convenient way of decontaminating the hands, say, between patients on a ward round.

It is not possible to wash the hands without removing the wrist watch and rolling up the sleeves. The number of organisms under a wrist watch band is very high and staff who have a wrist watch have higher counts of bacteria on the fingers of their dominant hand, compared with matched controls without a wrist watch.

Wearing gloves is an additional safety measure to reduce the likelihood of transferring micro-organisms to patients. When gloves are to be used, they must be subject to a proper set of guidelines and protocols. With sterile gloves on after a proper theatre hand 'scrub' with disinfectant, the anaesthetist must behave as though scrubbed for an operation and use a no-touch technique as far as possible. One danger with gloves is that they are assumed to remain sterile for as long as they are worn.

Before any invasive procedure in theatre or ICU, the patient's skin must be properly prepared with appropriate chlorhexidine or betadine solutions, preferably with 70% alcohol. For simple blood taking or temporary drip insertion, 70% isopropyl alcohol is probably sufficient but should preferably be applied twice and allowed to dry on each occasion. Spinal taps and anaesthesia require skin preparation with alcoholic betadine. The antiseptic should be allowed to dry and not be removed.

DECONTAMINATION OF ANAESTHETIC AND MONITORING EQUIPMENT

Decontamination of ICU equipment

The principles of decontamination of equipment in the ICU are as follows:

- patients are susceptible to infections mainly by virtue of breaks in the integument, bypass of the ciliary escalator and by having been given antibiotics that decrease colonization resistance and allow the proliferation of troublesome nosocomial organisms
- equipment that is placed in the body or used in any invasive procedure must be sterile
- the contamination of all ancillary equipment with environmental bacteria must be reduced as far as possible by regular cleaning
- humidification systems must be used that do not generate an aerosol of bacteria

When considering the equipment in the ICU (and this will apply perhaps more to new pieces of equipment than established ones), the first question to decide is whether it needs to be sterile.

Sterile equipment may be single-use. This is often heat sensitive and will have been sterilized by gamma-irradiation. Confidence in the sterility of the product is obtained by the quality assurance of the manufacturers and cannot be tested except by using the equipment in patients. The manufacturer takes product liability, providing the pack had not been opened at a time prior to the procedure. Single-use items should not be re-used. If some means of decontamination is employed, then the user takes product liability (which may be unlimited) for any subsequent event that may occur.

Sterile equipment that is reusable should be autoclaved under quality controlled conditions (as in Central Sterile Supply Departments (CSSD) or Theatre Sterile Supply Units (TSSU). Small stand-alone local autoclaves are to be discouraged.

Major problems arise over equipment that is re-usable and needs to be sterile but is heat sensitive. Ethylene oxide sterilization is very effective but is expensive and requires a long turnaround time. Stand-alone ethylene oxide units in local areas are dangerous, impossible to control and should be discarded.

The main alternative to autoclaving heat-sensitive equipment is chemical disinfection. Perhaps the only reliable sterilant is glutaraldehyde, which carries serious problems of toxicity to staff and restriction by CoSHH regulations.

If a method is to be employed for 'sterilization' of equipment, the protocol should be agreed with the microbiologist and incorporated in the standard operating procedures for the department. Staff will need to be trained and the system will have to be monitored in some way. Rarely will this involve microbial sampling; it will more often involve a check that the procedure is actually being carried out according to the agreed standard.

Equipment that does not have to be sterile must be clean. This is best achieved by simple detergent. Topical 'sterilants' are generally not required unless a room is to be cleaned which contained a patient shedding organisms such as *S. pyogenes*, methicillin-resistant *S. aureus*, multiply resistant coliforms or pseudomonads. Under these circumstances, surfaces should be wiped with a fresh solution of a phenolic such as 'Hycolin' 2%, *after* washing with detergent solution. Anaesthetic and electronic equipment can be satisfactorily decontaminated in a formalin aseptor.

Spillages of blood and other body fluids are naturally common in theatre and ICU. On the assumption that all such spills may constitute a high risk of infection to others, they should be decontaminated with fresh chlorine-releasing solution or granules. Unfortunately, this procedure often leads to the release of large amounts of free chlorine. The fixed surfaces in all clinical areas must be resistant to chlorine. If it has to be used on metal it must be carefully washed off to prevent corrosion.

CONCLUSION

Sterilization is best achieved by moist heat in an autoclave. Single-use items will be satisfactorily sterilized by gamma irradiation. There has been a gradual move away from using disinfectants widely in hospitals because of a rational approach to the perceived risks of specific practices to patients. Agreed disinfectants are used principally for skin preparation and handwashing. Handborne transmission of organisms represents the most important and efficient route of transfer from one patient to another.

REFERENCE

1 Babb JR, Davies JG, Ayliffe GAJ. A test procedure for evaluating surgical hand disinfection. *Journal of Hospital Infection* 1991; **18**: SB41–9.

FURTHER READING

Ayliffe GAJ, Lowbury EJL, Geddes AM, Williams JD. *Control of hospital infection*, London: Chapman & Hall Medical, 1992, 47–112.

Russell AD, Hugo WB, Ayliffe GAJ. *Principles and practice of disinfection, preservation and sterilization.* London: Blackwell Scientific, 1982.

Sanderson PJ, Newsom SWB (eds). Hand antiseptics – Efficacy and acceptability. *Journal of Hospital Infection* 1991; **18** (Suppl B): 1–71.

SECTION TWELVE

Adverse Effects of Drugs

37

Adverse Drug Reactions

M Pirmohamed, BK Park

INTRODUCTION

An adverse drug reaction may be defined as any undesirable drug effect beyond its anticipated therapeutic effects. Taken collectively, adverse drug reactions (ADR) are common accounting for a great deal of morbidity and occasional mortality. Estimates of ADR incidence vary widely (1–36%) between different studies because of differences in the definition, methods of detection and reporting of ADRs. However, most studies have shown that 3–5% of patients are admitted to hospital as a result of an ADR, while 10–20% of inpatients develop an ADR, often prolonging their stay. Drug-related deaths occur either as a result of therapeutic errors or because of unexpected and unpredictable drug effects. The incidence of drug deaths ranges from 0.01% (for surgical inpatients) to 0.1% for medical inpatients.

It has been estimated that 5% of general hospital beds in the UK and as high as 1 in 7 beds in the USA are occupied by patients who have had ADRs. Thus, the cost of drug toxicity is enormous; the direct costs include the cost of treatment, hospitalization, and prevention and detection of ADRs, while indirect costs include the lost contribution of the patient to the gross national product.

METHODS OF DETECTION OF ADVERSE DRUG REACTIONS

There are no operational diagnostic criteria for the diagnosis of an adverse drug reaction. Such a diagnosis depends on the suspicions of the doctor, often based on the temporal relationship between the start of therapy and the occurrence of the side-effect.

The first time a particular adverse event is associated with a new drug depends on the type (see classification below) and frequency of the adverse event. Thus, a side-effect that is related to the pharmacological action of the drug will be detected early on, either in the volunteer or patient studies before the drug is marketed. However, since the drug will have been taken by approximately 3000 individuals prior to being marketed, rare side-effects may not be detected until the drug is well established. In the latter case, various forms of postmarketing surveillance (Table 37.1) may identify a causal association between a drug and an adverse event.

One of the most important methods for detecting uncommon adverse effects is the 'yellow card' reporting system operated by the Committee on Safety of Medicines (CSM), which was first set up in 1964. All suspected reactions to newly introduced drugs (marked with a ▼ in the *British National Formulary*) and severe reactions associated with the older drugs should be reported to the CSM. Unfortunately, there is gross under-reporting of all adverse reactions, including drug fatalities, with only 10% of adverse reactions being reported to the CSM. However, this is a useful system which can alert to previously unsuspected reactions with new agents, for example cough associated with angiotensin-converting enzyme inhibitors, and allows continued safety monitoring of established compounds.

To encourage reporting by anaesthetists, a separate yellow card for reporting anaesthetic drug reactions was introduced in 1988.

CLASSIFICATION OF ADVERSE DRUG REACTIONS

ADRs can be classified into four main groups (Table 37.2). Although not every drug reaction can be neatly

TABLE 37.1 Forms of postmarketing surveillance and examples of adverse drug reactions (ADRs) detected

TYPE	EXAMPLE	
	DRUG	ADVERSE REACTIONS
Case reports	Practolol	Dermatitis, keratoconjunctivitis, sclerosing peritonitis
Cohort studies	Oral contraceptives (Royal College of General Practitioners Study)	Cardiovascular disease
Case-control studies	Aspirin	Reyes syndrome
Prescription event monitoring	Enalapril	Deafness
Yellow cards	Angiotensin-converting enzyme inhibitors	Cough, urticaria

TABLE 37.2 Classification of adverse drug reactions

TYPE	CHARACTERISTICS	INCIDENCE	MORBIDITY	MORTALITY
A	Dose-dependent, predictable from known pharmacology of drug	High	High	Low
B	Dose-independent, unpredictable, host-dependent	Low	High	High
C	Long-term effects	Low	High	High
D	Delayed effects, e.g. carcinogenicity and teratogenicity	Low	High	High

classified into the different groups, this is a useful clinical and mechanistic classification. Each type of ADR is discussed with relevant examples given, although the lists of drugs given for the different types of toxicity are by no means complete, and interested readers should consult the further reading listed at the end of the chapter.

TYPE A ADVERSE DRUG REACTIONS

Type A reactions account for 75% of all ADRs. Common examples of such reactions are listed in Table 37.3. Because these reactions are an augmentation of the normal pharmacological properties of the drug, they are predictable, and thus to a large extent preventable. They often have a clear dose-dependent relationship and are host independent. Type A reactions are usually mild, but by virtue of their common occurrence, they account for a great deal of morbidity. Factors that predispose to type A reactions often do so because of a change in the pharmacokinetic properties of the drug discussed below.

Since type A reactions are dose-dependent, reduction of the dose often results in alleviation of the adverse effect. The prevention of type A reactions depends on several factors, including careful clinical assessment of the patient prior to drug prescription, adequate knowledge of the pharmacological properties of the drug being used, use of appropriate patient-individualized dosages, adjusted as necessary for some drugs, such as digoxin and lithium, by serum concentration monitoring. Simplification of drug regimes and a reduction in the total number of drugs prescribed will also help in the prevention of type A reactions.

TYPE B ADVERSE DRUG REACTIONS

Type B reactions are also termed idiosyncratic adverse drug reactions. This term as used in this chapter describes adverse reactions that occur in only a minority of patients, and does not presume the mechanism of the ADR.

In contrast to type A reactions, type B reactions are unpredictable from the known pharmacology of the drug, show no simple relationship between dose and incidence, and are apparently host dependent. They are less common than type A reactions, and are therefore not detected by preclinical safety evaluation during drug development. They tend to be much more severe than type A reactions and account for the majority of drug-associated fatalities. A further frustrating factor for those involved in trying to determine the mechanisms of these reactions is the lack of a suitable animal model. Idiosyncratic drug reactions can be broadly divided aetiologically into immunological and non-immunological.

The role of metabolism in mediating idiosyncratic adverse drug reactions

Drug metabolism can normally be considered a detoxification process (Fig. 37.1). Its role is to convert lipophilic, active drugs by a combination of phase I (oxidation, reduction and hydrolysis) and phase II metabolic pathways into water-soluble compounds that can then be readily excreted from the body. However, in certain circumstances, phase I metabolism

TABLE 37.3 Examples of type A adverse drug reactions

DRUG/DRUG GROUPS		ADVERSE EFFECTS
Amiodarone		Hypo/hyperthyroidism
Antacids		
	Magnesium-containing	Diarrhoea
	Aluminium-containing	Constipation
Anti-asthmatics		
	β_2 agonists	Tachycardia, tremor, headache
	Inhaled steroids	Oral candida, hoarseness
	Theophylline	Tachycardia, nausea. arrhythmia, GIT disturbances
Antibiotics		Diarrhoea, vomiting
Anticoagulants		Haemorrhage
Anticonvulsants (Phenytoin, phenobarbitone, carbamazepine)		Drowsiness, dizziness, ataxia, lethargy
Antihypertensives		Hypotension
	β antagonists	Bronchospasm, bradycardia, heart block, heart failure
	Diuretics	Dehydration, electrolyte disturbances
	Calcium antagonists	Headaches, flushing, ankle oedema
	ACE inhibitors	Renal failure (in patients with renal artery stenosis)
Antipsychotics		Parkinsonism, acute dystonic reactions, tardive dyskinesia, antimuscarinic effects (dry mouth blurred vision, etc.), postural hypotension, hypothermia, galactorrhoea, gynaecomastia
Antithyroid drugs		Hypothyroidism
Aspirin/NSAIDs		GIT bleeding
Antiviral drugs (Vidarabine, zidovudine, ganiciclovir)		Bone marrow suppression
Benzodiazepines		Drowsiness, confusion, respiratory depression
Corticosteroids		Cushing's syndrome
Digoxin		Nausea, heart block, arrhythmias
L-DOPA		Nausea, tachycardia, postural hypotension
Immunosuppressants		Opportunistic infections
Nitrates		Hypotension, headaches, flushing, tachycardia
Opioids		Respiratory depression, constipation
Oral hypoglycaemics		Hypoglycaemia
Tamoxifen		Hot flushes, vaginal bleeding
Thrombolytics		Haemorrhage
Tricyclic antidepressants		Antimuscarinic effects, tremor, hypomania, sedation, arrhythmias, convulsions

ACE, angiotensin-converting enzyme; GIT, gastrointestinal tract.

by the cytochrome P-450 enzyme system can lead to the formation of chemically reactive, toxic metabolites (Fig. 37.1). If inadequately detoxified by phase II metabolism, the metabolites can bind irreversibly to cellular macromolecules inducing carcinogenicity (see below), cellular necrosis or hypersensitivity (Fig. 37.2).

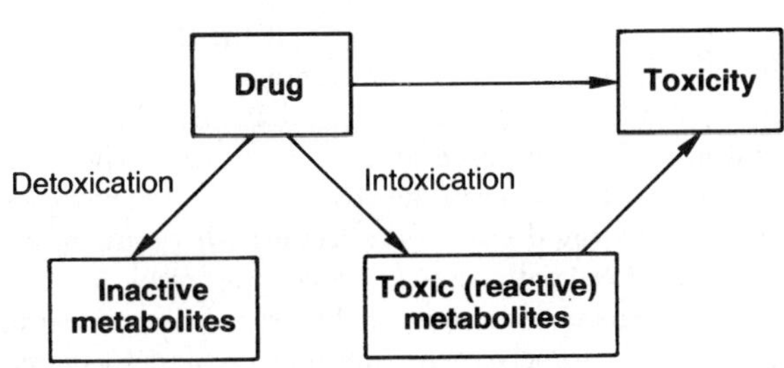

FIGURE 37.1 The role of metabolism in mediating idiosyncratic adverse drug reactions.

Metabolite-mediated direct toxicity

The chemical interaction of a toxic metabolite with cellular macromolecules, through either covalent bond formation or free-radical formation, can result in loss of cellular viability leading to tissue or organ necrosis. The toxic response to the initial challenge and to any subsequent rechallenge is often quite rapid, occurring with a few days, and is not accompanied by symptoms suggestive of an immunological response. The site of toxicity is dependent upon the

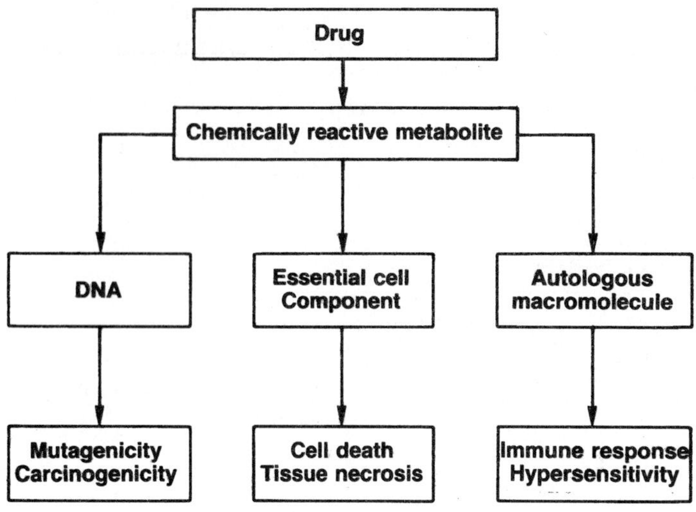

FIGURE 37.2 The possible mechanisms by which a chemically reactive metabolite can produce the different forms of drug toxicity.

site of generation of the toxic metabolite. Since the liver is the main site of drug metabolism in the body, this mechanism has been implicated in causing drug hepatotoxicity with certain drugs such as paracetamol, isonaizid, sodium valproate, ketoconazole and tacrine (an agent used in the treatment of Alzheimer's disease). The hepatotoxicity of alcohol may also be due to a similar mechanism.

Paracetamol in therapeutic doses is metabolized by sulphation, glucuronidation and oxidation to a chemically reactive metabolite which is normally detoxified by glutathione conjugation. However, after overdosage (10–15 g), the sulphation and glutathione pathways become saturated, allowing the reactive metabolite, N-acetyl-*p*-benzoquinoneimine, to bind covalently to essential hepatic proteins, with resultant necrosis. Thus, N-acetylcystine, which is used in the treatment of paracetamol overdosage, acts by increasing intracellular glutathione levels and thus restores detoxication of the reactive metabolite. Although the hepatic injury from paracetamol is predictable from the known pharmacology of the drug, and thus could be classified as a type A reaction, there is still considerable variation in host susceptibility; for example, children are less susceptible than adults to the hepatic damage, while chronic alcoholics (because of enzyme induction) are more susceptible.

Enzyme induction has also been shown to increase the incidence of isoniazid hepatotoxicity. Isoniazid given alone causes hepatitis in 1% of patients. The hepatitis is thought to be due to the formation of a reactive metabolite from a stable metabolite of isoniazid, acetylhydrazine. The use of isoniazid and rifampicin together, the mainstay in the treatment of tuberculosis, increases the incidence of hepatitis to 5–8%. It has been postulated that rifampicin, being a potent enzyme inducer, increases the formation of the reactive metabolite, thereby potentiating the isoniazid hepatotoxicity.

Drug hypersensitivity reactions

In this chapter, idiosyncratic (type B) ADRs which are immunologically mediated are termed drug hypersensitivity reactions. These reactions are thought to account for 20% of all ADRs.

It is well established that low molecular weight compounds (<1000 Da) – that is, drugs – cannot function as immunogens *per se*, but can initiate immune reactions only after covalent interaction with a macromolecular carrier, such as a protein, thereby acting as a hapten (Fig. 37.3). The covalent linkage is required for antigen processing by either macrophages or B lymphocytes, while antigen presentation and the resulting immune reaction involves a complex interaction between the major histocompatibility antigens (class II) and T and B lymphocytes. An immune response against a drug may be characterized by either specifically committed lymphocytes and/or antibodies directed against either the drug, the carrier protein (forming autoantibodies), or the neoantigen created by the combination of drug and protein. Drug hypersensitivity reactions can be classified into four types (Fig. 37.4), although these are not mutually exclusive.

Direct evidence for an immune-mediated mechanism is only available for a few drugs, such as penicillin, halothane and amodiaquine, while for the majority of drugs such evidence is lacking and the diagnosis has been based on clinical manifestations.

Typically, an induction period that varies between 2 and 6 weeks is required on first exposure to the drug before the occurrence of the adverse effect. On re-exposure to the drug the adverse effect usually occurs much sooner, often within 24 h, indicating prior specific immune sensitization against the drug. It is interesting to note that some patients develop immune-mediated reactions almost immediately despite not having a history of previous contact with the drug. In such cases,

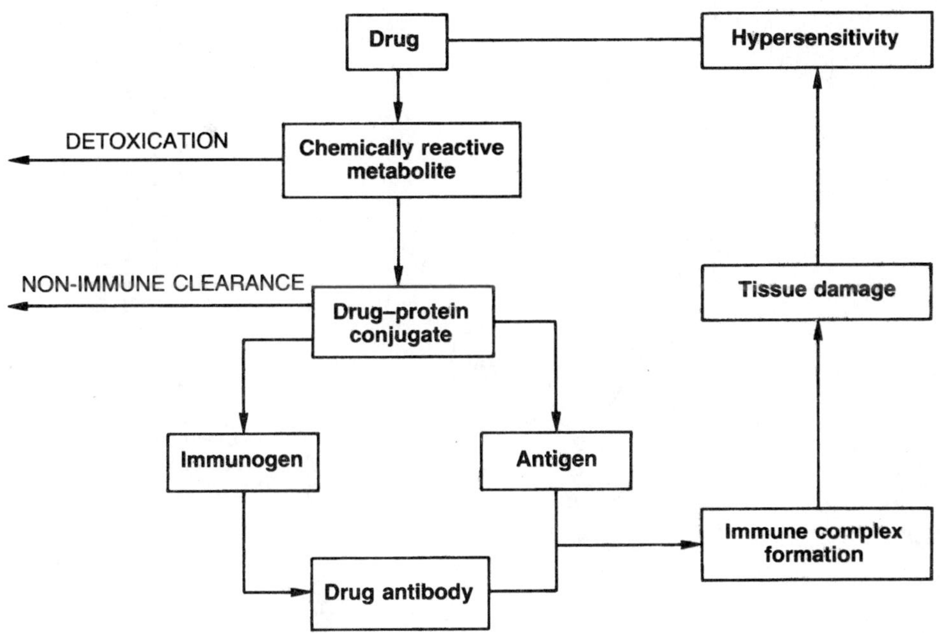

FIGURE 37.3 Schematic representation of the relationship between drug metabolism and drug hypersensitivity.

covert sensitization may have occurred; for example, with penicillin, sensitization may occur from drinking milk from animals treated with penicillin.

The clinical picture is highly variable, dependent not only on the drug, but also on the patient. The same drug can produce different toxic manifestations in different patients. However, most patients will develop symptoms and signs of drug hypersensitivity including fever, rash, arthralgia, lymphadenopathy and eosinphilia. Any other symptoms are dependent on the site of toxicity, the most commonly involved organs being the skin, liver and haematological system. An alternative presentation of drug hypersensitivity may be an anaphylactic reaction.

Sites of idiosyncratic toxicity

Anaphylaxis

Anaphylaxis is an example of a type I hypersensitivity reaction (Fig. 37.4). It usually occurs suddenly following exposure to the antigen and is manifested as breathlessness, urticaria and vomiting proceeding on to cardiovascular collapse with hypotension and shock. It is a medical emergency requiring immediate resuscitation of the patient and usually follows the second exposure to an antigen, although no history of previous exposure may be available. It is mediated by specific IgE antibodies, formed on previous exposure, cross-linking on a mast cell surface, resulting in the release of various chemical mediators including histamine, serotonin and leukotrienes. The mediators cause vasodilatation and increased permeability of the small blood vessels and bronchospasm, together with increased inflammatory cell infiltration.

A wide variety of insults ranging from bee stings to chemicals in strawberries can cause anaphylaxis. Drugs reported to cause anaphylaxis include antibiotics (particularly the penicillins), anaesthetic agents, radiocontrast media and non-steroidal anti-inflammatory drugs (NSAIDs) (see Chapter 38).

In anaesthesia, anaphylactic reactions to anaesthetic drugs are a major contributory factor to the overall morbidity and mortality. Part of the reason for this is that a large percentage of anaesthetic drugs have to be administered parenterally. In the past decade, three agents, propanidid, althesin and fazadinium, have been withdrawn because of an unacceptably high incidence of 'anaphylactoid reactions'. IgE-mediated type I allergic reactions to neuromuscular blocking drugs (NMBD) are well recognized. With these compounds, the specific IgE antibodies are directed towards the quaternary and tertiary ammonium groups on the drugs. Approximately 85% of patients who experience an anaphylactic reaction to NMBD have no history of prior exposure. It has been suggested that sensitization is due to drugs and chemicals containing tertiary or quaternary ammonium groups commonly encountered in the environment; for example, antiseptics, detergents, shampoos and throat lozenges to name a few. Prevention of such reactions depends on the identification of patients with specifically reactive IgE antibodies. Various assays are available (RAST, immunoassays and histamine release from basophil leucocytes), although further clinical research is required to determine their predictive value.

The cellular mechanisms and treatment of anaphylaxis are described in Chapter 38.

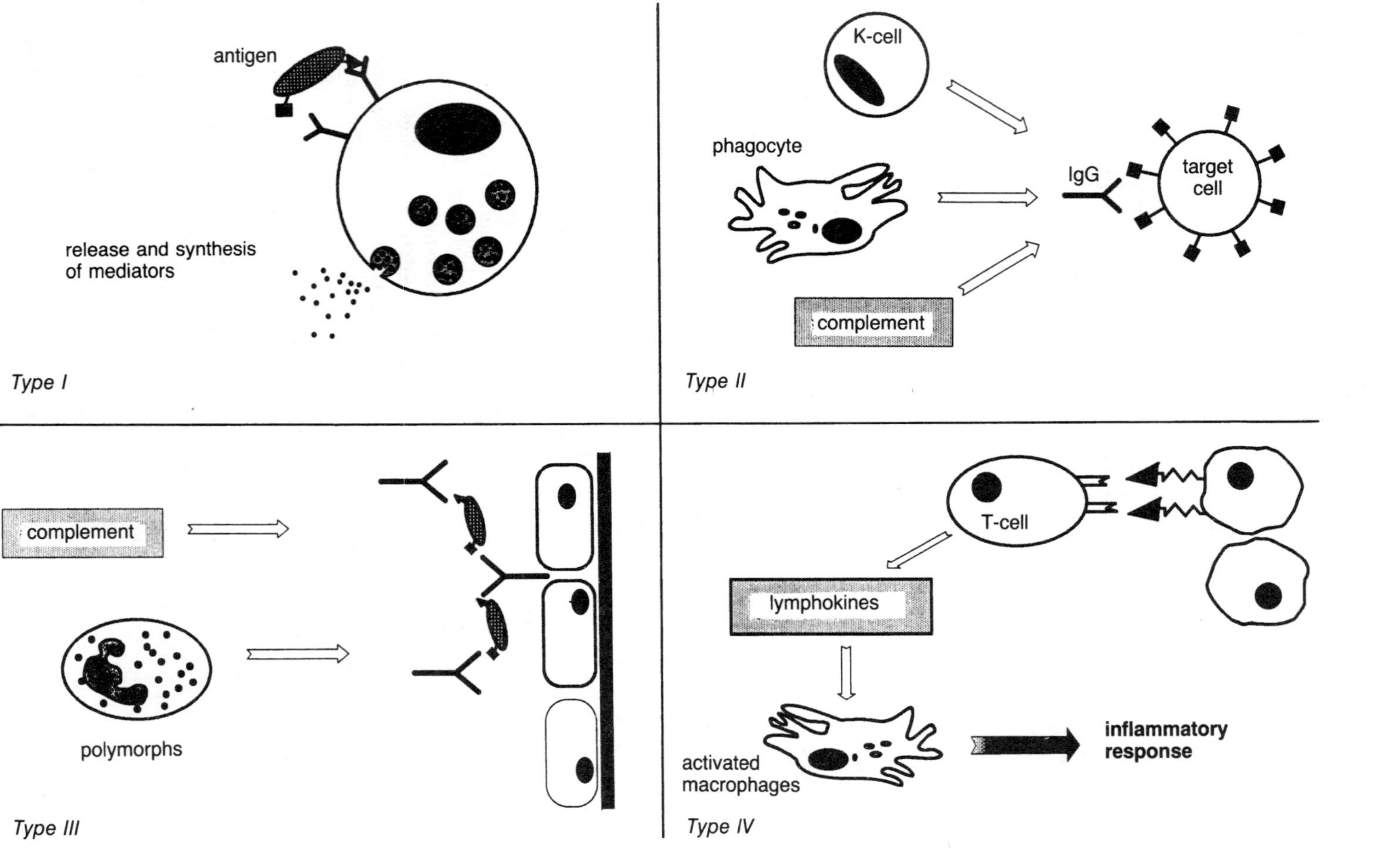

FIGURE 37.4 The four types of hypersensitivity reactions that can be induced by drugs. Type I; Specific IgE antibodies bind to mast cells via their F_c receptors. Binding of multivalent antigen to adjacent IgE induces degranulation and release of mediators, such as histamine and leukotrienes. Type II; Antibody (IgG, IgM) is directed against an individual's own cells. This may lead to cell destruction by killer T cells (K cells) or complement-mediated lysis. Alternatively, the cells may be removed by phagocytosis. Type III; Immune complexes are deposited in tissue (e.g. small blood vessels, glomerular basement membranes). Activation of complement leads to recruitment of polymorphs and a local inflammatory response. Type IV; Specific T cells bind to fixed antigen. Lymphokines are released that induce an inflammatory reaction and attract and activate macrophages, which release mediators.

Cutaneous reactions

Drug-induced cutaneous reactions are a common manifestation of idiosyncratic drug toxicity. These vary considerably in site, extent, severity, onset, and in time taken for improvement following drug withdrawal. The skin rash may be a primary manifestation of drug toxicity or may form part of a multisystem reaction. Drugs can cause any form of cutaneous reaction ranging from mild exanthematous eruptions to the severe, and occasionally fatal, toxic epidermal necrolysis (TEN). Two recent surveys have shown that the more severe cutaneous reactions such as erythema multiforme, Stevens–Johnson syndrome and TEN are rare, with incidence estimates of 7.0, 1.8 and 9.0 per 10^6 person-years, respectively. The drug groups most likely to cause such severe reactions are antibacterials (particularly co-trimoxazole), NSAIDs and the aromatic anticonvulsants (carbamazepine, phenytoin and phenobarbitone).

The mechanism of cutaneous reactions in most cases is unknown. With some drugs, for example phenytoin and to a lesser extent carbamazepine, the mild skin rashes may be dose-dependent. Such mild reactions are not accompanied by systemic manifestations. However, more severe rashes, particularly when accompanied by fever and circulating eosinophilia, are thought to be immune mediated. Evidence for the involvement of humoral immunity has been shown for some drugs, such as phenylbutazone, by the demonstration of antibody deposition in skin by immunofluorescence techniques. Cellular involvement may be of predominant importance in other cases, for example in ampicillin skin rashes in patients with infectious mononucleosis.

With some drug-induced rashes, it is not the drug itself that is the culprit, but the excipients used in the drug formulation. The best-known example of this is sensitivity to tartrazine, a yellow colouring used in many foodstuffs and drugs, which is manifested as urticaria and asthma.

Hepatotoxicity

Several hundred chemicals and drugs are known to cause hepatic injury, the pattern of which can mimic all patterns of non-drug-induced liver diseases described in man. A discussion of the classification and all the mechanisms of hepatic injury is beyond the scope of this section and interested readers are referred to the further reading at the end of this chapter.

Drug metabolite-mediated hepatic injury, either direct toxicity (see above) or immune-mediated, has been reported with a wide range of drugs (Table 37.4). Among the many causes of massive hepatic necrosis, drugs are responsible for 20–30% of cases, often having a case-fatality rate as high as 50%.

The severity of liver injury is variable ranging from asymptomatic elevation of liver enzymes to fatal hepatic failure. The histological picture can be either hepatocellular, mixed (hepatocellular and cholestatic), cholestatic or granulomatous (Table 37.4). The change in serum liver enzyme levels often reflects the histological pattern; thus, transaminases are elevated in hepatocellular injury, both transaminases and alkaline phosphatase (ALP) are raised in the mixed pattern, and ALP is raised in cholestatic and granulomatous liver injury.

The distinction between the two forms of idiosyncratic toxicity – that is, direct and immune-mediated toxicity – is often circumstantial, as has already been discussed. With immune-mediated hepatic damage, it is likely that both the humoral and cellular arms of the immune response are involved. In addition, it has been suggested that secondary involvement of the reticuloendothelial system is a factor in augmenting the hepatic damage.

Evidence for humoral immunity has been shown for some drugs, for example sera from patients with α-methyldopa-induced hepatitis have been shown to contain antibodies against drug-altered rabbit hepatocytes. Humoral immunity may also be manifested by the production of antibodies directed against the carrier protein – that is, autoantibodies (Fig. 37.5). Two types of drug-induced autoantibodies have been described: first, organ non-specific autoantibodies such as antinuclear antibodies. Antinuclear antibody has been shown in patients with hepatitis secondary to methyldopa, while a specific type of antimitochondrial antibody (termed anti-M_6) has been found in patients with

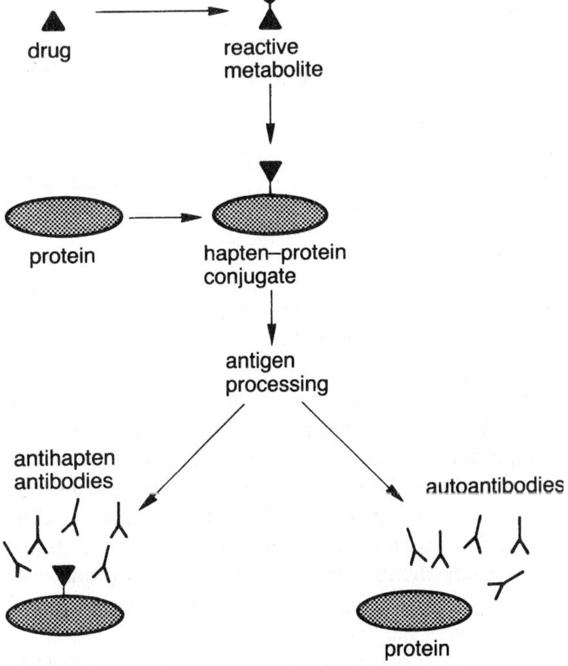

FIGURE 37.5 The postulated mechanism by which drugs can form autoantibodies.

TABLE 37.4 Some of the drugs reported to cause idiosyncratic hepatic damage

DRUGS	HISTOLOGY	COMMENTS
Anaesthetics		
Halothane	Hepatocellular hepatitis	Immune-mediated, reactive acyl halide (see text)
Enflurane	Hepatocellular hepatitis	Possible cross-reactivity with halothane
Antidepressants		
Monoamine oxidase inhibitors	Hepatocellular hepatitis Mixed	Immune-mediated
Tricyclic antidepressants	Hepatocellular Mixed Granulomatous	Hypersensitivity manifestations ? Genetic predisposition
Anticonvulsants		
Phenytoin	Hepatocellular	Hypersensitivity manifestations
Carbamazepine	Mixed Granulomatous	Thought to be due to arene oxide metabolites
Sodium valproate	Microvesicular steatosis	Direct toxicity Occurs in children
Antipsychotics		
Chlorpromazine	Cholestatic	1% incidence
Antithyroid drugs		
Carbimazole	Hepatocellular hepatitis	May be associated with leucopenia
Propylthiouracil	Mixed	
Cardiovascular agents		
Amiodarone	Phospholipidosis Alcoholic-like liver lesions	Mild and severe forms have been described
Calcium antagonists	Mixed	
Captopril	Mixed	
Dihydralazine	Hepatocellular hepatitis	Anticytochrome P-450 IA2 antibodies
Methyldopa	Hepatocellular hepatitis	See text
Infectious diseases		
Amodiaquine	Hepatocellular hepatitis	Reactive quinoneimine intermediate
Dapsone	Hepatocellular hepatitis Granulomatous	Reactive hydroxylamine metabolite
Erythromycin	Mixed	More common with estolate derivative
Isoniazid	Hepatocellular hepatitis	See text
Quinine	Granulomatous	Hypersensitivity manifestations may be present
Sulphonamides	Hepatocellular hepatitis Mixed	Reactive hydroxylamine metabolite
Tetracycline	Microvesicular hepatitis	Associated with pregnancy
Rheumatoid diseases		
Allopurinol	Hepatocellular hepatitis Mixed and granulomatous	May be associated with hypersensitivity manifestations
NSAIDs	Mixed	May be immune-mediated
Paracetamol	Hepatocellular hepatitis	Seen in overdosage Reactive metabolite

NSAIDs, non-steroid anti-inflammatory drugs.

hepatitis due to iproniazid, a monoamine oxidase inhibitor. The second type of autoantibody is specific for drug-induced disease, being virtually never found in spontaneous human diseases. For example, in patients with hepatitis induced by either tienilic acid or dihydralazine, specific anticytochrome P-450 antibodies have been demonstrated – these autoantibodies are directed against the P-450 enzyme that normally hydroxylates the drug.

Halothane hepatitis can be regarded as a model for immune-mediated hepatic damage caused by a drug metabolite. Two forms of hepatic injury have been reported; the first form occurs in 20% of patients and is characterized by a mild increase in the transaminase levels, but has no features of immune involvement. The second form is more severe and is thought to be immunologically mediated. It occurs in 1 in 35 000 patients on first exposure, and 1 in 3700 patients after multiple exposures. All animals and humans exposed to halothane are capable of generating hepatic neoantigens which correspond to distinct microsomal protein fractions that have been covalently modified by the reactive trifluoroacetyl halide metabolite of halothane, formed by P-450 mediated oxidation of the drug.

However, only patients with halothane hepatitis have circulating IgG antibodies that react with these neoantigens, suggesting that the predisposing factor to developing halothane hepatitis may be due to immune hyper-responsiveness to the neoantigens.

Haematological toxicity

All formed elements of the blood can be affected by idiosyncratic drug toxicity, either individually (resulting in anaemia, thrombocytopenia or granulocytopenia) or collectively resulting in aplastic anaemia. Such toxicity is relatively rare and is seen with a wide range of drugs (Table 37.5).

Aplastic anaemia

In aplastic anaemia, all cellular elements are depleted, suggesting that the haemopoietic pluripotential stem cell (HPSC) is the target cell. The mechanism of damage may involve either direct toxicity of a chemically reactive metabolite or immune-mediated destruction of HPSC via drug–antigen formation. With the former mechanism, the toxic metabolite may be produced either in the liver and then pass on to the bone marrow or may be produced locally in the vicinity of the progenitor cells. With chloramphenicol (incidence of aplastic anaemia 1 in 30 000), intermediary bacterial metabolism of the drug producing toxic metabolites is thought to be a predisposing factor for the development of aplastic anaemia (Fig. 37.6).

Immune-mediated bone marrow damage may involve antibody production against drug-altered cell surface antigens, as for example with amidopyrine and ibuprofen, and/or the induction of cytotoxic lymphocytes against bone marrow precursor cells; induction of cytotoxic lymphocytes has been shown in patients with amidopyrine-induced aplastic anaemia.

Agranulocytosis

Lowered circulating granulocytes may be a consequence of direct toxic damage or secondary to an immune reaction involving selective haptenation of the cell membrane. The former mechanism has been shown to occur with chlorpromazine where there is a gradual decrease in the neutrophil count; it may sometimes be associated with a mild decrease in the haemoglobin and platelet counts. The latter mechanism has been implicated for drugs such as propylthiouracil, although the numbers of patients found to have circulating antibodies has been small.

Haemolytic anaemia

Haemolysis may occur as a result of a genetically determined deficiency of intrinsic red cell enzymes such as glucose-6-phosphate dehydrogenase (G6PD) and methaemoglobin reductase (see section on pharmacogenetics). Alternatively, an immune mechanism involving either the production of antibodies against intrinsic erythrocyte antigens (i.e. autoantibodies, for example with methyldopa) or against the drug/metabolite adsorbed on to the red cell surface, as for example with penicillin and phenacetin, may be responsible.

Thrombocytopenia

Reduction in circulating platelets usually involves an immune mechanism of which three types have been hypothesized:

1 Drug and antibody bind to a specific receptor on the platelet surface, forming a tervalent complex, leading to damage of the platelet as an 'innocent bystander'. This mechanism has been shown with quinidine-induced thrombocytopenia.
2 Covalent binding of drug to platelet surface followed by antibody binding. No drug has yet consistently been shown to affect platelets by this mechanism.
3 Development of drug-induced platelet autoantibodies secondary to neoantigen formation on the platelet surface. Such a mechanism has been postulated for the thrombocytopenia associated with α-methyldopa, sodium valproate and L-DOPA.

TABLE 37.5 Some of the drugs reported to cause idiosyncratic haematological toxicity

APLASTIC ANAEMIA	AGRANULOCYTOSIS	HAEMOLYSIS	THROMBOCYTOPENIA
Amidopyrine	Amidopyrine	Cephalosporins	Carbamazepine
Carbamazepine	Amodiaquine	Mefenamic acid	Cotrimoxazole
Carbimazole	Carbamazepine	Methyldopa	Gold
Chloramphenicol	Carbimazole	Nomifensine	Heparin
Chlorpropamide	Clozapine	Penicillin	Methyldopa
Gold	Chlorpromazine	Procainamide	Mianserin
Penicillamine	Cotrimoxazole	Sulphonamides	Penicillamine
Phenothiazines	Imipramine		Procainamide
Phenylbutazone	Methyldopa		Quinidine
Phenytoin	Mianserin		Sulindac
Potassium perchlorate	Propylthiouracil		Sulphasalazine
Sulphonamides	Sulphasalazine		Valproate
Tricyclic antidepressants	Ticlopidine		

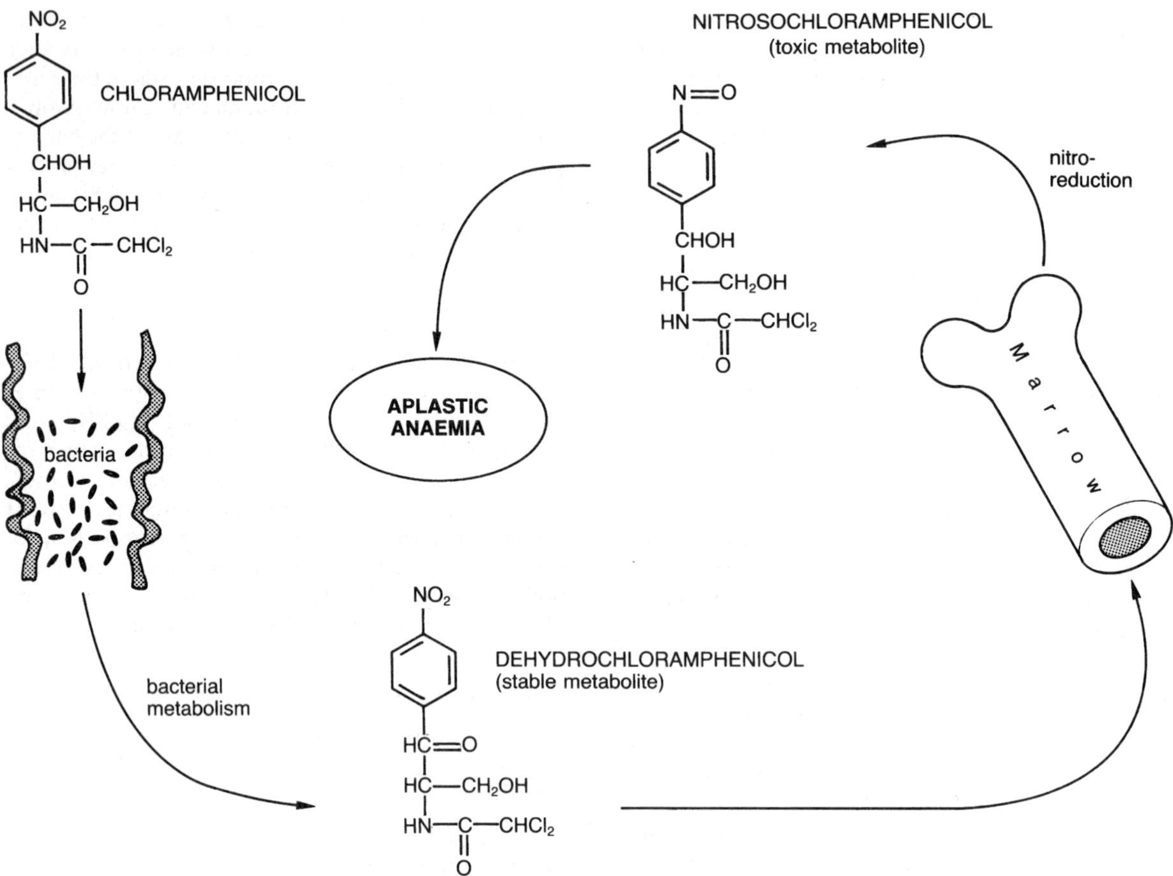

FIGURE 37.6 The role of intermediary bacterial metabolism in the pathogenesis of chloramphenicol-induced aplastic anemia.

Prevention of idiosyncratic drug reactions

Idiosyncratic drug reactions account for the majority of drug-associated fatalities. Currently, we have no consistent method of predicting which individual is likely to develop such a reaction, and thus, prevent it.

Two approaches could be used for the prevention of idiosyncratic drug reactions. First, synthesis of new drugs which would have the desired therapeutic effects without being converted to toxic metabolites. Unfortunately, this would not be possible for the majority of drugs since the structural features responsible for toxicity cannot always be defined, and in any extent may be essential for therapeutic efficacy.

The second method of prevention depends on developing *in vitro* genetic or biochemical tests to determine prospectively which individuals are likely to develop severe adverse effects. However, idiosyncratic drug reactions may be multifactorial in nature and thus, only when a single individual risk factor has been identified and shown to have a high correlation with the risk of toxicity would such a predictive test become feasible.

Clues to the understanding of individual susceptibility factors have come from research into the role of drug metabolism in drug toxicity. All individuals may be capable of bioactivating drugs into reactive metabolites to a greater or lesser extent. For the majority of the population, this would not represent a great hazard, as the bioactivation will be counterbalanced by the ability of the body to detoxify such metabolites allowing them to be harmlessly excreted from the body. In the minority of individuals who develop idiosyncratic drug toxicity, detoxification of a reactive metabolite may be deficient leading to an imbalance between activation and detoxication. Various factors, genetic and environmental, may be responsible for modulating the balance between activation and detoxication (Fig. 37.7).

A number of cellular detoxication systems have been described. These include:

1 Reduced glutathione (GSH), which is present intracellularly in concentrations as high as 10 mM. It is important in the direct inactivation of certain reactive metabolites, so-called 'soft' electrophiles. In addition, it is the primary substrate for GSH-S-transferases, an enzyme system required for the

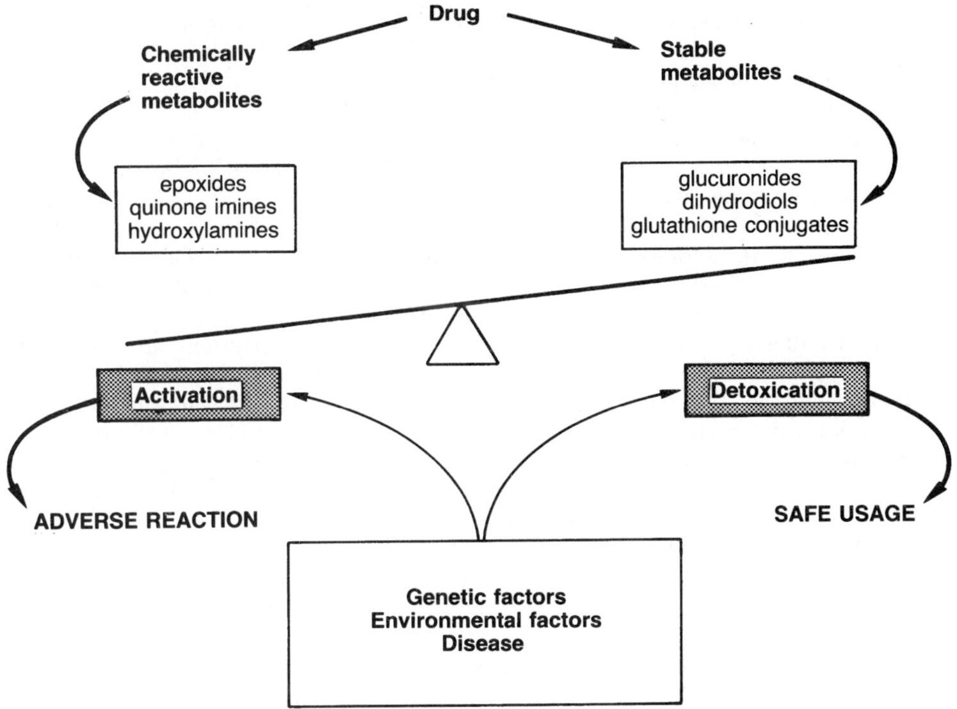

FIGURE 37.7 The importance of the balance between activation and detoxication in the predisposition to idiosyncratic adverse drug reactions.

inactivation of 'hard' electrophiles. It has been suggested that glutathione-deficient patients may be more susceptible to hepatotoxicity from paracetamol overdosage. Glutathione deficiency may be genetic in origin or environmentally acquired. For example, patients with AIDS have recently been shown to have a systemic deficiency of glutathione, which may partly account for their well-documented predisposition to drug hypersensitivity reactions.

2 Non-enzymic detoxication systems, which include ascorbate, tocopherols and β-carotene. β-Carotene is effective against singlet oxygen, while tocopherols are important intracellular radical scavengers, particularly effective in terminating lipid peroxidation reactions. Tocopherols are thought to be important in the detoxication of free radicals generated from nitrofurantoin. Ascorbic acid is important in the detoxication of superoxide anion radicals.

3 Enzymic detoxication systems, such as superoxide dismutase, catalase, catechol-*o*-methyltransferase and epoxide hydrolase. Of particular importance for toxic metabolites, such as arene oxides, may be the epoxide hydrolase enzyme system that is present in both the microsomal and cytosolic fractions of the cell.

Research in patients who have had hypersensitivity reactions to drugs may allow the identification of individual susceptibility factors, and thus the development of *in vitro* assays whereby idiosyncratic drug toxicity could be predicted and prevented. This can be illustrated by the example of primaquine, an antimalarial agent, which can cause life-threatening haemolysis in individuals deficient in G6PD. However, phenotyping of individuals for G6PD status prior to drug administration can eliminate the threat of haemolysis.

TYPE C ADVERSE DRUG REACTIONS

Type C ADRs occur with long-term therapy. In contrast to type B ADRs where only a minority of individuals are affected, with type C reactions the majority of individuals will be affected provided they take the drug for long enough. Typical examples include benzodiazepine dependence (see Chapter 38) and analgesic nephropathy.

Analgesic nephropathy is a cause of chronic renal failure in 15–22% of dialysis patients. It is the result of prolonged and excessive abuse of analgesic mixtures containing phenacetin, aspirin and caffeine. This mixture is more nephrotoxic than the drugs taken individually. The average nephrotoxic dose of analgesic mixtures contains about 5–10 kg of phenacetin. Some patients develop renal damage sooner than others, but all will develop renal failure if they continue to take the analgesic mixture for long enough. More recently, NSAIDs have also been shown to cause analgesic nephropathy.

The presentation of analgesic nephropathy is variable, ranging from co-incidental detection on routine urine testing to terminal renal failure. About 8% of patients develop uroepithelial tumours, most commonly in the bladder.

Paracetamol (the main metabolite of phenacetin), aspirin and caffeine seem to act synergistically to produce renal damage. Both paracetamol and aspirin are concentrated within the renal medulla. Aspirin acetylates components of cell membranes, uncouples oxidative phosphorylation and inhibits amino acid incorporation into cellular proteins. In addition, aspirin depletes intracellular glutathione, allowing the reactive metabolite of paracetamol to bind to tissue proteins, resulting in cytotoxicity. Caffeine by causing a diuresis and thus dehydration increases the concentration of aspirin and paracetamol in the renal medulla. Uroepithelial tumours occurring in analgesic nephropathy have an induction period of 20 years and may be related to the *o*-aminophenol and N-hydroxylated metabolites of phenacetin.

The removal of phenacetin from analgesic mixtures in several countries has been followed by a reduction in mortality and in the percentage of patients proceeding to terminal renal failure.

TYPE D ADVERSE DRUG REACTIONS

Drugs and teratogenicity

It is only since the 1960s (since the thalidomide disaster) that teratogenicity has been regarded as a serious hazard for man. It is thought that 1–5% of all congenital anomalies are caused by drugs. Prior to the establishment of the CSM, toxicological testing of new drugs was not legally required. Since 1964, all new drugs have to be screened for their teratogenic potential. Two species (usually rat or mouse and the rabbit) have to be administered the drug during the period of embryogenesis and the fetus subsequently examined for structural defects. In addition, in order to test the effects on fertility, males are treated with the drug for about 60 days prior to mating to cover all stages of spermatogenesis. Females are also administered the drug in the last trimester to assess the effects of drugs on fetal growth.

Any drug found to cause teratogenicity will be abandoned at an early stage of development. However, it must be emphasized that because of species differences in drug handling, a drug shown to be teratogenic in an animal species would not necessarily have caused the same or any defects in humans. Indeed, a large number of drugs currently on the market, for example aspirin, which are not known to be teratogenic in humans would not have passed the current safety requirements. Conversely, drugs that are not teratogenic in animals may cause birth defects in humans. The classic example of this is thalidomide where the rodent species are insensitive to its teratogenic effects, while humans and higher primates are susceptible. Therefore, despite these tests, postmarketing surveillance of new drugs is essential to identify such adverse effects as soon as possible after the introduction of the drug.

Importance of the stage of pregnancy

The effect of a drug on the fetus depends upon the stage of pregnancy at which it is administered. The most critical period is the period of organogenesis, which in humans is between the third week to the third month of pregnancy. During this period the major organs are formed and drugs interfering with this development may result in malformations such as spina bifida, phocomelia and so on. Exposure to drugs in the latter stages in pregnancy may result in fetal growth retardation or microcephaly and mental retardation.

Mechanisms of actions of teratogenic agents

For most drugs, the mechanism of teratogenicity is unknown. In some cases, known pharmacological actions of the drug may be responsible; for example, masculinization of the female fetus with administration of androgens. Some drugs, such as methotrexate and trimethoprim, are known inhibitors of the enzyme dihydrofolate reductase, which can result in folate deficiency, a known risk factor for congenital abnormalities.

More recently, analogous with the mechanisms proposed for the causation of type B adverse reactions, it has been increasingly realized that the parent drug *per se* may not be toxic to the fetus, but a reactive metabolite formed by the cytochrome P-450 enzyme system may be responsible. Such reactive intermediates formed from the drug could bind to essential cellular macromolecules – that is, proteins and nucleic acids – and mediate the teratogenic effects. Since drug metabolic pathways vary between different species, the involvement of reactive metabolites in the pathogenesis of drug teratogenicity, may explain interspecies differences in sensitivity to the same teratogenic agent.

The bioactivation of a drug to a reactive metabolite may occur either in the mother or in the fetus. The former mechanism presupposes that the reactive metabolite would be stable enough to pass from the maternal liver into the bloodstream and across the placenta before coming into contact with embryonic cells. However, this is unlikely for the majority of toxic metabolites as these are, by definition, unstable and have very short half-lives. Embryonic bioactivation of drugs to reactive metabolites is a strong possibility, which has been strengthened by the finding that bioactivation of known teratogens such as diethylstilboestrol does occur in rat embryos at early stages in development. For obvious reasons, it is not known what the cytochrome P-450 profile is in the human fetus, but studies in rats have shown that P-450 enzymes are present as early as the eleventh day of gestation.

The use of a potentially teratogenic agent will result in teratogenicity in only a minority of those exposed. Even with thalidomide the risk of fetal malformation has been estimated to be between 10 and 50%. Similarly, with alcohol, heavy maternal consumption leads to the fetal alcohol syndrome in 30–50% of the offspring. The reasons for individual susceptibility are not known, but as with type B adverse reactions, the ability of the fetus to detoxify reactive metabolites may be of paramount importance. However, very little is known about the detoxication mechanisms in the fetus, the time at which they are fully developed, and what factors modulate these mechansims. It is likely that the detoxication mechanisms that are important in predisposing to type B adverse drug reactions (discussed above) are also of importance.

In this context, of particular interest are the teratogenic effects of anticonvulsants, the overall risk of congenital anomalies being two to three times that in unexposed babies. The teratogenic effects of phenytoin and carbamazepine are thought to be caused by toxic, arene oxide intermediates. However, with phenytoin, only 5–10% of infants exposed to phenytoin *in utero* develop the full-blown fetal hydantoin syndrome. A genetic predisposition to developing birth defects with phenytoin has been shown, and a recent study has shown that affected infants have reduced levels of microsomal epoxide hydrolase, the enzyme required for detoxication of any arene oxide metabolites formed from phenytoin.

Table 37.6 lists some of the drugs that are known to be teratogenic in man. General anaesthetics have been reported to cause teratogenic effects in females working in operating theatres; there is scant evidence of their effects in pregnant women given an anaesthetic for an operation. It has been found by several studies that female anaesthetists and nurses working in operating theatres have a higher risk of spontaneous abortions, low-birthweight babies and offspring with congenital anomalies. Male anaesthetists may also be at risk; some studies have shown an increase in the rate of spontaneous abortions in the wives of anaesthetists and a 30% increase in 'minor' congenital malformations in the children of exposed fathers. The mechanism of teratogenicity is unclear, although it has been suggested that metabolites and breakdown products of anaesthetics may be responsible. Prevention will depend on better ventilation of theatres in order to reduce pollution and avoiding exposure at the time of pregnancy.

Drugs and carcinogenicity

Chemicals and drugs that induce cancer in an intact organism are referred to as carcinogens. The term does not differentiate between the various mechanisms by which a chemical compound can induce cancer. In a broad sense chemical carcinogens can induce neoplastic changes by acting either as genotoxic carcinogens (initiators), which damage DNA directly and cause mutations, or as epigenetic carcinogens (promoters), which accelerate the accumulation of critical spontaneous mutations.

Cancer has not been a common cause of drug toxicity to date, but is still of major concern in drug development for two reasons. First, a number of chemically and pharmacologically unrelated substances are carcinogenic in experimental animals. Second, cancer can take many years to develop, and in mammals this may correspond to half the natural lifespan. Appreciation of the fundamental mechanisms involved in chemical carcinogenesis is essential for the development of reliable screening systems for new drugs, and maintenance of vigilance for delayed effects in man.

Carcinogenic transformation is thought to occur primarily in cells that have the capacity to proliferate. Thus the target cells are most likely the so-called stem cells of the organ. Fully differentiated non-proliferating cells are unlikely to undergo malignant transformation. The

TABLE 37.6 Drugs reported to cause teratogenicity

DRUG	TERATOGENIC EFFECTS
Alcohol	Facial abnormalities (short palpebral fissures, hypoplastic upper lip, short nose); intrauterine growth retardation; microcephaly; mental retardation; increased risk with increased consumption; incidence 1 in 300–2000 live births
Androgens	Masculinization of female embryo. Dose-dependent effects
Carbamazepine	Craniofacial anomalies; growth retardation; spina bifida
Diethylstilboestrol	Masculinization of female; vaginal adenocarcinoma; anomalies of cervix and uterus; dose-dependent effects
Isotretinoin	Hydrocephalus; cardiovascular anomalies; microtia; micrognathia; cleft palate; retinal abnormalities; optic nerve defects
Phenytoin	Craniofacial anomalies; growth retardation; mental retardation; limb defects; cardiovascular anomalies; variable presentation; full-blown syndrome in 5–10%
Tetracycline	Hypoplastic tooth enamel, tooth and bone staining. Exposure during second or third trimester
Thalidomide	Bilateral limb defects, oesophageal or duodenal atresia, fetal ototoxicity, cardiovascular anomalies
Thyroid: antithyroid drugs	Fetal hypothyroidism; goitre
Valproate	Spina bifida

neoplasm that finally emerges is usually the progeny of a single cell. Carcinogenic cells differ from normal cells by their autonomous growth and invasive growth in a tissue. The hallmark of a cancer cell is immortality combined with uncontrolled growth. The new phenotype is a consequence of an irreversible, heritable change in the structure of the genetic material. A number of genes have now been identified in mammalian cells that are thought to be involved in the neoplastic process. These so-called proto-oncogenes can confer on a cell features of a cancerous phenotype and the gene products are related to pathways that determine the cell's response to growth-stimulating factors and/or differentiation, for example growth factors, growth factor receptors, cytoplasmic and nuclear regulatory proteins. Conversion of the proto-oncogenes into oncogenes (activation) can be effected by either a virus or a chemical.

Experimental and clinical evidence indicates that cancer is a multistep process, and that multiple genetic changes are required before a normal cell becomes fully neoplastic. The stages are broadly defined as initiation, promotion and progression. A number of environmental chemicals, food additives and hormones are proven carcinogens in animals and therefore potentially carcinogenic in man. With respect to therapeutic agents, the two main areas of concern that have emerged are the long-term use of hormones and drugs used in chemotherapy.

A number of anticancer drugs have been implicated in the occurrence of secondary acute myelogenous leukaemias arising in cancer patients several years after successful treatment. Prominent among these drugs are chlorambucil, cyclophosphamide and melphalan, all of which are alkylating agents that can bind covalently to DNA in a similar manner to established chemical mutagens.

The carcinogenic effects of hormones, such as oestradiol, are well established in animal models. It is thought that the mechanism is complex and that the oestrogen may well act as either initiator or promoter depending upon the circumstances and the tissue involved. Furthermore, it is now clear that a number of human cancers (breast, prostatic, thyroid, etc.) are hormone dependent, and thus respond to antihormone therapy or surgical ablation.

The relative risk of cancer associated with synthetic oestrogens administered at pharmacological doses, but for prolonged periods, is far more difficult to assess. Retrospective epidemiological studies are confused by the fact that individuals may have been exposed to a variety of hormonal preparations at different periods in their lives. Given the latency associated with cancer, it is difficult to establish cause and effect relationships.

The most widely studied aspect of drug-induced cancer in humans has been the relative risk associated with the use of the combined oral contraceptive. The effects observed have been modest and thus large cohorts of patients have required evaluation to obtain statistically significant results. Although the major studies have sometimes produced contradictory data, current opinion indicates that oral contraceptive use is associated with a moderately raised risk in younger nulliparous age groups and long-term users. However, the majority of these studies do not directly reflect the use of modern low-dose oral contraceptives pills. In view of this and the contradictory data, it is generally agreed that further, more carefully designed, studies are required. In the meantime, no revision of prescribing criteria has been recommended, although the low-dose oral contraceptive pill should be used wherever possible.

HOST FACTORS AND DRUG TOXICITY

Age

ADRs are more common at extremes of age. In the elderly, 10% of all hospital admissions may be due to drug side-effects. This is due to several factors: first, drugs are used much more frequently in the elderly than in any other age group. Second, multiple drugs are often prescribed in the elderly, increasing the risk of adverse drug interactions. Indeed, it has been shown that ADRs increase from 11% in those receiving one drug to 27% in those receiving six drugs. Third, changes in pharmacokinetics and pharmacodynamics, largely as a result of age-related changes in physiology (Table 37.7), contribute to the increased incidence of ADRs in the elderly. Metabolism of some drugs, particularly those with long half-lives, is impaired in the elderly, resulting in drug accumulation with consequent toxicity. This is illustrated by the experience with benoxaprofen, a NSAID withdrawn because of toxicity, which was more severe in the elderly. The half-life of benoxaprofen was found to be four times longer in the elderly than in young patients, resulting in drug accumulation and the reported toxic effects of kidney and liver damage. Finally, disease states which are more common in the elderly may alter the handling of a particular drug predisposing to an ADR. Thus, liver disease may be associated with impaired metabolism, while renal disease impairs drug excretion, both resulting in accumulation of the parent drug. The drugs that are particularly liable to cause ADRs in the elderly are listed in Table 37.8.

In neonates, certain drugs may cause ADRs not usually seen in adults because of poorly developed drug metabolism and elimination pathways. Chloramphenicol can cause a fatal grey syndrome in neonates characterized by vomiting, abdominal distension, grey pallor, shock and respiratory failure. This is thought to be due to failure of the drug to be conjugated with glucuronic acid (due to an inadequately developed glucuronyl transferase) and poor renal excretion of the conjugated drug. Similarly, with morphine, inadequate glucuronidation renders neonates very susceptible to its respiratory depressant effects. Sulphonamides, novobiocin, and vitamin K can lead to kernicterus in premature babies because of displacement of bilirubin

TABLE 37.7 Age-related changes in physiology

PHYSIOLOGICAL CHANGE	PHARMACOLOGICAL CONSEQUENCE	EXAMPLE OF AFFECTED DRUG
Decline in lean body mass Increase in body fat	Change in volume of distribution	Digoxin Diazepam
Intestinal mucosal atrophy	Altered absorption Altered intestinal wall enzyme activity	L-DOPA
Reduced hepatic blood flow	Reduced metabolism	Lignocaine
Reduced hepatic function	Reduced metabolism Reduced first-pass effect	Propranolol
Decreased glomerular filtration rate	Decrease in drug elimination	Digoxin
Decreased renal tubular secretion	Reduced drug elimination	Penicillins Aminoglycosides
Alteration of blood–brain barrier	Increased CNS drug entry	Nitrazepam
Reduction in number and altered sensitivity of β-receptors	Altered drug action	β-blockers Sympathomimetic amines

TABLE 37.8 Drugs particularly associated with adverse effects in the elderly

Antihypertensives
Antidepressants/tranquillizers/hypnotics
Diuretics
Anti-Parkinsonian drugs
Corticosteroids
Anticoagulants
Non-steroidal anti-inflammatory drugs
Digoxin
Insulin/hypoglycaemics

from plasma proteins. In contrast, there is a lower incidence of severe paracetamol hepatotoxicity in children which may be related to a greater ability of the young to metabolize paracetamol via non-toxic pathways.

Sex

ADRs are twice as common in women as in men, largely as a result of increased use of drugs in women.

Genetic constitution

This is discussed below in the section on Pharmacogenetics and drug toxicity.

Previous adverse reaction

Patients who have previous ADRs to a drug are more likely to have a further ADR when prescribed other drugs.

Disease

Disease may alter the handling and response to a drug predisposing to an ADR. Thus, renal or hepatic disease may impair elimination of a drug from the body resulting in accumulation of the parent drug. Other diseases, such as congestive cardiac failure, can reduce clearance of drugs like propranolol and lignocaine because of a reduction in hepatic blood flow. Atopic patients have a higher incidence of drug hypersensitivity reactions.

PHARMACOGENETICS AND DRUG TOXICITY

The considerable interindividual variation seen with drug response is due to a combination of environmental factors and host genetic constitution. The field of genetic variation in drug response has been termed pharmacogenetics. Genetic variation can either affect the metabolism of the drug (altering its rate and/or route of elimination) or response to the drug, both of which can predispose to drug toxicity. The abnormality is due to a mutant allele causing either a quantitative enzyme deficiency, or more commonly, a qualitative change in gene expression (i.e. structural abnormality with altered substrate specificity).

Table 37.9 lists some of the drugs where genetic influences are of prime importance in determining the incidence of toxicity.

Of the polymorphisms affecting drug metabolism, the classical examples are the hydrolysis of succinylcholine, the acetylator status and drug oxidation polymorphisms.

Succinylcholine, a neuromuscular-blocking agent, produces paralysis of short duration because of its rapid hydrolysis to the inactive succinylmonocholine by cholinesterases present in the plasma and liver. In about 1 in 3000 individuals, succinylcholine administration causes paralysis and apnoea lasting several hours, because of an atypical plasma cholinesterase which has a substrate affinity at least 100-fold less than the normal variant.

The acetylation of drugs is one of the major phase II metabolic inactivation pathways. It was first described

TABLE 37.9 Genetically determined variation in drug metabolism and drug response predisposing to drug toxicity

CONDITION	MECHANISM	INHERITANCE	FREQUENCY	DRUGS	EFFECT
Slow and fast acetylators	Variation in hepatic N-acetyltransferase	Slow: AR Fast: AD	Slow: 60% Fast: 40%	Isoniazid Procainamide (Table 37.12)	See text
Debrisoquine Hydroxylation Polymorphism	Lack of cytochrome P-450 2D6	Unknown	5–10% of population	Debrisoquine Phenacetin (Table 17.13)	See text
Suxamethonium sensitivity	Abnormal plasma cholinesterase with reduced substrate affinity	AR	1:3000	Suxamethonium	Prolonged paralysis and apnoea
G6PD deficiency	Inadequate protection against oxidative red cell damage	X-linked recessive	200 million people affected	See text	Haemolysis
Methaemoglobinaemia	Methaemoglobin reductase deficiency	AR	1:100 heterozygotes	Same drugs as for G6PD deficiency	Methaemoglobinaemia Haemolysis
Steroid-induced glaucoma	Unknown	AR	5% white population	Glucocorticoids	Raised intraocular pressure
Malignant hyperthermia	Defective ryanodine receptor	AD	1:20 000	Anaesthetics	Hyperthermia Muscle rigidity
Porphyria	Abnormal inducibility of δ-amino laevulinic acid synthetase	AD	Variable incidence dependent on type of porphyria	Barbiturates	Acute porphyria

G6PD, glucose-6-phosphate dehydrogenase; AR, autosomal recessive; AD, autosomal dominant.

in 1954, and it is now well documented that the ability to N-acetylate xenobiotics is under genetic control, the fast acetylator phenotype inherited as autosomal dominant and the slow acetylator phenotype as autosomal recessive. Slow acetylators have a deficiency in the cytosolic enzyme N-acetyltransferase. More recent studies have shown that there are two distinct loci for N-acetyl transferase, both of which have been mapped to chromosome 8 : one codes for the polymorphic N-acetyltransferase (NAT-2), which leads to variation in acetylation, while the second form is a monomorphic N-acetyltransferase (NAT-1) which does not vary in the population.

The frequency of the slow acetylator phenotype varies according to the population studied; 52% of the British population are slow acetylators, while less than 10% of the Japanese population are slow acetylators. A large number of xenobiotics undergo acetylation (Table 37.10). In general, slow acetylators tend to eliminate the drug more slowly, and thus have higher plasma levels of the parent drug and/or phase I oxidative metabolites which predisposes to dose-dependent toxicity (Table 37.10). Fast acetylators eliminate the drug more rapidly and have lower plasma levels after ingestion of equivalent doses than slow acetylators. This can occasionally lead to therapeutic failure, for example with isoniazid in the treatment of tuberculosis.

More recently, pharmacogenetic polymorphisms affecting phase I oxidative metabolic pathways have been described. The most widely studied of these is the polymorphism affecting debrisoquine hydroxylation and sparteine oxidation; in addition, independent polymorphisms have been reported for tolbutamide hydroxylation and mephenytoin hydroxylation.

Two distinct phenotypes can be distinguished in individuals given the antihypertensive drug, debrisoquine. The so-called 'extensive metabolizers' (EM) excrete 10–200 times more of the urinary metabolite 4-hydroxy debrisoquine than 'poor metabolizers' (PM). The PM phenotype behaves as an autosomal recessive trait and has a frequency of about 8% in the British population. Patients with PM phenotype have a deficiency of the cytochrome P-450 enzyme 2D6. Characterization at the DNA and mRNA level has shown that at least three forms of incorrectly spliced P-450 2D6 pre-mRNAs are present in the livers of PM.

Cytochrome P-450 2D6 has a broad substrate specificity and has been found to be involved in the metabolism of at least twenty commonly used drugs. A deficiency of this enzyme may lead to either therapeutic failure or drug toxicity. The former has been described with drugs, such as codeine, which need to be metabolized to their active components by the enzyme. Three types of adverse reactions are possible in PM: first poor metabolism of the drug will diminish first-pass metabolism, increase bioavailability and therefore result in an exaggerated pharmacological response, for example hypotension with debrisoquine. Second, diminished metabolism prolongs the half-life of a drug and leads to accumulation with consequent toxicity, for example neuropathy and hepatotoxicity with perhexiline were found to be much more common in PM. Third, the deficiency of the usual metabolic pathway can alter the route of metabolism of a drug, causing the formation of toxic metabolites, for example, phenacetin-induced methaemoglobinaemia. Some of the adverse reactions that have been associated with the PM phenotype are listed in Table 37.11.

Of the genetic polymorphisms affecting the response to a drug, perhaps the most important is G6PD deficiency which affects an estimated 200 million people worldwide. G6PD deficiency is inherited as X-linked recessive and therefore only affects males, with females' heterozygotes having two populations of red cells, deficient and normal. G6PD is essential for the detoxification of free radicals and peroxides by providing a source of reducing power that maintains sulphydryl groups. Thus, deficient cells are unable to reduce oxidized glutathione to reduced glutathione via the hexose monophosphate shunt, rendering them liable to oxidative damage from various insults including the ingestion of fava beans and certain drugs. Such patients may develop haemolysis, the severity of which varies according to the variant of the enzyme. Drugs reported to elicit haemolysis in deficient patients include the aminoquinolines (primaquine, chloroquine), sulphonamides (sulphapyridine, sulphamethoxazole, sulphamethoxypyridazine), dapsone, antimicrobials (nitrofurantoin, nalidixic acid) and doxorubicin. Simple avoidance of such drugs and/or phenotyping patients prior to drug administration should prevent the oxidative haemolysis.

TABLE 37.10 Effect of slow acetylator phenotype on xenobiotic toxicity

DRUG	ADVERSE REACTION
Isoniazid	Peripheral neuropathy and SLE
Procainamide	ANA and SLE
Hydralazine	ANA and SLE
Sulphasalazine	Nausea/vomiting
Arylamines	Bladder cancer

ANA, antinuclear antibodies; SLE, systemic lupus erythematosus.

TABLE 37.11 Association between debrisoquine hydroxylation poor metabolizer phenotype and drug toxicity

DRUG	ADVERSE REACTION
Debrisoquine	Hypotension
Perhexilene	Hepatotoxicity; neuropathy
Metoprolol	Excessive β-blockade
Nortryptiline	Confusion
Phenformin	Lactic acidosis
Phenacetin	Methaemoglobinaemia

DRUG INTERACTIONS AND DRUG TOXICITY

Many patients, particularly the elderly and those with chronic disease such as epilepsy and asthma, are often on polytherapy. The chance of a drug–drug interaction resulting in toxicity increases with the number of drugs prescribed; it has been estimated that if five drugs are given simultaneously, there is a 75% chance of causing an adverse drug interaction.

Although many types of drug interactions have been described, only a small proportion are clinically important. These usually involve drugs with a narrow therapeutic index, for example anticoagulants, anticonvulsants, theophylline, digoxin and lithium. The drug interaction may have two types of effects:

1 Elevation of plasma levels of the principal drug by the interacting drug resulting in drug toxicity (usually type A ADR).
2 Reduction in the plasma level of the principal drug because of the interaction resulting in therapeutic failure, and recurrence of the disease for which the drug was originally prescribed.

Drug interactions can be classified into pharmacokinetic and pharmacodynamic interactions. The pharmacokinetic interactions occur because of interference in the processes of absorption, distribution, metabolism or excretion; Table 37.12 lists some of the more important interactions, their mechanisms and toxic effects. With pharmacodynamic interactions, one drug alters the effect of another resulting in either synergism or antagonism (Table 37.13).

Rational prescribing based on a knowledge of the pharmacology of drugs prone to interactions, aided where appropriate by measurement of either circulating drug concentrations – for example, anticonvulsants, digoxin, lithium and theophyllines – or pharmacological effects, for example, monitoring of coagulation tests in patients on anticoagulants, will greatly increase the chances of avoiding adverse drug interactions.

TABLE 37.12 Important pharmacokinetic drug interactions that can result in drug toxicity

PRINCIPAL DRUG	INTERACTING DRUG(S)	EFFECT	MECHANISM
Azathioprine 6-Mercaptopurine	Allopurinol	Enhanced toxicity	Inhibition of xanthine oxidase
Carbamazepine	Sodium valproate	Increased carbamazepine levels	Inhibition of epoxide hydrolase
Carbamazepine	Isoniazid; verapamil; erythromycin	Increased carbamazepine levels	P-450 enzyme inhibitor
Cyclosporin A	Erythromycin; ketoconazole	Liver damage; kidney damage	Inhibition of cytochrome P-450IIIA
Digoxin	Quinidine; verapamil; amiodarone	Increased digoxin levels	Reduced renal clearance
Digoxin	K^+-losing diuretic	Digoxin toxicity	Hypocalcaemia
Lithium	Thiazides	Increased lithium levels	Increased tubular reabsorption
Lithium	NSAIDs	Increased lithium levels	Reduced excretion
Methotrexate	Aspirin; NSAIDs	Methotrexate toxicity	Reduced renal excretion + protein binding
Oral contraceptive	Phenytoin; phenobarbitone; carbamazepine; rifampicin	Pregnancy	Enzyme induction
Oral contraceptive	Broad-spectrum antibiotic, e.g. ampicillin	Pregnancy	Interruption of enterohepatic circulation
Phenytoin	Isoniazid; cimetidine; chloramphenicol	Increased phenytoin levels	P-450 enzyme inhibitor
Theophyllines	Cimetidine; erythromycin; ciprofloxacin	Theophylline toxicity	P-450 enzyme inhibitor
Warfarin	Phenytoin; phenobarbitone; carbamazepine; rifampicin	Therapeutic failure	P-450 enzyme induction
Warfarin	Cimetidine; sulphonamides; phenylbutazone	Excessive anticoagulation	P-450 enzyme inhibitor
Zidovudine (AZT)	Paracetamol	Increased bone marrow suppression	? Competition for glucuronidation

NSAIDs, non-steroid anti-inflammatory drugs.

TABLE 37.13 Important pharmacodynamic drug interactions which can result in drug toxicity

PRINCIPAL DRUG	INTERACTING DRUG(S)	EFFECT	MECHANISM
Synergistic drug interactions			
ACE inhibitors	K^+-supplement K^+-sparing diuretics	Hyperkalaemia	Decreased potassium excretion
β-Blockers	Verapamil	Heart failure	Negative inotropism
β-Blockers	Verapamil	Cardiac arrest	A-V node inhibition
Ethanol	Benzodiazepines Antihistamines Phenothiazines	Increased sedation	CNS depressants
Warfarin	Aspirin NSAIDs	Potentiation of anticoagulation	Inhibition of platelet function
Antagonistic drug interactions			
β-Blockers Thiazide diuretics ACE inhibitors	NSAIDs	Reversal of hypotensive effects	Unknown
Penicillin	Tetracycline	Reduced bactericidal activity of penicillin	Bacteriostatic effect of tetracycline

ACE, angiotensin-converting enzyme; NSAIDs, non-steroid anti-inflammatory drugs.

FURTHER READING

Assem ESK. Drug allergy. *Current Opinion in Immunology* 1989; **1**, 660–6.

Adkinson NF, Wheeler B. Risk factors for IgE-dependent reactions to penicillin. In: Kerr JW, Ganderton MA eds. *XI International Congress of Allergology and Clinical Immunology*. London: Macmillan, 1983: 55–9.

Baldo BA, Harle DG. Drug allergenic determinants. *Monographs in Allergy* 1990; **28**: 11–15.

Bateman DN, Chaplin S. Adverse reaction to drugs. In: Feely J ed. *New drugs*. London: British Medical Journal, 1991; 29–39.

Beutler E. Glucose-6-phosphate dehydrogenase deficiency. *New England Journal of Medicine* 1991; **324**: 169–74.

Boyd JA, Barrett JC. Genetic and cellular basis of multistep carcinogenesis. *Pharmacology and Therapeutics* 1990; **46**: 469–86.

Brodie MJ, Feely J. Adverse drug interactions. In: Feely J ed. *New drugs*. London: British Medical Journal, 1991; 40–55.

Brosen K. Recent developments in hepatic drug oxidation. Implications for clinical pharmacokinetics. *Clinical Pharmacokinetics* 1990; **18**: 220–39.

Brueton MJ, Lortan JE, Morgan DJR, Sutters CA. Management of anaphylaxis. *Hospital Update* 1991; **17**: 386–98.

Buehler BA, Delimont D, van Waes M, Finnell RH. Prenatal prediction of risk of the fetal hydantoin syndrome. *New England Journal of Medicine* 1990; **322**: 1567–70.

Chan HL, Stern RS, Arndt KA, Larglois J, Jick SS, Jick H, Walter AM. The incidence of erythema multiforme, Stevens–Johnson syndrome, and toxic epidermal necrolysis. A population based study with particular reference to reactions caused by drugs among outpatients. *Archives of Dermatology* 1990; **126**: 37–42.

Claas FHJ. Drug-induced immune granulocytopenia. *Baillière's Clinical Immunology and Allergy* 1987; **1**: 357–67.

Coleman JW. Allergic reactions to drugs: current concepts and problems. *Clinical and Experimental Allergy* 1990; **20**: 79–85.

Committee on Safety of Medicines. Oral contraceptives and breast cancer. *Current Problems* 1988; **21**.

D'Arcy PF, Griffin JP. *Iatrogenic diseases*. Oxford: Oxford University Press, 1986.

Davies DM. *Textbook of adverse drug reactions*. Oxford: Oxford University Press, 1991.

Denham MJ. Adverse drug reactions. *British Medical Bulletin* 1990; **46**: 53–62.

Habibi B. Drug-induced immune haemolytic anaemias. *Baillière's Clinical Immunology and Allergy* 1987; **1**, 343–55.

Hickman D, Sim E. Polymorphism in human *N*-acetyltransferase – the case of the missing allele. *Trends in Pharmacological Sciences* 1991; **12**: 211–13.

Juchau MR. Bioactivation in chemical teratogenesis. *Annual Review of Pharmacology and Toxicology* 1989; **29**: 165–87.

Lockridge O. Genetic variants of human serum cholinesterase influence metabolism of the muscle relaxant succinylcholine. *Pharmacology and Therapeutics* 1990; **47**: 35–60.

Lutz WK, Maier P. Genotoxic and epigenetic chemical carcinogenesis: one process, different mechanisms. *Trends in Pharmacological Sciences* 1988; **9**: 322–6.

Mach EP. Counting the cost of adverse drug reactions. *Adverse Drug Reaction Bulletin* 1975; **54**: 184–7.

Manns MP. Cytochrome P450 enzymes as human autoantigens. *Immunology Research* 1991 **10**: 503–7.

Meyer UA. The molecular basis of genetic polymorphisms of drug metabolism. *Journal of Pharmacy and Pharmacology* 1994; **46** (Suppl. 1): 409–15.

Mueller-Eckhardt C. Drug-induced immune thrombocytopenia. *Baillière's Clinical Immunology and Allergy* 1987; **1**: 369–89.

Nanra RS. Analgesic-associated nephropathies. In: Massry SG, Glassock RJ eds. *Textbook of nephrology* (Vol. 1). Baltimore: Williams & Wilkins, 1989: 842–8.

Neuberger J, Kenna JG. Halothane hepatitis: a model of immune-mediated drug hepatotoxicity. *Clinical Science* 1987; **72**: 263–70.

Park BK, Kitteringham NR. Drug-protein conjugation and its immunological consequences. *Drug Metabolism Reviews* 1990; **22**: 87–144.

Park BK, Coleman JW, Kitteringham NR. Drug disposition and drug hypersensitivity. *Biochemical Pharmacology* 1987; **36**: 581–90.

Park BK, Pirmohamed M, Kitteringham NR. Idiosyncratic drug reactions: a mechanistic evaluation of risk factors. *British Journal of Clinical Pharmacology* 1992; **34**: 377–95.

Pessayre D, Larrey D. Acute and chronic drug-induced hepatitis. *Baillière's Clinical Gastroenterology* 1988; **2**: 385–423.

Pirmohamed M, Park BK. Prediction of idiosyncratic drug reactions. *Adverse Drug Reaction Bulletin* 1993; **163**: 615–8.

Pirmohamed M, Kitteringham NR, Park BK. The role of active metabolites in drug toxicity. *Drug Safety* 1994; **11**: 114–44.

Pratt WB. Drug allergy. In: Pratt WB, Taylor P eds. *Principles of drug action.* New York: Churchill Livingstone, 1990: 775–95.

Roujeau JC, Guillaume JC, Fabre JP, Penso D, Flechet ML, Girre JP. Toxic epidermal necrolysis (Lyell syndrome). Incidence and drug etiology in France, 1981–1985. *Archives of Dermatology* 1990; **126**: 37–42.

Ruddon RW. Chemical teratogenesis. In: Pratt WB, Taylor P eds. *Principles of drug action.* New York: Churchill Livingstone, 1990: 775–95.

Saxon A (moderator). Immediate hypersensitivity reactions to β-lactam antibiotics. *Annals of Internal Medicine* 1987; **107**: 204–15.

Stricker BHC. *Drug-induced hepatic injury.* Amsterdam: Elsevier, 1992.

Strickler SM, Dansky LV, Miller MA, Seni MH, Andermann E, Spielberg SP. Genetic predisposition to phenytoin-induced birth defects. *Lancet* 1985; ii: 746–8.

Treleavan J, Barrett J. Drugs and the bone marrow. *British Journal of Hospital Medicine* 1990; **44**: 245–50.

Tucker GT. Clinical implications of genetic polymorphism in drug metabolism. *Journal of Pharmacy and Pharmacology* 1994; **46** (Suppl. 1): 417–24.

van Joost T, Ashgar SS, Cormane RH. Skin reactions caused by phenylbutazone. *Archives of Dermatology* 1974; **110**: 929–33.

Vincent PC. Drug-induced aplastic anaemia and agranulocytosis. Incidence and mechanisms. *Drugs* 1986; **31**: 52–63.

Winstanley P, Orme ML'E. Which adverse drug interactions are really important? *Adverse Drug Reaction Bulletin* 1988; **130**: 488–91.

38

Allergic Reactions and Anaphylaxis

PV Taberner

INTRODUCTION

Systemic anaphylaxis is one of the most dramatic and potentially life-threatening manifestations of acute hypersensitivity. It can be provoked by a number of exogenous stimuli including foods, foreign proteins, animal venoms and low molecular weight substances including drugs. The term was first introduced by Portier and Tichet in 1902 to describe the unexpected and untoward reaction that occurred in response to an immunization protocol that should have provided protection or resistance to a protein toxin. It can be regarded as the opposite of prophylaxis.

Allergic reactions to drugs are not that uncommon, but the term anaphylactic reaction is usually reserved for those which present an immediate threat to the survival of the patient, even though the cellular basis for the reaction is similar.

CLASSIFICATION OF ALLERGIC REACTION MECHANISMS

Four different mechanisms are generally recognized as mediating hypersensitivity; they are illustrated in Fig. 37.4.

Type I is characterized by local or systemic anaphylaxis; the latter characterized by an immediate acute reaction involving dyspnoea and hypotension, and occasionally uncontrolled urination and defecation. This is brought about by the stimulation of immunoglobulin E (IgE) antibodies which combine with the foreign molecule (the antigen) and bind to mast cells and basophils to evoke the release of histamine and other pharmacologically active mediators. Death usually occurs as a result of shock of peripheral vascular collapse, sometimes with additional respiratory symptoms, notably oedema of the upper airway and pulmonary hyperinflation. The classic example of this reaction occurs with penicillin-based antibiotics. Serious anaphylactic responses occur at about the rate of 1 in 5000 exposures, although less than 10% are normally fatal.

Type II reactions are often manifested by haemolytic anaemia, as a result of the production of drug-specific IgG or IgM antibodies which can react with red blood cell membranes. If an antipenicillin antibody binds to a red-cell bound penicillin molecule, for example, complement will become fixed and the cell will lyse. A similar haemolytic reaction is seen when incompatible blood transfusions take place (see Chapter 27). Other examples include methyldopa-induced haemolytic anaemia and sulphonamide-induced granulocytopenia.

Type III reactions (*Arthus* reaction) are mediated mainly by IgG and represent the most commonly observed form of drug allergy. Symptoms include joint pains (arthritis), fever, and gastrointestinal disorders. The antigen/antibody reaction in this case produces a protein complex that can bind complement and set up a destructive local inflammatory reaction in the tissue. Antigen–antibody complexes adhere to the vascular epithelium and are surrounded by an accumulation of fibrin that traps platelets and polymorphonuclear neutrophils. There follows an exudation of neutrophil-rich fluid into the surrounding tissues. The resultant inflammatory lesion, often manifested as an ulcer, is associated with oedema, haemorrhage, and eventually tissue necrosis in the most severe cases. Arthus reactions range from the localized and relatively mild skin reaction by which the suspected allergenic property of a drug can be tested by a skin prick to the more severe inflammation of the vascular epithelium (serum sickness) and the bronchial inflammation associated with farmer's lung (mycosis due to inhaled spores of *Aspergillus fumigatus*). Serum sickness is most commonly associated with sulphonamides and penicillins.

Type IV reactions (delayed hypersensitivity) are cell mediated and do not involve the production of antibodies; the reaction occurs directly between sensitized T lymphocytes and the antigen. This results in the production and release of lymphokines which cause local changes in immune cell recruitment and mobility and also capillary permeability. Allergic contact dermatitis is the most frequent manifestation of this type of hypersensitivity reaction. The clinical characteristics of the various allergic reactions are summarized in Table 38.1.

MEDIATORS INVOLVED IN ANAPHYLAXIS

The clinical features of systemic anaphylaxis can be easily understood in terms of the pharmacological effects of the endogenous mediators released from the mast cells (principally in the skin and lung) and the basophils (see Fig. 38.1). The principal mediator or autacoid is histamine, but leucotrienes C_4 and D_4, prostaglandin D_2, platelet-activating factor (PAF) and heparin are also released, together with a number of protease enzymes including tryptase and kinins. There are probably other, as yet unrecognized substances, also released. The direct actions of histamine can

TABLE 38.1 Clinical characteristics of allergic reactions

	TYPE I ANAPHYLAXIS	TYPE II CYTOTOXIC REACTION	TYPE III ARTHUS REACTION	TYPE IV DELAYED HYPERSENSITIVITY
Mediated by:	Mast cell and basophil passive sensitizing Ab	Antibody or cell-mediated	Precipitating antibody, complement	Cell-mediated
Associated with:	Drug allergy Protein allergy	Drug allergy Incompatible blood transfusion	Drug allergy Serum Infections	Transplant rejection Auto-allergies Infections
Clinical manifestations:	Hay fever, asthma, urticaria, gastroenteritis	Eczema, haemolytic anaemia	Skin rash, arthritis, serum sickness, fever, glomerulonephritis	Eczema, dermatitis

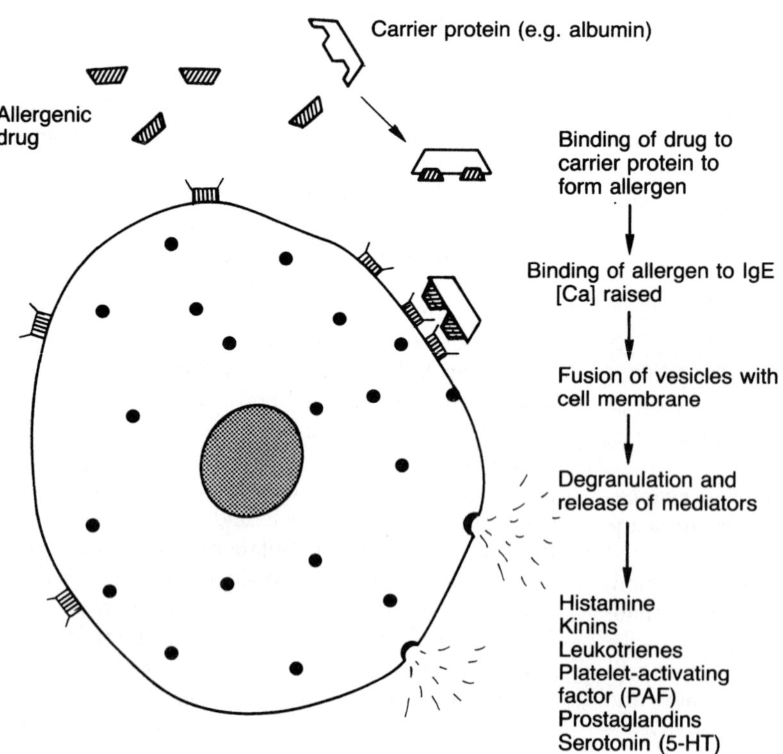

FIGURE 38.1 Sensitized mast cell response to exposure to allergen. 5-HT, 5-hydroxytryptamine.

account for the acute bronchoconstriction (H_1-receptor mediated); H_1/H_2-receptor mediated peripheral vasodilatation and increased vascular permeability resulting in a feeling of intense warmth, flushing of the skin and oedema; sensitization of peripheral nociceptive neurones leading to intense itching; a short-lasting fall in blood pressure and reflex tachycardia; and increased gastric acid secretion resulting in colic and abdominal pain. Histamine also activates postganglionic parasympathetic fibres which will increase bronchial secretion. Most of these symptoms can be mimicked by the infusion of histamine into normal volunteers. Histamine itself has a fairly short half-life in the plasma (less than 15 min), so the longer-lasting effects of anaphylaxis are presumably due to the other mediators. If the pooling of blood in the peripheral vessels and loss of fluid and plasma proteins by extravasation is sufficiently great there follows a profound fall in blood pressure resembling surgical or traumatic shock. Since the histamine that appears in the circulation in response to the anaphylactic reaction arises as a result of the explosive degranulation of the mast cells, these stores soon become depleted and the circulating histamine level falls. The main risk to the patient is therefore during this acute phase of the reaction.

TREATMENT OF ANAPHYLACTIC REACTIONS

The treatment of anaphylaxis is essentially symptomatic, with the main priorities being to maintain a patent airway and an adequate blood pressure. Adrenaline given by intravenous infusion at a rate of 0.5–5 μg/min or subcutaneous injection (0.25–0.5 mg every 10–20 min) is the first line of defence. This will restore the blood pressure by increasing peripheral vascular resistance and stimulating cardiac output. By stimulating β_2-adrenoceptors on bronchial smooth muscle, adrenaline will also relieve the bronchospasm. Selective β_2-adrenoceptor agonists may also be used; intravenous salbutamol being particularly useful in patients receiving non-cardio-selective β-blockers who may not respond to adrenaline. Intravenous fluids (saline, colloids) can be used to increase plasma volume and oxygen is also administered for hypoxia.

Secondary therapy includes corticosteroids (usually hydrocortisone 100-300 mg iv) to counteract the effects of the various mediators of the immune response (the late phase reactions); aminophylline to relieve bronchospasm; noradrenaline, in place of adrenaline; antihistamines such as diphenhydramine or chlorpheniramine to combat the urticaria, and cimetidine to counteract the effects of histamine on the peripheral vasculature and gastric acid secretion. The Association of Anaesthetists of Great Britain & Ireland publishes a data sheet on the emergency management of acute major anaphylaxis under general anaesthesia.

DRUG-INDUCED ANAPHYLAXIS

While intravenous contrast media and penicillin-related antibiotics represent the most frequent cause of drug-induced anaphylaxis, there are rarer instances of acute reactions to a number of drugs used in anaesthetic practice. Apart from a history of previous exposure, there is unfortunately no means of identifying patients likely to be at risk from these reactions. The most common non-medical cause of anaphylaxis is envenomation from a bee or wasp sting. However, a known sensitivity to hymenoptera venom does not indicate any increased risk of a subsequent drug-induced allergic reaction.

Penicillin allergy is the most widely studied form of drug allergy, and can be considered to be the classical model of drug allergy. Since its introduction in the 1940s, a wide variety of adverse effects affecting almost every organ system in the body, and mediated by all four types of hypersensitivity reactions (Fig. 38.2), have been reported with the penicillins. Anaphylaxis with penicillin occurs in 1 in 2000 patients and has a mortality of 1 in 500 000. Antibodies in these patients are not directed towards the penicillin molecule itself, but towards several haptenic structures formed by the reaction of the electrophilic groups on the penicillin molecule with nucleophilic groups on proteins (Fig. 38.2). One major antigenic determinant – the penicilloyl antigen – and several minor antigenic determinants have been described (Fig. 38.2). Antigen formation from the semisynthetic penicillins, such as amoxycillin, can involve either the penicillin nucleus or the synthetic side-chains. Because of the multiplicity of antigens, the various methods (skin tests, RAST, ELISA) that have been used to prospectively detect penicillin allergy are useful only when they yield positive results. A negative result does not totally exclude the possibility of an anaphylactic reaction to penicillin.

After the penicillins, sulphonamides and cephalosporins (to which 10–20% of the population have been estimated to be sensitized), the most frequent reactions occur in response to the administration of peptide or protein drugs. This would include tetanus antitoxin, enzymes such as trypsin and streptokinase, and human peptides such as insulin, corticotrophin and vasopressin. These agents all act through an IgE-mediated reaction with the protein itself, or a protein–hapten conjugate in the case of the antibiotics.

Opioids

The direct stimulation of mediator release from mast cells or basophils can also produce an anaphylactic response. This has been observed particularly with the opiates including morphine, which is well known to provoke mast cell histamine release by direct contact with the cell surface. Morphine can therefore

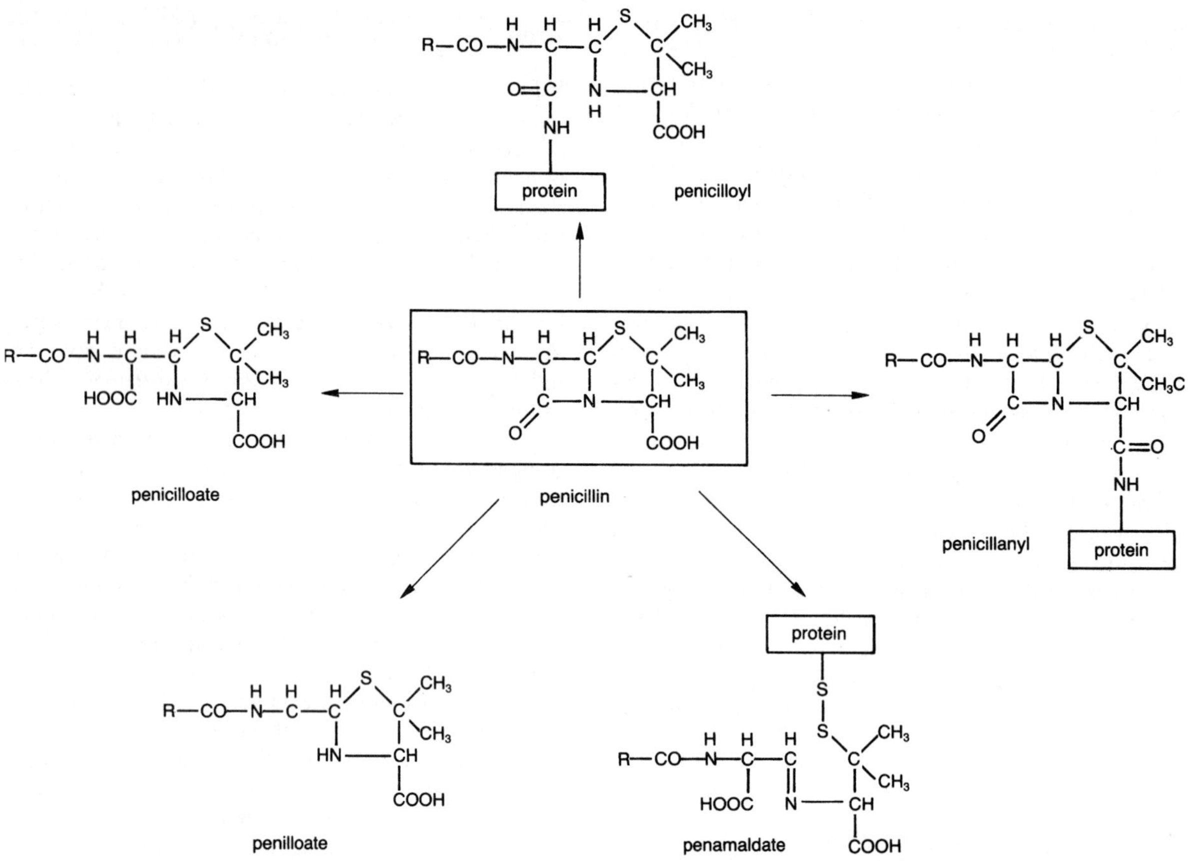

FIGURE 38.2 The allergenic determinants of penicillin.

TABLE 38.2 **Drugs particularly associated with hypersensitivity reactions**

Anaphylaxis:

- Penicillins (all tend to be cross-sensitizing)
- Cephalosporins (relatively contraindicated in penicillin sensitivity)
- Insulin (rare)
- Streptokinase (rare)
- Thiopentone (rare)

Fever, skin rashes and other hypersensitivity reactions:

- Allopurinol
- Anticonvulsants (carbamazepine phenytoin, phenobarbitone)
- Antipsychotics (chlorpromazine)
- Aspirin (and other salicylates)
- Fluoxetine
- Isoniazid
- Local anaesthetics (those that yield *p*-aminobenzoic acid as a breakdown product: benzocaine, procaine, tetracaine)
- Nitrofurantoin
- Omeprazole
- Streptokinase
- Sulphonamides
- Tricyclic antidepressants

Direct release of histamine from mast cells:

- *d*-Tubocurarine
- Pethidine (meperidine)
- Morphine
- Succinylcholine (rare)
- Atracurium (rare)
- Hypertonic radiocontrast media

precipitate an asthmatic attack in a sensitive subject. Fortunately, systemic anaphylactic reactions are rare, and the most frequently observed allergic response to morphine is urticaria or contact dermatitis. However, the vasodilator and respiratory depressant actions of morphine will tend to aggravate the immediate symptoms of the allergic response. Morphine-like opioids will also increase the severity of the circulatory collapse in hypovolaemic patients.

Neuromuscular-blocking drugs

Among the neuromuscular-blocking agents *d*-tubocurarine evokes histamine release, evidenced by bronchospasm, increased bronchial and salivary secretion, and a local skin reaction at the site of injection. Succinylcholine and atracurium also have this effect but to a lesser extent.

Other drugs

A number of non-steroidal anti-inflammatory drugs, including aspirin and indomethacin, and the steroids, progesterone and corticosterone, provoke anaphylaxis by a still unknown mechanism. Similarly, lidocaine and thiopentone have also been reported to produce anaphylaxis in rare instances. Hypertonic solutions, such as those used as radiocontrast media, also act directly to stimulate histamine release. The incidence of allergic reactions to the colloids used in blood transfusions are shown in Table 27.8. The drugs most frequently associated with anaphylactic reactions are listed in Table 38.2.

From the symptoms associated with anaphylactic reactions it should be evident that drugs which reduce blood pressure by acting to block β-adrenoceptors will constrict bronchial smooth muscle and thus have an exacerbating effect on the anaphylactic reaction. For this reason non-specific β-blockers, such as propranolol, should be discontinued or avoided if there is a significant risk of anaphylaxis.

FURTHER READING

Anaphylactic reactions associated with anaesthesia. London: Association of Anaesthetists, 1991.

Bochner BS, Lichtenstein LM. Anaphylaxis. *New England Journal of Medicine* 1991; **324**: 1785–90.

Duthie DJR, Nimmo WS. Adverse effects of opioid analgesic drugs. *British Journal of Anaesthesia* 1987; **59**: 61–77.

Pratt WB. Drug allergy. In: Pratt WB, Taylor P eds. *Principles of drug action*, 3rd edn. New York: Churchill Livingstone, 1990: 533–64.

Toogood JH. Risk of anaphylaxis in patients receiving beta-blocker drugs. *Journal of Allergy and Clinical Immunology* 1988; **81**: 1–5.

39

Drug Tolerance, Drug Dependence and Drug Abuse

PV Taberner

INTRODUCTION

Drug abuse is a rather imprecise term that is difficult to define and has significant emotional overtones. It is usually taken to refer to the non-medical or recreational use of a drug, but it can also be taken to include the misuse of anabolic steroids by athletes or β-blockers by professional snooker or darts players. In fact, drug misuse is probably a better expression, which can be applied to all instances where the use of a drug is medically unnecessary and non-drug alternatives are available. Both prescribed drugs and non-prescribed drugs obtained by illicit means can be misused. While some recreational drug use is regarded as socially acceptable and completely legitimate (alcohol, caffeine and nicotine for example), or illegal but relatively harmless (cannabis), there are both legal and illegal forms of drug misuse that present a very significant risk to the user. For example, sudden deaths from solvent abuse are an increasing problem among children and adolescents. While the proportion of the population who misuse illicit psychoactive drugs is still relatively small, the clinical implications of recreational drug use cannot exclude the very much larger populations of smokers and drinkers who present a distinctive pathophysiology as a direct consequence of their habit. The psychoactive drugs most commonly subject to misuse are listed in Table 39.1.

DEFINING THE TERMS

Drug tolerance, the need to increase the dose in order to maintain the same therapeutic response, is often but not exclusively associated with drugs that also have the potential to produce dependence. Many of these same drugs are also subject to compulsive abuse. Because of the confusion that has arisen over the indiscriminate use of terms such as abuse, addiction, habituation and dependence, it is probably worth defining the expressions used to describe these interrelated phenomena. The broadly accepted definitions, based on the WHO recommendations, are as follows.

Drug dependence

This is a syndrome that can vary in degree but is associated with:

- a recurrent compulsion to take the drug (which can usurp the normal social pattern of needs and desires)
- a tendency to increase the dose of the drug
- psychic and physical dependence on the continued presence of the drug, such that an abstinence syndrome occurs if the drug is withdrawn
- a detrimental effect on both the individual and society

TABLE 39.1 Drugs liable to abuse

DRUG CLASS	EXAMPLES
Alcohol	Ethanol
Amphetamines	Dextro-amphetamine (dexedrine, *speed*) Metamphetamine (methedrine) Methylenedioxyamphetamine (MDA), Methylenedioxymetamphetamine (MDMA, *ecstasy*)
Barbiturates	Amylobarbitone, pentobarbitone, hexobarbitone, etc.
Benzodiazepines	Diazepam, temazepam, etc.
Cannabis	Δ^9 tetrahydrocannabinol (*hash, grass, marijhuana, pot, weed*)
Cathinone	α-Aminopropriophenone (*khat*)
Cocaine	(*Coke, crack, snow, lady*)
Dissociative anaesthetics	Phencyclidine (PCP, *angel dust*), Ketamine (*Special K*) γ-Hydroxybutyrate (GBH)
Gases (propellents)	Butane, propane, nitrous oxide
Nitrites	Amyl nitrite, butyl nitrite (*poppers, bullet, locker room,* etc.)
Opiates	Heroin, morphine, methadone, etc.
Psychedelics	Lysergic acid diethylamide (LSD), mescaline, psilocybin, dimethyltryptamine (DMT)
Volatile solvents	Chloroform, ether, halothane, industrial solvents

Some representative street names are indicated in italics.

The non-specific term addiction is still widely employed in a general descriptive sense, but *physical dependence* is now preferred and denotes the neuro-adaptive changes that occur during the chronic use of drugs. Drug dependence can vary from the infrequent, mild and relatively non-toxic (caffeine, for example) to the more clinically important (alcohol, barbiturates, opiates, amphetamines and cocaine). Compulsive abuse is a social phenomenon that is difficult to relate to any specific neuronal mechanism. In general, the more pleasurable or hedonistic (i.e. rewarding) the immediate effects of the drug are, the more likely it is to be abused.

One of the important experimental clues to the dependency-producing potential of a drug is that it is self-administered by animals in a free-choice situation. In other words, the drug presents a strong reinforcing stimulus. This type of experiment constitutes one of the screening procedures employed during the development of new drugs for the market. However, it is not a completely reliable test; although nicotine and opiates are powerful reinforcers in a rodent model, amphetamine and cocaine are much weaker, and alcohol is markedly aversive in most non-primate species.

The dependence potential of any drug in an individual patient seems to be a function of both the level and frequency of dosing. (This became very apparent during investigations into the long-term use of benzodiazepines in patients, see below.) Even so, there are wide variations in individual susceptibility to dependence; not every social drinker will progress to becoming alcohol dependent, although the probability of developing dependence increases as the consumption increases. This variation in susceptibility has led to a number of theories proposing the idea of the *addictive personality*, implying that dependence could have a genetic, rather than environmental, basis. Those genetically susceptible individuals would in theory be more likely to progress from the occasional casual use of a recreational or prescribed drug to a more regular compulsive use. It is certainly true that multiple drug abusers are an increasingly common phenomenon and that drug dependence occurs across all social classes and most ethnic groups.

Sociologically, the predisposing factors for drug abuse can be summarized as A,B,C: availability, boredom and cash.

Habituation

This constitutes a desire, but not necessarily a compulsion, to continue taking the drug for the pleasure and sense of wellbeing it produces. It is sometimes described as psychological dependence and is associated with:

- little or no tendency to increase the dose
- an absence of any physical symptoms of withdrawal or abstinence syndrome
- detrimental effects, if any, are restricted to the individual

Abstinence syndrome

This describes the pattern of behavioural and physiological symptoms that occurs in response to withdrawal of the precipitating agent. As a general rule the withdrawal symptoms constitute a mirror image of the principal pharmacological actions of the drug. The withdrawal, from a dependent patient, of a sedative–hypnotic drug possessing anxiogenic and muscle-relaxant actions will result in an abstinence syndrome characterized by sleep disturbances, feelings of anxiety and increased muscle tension. The principal clinical features associated with withdrawal from the major classes of drugs that are subject to abuse are summarized in Table 39.2.

DRUG TOLERANCE

There are very many reasons why a drug may become less effective with continued use. Tolerance in its broadest sense can therefore be considered to encompass a number of widely differing mechanisms that can

TABLE 39.2 Signs and symptoms of abstinence syndromes associated with physical drug dependence

Alcohol	**Benzodiazepines**
Onset: 6–12 h	*Onset*: 2–28 days
Sweating	*(depends upon half-life and the nature of the drug)*
Moderate to severe tremor	Restlessness
Nausea	Anxiety
Anxiety	Irritability
Abdominal cramps	Sleep disturbances
	Insomnia
Duration: 12–72 h	Abdominal cramps
Sleep disturbances	Nausea
Visual hallucinations	Photophobia
Tonic–clonic seizures	Headache
Hyperthermia	Fatigue
Dehydration	Sweating
Delirium tremens	Muscular tension
Cardiovascular collapse	Muscle twitches
Barbiturates and other sedative–hypnotics	**Cocaine & Amphetamines**
Onset: 12–24 h	*Onset*: 12–24 h
(depends upon half-life of drug)	Depression
Restlessness	Anxiety
Anxiety	Dysphoria
Abdominal cramps	Feelings of weakness
Tremor	Anhedonia
Nausea	Hypotension
Duration: 1–7 days	**Opiates**
(depends upon half-life of drug)	*Onset*: 6–12 h
Sleep disturbances, nightmares,	Sweating
Insomnia	Lacrimation
Convulsions	Rhinorrhoea
(tonic–clonic seizures or even status epilepticus)	Yawning
Visual hallucinations	*Duration*: 12–72 h
Delirium	Agitation
	Restlessness
	Dilated pupils
	Anorexia
	Vomiting
	Pilomotor activity (gooseflesh)
	Feeling of cold
	Sleep disturbances
	Tremor
	Tachycardia
	Muscular spasms
	Dehydration
	Ketosis

involve either the pharmacokinetics of the drug (i.e. dispositional or metabolic tolerance), or the drug-receptor-signalling process (i.e. functional or cellular tolerance). Since the most commonly used drugs of abuse act in the central nervous system, functional tolerance to the actions of the drug is normally manifested as a behavioural tolerance. However, functional tolerance is not confined to the CNS and peripheral tissues can also exhibit tolerance.

Functional tolerance

The principal mechanisms include:

- a change in receptor function (desensitization)
- a reduction in the receptor number (down-regulation)
- exhaustion of the stores of mediators
- physiological adaptation (homoeostatic controls)
- immunological adaptation (antibody production)

Functional tolerance can occur fairly rapidly following the first exposure to the drug (tachyphylaxis) or require an extended period of exposure while the necessary adaptive changes take place. Examples of tolerance at the receptor level, manifested by either receptor desensitization (the signal transduction process has reduced efficacy so that the tissue response is correspondingly reduced) or receptor down-regulation (the number of available receptors becomes reduced), include the vasodilator response to nitrates, the bronchodilator response to β_2-adrenoceptor agonists, and the lipolytic response to insulin. Tachyphylaxis to the histamine-releasing effects of morphine can be explained in terms of depletion of the mast cell stores of histamine. Similarly, indirectly acting sympathomimetics, such as amphetamine, which act by releasing noradrenaline from sympathetic nerve endings, will also show decreased responses to repeated doses of the drug.

Intrinsic homoeostatic mechanisms are constantly operating to restore the *status quo*. For example, the actions of carbonic anhydrase inhibitors used as diuretics are not sustained because the increased excretion of bicarbonate results in a metabolic acidosis that limits the further excretion of bicarbonate. The production of antibodies to a drug (if it is a protein) or to its receptor site will also produce drug tolerance. This has been observed with drugs such as insulin (see Chapter 33).

Dispositional (pharmacokinetic) tolerance

This refers to the situation in which the metabolic degradation of the drug is increased. The hepatic microsomal drug-metabolizing enzymes (cytochrome P-450 system) are inducible. That is, an appropriate substrate for the enzymes can act to increase synthesis of the enzyme. A number of drugs including alcohol and some barbiturates have this ability (see Table 39.3) and increase their own rate of metabolism. The specifically-inducible enzymes include NADPH-cytochrome P-450 reductase, glucuronyl transferase, epoxide hydrolase, and glutathione-S-transferase. This form of tolerance will become apparent in terms of a shortened half-life for the drug as well as shortened half-lives for other drugs metabolized by the same enzymes.

It is important to recognize that dispositional tolerance is not necessarily associated with CNS tolerance; polycyclic aromatic hydrocarbons present in cigarette smoke, for example, can induce cytochrome P-450. As a consequence, the oxidation of the precarcinogen benzo-[α]-pyrene to potentially carcinogenic products is increased.

The route of administration of a drug is also important in determining whether dispositional tolerance affects its potency or duration of action to any clinically significant extent. An intravenously injected short-acting barbiturate will still be equally effective in a patient with increased hepatic P-450 capacity simply because the anaesthetic action is terminated by redistribution of the drug rather than by metabolic inactivation. On the other hand, the pharmacokinetics of a long-acting anticonvulsant barbiturate, administered chronically, would be significantly altered by induction of cyochrome P-450, possibly resulting in the need to adjust the dosage. Experimentally, phenobarbitone has been shown to increase the levels of the polysomal mRNA for cytochrome P-450 by 10-fold or more, probably by facilitating the transcription process. This increased oxidative capacity will significantly increase hepatic drug metabolism and increase the elimination of drugs inactivated by the P-450 system (see p. 531).

Cross-tolerance and dependence

This describes the situation in which tolerance to, or dependence upon, one particular drug bestows a degree of tolerance to other drugs with similar actions. Cross-tolerance gives rise to important clinical

TABLE 39.3 Substances that can increase the biotransformation of drugs by inducing metabolizing enzymes

DRUGS	XENOBIOTICS
Phenobarbitone	Aldrin
Phenytoin	Benzo-[α]-pyrene
Meprobamate	Dieldrin
Hexobarbitone	Polycyclic aromatic hydrocarbons
Chloral hydrate	
Carbamazepine	
Ethanol	
Phenylbutazone	
Rifampicin	

problems, particularly with regard to the use of anaesthetics and narcotic analgesics. The alcohol-tolerant patient will show some degree of cross-tolerance to nitrous oxide, barbiturates, benzodiazepines and other sedative–hypnotics. Cross-dependence within a class of drugs is perhaps not surprising: the synthetic opiate methadone, for example, can prevent a morphine or heroin abstinence syndrome. However, cross-dependence between different classes of drugs also occurs insofar as benzodiazepines can be used to diminish the severity of alcohol or barbiturate withdrawal. The treatment of withdrawal syndromes is usually based on a gradual detoxification process in which the symptoms are controlled by carefully regulated doses of a drug similar to that to which the patient has become dependent.

THERAPEUTIC IMPLICATIONS OF DRUG TOLERANCE AND DEPENDENCE

There are a large number of specialized journals and review articles that deal with the very large number of problems associated with drug tolerance and dependence, and the reader should refer to the further reading section at the end of this chapter for more detailed information on specific drugs. The following is only intended as a brief survey of the pharmacological characteristics associated with the principal drugs of abuse.

Alcohol

The pathophysiology of chronic heavy drinking is well documented and affects all the principal organs of the body as well as impairing the nutritional state of the patient. A heavy drinker who shows clinical symptoms of alcohol-induced tissue damage may not necessarily be alcohol dependent and alcoholism *per se* is only one of the many detrimental sequelae of excessive alcohol consumption. If alcohol dependence is also present then it will clearly be more difficult to ensure abstinence in the future in order to avoid exacerbation of the clinical condition.

Alcohol produces tolerance by a number of different mechanisms; a rapid behavioural tolerance develops within an hour or two of commencing drinking. This is evident from studies in which volunteers have self-assessed their inebriation while the blood alcohol concentration has been monitored. The results have shown that the subjects perceive themselves as progressively less intoxicated even though their blood alcohol levels may remain constant. Longer-term CNS adaptation also contributes to the development of functional tolerance. Regular heavy drinkers can still remain conscious and fairly alert at blood alcohol concentrations that would render an alcohol-naive subject heavily sedated or even comatose.

Alcohol can also induce one of the microsomal P450 cytochromes, P450 2E1 (CYP 2E1). At low concentrations alcohol is largely metabolized by a non-specific alcohol dehydrogenase, but this enzyme is easily saturable at the concentrations of alcohol associated with social drinking (15–45 mmols). Both cytochrome CYP 2E1 and catalase are capable of oxidizing ethanol to acetaldehyde and their contribution to alcohol metabolism become more important as the blood alcohol concentration rises. The most obvious pharmacological consequence of alcohol tolerance will be a resistance to the therapeutic effects of any sedative–hypnotic or anaesthetic drugs. On the other hand, if hepatic function is significantly impaired as a consequence of cirrhosis there will be a potentiation of the action of those drugs whose action is terminated by hepatic inactivation. The intrinsic blood-clotting process will also be impaired, leading to an increased risk of haemorrhage.

Amphetamines and cocaine

These drugs have already been mentioned in relation to the sympathetic nervous system (see Chapter 13). Behavioural tolerance to the psychostimulant properties of these drugs occurs with regular use. Since amphetamine acts mainly by provoking the release of noradrenaline from central and peripheral sympathetic nerve endings, closely repeated doses will demonstrate tolerance as a direct consequence of the depletion of stores of releasable noradrenaline. In contrast, the effect of cocaine, which acts by blocking noradrenaline re-uptake (uptake 1), will not be diminished with repeated use. The sensitivity of the myocardium to cocaine is maintained at the same time as CNS behavioural tolerance to the euphorigenic effect develops. For this reason, deaths from cocaine overdose are generally due to cardiac failure rather than CNS toxicity. However, both cocaine and amphetamine do have psychotoxic actions to which tolerance does not develop. The amphetamine-induced psychoses, which can resemble paranoid schizophrenia, are one example. There is still little information on the effects of regular use of the newer 'designer' amphetamines such as methylene dioxyamphetamine (MDA) and methylene dioxymetamphetamine (MDMA) (ecstasy), but the increasing incidence of reported deaths of drug users who have taken these substances suggests that they are no less toxic than amphetamine itself.

Benzodiazepines

The basic pharmacology of these drugs has been described earlier (see Chapter 21), but in terms of drug dependence, there are two principal sources of problems with these drugs:

- physical dependence following chronic regular use of benzodiazepines prescribed as anxiolytics

- abuse of short-acting hypnotic benzodiazepines obtained either on prescription or illicitly

The dangers associated with the overprolific prescribing of benzodiazepines for anxiety have now been recognized, and the chronic use of alprazolam, diazepam, lorazepam, etc. is actively discouraged. The dependence potential of these drugs was underestimated at first, partly because of their long duration of action and the presence of active metabolites. As a result, the abstinence syndrome tended to develop some time after dosing had ceased (see Table 38.2) and was not always recognized as being a drug-induced reaction.

Benzodiazepines, such as temazepam, have attracted drug users as alternatives or adjuncts to opiate use. Temazepam in particular is becoming widely abused because it is formulated in a liquid gel-filled capsule, which facilitates intravenous injection. The regular user of temazepam will be tolerant to the sedative effects of other benzodiazepines and will require higher doses in order to induce anaesthesia.

Cannabis

This drug, obtained from the Indian hemp plant, *Cannabis sativa*, is available in many forms on the black market, including dried leaf (grass), the compressed flowering heads of the plant (resin), and the more concentrated oily extracts prepared from the plant. The plant contains over forty different cannabinoids, but the principal active ingredient responsible for the psychotomimetic effects is Δ^9 tetra-hydrocannabinol (THC). The CNS effects of THC are principally sedation, relaxation, slight euphoria and a distorted perception of time, which is quite distinctive of the drug. Other effects include impairment of short-term memory and mental clouding. The expectation of the user is an important factor in determining the pattern of effects that are experienced. THC has been shown to have an anti-emetic action equivalent to that of metoclopramide in the treatment of the nausea associated with chemotherapy, and a synthetic cannabinoid, nabilone, has been licensed in the USA for this purpose.

Experiments *in vitro* have shown that brain tissue contains specific cannabinoid-binding sites, and the recent discovery and identification of a naturally occurring cannabinoid in the brain derived from arachidonic acid and christened anandamide has exciting implications for investigations of the neuropharmacology of this class of drugs.

THC also has peripheral effects, most notably on the cardiovascular system, producing tachycardia and postural hypotension. There is also a very characteristic reddening of the conjunctivae. Although there is some evidence that regular users become tolerant to the mood changes induced by THC, physical dependence and craving are not normally observed. The clearance of THC and its metabolites is relatively slow due to their high lipid solubility and sequestration in body fat. The half-life for the elimination of THC itself is about 30 h, and traces of metabolites may persist for weeks. Regular smokers of cannabis exhibit slightly increased rates of clearance, but this pharmacokinetic tolerance is of little clinical significance. It is difficult to assess the toxicity of THC itself, since most users are smoking the impure plant product. Many of the respiratory problems associated with cannabis use may be due to the admixture of tobacco with drug. Also, most cannabis users also smoke normal cigarettes.

Nicotine and tobacco

The pharmacology of nicotine, and the nicotinic acetylcholine receptor to which it binds, is well understood. Nicotine has CNS-stimulant properties in addition to its ganglionic stimulant action. The principal CNS effects of nicotine are suppression of appetite, increased alertness, stimulation of the chemoreceptor trigger zone and a mild euphoria. Nicotine is a potent reinforcing agent and is responsible for the craving experienced by smokers endeavouring to give up the habit. Regular smokers appear to be able to titrate their dosage of nicotine; if they switch to a brand containing less nicotine they will increase the number of cigarettes smoked in order to compensate. Peripheral effects of nicotine include increased blood pressure, pulse rate and fine tremor.

Nicotinic acetylcholine receptors show rapid desensitization (tachyphylaxis) to nicotine. Regular smokers become tolerant to the nausea and vomiting often associated with an individual's first experiences with smoking tobacco, but the cardiovascular effects tend to persist. More important from a clinical point of view is the ability of a number of other components of cigarette smoke to induce microsomal cytochrome P-450. The duration of action of a range of drugs, including imipramine, paracetamol, propranolol and theophylline, is shortened as a result. The analgesic response to opiates and the sedative actions of short-acting benzodiazepines is also reduced in smokers.

Tobacco provides a good example of a drug that produces a clearly differentiated physical dependence (to nicotine) as well as a psychological need for the cigarette. This is clearly shown by patients who have been treated with oral or transdermal nicotine to reduce the withdrawal symptoms of anxiety, irritability and hyperphagia and to aid abstinence. Although nicotine chewing gum or nicotine patches can deliver the equivalent dose of nicotine as that obtained by smoking a cigarette (typically 5–10 ng/ml plasma), patients still feel an urge to smoke. It is also worth noting that the withdrawal of these nicotine products can also provoke an abstinence syndrome.

The respiratory problems presented by the heavy smoker, and which are of immediate relevance to the anaesthetist, are mainly due to the toxicity of the many other components present in inhaled cigarette smoke. An extensive catalogue of tobacco-related disease can be compiled and ascribed variously to the carbon monoxide, particulate material, tars and other carcinogens present in the smoke.

Dissociative anaesthetics

Ketamine is the only drug of this type which has continued in clinical use, particularly in paediatric anaesthesia (see Chapter 5). The principal disadvantage of ketamine as an anaesthetic is the delirium often experienced on emergence. The first drug of this type to be introduced was phencyclidine (PCP). However, patients reported feeling dissociated from their environment following anaesthesia; some had 'out of body' experiences, others suffered hallucinatory flashbacks well after their apparent recovery from the anaesthetic. For these reasons the drug was withdrawn from use. A similar but less potent dissociative anaesthetic, γ–hydroxybutyrate, was widely used in France for a number of years. All three compounds have attracted illicit and non-medical drug use for the very reason of their psychogenic and hallucinatory effects. The principal danger associated with ketamine and phencyclidine is their potent analgesic action. The user becomes unaware of his or her environment (i.e. dissociated) and will also be unaware of any physical injury to themselves or others. At present there is insufficient information to determine whether functional tolerance or dependence occurs with regular use. The symptoms of ketamine or phencyclidine intoxication can resemble severe alcohol withdrawal but without the tremor.

CONCLUSIONS

The centrally acting drugs that are most commonly abused can be divided broadly into three classes: depressants (sedative–hypnotics and anaesthetics), stimulants, and psychotomimetics or hallucinogens. The choice of drug for abuse is largely a matter of their relative availability. The principal consequences of drug abuse are:

- physical dependence leading to an abstinence syndrome on withdrawal
- functional CNS tolerance which may result in cross-tolerance to the effects of other similar drugs
- dispositional or pharmacokinetic tolerance due to hepatic enzyme induction

The specific difficulties of dealing with a patient suspected of drug abuse are:

- the patient is very likely to be taking a number of different drugs
- the nature and state of purity of drugs obtained by illicit means is uncertain.

FURTHER READING

General texts

Bresnick E. Induction of cytochromes P 450 1 and 450 2 by xenobiotics. In: *Cytochrome P450*. Schenkman JB, Greim H eds *Handbook of experimental pharmacology* **105**. Berlin: Springer-Verlag, 1993; 503–26.

Cox BM. Drug tolerance and physical dependence In: Pratt WB, Taylor P eds. *Principles of drug action* 3rd edn. New York: Churchill Livingstone, 1990; 639–90.

Edwards G, Arif A, Hodgson R. Nomenclature and classification of drug and alcohol related problems. *Bulletin of the WHO* 1981; **59**: 225–42.

Finnegan LP. Influence of drug dependence on the newborn. In: Kacew S, Lock S eds. *Toxicologic and pharmacologic principles in paediatrics*. New York: Hemisphere Publishing, 1988; 183–98.

Goldstein A. *Addiction. From biology to drug policy*. New York: Freeman WH, 1994.

Jaffe JH. Drug addiction and drug abuse. In: Gilman AG, Rall TW, Nies AS, Taylor P eds. *The pharmacological basis of therapeutics*. 8th ed. Oxford: Pergamon Press, 1990; 522–73.

Koob GF, Bloom FE. Cellular and molecular mechanisms of drug dependence. *Science* 1988; **242**: 715–23.

Smith CM. The pharmacology of sedative/hypnotics, alcohol, and anaesthetics: sites and mechanisms of action. In: Martin WR ed. *Drug addiction I: Morphine, sedative/hypnotic and alcohol dependence. Handbuch der Experimentellen Pharmakologie* **45** (1). Berlin: Springer-Verlag, 1977; 413–587.

Wise RA. The neurobiology of craving — implications for the understanding and treatment of addiction. *Journal of Abnormal Psychology* 1988; **97**: 118–32.

Alcohol

Bloom FE. Neurobiology of alcohol and alcoholism. *Annual Reviews of Psychiatiatry* 1989; **8**: 347–60.

Doherty B, Webb M. The distribution of alcohol dependence severity among in-patients problem drinkers. *British Journal of Addiction* 1989; **84**: 907–14.

Goldstein DB. *Pharmacology of alcohol*. Oxford: Oxford University Press, 1983.

Barbiturates and benzodiazepines

Lader M. Clinical pharmacology of benzodiazepines. *Annual Review of Medicine* 1987; **38**, 19–28.

Rosenberg HC, Chiu TH. Time course for development of benzodiazepine tolerance and physical dependence. *Neuroscience and Biobehaviour Review* 1985; **9**: 123–31.

Wikler A. Diagnosis and treament of drug dependence of the barbiturate type. *American Journal of Psychiatry* 1968; **125**: 758–65.

Woods JH, Katz JL, Winger G. Abuse liability of benzodiazepines. *Phaqrmacological Reviews* 1987; **39**: 251–419.

Cannabis

Devane WA. New dawn of cannabinoid pharmacology. *Trends in Pharmacological Sciences* 1994; **15**: 40–1.

Hollister LE. Health aspects of cannabis. *Pharmacological Reviews* 1986; **38**: 1–20.

Matsuda LA, Lolait SJ, Brownstein MJ, Young AC, Bonner TL. Structure of a cannabinoid receptor and functional expression of the cloned cDNA. *Nature* 1990; **346**: 561–4.

Cocaine and amphetamines

Fischman MW. Behavioural pharmacology of cocaine. *Journal of Clinical Psychiatry* 1988; **49**: 7–10.

Gawin FH, Ellinwood EH. Cocaine and other stimulants: actions, abuse, and treatment. *New England Journal of Medicine* 1988; **318**: 1173–82.

Johanson C-E, Fischman MW. (1989) The pharmacology of cocaine related to its abuse. *Pharmacological Reviews* 1989; **41**: 3–47.

O'Brien CP, Childress AR, Arndt IO, McLellan T, Woody GE, Maany I. Pharmacological and behavioral treatment of cocaine dependence. *Journal of Clinical Psychiatry* 1988; **49**: 17–22.

Simpson DL, Rumack BH. Methylenedioxyamphetamine. Clinical description of overdose, death, and review of pharmacology. *Archives of Internal Medicine* 1981; **141**: 1507–9.

Nicotine

Breslau N, Kilbey M, Andreski P. Nicotine dependence, major depression, and anxiety in young adults. *Archives of General Psychiatry*, 1991; **48**: 1069–74.

Jaffe JH. Tobacco smoking and nicotine dependence. In: Wonnacott S, Russell MAH, Stolerman IP eds. *Nicotine psychopharmacology; molecular and behavioural aspects.* Oxford: Oxford University Press, 1990; 1–37.

Shiffman SM, Jarvik ME. Smoking withdrawal symptoms in two weeks of abstinence. *Psychopharmacology* 1976; **50**: 35–44.

Opiates

Johnson SM, Flemming WW. Mechanisms of cellular adaptive sensitivity changes — applications to opioid tolerance and dependence. *Pharmacological Reviews* 1989; **41**: 435–88.

Way EL. Opioid tolerance and physical dependence and their relationship. In: Herz A ed. *Opioids II. Handbook of Experimental Pharmacology* **104**. Berlin: Springer-Verlag, 1993; 573–96.

Psychotomimetics

Jansen KLR. Non-medical use of ketamine. *British Medical Journal* 1993; **306**: 601–2.

Johnson KM, Jones SM. Neuropharmacology of phencyclidine: basic mechanisms and therapeutic potential. *Annual Review of Pharmacology and Toxicology* 1990; **30**: 707–50.

Sonders MS, Keana JFW, Weber E. Phencyclidine and psychotomimetic sigma opiates: recent insights into their biochemical and physiological sites of action. *Trends in Neuroscience* 1988; **11**: 37–40.

Glossary of Pharmacological Terms

Adverse drug reaction A more or less unexpected harmful or unpleasant effect produced by a therapeutic dose of a drug that necessitates a reduction in dosage or withdrawal of the drug from the patient.

Affinity constant A numerical quantity (K_a) with the dimension of inverse concentration (M^{-1}), that indicates the tendency of a drug to bind to a protein.

Agonist A drug that binds to a receptor and activates it to produce a pharmacological response (depolarization, contraction, secretion, etc.). A full agonist has high efficacy.

Allergic reaction An immunologically mediated reaction to a foreign substance, often, but not necessarily, a protein. A severe systemic allergic reaction is termed anaphylaxis.

Antagonist A drug that blocks the effect of an agonist either competitively (surmountable) by binding at the same receptor site as the agonist, or non-competitively (not surmountable) at an alternative allosteric site.

AUC see Bioavailability

Autacoid A member of an unrelated group of substances naturally present in the body which produce potent pharmacological effects (e.g. histamine, 5-HT, prostaglandins, etc.).

Bioavailability A loose term that describes the fraction of the dose of an administered drug that is available to produce an effect after allowing for any loss during absorption. The area under the plasma concentration-time curve (AUC) is often used as a measure of bioavailability.

Bioequivalence A measure of the comparative bioavailability of a drug formulation relative to a standard or alternative formulation. It can be of importance to patients who are transferred from one formulation of a drug to another.

Clearance The rate of removal of a substance from the blood as it passes through an organ or tissue. It has the dimensions of volume per unit time (l/min).

Compartment A proportion of the body (blood, extracellular fluid, etc.) in which the concentration of a drug is taken to be uniform, and constant at equilibrium.

Competition The situation in which two drugs compete for the same binding site or receptor (see Antagonist).

Desensitization A phenomenon in which the tissue response to a given concentration of drug declines more or less rapidly (tachyphylaxis). No specific mechanism is implied, but it is often associated with decreased efficacy (q.v.) of the receptor.

Dissociation constant A numerical quantity (K_d), with the dimension of concentration, that indicates the tendency of a molecular species to dissociate. It is used to describe both drug–receptor and ionization equilibria. (N.B. The dissociation constant of an agonist at a receptor is often misleadingly represented as K_A.)

Down-regulation Desensitization due to a reduction in receptor density.

EC_{50} The molar concentration of an agonist that produces 50% of the maximum possible response for that agonist. The ED_{50}, where D = Dose, is often used as an alternative.

Efficacy A term that describes the ability of an agonist–drug receptor combination to elicit a pharmacological response in a tissue. A full agonist has high efficacy, a partial agonist has lower efficacy, an antagonist has zero efficacy.

Elimination The removal of the active form of a drug from the body by metabolic breakdown or excretion.

Equilibrium constant The rate constant derived from the Law of Mass Action. For drug receptor interactions the equilibrium rate constant is usually the dissociation constant (K_d).

False transmitter A chemical analogue of a normal neurotransmitter produced by the competitive incorporation of a drug precursor into the synthetic pathway for that transmitter. It is normally less effective than the natural transmitter (e.g. α-methylnoradrenaline produced from α-methyldopa).

First-pass effect The loss of a proportion of the dose of an orally administered drug before it can enter the general circulation as a consequence of intestinal or hepatic metabolism. This can significantly affect the bioavailability of drug.

IC_{50} The concentration of a drug that produces 50% of the maximum possible inhibition. It is often used as a means for comparing the potency of antagonists and enzyme inhibitors which do not produce a direct tissue response.

Inverse agonist A drug that produces an effect opposite to that of an agonist although it acts at the same receptor site.

LD_{50} The dose of drug which will kill, on average, 50% of animals in toxicity testing prior to clinical trials of a drug. It has little relevance to clinical medicine (see therapeutic index).

MAC The minimum alveolar concentration is that concentration necessary to suppress reflex response to skin incision in 50% of patients. The MAC for halothane is 0.76%, isoflurane 1.15%, enflurane 1.68%, desflurane 6%. These values are for the anaesthetic agent in oxygen and are less in the presence of nitrous oxide.

Occupancy The proportion of receptors to which a drug is bound. For a full agonist, 50% occupancy occurs at the EC_{50}, at which point the drug concentration is equal to its equilibrium dissociation constant (K_d).

Partial agonist An agonist that is unable to produce a maximal activation of the receptors, irrespective of the concentration applied.

pA_2 The negative logarithm of the molar concentration of an antagonist which necessitates the concentration of agonist to be doubled in order to produce the same response obtained in the absence of the antagonist. It is a measure of the potency of an antagonist.

pKa The negative logarithm (to the base 10) of the dissociation constant. Usually applied as a measure of the inherent acidity or alkalinity of a molecule. It is the pH at which an ionizable molecule will be 50% ionized.

Potency A vague term that roughly describes the concentration of a drug that is effective at producing a therapeutic response. It is a function of the drug's bioavailability, affinity constant and efficacy. It can be applied to agonists, antagonists and enzyme inhibitors. Defined measures of potency include the EC_{50}, IC_{50} pA_2.

Relative potency The ratio of the potency (e.g. the EC_{50}) of a test drug to that of a standard drug.

Second messengers A number of intracellular substances are now known to be important in transmitting the signal from the activated drug-receptor to the site which is responsible for the cell response. The best established 2nd messengers are cyclic AMP, cyclic GMP, inositol phosphates, and diacylglycerol.

Spare receptors Agonists possessing high efficacy (q.v.) often need only to occupy a small proportion of the total receptors available in order to produce a maximum response. The unoccupied receptors are the reserve, or spare receptors.

Tachyphylaxis The rapid desensitization of a tissue to the continued presence of a drug indicated by a progressive decline in the response to a standard dose.

Therapeutic index A measure of the ratio of the maximum tolerated dose of a drug to the minimum effective dose. It can be visualized as the goalposts between which the effective therapeutic concentration of drug has to be steered. (But beware: goalposts have a habit of moving unexpectedly.) In animal studies the ratio of the LD_{50} to the ED_{50} is often used.

Index